Mosby's

DENTAL
HYGIENE

Concepts, Cases, and Competencies

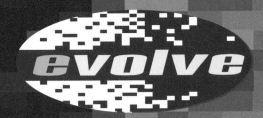

The Latest *Evolution* in Learning.

Evolve provides online access to free learning resources and activities designed specifically for the textbook you are using in your class.
The resources will provide you with information that enhances the material covered in the book and much more.

Visit the Web address listed below to start your learning evolution today!

▶▶ *LOGIN:* **http://evolve.elsevier.com/daniel/**

Evolve learning resources for Daniel/Harfst: *Mosby's Dental Hygiene: Concepts, Cases, and Competencies* offers the following features:

- **Before You Begin**
  Lists the software programs needed to use this website along with instructions for installation of each item.

- **Content Updates**
  Periodic updates are posted here to keep students apprised of new and/or revised book content without having to wait until a subsequent printing or later edition becomes available.

- **Feedback & Suggestions**
  Asks students to submit any feedback or suggestions that they have discovered as they use this learning package.

- **Frequently Asked Questions for Working With the CD-ROM**
  Students can get answers to frequently asked questions for working with the CD-ROM.

- **WebLinks**
  Three categories of direct links to hundreds of relevant websites: *United States Dental Hygiene Programs by State, Canadian Dental Hygiene Programs by Province,* and *Websites–Direct Links* (dentally focused websites)

Think outside the book...*evolve.*

Mosby's
DENTAL HYGIENE

Concepts, Cases, and Competencies

Editors

Susan J. Daniel, RDH, MS

Former Chairperson and Associate Professor, Department of Dental Hygiene
School of Health-Related Professions
The University of Mississippi Medical Center
Jackson, Mississippi;
Adjunct Associate Professor, Department of Dental Ecology
School of Dentistry
University of North Carolina
Chapel Hill, North Carolina;
President
Educational Visions
Ridgeland, Mississippi

Sherry A. Harfst, BSDH, MS

Adjunct Associate Professor, School of Dentistry
University of Detroit Mercy
Detroit, Michigan;
President
Oral Health Advantage
Lake Orion, Michigan

with 720 illustrations

Mosby

An Affiliate of Elsevier

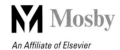

Publishing Director: Linda L. Duncan
Senior Acquisitions Editor: Penny Rudolph
Developmental Editor: Jaime Pendill
Project Manager: Linda McKinley
Production Editor: Rich Barber
Book Designer: Julia Dummitt

NOTICE

Pharmacology is an ever-changing field. Standard safety precautions must be followed, but as new research and clinical experience broaden our knowledge, changes in treatment and drug therapy may become necessary or appropriate. Readers are advised to check the most current product information provided by the manufacturer of each drug to be administered to verify the recommended dose, the method and duration of administration, and contraindications. It is the responsibility of the licensed healthcare provider, relying on experience and knowledge of the patient, to determine dosages and the best treatment for each individual patient. Neither the publisher nor the editor assumes any liability for any injury and/or damage to persons or property arising from this publication.

Mosby, Inc.
11830 Westline Industrial Drive
St. Louis, Missouri 63146

Printed in the United States of America

ISBN-13: 978-0-323-03062-5

ISBN-10: 0-323-03062-9

07 08 09 10 11 TG/RRD 9 8 7 6 5 4 3 2

CONTRIBUTORS

Cathy L. Backinger, MPH, PhD
Program Director
Tobacco Control Research Branch
National Cancer Institute
Bethesda, Maryland

Beckie M. Barry, RDH, MEd
Associate Professor
Department of Dental Hygiene
School of Health-Related Professions
The University of Mississippi Medical Center
Jackson, Mississippi

Kathy B. Bassett, BSDH, RDH, MEd
Clinic Coordinator and First-Year Lead Instructor
Department of Dental Hygiene
Pierce College
Lakewood, Washington

Thomas G. Berry, DDS, MA
Professor
Department of Restorative Dentistry
University of Colorado
School of Dentistry
Denver, Colorado;
Assistant Secretary
Academy of Operative Dentistry

Ann L. Brunick, RDH, MS
Chairperson and Associate Professor
Department of Dental Hygiene
University of South Dakota
Vermillion, South Dakota

Alan W. Budenz, MS, DDS, MBA
Associate Professor and Chair
Department of Diagnosis and Management
University of the Pacific School of Dentistry
San Francisco, California

Peggy W. Coleman, PhD
Professor
Department of Dental Hygiene
The University of Mississippi Medical Center
School of Health-Related Professions
Jackson, Mississippi

Marie A. Collins, RDH, MS
Chair and Assistant Professor
Associated Dental Sciences
Medical College of Georgia
Augusta, Georgia

Nora L. Cromley, MEd
Associate Dean for Admissions and Student Affairs
Department of Admissions/Student Affairs
Associate Professor/Associate Dean
Department of Educational Resoures/Administration
School of Dentistry
Oregon Health & Science University
Portland, Oregon

Susan J. Daniel, RDH, MS
Former Chairperson and Associate Professor
Department of Dental Hygiene
School of Health-Related Professions
The University of Mississippi Medical Center
Jackson, Mississippi;
Adjunct Associate Professor
Department of Dental Ecology
School of Dentistry
University of North Carolina
Chapel Hill, North Carolina;
President
Educational Visions
Ridgeland, Mississippi

Judith Ann Davison, JD, RDH
Attorney at Law
Windham, Maine

Christina B. DeBiase, BSDH, MA, EdD
Professor and Director
Division of Dental Hygiene
West Virginia University
Morgantown, West Virginia

Robert A. DeVille, DMD
Associate Professor
Department of Dental Hygiene
School of Health-Related Professions
The University of Mississippi Medical Center
Jackson, Mississippi

Cheryl H. DeVore, RDH, BS, MS, JD
Associate Professor and Director
Department of Dental Hygiene
Section of Primary Care
The Ohio State University
Columbus, Ohio;
Attorney at Law
Cheryl H. DeVore, Co., LPA
Dublin, Ohio

John D.B. Featherstone, MSc, PhD
Professor and Chair
Preventive and Restorative Dental Sciences
University of California at San Francisco
San Francisco, California

Bonnie Francis, RDH, MS
Regional Trainer
DentalView
Irvine, California

Joan I. Gluch, RDH, PhD
Director, Community Health
Dental Care Systems
University of Pennsylvania
School of Dental Medicine
Philadelphia, Pennsylvania

Mary Ann Haisch, RDH, MPA
Assistant Professor
Department of Dental Hygiene
Oregon Health & Science University
School of Dentistry
Portland, Oregon

Sherry A. Harfst, BSDH, MS
Adjunct Associate Professor
School of Dentistry
University of Detroit Mercy
Detroit, Michigan;
President
Oral Health Advantage
Lake Orion, Michigan

Margaret Hill, DMD
Associate Professor of Periodontology
Department of Periodontics, Endodontics, and Dental
  Hygiene
University of Louisville
School of Dentistry
Louisville, Kentucky

Lorie Holt, RDH, MS
Assistant Professor
Department of Dental Hygiene
School of Dentistry
University of Missouri—Kansas City
Kansas City, Missouri

Katherine Karpinia, RDH, MS, DMD
Assistant Professor
Department of Periodontology
University of Florida
College of Dentistry
Gainesville, Florida

Susan H. Kass, RDH, EdD
Program Director
Department of Dental Hygiene
Miami-Dade Community College
Miami, Florida

William Patrick Kelsey III, DDS
Associate Dean for Academic Affairs
Creighton University
School of Dentistry
Omaha, Nebraska

Darnyl King, RDH, MSDH
Instructor
Department of Dental Hygiene
Georgia Perimeter College
Dunwoody, Georgia

Michelle G. Klenk, RDH, EdD
Former Chairperson
Department of Dental Hygiene
West Virginia University Institute of Technology
Montgomery, West Virginia

Debbie Manne, RDH, RN, MSN, OCN
Coordinator/Oral Care Specialist
Oncology Dental Support Services
St. Louis, Missouri;
Clinical Assistant Professor
Division of Dental Hygiene
School of Dentistry
University of Missouri—Kansas City
Kansas City, Missouri

Jill Mason, MPH, RDH
Associate Professor
Department of Dental Hygiene
Oregon Health & Science University
School of Dentistry
Portland, Oregon

Deedee L. McClain, CDA, RDH, MS
Instructor
Department of Dental Assisting
Dental Assisting Academy of New Brunswick
Saint John, New Brunswick
Canada

Robert E. Mecklenburg, DDS, MPH
Coordinator, Tobacco and Oral Health Initiatives
Tobacco Control Research Branch
National Cancer Institute
Bethesda, Maryland

Shannon Mitchell, RDH, MS
Former Clinical Associate Professor
Department of Dental Ecology
School of Dentistry
University of North Carolina
Chapel Hill, North Carolina

Regan L. Moore, DDS, MSD
Associate Professor of Periodontology
Director of Predoctoral Periodontics
Department of Periodontics, Endodontics, and Dental
    Hygiene
University of Louisville
School of Dentistry
Louisville, Kentucky

Mary R. Pfeifer, RDH, MS, RN, CCRC
Manager, Clinical Research
Department of Medicine—Clinical Research Program
The University of Mississippi Medical Center
Jackson, Mississippi

Judith Qualtieri, RDH, BS, MS
Program Chair
Department of Dental Hygiene
Central Piedmont Community College
Charlotte, North Carolina

Dennis N. Ranalli, DDS, MDS
Professor of Pediatric Dentistry and Senior Associate
    Dean
University of Pittsburgh
School of Dental Medicine
Pittsburgh, Pennsylvania

Nelson L. Rhodus, DMD, MPH
Morse Distinguished Professor and Chair
Department of Oral Medicine
University of Minnesota
Minneapolis, Minnesota

Mary Kaye Scaramucci, RDH, MS
Associate Professor
Department of Dental Hygiene
Raymond Walters College
University of Cincinnati
Cincinnati, Ohio

Colleen R. Schmidt, RDH, MS
Former Assistant Professor and Junior Clinic Coordinator
University of Missouri—Kansas City
School of Dentistry
Division of Dental Hygiene
Kansas City, Missouri

Francis G. Serio, DMD, MS
Professor and Chairman
Department of Periodontics
The University of Mississippi Medical Center
School of Dentistry
Jackson, Mississippi;
Diplomate, American Board of Periodontology

Kenneth Shay, DDS, MS, FACD, FRCSEd, FASGD, FGSA
Director, Geriatrics and Extended Care Service Line
U.S. Department of Veterans Affairs
Veterans Integrated Service Network #11
Chief, Section of Dental Geriatrics
Affiliated Investigator, Geriatric Research, Education,
    and Clinical Center
Ann Arbor Veterans Healthcare System
Adjunct Associate Professor of Dentistry
Department of Periodontics, Preventive and Geriatric
    Dentistry
School of Dentistry
University of Michigan
Ann Arbor, Michigan

Robert Sherman, DMD
Captain, Dental Corps
United States Navy
Chairman
Oral Medicine Department
National Naval Dental Center
Naval Postgraduate Dental School
Bethesda, Maryland

Eric E. Spohn, DDS, FADI
Fellow, Academy of Dentistry International
Professor Emeritus
Department of Oral Health Science
University of Kentucky
College of Dentistry
Lexington, Kentucky

Cynthia A. Stegeman, RDH, MEd, RD, CDE
Assistant Professor
Department of Dental Hygiene
University of Cincinnati—Raymond Walters College
Cincinnati, Ohio

Katharine R. Stilley, RDH, MS
Assistant Professor
Department of Dental Hygiene
School of Health-Related Professions
The University of Mississippi Medical Center
Jackson, Mississippi

Deborah Studen-Pavlovich, DMD
Associate Professor and Interim Chair
Department of Pediatric Dentistry
University of Pittsburgh
School of Dental Medicine
Pittsburgh, Pennsylvania

George M. Taybos, DDS, MSEd
Associate Professor
Department of Diagnostic Sciences
The University of Mississippi Medical Center
School of Dentistry
Jackson, Mississippi

Peter T. Triolo Jr., DDS, MS
Associate Professor and Chairman
Department of Restorative Dentistry and Biomaterials
University of Texas Health Science Center at Houston
Dental Branch
Houston, Texas

Victoria C. Vick, RDH, BS
Former Adjunct Assistant Professor
Department of Periodontics
School of Dentistry
University of Louisville
Louisville, Kentucky

Kim Curbow Wilcox, PT, MS, NCS
Assistant Professor of Physical Therapy
Department of Physical Therapy
School of Health-Related Professions
The University of Mississippi Medical Center
Jackson, Mississippi

K. Joseph Wittemann, PhD
Professor Emeritus
Medical College of Virginia
School of Dentistry
Virginia Commonwealth University
Richmond, Virginia

William Woodall, MEd, PT, SCS
Associate Professor
Department of Physical Therapy
School of Health-Related Professions
The University of Mississippi Medical Center
Jackson, Mississippi

Douglas A. Young, DDS, MBA, MS
Associate Professor
Department of Diagnosis and Management
University of the Pacific
School of Dentistry
San Francisco, California

We dedicate this learning package to Irene R. Woodall for her years of dedication to the profession of dental hygiene, her determination in constantly challenging students and colleagues in the learning process, and her vision of integrating dental hygiene education and improved human health. Her affect and knowledge have changed the direction of dental hygiene education, setting goals and standards for objective and compassionate education. It is to her indomitable spirit, which partially lives within each of us, and to her personal honor that we dedicate this work. It is our hope that the work will continue the pattern of challenge and change to which she introduced us.

Also, this book is dedicated to the many great dental hygiene educators who have come before and who will come after us, for your unending patience, your determined dedication, and your personal unheralded joy in seeing the "light come on" for the student.

Susan J. Daniel
Sherry A. Harfst

*My personal dedication is to my husband, Hugo Newcomb, and my son, Daniel Austin,
for their support, encouragement, and understanding of my time and commitment.
You are the greatest!
SJD*

*My personal dedication of this text is to my friend, mentor, and husband, David,
whose encouragement, vision, and perspective helped make my participation
in this project even more enjoyable.
SAH*

PREFACE

STUDENTS

In choosing this learning package, your faculty has provided you with the most current educational material in dental hygiene in terms of content and educational technology. The textbook provides concepts, cases and competencies for the education of the competent dental hygienist; the interactive CD-ROM supports those elements with hundreds of interactive exercises; the web site provides updates and a wealth of additional resources.

FACULTY

By choosing to implement this learning package into your curriculum, you have elected the most contemporary dental hygiene text in terms of content and educational technology. The Faculty Guide details the chapter content and provides additional materials for teaching enhancement such as process performance forms and critical thinking skills assessments. It also contains a list of topics that can be used for class discussion, a thumbnail sketch of the case and case applications in each chapter, a full description of the CD-ROM exercises designed to support specific chapter content, patient profiles, teaching outlines and more.

Integrating all components of this learning package (text, CD-ROM, Evolve web site, and Faculty Guide) can assist in the development of a competent dental hygienist. This learning package promotes both self study and group learning experiences. The immediate feedback gained through the use of the CD-ROM activities, Critical Thinking Activities, and Review Questions in the textbook is most rewarding. More importantly, learning can be fun and somewhat self-paced with the ease of repeated review within the CD-ROM activities.

PRACTICING DENTAL PROFESSIONALS

This learning package is unique to the dental hygiene profession in that it contains not only concepts in text format but is supported by an interactive CD-ROM and a web site. The case-based approach to learning is certain to provide a new approach to your review of specific topics, and the CD-ROM will actively engage your clinical skills. Depending on the depth of your review, features that may prove useful to the practitioner (among others) are lesion description and identification, value identification and professional goal setting.

The following pages offer a detailed introduction to the textbook format, CD-ROM applications, and Evolve web site. We hope that this introduction is helpful to you as you begin to utilize this learning package to its full capacity, and that in accepting the challenge and exploration of new knowledge, each dental hygiene student will be more fully prepared to truly care for the health of those patients to whom they provide service.

Susan J. Daniel
Sherry A. Harfst

Mosby's Dental Hygiene: Concepts, Cases, and Competencies is a comprehensive and unique approach to the educational process of the dental hygienist because it offers a learning environment in a textbook, CD-ROM, and web site that support case-based and competency-based education. While this learning package is well-accepted and one of the most popular core dental hygiene textbooks, it is a distinct departure from the standard textbook format. An overview of its features is shown in the following diagram.

PHILOSOPHY OF CONTENT ORGANIZATION

HEALTHCARE PROFESSIONAL EDUCATION

Comprehensive textbooks such as this one are developed and presented around a central theme. In addition to providing the technical information with which to implement the varied clinical aspects of the dental hygiene profession, this text provides the learner with a clear understanding, beginning with the first chapter, of the full definition and meaning of becoming a healthcare professional.

While the sequencing of curricular content differs among schools, there are standards to which each accredited program must adhere. With this understanding, the textbook and CD-ROM are sequenced to parallel the components within a dental hygiene appointment: assessment, dental hygiene diagnosis, planning, implementation, and evaluation.

COMPETENCY INTEGRATION

Each of the nine distinct book divisions, or parts, were planned with attention to the sequence of dental hygiene curriculum. Each part opener page lists the competencies (ADEA, 2003) that correspond to the discussion of the chapters found within that part. You will notice that many of these are repeated for more than one book part. A full listing of the competency statements can be found in the appendix.

INTEGRATION OF HEALTH—ORAL AND SYSTEMIC

The content presented in the book, CD-ROM, and other supportive components address the biological, psychological, and sociological concerns of overall patient health. This learning package presents each element with clinical applications to assist in student understanding of their relevance to patient health. Understanding of the integration of the biological, psychological, and social concerns in assessment, diagnosis, planning, implementation, and evaluation is necessary for successful patient outcomes and clinician satisfaction.

PATIENT VS. CLIENT

While two schools of thought exist as to the name given those to whom we provide care, the co-authors believe that those in the healthcare professions are the only group

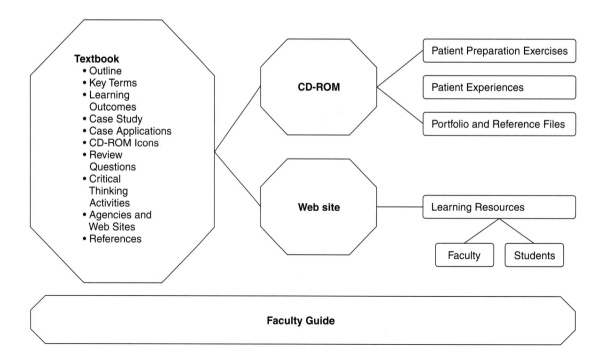

Textbook
- Outline
- Key Terms
- Learning Outcomes
- Case Study
- Case Applications
- CD-ROM Icons
- Review Questions
- Critical Thinking Activities
- Agencies and Web Sites
- References

CD-ROM
- Patient Preparation Exercises
- Patient Experiences
- Portfolio and Reference Files

Web site
- Learning Resources
  - Faculty
  - Students

Faculty Guide

that can refer to those individuals as *patients* and, further, that there is something sacred about the relationship between a healthcare provider and "patient" that other professions cannot claim. The concepts and applications within the text, CD, and other supportive materials surpass the "client/patient" issue and are appropriate for all who provide health care.

THE TEXTBOOK

The text content is based on the premise that the mouth, head, and neck are part of the body and as such affect overall human health. Decisions regarding care are made with this premise in mind.

The text is divided into Parts and the corresponding content on the CD-ROM is referred to as Sections. Chapters support the part title in the book.

Each chapter includes the following features:
- Outline
- Key Terms
- Learning Outcomes
- Case Study (to set up the chapter)
- Case Applications
- Review Questions
- Critical Thinking Activities
- Agencies and Web Sites
- References
- Additional Readings and Resources

Each of these features is designed to enhance your study of the chapter content. Possible uses for the various text elements are described below.

OUTLINE, KEY TERMS, LEARNING OUTCOMES

Once a chapter has been assigned, the Chapter Outline, Key Terms, and Learning Outcomes sections should be reviewed and a list made of the Key Terms. As the Key Term is encountered in the reading, take note of the definition or concept and usage. While reading the text, the Learning Outcomes can be recalled to identify ways each component of the text supports the outcome development.

CASE STUDY AND CASE APPLICATIONS

Each chapter presents at least one Case Study, reflecting the application of a portion of the content presented within the chapter. As the chapter further develops theory and concepts, Case Applications are presented. These elements relate directly to the Case Study and may require the learner to address an issue or respond to a question to reinforce certain concepts. Some chapters present more than one Case Study and may have multiple Case Applications. Others present one Case Study, but present several Case Applications throughout the chapter. For example, Chapter 4 (Communication) contains one complex Case Study, another smaller Case Study, numerous Case Applications, and additional case-related activities concerning communication.

INTERACTIVE CD-ROM ICONS

Icons are located throughout the text prompting the student to access interactive exercises to reinforce their learning.

REVIEW QUESTIONS

Review Questions appear at the end of each chapter and provide the learner with a method to assess his or her understanding of chapter content. These questions should be reviewed and a notation of the correct answer should be made after reading and reviewing all content within the chapter. At the completion of the review questions, the Answer Key in the back of the text can be referenced for correct responses and rationales for each question.

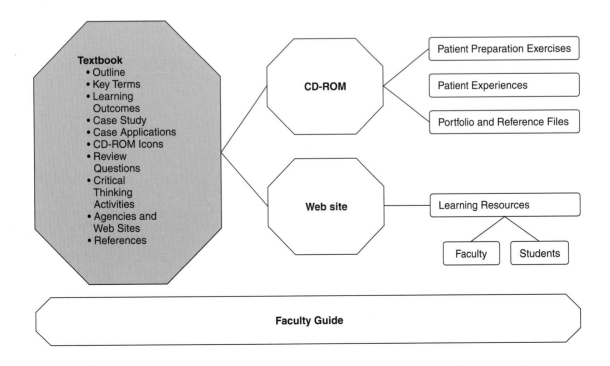

CRITICAL THINKING ACTIVITIES

At the end of each chapter is a section entitled, Critical Thinking Activities, which contains exercises designed to encourage the generation of thought, discussion, and application of ideas and concepts. Some activities are provided for independent learning, whereas others are designed for a peer partner or a small group activity. Review and completion of these activities will increase the student's critical thinking and problem-solving abilities by relating the content specifically to the chapter being studied.

SUGGESTED AGENCIES AND WEB SITES

An additional component to the development of competence and knowledge of each chapter's contents is the use of the Suggested Agencies and Web Sites section listed at the end of each chapter. Many entries are those of agencies that provide additional information on the chapter content. These web sites can help the learner develop a deeper understanding of the chapter content, for future use during patient care. Because of the ever-changing nature of the Internet, some of the web site listings may have changed since publication. We recommend referring to the Evolve site for the most current information.

ADDITIONAL READINGS AND RESOURCES

To further enhance the learner's knowledge of the chapter content, a listing titled Additional Readings and Resources at the end of each chapter provides a wealth of information. These references can be used at any time, but they may be particularly useful for a special project or paper related to the chapter content.

CD-ROM ORGANIZATION AND ACCESS

The Procter & Gamble Company, a valuable supporter of dental and dental hygiene education, provided an educational grant for the development of the accompanying interactive CD-ROM. The CD-ROM included with the book is an essential part of this total learning system designed to be used in conjunction with the text. This CD-ROM provides hundreds of case-based exercises for the immediate application of knowledge, to develop and retain critical thinking and problem-solving skills.

In the book, **CD-ROM** icons appear in the margins throughout each chapter. These icons indicate specific interactive exercises on the CD-ROM where content from the text is reinforced. Students can either access the portion of the CD-ROM identified by the icon as soon as it appears, or wait until completing all chapters in a section of the book to then work through the corresponding section on the CD-ROM. The user-friendly design and pull-down menus make it easy to navigate to all areas of the CD-ROM.

The CD-ROM is divided into 11 **Sections** that correlate with the 11 part divisions in the text. Each section of the CD-ROM is presented as a schedule of a typical work day for a dental hygienist. Beginning with **Patient Preparation Exercises**, students prepare for the **Patient Experiences** that occur throughout the day. Both of these features are explained in further detail throughout this introduction.

The CD-ROM includes a tutorial introduction that explains each of the learning applications.

FEATURES

You can build your own personal **Portfolio** when using the CD-ROM, tailoring it to include documentation of clinical and educational experiences. You are encouraged to continually add to and update their **Portfolio** as you progress through the dental hygiene curriculum. Personalized forms containing material unique to each student such as information pertaining to their particular state licensing agency, continuing education requirements and fulfillments, health history, prevention survey, health beliefs, and self-evaluation of their competence are powerful self-assessment tools that will be helpful throughout educational and professional career development.

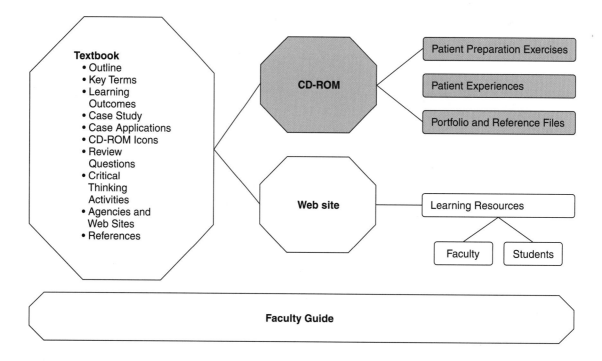

Another customizable feature of the **Portfolio** is the **Reference File**. At the completion of certain activities, you are given the option to place the form into your **Reference File**. If all of these forms are added to the file, you will end up with a very useful study tool and a handy chairside reference.

An extensive list of Internet resources in the **Direct Links** section connects you to hundreds of dentally focused websites, research and dental professional education associations, regional testing boards, worldwide oral health organizations, and government agencies.

The **Glossary** from the book also appears on the CD-ROM for quick location of key terms and their definitions.

The **Patient Preparation Exercises** are a fun yet challenging way to review and assess your comprehension of important concepts presented in the book. Included are video segments that demonstrate dental procedures followed by review questions, labeling activities, drag-and-drop exercises, fill-in-the-blank statements, identification activities, true/false drills, multiple-choice quizzes, and more.

The **Patient Experiences** further reinforce the concepts introduced in the text through practical application in patient-based reality. Nine patients are featured on the CD-ROM, each complete with their own profile, health history, prevention survey, intraoral photos, radiographs, examination forms, periodontal chart, dental chart, and 24-hour food diary. You must access and become acquainted with these elements in order to complete each patient exercise.

CD-ROM APPLICATIONS

The interactive portion of the learning package reinforces the key learning concepts in each chapter by engaging the student in one of three types of ways:

- PATIENT PREPARATION EXERCISES
  A direct application of the key learning concepts in a chapter
- PATIENT EXPERIENCES
  Accessed through a typical dental hygiene treatment schedule, these exercises apply the key concepts from each chapter to one of nine fully developed patients.
- PORTFOLIO
  Through these exercises, the student can track progress in all competency domains, compile materials for future self-evaluation, and build clinical chairside references.

PATIENT PREPARATION EXERCISES

By directly applying key concepts from chapter content, you will reinforce those concepts necessary for competent patient interaction. For this reason, we have called these "Patient Preparation Exercises."

In the more than 120 Patient Preparation Exercises, you will have the opportunity to order lists, determine correct definitions, review video and answer questions, identify correct and incorrect procedures, build decision trees, correctly order procedure steps, match terms and definitions, and label diagrams.

In reviewing these exercises it is important to keep in mind the following points:

- If a concept is not presented in a given chapter, it will not appear on the CD-ROM. These exercises are intended to reinforce, not to teach or test.

- Wherever possible, rationales and reasons for correct and/or incorrect responses are given to provide immediate feedback. Again, the purpose of the exercises is to reinforce, not to test.
- Once an exercise is completed, your work will be erased. This allows you to repeat any of the exercises for further reinforcement. The exception to this is contained in the next point.
- You can opt to SAVE certain predetermined exercises to a special feature on the CD called the Portfolio. These typically are references that can be printed and used as chairside guides and cover a wide range of clinical topics (see Portfolio below).
- You can select either Patient Preparation Exercises or Patient Experiences at any time for any given chapter. There are no "gates" built in to prevent students from accessing any of the components. The logic used for the educational structure and reinforcement, however, is best illustrated when the student first completes the Patient Preparation Exercises and then accesses the Patient Experiences for a given chapter.
- Patient records can be accessed from a drop down menu. This window does not have to be "closed" to continue the exercises but can simply be "downsized" for future access.

PATIENT EXPERIENCES

In selecting the Patient Experiences for a chapter, you will see a typical daily schedule for a dental hygienist. Built on an 8 AM to 5 PM treatment day, you select the patient from the treatment schedule and are then led through the patient experience. The richness of the patient interaction depends on working with patients of all ages. For this reason, we have provided patients ranging in age from 2 to 81 years, each with unique histories, complaints, and needs.

How are the patient-based experiences accessed?
Simply select the Patient Schedule for the book Part you are studying (Note: on the CD-ROM these divisions are termed sections but correspond directly to each book *part*.) You will see, via a drop-down menu, a schedule of patients, based on a typical 8-hour schedule. The chapter on which the patient-specific experience exercise is built is identified on the schedule.

What records can the student access?
The patient records can be accessed independently from any of the exercises, at any time. The Patient Records window can remain active by simply closing the *window only* and not the entire file.

What records are available to the student?
Each of the nine patients, ages 2 to 81 years, is detailed in the following records:

Patient Profile
Health History
Prevention Survey
Intraoral Photographs
Radiographs
Intraoral Exam
Extraoral Exam
Periodontal Chart
Dental Chart
24-hour Food Diary

You can select any of the patients on the schedule, although ideally they will begin at 8 AM and conclude with the last appointment at 5 PM. Intermingled throughout the sessions are a variety of additional patient experiences, such as a phone call, which will not appear on the schedule but will "interrupt" the day—typical of a day of practice and a bit more fun for the learner!

Why so many patient records?

Each patient has multiple uses, based on the chapter content. For example, (please see the accompanying Patient Experience Overview chart *in the appendix*) the student will interact with Mrs. Cronin's patient records in 29 of the exercises, Mr. Burkett's patients in 28 exercises, and so forth. There is a wealth of information built into each case, no different than if one were to review actual patient files. These exercises are intended to mimic clinical practice as much as possible and must therefore be as complete as possible. You and the students will become quite familiar with this patient family as you guide the student in transitioning into the professional domain.

In reviewing these exercises it is important for you, the faculty, to keep in mind the following points:

- The purpose of these **Patient Experiences** is to reinforce, not to test. Faculty, however, can use any of the nine fully developed patients as the basis for additional faculty-generated, case-based learning or testing. Not all records on all patients are used in these exercises. They are, however, fully developed and available for you to use as you deem appropriate. *For example, not all of the patient's radiographs are used in the evaluation exercise on the CD-ROM. You may elect to use another patient's radiographs, perhaps Mrs. Guri's, for an additional assignment or for discussion on technique or findings.*

- For many of the patient experiences, the student's answers are actually "recorded" (or appear to be recorded) on the patient record only *after* the student completes the exercise. *For example, the student is shown a photograph of angular cheilitis of patient Ann Cronin. Once the student correctly recognizes the lesion, a notation to that effect appears on Ann's intraoral exam form. Before that student interaction, if that patient form were accessed it would appear blank.*

- In each case, the Health History appears as it would have **at the initial patient visit;** if the patient is a returning patient, the health history update MUST be reviewed to see the *current* patient status just as in clinical practice. *For example, to see the current health status of Mr. Johnston, the student must check the Health history update form, which reveals that, in addition to the medications he listed initially, he is taking Cardizem and has a possible latex allergy.*

- You can select any of these patients from the Patient Records (a drop-down menu) to review patient records at any time for any CD-ROM exercise or for an independent faculty-assigned exercise.

PORTFOLIO

The PORTFOLIO is one of the first documents on the CD-ROM with which you will interact. While the use of the PORTFOLIO is not mandatory to the functioning of the CD, we encourage you to participate in the content.

As you progress through the curriculum, you can actually build a personal PORTFOLIO to contain information regarding your clinical experiences, community experiences, health beliefs, chairside references, philosophy of practice, and goal statements. A demonstration of how the PORTFOLIO functions can be seen on the Virtual Tour feature of the CD.

Initiating the PORTFOLIO

To initiate the PORTFOLIO feature, simply fill in the personalization screen.

PORTFOLIO Content

The PORTFOLIO is organized by competency headings, with forms for recording and collecting data in each category, as follows:

Core Competencies

- Descriptions of the core competencies are provided.
- You can use the form for recording what you feel is a demonstration of a core competence, noting the date, the demonstration event, the patient (if applicable), and your year of study.

Health Promotion Disease Prevention

- Descriptions of the Health Promotion Disease Prevention competencies are provided.
- You can use the form for recording what you feel is a demonstration of a core competence, noting the date, the demonstration event, the patient (if applicable), and your year of study.

Community Involvement

- Descriptions of the Community Involvement competencies are provided.
- You can use the form to record the community experience, the date, location, target audience, supervising faculty, the service provided, expected goals, outcomes, and comments/observations.

Patient/Client Care

- Descriptions of the Patient/Client Care competencies are provided.
- You can use the form to record patient/client care interface including the patient, age, classification, services rendered, date began, date completed, the goals, outcome, comments, and the year of study.

Professional Growth and Development

- Descriptions of the Professional Growth and Development are provided.

Legal Functions

A form is provided that lists many possible functions for which a dental hygienist could be licensed. From this list, you are asked to research and identify those functions for which you will be legally responsible, once licensed in a given state.

Professional Organizations

A form is provided for you to record the pertinent information for the national and state dental hygiene associations, as well as the state licensing agency.

Continuing Education Requirements

A form is provided for you to record the CE requirements for a given state.

Continuing Education Fulfillment

A form is provided for you to record CE fulfillment, including the date, topic, title, instructor location, and granted CE units.

Personal Health History

You are asked to complete a personal health history.

Prevention Survey

You are asked to complete a Prevention Survey.

Health Beliefs

You are asked to identify your currently held health beliefs.

Self-Evaluation

Periodic Review

Values

Needs

Philosophy of Practice

Career Goals

REFERENCE FILES

You can actually build these handy reference files that can then be printed and used for chairside reference. At the completion of the specific exercises (see list below), you will be asked if you want to place the form in the reference file in your PORTFOLIO. When you have completed the CD-ROM, you will have the following compendium of chairside references.

Extraoral Examination

Health History Questioning

Lymph Glands

Salivary Glands

Vital Signs

Temperature

Pulse

Respiration

Respiration Abnormalities

Blood Pressure

Intraoral Examination

Anatomical Landmarks

Lips

Labial Mucosa

Buccal Mucosa

Floor of Mouth (1)

Floor of Mouth (2)

Tongue (1)

Tongue (2)

Palate

Oropharynx

Common Sites of Oral Cancer

Oral Manifestations of Drug Therapy

Lesion Description

Elevated Lesion Descriptions

Depressed Lesion Descriptions

Flat Lesion Descriptions

Periodontal Examination

Periodontal Landmarks

Furcation Evaluation

Mobility Evaluation

Prevention Strategies

Chemotherapeutic Agents

Dentifrice Formulation Chart

Dentifrice Tube Ingredients

Interproximal Cleaning Aids

Life Stage Considerations

Care Modifications for Special

Needs Patients

Management of Dentinal Sensitivity

Mental and Emotional Disorders

Neurologic Conditions and Impairments

Xerostomia–Causes and Effects

Xerostomia–Possible Treatment

CD-ROM TROUBLE SHOOTING

Having trouble with the CD-ROM? Before contacting technical support, browse through the following answers to frequently asked questions for working with the CD-ROM.

- **Is it alright to keep other computer applications open while using the CD-ROM?** For optimal performance, close all other computer programs and applications before opening the CD-ROM.
- **I have used the CD-ROM several times. How can I skip the musical introduction?** Click the space bar on your keyboard to bypass the opening segment.
- **How can I get to my taskbar when the CD-ROM is running?** Simply press the Windows key on your keyboard (usually located between the ALT and CTRL keys). If you don't have a Windows key, you can also hold down CTRL and tap ESC to bring up the START menu.
- **I forgot my password. How can I retrieve it without having to reinstall the program and losing all my information?** Navigate to the folder containing the Dental Hygiene CD-ROM's executable program. Here you'll find a file called "userinfo.txt." Open it up (in Notepad on Windows or SimpleText on Macintosh). Look through the file until you see the word "password" immediately followed by a colon (:). Your password will appear in quotation marks immediately after that.
- **Does the Portfolio have to be completely filled out in order to retrieve it later?** No. To view your partially completed Portfolio, go to Section 1 and click "Portfolio Initiation."
- **How can I adjust the volume of the audio narration?** You have two options: (1) Click the audio icon in the upper right-hand corner of each screen to turn off the narration. (2) Go to "CD Setup" (located in the pull-out menu on the left) and minimize or maximize the Master Volume to your desired level.
- **Do I have to keep opening and closing the Patient Records as I work through the exercises?** No. Simply minimize and maximize the Patient Records window as needed.
- **Why can't I always see the Glossary?** Sometimes the glossary appears behind the active window. With your mouse, move or minimize the active window to view the glossary.
- **When I open a link from Direct Links, my browser is launched and the site displays fine. However, when I click on another link, nothing seems to happen. What should I do?** Your browser is most likely still running in the background as another task. Hold down the ALT key and hit TAB to cycle through all applications that are running. You will see that the new site has already been loaded into one of the existing browser windows.
- **What program do I need to access the PDF files?** To view, print, and work with PDF files, you must have Adobe Acrobat Reader installed. This program can be downloaded for free from the Internet and can be accessed at the Adobe site: www.adobe.com
- **Why do some of the videos seem jumpy while playing?** Some video segments are intended to freeze-frame at times. This is not a problem with the videos or your system.
- **Why does it take so long to exit this program?** Because of the tremendous amount of media that is loaded

into your system's memory as the program runs, when exiting, it may take some time to return that memory to its original state.

- **How can I get specific instructions on how to install and run this program?** Refer to the booklet located inside the CD-ROM envelope. If you require technical support, please call the Technical Support Hotline between 9 A.M. and 5 P.M. Central Standard time, Monday through Friday. Inside the United States, call 1-800-692-9010. Outside the United States, call 314-872-8370. You may also contact Customer Support online at http://www.elsevier.com/homepage/support/. Click the link "Electronic Product and CD-ROM Help Desk."

EVOLVE WEB SITE ORGANIZATION AND ACCESS

Faculty and students will benefit from the many features of the accompanying Evolve web site, another valuable component of this learning package. If you are familiar with the Merlin web site that launched when the textbook originally published in 2002, you will find that the newly developed Evolve site offers the same features of Merlin plus additional information presented in a new and improved format. Although the look and feel may be different, it won't take long to acclimate to the contemporary design and enhanced features of Evolve. Unlike before, no passcode is required to gain access to the website. Instructions for faculty and students as well as a list of the site features are outlined below:

TO ACCESS THE EVOLVE WEB SITE LEARNING RESOURCES

FACULTY

At the front of the textbook is a page introducing the Evolve web site. All you need to get started is a computer with an Internet connection:

1. Go to http://evolve.elsevier.com/daniel
2. Click the "Instructor" button under the "Learning Resources" heading.
3. On the Login page you can either enter your established Evolve username and password or create a new account by clicking on the "Click here to register" link. If you need to create a new account, follow the on-screen instructions.
4. After logging in or creating an account, fill out all the required fields on the Verification Form and click the "Submit Form" button.

Wait approximately 2 to 3 business days for verification. After you have been verified as an adopting instructor, you will receive an email from the Evolve Administrator indicating the resources have been added to your account.

EVOLVE WEB SITE FEATURES FOR FACULTY

- **Before You Begin**—This page lists the software programs needed to use this web site along with instructions for installation of each item.
- **ADEA-Based Competency Statements**—This page provides access to the American Dental Education Association (ADEA)'s *Competencies for Entry into the Profession of*

Dental Hygiene. Additionally, you will find a document that demonstrates how these various competencies are related to content in the CD-ROM and the textbook.

- **Content Updates**—Periodic updates are posted here to keep you apprised of new and/or revised book content without having to wait until a subsequent printing or later edition becomes available.
- **Faculty Resource**—Perhaps the most valuable part of the web site, this section thoroughly explains how the content of the textbook, CD-ROM, and Evolve site all work together. Suggestions for the integration of these materials into the dental hygiene curriculum serve as a helpful guide for faculty.
- **Feedback & Suggestions**—This area asks you to submit any feedback or suggestions that you have discovered as you use this learning package.
- **Image Collection**—Here you will find a complete electronic image collection of every figure in the book. You can download the images of your choice into a PowerPoint program for effective classroom presentations.
- **Process Performance Forms**—These forms are intended as worksheets for your use with many of the clinical procedures described in the text. It is acknowledged that each dental hygiene program will have these types of documents already in place; however, these closely follow the procedures as described in the text and are intended for your personal edit and application.
- **Textbook Elements**—The *Chapter Outline, Key Terms,* and *Learning Outcomes* are listed for each chapter in the book for quick reference.
- **Teaching Tips for CD-ROM**—Get answers to frequently asked questions and teaching tips for working with the CD-ROM.
- **Test Bank**—Click on this item to view the instructions for downloading the test bank located in the **Downloads** folder (see below).
- **WebLinks**—Three categories of direct links to hundreds of relevant web sites: *United States Dental Hygiene Programs by State, Canadian Dental Hygiene Programs by Providence,* and *Web sites–Direct Links* (dentally focused web sites)
- **What Works For You**—Send your ideas that work well in the classroom as you incorporate this learning package into your curriculum. By sharing your tips with each other, we can make your teaching experience easier and more effective for your students.
- **Downloads**—Here is where you can download all of the above-listed items, including a comprehensive test bank of multiple-choice questions divided into two categories: Part Questions (related to important concepts from the book) and Case-Based (related to the specific patients featured on the CD-ROM). Additional sets of questions are periodically posted to the test bank, so check back often.

TO ACCESS THE EVOLVE WEB SITE LEARNING RESOURCES

STUDENTS

1. Go to http://evolve.elsevier.com/daniel
2. Click the "Student" button under the "Learning Resources" heading.

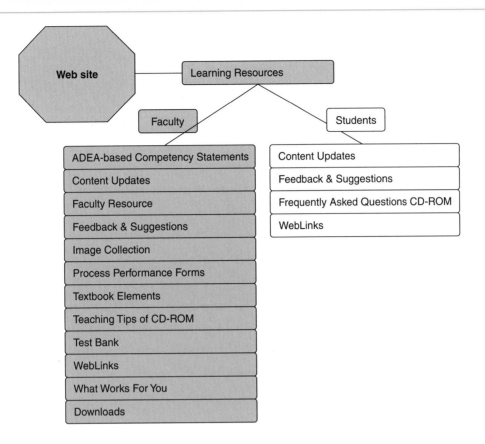

3. On the Login page you can either enter your established Evolve username and password or create a new account by clicking on the "Click here to register" link. If you need to create a new account, follow the on-screen instructions.

EVOLVE WEB SITE FEATURES FOR STUDENTS

- **Before You Begin**–This page lists the software programs needed to use this web site along with instructions for installation of each item.
- **Content Updates**–Periodic updates are posted here to keep students apprised of new and/or revised book content without having to wait until a subsequent printing or later edition becomes available.
- **Feedback & Suggestions**–This area asks students to submit any feedback or suggestions that they have discovered as they use this learning package.
- **Frequently Asked Questions for Working With the CD-ROM**–Students can get answers to frequently asked questions for working with the CD-ROM. (This is the same document as **Teaching Tips for CD-ROM** in the Instructor section.)
- **WebLinks**–Three categories of direct links to hundreds of relevant web sites: *United States Dental Hygiene Programs by State, Canadian Dental Hygiene Programs by Providence,* and *Web sites - Direct Links* (dentally focused web sites)

EVOLVE TROUBLE SHOOTING

We encourage you to explore the various support options available to you as an Evolve user. There are several ways to get answers to your questions.

Easy-to-read documentation, online answers to commonly asked questions, e-mail and technical support contacts, sales representative and customer support information, and centralized links to plug-in enhancements for your browser of choice highlight the variety of material that you will encounter as you explore the site.

Our continued effort to provide you with an unprecedented level of customer service depends on your input. Within all Evolve courses and resources is a Feedback link in the top frame that allows you to get in touch with us quickly and efficiently.

Please e-mail any suggestions on how we can improve this and other areas of our site to evolvefeedback @elsevier.com.

Evolve Technical Support:
Web: http://evolve.elsevier.com/TechSupport
Phone: 1-800-692-9010

FAQs (Frequently Asked Questions)–A listing of commonly asked questions and their answers regarding the Evolve Learning System and courses in general, a valuable knowledge resource. The FAQs are located in the "Support" section of the Evolve Portal (http:// evolve.elsevier.com).

Plug-Ins–Links to the most common content readers, media players, and browsers to make sure that you and your students get the most out of your courses and the Internet as a whole. The Plug-Ins page is located in the "Support" section of the Evolve Portal (http://evolve. elsevier.com).

ACKNOWLEDGMENTS

I would like to thank the many people who assisted in making this learning package possible. To the many students who have provided insight into what would make learning better—without you, this learning package would have no purpose. To faculty members and former colleagues who contributed and provided encouragement, I thank you. For their assistance with administrative and clerical matters, I would especially like to thank Earline Fitzhugh and Allyson Lowman.

I wish acknowledge two people who profoundly influenced my teaching and educational philosophy. First is Mary George for her guidance, support, and encouragement throughout the years; for teaching me how to use a Gracey curet and requiring me to develop a task analysis;

and for the confidence she instilled in me. Second, I wish to acknowledge Margaret Cain, who by example showed me how to operate a clinic and taught me how to embrace students and nurture them beyond the development of professional knowledge and skills.

Finally, I want to thank my father, John David Daniel, for teaching me about the mechanical world, logic, how to drive a manual transmission, and much more. I also want to thank my mother, Janice Daniel, for showing me how to operate a business and prepare a meal and for demonstrating faith during those last days.

Susan J. Daniel

To the faculty and countless students whose paths I have crossed, to you I owe a debt of honesty and self-evaluation. To those mentors whose images I have held as a beacon and whose challenges I have accepted in taking a "different" direction, I owe you gratitude beyond description. To my staff members, Rachael Newingham and three dental hygienists—Sue Cieslak, Donna Napiorkowski, and Palbina McNabney—whose insights and creativity were instrumental in the CD-ROM development, I owe a deep appreciation that only teamwork can speak to. To James Hull, DDS, FADI, and The Procter & Gamble Com-

pany, whose unyielding support and funding made the interactive CD-ROM portion of this learning package a reality. To my husband, David, my family, and dear friends who have supported my work schedule and understood the demands of this project, your kindness and encouragement can never be repaid. And finally, to Susan Daniel—visionary, colleague, and friend—I owe an unending gratitude for allowing me the opportunity to work on such an exciting, challenging, and significant project.

Sherry A. Harfst

To Penny Rudolph, Senior Acquisitions Editor, Kimberly Alvis, Developmental Editor, and Kristin Hebberd, Production Editor, who made these thoughts and concepts understandable, credible, and workable, your dedication to this project has been nothing short of an inspiration. To Victoria Vick for recognizing the value of case-based instruction in dental hygiene education and the initiation of the interactive portion of this project.

Also, thanks to all dental hygiene faculty members who strive for excellence in dental education. We hope our vision meets your dreams.

Susan J. Daniel
Sherry A. Harfst

CONTENTS

PART I

The Dental Hygiene Professional 1

1 Dental Hygiene—Then and Now 2
Development of the Profession of Dental
Hygiene 3
Case Study: Advances in Dental Technology 3
History of Dentistry 3
Education 5
Clinical Practice Patterns 7
Licensure and Regulation 9
Career Mobility and Career Choices 11
Maintaining Competence 12

2 Health Promotion: A Basis of Practice 16
Case Study: Expanding the Definition of Health 17
The Link between Dentistry and Human
Health 17
Historical Perspective on Health Promotion 17
Health Promotion: Broadening the Paradigm 18
The Oral Cavity in the Equation of Health
and Disease 19
Burden of Oral Disease 21
Health Promotion Guidelines 29

3 Legal and Ethical Considerations 40
Patients' Rights and Responsibilities in Dental
Care 41
Case Study: Ethics and the Law 42
Dental Hygienists' Responsibilities in Providing
Dental Hygiene Care 52

4 Communication 57
Self-Evaluation 58
Case Study 1: Team Approach
to Communication 59
A Working Definition 60
Steps toward Changing Communication
Behaviors 60
Key Elements of Communication 61
Case Study 2: Effective Communication—
Attending 62

PART II

Environmental Ergonomics 72

**5 Exposure Control and Prevention of Disease
Transmission 74**
Case Study: Infection Control and Disease
Prevention 75
Theory (Literature) 75
Techniques, Procedures, and Supportive
Evidence 89

6 Workstation Design and Positioning 115
Case Study: Musculoskeletal Problems Resulting
from Equipment 116
Workstation Design and Positioning for the
Dental Hygienist 116
Musculoskeletal Problems 116
Normal Anatomy and Anatomical Changes 118
Positioning 120
Reducing Fatigue 127
Treatment and Exercises 128

**7 Instrument Design and Principles
of Instrumentation 137**
Evolution of Instruments 138
Parts of the Instrument 138
Instrument Identification 141
Case Study: Instrument Selection Evaluation 149
Fundamentals of Instrumentation 150

8 Instrument Sharpening 158
Case Study: Disadvantages to the Use of Dull
Instruments 159
Goals for Maintenance of Sharp
Instruments 159
Sharpening Needs 160
Testing Sharpness 160
Sharpening Technique 161
Devices Used to Sharpen Instruments 161
Workstation and Equipment 163
Manual Sharpening Methods 163
Specific Instruments 166
Common Technique Errors 170
Care and Maintenance of a Sharpened
Instrument 171

PART III

Patient Assessment 174

9 Life Stage Changes 176
Case Study: Appreciating Lifestyle Changes to Build
Rapport and Guide Treatment 177
Life Stages 178
Early Childhood (Birth to 6 Years) 178
Later Childhood (7 to 12 Years) 180
Adolescence to Young Adulthood
(13 to 20 Years) 181
Early Adulthood (21 to 39 Years) 183
Mature Adulthood (40 to 60 Years) 184
Late Adulthood (61 Years and Older) 186

10 Comprehensive Health History 192
Essential Elements of a Health History 193
Case Study: Significance of a Thorough Health History 194
Review of Organ Systems 198
Dental History 209

11 Physical and Extraoral Examinations 214
Case Study: The Examination Process 215
Physical Evaluation 215
Principles and Techniques of Physical Evaluation 215
Vital Signs 222
Referrals and Consultations 225

12 Tobacco and Chemical Dependencies 228
Seduction 229
Addiction 229
Intended Consequences 229
Case Study: Helping a Patient Quit Tobacco Use 230
Results 230
Costs of Tobacco Habit 230
Smokeless/Spit Tobacco 231
Other Tobacco Products 231
Essential Elements of Patient History 232
Techniques, Procedures, and Supportive Evidence 234
The Team Approach 240

13 Intraoral Examination 245
Case Study: Thorough Intraoral and Extraoral Examination 246
Examination of the Lips and Labial Mucosa 246
Examination of the Buccal Mucosa and Vestibular Folds 252
Examination of the Floor of the Mouth 254
Examination of the Tongue 256
Examination of the Hard and Soft Palates 259
Examination of the Oropharynx and Palatine Tonsils 261

14 Clinical Manifestations of Common Medications 267
Erythema Multiforme 268
Case Study: Erythema Multiforme 269
Xerostomia 271
Lichenoid Drug Reaction 272
Gingival Hyperplasia 273
Dysgeusia 274
Oral Pigmentation 275
Hairy Tongue 276
Angioedema 276
Candidiasis 277

15 Periodontal Examination 282
Case Study: Completing the Periodontal Examination 283
Periodontal Anatomy 285
Anatomical Landmarks of the Periodontium 285
Attachment Mechanisms 287

Components of the Periodontal Examination 289
Periodontal Pocket Probing 290
Location of the Free Gingival Margin in Relation to the CEJ 291
Calculation of Attachment Loss 293
Amount of Keratinized or Attached Gingiva 293
Detection of Marginal and Deep Bleeding on Probing 293
Detection of Suppuration 294
Exploration of Furcations 294
Detection of Mobility 295
Assessment of Plaque and Calculus 296
Indices 298
Dental Factors in Periodontal Disease Risk 301
Examination and Evaluation of Dental Implants 303
Technology in the Periodontal Examination 303
Classification of Periodontal Disease 304

16 Hard Tissue Examination 309
Case Study: Examination and Recording of Dental Findings 310
Comprehensive Hard Tissue Charting 310
Types of Charting Forms 310
Tooth Numbering Systems 311
Infection Control 311
Caries-Classification Systems and Cavity Design 311
Charting Existing Conditions 316
Other Conditions that Modify Teeth 316
Types of Tooth Fracture 318
Charting Caries 319
Defining Dental Caries and Related Terms 319
New Caries-Classification Systems 320
Current Methods of Caries Detection 323
Recurrent or Secondary Caries 324
Color Changes in Enamel 325
Color Changes in Dentin and Cementum 325
Caries-Indicating Dyes 326
Detection with Dental Radiographs 326
Future Caries-Detection Technologies 327
Occlusal Analysis 328

17 Radiographic Evaluation and Utilization 333
Selection of Radiographs 334
Case Study: Radiographic Evaluation: Essential to Patient Care 334
Radiographic Evaluation 334
Patient Assessment 338
Treatment Planning 340
Patient Education 340
New Radiographic Techniques 340

18 Nutritional Assessment 344
Case Study: Effects of Nutrition on Oral Health 345
Nutrition in Dental Hygiene Practice 345
Effects of Nutrition on the Oral Cavity 345
Effects of Oral Complications on Nutrition 348

Diet and Dietary Habits Contributing to Dental
Caries 348
Nutritional Assessment 351

19 Intraoral Photographic Imaging 355
Theory 356
Case Study: Intraoral Images Enhance Treatment
Acceptance 356
Types of Intraoral Photographic Imaging Systems
356
Selection Process for an Intraoral Photographic
Imaging System 360
Photographic Accessories 360
Photographic Exposures 361
Future Trends 361

20 Supplementary Aids 366
Review of Examination Techniques 367
Case Study: Role of Supplementary Aids
in Diagnosis 367
Supplementary Aids 368
Tooth Sensitivity 368
Oral Mucosa 370
Systemic Diagnostic Aids 371

PART IV

Disease-Prevention Therapy: Professional and Self-Care 376

21 Devices for Oral Self-Care 378
General Guidelines for Oral Self-Care
Recommendations 378
Case Study: Specific Oral-Care
Recommendations 379
Toothbrushes 380
Interdental Cleaning 383
Tongue Cleaning 386
Evaluating Effectiveness of Oral Self-Care
Devices 386

22 Fluoride and the Reversal of Dental Caries 390
Caries and Oral Hygiene 391
The Caries Process 391
Case Study: Remineralization of the Early Carious
Lesion 391
Fluoride 393
Management of Dental Caries 395
Clinical Implications: Fluoride-Delivery
Systems 399
Professional Applications 400
Fluoride Toxicity 401
Self-Applied Topical Fluoride Products 401
Fluoride Supplements in Caries Prevention 402

23 Dentifrices 406
Composition of Dentifrice 407
Adverse Effects 407
Safety and Efficacy 407
Case Study: Selecting the Correct Dentifrice 407
Evaluating Clinical Studies 409
Dentifrice Formulations 409

24 Chemotherapeutics 416
Delivery Systems 417
Case Study: Selecting a Chemotherapeutic Agent
Based on Patient Need 417
Antimicrobials: General Considerations and
Specific Agents 420
Agents 420
Controlled Drug-Delivery Systems 423
Systemic Delivery 424
Quality Assurance 425
Evaluation of Success 425

25 Dentinal Sensitivity 429
Etiology 429
Case Study: Treatment of Dentinal Sensitivity to
Cold Stimuli 430
Stimuli that Elicit Pain Response 430
Natural Defense Mechanisms 431
Treatment of Sensitivity 432

26 Sealants 440
Action and Effectiveness of Sealants 441
Case Study: Pediatric Considerations for Sealant
Application 441
Sealant Composition and Types 443
Armamentarium and Application 443
Retention, Wear, and Replacement 446
Potential Estrogenicity 447
Future Applications 447

**27 Prevention and Emergency Management
of Dental Trauma 452**
Epidemiology 453
Case Study: Sports-Related Dental Trauma 453
Developmental Etiology 453
Sports-Related Injury 454
Emergency Management of Dental Trauma 456
Child Abuse and Neglect 458
Prevention of Sports-Related Injury 463
Strategies for the Dental Hygienist 464

**28 Care of Appliances and Dental
Prostheses 469**
Role of the Dental Hygienist 470
Overview of Dental Appliances 470
Case Study: Caring for the Prosthodontic
Patient 471
Evaluating Oral Tissues Associated with
Appliances 476
Care and Cleaning of Dental Appliances 478

PART V

Health Promotion and Disease Prevention 484

**29 Oral Risk Assessment and Intervention
Planning 486**
Patient-Specific Approach to Oral Care 487
Case Study: Therapeutic Intervention with Risk
Assessment 487

ORA System   488
ORA Application to Case Study   498
Case Summary   502

30   Individualizing Preventive and Therapeutic Strategies   507
The Patient as a Clinical Partner   507
Case Study: Individualizing Prevention Strategies   508
Step 4: Recommend   508
Prevention Strategy Implementation   511
Step 5: Reevaluation   514

PART VI

Therapeutic Implementation   520

31   Powered Instrumentation in Periodontal Debridement   522
Periodontal Debridement   523
Case Study: Therapeutic Selections for the Periodontal Patient   524
Review of Pathogenesis and Wound Healing   526
Powered Scaling Instruments   527
Tip Selection and Application   530
Preparation of Powered Instruments   532
Fundamentals of Powered Instrumentation   533
Evaluation of Debridement   536
Coding for Periodontal Debridement   537

32   Cosmetic and Therapeutic Polishing   541
Assessment of Need   542
Case Study: Selecting the Appropriate Polishing Method   542
Theory   542

33   Periodontal Dressings and Suturing   563
Suture Materials   563
Case Studies: Suturing—Three Specific Procedures   564
Suture Needles   566
Suture Size   566
Suture Packaging   566
Suturing Techniques   567
Suture Removal   570
Periodontal Dressings   570

PART VII

Anxiety and Pain Control   574

34   Anxiety Control   576
Definition   577
Case Study: Identification and Management of Dental Anxiety   577
Etiology   577
Anxiety Related to Dental Hygiene Care   578
Psychological Management   580
Management of Fearful Children   582

35   Chemistry and Pharmacology of Anesthetics   585
History of Anesthetics   586
Physiology of Nerve Conduction   586
Case Study: Considerations in the Selection of Dental Anesthetic   586
Mechanism of Action   588
Chemistry   588
Ionization Factors   588
Pharmacokinetics   589
Systemic Actions of Local Anesthetics   589
Vasoconstrictors in Anesthetic Solutions   590
Clinical Action of Specific Local Anesthetic Agents   591

36   Local Anesthetics: Injectable and Topical   595
Equipment   596
Case Study: Administering Local and Topical Anesthetic Agents   596
Topical Anesthetics   598
Local Anesthesia Techniques   599
Myths about Injection Techniques   606

37   Nitrous Oxide/Oxygen Sedation   610
Case Study: Administration of Nitrous Oxide/Oxygen Sedation   611
Analgesic and Other Effects   611
Pharmacology   611
Indications   612
Relative Contraindications   612
Equipment   612
Administration   614
Recovery   617
Biological Effects and Issues   618

PART VIII

Operative Therapies   622

38   Operative Procedures   624
Classification and Nomenclature   625
Case Study: Application of Operative Therapies   625
Minimally Invasive Dentistry   630
Aesthetic Dentistry   632
Isolation of Teeth   632
Evaluation Criteria   638
Restorative Materials   638
Restorative Procedures   639

39   Cosmetic Whitening   650
Case Studies: Cosmetic Whitening   651
Evolution of Bleaching   653
Dental Bleaching Agents: Composition and Mode of Action   654
Patient Selection: Indications and Contraindications   655
Data Collection: The Clinical Examination   656
Patient Instructions   656
Modes of Delivery: Bleaching Techniques   656

Side Effects of Bleaching   658
Role of the Dental Hygienist   658

PART IX

Care Modifications for Special Needs Patients   662

40 Salivary Dysfunction   664
Development of Salivary Glands   664
Classification of Salivary Glands   664
Case Study: Dental Management of Salivary Gland
   Dysfunction   665
Salivary Gland Dysfunction   665
Dental Management of Salivary Gland
   Dysfunction   666
Clues to Determine the Presence
   of Xerostomia   667

41 Neurological and Sensory Impairment   671
Case Study: Supportive Care Challenges
   in the Treatment of the Quadriplegic
   Patient   672
Selected Conditions   672
Impairments, Level of Severity, and Effect
   on Dental Care   677

42 Hormonal Imbalances   687
Female Sex Hormones   687
Case Studies: Hormonal Considerations
   in the Female Dental Patient   688
Clinical Manifestations   689
Hormone Replacement Therapy   691
Osteoporosis   691
Dental Hygiene Supportive Care Plan   691

43 Mental and Emotional Disturbances   694
Case Study: Fear and Anxiety in the Dental
   Patient   695
Definitions and Classification   696
Anxiety Disorders   698
Mood Disorders   703
Personality Disorders   705
Eating Disorders   707
Schizophrenia   709

44 Immune System Dysfunction   715
Immune System Function   716
Immune System Dysfunction   716
Case Study 1: Oral Care Considerations
   for the Cancer Patient   718
Cancer   719
Acquired Immunodeficiency Syndrome   725
Case Study 2: Oral Care Considerations
   for the HIV-Positive Patient   725

45 Head and Neck Cancer and Radiation   731
Case Study: Intraoral Considerations in the Dental
   Treatment of a Patient with Head and Neck
   Cancer   732
Etiology and Contributing Factors   732

Clinical Diagnosis   733
Staging   733
Early Detection   733
Treatment   734
Oral Care Protocol   741

PART X

Evaluation of Care   744

46 Evaluation and Supportive Care   746
Case Study: Evaluating Periodontal
   Outcomes   747
Risk Assessment   747
Rationale for Supportive Care   748
Patient Compliance   748
Evaluation of Initial Therapy   749
Supportive Care Intervals for Periodontal
   Patients   750
Review of Patient Record   750
Elements of the Periodontal Supportive Care
   Appointment   751
Responsibility for Periodontal Supportive Care
   Appointments   752
Supportive Care for Caries and Other Chronic
   Oral Conditions   752

**47 Case Development, Documentation,
   and Presentation   756**
Uses and Applications   756
Case Study: Use of Patient Case Documentation
   for Extended Learning   757
Theory   757
Example of Case Development and
   Documentation Guidelines   759

PART XI

Professional Development and Vision   768

48 Professional Development   770
Professional Self   770
Case Study: Embracing the Dental Hygiene
   Profession   771
Working with Other Professionals   772
Maintaining Competence   772

49 Insight and Commitment   775
Disease Prevention and Health Promotion   775
Future Direction   776
Case Study: Vision of Oral Care in 2010   776
The Future   778

ANSWER KEY   781

GLOSSARY   797

APPENDICES   821

CD-ROM Exercises Related to Text Discussions

Exercise number	Text page	Exercise name
1-A	7	Educational Opportunities
1-B	10	Legal Duties
1-C	11	Career Opportunities
1-D	12	Continuing Education
1-E	12	Professional Opportunities
1-F	12	Portfolio Initiation
1-G	14	Internet Resources
2-A	19	Portfolio Introduction and Initiation
3-A	41	Legal and Ethical Principles
3-B		
3-C		
3-D		
4-A	61	Communication
4-B		
4-C		
5-A	90	Universal Precautions
5-B	94	Selection of Personal Protective Equipment (PPE)
5-C	102	Surface Disinfection
5-D		
5-E	104	Sterilization Sequence
5-F	109	Waste Disposal
6-A	117	Identifying Repetitive Strain Injuries (RSIs)
6-B	120	Detemining Repetitive Strain Injuries (RSIs)
6-C	120	Operator Positioning
7-A	150	Principles of Instrumentation
7-B		
7-C	155	Instrument Correlation to Activation Stroke
8-A	163	Instrument Sharpening
8-B		
8-C		
8-D		
8-E	170	Determining Sharpening Error
9-A	178	Life Stage Identification
10-A	196	OPQRST Questioning
11-A	216	Palpation Technique
11-B		
11-C	217	Lymph Nodes
11-D	218	Salivary Glands
11-E	223	Vital Signs—Temperature
11-F	223	Vital Signs—Pulse
11-G	224	Vital Signs—Respiration
11-H	224	Vital Signs—Blood Pressure
12-A	235	Tobacco Cessation
13-A	246	Intraoral Examination
13-B	246	Lesion Description
13-C		

Exercise number	Text page	Exercise name
13-D	246	Intraoral Landmarks—Lips
13-E	246	Intraoral Landmarks—Labial Mucosa
13-F	252	Intraoral Landmarks—Buccal Mucosa
13-G	254	Intraoral Landmarks—Floor of the
13-H		Mouth
13-I	256	Intraoral Landmarks—Tongue
13-J		
13-K	259	Intraoral Landmarks—Palate
13-L	261	Intraoral Landmarks—Oropharynx
14-A	268	Oral Manifestations of Common Medications
15-A	285	Identification of Periodontal Landmarks
15-B	289	Gingival Description
15-C	289	Gingival Disease Recognition
15-D	290	Calculating Loss of Attachment
15-E	294	Furcation Classification
15-F	294	Furcation Identification
15-G	295	Mobility Classification
15-H	295	Evaluating Mobility
15-I	303	Periodontal Charting
16-A	310	Hard Tissue Examination
17-A	334	Radiographic Evaluation
17-B		
18-A	351	Nutritional Assessment
18-B		
19-A	356	Intraoral Imaging
19-B		
20-A	368	Supplementary Aids
20-B		
21-A	380	Toothbrush Characteristics
21-B	381	Tooth-Brushing Methods
21-C	381	Brushing Recommendations
21-D	383	Interproximal Cleaning
22-A	395	Management of Dental Caries
22-B	396	Caries Risk Assessment
23-A	407	Dentifrice Ingredients
23-B	409	Dentifrice Formulation
24-A	420	Chemotherapeutic Agents
25-A	430	Theory of Dentinal Sensitivity
25-B	432	Management of Dentinal Sensitivity
26-A	443	Sealant Procedure
26-B	443	Sealant Armamentarium
27-A	453	Prevention and Emergency Management of Dental Trauma
27-B	454	Risk-Prone Profiles
27-C	454	Physical Evaluation of Trauma
27-D	458	History of the Protection of Children
28-A	478	Care of Dental Appliances
29-A	487	Oral Risk Assessment

Exercise number	Text page	Exercise name
30-A	508	Oral Risk Assessment
31-A	526	Wound Healing
31-B	526	Healing Rate of Periodontal Tissues
31-C	527	Powered Instruments
31-D	530	Correct Tip Angulation
31-E	532	Patient Selection
32-A	542	Stain Classification
32-B	549	Selection of a Polishing Method and Agent
33-A	563	Suture Identification
33-B	570	Steps in Suture Removal
34-A	580	Methods of Controlling Anxiety
35-A	591	Types of Anesthetic
36-A	599	Sites of Injection
37-A	612	Contraindications
37-B	614	Identifying the Level of Sedation
37-C	614	Nitrous Oxide/Oxygen Sedation— The Facts
38-A	625	Identifying G.V. Black Classification
38-B	627	Labeling the Cavity Preparation
38-C	638	Advantages and Disadvantages of Restorative Materials
39-A	658	Cosmetic Whitening
40-A	665	Xerostomia: Causes and Effects
40-B	666	Management of Salivary Gland Dysfunction

Exercise number	Text page	Exercise name
41-A	672	Neurological Conditions and Related Impairments
41-B	677	Impairments and their Impact on Dental Care
42-A	687	Female Hormone Effects on the Body
42-B	689	Female Life Stages and Clinical Oral Manifestations
43-A	696	Dental Treatment Considerations
44-A	722	Oral Management of the Patient in Chemotherapy
45-A	733	Common Sites for Oral Cancer
45-B	733	Classification and Staging of Tumors
45-C	738	Oral Complications of Radiation Therapy
46-A	747	Identifying Periodontal Disease Risk in Reevaluation
46-B	752	Identifying Caries Risk in Reevaluation
47-A	759	Patient Selection
47-B	759	Topic Selection
48-A	770	Values Assessment
48-B	770	Philosophy of Practice
48-C	771	Needs Assessment
48-D	771	Career Goals
48-E	771	Evaluation of Career Paths
48-F	772	Portfolio Review
48-G	773	Evaluating Areas of Learning

Mosby's

DENTAL
HYGIENE

Concepts, Cases, and Competencies

PART I

Chapter 1
Dental Hygiene—Then and Now

Chapter 2
Health Promotion: A Basis of Practice

Chapter 3
Legal and Ethical Considerations

Chapter 4
Communication

Competency Statements

The learner is expected to possess knowledge, skills, judgments, values, and attitudes to develop the listed competencies.

Core Competencies

- Apply a professional code of ethics in all endeavors.
- Adhere to state and federal laws, recommendations, and regulations in the provision of dental hygiene care.
- Provide dental hygiene care to promote patient health and wellness using critical thinking and problem solving in the provision of evidence-based practice.
- Use evidence-based decision making to evaluate and incorporate emerging treatment modalities.
- Assume responsibility for dental hygiene actions and care based on accepted scientific theories and research as well as the accepted standard of care.

Courtesy American Dental Education Association, Washington, DC.

The Dental Hygiene Professional

- Continuously perform self-assessment for lifelong learning and professional growth.
- Promote the profession through service activities and affiliations with professional organizations.
- Provide quality assurance mechanisms for health services.
- Communicate effectively with individuals and groups from diverse populations both verbally and in writing.
- Provide accurate, consistent, and complete documentation for assessment, diagnosis, planning, implementation, and evaluation of dental hygiene services.
- Provide care to all patients using an individualized approach that is humane, empathetic, and caring.

Health Promotion and Disease Prevention

- Promote the values of oral and general health and wellness to the public and organizations within and outside the profession.
- Respect the goals, values, beliefs, and preferences of the patient while promoting optimal oral and general health.
- Evaluate factors that can be used to promote patient adherence to disease prevention and/or health maintenance strategies.

Patient Care

- Establish a collaborative relationship with the patient in the planned care to include etiology, prognosis, and treatment alternatives.
- Make referrals to other healthcare professionals.
- Obtain the patient's informed consent based on a thorough case presentation.

Professional Growth and Development

- Identify alternative career options within health care, industry, education, and research and evaluate the feasibility of pursuing dental hygiene opportunities.
- Access professional and social networks and resources to assist entrepreneurial initiatives.

CHAPTER 1

Dental Hygiene—Then *and* Now

Susan J. Daniel

Chapter Outline

Development of the Profession of Dental Hygiene
Case Study: Advances in Dental Technology
History of Dentistry
Education
    Development of formal education
    Institutional settings of programs and
      accreditation
    Entry level to profession and types of degrees
Clinical Practice Patterns
    Changes in practice environment
    Changes in caries detection and prevention
    Changes in etiology of periodontal disease
    Changes in treatment of periodontal disease
    Risk assessment: disease prevention and health
      promotion
    Informed consent and documentation
    Technology changes: computers
    Research

Licensure and Regulation
    National and state/regional
    Licensure by credentials or reciprocity
Career Mobility and Career Choices
    Private practice
    Education
    Public health
    Dental product sales and marketing
    Insurance industry
    Dental research
Maintaining Competence
    Continuing education
    Professional organizations
    Professional portfolio

Key Terms

Accreditation
Calculus
Competence
Debridement

Disease prevention
Evidence-based practice
Evidence-based teaching

Health promotion
Licensure
Plaque

Regulation
Risk assessment
Ultrasonic

Learning Outcomes

1. Appreciate the value of the history of the dental hygiene profession.
2. Understand the process necessary to become a licensed professional.
3. Develop educational goals for the first term of dental hygiene.
4. Identify the best way to maintain a professional portfolio.
5. Become aware of the career and professional opportunities available to the dental hygienist.

6. Explore the components of the dental practice act in your jurisdiction.
7. Perform literature searches using Pub Med or another search engine on topics related to dental hygiene.
8. Recognize change in the dental environment and profession.
9. Develop an appreciation for the different roles that dental hygienists play in the development of the profession and direction for the future.

DEVELOPMENT OF THE PROFESSION OF DENTAL HYGIENE

Historical accounts detail oral care regimens that have included cleansing of the teeth and gingiva (gums) with various ingredients. The theory that oral uncleanness or oral diseases resulted in oral and systemic disease drove modern dentistry to devise methods to rid the mouth of disease-causing agents.

Early records indicate mechanical and chemical methods of tooth deposit removal had been used throughout time to help prevent oral diseases. Some of the earliest recorded solutions for oral rinsing included alum and vinegar and even myrrh.[22] Hippocrates also advocated the use of whitstone (chalk) as an abrasive. Chalk is still an ingredient in today's dentifrices. Although some of these cleaning protocols seem extreme by today's standards, the use of abrasives and instruments to remove deposits forms the basis of many of today's oral care products (Box 1-1).

Modern dentistry has seen intermittent exploration but little acceptance of the theory or hypothesis of gum disease causing or compounding systemic disease. Consideration of diseases of the oral cavity has been just that—a disease state considered isolated only to the oral cavity. Systemic sequela was not part of the equation. Beginning in the late 1980s, researchers began to explore the relationship between oral and systemic health, reuniting the oral cavity and head with the rest of the body.* The renewed interest in this integrated concept clearly makes sense; the blood that passes through the oral tissues also circulates to the rest of the body. The humoral response found in host immunity is responsible for circulating antibodies effective against bacterial, parasitic, and viral infections. Thus an approach to *disease prevention* and *health promotion* is exciting and will certainly affect the practice of dental hygiene. Chapter 2 explores this concept in greater depth.

This chapter explores the past and present in dental hygiene education and *accreditation;* practice behaviors, clinical environment, technology, *licensure,* and *regulation;* career opportunities; and continued *competence.*

HISTORY OF DENTISTRY

Fig. 1-1 highlights of the development of dentistry. History provides a perspective on the richness of the dental hygiene profession.

Archeological finds have given dentistry a visual account from ancient cultures.[40] One of the earliest finds is a vanity set that includes a toothpick (Fig. 1-2).[34] As civilization continued to develop and became more educated, the use of instruments for deposit removal on the teeth was developed. Albucasis was the first to develop a set of instruments and instructions to remove deposits (Fig. 1-3[34] and Box 1-2). Albucasis was an extremely religious Moorish surgeon in Spain and, in the Latin treatise *De Chirurgia*, the first individual to recommend a thorough cleaning of the mouth.

Even though dentistry has been a surgically oriented profession, its history contains many references to cleaning of the mouth and prevention of disease, specifically in the early decades of the 1900s in America.[30] With the

 Case Study   **Advances in Dental Technology**

Pretend for a moment that Irene Newman, the first dental hygiene graduate of Dr. Fones' school in Connecticut, has an opportunity to encounter today's new, modern clinical dental environment. The following section describes the setting that Irene encounters.

Irene arrives at her place of employment and opens the door; her world has been transformed. The area where patients wait is no longer stark with hard, wooden chairs lining the perimeter of the room. Instead, the room is attractive and inviting, with light-colored, soft upholstered chairs. A small sofa, side tables with magazines, and live plants are located strategically in the room. Pleasant artwork adorns the walls, and a dental-related video and monitor for patient viewing occupies a cozy corner.

In awe, Irene proceeds to her work area only to see a totally strange sight. The equipment appears completely foreign. She recognizes what she assumes to be a patient chair, but what is the other chair? She looks at the dental unit and cannot identify the components. She finds neat, small labeled packages containing odd-looking instruments. Next to the unit is a strange boxlike apparatus with a pedal and some type of metal probe protruding from the end of a hose. She notices a large, square box with a glass side attached to something that resembles a typewriter. She is lost in an unfamiliar world.

BOX 1-1

First Dentifrice Prescribed by Hippocrates

When a woman's mouth smells and her gums are black and unhealthy; one burns, separately, the head of a hare, and three mice, after having taken out the intestines of two of them (not however the liver or kidneys): one pounds in a stone mortar some marble and whitstone, and passes it through a sieve; one then mixes equal parts of these ingredients and with this mixture one rubs the teeth and the interior of the mouth; afterward one rubs them again with greasy wool and one washes the mouth with water. One soaks the dirty wool in honey and with it rubs the gums inside and outside. One pounds dill and anise seeds, 2 aboles (1 abole = ¾ gram) of myrrh: one immerses these substances in half a cotyle (1 cotyle = ¼ liter) of pure white wine; one then rinses the mouth with it, holding it in the mouth for some time; this is to be done frequently and the mouth to be rinsed with said preparation fasting and after each meal. The medicament described above cleans the teeth and gives them a sweet smell.

From Hippocrates: *De Morbis Mulerum,* Lib II, 606.

---

*References 4-6, 9, 10, 18, 19, 25-30, 32-36, 41.

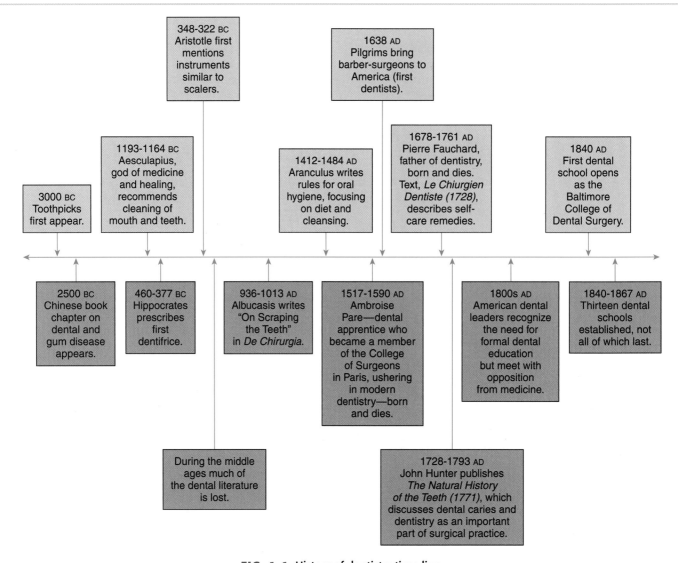

348-322 BC Aristotle first mentions instruments similar to scalers.

1638 AD Pilgrims bring barber-surgeons to America (first dentists).

1193-1164 BC Aesculapius, god of medicine and healing, recommends cleaning of mouth and teeth.

1412-1484 AD Aranculus writes rules for oral hygiene, focusing on diet and cleansing.

1678-1761 AD Pierre Fauchard, father of dentistry, born and dies. Text, *Le Chiurgien Dentiste (1728)*, describes self-care remedies.

1840 AD First dental school opens as the Baltimore College of Dental Surgery.

3000 BC Toothpicks first appear.

2500 BC Chinese book chapter on dental and gum disease appears.

460-377 BC Hippocrates prescribes first dentifrice.

936-1013 AD Albucasis writes "On Scraping the Teeth" in *De Chirurgia*.

1517-1590 AD Ambroise Pare—dental apprentice who became a member of the College of Surgeons in Paris, ushering in modern dentistry—born and dies.

1800s AD American dental leaders recognize the need for formal dental education but meet with opposition from medicine.

1840-1867 AD Thirteen dental schools established, not all of which last.

During the middle ages much of the dental literature is lost.

1728-1793 AD John Hunter publishes *The Natural History of the Teeth (1771)*, which discusses dental caries and dentistry as an important part of surgical practice.

FIG. 1-1 History of dentistry time line.

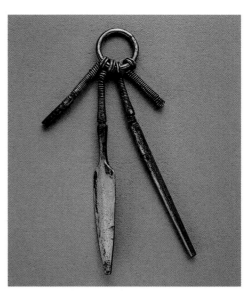

FIG. 1-2 An early archeological find of a vanity set includes a toothpick. (Courtesy University of Pennsylvania Museum of Archaeology and Anthropology, Philadelphia.)

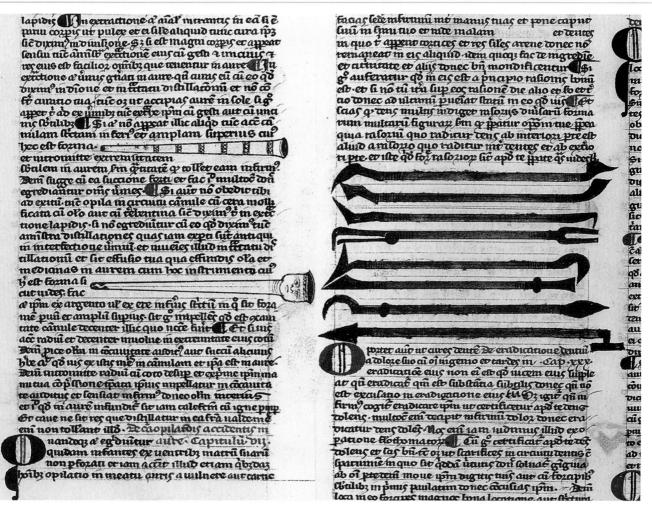

FIG. 1-3 A twelfth-century Latin translation of Albucasis' instruments for scaling teeth. (From Staatsbibliothek, Bamberg Ms. 91, fol. 75. In: Ring ME: *Dentistry: an illustrated history,* New York, 1985, Harry N. Abrams.)

BOX 1-2

Albucasis' Written Instructions "On the Scraping of the Teeth"

Sometimes on the surface of the teeth, both inside and outside, as well as under the gums, are deposited rough scales, of ugly appearance, and black, green or yellow in color, thus corruption is communicated to the gums, and so the teeth are in process of time denuded. It is necessary for you to lay the patient's head upon your lap and to scrape the teeth and molars, on which are observed either true encrustations, or something similar to sand, and this until nothing more remains of such substances, and also until the dirty color of the teeth disappears, be it black or green or yellowish, or nay other color. If a first scraping is sufficient, so much the better, if not, you shall repeat it on the following day or even on the third or fourth day, until the desired purpose is obtained.

Albucasis A: *De Chirurgia* (translated from Latin by Channing S), Oxford, England, 1778.

---

focus on disease prevention and mouth cleaning, early leaders in dentistry realized the need for other dental personnel to perform these tasks. By 1906 women were trained to be *dental nurses.* Dr. Alfred Fones did not like this name because it carried the connotation of disease. In 1913 he provided a more descriptive name, *dental hygienist;* a hygienist is one versed in the science of health and the prevention of disease.[17,30]

EDUCATION

Formal education of dental hygienists began in the early 1900s with a program for dental nurses at the Ohio College of Dental Surgery. However, in 1911, because of opposition from the Ohio dentists, the program closed and the graduates were never allowed to practice. Fig. 1-4 highlights events leading to the prevention movement and the development of dental hygiene. The term *prevention movement* was given to the efforts of a group of prominent dentists who believed in the prevention of oral disease, defined methods for prevention, and wrote and spoke on the subject.

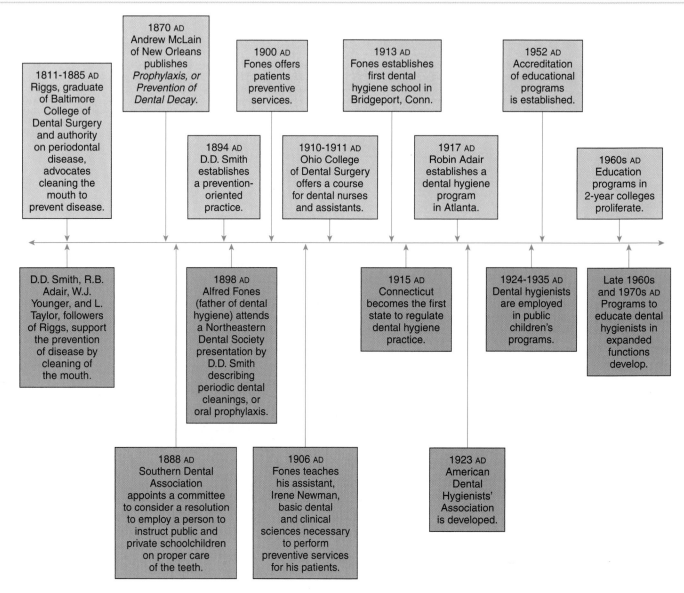

FIG. 1-4 History of dental hygiene time line.

DEVELOPMENT OF FORMAL EDUCATION

After attending a lecture on the benefits of periodic oral prophylaxis, Dr. Alfred C. Fones added this service to his practice. He soon realized the many benefits to his patients' oral health. In 1906 Dr. Fones trained his dental assistant, Irene Newman (the first dental hygiene graduate of his Connecticut school), to scale and polish teeth and to provide general oral self-care instructions to patients. Her education included reading basic and dental science texts and developing scaling and polishing skills.[16,17] The majority of the 27 women in Dr. Fones' first dental hygiene graduating class were employed by the Bridgeport, Connecticut, Board of Education. These first dental hygienists were credited with helping reduce dental caries by 75% in children participating in their oral care/prevention program. In 1917 Connecticut became the first state to pass licensure laws governing dental hygienists. During this same period, dentists in several other states became disciples of preventive

services, including the removal of **plaque** and hard deposits with specially designed instruments.[16,17]

Many of the early dental hygienists were employed in the public school system and provided educational and preventive services to children.[16] Public health was the primary employment setting for dental hygienists and private practice secondary, whereas the opposite is true today. The original role of the dental hygienist was that of disease prevention; the same role forms the basis of current practice.

INSTITUTIONAL SETTINGS OF PROGRAMS AND ACCREDITATION

The educational requirements for dental hygienists have changed over the years. Subjective curriculums were replaced with standards and most recently with competencies.[1] Originally, programs were housed in university settings and later in community colleges. In the 1960s the number of programs in 2-year institutions multiplied drastically. A minimum entry level of education was established as 2 years of a college education. The Commission on Dental Education established standards requiring course work in general education; basic, dental, and clinical sciences; and community dental health.

Accredited schools are reviewed every 7 years through a program self-study by the institution, culminating in a site visit by accreditation members. Meeting specified standards grants a program accreditation.

ENTRY LEVEL TO PROFESSION AND TYPES OF DEGREES

1-A

Although the minimum educational requirement is 2 years of college with specific standards set forth by the American Dental Association (ADA) Commission on Dental and Allied Dental Accreditation, not all dental hygiene programs award the same degree. The entry-level dental hygienist can earn a certificate, an associate's degree, or a bachelor's degree. The type of degree awarded depends on the institution and curriculum. Although some 4-year programs might offer expanded functions, no special licensure or functions differentiate a graduate with a certificate or an associate's degree from one who has 4 years of education culminating in a bachelor's degree.

Most dental hygiene programs awarding an associate's degree require more than 2 years of college education. Some require a full year of prerequisite courses followed by 2 years of dental hygiene courses. Certificates in dental hygiene often are awarded by an institution (university or college) that recognizes the bachelor's degree as the minimal degree awarded. In the university setting, any less than 4 academic years or equivalent hours usually results in a certificate.

CLINICAL PRACTICE PATTERNS

CHANGES IN PRACTICE ENVIRONMENT

Although dental hygiene remains a prevention-oriented profession, clinical practice behaviors—such as educational requirements—have changed over the years. Approaches to patient education and therapy based on knowledge of etiology and treatment modalities have altered the way preventive care is delivered. The practice environment also has changed. Fig. 1-5 is an early dental chair. Dentistry has evolved from the dental professionals working in a standing position (Fig. 1-6) to the ergonomically sound, seated position during patient care (Fig. 1-7). Dental equipment has been modified significantly to accommodate this change. Equipment modifications to the patient chair allow the patient to be placed in a supine position for the delivery of care by a seated operator.

The dental unit was redesigned to allow the seated operator access to the handpiece, suction, and air/water syringe. These components also have undergone modifications. Some equipment changes, known as *engineering controls*, have been developed to protect the operator from infectious diseases, whereas others have been made for operator and patient comfort (ergonomics). More information about engineering controls and ergonomic changes is presented in Chapters 5 and 6.

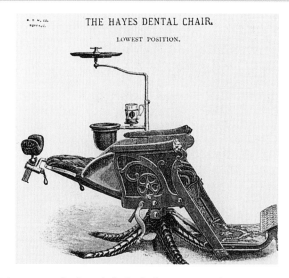

FIG. 1-5 Early dental chair, dating to 1875. (Courtesy James Ulrich, State University of New York, Buffalo, N.Y.)

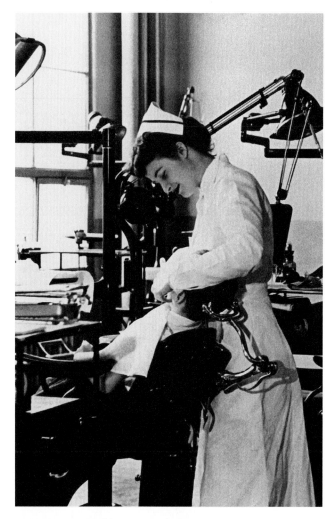

FIG. 1-6 Dental hygienist during the 1960s working in a standing position. (Courtesy Fr. Edward J. Dowling, S.J. Marine Historical Collection, University of Detroit Mercy, Detroit.)

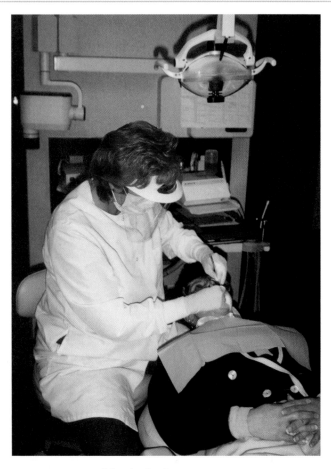

FIG. 1-7 Seated hygienist in a contemporary treatment room.

CHANGES IN CARIES DETECTION AND PREVENTION

Positioning of the operator, patient, and equipment reflects environmental alterations in the practice setting. Terminology, etiology, detection, prevention, intervention, and treatment of oral diseases also have changed.

Protocols used to diagnose oral disease likewise have changed. A dental explorer and radiographs were originally the primary tools used to detect dental caries. Because microbes responsible for caries have been identified at different stages during lesion development, current literature suggests less use of the explorer and more visual examination with the use of dyes, special illumination, and microbial testing.* Laser technology has been developed for early caries detection and can be operated by the dental hygienist for detection of carious lesions.[24] Prevention and intervention of caries development has improved with the use of caries *risk assessment* tools, microbial testing, systemic and topical fluorides, and knowledge of the remineralization and demineralization processes. Treatment has become more conservative with less emphasis on removal of tooth structure and more emphasis on retention of tooth structure, use of dental sealants, and placement of preventive resins.

---

*References 8, 12, 21, 24, 37, 38.

CHANGES IN ETIOLOGY OF PERIODONTAL DISEASE

Periodontal diseases used to be viewed as one singular disease. Before the late 1960s, only two identified diseases of tooth-supporting structures existed: periodontitis (an inflammatory process requiring gingival tissue or tooth removal) and periodontosis (of unknown etiology but degenerative, with no treatment other than tooth loss).

Knowledge of etiology (quantitative versus qualitative plaque theory), differentiation between several forms of gingival and periodontal diseases, and preventive and conservative therapies have been developed. Today many known forms of periodontal diseases exist and can be differentiated by clinical, microbiological, and patient history assessments.

CHANGES IN TREATMENT OF PERIODONTAL DISEASE

More definitive treatment modalities for periodontal diseases now exist. After the specific form of periodontal disease has been identified based on oral risk parameters, the appropriate patient-specific prevention, intervention, and therapeutic strategies can be developed. Removing or lowering the bacterial load in the periodontal environment to enable the immune system to trigger wound healing is still the primary therapeutic focus.

Not long ago (in the 1970s and 1980s), dental professionals thought removal of all hard deposits *(calculus)* and elimination of bacterial plaque were necessary to prevent gingivitis and periodontitis. This theory did not take into account each individual's immune response to infection. Some individuals with little bacterial plaque or calculus had a higher rate of gingival and periodontal infections than did those with greater amounts of plaque and calculus. Additional research indicated that lowering of the amount of deposits is not the key to treatment success. The key is to reduce the bacterial load to a level at which the individual's immune system can manage the infection, which improves periodontal health.

Current understanding of the disease process and the immune system has changed professional therapeutic strategy. *Ultrasonic* instrumentation is more frequently used to gain a better healing response than is hand instrumentation. As a result of research and clinical evidence, the terms *scaling* and *root planing* are being replaced by the term *debridement.* Patient self-care habits, the use of chemotherapeutics, and professional intervention provide greater options in the development of individual strategies to assist the immune response.

RISK ASSESSMENT: DISEASE PREVENTION AND HEALTH PROMOTION

Although the practice of dental hygiene always has focused on prevention, the prevention aspect has expanded to whole-body health. The removal of deposits may be the primary concern of the patient, but the practice of dental hygiene is centered on treatment of the patient as a whole. Careful review of the patient's medical/health history, assessment of medications, and interview for signs and symptoms of systemic disease, along with education in the prevention of oral disease, is a part of today's supportive care appointment.

A total risk assessment is essential to disease prevention and health promotion. Inclusion of all aspects of the patient's health, medical, and dental history; fluoride history; behaviors and beliefs; clinical and radiographic findings; current medications; oral care routine; and nutritional habits provide an insight into the patient's well-being (Box 1-3).

Oral Health in America: A Report of the Surgeon General states the following:[39]

> *The terms* oral health *and* general health *should not be interpreted as separate entities. Oral health is integral to general health.*

Recently research has linked several systemic conditions with periodontal disease. Lifestyle behaviors such as alcohol use, tobacco use, and improper nutrition affect oral health. Oral infections can be the source or first sign of systemic infections.

The role of the dental hygienist has evolved from that of a tooth cleaner/educator to that of a disease prevention and health promotion specialist. The dental hygienist's role is well suited to monitoring the patient's general health. A dental patient usually sees the dental hygienist periodically for supportive care. Dental hygienists have been educated to note variations from the normal and understand the implications of abnormalities. In addition, dental hygienists develop a rapport with their patients, instilling trust and confidence.

INFORMED CONSENT AND DOCUMENTATION

Medical legal considerations have received greater emphasis over the years, and informed consent of the patient has become an important issue. Treating humans without providing them adequate information about procedures, options, untoward events, and costs is illegal. Informing a patient of the above is not enough; the patient or guardian must *understand,* and that individual's signature must be obtained before the initiation of procedures.[23] Documentation in the patient record of all pertinent findings and procedures and the form of documentation is critical. Failure to meticulously document patient care can result in significant legal ramifications. Chapter 3 presents more on ethical and legal considerations.

TECHNOLOGY CHANGES: COMPUTERS

The introduction of computers to dentistry has evolved some clinical practices into paper-free zones. What originally began as a business management tool (appointment scheduling, patient and insurance billings) has moved into the treatment room. Current use of chairside computers includes all patient record keeping, charting, digital radiography, and voice-activated periodontal recording. Care must be taken to preserve these computer files as permanent documentation of the patient's treatment history.

RESEARCH

The body of scientific knowledge of dentistry and medicine is growing rapidly. Continued research to identify the disease process and components of the immune response in healing provides evidence for education and practice. Ultimately, the goal is to preserve the oral tissues (hard and soft) in health. ***Evidence-based teaching*** and ***evidence-based practice*** will be the ways for the dental professional to attain this goal. Treatment options must be based on assessment of the patient's needs and expectations, the care providers' clinical experience and scope of expertise, and sound scientific evidence based on successful treatment outcomes. Evidence-based protocols require the use of rapidly changing technology through the evaluation of literature and continued professional education.

LICENSURE AND REGULATION

NATIONAL AND STATE/REGIONAL

Successful progress toward completion of an ADA-accredited dental hygiene program permits a candidate to sit for the Dental Hygiene National Board Examination, a written, comprehensive, and objective test required for licensure in all states except Alabama. On successful completion of an accredited program and successful performance on the national board examination, a graduate then can sit for a state licensure examination that covers the evaluation of a candidate's practical application of dental hygiene skills. A regional or state board of examiners administers this licensure examination. Passing a regional board allows a candidate to apply for licensure in any participating state (Box 1-4). All states require the successful completion of a jurisprudence examination before issuing a dental hygiene license. Passing a state-administered board examination and jurisprudence examination completes the requirements for licensure in that respective state *only.*

LICENSURE BY CREDENTIALS OR RECIPROCITY

Previously, single-state licensing practices required the state-licensing applicant to take another board examination before procuring a license to practice. Realizing the limitations this law created for relocation of dental professionals, some state boards have established licensing by credentials and reciprocity avenues as alternatives to a repeat of the practical examination. However, licensing boards still require the candidate to sit for the practical examination for licensure, regardless of how many jurisdictions in which that individual is licensed or the number of

---

BOX 1-4

Membership in the Four Regional Testing Agencies in the United States*

NERB: North East Regional Board
The first regional board examination, and the largest with 15 states enrolled, began in the late 1960s. Participating states include the following:
    Connecticut
    District of Columbia
    Illinois
    Maine
    Maryland
    Massachusetts
    Michigan
    New Hampshire
    New Jersey
    New York
    Ohio
    Pennsylvania
    Rhode Island
    Vermont
    West Virginia

CRDTS: Central Regional Dental Testing Service
The second regional board examination, formed in the mid-1970s, includes the following 11 states between the Rocky Mountains and the Mississippi River:
    Colorado
    Illinois
    Iowa
    Kansas
    Minnesota
    Missouri
    Nebraska

    North Dakota
    South Dakota
    Washington (dental only)
    Wisconsin
    Wyoming

SRTA: Southern Regional Testing Agency
Formed in the mid 1970s, this board now includes the following:
    Arkansas
    Georgia
    Kentucky
    South Carolina
    Tennessee
    Virginia
    West Virginia

WREB: Western Regional Examining Board
Established in the late 1970s, this board has grown from three to the following eight states:
    Alaska
    Arizona
    Idaho
    Montana
    New Mexico
    Oklahoma
    Oregon
    Texas
    Utah
    Washington
    Wyoming

---

*Memberships in the boards can fluctuate as states join or withdraw.

years of practice experience. Additionally, Florida has a statute of limitations on the number of years allowed after national board certification to qualify for state licensure.[11] If more than 10 years have elapsed since passing the Dental Hygiene National Board Examination, the candidate must retake the examination before being allowed to take the Florida clinical examination for licensure.

Groups of educators, practitioners, and examiners believe clinical board examinations are unnecessary if the student graduated from an ADA-accredited program.* In other words, competence as judged by the educational program through the documentation of successful performance should be sufficient to obtain licensure to practice without sitting for a clinical examination.

An alternative course of action for dental licensure under consideration is the use of simulated clinical examinations.[2,12] Currently, each applicant for licensure is required to present one or more patients meeting specific criteria. Selecting appropriate patients and paying transportation, meals, and sometimes lodging and a day's wages are difficult and expensive for the licensure applicant. Using a simulation manikin for the examination sets criteria-based standards, allowing the examination to more objectively assess clinical performance. The Dental Interactive Simulation Corporation (DISC) is working on the development of an interactive simulated national and clinical board examination.[12]

Types of Supervision

Few states allow dental hygienists to practice independently. In most states the practice of dental hygiene is allowed under the supervision of a licensed dentist. Supervision can range from direct to general. States with general supervision language in the practice act may have additional criteria for this form of supervision. Definitions of supervision and business arrangements are identified in Box 1-5.[3]

Functions

A dental hygienist's duties vary by state. Universally, dental hygienists remove deposits on the teeth, expose dental radiographs, place topical fluoride and dental sealants, and teach patients self-care techniques. In more than half the United States, dental hygienists are licensed to provide local anesthesia. Other functions delegated to the dental hygienist may include operative procedures, such as placing restorations, performing cosmetic whitening, placing and/or removing sutures, making impressions, administering nitrous oxide and oxygen analgesia, and placing subgingival preventive agents. Delegation of procedures varies among the states. Dental hygienists must become familiar with the dental practice act in the states in which they wish to practice.

Will universal licensure, simulated examinations, or licensure by competence ever be administered directly by a dental hygiene program? Which functions will the dental hygienist perform 50 years from today? The future holds many secrets. Chapters 48 and 49 explore these questions.

1-B

---

*References 2, 7, 14, 15, 20, 25, 31.

BOX 1-5

Types and Definitions of Dental Supervision

Direct supervision: A dentist must be present in the facility when a dental hygienist performs procedures.

General supervision: A dentist has authorized a dental hygienist to perform procedures but does not need to be present in the treatment facility during the performance of those procedures. More than 70% of the states have some form of general supervision in the dental practice act.

Independent practice: In this business arrangement the dental hygienist owns a dental hygiene practice—a recognizable incorporated or unincorporated business structure that can be bought and sold. An independent practitioner may have a supervisory relationship with a dentist. An unsupervised dental hygienist may be employed to work in a dental office or other entity.

Independent contracting: With this tax status, the dental hygienist does not maintain an employee relationship with a dentist for whose patients the hygienist provides dental hygiene services. As non-employees the dental hygienists pay their own withholding taxes and Social Security, and the dentist does not pay worker's compensation or unemployment insurance on their behalf.

BOX 1-6

Specialty Practices in Dentistry

Endodontics	Oral and maxillofacial surgery
Periodontics	Oral and maxillofacial
Pediatric dentistry	radiology
Prosthodontics	Oral pathology
Orthodontics	Dental public health

CAREER MOBILITY AND CAREER CHOICES

1-C   Dental hygienists are part of an exciting and expanding healthcare environment. Growth in knowledge and technology are being transferred to the educational and career environment. Licensed dental hygienists have many professional career options, from private practice to consulting.

PRIVATE PRACTICE

The private dental practice employs the most dental hygienists. In private practice the hygienist typically functions as a clinician and patient educator, providing preventive services to patients. Dental hygienists are most often employed in a general dental practice, but some choose to work in a dental specialty practice (Box 1-6). In some private offices the dental hygienist assumes the role of the practice manager or office manager. Frequently this role is in addition to the clinical responsibilities and requires specific skills and knowledge in business management.

EDUCATION

Dental hygienists holding advanced degrees also serve as dental hygiene educators. The type of institution and dental hygiene degree being awarded by the program dictate the level of degree required of full-time faculty members. Academic responsibilities of a dental hygiene faculty member vary according to the type of institution (community college and university) and its mission. In some institutions, faculty members are required to teach, provide community service, and perform scholarly activities. Clinical patient care also is required by some in-

stitutions. Continued activity in these areas assists the dental hygiene educator in maintaining competence. Students are only as competent as the educators who facilitate learning.

PUBLIC HEALTH

Some dental public health divisions of state governments employ hygienists to perform oral screenings of school children for dental diseases and provide preventive services in local clinics.

The U.S. Public Health Service and Indian Health Service Branch of the federal government employ dental hygienists to work in dental clinics nationwide. Dental hygienists with bachelor's degrees can become commissioned officers in the U.S. Public Health Service. Other employment opportunities are available within the Veteran's Administration Hospitals' dental clinics and the federal and state prison systems. Many larger institutions have dental clinic facilities on their premises.

DENTAL PRODUCT SALES AND MARKETING

Corporations employ dental hygienists to market products to private offices, retail stores, and institutions. The dental hygienist's knowledge and use of preventive products is most beneficial for the companies that employ them. Pharmaceutical and medical sales are also options for the dental hygienist. The basic science foundation within the hygienist's educational curriculum provides the understanding needed to effectively market these types of products.

INSURANCE INDUSTRY

Hygienists have been employed in the insurance industry as dental claim reviewers. The knowledge of radiographic imaging (pathology), treatment need, treatment codes, and ethical behavior provides the dental hygienist the background to enter the insurance industry.

DENTAL RESEARCH

The quest for new knowledge provides another opportunity for employment and career extension. Investigation of ideas and questions is the genesis of tomorrow's education and practice—evidence supporting which treatment to provide, when, why, and how. Dental hygienists are employed as researchers. Some work independently; others are part of a group of investigators. Most dental hygiene researchers have obtained the advanced degrees necessary to understand the research process and to open the doors to become a respected researcher. Research activity without publication of the findings is of little value to anyone other than perhaps those directly involved in the investigative activity. Publishing research findings adds to the body of literature and supports educational and clinical practice knowledge and techniques. Using research findings in education and practice assists in the quest for continued competence.

MAINTAINING COMPETENCE

 ### *CONTINUING EDUCATION*

1-D Although maintaining competence is necessary in all fields, it is especially important in health care. Healthcare providers should desire continued learning. The knowledge and technology changes in medicine and dentistry are rapid. One measure of competence is to assess continually or annually the amount (in hours) and content of education a healthcare provider receives. Continuing education hours have been specifically mandated for a given time period by almost all state dental licensing boards to allow for the licensee to retain active licensure and practice. Continuing education hours may be obtained in many forms, and each state identifies the type of format it will accept, which include class sessions or workshops, courses on video, and CD or online and courses within professional journals.

 ### *PROFESSIONAL ORGANIZATIONS*

1-E Maintaining competence can be time consuming. Isolation allows complacency and satisfaction with the care being rendered and its outcomes. Dental hygienists often report feeling isolated when working in a solo dental practice. Becoming a member and participating in a professional organization facilitates discussion among peers who frequently experience or have experienced similar situations. Professional organizations allow for the sharing of ideas, support, and encouragement and provide a forum for formal learning experiences through seminars and other continuing educational activities. Membership is important for a sense of belonging in the healthcare profession.

Dental hygienists have various professional associations from which to choose, and many dental hygienists have membership in more than one professional association. The American Dental Hygienists' Association (ADHA) was organized in 1923 and is the professional association representing dental hygienists only. The association offices are located in Chicago, Illinois. Members, officers, and staff members provide representation for dental hygiene in national governmental affairs and in other associations, especially on the American Dental Association's (ADA's) Commission on Dental and Allied Dental Accreditation and the American Dental Education Association (ADEA). The ADHA develops recommendations for dental hygiene practice and supports dental hygiene activities nationwide.

Many countries have national professional organizations for dental hygienists. An international association exists for national organizations and individual members. The International Federation of Dental Hygiene comprises 21 national organizations (Box 1-7).

ADEA is the professional association representing educators. The association provides continuing education opportunities for dental, dental hygiene, dental assisting, and dental laboratory technology faculty and supports dental and allied dental education in other healthcare and governmental affairs. Educators have an opportunity to share and learn what other educators are doing in their respective programs. Additionally, members of the association, through committees, develop subject guidelines for program curricula.

The American Association for Dental Research (AADR) is the research association for dental and allied dental researchers in the United States. Other countries also have their own dental research associations. Membership in the AADR has reciprocal membership with the International Association for Dental Research (IADR). Like the other professional organizations, the AADR/IADR provide a forum to showcase dental research. This exchange of ideas, theories, and original research findings assists with the development of improved treatment and prevention regimens and forms the basis of future educational curricular change.

The American Association of Public Health Dentistry and the American Public Health Association are organizations providing support and innovations in dental public health and public health, respectively. These associations address general and oral health issues, their effect on the population, and measures to alleviate and prevent disease.

Other professional associations and organizations in which dental hygienists can become members include the National Dental Hygienists' Association and the Hispanic Dental Association. These organizations support and encourage oral health promotion in their respective minorities. The important aspect is to remain a part of a professional organization that promotes oral and systemic health and supports the role of dental hygienists in the pursuit of better oral health care for all.

PROFESSIONAL PORTFOLIO

Documentation of continuing education or other activities to maintain competence is necessary for a career in dental hygiene. A mechanism used to document this process is the professional portfolio. Portfolios have been used in art and journalism to demonstrate ability or competence. The dental hygienist portfolio can include information about all forms of continuing education received, information on community service activities performed individually or with other professionals, and professional meetings attended. The portfolio can provide a place to **1-F** document patient cases with various systemic and oral diseases, oral risks identified, strategies employed, and treatment successes. This information will assist with future patient care and self-evaluation of effectiveness and perhaps provide the information required for a salary increase or for a change in employment settings. Of the many responsibilities of being a healthcare provider, maintaining competence is possibly the most important. Many avenues exist for documentation, but the most comprehensive is the professional portfolio.

This chapter presents an overview of the history of den-

tal hygiene and current trends in the field, modifications to licensure, education, and current challenges. The remainder of the text details the information necessary to become a dental hygienist. Providing preventive oral health care is becoming increasingly important as more links are discovered between oral and systemic health. This is an exciting time to embark on a career in dental hygiene. Dental hygienists always should look for ways to improve themselves and those they serve, goals for which this text and its accompanying CD-ROM provide a rich foundation.

 CRITICAL THINKING ACTIVITIES

1. Through conversation with faculty, colleagues, your dentist/dental hygienist, and/or local dental hygiene society, identify a local dental hygienist that has been in practice for more than 20 years. Call and introduce yourself and ask for an interview on the topic of dental hygiene: then and now. Determine the nature of the changes the dental hygienist has witnessed in the following areas: sterilization, staffing, staff interaction, uniforms, equipment, use of technology, emphasis in practice, educational requirements, and licensing process.
   Which areas have seen the most change?
   Which areas have seen the least change?
   Compare your findings with those of a classmate who has interviewed a different hygienist with a similar career history.
2. Review the concept of the dental hygiene portfolio in this chapter. Make a list of potential portfolio folders from your most recent education accomplishments. Would such a portfolio have been helpful to your interview process on entering the dental hygiene program?

3. Investigate dental hygiene practice/application in any of the following areas that appeal to you and list the advantages and disadvantages involved:
   Clinician
   Administrator/manager
   Educator
   Researcher
   Consumer advocate
   Change agent
   Public health dental hygienist
4. Are you interested in pursuing a career in areas other than clinical dental hygiene? Do you think a mentor, someone already accomplished in that area of dental hygiene practice, would be helpful to you? If yes, how do you see that relationship starting?
5. Determine your state's continuing education requirements. Which continuing education courses are offered at your school? Is a college or university within driving distance at which you could attend a course? Does your school require you to keep track of any continuing education (CE) courses you take? Do you see any benefit to doing so as a student?
6. If your school has provided you with competency statements specific to your program, which of those competencies does Chapter 1 address?

 REVIEW QUESTIONS

1. All of the following components of dentistry have changed dramatically since the 1900s *except* which one?
   a. Professional attire
   b. Patient and operator positioning
   c. Equipment
   d. Need for better communication
2. Which of the following individuals is credited with being the founder of dental hygiene?
   a. Irene Newman
   b. Alfred Fones
   c. D.D. Smith
   d. Robin Adair

3. In which of the following areas of dentistry are most dental hygienists employed?
   a. Periodontal practices
   b. General dental practices
   c. Public health dentistry
   d. Pediatric dentistry
4. Dental hygienists practice under all *except* which of the following?
   a. Independent
   b. Direct
   c. Modified direct
   d. General

Continued

REVIEW QUESTIONS—cont'd

5. Oral and systemic health are related by which of the following mechanisms?
   a. Immune components
   b. Treatments
   c. Prevention strategies
   d. Diseases

6. Dental hygiene programs can be found in which of the following institutions?
   a. Universities
   b. Community colleges
   c. Technical institutes
   d. All of the above

 SUGGESTED AGENCIES AND WEB SITES

1-G

Because of the ever-changing nature of the Internet, some of the web sites listed here may have changed since publication. Please refer to Mosby's Evolve web site for the most current information.

American Dental Association: http://www.ada.org
American Dental Education Association: http://www.adea.org
Hu-Friedy Manufacturing Company, Inc.: http://www.hufriedy.com
Indian Health Service: http://www.ihs.gov

International Federation of Dental Hygienists: http://www.ifdh.org
KaVo America Corporation: http://www.kavo.com
Public Health Service: http://www.phs.os.dhhs.gov
The American Dental Hygienists' Association: http://www.adha.org

 REFERENCES

1. *Accreditation Standards for Dental Hygiene Education,* Chicago, 1998, Commission on Dental Accreditation, American Dental Association.
2. American Dental Association House of Delegates: Resolution 64RC, 2000.
3. American Dental Hygienists' Association: *House of Delegates manual: definition of commonly used terms,* Chicago, 1999, The Association.
4. Beck JD et al: Evaluation of oral bacteria as risk indictors for periodontitis in older adults, *J Periodontol* 63:93-9, 1992.
5. Beck J et al: Periodontal disease and cardiovascular disease, *J Periodontol* 67:1123-37, 1996.
6. Beck JD et al: Periodontitis: a risk factor for coronary heart disease, *Ann Periodontol* 3(1):127-41, 1998.
7. Buchannan RN: Problems related to the use of human subjects in clinical evaluation/responsibility for follow-up care, *J Dent Educ* 55:797-8, 1991.
8. Coleston BW et al: Imaging of hard and soft-tissue structure in the oral cavity by optical coherence tomography, *Applied Optics* 37:3582-5, 1998.
9. Dasanayake AP: Poor periodontal health of the pregnant woman as a risk factor for low birth weight, *Ann Periodontol* 3(1):206-11, 1998.
10. Davenport ES et al: The East London study of maternal chronic periodontal disease and preterm low birth weight infants: study design and prevalence data, *Ann Periodontol* 3(1):213-21, 1998.
11. Department of Health, Board of Dentistry, Division of Medical Quality Assurance: Chapters 466 & 455. Florida Statutes and Rule 64B5, Florida Administrative Code, Feb. 2000, p. 7.
12. Dental Interactive Simulation Corporation: *DISC dental simulations* [Internet], Aurora, Colo, 2001, The Corporation [http://www.uiowa.edu/dentistry-disc/index.html].
13. Everett MJ et al: Non-invasive diagnosis of early caries with polarization sensitive optical tomography (PS-OCT). In Featherstone JD, editor: *Lasers in Dentistry v. Proceedings of SPIE,* Bellingham, Wash, 1999, SPIE.
14. Feil P, Meeske J, Fortman J: Knowledge of ethical lapses and other experiences on clinical licensure examinations, *J Dent Educ* 63:453-8, 1999.

15. Field MJ, editor: *Dental education at the crossroads: challenges and change,* Washington, DC, 1995, National Academy Press.
16. Fones AC: *Mouth hygiene,* ed 2, Philadelphia, 1921, Lea & Febiger.
17. Fones AC: The origin and the history of the dental hygiene movement, 12:1816, 1920.
18. Grau AJ et al: Association between acute cerebrovascular ischemia and chronic and recurrent infection, *Stroke* 28:1724-9, 1997.
19. Grossi SG, Genco RJ: Periodontal disease and diabetes mellitus: a two-way relationship, *Ann Peridontol* 3(1):51-61, 1998 (review).
20. Guarino KS: Licensure and certification of dentists and accreditation of dental schools, *J Dent Educ* 59:205-236, 1995.
21. Hall FA et al: Dye-enhanced laser fluorescence method. In *Early detection of dental caries: proceedings of the 1st Annual Indiana Conference,* Indianapolis, 1996, Indiana University.
22. Hippocrates: *De Morbis Mulerum,* Lib II, 606.
23. Justice Cardozo BN: Doctrine of Informed Consent. *Schloendorff v. Society of New York Hospital,* 211 N.Y. 125, 105 N.E. 92, 1914.
24. KaVo Corporation: [Internet], Lake Zurich, Ill, 2001, kavo.com [http://www.kavo.com].
25. Linz AM: Dental licensure, *J Am Dent Assoc* 123:9-10, 1992.
26. Loesche W, Pohl A, Karapetow F: Plasma lipids and blood glucose in patients with marginal periodontitis, *J Dent Res* 76(special issue):408, 1997.
27. Mattila KJ et al: Association between dental health and acute myocardial infarction. *Br Med J* 298:779-81, 1989.
28. Mattila KJ et al: Dental infections and coronary atherosclerosis, *Atherosclerosis* 103:205-11, 1993.
29. Mattila KJ et al: Dental infection and the risk of new coronary events: prospective study of patients with documented coronary artery disease, *Clin Infect Dis* 20:588-92, 1995.
30. Motley WE: *History of the American Dental Hygienists' Association 1923-1982,* Chicago, 1983, American Dental Hygienists' Association.
31. Meskin LH: Dental licensure revisited, *J Am Dent Assoc* 127:292-294, 1996.

32. Offenbacher S et al: Periodontal infection as a possible risk factor for preterm low birth weight, *J Periodontol* 67:1103-13, 1996.

33. Offenbacher S et al: Potential pathogenic mechanisms of periodontitis-associated pregnancy complications, *Ann Periodontol* 3(1):233-50, 1998.

34. Ring ME: *Dentistry: an illustrated history,* St Louis, 1985, Mosby.

35. Schlossman M et al: Type 2 diabetes mellitus and periodontal disease, *J Am Dent Assoc* 121:532-6, 1990.

36. Syrjanen J et al: Dental infections in association with cerebral infarction in young and middle-aged men, *J Intern Med* 25:179-84, 1989.

37. ten Bosch JJ: General aspects of optical methods in dentistry. *Adv Dent Res* 1:5-7, 1987.

38. ten Bosch JJ, Angmar-Mansson B: A review of quantitative methods for studies of mineral content of intra-oral incipient caries lesions, *J Dent Res* 70:2-14, 1991.

39. US Department of Health and Human Services: *Oral health in America: a report of the surgeon general.* Rockville, MD, 2000, The Department, National Institute of Dental and Craniofacial Research, National Institutes of Health.

40. Weinberger BW: *An introduction to the history of dentistry in America,* vol. I, St Louis, 1948, Mosby.

41. Zambon JJ et al: Identification of periodontal pathogens in atheromatous plaques, *J Dent Res* 76(special issue):408, 1997.

CHAPTER 2

Health Promotion:
A Basis *of* Practice

Sherry A. Harfst

Chapter Outline

The Link Between Dentistry and Human Health
Case Study: Expanding the Definition of Health
Historical Perspective on Health Promotion
    Milestones
    Definition of health
Health Promotion: Broadening the Paradigm
    The evidence
    Obstacles to health promotion
    Definition of health promotion
    The challenge
The Oral Cavity in the Equation of Health
  and Disease
    First port of entry for potential pathogens
    Extraoral and intraoral findings

Periodontal disease and diabetes
Oral infection, heart disease, and stroke
Periodontal disease and adverse birth outcomes
Burden of Oral Disease
    Data-gathering methods
    Findings
Health Promotion Guidelines
    Healthy People 2010
    Surgeon general's report

Key Terms

Burden of disease
Causal factors

Epidemiological survey
Health

Health promotion
Risk factors

 ## *Learning Outcomes*

1. Determine working definitions for *health* and *health promotion.*
2. Discuss the paradigm shift with regard to health promotion in dentistry.
3. Become familiar with the demographic parameters of an epidemiological survey.
4. Give general impressions of the burden of oral disease in the U.S. population.

5. Establish an opinion of at least one of the national health promotion initiatives.
6. Discuss the significance of a causal relationship.
7. Become aware of your personal health beliefs and values while working through health assessment surveys used in patient care.
8. Explore your values and methods for promoting health and preventing disease.

Case Study

Expanding the Definition of Health

Elizabeth Marino, age 57, visits her dental office for a routine supportive care appointment, during which she expects to have a dental prophylaxis, radiographs, and intraoral and extraoral examinations. Ms. Marino presents for her appointment with a runny nose, a scratchy throat, and a slight cough, which she has had for about 5 days. She states that she feels she has caught a cold, although she does report feeling much better than she did at the beginning of the onset of the symptoms. Ms. Marino's health history indicates frequent upper respiratory infections, occasionally bronchitis. She takes two over-the-counter cough syrups—one to suppress her cough during the day and another with a formula advertised to help her sleep.

Her vital signs, taken at the appointment, indicate a blood pressure of 160/93 with a faint pulse of 86 beats per minute. She reports no additional illness or medication. Her personal history indicates that she is overweight (5 feet tall and 155 pounds), lacks daily physical exercise, and smokes nine 1½ pack years (which means she has smoked 1½ packs of cigarettes for 9 years.) On reviewing her chart before the appointment, you notice that she has several areas of attachment loss, generalized bleeding on probing, and areas along her gumline where incipient caries (beginning dental decay) has been noted.

Because Ms. Marino is uncomfortable and her cough increases when she is reclined in the dental chair, you and she agree to suspend treatment until the she returns to "health." In what ways have you promoted concepts of health to Ms. Marino?

THE LINK BETWEEN DENTISTRY AND HUMAN HEALTH

One of the many benefits of becoming a member of a healthcare profession is the personal and professional satisfaction gained in patient interaction. As a member of the dental healthcare team, the dental hygienist's role is critical in the *promotion* of **health.**

As healthcare providers, dental hygienists are in a key position to promote health. They have an opportunity to discuss and promote oral health, systemic health, and general well-being. Some populations of patients are seen by dental hygienists on a more consistent basis and at a more constant frequency than by most other healthcare professionals. Dental hygienists have the opportunity to touch a patient's life and, through a thorough assessment and patient-specific intervention, to significantly affect the behaviors and beliefs of those seeking care.

HISTORICAL PERSPECTIVE ON HEALTH PROMOTION

MILESTONES

Significant progress in the reduction of the incidence, prevalence, and severity of common oral diseases clearly heralded the age of *prevention* in dentistry. Beginning with the successful adoption of preventive methods to control dental caries, led by dental professionals, the United States

---

BOX 2-1

Improvements in Oral Health Based on Prevention

The United States was once a nation at risk for a legion of ineligible draftees because of poor and serious oral conditions. Now the majority of young adults have fewer than one area of dental caries. In the early 1900s most Americans could expect to lose their teeth by age 45. These facts testify to the full impact of one aspect of health promotion.

BOX 2-2

Community Strategies for Primary Prevention of Key Oral Diseases and Conditions

Dental Caries
Communitywide health promotion interventions*
Fluoride use
   Community water fluoridation
   School-based dietary fluoride tablets
   School-based fluoride mouthrinse
School-based/linked sealant programs
School-linked screenings and referrals
Periodontal Disease
Communitywide health promotion interventions*
   School-based personal hygiene
      Reinforcement of personal and oral hygiene habits
       in Head Start or primary school classrooms
   School-linked screenings and referrals
Head and Neck Cancers
Communitywide health promotion interventions*
   Cancer screening programs (such as health fairs)
Inherited Disorders
Early detection programs
Trauma
Communitywide health promotion interventions*
   Mouth protector fittings for entire sports teams

Modified from US Department of Health and Human Services: Community, provider, and individual strategies for primary prevention of key oral diseases and conditions, *Oral Health in America: a report of the surgeon general,* Rockville, Md, 2000, The Department, National Institute of Dental and Craniofacial Research, National Institutes of Health. *Communitywide health promotion interventions (education, political, regulatory, and organizational) are directed toward the public, practitioners, and policymakers to create a healthy environment, reduce risk factors, inform target groups, and improve knowledge and behaviors.

---

has benchmarked significant improvement in oral health (Box 2-1).

Community water fluoridation clearly can be cited as one of the greatest achievements of public health in the twentieth century—an inexpensive means to improve oral health that benefits all community residents, regardless of age or socioeconomic status. Other community strategies for primary prevention of dental caries have included school-based programs of fluoride use (mouthrinse and dietary fluoride tabs), sealant programs, and screening and referral programs. This type of science application to a generalized, severe oral health problem gave the profession an opportunity to evaluate methods to positively affect human health in other areas (Box 2-2).

DEFINITION OF HEALTH

In the current era focused on whole health, in which dental professionals assume an expanded role in *health promotion,* the definition of health takes on a new meaning as well. Health can no longer be defined as the mere absence of disease. As defined by noted scholars in health promotion, health is the quality of life with social, mental, emotional, spiritual, and physical functions.[26] The observation can be made that in the past, the focus of all health care has been on the physical aspect to the exclusion of those aspects that are clearly more difficult to assess.

HEALTH PROMOTION: BROADENING THE PARADIGM

The traditional role of the dental hygienist as primarily an educator has once again cycled to the lead. Although the promotion of oral health through patient education has provided an underlying philosophy of the practice of dentistry and dental hygiene over the past century, the reality of practice has been in the delivery of services—hands-on treatment rendered by the dental professional. Examining the shift in focus for the dental professional includes a vision of total health promotion, including both systemic and oral health.

In recent years the impact of the relationship between oral and systemic health has been more fully analyzed. Studies linking chronic oral infection with heart and lung diseases, stroke, and preterm, low–birth-weight births are being indexed in medical and dental literature. Included in this growing knowledge base are emerging relationships between diabetes and periodontal disease and between oral and pharyngeal cancers and alcohol and tobacco use, studies detailed in subsequent chapters in this text.

THE EVIDENCE

Systemic Disease: Oral Manifestation

Knowledge that systemic disease can cause oral manifestations is clearly documented in medical and dental literature. The list of *risk factors* for oral disease has grown in recent years to include both *causal factors* known to induce the infectious diseases of dental caries, periodontal diseases, and the pharmacological and psychosocial-cultural element of behaviors and values specific to an individual that contribute to oral disease.[69] Correlations between smoking and periodontal diseases and between diabetes and periodontal diseases have been well-documented.* Only recently has the reverse relationship been examined.

Oral Disease: Systemic Manifestation

Scientific knowledge of the connection between dentistry and human health is growing to encompass oral infection, which can correlate to systemic disease. The relationship between periodontal disease and the risk of stroke, pre-

*References 4, 7, 8, 9, 11, 12, 18-20, 22, 23, 27-29, 34, 40, 59, 60, 62, 65.

> **BOX 2-3**
>
> **Barriers to Health Care**
>
> Lack of access to care that still plagues the United States
> Limited income
> Limited or no insurance benefits
> Lack of transportation
> Inability to schedule free time for health issues
> Complex issues surrounding medical conditions
> Physical, emotional, and mental disabilities
> Low priority with policymakers

term, low–birth-weight babies, and cardiovascular disease is evidenced in medical literature.*

Further investigation into the causal nature of the relationship will be the subject of future studies. With each new discovery comes the reality that the dental professional is in a key role to affect the quality of life through a process called *risk assessment and health promotion,* the subject of Part V of this text, Health Promotion and Disease Prevention.

The full impact of oral health and its significance to general health will lead the coming decade of scientific research. Just as this text will clearly identify those factors known to place an individual at risk for developing oral disease, so too will future texts be able to more clearly identify oral risk factors that place an individual at risk for developing systemic disease.

OBSTACLES TO HEALTH PROMOTION

This growing body of knowledge does not guarantee a higher quality of life for patients. It is worthless if not shared with the patient by healthcare professionals. Regardless of the effectiveness of any preventive measure, the uninformed patient cannot reap its benefit. Furthermore, simply imparting information is not enough to overcome barriers to a change in health behavior. Disparity exists between *knowledge* about prevention of disease and prevention *actions taken* (Box 2-3).[36,52] Compounding this complex interaction between patient and oral healthcare provider are the variety of patient habits, practices, values, beliefs, and attitudes toward their teeth, oral care, and oral healthcare providers.[45,64,70]

DEFINITION OF HEALTH PROMOTION

Health promotion is the bridge between the health knowledge, supported by science, and its application to the patient.[36] The past decade has witnessed a significant increase in interest in the concept of health promotion in dentistry, especially in the incorporation of the biopsychosocial aspects of well-being.

Among the reasons for this renewed interest are the following:
- An increase in healthcare costs associated with the treatment of preventable diseases

*References 3, 5, 6, 13-16, 24, 25, 30, 31, 35, 37, 42-44, 46-48, 53, 54, 67, 71.

- A growing body of literature demonstrating that many chronic diseases are the direct result of chosen personal health behaviors
- A growing body of literature and ongoing studies linking oral heath with systemic health[1]

Oral health is essential to the meaning of general health and well-being. As defined more than 50 years ago by the World Health Organization, the expanded definition of health means "a complete state of physical, mental, and social well-being, and not just the absence of infirmity."[69] The integration of oral health to general health cannot be ignored in a review of the application of science to improve health. The 1950s and 1960s witnessed a surge in the idea of prevention; research demonstrating the infectious nature of both dental caries and periodontal disease led to a new era in treatment and measures of successful treatment. Led by the dental professional, the prevention theme continues to be the cornerstone of practice today.

 THE CHALLENGE

2-A   Separating oral health and general health is no longer appropriate. Oral health and general health are mutually exclusive terms; one cannot exist without the other. As supported by a report on the oral health status in the United States published in 2000, the full realization that oral health can have a significant impact on overall health and well-being presents a challenge to the profession to focus on *producing* health rather than merely *restoring* health.[68] However, a continuum of care exists in which restoration many times must precede a state of health promotion.

A good working definition of health promotion is any combination of educational, organizational, economic, and environmental supports for behavior conducive to health. Careful examination of this definition reveals roles for dental health professionals in both patient and community service.[26]

 Case Application

Revisit the case presented at the beginning of the chapter. You and Ms. Marino mutually agreed to suspend treatment until she felt healthier. At the time of the initial case presentation, did any additional aspects of health, such as long-term objectives for the promotion and maintenance of health, come to mind? Might you suggest ways in which the hygienist could adapt to a newer definition of health and see beyond the acute symptoms presented in this case to determine health topics for discussion that could promote a healthier lifestyle?

THE ORAL CAVITY IN THE EQUATION OF HEALTH AND DISEASE

FIRST PORT OF ENTRY FOR POTENTIAL PATHOGENS

At the turn of the century, one of the physician's diagnostic procedures was to examine the patient's tongue. The phrase "Stick out your tongue; let me see how you are," was closer to the truth than once was thought. Perhaps the physician was looking for the color of the tongue. A pale tongue might indicate anemia; a bright-red tongue might indicate a nutritional deficiency. The tongue might have been observed for texture or for a coating, or perhaps a clearer view of the throat was needed. Whatever the diagnostic rationale, exploring the relationship between oral and systemic health is not far from today's experience—discovering the link between oral and systemic health.

As a portal of entry, the mouth serves as a gateway though which pass any number of potential pathogens, namely bacteria, viruses, parasites, and fungi. More than 500 strains of bacteria have been identified in dental biofilm and 150 strains in bacterial plaque, and more recently 37 unknown bacterial strains have been isolated from infections involving the nerve of the tooth (pulpal tissues).[38] Once the pathogen enters the oral cavity, protective mechanisms are immediately released. When the oral tissues are not compromised, the invader is swiftly defeated. Most dental infections are opportunistic in that they are caused by microorganisms commonly found in the mouth. If, however, oral tissues are compromised, an opportunity for infection is present. In this way, the mouth can actually serve as a source for diseases and pathological processes that can affect other organ systems, as well as a source for contagion to others.

EXTRAORAL AND INTRAORAL FINDINGS

One of the basic examination procedures performed on every dental patient is the extra- and intraoral examination. The extraoral examination of the head and neck can reflect signs of malignancy, symptoms associated with diseases or conditions such as neoplasm, and endocrine disorders. Swollen glands can accompany mumps, HIV infection, Sjögren's syndrome, tuberculosis, and histoplasmosis infections.

At the least, an intraoral examination can reveal signs and symptoms associated with some viral, bacterial, and fungal infections (Boxes 2-4, 2-5, and 2-6).

The most prevalent diseases caused by this host of invaders are dental caries and periodontal disease; the direct relationship can be inferred. Most systemic diseases, notably diabetes, arthritis, osteoporosis, autoimmune deficiency syndromes, along with the associated therapies for each, can have a direct or indirect impact on oral tissues. The World Health Organization's *International Classification of Diseases and Stomatology* lists more than 120 diseases, distributed in 10 or more classes, reporting oral manifestations.[69]

PERIODONTAL DISEASE AND DIABETES

In 1993 Dr. Harald Löe defined periodontitis as the sixth complication of diabetes.[40] Insulin-dependent diabetes mellitus (IDDM) is a condition that typically begins in childhood or adolescence in which the pancreas produces little or no insulin. Non–insulin-dependent diabetes mellitus (NIDDM) is a condition that usually develops after the age of 30 in which insulin production and absorption are deficient. Together, these diseases affect an estimated 15.7 million people in the United States.[51] The correlation in literature of periodontal disease to IDDM appears quite high. Reasons cited include altered vascular functions, exaggerated host immunological and inflammatory response, changes in the crevicular fluid and connective tissue metabolism, and hereditary patterns. Although a direct causal relation has yet to be completely established, diabetes is a risk factor for the occurrence and prevalence of periodontal diseases.

BOX 2-4

Diseases and Conditions Causing Lesions of the Oral Mucosa

Viral
Primary acute herpetic gingivostomatitis (herpes simplex type 1; rarely type 2)
Recurrent herpes labialis
Recurrent intraoral herpes simplex
Chicken pox (varicella-zoster virus)
Herpes zoster (reactivation of the varicella-zoster virus)
Infectious mononucleosis
Warts (papillomavirus)
Herpangina (coxsackie virus A; also possibly coxsackie virus B and echovirus)
Hand, foot, and mouth disease (type A coxsackie virus)
Primary human immunodeficiency virus infection
Bacterial or Fungal
Acute necrotizing ulcerative gingivitis (trench mouth, Vincent's infection)
Prenatal (congenital) syphilis
Primary syphilis (chancre)
Secondary syphilis
Tertiary syphilis
Gonorrhea
Tuberculosis
Cervicofacial actinomycosis
Histoplasmosis
Candidiasis
Dermatological
Mucous membrane pemphigoid
Erythema multiforme (Stevens-Johnson syndrome)
Pemphigus vulgaris
Lichen planus
Other
Recurrent aphthous ulcers
Behçet's syndrome
Traumatic ulcers

Modified from Greenspan JS: Oral manifestation of disease. In Fauci AS et al: *1998 Harrison's principles of internal medicine*, ed 11, New York, 1998, McGraw-Hill.

BOX 2-5

Examining the Oral Cavity

An examination of the oral cavity can reveal the following:
Signs of disease
Drug use
Domestic physical abuse
Harmful habits, such as tobacco addiction

BOX 2-6

Examining Radiographs

Radiographs can reveal the following:
Skeletal changes associated with osteoporosis
Musculoskeletal disorders
Salivary, congenital, neoplastic, and developmental disorders

---

Dental science is beginning to establish whether a causal relationship also might exist in the reverse. Periodontal disease may be a risk factor for inappropriate glycemic control in the patient with diabetes. Although the preliminary evidence only suggests a connection and does not support that treatment of periodontal disease can manage glycemic control in the individual with diabetes, studies using systemic antibiotic treatment for periodontal disease have demonstrated a favorable glycemic control.

ORAL INFECTION, HEART DISEASE, AND STROKE

Studies suggest a link between oral infections and the risk for cardiovascular disease.

Studies initiated in the 1980s[32] and recently confirmed[3,31,32,47,48] suggest a correlation between periodontal disease and cardiovascular disease. Specific organisms of *Streptococcus sanguis* and *Porphyromaonas gingivalis,* identified as two pathogens in the complex etiology of periodontal disease, have the potential to produce platelet aggregation, promoting thrombus formation.[30]

Mechanisms of action that have been examined include a direct infection of the blood vessel walls with bacteria or viruses originating in tissues such as the oral mucosa, causing local inflammation and injury contributing to atherosclerosis. White blood cells or platelets become integrated into the atherosclerotic plaque, triggering inflammatory pathways (the release of prostaglandins, interleukins, thromboxane, and tumor necrosis factor alpha). Under these conditions, the liver may be stimulated to produce additional inflammatory responses. Tissue factor, another proinflammatory element released by the presence of bacteria in the blood, is responsible for coagulation. During coagulation, more platelets become entrapped by the developing thrombus. As the lumen of the coronary vessels becomes narrower, blood supply to the cardiac muscle diminishes. When the artery fully occludes, a myocardial infarct, or heart attack, occurs. If blood supply is not returned, the cardiac muscle dies, resulting in profoundly diminished cardiac function, or death.

PERIODONTAL DISEASES AND ADVERSE BIRTH OUTCOMES

Prematurity and low birth weight threaten to increase infant mortality rates[61] and for survivors, to contribute to a wide variety of functional disorders.

Examinations of the inflammatory pathways involved in the preterm delivery of low–birth-weight babies have found them to be consistent with the inflammatory pathways brought about by the gram-negative infections of periodontal disease.* These early associations between oral disease and systemic health require comprehensive, indepth studies to determine whether a causal relationship exists and will thus be the next dental frontier.

 Case Application
Review the brief health history notes in the initial case presentation. Which specific topic would you elect to discuss when Ms. Marino returns for supportive care?

---

*References 13, 14, 15, 24, 35, 46, 53, 54.

BURDEN OF ORAL DISEASE

Those considering the cost of dental care in our nation may tend to figure the cost of the placement and replacement of fillings, tooth extractions, and treatment of gum disease. However, closer evaluation allows appreciation of oral disease as progressive, cumulative, and complex. Strictly based on dental needs, our nation's dental bill exceeded $60 billion in 2000.[68] Added to that initial figure are tens of billions of dollars in medical care associated with chronic craniofacial pain from conditions such as the following: temporomandibular disorders, trigeminal neuralgia, shingles, burning mouth syndrome, cleft lip, cleft palate, oral and pharyngeal cancers, autoimmune diseases, and injury. To that bill is added the cost of social, psychological, and economic consequences.

Although major oral health improvements have been made in the past 50 years, disparities remain in some subgroups as classified by sex, income, age, and race/ethnicity. One means to capture a picture of the state of the nation's oral health is through the evaluation of epidemiological data for specific oral conditions.

DATA-GATHERING METHODS

To evaluate the health of a nation, and then to determine which health promotion actions should be taken, is a huge task involving thousand of subjects, volunteers, and hours. Several of the major studies from which status data are drawn are listed in the following sections. Population samples from which this type of data are drawn are usually large, nationally representative surveys of the United States civilian, noninstitutionalized population and are referred to as *epidemiological surveys.*

National Health and Nutrition Examination Survey

The most recent survey, National Health and Nutrition Examination Survey (NHANES) III, was conducted between 1988 and 1994 by the National Center for Health Statistics of the Centers for Disease Control. Demographic and related health data were gathered by trained interviewers. Selected individuals then were invited to a mobile examination center for health assessments, including an oral examination by a trained dentist.

National Health Interview Survey

Conducted in 1989, the most recent National Health Interview Survey (NHIS) included data on orofacial pain conditions, data on dental visits, socioeconomic data, and data on reasons individuals do not visit a dentist.

National Institute of Dental and Craniofacial Research

In both 1979 to 1980 and 1986 to 1990, the National Institute of Dental and Craniofacial Research (NIDCR) conducted a probability sample of U.S. schoolchildren, in a sample manner similar to the NHANES.

FINDINGS*

Dental Caries

In Children

One of the most common childhood diseases, dental caries, is five times more common than asthma and seven times more common than hay fever. The majority of children ages 5 to 9 years have at least one carious lesion or filling in the coronal portion of a primary or a permanent tooth. The proportion increases to 77.9% in the 17-year-old age range, and 84.7% for adults ages 18 and older. Poverty and race/ethnicity affect the disease occurrence and treatment incidence (Figs. 2-1 through 2-3 and Box 2-7).

In Adults

Over the past 30 years the average number of teeth per person affected by dental caries has decreased; the average number of teeth per person showing no signs of infection and the proportion of the population without dental caries has increased. The number of untreated decayed teeth per person across all age groups also has declined. As with children, poverty affects treated and untreated dental caries (Figs. 2-4 and 2-5 and Boxes 2-8 and 2-9). Poor adults have a higher percentage of untreated decayed teeth than do adults living above the poverty level.

Periodontal Diseases

One method used to clinically measure periodontal disease is through calculation of attachment loss, which accounts

---

*All findings are gleaned from the NHANES III.[68]

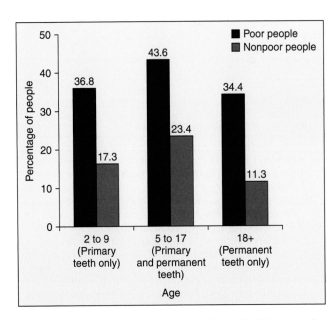

FIG. 2-1 A higher percentage of people living at the poverty level have at least one untreated decayed tooth. (Modified from U.S. Department of Health and Human Services, National Center for Health Statistics: *Third national health and nutrition examination survey, 1988-94.* Public use Data File No. 7-0627. Hyattsville, Md, 1997, [U.S.] Centers for Disease Control and Prevention.)

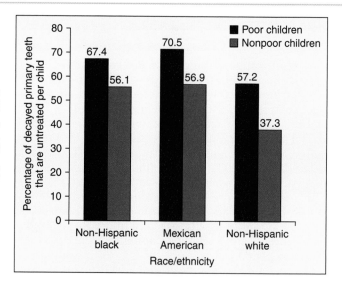

FIG. 2-2 Children ages 2 to 9 years living in poverty in each racial/ethnic group have a higher percentage of untreated decayed primary teeth in comparison with other children. (Modified from U.S. Department of Health and Human Services, National Center for Health Statistics: *Third national health and nutrition examination survey, 1988-94.* Public use Data File No. 7-0627. Hyattsville, Md, 1997, [U.S.] Centers for Disease Control and Prevention.)

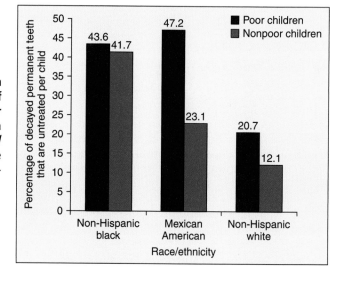

FIG. 2-3 Children and teenagers ages 12 to 17 years living in poverty in each racial/ethnic group have a higher percentage of untreated decayed permanent teeth in comparison with other children. (Modified from U.S. Department of Health and Human Services, National Center for Health Statistics: *Third national health and nutrition examination survey, 1988-94.* Public use Data File No. 7-0627. Hyattsville, Md, 1997, [U.S.] Centers for Disease Control and Prevention.)

BOX 2-7

Burden of Disease in Children

Cleft lip/palate affects an estimated 1 of 600 live births for whites; 1 out of 1,850 live births for African Americans.

Other devastating birth defects, such as ectodermal dysplasia, cause ongoing, lifetime problems.

Dental caries is the single most common chronic childhood disease—five times more common than asthma and seven times more common than hay fever.

More than 50% of 5- to 9-year-olds have at least one area of dental caries or filling. That figure increases to 78% among 17-year-olds.

Income levels create disparities in dental disease. Poor children suffer twice as much from dental caries, and their diseases are more likely to be untreated. One of four children is born into poverty; children living below the poverty line (annual income of $17,000 for a family of four) have more severe and/or untreated dental caries.

Head, neck, and mouth are common sites of unintentional injuries in children.

Tobacco-related oral lesions are prevalent in adolescents who use smokeless (spit) tobacco.

Professional care is necessary to maintain oral health. Approximately 25% of poor children have not seen a dentist before entering kindergarten.

Uninsured children are 2.5 times less likely to receive dental care and have 3 times the dental needs than children with public or private insurance. For every child with medical insurance, 2.6 children exist without.

More than 41 million school hours are lost each year to dental-related illness. Poor children suffer 12 times more restricted-activity days than children from higher-income families.

From U.S. Department of Health and Human Services: *Oral health in America: a report of the surgeon general,* Rockville, Md, 2000, The Department, National Institute of Dental and Craniofacial Research, National Institutes of Health.

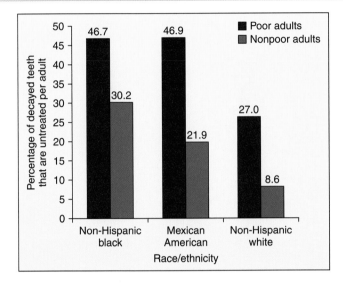

FIG. 2-4 Adults ages 18 years and older living in poverty have a higher percentage of untreated decayed teeth than other adults. (Modified from U.S. Department of Health and Human Services, National Center for Health Statistics: *Third national health and nutrition examination survey, 1988-94.* Public use Data File No. 7-0627. Hyattsville, Md, 1997, [U.S.] Centers for Disease Control and Prevention.)

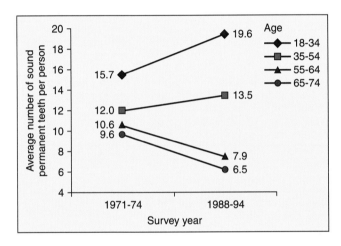

FIG. 2-5 Since 1971 to 1974 the average number of permanent teeth without decay or fillings has increased among 18- to 54-year-olds. (Modified from U.S. Department of Health and Human Services, National Center for Health Statistics: *Third national health and nutrition examination survey, 1988-94.* Public use Data File No. 7-0627. Hyattsville, Md, 1997, [U.S.] Centers for Disease Control and Prevention.)

BOX 2-8

Adults: Summary Findings

Most adults show signs of periodontal or gingival disease.

Clinical symptoms of viral infections (herpes labialis and oral ulcers) are common in adulthood, affecting about 19% of adults ages 25 to 44.

Chronic disabling diseases, such as the following, affect millions of Americans, compromising oral health and function:
Temporomandibular disorders
Sjögren's syndrome
Diabetes
Osteoporosis

Approximately 22% of adults reported some form of chronic craniofacial pain with the previous 6-month period.

Of the patients undergoing treatment for oral and pharyngeal cancers, more than 400,000 will develop complications annually.

Immunocompromised patients are at greater risk for oral problems.

Employed adults lose more that 164 million hours of work each year as a result of dentally related problems (treatments or diseases).

For every adult age 19 years or older without medical insurance, three are without dental insurance.

Fewer than two thirds of adults visited a dentist in the previous 12-month period.

Approximately 23% of 65- to 74-year-olds have severe periodontal disease.

From U.S. Department of Health and Human Services: *Oral health in America: a report of the surgeon general,* Rockville, MD, 2000, The Department, National Institute of Dental and Craniofacial Research, National Institutes of Health.

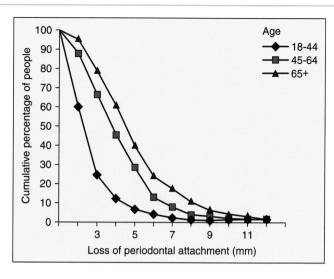

FIG. 2-6 Although older adults have more periodontal attachment loss than younger adults, severe loss is seen among a small percentage of individuals at every age. (Modified from U.S. Department of Health and Human Services, National Center for Health Statistics: *Third national health and nutrition examination survey, 1988-94.* Public use Data File No. 7-0627. Hyattsville, Md, 1997, [U.S.] Centers for Disease Control and Prevention; Burt BA, Eklund SA: *Dentistry, dental practice and the community,* Philadelphia, 1999, WB Saunders.)

BOX 2-9

Older Adults: Summary Findings

Approximately 30% of adults 65 years and older are edentulous (compared with 46% 20 years ago). For those living at the poverty level, higher percentages are noted.

Primarily diagnosed in the elderly, oral and pharyngeal cancers are diagnosed in about 30,000 Americans annually; 8000 die from these diseases annually. Survival rate is 56% for white patients and 34% for blacks.

Most older adults take both prescription and over-the-counter medications. Most likely, at least one will cause dry mouth, increasing the risk for increased oral disease. Long-term-care residents are prescribed an average of eight medications.

Approximately 5% of Americans ages 65 and older are living in long-term-care facilities where dental care is problematic.

Most older adults lose their dental insurance at retirement.

From U.S. Department of Health and Human Services: *Oral health in America: a report of the surgeon general,* Rockville, Md, 2000, The Department, National Institute of Dental and Craniofacial Research, National Institutes of Health.

---

for the way in which much of the supporting structure has been lost. The greater the attachment loss is, the more severe the disease. Attachment loss varies by age, sex, and racial/ethnic group. Most adults 25 years and older have at least one site of 2 mm or more loss of attachment. The percentage of adults with 6 mm or more of attachment loss increases with age (Fig. 2-6); 19% percent of 55- to 64-year-olds and 23.4% of 65- to 74-year-olds showed an attachment loss of 6 mm or more at one or more sites.

More men than women are likely to have at least one tooth exhibiting a 6 mm loss of attachment (Fig. 2-7). More non-Hispanic blacks had at least one tooth site exhibiting 6 mm or more of attachment loss as compared with Mexican Americans and non-Hispanic whites (Fig. 2-8). Those of the lowest socioeconomic status demonstrated at least one site with attachment loss of 6 mm or more, compared with those at a higher socioeconomic standing (Fig. 2-9).

Tooth Loss and Edentulism

Edentulism affects men and women equally. Those living below the poverty level are more likely to be edentulous than those living above. By age 17, more than 7.3% of U.S. children have lost at least one permanent tooth because of dental caries. By age 50, Americans have lost an average of 12.1 teeth, including their third molars. Complete tooth loss varies by race/ethnicity and poverty status (Fig. 2-10).

Oral and Pharyngeal Cancers

Oral and pharyngeal cancers account for about 30,200 annual cases, or 2.4% of all cancers. Approximately 7800 die from these cancers annually.[2] The median age of diagnosis is 64 years, and occurrence increases with age. The overall 5-year survival rate for individuals with oral and pharyngeal cancers is 52%. Although the 5-year survival rate is 81.3% for individuals with oral cancers detected at an early stage, only 35% of oral and pharyngeal cancers are diagnosed at this stage.

The incidence of oral and pharyngeal cancer is higher for black individuals than for whites. Males have a slightly higher incidence than do females, and the incidence rate for oral and pharyngeal cancers for black males is 39.6% higher than for white males (Fig. 2-11).

Overall, the incidence rate of oral and pharyngeal cancer is decreasing. The largest annual decline in incidence rates was noted for lip cancers. The incidence of tongue cancer, however, may be increasing among young males.[68]

Tobacco-Related Lesions

The most related risk factor for cancers of the oral cavity and pharynx is the use of tobacco. Both smoking and smokeless (spit) tobacco account for more than 90% of cancers of the oral cavity and pharynx. Tobacco-related oral lesions are common in school-aged children (Fig. 2-12).

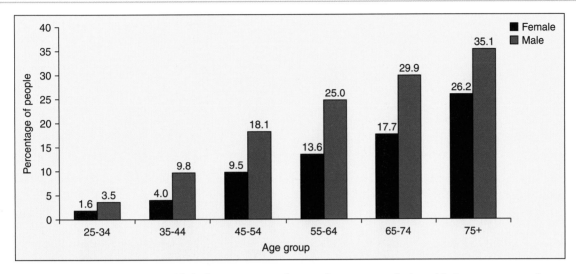

FIG. 2-7 Men are more likely than women to have at least one tooth site with 6 mm or more of periodontal loss of attachment. (Modified from U.S. Department of Health and Human Services, National Center for Health Statistics: *Third national health and nutrition examination survey, 1988-94.* Public use Data File No. 7-0627. Hyattsville, Md, 1997, [U.S.] Centers for Disease Control and Prevention; Burt BA, Eklund SA: *Dentistry, dental practice and the community,* Philadelphia, 1999, WB Saunders.)

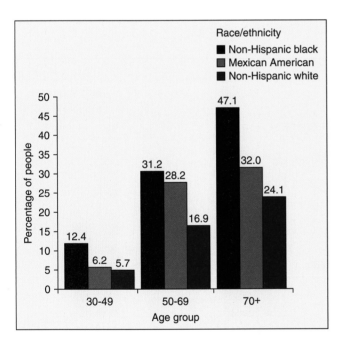

FIG. 2-8 Non-Hispanic blacks are more likely than other groups to have at least one tooth site with 6 mm or more of periodontal loss of attachment. (Modified from U.S. Department of Health and Human Services, National Center for Health Statistics: *Third national health and nutrition examination survey, 1988-94.* Public use Data File No. 7-0627. Hyattsville, Md, 1997, [U.S.] Centers for Disease Control and Prevention.)

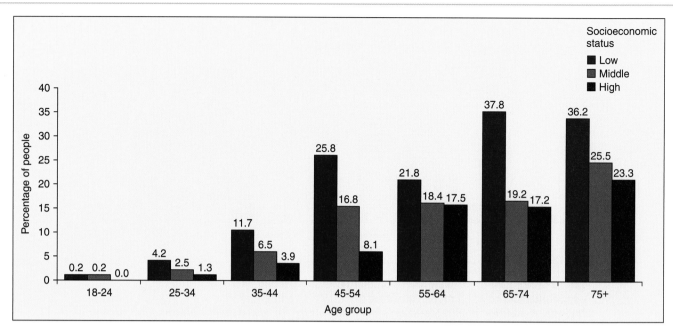

FIG. 2-9 The percentage of adults with at least one tooth site with 6 mm or more of periodontal attachment loss is greater among persons of low socioeconomic status at all ages. (Modified from U.S. Department of Health and Human Services, National Center for Health Statistics: *Third national health and nutrition examination survey, 1988-94.* Public use Data File No. 7-0627. Hyattsville, Md, 1997, [U.S.] Centers for Disease Control and Prevention; Burt BA, Eklund SA: *Dentistry, dental practice and the community,* Philadelphia, 1999, WB Saunders.)

FIG. 2-10 Complete tooth loss varies by race/ethnicity and poverty status; a higher percentage of poor and nonpoor non-Hispanic white adults (18 years and older) have no teeth, compared with non-Hispanic blacks and Mexican Americans. (Modified from U.S. Department of Health and Human Services, National Center for Health Statistics: *Third national health and nutrition examination survey, 1988-94.* Public use Data File No. 7-0627. Hyattsville, Md, 1997, [U.S.] Centers for Disease Control and Prevention.)

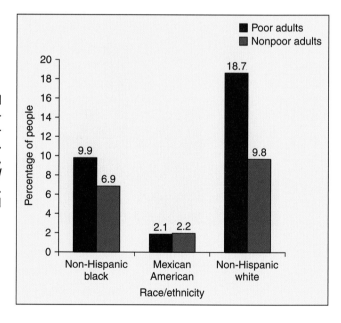

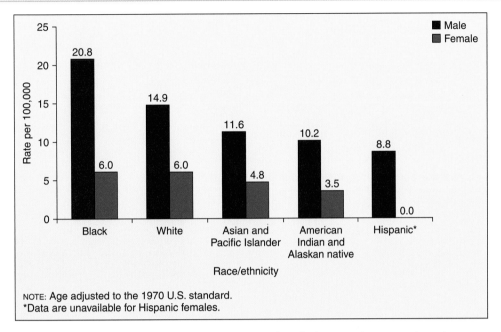

FIG. 2-11 Men have higher incidence rates of oral and pharyngeal cancers than do women. (Modified from Wingo PA et al: Annual report to the nation on the status of cancer, 1973-1996, [with a special section on lung cancer and tobacco smoking], *J Natl Cancer Inst* 91:675-90, 1999.)

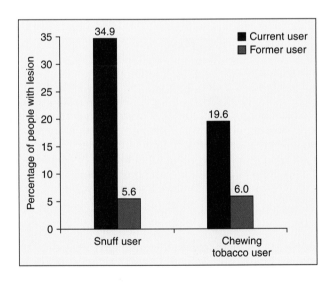

FIG. 2-12 Tobacco-related oral lesions are more common in 12- to 17-year-olds who currently use spit tobacco. (Modified from Tomar SL et al: Oral mucosal smokeless tobacco lesions among adolescents in the United States, *J Dent Res* 76[6]:1277-86, 1997.)

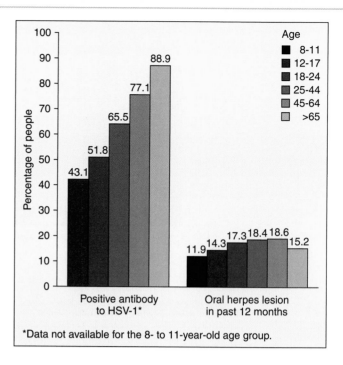

FIG. 2-13 Herpes simplex type 1 virus infection is widespread, and oral herpes lesions (cold sores/fever blisters) are common. (Modified from U.S. Department of Health and Human Services, National Center for Health Statistics: *Third national health and nutrition examination survey, 1988-94.* Public use Data File No. 7-0627. Hyattsville, Md, 1997, [U.S.] Centers for Disease Control and Prevention.)

Oral Herpes Simplex Virus Infections

The prevalence of antibodies and the occurrence of herpetic lesions is approximately 15% to 40%, varies by age group, and is related to socioeconomic factors.[63] Of individuals from lower socioeconomic populations, 75% to 90% develop antibodies by the age of 10 years. The frequency of recurrence ranges from a single episode to several times per year (Fig. 2-13).

Recurrent Aphthous Ulcers

The prevalence of recurrent aphthous ulcers varies from 5% to 60%. Data from the NHANES III indicate that the occurrence is most common among young adults, 18 to 24 years of age.

Other Mucosal Lesions

The most common mucosal conditions contributing to oral disease burden are oral candidiasis, denture stomatitis, and oral human papillomavirus infection.

Oral Candidiasis
Oral candidiasis is seen most frequently in patients with impaired immune function, such as patients with renal transplants and individuals with human immunodeficiency virus (HIV).

Denture Stomatitis
Denture stomatitis is seen in approximately one quarter of persons ages 18 years and older who have both an upper and lower full denture. Of those with one full denture, 32% report denture stomatitis.[68]

Oral Human Papillomavirus Infections
Oral human papillomavirus infections are common among patients who are HIV-positive and may be associ-

ated with some oral leukoplakias with a high risk for malignant transformation.[56]

Developmental Disorders

Oral clefts occur in the general population at a rate of 1.2 per 1000 births for cleft lip (with or without cleft palate) and 0.56 per 1000 births for cleft palate. Whites are affected greater than three times more than blacks, and North American Indians show the greatest incidence. Cleft palate appears more frequently in females; cleft lip or lip/palate appears more frequently in males.[10,21,41,55,58]

Malocclusions (crowding) can occur in more than 75% of the U.S. population, 11% with severe crowding.

Injury

Head, face, and tooth injury are most often reported in the young and old. Exact data are limited, and most information comes from those injuries resulting in emergency room services. Between 1993 and 1994 craniofacial injury accounted for approximately 20 million emergency room (ER) visits. Of persons aged 6 to 50, 25% have had an orofacial injury resulting in damage to one or more anterior teeth. Of the 2.9 million ER visits for tooth-related injuries between 1997 and 1998, 25% were seen in children younger than 4 years of age.[49] The leading causes of injury include falls, assaults, sports injuries, and motor vehicle collisions.[17,57]

Chronic and Disabling Conditions

Orofacial Pain
Estimated from a national survey[66] during a 6-month period, 1 adult in 8 experiences toothache pain, 1 in 12 a painful oral sore, 1 in 19 jaw joint pain, and 1 in 71 face and cheek pain. Prevalence of toothache pain and oral sores increases with age. Twice as many women as men re-

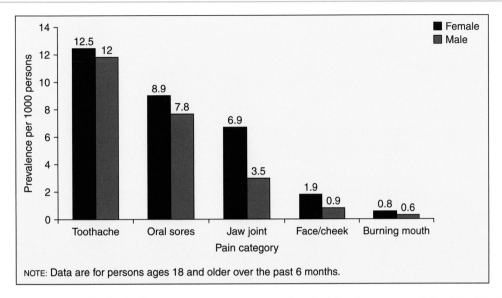

FIG. 2-14 Toothache is the most common source of orofacial pain among adults. (Modified from Lipton JA, Ship JA, Larach-Robinson D: Estimated prevalence and distribution of reported orofacial pain in the United States, *J Am Dent Assoc* 124[10]:115-21, 1993.)

port jaw joint pain and face/cheek pain.[39] Poverty affects the incidence of toothache[50] (Fig. 2-14).

Temporomandibular Disorders
Approximately 10 million Americans experience pain from temporomandibular disorders (TMD). Men and women are equally affected; however, women aged 30 to 49 are more likely than men of the same age to seek care for TMD.

Sjögren's Syndrome
An autoimmune disorder, Sjögren's syndrome affects more women than men. The symptoms include xerostomia, difficulty in swallowing, and xerophthalmia, and the condition affects an estimated 1 to 2 million people in the United States.[44]

Case Application
Considering the **burden of disease** in the U.S. population, should you discuss any additional health promotion topics with Ms. Marino? Is she possibly at risk for oral manifestations of reported diseases and medications? Is she at risk for systemic manifestation as a result of oral disease?

HEALTH PROMOTION GUIDELINES

As the focus and definition of oral health change from the restoration of teeth and support of oral structures to the recognition that the mouth is the center of vital tissues and critical to the restoration of health and well-being across all individuals, the role of the dental hygienist is clarified. Dental hygienists continue to provide necessary dental services to restore health. Their primary focus, however, is on the promotion of health.

The dental professional has an ideal background from which to promote health: training and education in clin-ical skills, behavioral and social sciences, public health, and health education. Two sources from which the dental professional can gain direction in setting professional and community goals are from *Healthy People 2010* and from the surgeon general of the United States.

HEALTHY PEOPLE 2010

Healthy People 2010 is a national health promotion and disease prevention initiative that brings together national, state, and local government agencies; nonprofit, voluntary, and professional organizations; business; communities; and individuals to improve the health of all Americans, eliminate disparities in health, and improve the quality of the years of a healthy life. The nation's progress in achieving the two overarching goals of *Healthy People 2010* is monitored through 467 objectives in 28 focus areas (Box 2-10). Many objectives focus on interventions designed to reduce or eliminate illness, disability, and premature death among individuals and communities. Others focus on broader issues, such as improvement in access to quality health care, strengthening of public health services, and improvement in the availability and dissemination of health-related information. Each objective has a target for specific improvements to be achieved by the year 2010. To-gether, these objectives reflect the depth of scientific knowledge and the breadth of diversity in the nation's communities. More importantly, they are designed to help the nation achieve its two platform goals and realize the vision of healthy people living in healthy communities.

Oral Health Goals for 2010

The overall *oral health goal* of *Healthy People 2010* is to pre-vent and control oral and craniofacial diseases, condi-tions, and injuries and improve access to related services.

BOX 2-10

Healthy People 2010 Focus Areas

Access to quality health services
Arthritis, osteoporosis, and chronic back conditions
Cancer
Chronic kidney disease
Diabetes
Disability and secondary conditions
Educational and community-based programs
Environmental health
Family planning
Food safety
Health communication
Heart disease and stroke
Human immunodeficiency virus
Immunization and infectious diseases
Injury and violence prevention
Maternal, infant, and child health
Medical product safety
Mental health and mental disorders
Nutrition and the overweight
Occupational safety and health
Oral health
Physical activity and fitness
Public health infrastructure
Respiratory diseases
Sexually transmitted diseases
Substance abuse
Tobacco use
Vision and hearing

Specific to that goal, the Healthy People 2010 Conference established 17 distinct objectives, as follows:

1. Reduce the proportion of children and adolescents who have dental caries experience in their primary or permanent teeth.

	Baseline	*Target goal*
Young children, primary teeth	18%	11%
Young children, primary and permanent teeth	52%	42%
Adolescents, permanent teeth	61%	51%

2. Reduce the proportion of children, adolescents, and adults with untreated dental decay.

	Baseline	*Target goal*
Young children, primary teeth	16%	9%
Young children, primary or permanent teeth	29%	21%
Adolescents, permanent teeth	20%	15%
Adults, permanent teeth	27%	15%

3. Increase the proportion of adults who have never had a permanent tooth extracted because of dental caries or periodontal disease.

	Baseline	*Target goal*
Adults	31%	42%

4. Reduce the proportion of older adults who have had all their natural teeth extracted.

	Baseline	*Target goal*
Older adults	26%	20%

5. Reduce periodontal disease.

	Baseline	*Target goal*
Gingivitis	48%	41%
Destructive periodontal disease	22%	14%

6. Increase the proportion of oral and pharyngeal cancers detected at the earliest stage.

	Baseline	*Target goal*
All	35%	50%

7. Increase the proportion of adults who, in the past 12 months, report having had an examination to detect oral and pharyngeal cancer.

	Baseline	*Target goal*
Adults	14%	35%

8. Increase the proportion of children who have received dental sealants on their molar teeth.

	Baseline	*Target goal*
Children age 8 years	23%	50%
Adolescents age 14 years	15%	50%

9. Increase the proportion of the U.S. population served by community water systems with optimally fluoridated water.

	Baseline	*Target goal*
All	62%	75%

10. Increase the proportion of children and adults who use the oral healthcare system each year.

	Baseline	*Target goal*
Children and adults	65%	83%

11. Increase the proportion of long-term-care residents who use the oral healthcare system each year.

	Baseline	*Target goal*
Long-term-care residents	19%	25%

12. Increase the proportion of children and adolescents under age 19 years at or below 200% of the federal poverty level who received any preventive dental service during the past year.

	Baseline	*Target goal*
Children and adolescents under age 19	20%	57%

13. Attain a developmental increase in the proportion of school-based health centers with an oral health component.

	Baseline	*Target goal*
None available	N/A	N/A

14. Increase the proportion of local health departments and community-based health centers, including community, migrant, and homeless health centers that have an oral health component.

	Baseline	*Target goal*
Community-based health centers	34%	75%

15. Increase the number of states and the District of Columbia that have a system for the recording and referral of infants and children with cleft lips, cleft palates, and other craniofacial anomalies to craniofacial anomaly rehabilitative teams.

	Baseline	*Target goal*
All states	23 States	All states

16. Increase the number of states and the District of Columbia that have an oral and craniofacial health surveillance system.

	Baseline	*Target goal*
All states	0	All states

17. Attain a developmental increase in the number of tribal, state (including the District of Columbia), and local health agencies that serve jurisdictions of 250,000 or more persons that have in place an effective dental health program directed by a dental professional with public health training.

	Baseline	*Target goal*
In development	In development	In development

SURGEON GENERAL'S REPORT

The first-ever Surgeon General's Report on Oral Health, in May 2000, was designed to alert Americans to the full meaning of oral health and its importance to general health and well-being. The in-depth report covered topics from *What is oral health?* to *What are the needs and opportunities to enhance oral health?* It included a summary document of findings at the conclusion of most chapters. (See the boxes beginning on p. 32 discussing the major findings in this report.)

The report offered a framework for action, outlining needs and opportunities to enhance oral health, as follows:

- *Change the perceptions regarding oral health and disease so that oral health becomes an accepted component of general health.* Perceptions need to change on three levels: public perceptions, policymakers' perceptions, and health providers' perceptions.
- *Accelerate the building of the science and evidence base and apply science effectively to improve oral health.* The acceleration of research and effective transfer of research findings to the public and health professions are key to this part of the plan.
- *Build an effective health infrastructure that meets the oral health needs of all Americans and integrates oral health effectively for all.* Because of cutbacks, limited personnel, equipment, and facilities, disease prevention programs are not being implemented in many communities. Coupled with the lack of racial and ethnic diversity in the oral health workforce, those populations most in need of health promotion receive the least. Shortages also exist in oral health education, research, and practice.
- *Remove known barriers between people and oral health services.* Use public-private partnerships to improve the oral health of those who still suffer disproportionately from oral disease.

Specifically, the dental professional was charged with the following responsibilities:

- Stay abreast of technological advances in dental and medical science.
- Continue to be responsive to the expectations of patients.
- Explore partnerships with medicine as the knowledge base regarding the relationship between oral health and systemic health increases.
- Expand the community disease-based prevention programs to meet emerging needs.
- Continue to seek solutions to questions of access and barriers to care.
- Understand the profound relationship between oral health and quality of life.

The dental hygienist's ability to touch a life and to promote health, not just restore oral health, will be shaped by the faculty members of academic programs, appreciated by patients, and respected by colleagues. Students must accept the challenge of embracing a broadened view of health and health promotion and understand the vast opportunity in dentistry to promote optimal health for all.

Case Application

Dismissing Ms. Marino until she felt healthier might have been done for the right reasons (coughing when reclined/runny nose), but not taking the opportunity to discuss at least one additional aspect of health with her clearly missed an opportunity to promote health. Additionally, implying that the absence of disease (focusing only on the acute upper respiratory infection) is synonymous with health does not fit with the newer, broader health paradigm. The topics from which you, the dental hygienist, might have chosen include the relationships between the following:

- Smoking and health
- Smoking and gingival inflammation
- Gingival inflammation and heart disease
- Hypertension and general well-being
- Periodontal disease and increased risk of stroke
- Over-the-counter drugs and prescription drugs and xerostomia
- Xerostomia and dental caries
- Cough syrup contents and dental caries
- Smoking and lung disease
- Smoking cessation

Clearly, when a patient is not feeling well, a long discussion of any nature is not appropriate. However, an initial thought or two might be planted, which could then be expanded at the next visit. The opportunity to ask Ms. Marino whether she would like to feel better all the time, not just when she gets rid of her cold, would have been one way to initiate discussions and then to plan a health promotion strategy targeted to her specific needs.

- *Oral disease and disorders in and of themselves affect health and well-being throughout life.* Dental disease affects patient life. The patient may be among a particularly vulnerable population. The burden of disease is extensive and may include the following:

  Oral lesions

  Candidiasis

  Birth defects

  Chronic facial pain

  Oral cancers

  Many of these conditions and their treatments may undermine self-image and self-esteem, discourage normal social interaction, cause other health problems, lead to chronic stress and depression, and incur great financial cost. They also may interfere with vital functions, such as breathing, food selection, eating, swallowing, and speaking, as well as with activities of daily living, such as work, school, and family interactions.

- *Safe and effective measures exist to prevent the most common dental diseases—dental caries and periodontal diseases.* Community water fluoridation is safe and effective in the prevention of dental caries in both children and adults. Water fluoridation benefits all residents served by community water supplies, regardless of their social or economic status. Professional and individual measures, including the use of fluoride mouthrinses, gels, dentifrices, and dietary supplements and the application of dental sealants, are additional means use to prevent dental caries. Gingivitis can be prevented with good personal oral hygiene, including brushing and flossing.

- *Lifestyle behaviors that affect general health, such as tobacco use, excessive alcohol use, and poor dietary choices, affect oral and craniofacial health as well.* These individual behaviors are associated with increased risk for craniofacial birth defects, oral and pharyngeal cancers, periodontal disease, dental caries, and candidiasis, among other oral health problems. Opportunities exist to expand the public's oral disease prevention and health promotion knowledge and practices through community programs and in healthcare settings. All healthcare providers can help promote healthy lifestyles by incorporating tobacco-cessation programs, nutritional counseling, and other health promotion efforts into their practices.

- *Profound and consequential oral health disparities exist within the U.S. population.* Disparities for various oral conditions may relate to income, age, sex, race or ethnicity, or medical status. Although common dental diseases are preventable, not all members of society are informed about or able to use appropriate oral health–promoting measures. Similarly, not all healthcare providers may be aware of the services needed to improve health. In addition, oral healthcare is not fully integrated into many care programs. Social, economic, and cultural factors and changing population demographics affect the ways in which health services are delivered and used, as well as the ways in which people care for themselves. Reducing disparities requires wide-ranging approaches that target populations at highest risk for specific oral diseases and the improvement of access to existing care. One approach includes more available dental insurance for Americans. Public coverage for dental care is minimal for adults, and programs for children have not reached the many eligible beneficiaries.

- *More information is needed to improve America's oral health and eliminate health disparities.* Adequate data do not exist for health, disease, and health practices and care use for the U.S. population as a whole and its diverse segments, including racial and ethnic minorities, rural populations, individuals with disabilities, the homeless, immigrants, migrant workers, the very young, and the frail elderly. Nor do sufficient data exist that explore health issues in relation to sex or sexual orientation. Data on state and local populations, essential for program planning and evaluation, are rare or unavailable and reflect the limited capacity of the U.S. health infrastructure for oral health. Health services research, which could provide much-needed information on the cost, cost-effectiveness, and outcomes of treatment, is also sorely lacking. Finally, measurement of disease and health outcomes is needed. Although progress has been made in the measurement of oral health–related quality of life, more needs to be done, and measures of oral health *per se* do not exist.

- *The mouth reflects general health and well-being.* The mouth is a readily accessible and visible part of the body and provides healthcare providers and individuals with a window to their patients' general health status. As the gateway of the body, the mouth senses and responds to the external world and at the same time reflects what is happening deep inside the body. The mouth may show signs of nutritional deficiencies and serve as an early warning system for diseases such as human immunodeficiency virus (HIV) infection and other immune system problems. The mouth also can show signs of general infection and stress. As the number of substances that can be reliably measured in saliva increases, it may well become the diagnostic fluid of choice, enabling the diagnosis of specific disease and the measurement of the concentration of a variety of drugs, hormones, and other molecules of interest. Cells and fluids in the mouth also may be used for genetic analysis to help uncover risks for disease and predict outcomes of medical treatments.

- *Oral diseases and conditions are associated with other health problems.* Oral infections can be the source of systemic infections in people with weakened immune systems, and oral signs and symptoms often are part of a general health condition. Associations between chronic oral infections and other oral health problems, including diabetes, heart disease, and adverse pregnancy outcomes, also have been reported. Ongoing research may uncover mechanisms that strengthen the current findings and explain these relationships.

- *Scientific research is key to further reduction in the burden of diseases and disorders that affect the face, mouth, and teeth.* The science base for dental diseases is broad and provides a strong foundation for further improvements in prevention; for other craniofacial and oral health conditions, the base has not yet reached the same level of maturity. Scientific research has led to a variety of approaches to improve oral health through prevention, early diagnosis, and treatment. These prevention measures can be taken further through investigation into the ways to develop more targeted and effective interventions and devise ways to enhance their appropriate adoption by the public and the healthcare professions. The application of powerful new tools and techniques is important. Their use in research into genetics and genomics, neuroscience, and cancer has permitted rapid progress in these fields. An intensified effort to understand the relationships between oral infections and their management and other illnesses and conditions is warranted, along with the development of oral-based diagnostics. These developments hold great promise.

The Craniofacial Complex

Oral health in America: a report of the surgeon general

Natural selection has served *Homo sapiens* well in the evolution of a craniofacial complex with remarkable functions and abilities to adapt, enabling the organism to meet the challenges of an ever-changing environment. An examination of the various tissues reveals elaborate designs that have evolved to serve the basic needs and functions of a complex mammal, as well as those that are uniquely human, such as speech. The rich distribution of nerves, muscles, and blood vessels in the region and extensive endocrine and immune system connections indicates the vital role of the craniofacial complex in adaptation and survival over a long life span. The following features are of particular interest:

- Genes controlling the basic patterning and segmental organizations of human development, and specifically the craniofacial complex, are highly conserved in nature. Mutated genes affecting human development have counterparts in many simpler organisms.
- Considerable reserve capacity or redundancy exists in the cells and tissues of the craniofacial complex so that if they are properly cared for, the structures should function more than a lifetime.
- The salivary glands and saliva subserve tasting and digestive functions and also participate in the mucosal immune system, a main line of defense against pathogens, irritants, and toxins.
- Salivary components protect and maintain oral tissues through antimicrobial components, buffering agents, and a process by which dental enamel can be remineralized.

The Magnitude of the Problem

Oral health in America: a report of the surgeon general

Over the past five decades, major improvements in oral health have been noted nationally for most Americans.

Despite improvements in oral health status, profound disparities remain in some population groups as classified by sex, income, age, and race or ethnicity. For some disease and conditions, the magnitude of the differences in oral health status among population groups is striking.

Oral diseases and conditions affect persons throughout their life spans. Nearly every American has experienced the most common oral disease, dental caries.

Conditions that severely affect the face and facial expression, such as birth defects, craniofacial injuries, and neoplastic diseases, are more common in the young and elderly.

Orofacial pain can greatly reduce quality of life and restrict major functions. Pain is a common symptom for many of the conditions affecting orofacial structures.

National and state data for many oral and craniofacial diseases and conditions and for population groups are limited or nonexistent. Available state data reveal variations within and among states in patterns of oral health and disease among population groups.

Research is needed to develop improved measures of disease and health, to explain differences among population groups, and to develop interventions targeted at eliminating disparities.

Diseases and Disorders

Oral health in America: a report of the surgeon general

Microbial infections, including those caused by bacteria, viruses, and fungi, are the primary cause of the most prevalent oral diseases. These include dental caries, periodontal diseases, herpes labialis, and candidiasis.

The etiology and pathogenesis of diseases and disorders affecting the craniofacial structures are multifactorial and complex, involving an interplay among genetic, environmental, and behavioral factors.

Many inherited and congenital conditions affect the craniofacial complex, often resulting in disfigurement and impairments that may involve many body organs and systems and affect millions of children worldwide.

Tobacco use, excessive alcohol use, and inappropriate dietary practices contribute to many diseases and disorders. In particular, tobacco use is a risk factor for oral cavity and pharyngeal cancers, periodontal diseases, candidiasis, and dental caries, among other diseases.

Some chronic diseases, such as Sjögren's syndrome, manifest with primary oral symptoms.

Orofacial pain conditions are common and often have complex etiologies.

Linkages with General Health

Oral health in America: a report of the surgeon general

Many systemic diseases and conditions have oral manifestations that may be the initial sign of clinical disease and as such serve to inform clinicians and individuals of the need for further assessment.

The oral cavity is a portal of entry and the site of disease for microbial infections that affect general health status.

The oral cavity and its functions can be adversely affected by many pharmaceuticals and other therapies commonly used to treat systemic conditions. The oral complications of these therapies can compromise patient compliance with treatment.

Immunocompromised and hospitalized individuals are at greater risk for general morbidity because of oral infections.

Individuals with diabetes are at greater risk for periodontal diseases.

Animal and population-based studies have demonstrated associations between periodontal diseases and diabetes, cardiovascular disease, stroke, and adverse pregnancy outcomes.

Further research is needed to determine the extent to which these associations are causal or coincidental.

Effects on Well-Being and Quality of Life

Oral health in America: a report of the surgeon general

Examination of efforts to characterize the functional and social implications of oral and craniofacial disease reveals the following findings:

Oral health is related to well-being and quality of life as measured along functional, psychosocial, and economic dimensions. Diet, nutrition, sleep, psychological status, social interactions, school, and work are affected by impaired oral and craniofacial health.

Cultural values influence oral and craniofacial health and well-being and can play an important role in care use practices and in the perpetuation of acceptable oral health and facial norms.

Oral and craniofacial diseases and their treatment place a burden on society in the form of lost days and years of productive work. Acute dental conditions contribute to a range of problems for employed adults, including restricted activity, bed days, and work loss, with children losing days of school. In addition, conditions such as oral and pharyngeal cancers contribute to premature death and can be measured by years of life lost.

Oral and craniofacial diseases and conditions contribute to compromised abilities to bite, chew, and swallow foods; limitations in food selection; and poor nutrition. These conditions include tooth loss, diminished salivary functions, orofacial pain conditions such as temporomandibular disorders, alterations in taste, and functional limitations of prosthetic replacements.

Orofacial pain, as a symptom of untreated dental and oral problems and as a condition in and of itself, is a major source of diminished quality of life. It is associated with sleep deprivation, depression, and multiple adverse psychosocial outcomes.

Self-reported impacts of oral conditions on social function include limitations in verbal and nonverbal communication, social interaction, and intimacy. Individuals with facial disfigurements resulting from craniofacial diseases and conditions and their treatments may experience loss of self-image and self-esteem, anxiety, depression, and social stigma; these in turn may limit educational, career, and marital opportunities and affect other social relations.

Reduced oral–health-related quality of life is associated with poor clinical status and reduced access to care.

Community and Other Approaches to Promote Oral Health and Prevent Oral Disease

Oral health in America: a report of the surgeon general

Community water fluoridation, an effective, safe, and ideal public health measure, benefits individuals of all ages and socioeconomic strata. Unfortunately, more than one third of the U.S. population (100 million persons) are without this critical public health measure.

Effective disease prevention measures exist for use by individuals, practitioners, and communities. Most of these focus on dental caries prevention, such as fluorides and dental sealants, in which a combination of services is required to achieve optimal disease prevention. Daily oral hygiene practices, such as brushing and flossing, can prevent gingivitis.

Community-based approaches for the prevention of other oral diseases and conditions, such as oral and pharyngeal cancers and orofacial trauma, require intensified developmental efforts.

A gap exists between research findings and the oral disease prevention and health promotion practices and knowledge of the public and the health professions.

Disease prevention and health promotion approaches, such as tobacco control, appropriate use of fluoride for caries prevention, and folate supplementation for neural tube defect prevention, highlight opportunities for partnerships between community-based programs and practitioners and collaborations among healthcare professionals.

Many community-based programs require a combined effort among social service, health care, and education services at the local or state level.

Personal and Provider Approaches to Oral Health

Oral health in America: a report of the surgeon general

Achieving and maintaining oral health require individual action, complemented by professional care and community-based activities.

Individuals can take actions for themselves and for persons under their care to prevent disease and maintain health. Primary prevention of many oral diseases is possible with appropriate diet, nutrition, oral hygiene, and health-promoting behaviors, including the appropriate use of professional services. Individuals should use a fluoride dentifrice daily to help prevent dental caries and should brush and floss daily to prevent gingivitis.

All primary care providers can contribute to improved oral and craniofacial health.

Interdisciplinary care is needed to manage the oral health–general health interface. Dentists, as primary care providers, are uniquely positioned to play an expanded role in the detection, early recognition, and management of a wide range of complex oral and general diseases and conditions.

Nonsurgical interventions are available to reverse disease progression and to manage oral diseases as infections.

New knowledge and the development of molecular and genetically based tests will facilitate risk assessment and management and improve the ability of healthcare providers to customize treatment.

Healthcare providers can successfully deliver tobacco-cessation and other health-promotion programs in their offices, contributing to both overall health and oral health.

Biocompatible rehabilitative materials and biologically engineered tissues are being developed to greatly enhance the treatment options available to providers and their patients.

Provision of Oral Health Care

Oral health in America: a report of the surgeon general

Dental, medical, and public health delivery systems each provide services that affect oral and craniofacial health in the U.S. population. Clinical oral health care is predominantly provided by a private practice workforce.

Dental services alone made up 4.7% of the nation's health expenditures in 1998, $53.8 billion of $1.1 trillion. These expenditures underestimate the true costs to the nation, however, because data are unavailable to determine the extent of the expenditures and services provided for craniofacial health care by other providers and institutions.

The public health infrastructure for oral health is insufficient to address the needs of disadvantaged groups, and the integration of oral and general health programs is lacking.

Expansion of community-based disease prevention and lowering of barriers to personal oral health care are needed to meet the needs of the population.

Insurance coverage for dental care is increasing but still lags behind medical insurance. For every child age 18 or younger without medical insurance are at least two children without dental insurance; for every adult 19 years or older without medical insurance are three without dental insurance.

A narrow definition of the phrase *medically necessary dental care* currently limits oral health services for many insured persons, particularly older adults.

The dentist-to-population ratio is declining, creating concern as to the capability of the dental workforce to meet the emerging demands of society and provide required services efficiently.

An estimated 25 million individuals reside in areas lacking adequate dental care services, as defined by Health Professional Shortage Areas (HPSA) criteria.

Educational debt has increased, affecting both career choices and practice location.

Disparities exist in the oral health profession workforce and career paths. The number of underrepresented minorities in the oral health professions is disproportionate to their distribution in the general population.

Current and projected demand for dental school faculty positions and research scientists is not being met. A crisis in the number of faculty members and researchers threatens the quality of dental education; oral, dental, and craniofacial research; and, ultimately, the health of the public.

Reliable and valid measures of outcomes for oral health care need to be developed, validated, and incorporated into practice and programs.

Factors Affecting Oral Health Over the Life Span

Oral health in America: a report of the surgeon general

The major factors that determine oral and general health and well-being are individual biology and genetics; the environment, including its physical and socioeconomic aspects; personal behaviors and lifestyle; access to care; and the organization of health care. These factors interact over the life span and determine the health of individuals, population groups, and communities—from neighborhoods to nations.

The burden of oral disease and conditions is disproportionately borne by individuals with low socioeconomic status at each life stage and by those who are vulnerable because of poor general health.

Access to care makes a difference. A complex set of factors underlies access to care and includes the need to have informed public and policymakers, integrated and culturally competent programs, and resources to pay and reimburse for the care. Among other factors, the availability of insurance increases access to care.

Preventive interventions, such as protective head and mouth gear and dental sealants, exist but are not uniformly used or reinforced.

Nursing homes and long-term-care and other institutions have a limited capacity to deliver necessary oral health services to their residents, most of whom are at increased risk for oral diseases.

Anticipatory guidance and risk assessment and management facilitate care for children and for the elderly.

Federal and state assistance programs for selected oral health services exist; however, the scope of services is severely limited, and their reimbursement level for oral health services is low compared with the usual fee for care.

RITICAL THINKING ACTIVITIES

1. With a study partner, review the medical histories of several clinic patients. Select several health promotion topics and present your conclusions to a faculty member and a fellow student. What is the nature of their feedback?

2. Develop a personal philosophy of practice. Include such topics as services you will provide, processes you will use to determine the best approach to health promotion for the patient, and the exact ways you plan to promote health.

3. "You have the ability to touch a life." In the context of this chapter, what is the meaning of this phrase?

4. Oral health is related to well-being and quality of life as measured by functional, psychosocial, and economic dimensions. What does this statement mean to clinical practice?

5. Survey 10 classmates. Ask whether in the past 6 months they have experienced orofacial pain in any of the following categories:
   Toothache
   Oral sores
   Jaw joint
   Face/cheek
   Burning mouth
   How consistent are your findings with those reported in the text?

6. With a group of four classmates, select one of the goals from *Healthy People 2010* and one of the action steps from the surgeon general's report. Develop an action plan for your class as to how you would execute those strategies.

REVIEW QUESTIONS

1. Significant progress in the reduction of the incidence, prevalence, and severity of dental caries has been the result of which of the following community-based programs?
   a. Community water fluoridation
   b. Dental sealants
   c. School-based topical fluoride programs
   d. *a* and *b*
   e. All the above

2. Health can be defined as which of the following?
   a. Quality of life
   b. Absence of disease
   c. A complete state of physical, mental, and social well-being
   d. All the above

3. In which ways are oral infections opportunistic?
   a. Oral infections are caused by extrinsic pathogens.
   b. Oral infections are caused by microorganisms commonly found in the oral cavity.
   c. Oral infections occur when oral tissues are compromised.
   d. *b* and *c*
   e. All the above

4. Periodontitis is defined as the sixth complication of diabetes.
   a. True
   b. False

REVIEW QUESTIONS—cont'd

5. Examples of a suspected causal relationship between oral disease and systemic health has been noted in which of the following?
   a. Periodontal disease and oral cancer
   b. Periodontal disease and preterm, low–birth-weight babies
   c. Periodontal disease and stroke
   d. Periodontal disease and diabetes
   e. *b* and *d*
   f. All the above
6. The most recent national health survey (NHANES III, 1988-1994) validates which of the following statements?
   a. Dental caries is five times more common than asthma.
   b. Dental caries is equally evident across all socioeconomic guidelines.

   c. Dental caries represents the single-most chronic childhood disease.
   d. *a* and *c*
   e. All the above
7. Which of the following statements is *true?*
   a. The mouth reflects the general health and well-being of an individual.
   b. Oral diseases and conditions are associated with general health problems.
   c. Despite improvements in oral health status, profound disparities still exist in some population groups.
   d. Many systemic diseases and conditions have oral manifestations.
   e. *a, c,* and *d*
   f. All the above

 SUGGESTED AGENCIES AND WEB SITES

Because of the ever-changing nature of the Internet, some of the web sites listed here may have changed since publication. Please refer to Mosby's Evolve web site for the most current information.

American Academy of Pediatrics: http://www.aap.org
American Academy of Pediatric Dentistry: http://www.aapd.org
CancerNet: http://www.icic.nci.nih.gov
CDC National Prevention Information Network: http://www.cdcnpin.org
Census Bureau of the United States: http://www.census.gov
Centers for Disease Control and Prevention: http://www.healthlinkusa.com
Health Direction National Associations and Healthcare Links: http://www.healthdirection.com
HealthLinks: http://healthlinks.washington.edu
Health Objectives for the Nation Progress Toward Achieving Health: http://www.cdc.gov
National Cancer Institute: http://www.nci.nih.gov
National Center for Education in Maternal and Child Health: http://www.ncemch.org
National Center for Health Statistics: http://www.cdc.gov/nchs
National Center for Prevention Services, Chronic Disease Prevention: http://www.cdc.gov
National Health Information Center: http://nhic-nt.health.org

National Health Service Corps: http://www.bphc.hrsa.dhhs.gov
National Human Genome Research Institute, National Institute: http://nhic-nt.health.org
National Institute of Dental and Craniofacial Research: http://www.nidr.nih.gov
National Institute of Diabetes and Digestive & Kidney Diseases: http://www.niddk.nih.gov
National Institutes of Health: http://www. nih.gov
National Oral Health Information Clearinghouse: http://www.aerie.com
National Oral Health Information Clearinghouse: http://www.health.org
NIH Web Search: http://search.info.nih.gov
Oral Health Promotion Research: http://www.nidcr.nih.gov
Perspectives in Disease Prevention and Health Promotion: http://www.cdc.gov
U.S. Bureau of Census: http://www.census.gov
U.S. Department of Health and Human Services: http://www.os.dhhs.gov
U.S. Preventive Services Task Force: http://cpmcnet.columbia.edu

 ADDITIONAL READINGS AND RESOURCES

Burt BA, Eklund SA: *Dentistry, dental practice and the community,* Philadelphia, 1999, WB Saunders.
Gluck GM, Morganstein WM: *Jong's community dental health,* ed 5, St Louis, (in press), Mosby.
Institute of Medicine: *Dental education at the crossroads: challenges and change,* Washington, DC, 1995, National Academy Press.
National Institute of Dental Research: *Oral health of United States children: the national survey of dental caries in U.S. school children 1986-1987.* DHHS pub no (PHS) 89-2247. Bethesda, Md, 1989, U.S. Department of Health and Human Services.

Pamuk E, Makuc D, Heck K, et al: *Socioeconomic status and health chartbook.* Health, United States. 1998. Hyattsville, Md, 1998, National Center for Health Statistics.
Schol L, Blinkhorn AS, editors: *Oral health promotion,* New York, 1993, Oxford.
U.S. Department of Health and Human Services (USD-HHS): *Healthy People 2000 Review 1995-96.* Pub. no. 96-1256. Washington, DC, 1996, The Department.
U.S. Department of Health and Human Services (USD-HHS): *Healthy People 2010: conference edition in two volumes,* Washington, DC, 2000, The Department.

Continued

ADDITIONAL READINGS AND RESOURCES—cont'd

U.S. Department of Health and Human Services (USD-HHS): *Healthy People 2010: understanding and improving health*, Washington, DC, 2000, The Department.

U.S. Department of Health and Human Services: *Oral Health in America: a report of the surgeon general*, Rockville, Md, 2000, The Department, National Institute of Dental and Craniofacial Research, National Institutes of Health.

U.S. Department of Health and Human Services (USD-HHS): Public Health Service, National Institutes of Health. *Agenda for research on women's health for the 21st century. A report of the Task Force on the NIH Women's Health Research Agenda for the 21st Century*, vol 2, Bethesda, Md, 1999, National Institutes of Health.

World Health Organization: *International classification of disease and stomatology*. IDC-OA, ed 3, Geneva, 1992, The Organization.

REFERENCES

1. Allukian M Jr, Horowitz AM: Effective community prevention programs for oral disease. In Gluck G, Morganstein W, editors: *Jong's community dental health*, ed 4, St Louis, 1998, Mosby.
2. American Cancer Society (ACS): *Cancer facts and figures*. Atlanta, 1999, The Society.
3. Asikainen S et al: Age, dental infections, and coronary artery disease, *J Dent Res* 79:756-60, 2000.
4. Barbour SE et al: Tobacco and smoking: environmental factors that modify the host response (immune system) and have an impact on periodontal health, *Crit Rev Oral Biol Med* 8(4):437-60, 1997.
5. Beck JD et al: Periodontal disease and cardiovasvular disease, *J Periodontol* 67(10 Suppl):1123-37, 1996.
6. Beck JD et al: Periodontics: a risk factor for coronary heart disease? *Ann Periodontol* 3(1):127-41, 1998.
7. Belting CM, Hiniker JJ, Dummett CO: Influence of diabetes mellitus on the severity of periodontal disease in diabetics. *J Periodontol* 35:476-80, 1964.
8. Benveniste R, Bixler D, Conneally PM: Periodontal disease in diabetics. *J Periodontol* 38(4):271-9, 1967.
9. Bridges RB et al: Periodontal status of diabetic and non-diabetic men: effects of smoking, glycemic control, and socioeconomic factors. *J Periodontol* 67(11):1185-92, 1996.
10. Burman NT: A case: control study of orofacial clefts in Western Australia, *Aust Dent J* 30(6):423-9, 1985.
11. Campbell MJ: Epidemiology of periodontal disease in the diabetic and the non-diabetic, *Aust Dent J* 17(4):274-8, 1972.
12. Cohen DW et al: Diabetes mellitus and periodontal disease: two-year longitudinal observations. I. *J Periodontol* 41(12):709-12, 1970.
13. Collins JG et al: Effects of *Escherichia coli* and *Porphyromonas gingivalis* lipopolysaccharide on pregnancy outcome in the golden hamster, *Infect Immun* 62(10):4652-5, 1994.
14. Dasanayake AP: Poor periodontal health of the pregnant woman as a risk factor for low birth weight, *Ann Periodontol* 3:206-12, 1998.
15. Davenport ES et al: The east London study of maternal chronic periodontal disease and preterm low birth weight infants: study design and prevalence data, *Ann Periodontol* 3:213-21, 1998.
16. DeStefano F et al: Dental disease and risk of coronary heart disease and mortality, *Br Med J* 306(6879):688-91, 1993.
17. DeWet FA: The prevention of orofacial sports injuries in the adolescent, *Int Dent J* 31:313-9, 1981.
18. Emrich LJ, Shlossman M, Genco RJ: Periodontal diseases in non–insulin-dependent diabetes mellitus, *J Periodontol* 62(2):123-21, 1991.
19. Finestone AJ, Boorujy ST: Diabetes mellitus and periodontal disease, *Diabetes* 16(5):336-40, 1967.
20. Firatli E: The relationship between clinical periodontal status and insulin-dependent diabetes mellitus. Results after 5 years, *J Periodontol* 68(2):136-40, 1997.
21. Fraser BR, Calnan JS: Cleft lip and palate: seasonal incidence, birth weight, birth rank, sex, site, associated malformations and parental age. A statistical survey, *Arch Dis Childhood* 36:420-3, 1961.
22. Galea H, Aganovic I, Aganovic M: The dental caries and periodontal disease experience of patients with early onset insulin-dependent diabetes, *Int Dent J* 36(4):219-24, 1986.
23. Genco RJ: Current view of risk factors for periodontal diseases, *J Periodontol* 67(10 Suppl):1041-9, 1996.
24. Gibbs RS et al: A review of premature birth and subclinical infection, *Am J Obstet Gynecol* 166(5):1515-28, 1992.
25. Grau AJ et al: Association between acute cerebrovascular ischemia and chronic and recurrent infection, *Stroke* 28(9):1724-9, 1995.
26. Greenberg JS: *Health education*, Dubuque, Iowa, 1989, Brown.
27. Grossi SG, Genco RJ: Periodontal disease and diabetes mellitus: a two-way relationship, *Ann Periodontol* 3(1):51-61, 1998.
28. Grossi SG et al: Response to periodontal therapy in diabetics and smokers, *J Periodontol* 67(10 Suppl):1094-102, 1996.
29. Haber J: Cigarette smoking: a major risk factor for periodontitis, *Compend Cont Educ Dent* 15:1002-14, 1994.
30. Herzberg MC, Myer MW: Dental plaque, platelets, and cardiovascular diseases, *Ann Periodontol* 3(1):151-60, 1998.
31. Herzberg MC, Myer MW: Effects of oral flora on platelets: possible consequences in cardiovascular disease, *J Periodontol* 67(10 suppl):1138-42, 1996.
32. Herzberg MC et al: The platelet as an inflammatory cell in periodontal diseases: interactions with *Porphyromonas gingivalis*, In Genco R et al, editors: *Molecular pathogenesis of periodontal disease*, Washington, DC, 1994, American Society for Microbiology.
33. Herzberg MC, Brintzenhofe KL, Clawson CC: Aggregation of human platelets and adhesion of *Streptococcus sanguis*, *Infect Immun* 39(3):1457-69, 1983.
34. Hildebolt CF et al: Attachment loss with postmenopausal age and smoking, *J Periodontal Res* 32(7):619-25, 1997.
35. Hillier SL et al: Association between bacterial vaginosis and preterm delivery of a low-birth-weight infant. The vaginal infections and prematurity study group, *N Engl J Med* 333(26):1737-42, 1995.
36. Horowitz AM: The public's oral health: the gaps between what we know and what we do, *Adv Dent Science* 9:91-5, 1995.
37. Joshipura KJ et al: Poor oral health and coronary heart disease, *J Dent Res* 75(9):1631-6, 1996.
38. Kroes I, Lepp PW, Relman DA: Bacterial diversity within the human subgingival crevice, *Proc Natl Acad Sci USA* 7:96(5):14547-52, 1999.
39. Lipton JA, Ship JA, Larach-Robinson D: Estimated prevalence and distribution of reported orofacial pain in the United States, *J Am Dent Assoc* 124(10):115-21, 1993.

40. Löe H: Periodontal disease—the sixth complication of diabetes mellitus, *Diabetes Care* 16(1):329-34, 1993.

41. Lowry RB, Thunem NY, Uh SH: Birth prevalence of cleft lip and palate in British Columbia between 1952 and 1986: stability of rates. *Can Med Assoc J* 15;140(10):1167-70, 1989.

42. Mattila KJ: Dental infections as a risk factor for acute myocardial infarction, *Eur Heart J* 14 (Suppl):51-3, 1993.

43. Mattila KJ et al: Association between dental health and acute myocardial infarction, *Br Med J* 298(6676):779-81, 1989.

44. Mattila KJ et al: Dental infection and the risk of new coronary events: prospective study of patients with documented coronary artery disease, *Clin Infect Dis* 20(3):588-92, 1995.

45. McCaul KD, Glasgow RE, Gustafson C: Predicting levels of preventive dental behaviors, *J Am Dent Assoc* 111:601-5, 1985.

46. McCormick MC: The contribution of low birth weight to infant mortality and childhood morbidity, *N Engl J Med* 312(2):82-90, 1985.

47. Meyer DH, Fives-Taylor PM: Oral pathogens: from dental plaque to cardiac disease, *Curr Opin Microbiol* 1(1):88-95, 1998

48. Morrison H.I., Ellison LF, Taylor GW: Periodontal disease and risk of fatal coronary heart and cerebrovascular diseases, *J Cardiovasc Risk* 6:7-11, 1999.

49. National Center for Health Statistics (NCHS): Preliminary data from the Centers for Disease Control and Prevention, *Mon Vital Stat Rep* 46 (Suppl 2), 1997.

50. National Center for Health Statistics (NCHS): *Prevalence of selected chronic conditions: United States 1990-92.* DHHS Pub. no PH-S97-1522. Hyattsville, Md, January 1997, U.S. Department of Health and Human Services, Centers for Disease Control and Prevention.

51. National Institute of Diabetes and Digestive and Kidney Diseases (NIDDK): *Diabetes statistics.* Pub. no. 99-3892. Bethesda, Md, 1999, National Institutes of Health.

52. O'Neill HW: Opinion study comparing attitudes about dental health, *J Am Dent Assoc* 109:910-5, 1984.

53. Offenbacher S et al: Periodontal infection as a possible risk factor for preterm low birth weight, *J Periodontol* 67(10 Suppl):1103-3, 1996.

54. Offenbacher S et al: Potential Pathogenic mechanisms of periodontitis-associated pregnancy complications, *Ann Periodontol* 3(1):233-50, 1998.

55. Owens JR, Jones JW, Harris F: Epidemiology of facial clefting, *Arch Dis Child* 60(6):521-4, 1985.

56. Palefsky JM et al: Association between proliferative verrucous leukoplakia and infection with human papillomavirus type 16, *J Oral Pathol Med* 24:193-7, 1995.

57. Sane J: Comparison of maxillofacial and dental injuries in four contact team sports: American football, bandy, basketball, and handball, *Am J Sports Med* 16(6):647-51, 1988.

58. Schulman J et al: Surveillance for and comparison of birth defect prevalences in two geographic areas—United States, 1983-1988, *MMWR Morb Mortal Wkly Rep* 19;42(1):1-7, 1993.

59. Seppala B, Almamo J: A site-by-site follow-up study on insulin-dependent diabetes mellitus, *J Clin Periodontol* 21(3):161-5, 1994.

60. Seppala B, Seppala M, Ainamo J: A longitudinal study on insulin-dependent diabetes mellitus, *J Clin Periodontol* 21(3):161-5, 1994.

61. Shapiro S et al: Relevance of correlates of infant deaths for significant morbitidy at 1 year of age, *Am J Obstet Gynecol* 136(3):363-73, 1980.

62. Shlossman M et al: Type 2 diabetes mellitus and periodontal disease, *J Am Dent Assoc* 121(4):532-6, 1994.

63. Skully C: Herpes simplex virus (HSV). In Millard HD, Mason DK, editors: *World workshop on oral medicine,* Chicago, 1989, Year Book.

64. Sogaard AJ: Theories and models of health behavior in oral health promotion. In Schol L and Blinkhorn AS, editors: *Oral health promotion,* New York, 1993, Oxford.

65. Szpunar SM, Ismail AI, Eklund SA: Diabetes and periodontal disease: analyses of NHANES I and HHANES, *J Dent Res* 68(SI):164-438, 1989.

66. Talal N: Sjögren's syndrome: historical overview and clinical spectrum of disease, *Rheum Dis Clin North Am* 18(3):507-51, 1992.

67. Trevisan M et al: Examination of the relation between periodontal health status and cardiovascular risk factors: serum total and high density lipoprotein, cholesterol, C-reactive protein, and plasma fibrinogen, *Am J Epidemiol* 151:273-82, 2000.

68. U.S. Department of Health and Human Services: *Oral Health in America: a report of the surgeon general,* Rockville, Md, 2000, U.S. Department of Health and Human Services, National Institute of Dental and Craniofacial Research, National Institutes of Health.

69. World Health Organization (WHO): *World Health Organization's International classification of diseases and stomatology,* IDC-DA, ed 3, Geneva, 1995, The Organization.

70. Wright FA: Children's perception of vulnerability to illness and dental disease, *Community Dent Oral Epidemiol* 10:29-32, 1982.

71. Wu T et al: Periodontal disease and risk of cerebrovascular disease: a prospective study of a representative sample of U.S. adults, *Am J Epidemiol* 149(11 suppl):290, 1999.

CHAPTER 3

Legal *and* Ethical Considerations

Judith Ann Davison, Cheryl H. DeVore

Chapter Outline

Case Study: Ethics and the Law
Patients' Rights and Responsibilities in Dental Care
    Informed consent
    First Amendment rights
    Patient self-determination
    Patient duties and responsibilities
    Abandonment
Dental Hygienist's Responsibilities in Providing
  Dental Hygiene Care
    Proper licensure and education
    Practice within the limits of the law

Continuing dental hygiene education
Risk management for the dental hygiene
    practitioner
Effective communication
Documentation
Ownership and access to dental treatment
    records
Respect for the patient/practitioner relationship

Key Terms

Battery
Beneficence

Confidentiality
Ethics

Informed consent
Liability

Nonmaleficence
Practice act

Statutes
Tort

Learning Outcomes

1. Develop an understanding and appreciation for *informed consent* in the healthcare environment, and when it need not be obtained.
2. Identify the elements a plaintiff must prove in a lawsuit based on tort law.
3. Possess an understanding of legal terms such as battery, medical directives, risk management, and standard of care.
4. Describe how the First Amendment to the U.S. Constitution may relate to the medical care an individual receives.
5. State the steps that must be taken in the termination of a patient from care to protect the healthcare provider from charges of abandonment.

6. Become knowledgeable of the legal risks involved in dental hygiene.
7. Describe key points in documentation of the dental hygiene treatment process.
8. Discuss how a license to practice dental hygiene is obtained.
9. Discuss the role of the regulatory agency in dental hygiene practice.
10. Evaluate whether ethical principles and legal duties have been upheld.

ealth care cannot be provided in a manner that does not comply with the laws that govern it. These laws are enforced today perhaps with more vigor than they were historically. Consumers are more aware of reasonable expectations from their healthcare providers. When treatment does not go as planned, consumers who believe they have been wronged may take legal action by filing suit against the practitioner or by filing a complaint with the appropriate regulatory agency. Consequently, dental healthcare providers must be aware of and consistently apply the laws that govern their practice, ensuring they are always in compliance.

Dental hygienists are fully responsible healthcare providers. Although dental hygienists have often perceived that their own exposure to **liability** is significantly less than that of the dentist or is nonexistent, this is not true. The scope of dental hygiene practice has changed and expanded; therefore dental hygiene practitioners must accept their legal responsibility in providing care and hold themselves legally accountable.

The laws that affect dental and dental hygiene practice come from several sources. Statutory laws are created by a legislative body and regulate the practice of dentistry and dental hygiene in every state. Federal and local laws also affect dental hygiene care. In addition to these laws, administrative laws are enacted by the agencies empowered to license and monitor the profession in their tasks. For example, professional boards are empowered to prescribe laws to help enforce statutory laws among the professional group. The combined state statutory regulations and the agency law are often referred to as a **practice act.** Additionally, law evolves from court decisions over time and is known as *common law.*

All these laws affect and control the direct delivery of dental and dental hygiene services, the manner in which communication among healthcare professionals and between dental hygienists and patients transpires, and the way in which information learned during those communications is used. Much of the patient/practitioner relationship is shaped by these laws.

Generally, discussions of the dental hygienist's legal responsibility in providing dental hygiene care are impossible without some incorporation of the ethical responsibility. Although law denotes the legal practice of the profession, the ethical code of a profession tends to lend guidance and force when a direct legal component does not exist.

Dental hygienists must assess and minimize their exposure to risk in practice. They must manage risks through improved patient practitioner communication, informed consent, and care that always meets or exceeds the standard. Thorough and accurate documentation is also a critical component of any risk management program.

This chapter reviews the legal responsibilities of both the patient in the receipt of care and the dental hygienist in the provision of dental hygiene care.

PATIENTS' RIGHTS AND RESPONSIBILITIES IN DENTAL CARE

3-A
3-B
3-C
3-D

Duties or responsibilities are integral to any discussion of patient rights because each patient right creates a duty on the part of a healthcare provider. Dental healthcare providers have the ethical and legal duty to ensure that their patients' rights are protected. Lawsuits regarding these duties often refer to physicians; however, these legal principles are just as applicable to all healthcare providers, including the dental hygienist or the dentist.

INFORMED CONSENT

Informed consent is an ethical and legal doctrine that has roots in the early part of the century but did not gain a great deal of attention in the legal and medical community until the 1960s and 1970s. During the 1960s, many in American society began to question authority, and this included the authority of medical professionals to dictate the type of health care that each should receive. In the 1960s through 1980s the number of lawsuits increased against physicians and medical institutions, alleging failure to disclose the risks and alternatives for medical procedures performed. Because healthcare providers have greater medical knowledge than patients, and patients may be anxious (in addition to lack of understanding of medical or dental terminology), courts have found that healthcare providers have an obligation to keep patients informed and allow them to make choices regarding the medical or dental care they receive.

A 1905 court case[13] declared that employment of physicians does not give them implied license to perform whatever treatment, in the exercise of their judgment, is necessary. It further stated that each free citizen in a free government has a right that underlies all others, the right to himself or herself. This right, "forbids a physician or surgeon, however skillful or eminent, who has been asked to examine, diagnose, advise and prescribe, to violate without permission the bodily integrity of his patient by a major or capital operation, placing him under anesthetic for that purpose, and operating on him without his consent or knowledge."[13]

In 1914 a New York court decision written by Justice Cardozo[15] stated:

Every human being of adult years and sound mind has a right to determine what shall be done with his own body.

In 1972 *Canterbury v Spence*[4] became a landmark case articulating the parameters of informed consent. The court in Canterbury declared that because the average patient has little or no understanding of medicine, the physician's duty is to provide information to the patient relative to the alternatives and risks of treatment. This obligation to communicate information to the patient arises when reasonable care calls for it. True informed consent occurs only when the patient understands alternatives to and risks of medical or dental treatment. The professional's obligation is to inform the patient "in nontechnical terms as to what is at stake: the therapy alternatives open to him, the goals expectably to be achieved, and the risks that may ensue from particular treatment and no treatment."[5]

In 1973 the American Hospital Association adopted the first Patient's Bill of Rights (Box 3-1).

In 1981 The World Medical Association adopted a statement on the rights of patients that reads, in part:

The patient has the right to accept or refuse treatment after receiving adequate information.

The 1998-1999 Code of Ethics for the American Dental Hygienists' Association (ADHA; Box 3-2), Section 7,

Text continued on p. 46

Gloria Allen has been a dental hygienist for 15 years. She is presently working in a general practice for Dr. Randolph Peters in a state in which the dental practice act permits the following tasks to be performed by a dental hygienist:

1. A complete prophylaxis, including removal of all hard and soft deposits from all surfaces of human teeth to the epithelial attachments, polishing of natural and restored teeth, root planing, and performance of curettage
2. Preventive measures such as an oral prophylaxis and the application of fluorides and other recognized topical agents for the prevention of oral disease or discomfort
3. Examination of soft and hard tissue of the head, neck, and oral cavity; notation of deformities, defects, and abnormalities
4. Application of pit and fissure sealants
5. Fabrication of athletic mouthguard appliances
6. Polishing of amalgam restorations
7. Removal of excess cement from crown/orthodontic bands
8. Exposure and processing of radiographs

Before accepting her current position, Gloria worked for Dr. Samuel Ray in a state in which the dental practice act permits the following tasks to be performed by a dental hygienist:

1. Oral prophylaxis, including scaling and polishing of the dentition
2. Application of pit and fissure sealants
3. Information gathering for patients' medical histories
4. Application of topical fluoride
5. Instruction of patients in oral hygiene techniques
6. Placement and condensing of amalgam and tooth-colored restorations
7. Impressions for diagnostic models
8. Preparation of teeth for bonding
9. Exposure and processing of radiographs
10. Application of topical anesthetic agents
11. Record of patient's vital signs
12. Placement and removal of a rubber dam
13. Administration of local anesthetics and nitrous oxide
14. Placement of periodontal sutures

Breach of Duty: Confidentiality

Gloria is an excellent clinician who enjoys chatting with all her patients. On Monday, her third patient was Mr. Alex Fenten, a 54-year-old architect for whom she has provided dental hygiene services during the past 5 years. She complimented Mr. Fenten on his excellent oral hygiene. She cited her first patient of the day, Mrs. Amelia Gray, a nurse. Gloria described Mrs. Gray's terrible periodontal disease resulting from improper care of her oral tissues. She also told Mr. Fenten that Mrs. Gray was going through an awful divorce after her husband had run off with his secretary and that Mrs. Gray was recently diagnosed with cancer.

After listening to Gloria describe Mrs. Gray's plight, Mr. Fenten explained that Mrs. Gray is his sister. Gloria expressed surprise, changed the subject, and completed her work.

Practicing in Violation of State Law

The next Friday afternoon, Gloria was completing a prophylaxis for her last patient of the day, Mrs. Betty Lou Walters. Dr. Peters was out of town attending a continuing dental education program. As Gloria was scaling Mrs. Walters' anterior teeth, she accidentally removed the restoration on tooth #8, leaving a rather unsightly gap between teeth #8 and #9. Gloria explained to Mrs. Walters what happened and that she would

have to return on Monday to have Dr. Peters replace the restoration. Mrs. Walters saw her smile in the mirror and was horrified. She explained that she and her husband were attending a dinner party that evening at the home of her husband's employer and that she absolutely could not attend with her tooth in such a condition. She then pleaded with Gloria to fix the tooth. Feeling responsible for Mrs. Walters' dilemma and knowing that she had completed such restorations in the past, Gloria used Dr. Peters' treatment room to replace a restoration on tooth #8. She then explained to Mrs. Walters that this was only a temporary measure and she would have to return to the office to have Dr. Peters replace the filling.

Illegal and Unethical Behavior

The following week Gloria had lunch with her friend Elisa Jensen. Elisa is also a dental hygienist who works for another dentist in the same office complex. Elisa told Gloria that her mother has been seriously ill for the past 6 months. She explained that she has been so busy caring for her mother that she did not have the time to attend continuing dental hygiene education courses and feared the loss of her license. In an attempt to console her friend, Gloria explained that she had attended far more dental hygiene education programs than she needed for relicensure and would be happy to give Elisa the documentation of attendance for them.

Negligence, Practicing below the Standard of Care, and Violating the ADHA Code of Ethics

After lunch Gloria's first patient was Mr. Jonas Black, whom she had not seen for 3 years. An oral assessment indicated that Mr. Black has advanced periodontal disease. Heavy generalized calculus deposits were on both maxillary and mandibular arches. His oral tissue was edematous, with profuse bleeding on probing, which revealed 5- to 8-mm pocketing on teeth #2, #3, #14, #15, #16, #18, #19, #30, and #32, and 4- to 6-mm pocketing on teeth #6, #9, #23, #27, and #28. Gloria, fearing that she did not have adequate time to treat Mr. Black, immediately began scaling with the ultrasonic scaler on the maxillary right quadrant but did not scale any teeth to completion. When she finished, Gloria explained to Mr. Black that because he had not received a dental prophylaxis in more than 3 years it had taken her longer than normal to complete; therefore the charges for his appointment would be higher than the usual cost. Gloria also explained that she was able to complete only one quadrant of his mouth and that he must return for at least four visits to complete the treatment. Mr. Black left, announcing he was on his way to his attorney's office.

Answer the following questions regarding this case. After reading the chapter, assess your answers to see whether you would change any of your responses. Refer to the case application for these questions near the end of the chapter.

1. Is there a breach of duty reagarding Gloria's conversation with Mr. Fenten? If so, describe the breach. Was this a breach of **ethics** or a legal duty?
2. In view of Mrs. Walters' dilemma and Dr. Peters' absence, was Gloria justified in placing the restoration? If so, by what authority? If not, what was the violation?
3. Was the friendly exchange between Gloria and Elisa illegal, unethical, or neither?
4. Considering Mr. Black's periodontal disease, was Gloria justified in proceeding with treatment? Why would Mr. Black consult his attorney? What advice will Mr. Black's attorney give him?

BOX 3-1

A Patient's Bill of Rights

A Patient's Bill of Rights was first adopted by the American Hospital Association (AHA) in 1973. This revision was approved by the AHA Board of Trustees on October 21, 1992.

Introduction

Effective health care requires collaboration between patients and physicians and other healthcare professionals. Open and honest communication, respect for personal and professional values, and sensitivity to differences are integral to optimal patient care. As the setting for the provision of health services, hospitals must provide a foundation to understand and respect the rights and responsibilities of patients, their families, physicians, and other caregivers. Hospitals must ensure a healthcare ethic that respects the role of patients in decision making about treatment choices and other aspects of their care. Hospitals must be sensitive to cultural, racial, linguistic, religious, age, gender, and other differences, as well as the needs of persons with disabilities.

The American Hospital Association presents *A Patient's Bill of Rights* with the expectation that it will contribute to more effective patient care and be supported by the hospital on behalf of the institution, its medical staff, employees, and patients. The American Hospital Association encourages healthcare institutions to tailor this bill of rights to their patient communities by translating and/or simplifying the language of this bill of rights as may be necessary to ensure that patients and their families understand their rights and responsibilities.

Bill of Rights

The following rights can be exercised on the patient's behalf by a designated surrogate or proxy decision maker if the patient lacks decision-making capacity, is legally incompetent, or is a minor:

1. The patient has the right to considerate and respectful care.

2. The patient has the right to and is encouraged to obtain from physicians and other direct caregivers relevant, current, and understandable information concerning diagnosis, treatment, and prognosis.

   Except in emergencies when the patient lacks decision-making capacity and the need for treatment is urgent, the patient is entitled to the opportunity to discuss and request information related to the specific procedures and/or treatments, the risks involved, the possible length of recuperation, and the medically reasonable alternatives and their accompanying risks and benefits.

   Patients have the right to know the identity of physicians, nurses, and others involved in their care, as well as when those involved are students, residents, or other trainees. The patient also has the right to know the immediate and long-term financial implications of treatment choices, insofar as they are known.

3. The patient has the right to make decisions about the plan of care prior to and during the course of treatment and to refuse a recommended treatment or plan of care to the extent permitted by law and hospital policy and to be informed of the medical consequences of this action. In case of such refusal, the patient is entitled to other appropriate care and services that the hospital provides or transfer to another hospital. The hospital should notify patients of any policy that might affect patient choice within the institution.

4. The patient has the right to have an advance directive (such as a living will, healthcare proxy, or durable power of attorney for health care) concerning treatment or designating a surrogate decision maker with the expectation that the hospital will honor the intent of that directive to the extent permitted by law and hospital policy.

   Healthcare institutions must advise patients of their rights under state law and hospital policy to make informed medical choices, ask whether the patient has an advance directive, and include that information in patient records. The patient has the right to timely information about hospital policy that may limit its ability to implement fully a legally valid advance directive.

5. The patient has the right to every consideration of privacy. Case discussion, consultation, examination, and treatment should be conducted so as to protect each patient's privacy.

6. The patient has the right to expect that all communications and records pertaining to his or her care will be treated as confidential by the hospital, except in cases such as suspected abuse and public health hazards when reporting is permitted or required by law. The patient has the right to expect that the hospital will emphasize the confidentiality of this information when it releases it to any other parties entitled to review information in these records.

7. The patient has the right to review the records pertaining to his or her medical care and to have the information explained or interpreted as necessary, except when restricted by law.

8. The patient has the right to expect that, within its capacity and policies, a hospital will make reasonable response to the request of a patient for appropriate and medically indicated care and services. The hospital must provide evaluation, service, and/or referral as indicated by the urgency of the case. When medically appropriate and legally permissible, or when a patient has so requested, a patient may be transferred to another facility. The institution to which the patient is to be transferred must first have accepted the patient for transfer. The patient must also have the benefit of complete information and explanation concerning the need for, risks, benefits, and alternatives to such a transfer.

9. The patient has the right to ask and be informed of the existence of business relationships among the hospital, educational institutions, other healthcare providers, or payers that may influence the patient's treatment and care.

10. The patient has the right to consent to or decline to participate in proposed research studies or human experimentation affecting care and treatment or requiring direct patient involvement and to have those studies fully explained prior to consent. A patient who declines to participate in research or experimentation is entitled to the most effective care that the hospital can otherwise provide.

11. The patient has the right to expect reasonable continuity of care when appropriate and to be informed by physicians and other caregivers of available and realistic patient care options when hospital care is no longer appropriate.

Continued

BOX 3-1

A Patient's Bill of Rights—cont'd

12. The patient has the right to be informed of hospital policies and practices that relate to patient care, treatment, and responsibilities. The patient has the right to be informed of available resources for resolving disputes, grievances, and conflicts, such as ethics committees, patient representatives, or other mechanisms available in the institution. The patient has the right to be informed of the hospital's charges for services and available payment methods.

The collaborative nature of health care requires that patients, or their families/surrogates, participate in their care. The effectiveness of care and patient satisfaction with the course of treatment depend, in part, on the patient fulfilling certain responsibilities. Patients are responsible for providing information about past illnesses, hospitalizations, medications, and other matters related to health status. To participate effectively in decision making, patients must be encouraged to take responsibility for requesting additional information or clarification about their health status or treatment when they do not fully understand information and instructions. Patients are also responsible for ensuring that the healthcare institution has a copy of their written advance directive if they have one. Patients are responsible for informing their physi-

cians and other caregivers if they anticipate problems in following prescribed treatment.

Patients should also be aware of the hospital's obligation to be reasonably efficient and equitable in providing care to other patients and the community. The hospital's rules and regulations are designed to help the hospital meet this obligation. Patients and their families are responsible for making reasonable accommodations to the needs of the hospital, other patients, medical staff, and hospital employees. Patients are responsible for providing necessary information for insurance claims and for working with the hospital to make payment arrangements, when necessary.

A person's health depends on much more than healthcare services. Patients are responsible for recognizing the impact of their lifestyle on their personal health.

Conclusion
Hospitals have many functions to perform, including the enhancement of health status, health promotion, and the prevention and treatment of injury and disease; the immediate and ongoing care and rehabilitation of patients; the education of health professionals, patients, and the community; and research. All these activities must be conducted with an overriding concern for the values and dignity of patients.

From American Hospital Association: *A Patient's Bill of Rights,* Chicago, 1992, The Association.

BOX 3-2

Code of Ethics for Dental Hygienists

1. Preamble
As dental hygienists, we are a community of professionals devoted to the prevention of disease and the promotion and improvement of the public's health. We are preventive oral health professionals who provide educational, clinical, and therapeutic services to the public. We strive to live meaningful, productive, satisfying lives that simultaneously serve us, our profession, our society, and the world. Our actions, behaviors, and attitudes are consistent with our commitment to public service. We endorse and incorporate the Code into our daily lives.

2. Purpose
The purpose of a professional code of ethics is to achieve high levels of ethical consciousness, decision making, and practice by the members of the profession. Specific objectives of the Dental Hygiene Code of Ethics are as follows:
- To increase our professional and ethical consciousness and sense of ethical responsibility
- To lead us to recognize ethical issues and choices and to guide us in making more informed ethical decisions
- To establish a standard for professional judgment and conduct
- To provide a statement of the ethical behavior the public can expect from us

The Dental Hygiene Code of Ethics is meant to influence us throughout our careers. It stimulates our continuing study of ethical issues and challenges us to explore our ethical responsibilities. The Code establishes concise standards of behavior to guide the public's ex-

pectations of our profession and supports dental hygiene practice, laws and regulations. By holding ourselves accountable to meeting the standards stated in the Code, we enhance the public's trust, on which our professional privilege and status are founded.

3. Key Concepts
Our beliefs, principles, values, and ethics are concepts reflected in the Code. They are the essential elements of our comprehensive and definitive code of ethics and are interrelated and mutually dependent.

4. Basic Beliefs
We recognize the importance of the following beliefs that guide our practice and provide context for our ethics:
- The services we provide contribute to the health and well-being of society.
- Our education and licensure qualify us to serve the public by preventing and treating oral disease and helping individuals achieve and maintain optimal health.
- Individuals have intrinsic worth, are responsible for their own health, and are entitled to make choices regarding their health.
- Dental hygiene care is an essential component of overall health care, and we function interdependently with other healthcare providers.
- All people should have access to health care, including oral health care.
- We are individually responsible for our actions and the quality of care we provide.

BOX 3-2

Code of Ethics for Dental Hygienists—cont'd

5. Fundamental Principles

These fundamental principles, universal concepts, and general laws of conduct provide the foundation for our ethics.

Universality

The principle of universality expects that if one individual judges an action to be right or wrong in a given situation, other people considering the same action in the same situation would make the same judgment.

Complementarity

The principle of complementarity recognizes the existence of an obligation to justice and basic human rights. In all relationships, it requires considering the values and perspectives of others before making decisions or taking actions affecting them.

Ethics

Ethics are the general standards of right and wrong that guide behavior within society. As generally accepted actions, they can be judged by determining the extent to which they promote good and minimize harm. Ethics compel us to engage in health promotion and disease prevention activities.

Community

This principle expresses our concern for the bond among individuals, the community, and society in general. It leads us to preserve natural resources and inspires us to show concern for the global environment.

Responsibility

Responsibility is central to our ethics. We recognize that there are guidelines for making ethical choices and accept responsibility for knowing and applying them. We accept the consequences of our actions or the failure to act and are willing to make ethical choices and publicly affirm them.

6. Core Values

We acknowledge these values as general for our choices and actions.

Individual autonomy and respect for human beings

People have the right to be treated with respect. They have the right to informed consent prior to treatment, and they have the right to full disclosure of all relevant information so that they can make informed choices about their care.

Confidentiality

We respect the confidentiality of client information and relationships as a demonstration of the value we place on individual autonomy. We acknowledge our obligation to justify any violation of a confidence.

Societal trust

We value client trust and understand that public trust in our profession is based on our actions and behavior.

Nonmaleficence

We accept our fundamental obligation to provide services in a manner that protects all clients and minimizes harm to them and others involved in their treatment.

Beneficence

We have a primary role in promoting the well-being of individuals and the public by engaging in health promotion and disease prevention activities.

Justice and fairness

We value justice and support the fair and equitable distribution of healthcare resources. We believe all people should have access to high-quality, affordable oral health care.

Veracity

We accept our obligation to tell the truth and expect that others will do the same. We value self-knowledge and seek truth and honesty in all relationships.

7. Standards of Professional Responsibility

We are obligated to practice our profession in a manner that supports our purpose, beliefs, and values in accordance with the fundamental principles that support our ethics. We acknowledge the following responsibilities.

To ourselves as individuals . . .

- Avoid self-deception and continually strive for knowledge and personal growth.
- Establish and maintain a lifestyle that supports optimal health.
- Create a safe work environment.
- Assert our own interests in ways that are fair and equitable.
- Seek the advice and counsel for others when challenged with ethical dilemmas.
- Have realistic expectations for ourselves and recognize our limitations.

To ourselves as professionals . . .

- Enhance professional competencies through continuous learning in order to practice according to high standards of care.
- Support dental hygiene peer-review systems and quality-assurance measures.
- Develop collaborative professional relationships and exchange knowledge to enhance our own lifelong professional development.

To family and friends . . .

- Support the efforts of others to establish and maintain healthy lifestyles and respect the rights of friends and family.

To clients . . .

- Provide oral health care, using high levels of professional knowledge, judgment, and skill.
- Maintain a work environment that minimizes the risk of harm.
- Serve all clients without discrimination and avoid action toward any individual or group that may be interpreted as discriminatory.
- Hold professional client relationships confidential.
- Communicate with clients in a respectful manner.
- Promote ethical behavior and high standards of care by all dental hygienists.
- Serve as an advocate for the welfare of clients.
- Provide clients with the information necessary to make informed decisions about their oral health and encourage their full participation in treatment decisions and goals.
- Refer clients to other healthcare providers when their needs are beyond our ability or scope of practice.
- Educate clients about high-quality oral health care.

To colleagues . . .

- Conduct professional activities and programs and develop relationships in ways that are honest, responsible, and appropriately open and candid.
- Encourage a work environment that promotes individual professional growth and development.
- Collaborate with others to create a work environment that minimizes risk to the personal health and safety of our colleagues.

Continued

Code of Ethics for Dental Hygienists—cont'd

- Manage conflicts constructively.
- Support the efforts of other dental hygienists to communicate the dental hygiene philosophy and preventive oral care.
- Inform other healthcare professionals about the relationship between general and oral health.
- Promote human relationships that are mutually beneficial, including those with other healthcare professionals.

To employees and employers . . .
- Conduct professional activities and programs, and develop relationships in ways that are honest, responsible, open, and candid.
- Manage conflicts constructively.
- Support the right of our employees and employers to work in an environment that promotes wellness.
- Respect the employment rights of our employers and employees.

To the dental hygiene profession . . .
- Participate in the development and advancement of our profession.
- Avoid conflicts of interest and declare them when they occur.
- Seek opportunities to increase public awareness and understanding of oral health practices.
- Act in ways that bring credit to our profession while demonstrating appropriate respect for colleagues in other professions.
- Contribute time, talent, and financial resources to support and promote our profession.
- Promote a positive image for our profession.
- Promote a framework for professional education that develops dental hygiene competencies to meet the oral and overall health needs of the public.

To the community and society . . .
- Recognize and uphold the laws and regulations governing our profession.
- Document and report inappropriate, inadequate, or substandard care and/or illegal activities by a healthcare provider to the responsible authorities.
- Use peer review as a mechanism to identify inappropriate, inadequate, or substandard care provided by dental hygienists.
- Comply with local, state, and federal statutes that promote public health and safety.
- Develop support systems and quality-assurance programs in the workplace to assist dental hygienists in providing the appropriate standard of care.

- Promote access to dental hygiene services for all, supporting justice and fairness in the distribution of healthcare resources.
- Act consistently with the ethics of the global scientific community, of which our profession is a part.
- Create a healthful workplace ecosystem to support a healthy environment.
- Recognize and uphold our obligation to provide *pro bono* service.

To scientific investigation . . .
We accept responsibility for conducting research according to the fundamental principles underlying our ethical beliefs in compliance with universal codes, governmental standards, and professional guidelines for the care and management of experimental subjects. We acknowledge our ethical obligations to the scientific community:
- Conduct research that contributes knowledge that is valid and useful to our clients and society.
- Use research methods that meet accepted scientific standards.
- Use research resources appropriately.
- Systematically review and justify research in progress to ensure the most favorable benefit-to-risk ratio to research subjects.
- Submit all proposals involving human subjects to an appropriate human subject review committee.
- Secure appropriate institutional committee approval for the conduct of research involving animals.
- Obtain informed consent from human subjects participating in research that is based on specification published in Title 21 Code of Federal Regulations Part 46.
- Respect the confidentiality and privacy of data.
- Seek opportunities to advance dental hygiene knowledge through research by providing financial, human, and technical resources whenever possible.
- Report research results in a timely manner.
- Report research findings completely and honestly, drawing only those conclusions that are supported by the data presented.
- Report the names of investigators fairly and accurately.
- Interpret the research and the research of others accurately and objectively, drawing conclusions that are supported by the data presented and seeking clarity when uncertain.
- Critically evaluate research methods and results before applying new theory and technology in practice.
- Be knowledgeable concerning currently accepted preventive and therapeutic methods, products, and technology and their application to our practice.

Approved and ratified by the ADHA House of Delegates, 1995.

Standards of Professional Responsibility, includes the following:[1]
- Provide patients with the information necessary to make informed decisions about their oral health and encourage their full participation in treatment decisions and goals.
- Refer patients to other healthcare providers when their needs are beyond our ability or scope of practice.
- Educate patients about high-quality oral health care.

The ADHA Code of Ethics also incorporates the core values of individual autonomy and respect for human be-

ings: nonmaleficence, beneficence, justice, and fairness.[1] These core values are acknowledged as general for the dental hygienist's choices and actions in providing care. **Nonmaleficence** dictates that the dental professional has a fundamental obligation to provide services in a manner that protects the patient and results in minimal harm; **beneficence** is the promotion of well-being of both individuals and the public by engaging in health promotion and disease prevention activities. Furthermore, justice and fairness emphasize the fair and equitable distribution of healthcare resources and incorporate a belief that all people should have access to high-quality, affordable oral health care. The individual autonomy and respect provision in the ADHA Code of Ethics addresses the fact that people have the right to be treated with respect. This code includes the patient's right to informed consent before receiving any treatment and that patients have the right to full disclosure of all relevant information for them to make informed decisions.

Today, most litigation involving medical or dental care comes within the purview of tort law. *Tort* is a civil wrongdoing. The elements of a tort that must be proved in a court of law are the following:

1. *Duty:* The defendant/healthcare provider owed a duty to the plaintiff/patient.
2. *Breach of duty:* The defendant/healthcare provider must have breached that duty owed the plaintiff/patient.
3. *Harm:* The plaintiff/patient suffered injury or harm.
4. *Causation:* The breach of duty caused the injury or harm.

In attempting to dispense justice for all individuals before the court in a tort action, the court uses a standard called the *reasonably prudent person* or *reasonably prudent professional.* The court then compares what a reasonably prudent person or professional in the shoes of the plaintiff/patient or defendant/healthcare provider would do in a similar situation.

In a lawsuit based on failure to provide informed consent before dental treatment, the plaintiff/patient must prove, as follows, by a *preponderance of the evidence* (more likely than not that the claims of the plaintiff are true) that:

1. The dental healthcare provider had a duty to disclose treatment related information to the patient.

and

2. The dental healthcare provider failed to provide the patient with material information regarding the risks and alternatives to treatment.

and

3. Disclosure of the risks would have led a reasonable patient in the plaintiff's position to reject the procedure or choose a different course of treatment.

and

4. The patient suffered harm or injury as a result of the dental healthcare provider's failure to provide the information.

All four elements must be present.

Healthcare professionals have an obligation or duty of *due care,* or care that a reasonably prudent healthcare provider would give to a patient. This due care includes advising the patient of any alternative treatment that may provide greater benefits than the treatment recommended and warning the patient of any risks to the recommended treatment, alternative treatment, or no treatment. This duty also exists when the medical or dental needs of the patient are beyond the skills of the practitioner and the patient must be referred to a specialist. For example, in dentistry, patients expect to be referred to an orthodontist, oral surgeon, or endodontist when the requirements of their particular treatment go beyond the scope of the general dentist. The larger issue for the dental hygienist is usually whether or not to recommend to the dentist that a patient be referred to a periodontist. Assessing the risk of a patient's loss of their dentition because of periodontal disease is a necessary skill for all dental hygienists.

A healthcare provider must secure the patient's informed consent before treatment that would involve a risky or invasive procedure or is potentially harmful. Most courts require that the patient be given information that the reasonable person would understand. Patients may not be coerced or manipulated in any way into providing their consent; the consent must be voluntary. If unauthorized treatment is provided for a patient, the individual rendering the treatment has committed a tort called a **battery** and may be held liable in a court of law. A battery is the intentional infliction of a harmful or offensive bodily contact. Therefore a battery includes bodily contacts that cause pain or bodily harm or bodily contacts that are simply offensive (damaging to a reasonable sense of dignity). The latter (offensive touching) applies to instances of failure to provide informed consent. For patients to prevail in a court of law, patients are required to show that they were not informed of the nature of the medical or dental procedure performed. Demonstrating physical injury is not necessary. Patient consent applies only to the specific procedure to which they have consented. Performing any additional treatment not consented to regardless of whether or not the patient needed the treatment would place the healthcare provider at risk of liability.

When a patient is not capable of consenting (for instance, if the patient is a minor or under guardianship for other infirmities), consent must obtained from someone entitled to speak for the patient. In the case of a minor, consent must be obtained from a custodial parent. Dental hygienists often expose radiographs and apply fluoride in conjunction with providing a prophylaxis for minors. The dental hygienist must obtain parental consent for all procedures. It cannot be assumed that the parent agrees to treatment deemed necessary by a dental professional. The courts have found two exceptions to the duty to disclose and obtain informed consent before treatment. One occurs when the patient is unconscious or otherwise incapable of consenting (e.g., disoriented from an incorrect dosage of a prescription drug) and harm from failure to treat the patient outweighs any harm threatened by the recommended treatment. The second occurs when risk of disclosure poses a threat to the emotional well-being of the patient and that such disclosure is contraindicated from a medical point of view.

This exception to informed consent is commonly called therapeutic privilege. In such cases talking with an appropriate family member is usually wise. Because most dental procedures represent elective treatment, it would be rare for these exceptions to exist in the dental setting unless a medical emergency occurred. However, if the patient is incapable of consenting, the practitioner must attempt to obtain consent of a person who may provide consent for the incompetent person. Laws differ from state to state regarding age and specific treatment in situations in which a minor may legally give consent. State laws also address who may consent for an incompetent individual. Dental hygienists need to know the law of the state where they provide patient services.

If patients have consented to treatment to remedy their condition, patients are presumed to have consented to all procedures required for such treatment. This is called *implied consent.* Implied consent also is presumed for noninvasive treatment such as dental examinations and prophylaxis. When in doubt as to whether implied consent will be presumed, practitioners should always err on the side of obtaining informed consent. Legally, patients may waive their right to give informed consent. The waiver must be made freely and with full information. This makes it difficult to determine how much disclosure is required. In final analysis, no bright line exists between informed consent and a waiver for informed consent.

Informed consent can be written or oral. Generally, in dentistry, patients are presented with a treatment plan and they agree or refuse the recommended treatment. For the protection of both clinician and patient written consent is essential. Patients alleging a lack of informed consent will not remember to what they agreed. Taking a seat in the dental chair is often an intimidating event. Expectations that patients will remember what is said to them before, during, or after their treatment are simply not realistic. Nothing replaces a written document to remind both parties of the agreement regarding specific treatment. Fig. 3-1 is an example of an informed consent agreement. Informed consent agreements should be written specifically for the treatment needs of the individual patient as opposed to the use of a blanket consent form.

Many factors should be considered regarding whether adequate information was disclosed to the patient to deem the patient's consent truly informed. Basically, patients need to know whether they are vulnerable to significant risks before consenting to recommended treatment. In general, patient rights include a reasonable understanding of the following:

- Patients have the right to be informed of a diagnosis of their condition requiring treatment. This includes the right to obtain the results of diagnostic tests. Common examples are diagnostic procedures such as radiographs, pulp testing, and microscopic examinations, commonly used in dentistry.
- Patients have the right to be informed of the type and purpose of treatment proposed. This information should include the probability of success. If the treatment is experimental, the healthcare provider has the duty to inform the patient of the experimental nature of the proposed procedure, including the most likely risks.
- Patients have the right to be informed of the risks of treatment. This is an important right as risks may be the sole determiner of the patient's decision making regarding treatment. If risks are remote or commonly known (e.g., the risk of infection) they need not be disclosed. In *Canterbury v Spence*[5] the court held that the threshold of disclosure varies with the probability and severity of the risk. If the probability was 1%, the risk need not be disclosed. However, if that 1% risk was the probability of death, the risk should be disclosed. There-

---

INFORMED CONSENT

I hereby request that _____ provide treatment for me for the following condition: _____. I have been afforded the time and opportunity to discuss this proposed treatment, the alternatives, and risks with _____, and I understand:

1. The means of treatment will be:

2. The alternative means of treatment are:

3. The advantages of proposed treatment over alternative treatment are:

4. That all treatments including the one proposed have some risks. The risks of importance involved in my treatment have been explained to me, and they are:

5. The risks of nontreatment are:

_____
Signature of Patient

_____
Date

_____
Signature of Witness

_____
Signature of Health Practitioner

FIG. 3-1 Informed consent form.

fore informed consent is required if potential harm is serious, whether or not the likelihood of the harm is slight. If the patient inquires about specific risks, the duty to disclose and the patient's right to know expand. The patient's inquiries need to be addressed.

- Patients have the right to be informed as to the level of skill or status risk.

The prevalence of health/dental care insurance data, managed care, data from hospitals and other institutions (such as success rates), state and federal procedures to curtail healthcare fraud and abuse, and computerization in general have contributed to the proliferation of medical and dental healthcare data that were not available to previous generations. Legal rights have expanded as a result of the volume of information now widely available. In *Hales v Pittman*,[8] the court suggested that physicians should disclose both the general statistical success rate for a given procedure and their particular experience with that procedure.

In addition, courts have held that failure to inform patients of a physician's physical condition would violate informed consent because it would affect the patient's decision whether or not to proceed with treatment. In *Hidding v Williams*[6] the court found that the physician's failure to disclose his alcoholism addiction negated the patient's consent to surgery. Because alcoholism created a material risk associated with the physician's ability to perform, which if disclosed would have obligated the patient to elect another treatment, the nondisclosure of alcohol addiction violated the informed consent doctrine. Also, *Behringer v The Medical Center at Princeton*[3] explored the issues of a hospital's obligation to protect the **confidentiality** of an AIDS diagnosis of a healthcare worker and a hospital's right to regulate and restrict the surgical activities of an HIV-positive doctor. The court held that:[3]

> . . . the risk of accident and implications thereof would be a legitimate concern to the surgical patient, warranting disclosure of this risk in the informed consent setting.

These cases raise legal and ethical issues that, to date, remain unanswered. Whose rights take precedence? How are the rights of the patient weighed versus the rights of the healthcare provider? What represents a material risk? What must be disclosed? Who decides these issues: legislative bodies, the courts, or the professional organizations? If human immunodeficiency virus (HIV) status must be disclosed, what other conditions or diseases must be disclosed? Policies of the American Dental Association, the American Medical Association, and other organizations presently state that those professionals who are HIV-positive may either cease performing invasive procedures or disclose their HIV status to their patients. Most dental hygiene services are considered invasive procedures; therefore these questions are relevant to the practicing dental hygienist. Following are patient rights concerning such topics:

- The patient has the right to be informed of any conflict of interest involving the healthcare provider. This occurs when a healthcare provider stands to benefit from the patient's treatment. This benefit is due to a financial interest other than the fee charged to the patient. For instance, a conflict of interest would exist if a dental hygienist refers all patients whose examination indicates periodontal disease to a periodontal specialty practice owned by her husband.
- The patient has the right to be informed of the alternatives to recommended methods of diagnosis and/or treatment, including their risks and probability of success. The need for disclosure of these alternative diagnostic measures or treatment modes relate only to those that are generally accepted in the medical/dental community. All dental offices do not necessarily utilize more recent or expensive techniques. Available continuing education courses, professional journals, and the Internet provide information relating to new procedures for all dental professionals. Dental professionals need to be aware of new alternative treatment modalities whether or not they perform these services. If these treatment alternatives are commonly provided in other dental offices, they must be presented to the patient. To do otherwise could be considered negligence in a court of law. The alternative treatment must be accepted by the profession and not considered an experimental procedure. For instance, not all dental practices offer dental implants to replace missing teeth. However, not suggesting an implant as a possible treatment alternative could be deemed negligent. In addition, patients need to be informed of the costs of alternative procedures before beginning treatment.
- Patients have the right to be informed of their prognosis if testing or treatment is refused. In *Truman v Truman*, the court held:[16]

> If a patient indicates that he or she is going to decline the risk-free test or treatment, then the doctor has the additional duty of advising of all material risks of which a reasonable person would want to be informed before deciding not to undergo the procedure.

The right to informed refusal mandates that a healthcare provider explain the risks of such refusal. Because healthcare providers control information unavailable to a patient, their duty is to convey this information to the patient and avoid decisions that would medically compromise the patient. Informed refusal should be documented in the patient's record. Documentation should include all information provided to the patient. This includes treatment recommendations. Both the patient and dental healthcare provider should sign the document. This serves to avoid later claims by the patient that he or she was not informed of the need for the diagnostic test or treatment. Dental healthcare providers must seriously consider whether they wish to continue to care for the patient because the patient cannot give the healthcare provider permission to commit malpractice via such a refusal.

- The patient has the right to be informed of his or her prognosis if treatment is accepted.
- The patient has the absolute right to refuse medical or dental treatment even if the act of refusal is life threatening as long as the individual is competent. Competence is judged by the following:
  1. Understanding of the illness, options for treatment, and their consequences
  2. Decision making based on rational reasoning (altered if the decision is based on religious faith)

FIRST AMENDMENT RIGHTS

Because the First Amendment protects religious beliefs, courts have found that the decision to refuse medical treatment need not be rational but the reasoning process should be. What seems to be irrational reasoning is protected if it is based on a religious belief. The belief must be held by a sufficient number of people, for an extended time period, or be similar to beliefs held by other religious groups considered to be orthodox. In a 1965 case, *Aste v Brooks*, a woman informed her physician that she would not permit a blood transfusion because of her faith, despite the consequences of her refusal. The court held:[2]

> *Even though we may consider the appellant's beliefs unwise, foolish, or ridiculous, in the absence of an overriding danger to society we may not permit interference . . . in the waning hours of her life for the sole purpose of compelling her to accept medical treatment forbidden by her religious principles and previously refused by her with full knowledge of the probable consequence.*

The First Amendment to the U.S. Constitution provides that:

> *Congress shall make no law respecting an establishment of religion, or prohibiting the free exercise thereof*

(referred to as the *establishment clause* or the *free exercise clause*). Historically, in Europe and in the early days of America, individuals were punished in cruel and inhumane ways if they did not conform their religious beliefs to those held by the most powerful in society. Constitutional separation of church and state protected religious freedom from government control and was a critical component of the concept of individual freedom, which the drafters of the United States Constitution sought to preserve.

Countless court decisions have addressed the issues surrounding First Amendment protection. One of these decisions was *Cantwell v Connecticut*.[6] The court addressed the free exercise clause by stating:[6]

> *The Amendment embraces two concepts, freedom to believe and freedom to act. The first is absolute but, in the nature of things, the second cannot be. Conduct remains subject to regulation for the protection of society.*

For instance, the courts upheld decisions to require vaccinations[11] and prohibit polygamous marriages[14] despite claims of interference with the free exercise clause because society has an overriding interest in protecting the lives of its citizens, and conduct may be regulated to ensure this protection.

Another example of the way in which conduct may be regulated relates to the protection of children. Members of religious groups that restrict medical care are not always permitted to do so on behalf of their children. Courts have held that parents may not exercise the power of life and death over their children. The court will often appoint a guardian *ad litem* for the purpose of making medical decisions on behalf of the child and for the best interest of the child. The child sometimes is removed from the home but usually is not. With the exception of decision making regarding medical treatment, parents maintain control of the child. Parents' authority to control their children is also restricted under state child abuse and neglect **statutes.** Parents may not deprive their children of the basic necessities of life, including housing, clothing, food, education, and medical care. Neglect regarding medical care may be extended to dental care. The state may exercise its authority and take custody of a child to ensure basic needs are met, or in the case of abuse, the child may be removed from a harmful environment. Therefore children have a right to the protection of society for basic needs, and dental healthcare providers have a duty to report suspected cases of child abuse to the appropriate state authorities.

PATIENT SELF-DETERMINATION

Patients have the right to direct the medical or dental care they receive, and this direction includes the participation in treatment choices. When professionals provide material information regarding treatment choices communication is enhanced. Increased communication and participation of patients in making informed decisions relating to dental treatment is beneficial. First and foremost is patient satisfaction with care. This satisfaction produces a harmonious patient/provider relationship. Healthcare providers do not have a duty to continue to treat a patient who repeatedly refuses to follow their recommendations.

In the past, patients with terminal diseases have not always been informed that recommended treatment might not greatly expand their life expectancy. Nor were they informed of their fatal condition. The courts and members of society now generally agree that withholding of this information is not ethical or legal. A physician may not exercise control over decisions relating to the life and death of a patient. For personal and/or religious reasons, patients must have the opportunity to control their last hours, days, weeks, months, or years.

The United States Congress determined that a patient's right of self-determination regarding health care is an essential individual right to be upheld throughout their lives, if so desired. In 1990 Congress passed the Patient Self-Determination Act. This law was enacted to require healthcare institutions to inform patients regarding their rights under state law in making decisions related to medical care (e.g., the right to accept or refuse medical treatment and to execute advanced directives). An advanced directive is a living will or durable power of attorney for health care (called *healthcare surrogates* in some states). Each institution must have a written policy regarding the implementation of these rights and must provide the patient a copy of such policy. Each patient's record must include information as to whether or not the patient has executed an advanced directive of any kind. Under a durable power of attorney, an agent (usually a trusted friend, family member, or spouse) is designated to make decisions relating to medical treatment when the person is unable to make such decisions. A living will defines an individual's wishes regarding the termination of life-sustaining treatment (Figs. 3-2 and 3-3). These are included to demonstrate the difference between the two documents and are not meant to be legal documents; the legal requirements regarding content vary from state to state.

DURABLE POWER OF ATTORNEY FOR HEALTH CARE

If I should have an incurable and irreversible condition that will, without the administration of life-sustaining treatment, in the opinion of my attending physician, cause my death within a relatively short time, and I am no longer able to make or communicate decisions regarding my medical treatment, I appoint _____, whose address is _____, or, if he or she is not reasonably available or is unwilling to serve, _____, whose address is _____, to act as my attorney in fact to make decisions on my behalf regarding any and all healthcare decisions, including the type of treatment, location of treatment, and in addition, the right to refuse or decline life-prolonging treatment and to decide whatever care I receive solely to alleviate pain.

Signed this _____day of _____,_____.

Signature:_____

Address:_____

Witness to Signature:_____Address:_____

Witness to Signature:_____Address:_____

STATE OF _____

COUNTY OF _____

_____personally appeared before me and acknowledged the execution of this power of attorney for the purposes set forth therein.

Dated:_____

_____

Notary Public

FIG. 3-2 Durable power of attorney form for health care.

LIVING WILL DECLARATION

If I should have an incurable and irreversible condition that will, without the administration of life-sustaining treatment, in the opinion of my attending physician, cause my death within a relatively short time, and I am no longer able to make or communicate decisions regarding my medical treatment, I direct my attending physician to withhold or withdraw treatment which only prolongs the process of dying and is not necessary for my comfort or to relieve pain.

If it is permissible under the laws of the jurisdiction in which I may be hospitalized, I direct that the physicians supervising my care upon a terminal diagnosis to discontinue artificially administered nutrition and/or hydration should the continuation of either or both be judged to result in prolonging a natural death.

I release any and all hospitals, physicians, and others both for myself and for my estate from any and all liability for complying with this declaration to the fullest extent provided by law.

I authorize my spouse,_____, or any individual who may become responsible for my health to effectuate my transfer from any hospital or other healthcare facility in which I may be receiving care should that facility decline or refuse to effectuate the instructions given herein.

Signed this _____day of _____, _____.

Signature:_____

Address:_____

Social Security Number:_____

Witness to Signature:_____Witness to Signature:_____

Address:_____Address:_____

FIG. 3-3 Living will declaration form.

PATIENT DUTIES AND RESPONSIBILITIES

The bulk of what has been said refers to the rights of the patient. Patients also have duties or responsibilities in the healthcare provider/patient relationship. Because the professional is responsible for informed consent, the patient bears the duty to ask questions and address any concerns relating to treatment so that consent may be truly informed. Also, the patient owes a duty to disclose personal medical information. Treatment risks may be determined only by a full disclosure of the patient's health. Patients have the duty to comply with professional recommendations relating to their health. A patient has the duty to pay the healthcare provider a fee for services rendered. A patient's refusal to comply with any of these duties may be the basis for the termination of the healthcare provider/patient relationship by the healthcare provider.

ABANDONMENT

A healthcare provider generally has no legal or ethical duty to provide care and may refuse to provide care for any reason except the reason may not be based on discriminatory reasons. However, once the patient/healthcare provider relationship is created, the healthcare provider has a duty not to abandon the patient.

In *Domurad v Hill,*[7] the court held that a dentist is held to the same standard as a physician. More specifically, when a dentist terminates a dentist/patient relationship, the dentist must provide due notice to the patient and give the patient an opportunity to secure other dental services. Such notice should be in writing and include the reason for the termination. A copy should be retained for the patient's file. All patient treatment started should be completed. Therefore between the time that notice is given and the termination date, the dentist should try to complete any dental treatment in progress. The dentist also should be available to provide emergency care during this time so that the patient's oral health is not compromised by the transition to a new dentist. In addition dental professionals are strongly urged to contact their lawyers to ensure that all of their state's legal requirements are met.

DENTAL HYGIENISTS' RESPONSIBILITIES IN PROVIDING DENTAL HYGIENE CARE

PROPER LICENSURE AND EDUCATION

The regulation of dental hygiene practice continues today to be under the purview of the individual states. The result has been the requirement that dental hygienists must obtain licensure in each state in which they intend to practice. Although some individuals continue to pursue the elimination of the state licensure requirement for a more national approach to credentialing for dental hygiene practice, as of this writing, licensure is still required. Licensing in each state in the nation is generally under the direct control and authority of a regulatory agency. These agencies are given the authority to prescribe administrative laws that generally compliment and further interpret the statutory laws created by the state legislature pertaining to dental hygiene. Dental hygiene is still most fre-

quently regulated by dentistry through state boards of dentistry. For example, in the state of Ohio[12] and the state of Indiana,[10] a State Dental Board of Dentistry has the authority to license, regulate, supervise, and discipline dental hygiene in addition to dentistry and in some cases, certain aspects of dental assisting.

These boards generally comprise dentists, dental hygienists, and nondental professional consumers as board members. These members are appointed by a political body in each state. The total number of board members, including the number of dental hygienists and dentists, varies from state to state. Presently, Ohio has a total of seven board members, with five dentists, one dental hygienist, and one consumer. In contrast the State of Indiana's Board of Dentistry consists of nine practicing dentists, one practicing dental hygienist, and one consumer who is not associated with dentistry.

At least 10 states have some degree of self-regulation or have implemented dental hygiene advisory committees. For instance, California has a Committee on Dental Auxiliary created by statute to advise the California Dental Board and perform administrative functions with respect to dental hygienists and unlicensed and licensed dental assistants. Also, the state of Washington has a separate practice act for dentistry and dental hygiene.

These regulatory agencies are generally authorized to do some or all of the following: set the standard and the manner in which a dental hygiene license is obtained, monitor dental hygiene practice, and discipline licensed dental hygienists for actions in violation of law.

Presently, every state requires dental hygienists to be licensed to practice in that state. To be eligible for state licensure many states require candidates to sit for licensing examinations, regardless of whether the applicant is licensed in other states. In addition, many states still require eligible candidates for examination to graduate from an accredited educational program of dental hygiene. This requirement has prohibited dental hygienists who have received their education in programs not accredited by the standards currently implemented by the accreditation body known as the *American Dental Association Council on Dental Education* from taking the exam. This applies to dental hygienists who received their dental hygiene education in countries other than the United States and also affects dental hygienists graduating from nonaccredited programs of dental hygiene like preceptorship programs in the state of Alabama.

Not all states require that candidates sit for examinations to be licensed. Some states allow for reciprocity among states. For example, dental hygienists who hold a valid license to practice dental hygiene in one state may be eligible to become licensed in another state without examination. This is generally a formal or informal arrangement made between two states in which the initial licensing requirements are essentially equivalent.

Another example of licensure without examination is licensure by credentials. In this case, a candidate becomes eligible for licensure based on a review of the candidate's previously granted license. Candidates' licensure "credentials" are reviewed by the appropriate regulatory agency and in some cases the candidate may also be interviewed. Based upon this type of an evaluation of the candidate, the agency determines whether or not to grant licensure. Other state requirements may be separate from reciprocity, licensing by credentials, or licensing by examination. Candidates for licensure must become familiar with these requirements in the state in which they are applying for licensure.

PRACTICE WITHIN THE LIMITS OF THE LAW

Individuals who meet all the criteria for licensure in a particular state and are granted a valid license must recognize that licensure is a privilege, not a legal right. To maintain that privilege, the dental hygienist must practice within the law. The dental hygiene practitioner cannot exceed the legally delegable scope of practice for dental hygiene in a particular state.

Additionally, dental hygienists must practice with the legally required level of supervision. Presently, the majority of states have some form of relaxed or general supervision allowed for dental hygiene practice. Only the state of Colorado allows the dental hygienist to practice without any supervision by a dentist.

Dental hygienists, as licensed dental professionals, must accept their legally delegated responsibility to provide competent dental hygiene care. This requires that contemporary dental hygiene care always meet or exceed the standard of care. The standard of care is generally recognized as that degree of skill, care, and knowledge possessed and exercised by dental hygienists in similar situations. This standard may be affected by and derived from a multitude of professional sources, including criteria developed in educational programs for health professionals and professional organizations. For instance, A Patient's Bill of Rights developed by the American Hospital Association (see Box 3-1) establishes a basis for the standard of care relating to patient services.

A court may find healthcare professionals liable for harm to patients when the services they provide fall below the standard of care. Historically, tracking lawsuits against dental hygienists has been difficult because many complaints filed ended in settlement and were not concluded in trial. Case law demonstrates that dental hygienists have been held accountable for their actions in addition to their dentist employers by patients who believed they sustained injury as a result of the dental hygiene care received.[16] Patients are also more likely than in the past to file complaints against dental hygiene licensees, complaining about the care they received. A national unpublished survey completed by the ADHA Governmental Affairs Division during 1987 and 1988 indicated that the complaints most often filed against dental hygienists were based on the following: practice without a license, performance of procedures beyond the role of practice, substance abuse/dependency and practicing while under the influence, and performance of duties outside of required supervision.

Adverse action (e.g., revocation or suspension) against a healthcare professional's license to practice and legal action against the healthcare professional, must be reported to the National Data Bank. The National Data Bank is a result of the Health Care Quality Improvement Act of 1986. The purpose of the Bank is to monitor professional practice so that healthcare professionals who have been disciplined in one state will not find it easy to obtain a license in another state. The Data Bank may be accessed for information by state licensing agencies and professional societies. An individual practitioner may access the Data Bank only as it relates to actions taken against that practitioner.

CONTINUING DENTAL HYGIENE EDUCATION

As professionals, dental hygienists must assume the responsibility for keeping themselves apprised of changes in professional practice. As state laws change, the dental hygienist is responsible for knowledge of these changes. Some of the best ways to do this are for the practitioner to participate in professional meetings and organizations. Often members of organized dental hygiene will specifically receive notification of such changes in the laws affecting practice through the association newsletters or as a part of a continuing dental hygiene education (CE course). The number of hours for renewal varies from state to state. Some states additionally require that a portion of the hours be directed toward certain topics, such as infection control, or that all courses be related to clinical care. As the scope of practice for dental hygiene changes and/or increases in various states, the CE requirements often increase.

RISK MANAGEMENT FOR THE DENTAL HYGIENE PRACTITIONER

In everyday practice, dental hygienists should exercise appropriate risk management. Risk management involves recognition and reduction of one's exposure to risks in professional practice. Functions that can place the dental hygienist at risk include the following: assessment of a patent's oral condition, the delivery of care, communication with patients, and maintenance of confidentiality.

EFFECTIVE COMMUNICATION

Effective communication in practice is essential to maintain good patient relations, minimize misunderstanding between the parties, and prevent unrealistic expectations. Patients who are adequately informed in an honest and caring manner are far less likely to harbor unrealistic expectations regarding the progression and/or outcome of their treatment. In the event of an undesired outcome, which can happen in the face of excellent technique and adequate patient compliance, a patient who has had the opportunity to make an informed decision about care through an informed consent process will be more likely to continue to work with the practitioner. As a result, this patient will be less likely to pursue administrative or legal recourse against a practitioner or the practice in which the dental hygienist is employed. The practitioner should keep patients apprised of the progress of their treatment, including unforeseen consequences, rather than misinform or fail to inform them.

DOCUMENTATION

Although good communication begins with the interaction between the patient and the practitioner, the result of those communications and the decisions made should be thoroughly documented in the patient record. The entire process from assessment of the patient's presenting condition, including the treatment provided and the evaluation after treatment, should be documented in the patient treatment record. This record should reflect what was done, how it was done, and why it was done in as complete and understandable manner as possible, making the occurrences clear to any third party. A standard system of documentation should be developed for the dental office, and all providers should adhere to that system. Failure to implement such a system usually results in an unorganized and incomplete document. The patient treatment record is significant because it documents treatment provided and is a legal document that may be used in the event of a future dispute between practitioner and patient. Poorly documented and/or inaccurate patient records are one of the major problems in litigation against dental hygienists or dentists.

Dental hygienists must accurately record in the dental treatment record and avoid any attempt to alter an entry. If an error is made during the entering of information into the record, it should be acknowledged as an entry and the correct information entered. For example, a practitioner forgets to enter pertinent information regarding patient assessment or treatment and remembers it at a later date. In this case, the dental hygienist should date and enter the information when remembered. All entries should be clearly signed, with the full name, by the dental hygienist.

Because the treatment record is a legal document, it must accurately reflect all aspects of patient assessment, treatment, and compliance and must be written in a professional, factual manner. For example, including subjective comments about a patient's psychological state or derogatory statements about the patient is inappropriate. Entries should be factual and describe as objectively as possible the circumstances surrounding the care received.

OWNERSHIP AND ACCESS TO DENTAL TREATMENT RECORDS

As in all healthcare records, ownership of the dental treatment record lies with the owner dentist of the practice. Patients have a legal right to access a copy of their record at their request. The Health Insurance Portability and Accountability Act of 1996 (HIPAA), effective October 2002, covers three primary areas: privacy standards, patients rights, and administrative requirements (see Appendix). The release of patient records for those persons with HIV/AIDS may be further restricted by specific laws in each state. Patients may be charged a reasonable fee for copying their records but cannot legally be denied access to those records because they have outstanding balances for treatment received.

RESPECT FOR THE PATIENT/PRACTITIONER RELATIONSHIP

A professional relationship exists between patient and dental hygienist that requires the dental hygienist to keep the information learned as a part of the relationship in confidence. Improper disclosure of information learned as part of this relationship may lead to liability for breach of confidentiality on the part of the dental healthcare provider.

Case Application

The case study presented at the beginning of the chapter incorporates many of the legal and ethical issues addressed in this chapter regarding dental hygiene practice. The following summary comments will address each of the questions presented at the end of the case study and discuss the legal and ethical implications associated with each:

1. Gloria (the dental hygienist) breached her duty to keep all information learned as a part of the patient/dental hygienist relationship confidential when she disclosed information regarding one patient to another without legal authority to do so. She had not received written consent to disclose this information, nor was she required to disclose it under the law. The breach represents both a violation of law and a breach of ethics.

2. Dental hygienists must practice within the law in the state in which they practice regardless of their educational preparation or prior experience. Although Gloria may have the expertise to provide dental therapies not legally allowed, she practices in violation of the law when she provides these services when such responsibilities are not legally delegable. Arguably, Gloria was attempting to assist the patient in the dilemma that had occurred—the loss of a restoration. Ethically, she may have considered what she was doing as a service to the patient, specifically because she felt adequately trained to perform the procedure.

3. The friendly exchange between the two dental hygienists involving the renewal of their licenses and the continuing dental education requirement for nonrenewal was both illegal and unethical. Although Gloria may have thought she was helping a colleague, she was in fact assisting her in committing misrepresentation to the state board. State dental boards often perform audits or reviews of this documentation, and if the board discovered that Elisa had falsified her information regarding renewal, her actions would be considered fraud. Misrepresentation and fraud are illegal and unethical. The requirement for continuing education is in place to promote additional education for the dental hygienist to assist these practitioners in practice. Gloria was promoting a behavior inconsistent with certain principles of the ADHA Code of Ethics (see Box 3-2).

4. The situation that occurred with Mr. Black presents several issues. Gloria's oral assessment indicated significant disease in Mr. Black's mouth. The disease may have been so severe that its treatment warranted an immediate referral to a periodontist for a complete diagnosis before the initiation of treatment. Without proper diagnosis, an appropriate treatment plan cannot be developed. Dental hygiene care provided without this accurate diagnosis may fall below the standard of care.

Another issue is whether Mr. Black's periodontal problem has gone undiagnosed and treated because of the negligence of the office, including Gloria, over the course of the past 3 years. If this has occurred, then the patient may have a legal cause of action based on negligence, in this case a concept known as *supervised neglect*. These may be reasons that Mr. Black would see an attorney.

Finally, the increase in cost assessed Mr. Black because the treatment took longer is not illegal. However, the manner in which this information was presented to the patient did not promote patient acceptance and understanding. Gloria should have developed a treatment plan based on an accurate diagnosis and presented this to the patient for acceptance before the implementation of any treatment. She should have made a full disclosure to Mr. Black and obtained informed consent before proceeding with dental hygiene care. Mr. Black's attorney may review this issue in considering whether Mr. Black actually owes the office the fee charged.

In addition, this scenario involves ethical considerations. By starting treatment immediately, Gloria may actually have done harm to Mr. Black. This action is in direct violation with the ADHA Code of Ethics because dental hygienists are to practice nonmaleficence and promote beneficence to the patients whom they provide dental hygiene care.

RITICAL THINKING ACTIVITIES

1. In a small group of three to five students, review clinical case studies containing ethical and legal issues. Identify the nature of the ethical and legal issue(s) and discuss the process you would follow to handle these issues.
2. Obtain a dental hygiene plan from a clinical record or develop one. Role-play with a peer the presentation you would make to inform the patient of the procedures planned and obtain consent to begin care.
3. Role-play the presentation of the patient's bill of rights and have peers critique your presentation.
4. Develop a patient's bill of rights for your clinic.
5. Critique informed consent documents obtained from various healthcare facilities.
6. Review your state practice act and discuss the role of the regulatory body in enforcing these laws.
7. Discuss the process used to introduce change to the practice act either by the regulatory body or other entity.

REVIEW QUESTIONS

1. Which of the following describes the basis of informed consent?
   a. Protecting the dentist or dental hygienist from a lawsuit initiated by an angry patient
   b. Explaining the costs of dental care
   c. Reviewing the practitioner's credentials
   d. Providing the patient will all material facts regarding his or her proposed treatment
2. Which of the following elements must be proven in court for a plaintiff to prevail on a tort claim?
   a. Mutual agreement, consideration, and breach
   b. Duty owed, breach of duty, harm, and causation
   c. Breach of duty
   d. Injuries and costs
3. Informed consent is required in which case *only?*
   a. For surgical procedures
   b. If proposed treatment involve a risky or invasive procedure
   c. For those over age 21
   d. If the patient is coerced into accepting the treatment
   e. When a patient is incompetent
4. Informed consent requires that a patient be told which of the following?
   a. Alternative means of treatment
   b. Cost of treatment and alternatives
   c. Prognosis of treatment and alternatives
   d. *a* and *b* only
   e. *a* and *c* only
   f. All the above
5. A patient's right to self-determination may be expressed as which of the following?
   a. The patient's right to demand the treatment he or she wishes to receive
   b. The patient's right to direct his or her medical care
   c. The patient's right to participate in treatment choices
   d. None of the above
   e. All the above
6. Thorough documentation of the treatment record should include which elements?
   a. What treatment was provided
   b. Why treatment was provided
   c. How treatment was provided
   d. *a* and *b*
   e. All the above
7. The practice of dental hygiene is affected by which of the following laws?
   a. Statutory laws
   b. Common law
   c. Federal law
   d. Local law
   e. All the above
8. In most states in the United States, dental hygiene is regulated by which of the following?
   a. State boards of dental hygiene
   b. Dental hygiene committees
   c. State boards of dentistry
   d. None of the above

Continued

REVIEW QUESTIONS—cont'd

9. Dental hygiene treatment should always be provided in a manner that _____ or _____ the standard of care.
   a. Equals/comes close to
   b. Meets/falls just below
   c. Is superior/exceeds
   d. Meets/exceeds

10. The dental hygienist discusses a patient's assessment results with another dental hygienist in the office, one who is not involved in the care of the patient. The dental hygienist may be liable for which of the following?
    a. Failure to disclose
    b. Breach of confidentiality
    c. Failure to obtain informed consent
    d. Falling below the standard of care

 SUGGESTED AGENCIES AND WEB SITES

Because of the ever-changing nature of the Internet, some of the web sites listed here may have changed since publication. Please refer to Mosby's Evolve web site for the most current information.

American Bar Association: http://www.lawtechnology.org
American Society of Law, Medicine and Ethics (Boston): http://www.aslme.org
Hastings Center: http://www.thehastingscenter.org

Kennedy Institute of Ethics (at Georgetown University in Washington, DC): http://www.georgetown.edu
Park Ridge Center (Chicago): http://www.parkridgecenter.org

 ADDITIONAL READINGS AND RESOURCES

Bailey BL: Informed consent in dentistry, *J Am Dent Assoc* 110: 709, 1985.
Beauchamp TL, Childress JF: *Principles of biomedical ethics,* Oxford, England, 1994, Oxford University Press.
Christensen GJ: Educating patients about dental procedures, *J Am Dent Assoc* March:371, 1995.
Darby ML, Walsh MM: *Dental hygiene theory and practice,* Philadelphia, 1994, WB Saunders.
Davison JA: *Legal and ethical considerations for the dental hygienist and dental assistant,* St Louis, 2000, Mosby.

DeVore CH: Legal risk management for the dental hygienist, *Pract Dent Hyg* 6(4):59-61, 1997.
Edge RS, Groves JR: *The ethics of healthcare: a guide for clinical practice,* Albany, NY, 1994, Delmar.
Furrow B et al: 1997 *Health law,* ed 3, American case book series. Eagan, Minn, 1997, West.
Pozgar GD: *Legal aspects of healthcare administration,* Gaithersburg, Md, 1999, Aspen.
Roach WH: *Medical records and the law,* ed 3, Gaithersburg, Md, 1998, Aspen.

 REFERENCES

1. American Dental Hygienists' Association: *Code of ethics,* Chicago, 1998-1999, The Association.
2. *Aste v Brooks,* 32 Ill 2d 361, 205 NE 2d 435 (Ill 1965).
3. *Behringer v The Medical Center at Princeton,* 592 A2d 1251 (NJ Super Law Div 1991).
4. *Campbell v Pommier,* 5 Conn App 29, 496 A2d 975, 1985.
5. *Canterbury v Spence,* 464 F2d 722 (DC Cir 1972).
6. *Cantwell v Connecticut,* 310 U.S. 296, 60 SCt 900 (Conn 1940).
7. *Domurad v Hill,* 605 NE 2d 858 (Mass 1993).
8. *Hales v Pittman,* 576 P2d 493 (Ariz 1978).
9. *Hidding v Williams,* 578 So 2d 1192 (La App 1991).
10. Ind Code §25-13-1-5 (1998).
11. *Jacobson v Massachusetts,* 25 SCt 358 (Mass 1905).
12. Ohio Rev Code Ann §4715.03.
13. *Pratt v Davis,* 118 Ill App 161 (Ill 1961).
14. *Reynolds v United States,* 98 U.S. 145 (U.S. 1978).
15. *Schloendorff v Society of New York Hospital,* 211 NY 125, 105 NE 92 (NY 1914).
16. *Truman v Truman,* 165 Cal Rptr, 611 P2d 902 (Cal 1980).

CHAPTER 4

Communication

K. Joseph Wittemann, Susan H. Kass

Chapter Outline

Self-Evaluation
Case Study: Case 1: Team Approach
   to Communication
A Working Definition
Steps Toward Changing Communication Behaviors
   Influential communicators: models for learned
      communication
   Communication assets
   Unlearning poor communication habits
   Recognizing the need for better communication
   Interest
   Belief
   Commitment
   Action
   Repeated action and habituation
Key Elements of Communication

Case Study: Case 2: Effective Communication—
   Attending
   Listening
   Observing
   Establishing rapport
   Deepening rapport and establishing ongoing
      relationships
   Responding with empathy
   Demonstrating respect
   Expressing emotional warmth
   Being direct
   Being concrete
   Being genuine
   Practicing self-disclosure
   Providing feedback using the "I" message

Key Terms

Attending   Distance   Jargon   Public distance
Communication   Empathy   Listening   Rapport
Cultural sensitivity   Intimate distance   Observing

Learning Outcomes

1. Recognize that effective communication skills can be learned.
2. Identify the stages in the acquisition of new skills: knowledge, interest, belief, commitment, practice, and habituation.
3. Distinguish between the three key attributes to effective communication: listening, observing, and attending.
4. Explain the function of space, time, culture, context, and language in the establishment of rapport.
5. Identify and explain the importance of core nonverbal behaviors such as facial expression, body language, and eye contact.
6. Explain and demonstrate key elements of deepening rapport: empathy, respect, warmth, concreteness, genuineness, and self-disclosure.
7. Become a better communicator by providing positive feedback, using "I" messages and practicing active listening.
8. Evaluate with discernment principles of communication.

ommunication poses many frustrating challenges. Unclear communication can be unproductive and sometimes offensive. Clear communication is difficult to achieve at times but ultimately satisfying to all parties involved.

The purpose of this chapter is to better understand the art of communication, in both professional and personal relationships. Effective, healthy, forthright, and clear *communication* is the catalyst used to establish, maintain, and enhance relationships, wherever they may be found.

SELF-EVALUATION

Fig. 4-1 lists 10 questions to consider about communication. This survey has no right or wrong answers. Individuals should read each question in the context of their natural communication style and circle the number corresponding to the degree that best describes them. The score is derived as follows: points are totaled and divided by 10. A score below 2.5 is associated with a successful communication style. However, a score of 4.5 and greater

1. Is it difficult for you to talk comfortably with other people?

1	2	3	4	5	6
It is very easy for me.					It is very difficult for me.

2. Are you aware of how your tone of voice may affect others?

1	2	3	4	5	6
I am conscious of my tonality.					I am not aware at all.

3. Is it difficult for you to accept constructive criticism from others?

1	2	3	4	5	6
It is not a problem.					I do not do well with it at all.

4. When you are working with a patient, are you able to put yourself in his or her shoes?

1	2	3	4	5	6
I do so all the time.					What shoes?

5. Do you become uncomfortable when a patient asks you a difficult question?

1	2	3	4	5	6
Not at all					Usually

6. Do you find yourself becoming impatient with people who don't seem to understand what you are trying to explain?

1	2	3	4	5	6
I am very patient.					I get really frustrated.

7. Do your patients and other team members listen to you when you are talking?

1	2	3	4	5	6
I believe that others listen to me.					Many times I feel as if I am not heard.

8. In conversation with a patient, can you tell the difference between what a person is saying and what that person may be feeling?

1	2	3	4	5	6
Yes, readily.					I usually misperceive.

9. In conversation, do you let the other person finish talking before responding to what he or she says?

1	2	3	4	5	6
Always					Never happens

10. Generally, are you able to trust others?

1	2	3	4	5	6
Almost always					Almost never

FIG. 4-1 Self-evaluation on communication skills.

Andrea Miller is a dental hygienist and has worked in Dr. Justin Joy's dental practice for 10 years. During that time she has developed exceptional professional and interpersonal skills. As a result of Andrea's and Dr. Joy's attention to both patients and other dental team members, the practice has grown.

Together with the dental team, Andrea has helped Dr. Joy create a philosophy of practice and patient care that demonstrates high professional standards. Patients are at the heart of the mission of the practice, and the values displayed on a daily basis attest to it.

Today Andrea is running 30 minutes behind schedule with her morning patients. A family of four was scheduled for the day's first set of appointments but they arrived late. Andrea has been trying to catch up but she is still behind schedule. Andrea's next patient, Todd McPherson, has arrived, and Andrea is not ready to seat him. Mr. McPherson is getting a bit irritated. How might his needs be satisfied as well as the needs of the family members that Andrea is treating without creating additional stress and still maintaining the integrity of the office?

A different scenario may control a potentially volatile situation. When Mr. McPherson arrives, the receptionist, Julie Rodriguez, has the appointment schedule in front of her and has anticipated his arrival. Julie leaves her desk and greets Mr. McPherson in the reception room:

Julie: Hi, Mr. McPherson. Thank you for being prompt. I know how difficult it can be to get away from work and make it downtown at this time of day. I need to let you know that I tried calling you earlier, but your secretary told me that you had already left your office. She gave me your cell phone number but I was unable to get through to you. The reason for the call was to let you know that Andrea is running about 30 minutes behind schedule today.

Mr. McPherson: Oh swell. Just when I have a critical lunch meeting on the other side of town. I do appreciate the attempts to call, but what are we going to do now?

Julie: I am terribly sorry for this inconvenience. I'm sure that this is very frustrating for you. I know it would be the same for me *[with empathy in her voice]*. What I would suggest, Mr. McPherson, is that we get you settled into the treatment room right away and have Ann Jenkins get all the necessary paperwork completed. Ann, our assistant, as you know, has worked with you before. Andrea can check on you and as soon as she is finished with her current patient and can pick up where Ann left off. I think we would save quite a bit of time, and depending on the time you have available at that point, we can make a decision as to how far to take your treatment today. Is this agreeable with you.

Mr. McPherson: What are my other options?

Julie: The alternative that I see is that we reschedule your appointment for another time, perhaps the same time next week. I would feel bad if all this effort were wasted, however.

Julie is quietly looking at Mr. McPherson while he considers what she has said. He seems perplexed and still a bit upset.

Julie: Why don't you have a glass of water and think about it for a moment or two. I'll go see how Ann and Andrea are progressing and then come back to see what you want to do. It is your choice, whatever suits you best.

Julie brings Mr. McPherson a glass of water and makes sure that he is comfortable in a chair in the reception area.

She looks at him again to see how he is doing as she walks to the door and back to the treatment room. She quickly confers with Andrea. Julie tells her about her conversation with Mr. McPherson and the options that she has offered him. Andrea agrees with the plan (it is consistent with their philosophy) and asks Julie to check with Ann regarding her readiness to help. Ann has been in this situation before and knows what needs to be done.

Julie returns to the reception area. Mr. McPherson is sitting there deep in thought.

Julie: Well, Mr. McPherson, what would you like to do?

Mr. McPherson: [standing up and squaring his shoulders, looking Julie in the eyes and smiling] Why don't we go with plan A. I know how efficient Ann is, and I am certain that Andrea will get to me just as soon as she can.

Julie smiles back at Mr. McPherson and asks him to accompany her to the treatment room. She allows him to lead the way while she accompanies him with an attending manner.

As they arrive at the treatment room, Ann is already waiting. Ann greets Mr. McPherson and expresses her appreciation for being flexible with his schedule. She makes sure that he comfortably gets into the chair and asks him whether he would like a magazine. He states that everything is fine. As Mr. McPherson reclines in the chair, he notices the absence of a lot of equipment and instruments and recognizes the enlarged pictures of the staff's family members.

Mr. McPherson: Nice photos. *[gazing around the room]* Which family is yours.

Ann: [taking a color picture down from the wall] This is my family—my two sons, my daughter, and my husband, Tom. The boys are 11 and 12 years old, and Emily is 14. Tom works at the local bank.

Mr. McPherson: Nice-looking family. I also deal with the bank where your husband works.

Placing the picture back on the wall, Ann gets Mr. McPherson settled into the chair. Andrea walks in, greets her patient, and states how happy she is that he decided to keep the appointment. She adjusts her stool to ensure that she is at a comfortable eye level with him:

Andrea: I realize how busy you are and what an inconvenience even 15 minutes can be in your schedule.

As she is speaking with him, she observes his face to see that he is attending to her and recognizing that she is being sincere.

Andrea: I am so sorry about the delay, Mr. McPherson. We will do everything feasible to get back on schedule. I need to spend another 5 minutes with my previous patient, and then we can begin. Ann will be sure to have everything ready so that we can finish in ample time for your lunch appointment.

She tells them this while she is scanning his face, again making sure that she is exuding sincerity.

Mr. McPherson: Andrea, thanks for taking a moment to be with me. I'm sure Ann will take good care of me. I will be ready when you come back. I wonder though, can I call my office and let them know the situation?

Andrea: Certainly. Let me get our portable phone, so you don't have to get up. [moving the overheard light and getting the phone].

Continued

Case 1: Team Approach to Communication—cont'd

Just as Andrea begins her assessment, Dr. Joy comes into the room.

Dr. Joy: Hi, Mr. McPherson, good of you to be so patient with us. I'm certain Andrea will do everything she can to get your treatment completed thoroughly in comfort and in a reasonable time frame. If there is anything we can do for you, let me know. I'll stop in before you leave.

The treatment continues. Julie and Ann did what they needed to do to minimize Mr. McPherson's stress. Andrea re-

assured him that they can get quite a bit accomplished, and Dr. Joy appreciated his patience and understanding. Mr. McPherson apparently felt he was treated well. His needs were recognized, options were provided, comfort was ensured, and he was made to feel like he was the integral person to several successful outcomes.

Which elements of this case demonstrate effective communication?

---

suggests a need to pay particular attention to the concepts in this chapter and to practice the lessons that follow with a peer. A score between 2.5 and 4.5 is typical; however, as the score approaches 4.5, more attention is required to that individual's communication.

After completing this brief questionnaire, readers should review their responses, asking, "How do I know this is true?" Capturing examples and feelings can bring personal insight to behavior that can pave the way for change.

A WORKING DEFINITION

Adler and Towne[1] state the following:

> . . . *all that ever has been accomplished by humans and all that ever will be accomplished involves communication with others. Many social and organizational problems derive from unsatisfactory relationships brought about by inadequate communication between people.*

Communication is a process between at least two people beginning with one person's desire to convey some information. It originates as a mental image, such as a picture, idea, thought, or emotion. However, what is communicated is not always what was intended.

Effective communication is dynamic; that is, messages and images flow almost instantaneously between the sender and the receiver. Communication involves a vast range of sounds, words, pictures, and gestures; some clearly articulated and some perceived only subtly. A message stated in one context may be perceived differently in another context. The context of the dental office generates a message of its own. This can include the colors chosen for a treatment room, the textures of fabric for the chair in the reception room, the paintings hanging on the wall, or the dental instruments on the tray.

Both nonverbal and verbal actions relay important messages. Sometimes these messages are misunderstood.

STEPS TOWARD CHANGING COMMUNICATION BEHAVIORS

INFLUENTIAL COMMUNICATORS: MODELS FOR LEARNED COMMUNICATION

Can a person really learn how to communicate more effectively, or is it a skill that is predominantly inborn? Actually, the skills pertaining to effective communication can be learned. Helen Keller—a girl unable to hear, see, or

speak—became an influential figure in the twentieth century. She was able to communicate using tactile and kinetic symbols and acquired speech. Her writings were published. Helen Keller influenced the lives of many people living with physical challenges today.

Mother Teresa of Calcutta is another example—a small woman of immense stature who communicated her message of love for the poor through the use of her physical size, actions, and deeds without a lot of words. She was and still is the symbol of the powerful message she delivered to the world.

Think, too, of Stephen Hawking, the renowned physicist who is confined to a wheelchair because of a motor neuron disease (amyotrophic lateral sclerosis [ALS]) and yet has been hailed as the most brilliant theoretical physicist since Einstein. In 1985 after finishing the first draft of his best selling book *A Brief History of Time,*[7] Hawking developed pneumonia, resulting in a tracheotomy that removed his ability to speak. Although Hawking is neither able to move his body nor able to speak except through a synthesized program, he continues to communicate effectively to audiences on the issues of time and space.

Thousands of inspirational stories attest to the courage of the human spirit and show how, given the determination, time, and practice, anyone can become more effective in our communication.

COMMUNICATION ASSETS

Considering the examples mentioned above, are seeing, hearing, vocalizing, and moving essential to communication? Obviously, the answer is no, but they make communication a lot easier. Some basic physical structures are helpful to the communication process: ears, complete with intact inner ear structures; a larynx with a functional set of vocal chords; eyes, with the attending rods, cones, and nerve endings; and an intact set of neural pathways and an alert and conscious brain. The ability to move arms, hands, fingers, head, shoulders, or the whole body helps create gestures to support (or not support) verbal communication.

Assuming that the physical structures used to communicate are intact and fully functioning, what can improve communication skills? The following model is helpful; it has been used to explain how behaviors are learned. This model suggests an upward, stepwise approach toward communication. The first step is acknowledgment of the need for change. The next step is a willingness to act on

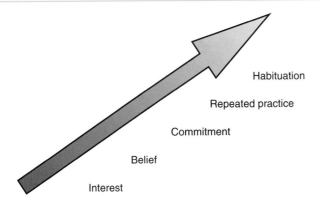

Habituation

Repeated practice

Commitment

Belief

Interest

Knowledge and understanding

FIG. 4-2 Model for communication enhancement.

this knowledge. The desire to act and improve one's communication skills must be a conscious decision.

UNLEARNING POOR COMMUNICATION HABITS

Improving a skill may mean "unlearning" an old skill. In other words, an existing behavior must be replaced with a new behavior. For example, to improve communication skills, a shy person should try to make direct eye contact, a difficult task for such a person. In a different example, when someone makes sounds while speaking that others find distracting to the conversation, this individual first must become aware of the distracting habit so that effective communication can be maintained. Fig. 4-2 is a model for communication, listing the steps to better communication.

RECOGNIZING THE NEED FOR BETTER COMMUNICATION

Recognizing communication skills need improvement is an important first step. Patients' facial expressions may communicate, "What in the world are you talking about?" A child's blank stare may say, "You're not making sense again." Rolling of the eyes may indicate a lack of communication.

Communication breakdown may occur when either the right message is not sent or the right message is sent in an unclear manner, whether by spoken words, written words, or gestures. Communication requires constant monitoring to ensure the receiver of the message is indeed receiving the correct message.

INTEREST

Mere recognition of a communication breakdown is not enough to inspire a change in communication tactics. Interest is also required. Individuals must intensify their interest in how others perceive their communication message.

A realistic assessment of communication skills is necessary, in different settings, under different conditions, and with different people. What are the strengths and weaknesses of an individual's communication skills?

BELIEF

Believing in positive results is necessary for anyone desiring to change a behavior. Belief reflects personal values. Where communication is concerned, values of family, satisfaction in work, good friendships, and professional growth are critical.

COMMITMENT

Commitment describes a pledge of devotion to something. Verbalizing intent to improve communication states a person's commitment. The next step is preparation for action.

ACTION

This is the quantum leap in the acquisition of new skills or the enhancement of old skills. All the knowledge, interest, belief, and commitment mean little without action. Being proactive may include the purchase of a book on more effective communication, a request for input from colleagues, a request for feedback from a spouse, a request for the boss to restate the intended message, or the checking up on children to see whether they followed instructions.

REPEATED ACTION AND HABITUATION

Effective change demands repeated practice. Performing a new skill once does not ensure mastery. Every interaction is an opportunity to practice new skills. Conscious attention to the need for change and method of change will help.

KEY ELEMENTS OF COMMUNICATION

4-A
4-B
4-C

Using three key elements of communication ensures effective communication and supports the development of working relationships. These important ingredients are *listening*, *observing*, and *attending*. These interrelated behaviors occur almost simultaneously in an effective interpersonal exchange.

LISTENING

In dealing with dental staff who have poor communication skills, patients may say, "You are not listening to me," or "You didn't hear a thing I said." Sometimes patients speak softly and some sounds are not heard as clearly as others. Low-pitch sounds tend to fade. Soft voices compete with background noise. On the other hand, excitement results in a loud speaking voice. The "noise" is so profound that the other person is unable to hear us. Listening and speaking are inextricably linked, and both are important elements in effective communication.

OBSERVING

Listening well is an art. For example, Sally, a dental hygienist and an effective listener, attends to the speaker. She acknowledges the person's comments with a nod of her head or by verbally rephrasing what she believed the other person said. In doing so, Sally engenders warmth and

Case 2: Effective Communication— Attending

Jorges Selinta, a dental hygienist employed in a periodontal practice, is attentive to his patients. After a patient is greeted by the receptionist and made comfortable, Jorges appears to prepare her for treatment. Jorges greets her warmly, politely using her surname, and asks about her preparedness for the appointment. Jorges observes the patient as she walks toward the room. He is noting any particular postural or gait issues that might foretell problems getting into the chair. While walking back to the room, Jorges may assist the patient if he notes gait issues by allowing his patient to hold his arm for stability while Jorges guides him to the treatment room. Once there he helps the patient into the chair and makes sure that she is comfortably settled in before proceeding. Then, Jorges ensures he is at the patient's eye level while asking her questions about her health and any concerns she has.

What does Jorges do that sets him apart from other professionals? He is actively involved with his patients. This is perhaps the key dimension in effective communications. Active involvement means being in communication *with* another. It is not communicating *to* another. The "in" communication denotes empathy for and with another person. *Rapport* is established.

---

empathy. She watches her communication partners, looks at their eyes, and stands far enough back to observe their posture. Sally knows when she has been heard. If she believes that she hasn't been heard, she asks for comments. She chooses easily understood words and ensures that the background noise is not overwhelming. She gestures to support her words but makes sure not to be overbearing with them. Her colleagues leave a meeting feeling certain that they were heard. Sally builds relationships.

ESTABLISHING RAPPORT

Miller and Steinberg[10] describe rapport as a state of being with mutual openness, trust, and spontaneity. Rapport is characterized by an "absence of defensiveness and freedom from censored speech."[10] Developing rapport is critical to the maintenance of effective patient management, the performance of treatment, and the obtaining of patient compliance. Patients have a better sense of how they are being treated than they do of the actual procedures.

Communication is easier in an accepting, noncritical environment. With friendships, rapport develops over time through many varied experiences. In the dental setting the time is brief, and the setting is consistently within the practice. Achieving rapport in the dental setting is demanding. How can this be accomplished in a short period of time and in a potentially stressful environment (Box 4-1)?

Personal Space

The dental hygienist should find a *distance* from the other person that is neither threatening nor too distant so as not

to be heard. Hall, in his book *The Hidden Dimension,*[6] discusses four distances and their appropriateness for certain relationships. He asserts that violation of the distance or inappropriate encroachment on another person's space results in tension. The four zones are as follows:

1. *Intimate distance* (0 to 18 inches) is usually reserved for individuals who know one another well. One's physical presence tends to be powerful within this space. Trying to communicate within this proximity is extremely difficult unless the communication conforms to or mirrors the space. Listening is hard within close proximity.
2. *Personal distance* (18 inches to 4 feet) is typically reserved for close friends. Physical presence is not a problem between them. They are able to listen attentively with seemingly little effort. (Various cultures may have different categories or definitions for personal space.)
3. *Social distance* (4 to 7 feet) is apparent when in public places. An example is the distance between groups of people in shopping malls or cafeterias. It is a comfortable distance between strangers. Interestingly, most restaurants, movie theaters, and many other public places do not provide this amount of space.
4. *Public distance* (more than 12 feet) suggests formality and status. However, it is rarely found in professional offices or public settings.

Each person has a unique need for personal space. Individuals do not like to have others "invade their space." They know when they feel encroached and when others are getting too close for comfort. People request tables in the backs of restaurants to ensure added privacy. They walk around groups of people to give themselves and others more room; they push away from overwhelming hugs or pull closer when they are feeling comfortable.

In the dental setting, the professional is continuously invading the patient's space. The nature of dental work does not allow for public distance. On entering the practice, the patient begins to lose personal space. When seated in the dental chair, the patient has personal space of only a few inches.

To minimize tension, personal space should be reduced slowly.

Case #2 Application—Rapport

Jorges greeted his seated patient and knelt down to achieve eye contact. Distance was close as they moved to the treatment room. Jorges realized that he would be invading the intimate space as demanded by dental treatment and wanted to take some time to ensure the patient's comfort.

Patients realize that dental treatment demands close physical proximity. They are willing to tolerate this briefly, until the need for more space becomes too great. Providing time between treatment phases can relieve tension during the intense encounter.

Cultural Sensitivity

Culture plays an important role in the way people attend to one another. Some cultures are more reserved than others. *Cultural sensitivity,* as part of communication, implies an awareness and an accounting for cultural differences during human interaction. Cultures differ in dynamic ways (e.g., differences in expression, gender roles, dress, dietary intake, etc.), which can affect interpersonal communication.

Linguistic differences are also a consideration. The number of individuals who speak English as a second language is increasing. Language may be only one barrier to overcome. Other considerations may include issues of gender, attitudes toward preventive medicine/dentistry, wellness and health promotion, territoriality, eye contact, nutrition, and temporal issues.

A culture exists within the dental practice. The dental environment has a language with a set of norms and customs that govern behavior and a unique physical context. The members of the staff take this culture for granted. They know their roles, their responsibilities, and their colleagues' dispositions and expectations. Practices that have maintained the same staff for a long period of time become like families in which behaviors are taken for granted. Communication flows with the ease of a family gathering and few words are necessary to make requests or explain actions.

Members of the dental culture typically share similar values. Beliefs about professionalism, family, community, well-being, and patient care are readily shared. These values are visible in the décor of the office, the information given to patients as they arrive (such as *A Patient's Bill of Rights)* or leave, the information posted on walls, pictures, and patient information. When the behaviors that reflect those values are evident to patients, the culture becomes a powerful ally to the technical care of the patient.

Cultures do not spring into existence overnight. They must be built with care over time. Discussing the evolving culture helps focus its energies on those areas where values are in conflict or where personal action is not consistent with the value expressed. Developing a consistent practice philosophy should be an ongoing activity.

The language of the dental office culture includes unique terminology, or *jargon.* This vocabulary is necessary to convey critical information between the professional staff. Although the dental team understands dental terminology, it can be confusing to a patient. Disease processes such as gingivitis or periodontitis, or treatment modalities such a pulpectomy, hold specific meaning to the professional. They may, however, convey a different meaning to the patient and may carry emotional overtones. Therefore practitioners should select words that patients will understand. Using more common terms and ensuring that the terms are understood enhances positive patient comprehension and subsequent behavioral compliance.

Context

Social conversation differs from professional conversation. Maintaining communication consistent with the context in which it takes place helps ensure active listening and enhance understanding. For example, a dental professional should not discuss items of intimate personal interest or share inappropriate jokes.

The dental team members can create the context they believe necessary to reflect their culture. How an office and its treatment rooms are decorated speaks volumes to the values that the office shares. Cool colors create a sense of warmth and well-being. Comfortable chairs in the reception room help minimize anxiety. Appropriate reading material can help the patient focus on personal health-related interests. An orderly, clean treatment room reflects the cleanliness values of the staff members.

Time

The duration of the appointment is less important than the quality of the interaction during that visit. However, respecting the time set for an appointment helps ease patients' anxiety. Effective use of time can ease the patient into the treatment setting. A receptionist who is quick to attend to the patient can set the tone for what follows. Visiting with the patient briefly before movement to the treatment room helps stage the visit. Taking time to become acquainted with what has occurred during the interval between visits eases the transition to treatment. Effectively and judiciously suggesting the time needed to devote to a particular treatment will help frame the patient's expectations.

Zunin,[11] writing about the importance of time, particularly short periods of time, proposes that relationships grow or fail depending on what occurs in the first 4 minutes of the encounter. Zunin asserts that each new encounter has the potential to create a new relationship or enhance an existing one, regardless of age, gender, status, profession, or occupation.

Communication encounters are influenced by outside events. For example, a staff member has a fight with his spouse and is still fuming when he arrives at work. An employer misplaced a dental record she took home with her over the weekend and realizes that the file belongs to the first patient of the day. The second patient of the day is 15 minutes late, and the dental hygienist realizes she is already running behind schedule. A patient needs to make an emergency appointment although the schedule includes no available time. How these common and human experiences are expressed in the first few seconds will set the tone for the day.

The following are ways dental hygienists can make use of this time concept:

- Attending to patients more quickly
- Smiling at colleagues even when it is difficult
- Withholding criticism or derogatory comments about a colleague rather than engaging in gossip
- Opening the conversation with a patient in a friendly, warm manner

The response may be surprising. The expressed behavior in the first few seconds and minutes within an encounter can make or break the chance to establish rapport.

Language

A previous section highlighted the importance of the use of words patients understand and the avoidance of the profession's jargon. Consideration should also be given to words that may convey strong emotion. Words such as *needle, drill, explore, bleed, scalpel, probe, cut,* and *oops* may result in strong emotional reactions. Although avoidance of these words is not always possible, observance and attendance to patients' responses to them can help manage the emotion. Momentary pausing in a procedure or discussion to validate the response also reduces the emotional potential.

Words that are relative or equivocal also can be confusing. Consider the phrase, "It's only a small amount of decay." The word *only* minimizes the importance of the problem, and the patient has no reference point for the word "small." Relative words need further explanation. Being specific is a better tactic. Practitioners should break down complex thoughts and messages into smaller and understandable segments. Being clear, specific, and forthright helps build trust and compliance.

Other words and expressions make people immediately defensive. When a person is contradicted, criticized, ridiculed or shamed, threatened, or lectured, the person tends to "turn off and tune out" what is being said. For example, patients are not likely to improve their toothbrushing technique based on a dental hygienist's condescending statement, "Gee, you haven't gotten it right yet."

Nonverbal Cues

Effective listening is not a passive process. It involves attendance to both verbal and nonverbal cues throughout the encounter. The sender of the message must be acknowledged. Restating words spoken in a questioning tone can enhance the meaning of what has been said. Asking open-end questions rather than closed-end questions will allow the speaker to provide more information than "yes" or "no." Nonverbal cues such as a nod of the head or the turn of one's face toward the person speaking can encourage elaboration. Responses such as "I don't understand what you mean," "Oh, I see," and "Hmmm" also can encourage a person to provide additional information.

Even though much information is transmitted through vocalization, only a limited amount of meaning about the information comes from the spoken word. Nonverbal cues fill in the blank spaces. Tilting the head toward the communication partner elicits attention, whereas tilting it away lessens the demand for attention. Arm and hand gestures provide considerable information about the importance of the message. Too many gestures are bewildering, and gestures that appear to be incongruous with what is being said are confusing. The dental hygienist providing feedback while looking out the window shows a lack of interest in the patient.

Facial expressions tend to provide the most information about people's attitudes, beliefs, and emotions.

Knapp suggests that in normal conversation between two people, nonverbal behaviors provide almost two thirds of the total social meaning expressed by them.[8] And Ekman states that "the primary emotions of anger, sadness, happiness, surprise, fear, and disgust are communicated by means of facial expression that are quite uniform across cultures."[2]

Becoming reasonably adept at the understanding of body language and facial cueing is an important skill in the professional setting, particularly when the ability to obtain patients' verbal responses is often difficult. The concept of verbal-nonverbal congruity is essential to understanding. Congruity implies that a patient's nonverbal response supports or is in alignment with what is vocalized. For example, a dental hygienist asks, "Is this hurtful to you?" The patient replies, "No!" but the patient's fingers may be wrapped tightly on the arm of the chair and the patient is wincing. These nonverbal cues suggest incongruity.

Of all the nonverbal cues, eye contact is perhaps the most important and the most difficult to sustain over long periods of time. Ekman and Friesen suggest that the average length of eye contact in an interpersonal setting last about 3 seconds.[3] The speaker usually maintains eye contact twice as long as the listener does. As distance between people increases, so will eye contact.

Eye contact is also cultural. People from more introverted cultures tend to display less eye contact.[3] Eye contact is also gender based; women tend to gaze into space more and more quickly avoid mutual eye contact. Eye contact, according to these authors, regulates verbal communication, reflects interest in what is being discussed, mediates and helps build rapport, expresses emotions, reflects status, and reflects personal characteristics.[3] Maintaining eye contact is particularly important in the dental environment because of the use of personal protective barriers. Face masks worn during treatment obstruct the patient from observing the dental hygienist's smile. Therefore the expression in a dental hygienist's eyes is a critical asset to the development of rapport.

Regulating Verbal Communication

The clues are obvious when a person becomes disinterested in a conversation and stops listening. The person's eyes glaze over and begin drifting away. As this happens, the dental hygienist may wonder whether the person is confused or just not paying attention. Was the patient upset by something that was said? Was the dental hygienist using words that were not understood? Was the dental hygienist's rate of speaking too fast? Is the patient tired? Answers to these questions will affect the outcome of the interaction.

Reflecting Interest in the Discussion

Dental hygienists have the challenge of conveying instructions for mundane tasks with interest. For example, when providing tooth-brushing instructions to a teenager, a dental hygienist may observe the teen's lack of eye contact or fidgeting. As the patient's eyes glaze over, the importance of the message is lost. The dental hygienist relays this information frequently; however, expressing it with interest is more effective. The patient's continued focused gaze and nodding head suggest interested and attention. Only time will tell whether that interest leads to commitment or subsequent action.

Expressing Emotion

A common saying is, "The eyes are the windows to the soul." This is true in the dental office. Expression in the eyes tells the dental staff how the patient is feeling. Pupils constricting and eye muscles tightening are evidence of pain. The dental hygienist should observe the patient's eyes while explaining the treatment planned for the day, particularly when using words such as *drill, needle, prophylaxis, decay,* or *gingivitis,* or the phrase, "This may hurt a little." The dental hygienist should immediately pause, identify, and attempt to assuage negative emotions.

Reflecting Status and Describing Personal Characteristics

Extroverted, more self-confident people tend to be more direct in their eye contact than introverted, more self-conscious people. Authority figures tend to maintain eye contact. People who are in trouble or frightened look away.

The previous statements are generalizations. However, recognition of these characteristics within the dental practice may be helpful. Some patients like to be in control. Their eyes are penetrating, which may make others, including dental staff members, uncomfortable. Dental professionals can deal with this by taking a deep breath while maintaining eye contact.

DEEPENING RAPPORT AND ESTABLISHING ONGOING RELATIONSHIPS

In 1975 George Gazda and his colleagues presented information on the importance of six interpersonal skills needed to create and enhance positive relationships.[4] These skills are empathy, respect, warmth, concreteness, genuineness, and self-disclosure. Twenty-five years later these skills seem more important than ever. Practicing these skills deepens the hygienist-patient relationship. A description of and practice scenarios for these techniques follow.

RESPONDING WITH EMPATHY

Empathy means a deep understanding of another person's feelings, thoughts, or attitudes. In the dental setting, empathy is often shared between team members. For example, one team member displays emotions, which others recognize, label, and respond to appropriately. Empathy also should be present in the treatment room. For example, a dental hygienist demonstrates empathy by pausing to reassure a patient who is gripping the arms of the dental chair.

In addition to attending to patients, dental hygienists must also be conscious of themselves and their environment.

 Effective Communication Application— Empathy

A comment to a seemingly anxious co-worker demonstrates empathy: "Mary, you seem so upset about misplacing Mr. Randolph's chart. Let me help you look for it. Where should we begin to look for it?" This comment shows concern for Mary's feelings and a willingness to help her resolve the problem. The following statements demonstrate empathy among dental office team members and patients:

1. *Hygienist to receptionist:* Boy, am I tired today; my son was up all night with a fever. I finally got the fever down, and he fell asleep. My sitter was able to come over early, but I don't know how things are going to work out this afternoon.

   What words could be used to describe the hygienist's feelings?

2. *Hygienist to dentist:* Dr. Jankowski, this is the fourth time someone has misplaced Mr. Randolph's charts. How in the world does something like this happen in this office? I thought we had a good system for chart management. We should have a meeting on this. What do you think?

   What words could be used to describe the hygienist's feelings?

3. *Patient to hygienist:* I want you to know that I think you do a great job. When I leave this office, my teeth feel cleaner that they ever did before. Dr. Joy is lucky to have such a terrific hygienist. I'm going to tell everybody I know about you and this office.

   What words could be used to describe the patient's feelings?

DEMONSTRATING RESPECT

Respect is not automatic; it is earned. Respect for the skills of others on the dental team involves verbal acknowledgment of tasks well performed and other non–work-related activities that help create the desired office culture. Respect is earned when patients are greeted in a timely manner, treated with utmost sensitivity, and listened to empathetically. Gossip and lack of interest diminish respect.

 Effective Communication Application— Respect

The following sample statements demonstrate ways the dental team members can show respect for one another and toward their patients. The following statements demonstrate ways in which the dental team members can demonstrate respect amongst themselves and toward their patients:

1. *Hygienist to patient:* Mr. Brownstein, I am delighted to see that your oral hygiene has improved since your last visit. You have been able to maintain a plaque-free condition, and your gums look super. You have really spent time with your brush and floss these past 3 months, haven't you?

   What has the hygienist said to demonstrate respect?

2. *Hygienist to patient:* Hi, Tommy! I'm so happy to see you again. How is that throwing arm doing? Your mom told me that you were getting ready to play first base on your T-ball team. Sounds exciting, good for you! Let me sit down to get a good look at you so I can see that handsome smile of yours.

   What has the hygienist said to demonstrate respect?

3. *Dentist to hygienist:* Maria, I am delighted with the progress of the Martin family's oral hygiene. The whole family seems to have taken your instructions very well. Now that they are responding, I am sure there is even more we can do for them if other members of the team can get involved. Why don't you get the group together to discuss this and report back at our next regularly scheduled office meeting?

What has the dentist said to demonstrate respect?

EXPRESSING EMOTIONAL WARMTH

Warmth is actively demonstrated through facial expression, gestures, and touch. As the dental team members become more comfortable with one another, they more readily disclose their feelings and thoughts.

Touch is one of the most sensitive means of communication, conveying feelings impossible to express verbally. A light touch on someone's arm during a heated exchange demonstrates understanding and eases tension. A firm hand on the back of a frail patient engenders reassurance.

 Effective Communication Application— Emotional Warmth

How could the dental hygienist demonstrate warmth in the following situations?

1. While the hygienist is cleaning his teeth, an adult patient suddenly digs his hands into the sides of the chair, and his eyes become closed tight.
2. A patient is arguing with the receptionist. Both people are standing by the counter. Neither seems to be listening to the other.
3. One of the dental assistants in the office was visibly upset by a particularly difficult procedure. Now she is about to set up your treatment room. The hygienist's patient is waiting.
4. A 10-year-old is squirming in the chair. He is restless but not belligerent.

BEING DIRECT

The possibility of misperceiving, mistaking, misrepresenting, misstating, and misunderstanding is always present. These errors usually occur as a result of incomplete, insufficient, or unclear information. It is important to use language consistent with the level of understanding of the patient. Providing new information in small amounts helps patients listen. Giving examples and showing pictures or models reinforce the verbal messages and make difficult concepts understandable. For example, a straightforward, stepwise approach helps ensure patient compliance with oral hygiene techniques. Dental hygienists should start at the beginning and "walk" the patient through the experience. Requesting the patient demonstrate the behavior in the dental office allows for correction of any mistaken ideas.

BEING CONCRETE

In a similar manner, being clear and precise with each dental team member helps enhance the team member's job performance. Clarity of expression also promotes a healthy work culture. For example, when asked where Mr. Randolph's chart is located, a dental hygienist could respond with a precise location rather than stating, "It's somewhere in the treatment room."

 Effective Communication Application—Being Direct and Concrete

The following statements help demonstrate how the patient and dental team member can be direct and concrete:

1. *Patient to hygienist:* I have been coming to see you on a regular basis for the past 2 years, but my gums are still bleeding. Do you think I should be using a different toothbrush or brushing a new way?

What should the hygienist say? What should he or she do?
2. *Hygienist to dental assistant:* Mary is really a pill today. I've never seen her so worked up! If we don't get her under control, we'll have our hands full for the rest of the day. She is going to drive us all crazy.

What could the hygienist do to find out what is bothering Mary? What words might the hygienist choose to ensure that Mary hears and understands?

BEING GENUINE

Each person is unique. Dental hygienists each carry their own special set of values, beliefs, attitudes, likes, dislikes, wishes, and dreams. Sharing them appropriately with patients and colleagues helps build an interpersonal rapport.

Humans are fallible, and dental hygienists are of course no exception. Making mistakes and learning from them is an important part of life. Dental staff members should not feel obligated to hide errors but rather to be genuine, admitting errors and finding remedies as soon as possible.

Being genuine also demands caring about the whole person—the patient's general health and health of the patient's family is critical. Dental hygienists should be interested in the work patients do, where they live, what schools they attend, what they like to do for recreational activities, and what they don't like. They respect patients' intelligence and their ability to make choices. Dental hygienists should recognize they are not superior to patients, but they simply have an expertise different from that of the patients.

 Effective Communication Application— Being Genuine

The following statements help demonstrate ways in which the patient and dental team member can be genuine in their interactions:

1. *Patient to hygienist:* You know every time I make an appointment here, I am kept waiting. It's not your fault, but I get so frustrated and you know how stressed I get about being here anyway.

What could the hygienist say to the patient to let her know that the hygienist is empathetic and genuine?
2. *Hygienist to patient:* The patient has not followed any of oral hygiene instructions. His oral condition has deteriorated significantly since his last visit. The patient has been provided with ample instruction and feedback in the past.

How should the hygienist introduce this observation?

What words could the hygienist use to demonstrate the extent of the problem?

What other communication aids might be useful?

PRACTICING SELF-DISCLOSURE

Luft, in his book *Of Human Interaction,* suggests that openness engenders openness in others.[9] It is a reciprocal and dynamic experience. Sharing a tale of joy or sorrow inspires others to share similar stories.

Establishing relationships in the practice community introduces the opportunity and risk of exposing the true self. For example, sharing too much personal information too quickly may be somewhat disconcerting to others. Therefore the level of existing and growing trust in the practice setting governs the rate at which patients and dental professionals share personal information.

 Effective Communication Application—Self-Disclosure

The following statements help demonstrate ways in which the dental team member and the patient can disclose personal information to facilitate communication:

1. *Patient to hygienist:* Mary, I am so glad you are my dental hygienist. You always seem to care about me. You know, when I was younger I was really very scared of going to the dentist. Now I'm not fearful at all.

   How could the hygienist share personal experiences this patient?

2. *Patient to hygienist:* Time is so crucial for me. I'm pleased that this office respects that. Some offices keep you waiting forever. Life is so hectic nowadays, and I always feel so rushed.

   How could the hygienist share personal experiences with this patient?

3. *Pediatric patient to hygienist:* This a neat place. You have some great stuff for me to play with while I'm waiting. I really like the Legos.

   How could the hygienist share personal experiences with this patient?

Developing these skills helps to deepen the rapport between the dental team members and their patients. Carefully providing feedback, actively listening, and using appropriately framed "I" messages that are complemented by congruent nonverbal cues of facial expression, gestures, and touch enhance relationships.

PROVIDING FEEDBACK USING THE "I" MESSAGE

Critical to a healthcare professional's success is the ability to effectively provide personal and professional feedback. Feedback should both enhance relationships and correct problems. This term is borrowed from the early days of rocket engineering, when an intricate feedback loop was designed to control rocket operations.

Feedback occurs constantly, in a variety of situations. In the professional environment, feedback occurs either between members of the dental team or between the dental professional and the patient. For example, the dental hygienist is discussing a new concept in oral hygiene practice and the dental assistant wants a more detailed description. The dental hygienist stops and provides the description. Another example is a patient interrupting the practitioner's presentation on tooth-brushing techniques to ask a question about a new mechanical brush she has heard about. The dental hygienist stops talking about tooth-brushing techniques and discusses the benefits of these devices.

This exchange of information has all the risks involved in any other communication. The following guidelines are useful in adequately providing feedback in the professional setting (Box 4-2):

- *Consider the needs of others.* Although this maxim sounds relatively easy, it is among the most difficult of guidelines to keep in mind. Often the dental hygienist is so intent on procedure that the patient's needs are ignored. Instructions on oral health should consider the patient's frame of reference. How knowledgeable is the patient about dental disease and the ability to control it? Does he seem to care? What values drive the patient to better oral health? Is she concerned more with function than cosmetics? How does his cultural values affect his behavior? What emotions are expressed during the discussion on oral self-care? How can the dental hygienist assuage negative emotion? Is the dental hygienist choosing words that are appropriate to the patient's level of knowledge?

  The dental professional should begin with the patient's frame of reference. If the professional has truly taken time to understand the patient's background, emotion, and level of understanding, the interaction should be successful. Emotion can make or break the success of an interaction. When patients are feeling anxious or fearful, they will not fully attend to instructions.

- *Avoid using jargon.* Dental staff members should use words the patient understands. Although patients may be impressed with the dental vocabulary of the dental profession, it often interferes with successful feedback. Less complicated words facilitate understanding.

- *Use straightforward language to describe only the patient's behaviors—not attitudes, beliefs, or faults—when attempting to interpret them.* Dental hygienists should be descriptive rather than interpretive. Visual aids may help descriptions. Examples help clarify answers to questions.

BOX 4-2

Providing Feedback

Consider the needs of others.
Avoid using jargon.
Use straightforward language to describe only the patient's behaviors—not attitudes, beliefs, or faults—when attempting to interpret them.
Focus on behaviors that can be changed.
Be specific.
Wait for feedback to be solicited.
Be nonjudgmental.
Provide feedback immediately after the behavior has been exhibited.
Allow freedom to change or not to change.
Define expectations.
Specify the value of the acquisition of the new behavior in real terms.
Structure the skill in manageable steps.
Coach for success.
Provide rewards for successful outcomes.
Express feelings directly.

- *Focus on behaviors that can be changed.* Attempting to help patients overcome unsurpassable obstacles is frustrating. Breaking large-scale changes into smaller, achievable steps will enhance the patient's ability to acquire the new skill. The change will probably not be immediate. Acquiring fine motor skills related to effective flossing, for example, takes time and practice just as changing one's diet does. The professional has to consider whether or not the patient can adopt the new behavior, identify the patient's interest level in changing behavior, and determine whether or not the patient will practice the new behavior.

- *Be specific.* Using vague descriptions and explanations will not be helpful. Patients' questions should be answered thoroughly within the practitioner's knowledge base. This is particularly important with young patients. The more specific and direct you are with children, the better they will follow direction.

- *Wait for feedback to be solicited.* When possible, the practitioner should wait for the patient to make the first move. This may be as blatant as the question, "What should I do?" However, the feedback may be solicited without words, such as a quizzical look or confused frown. These nonverbal cues can be used to advance discussion and instruction.

- *Be nonjudgmental.* Patients flee from criticism. They are willing to hear the "bad" news but do not want to be judged as being "bad." Focusing on behavior, skills, and conditions in understandable language with gentle tones allows patients to remain open to the communication. Harsh criticism is an obstacle to communication and rapport. Defensive patients will not respond well to instruction or advice.

- *Provide feedback immediately after the behavior has been exhibited.* Flossing skills can be taught and evaluated in the dental office. Providing feedback immediately corrects any errant flossing behaviors before they become habitual. Allowing too much time to intervene between the behavior and the feedback diminishes learning potential.

- *Allow freedom to change or not to change.* Most dental professionals probably have strong beliefs about oral hygiene and oral health. Understandably they desire positive outcomes from patient education. However, patients will typically behave in ways that are comfortable to them. They may not want to change their behaviors in the direction prescribed. The patient always has choices and they should be honored. However, to maximize the chance of changing the patients' oral health/hygiene behaviors, the following guidelines are recommended:
  1. *Define expectations.* Dental personnel should be explicit and help the patient set goals relative to the expectations. Patients should participate in setting goals.
  2. *Specify the value of the acquisition of the new behavior in real terms.* Dental hygienists may want to discuss what will happen to the patient's dentition without a behavior change. Contrasting the consequence of no change in the behavior with the adoption of the new (different) technique may be a helpful persuasive tool. Pictures, diagrams, and/or models enhance the discussion.

  3. *Structure the skill in manageable steps.* Breaking down instruction into manageable elements makes it easier for the patient to follow.
  4. *Coach for success.* Positive feedback, "I" statements that reflect success and approval, specific feedback during the learning process, and continuing support are effective "coaching" techniques.
  5. *Provide rewards for successful outcomes.* Meeting a challenge does provide its own internal reward. A small token may help reinforce the new behavior. It can be something as simple as a certificate showing successful completion of an oral self-care program, complete with the name of the patient and signature of dentist or dental hygienist.
  6. *Express feelings directly.* Using "I" messages allows ownership of feelings without excessive emotionality. The listener's feedback will determine what is said next. Expressing feelings to patients may be more difficult, but appropriate phrasing and avoidance of harsh criticism should help.

The concept of active listening and the use of "I" messages was best described in a book by Thomas Gordon published in 1970. In the book *Parent Effectiveness Training* and its several sequels, Gordon presented a very powerful model for communication with children and adults.[5] This model is particularly useful when the message that needs to be conveyed is negative or unpleasant. Gordon challenges the senders of messages to focus on themselves as the "owners" of the attending feeling, rather than on the explicit behavior of the other person. The "I" message contains the following four components:

1. A description of unpleasant or uncomfortable behavior
2. A statement of feelings concerning the effects of the unpleasant behavior
3. A description of the consequence the behavior
4. A statement of the request or preference

In the professional setting unpleasant behavior may relate to a patient's continuous refusal to floss after meals, or it may relate to the receptionist's unwillingness to avoid scheduling a supportive care appointment during the hygienist's lunch break.

In brief, the "I" message reads as follows:
1. When I . . .

   Dental professionals should state the unpleasant feeling, behavior, or situation/condition. For example, "When I look into your mouth and see all the plaque accumulated around your teeth and your gums bleeding as I probe around them, I . . ."
2. I feel (sense, experience, believe, understand, think, etc.) . . .

   Dental professionals should state what is felt, experienced, believed, understood, or thought. For example, "I feel worried."
3. Because . . .

   Dental professionals should state the consequence of the feeling, behavior, situation, or condition. For example, "I am at a loss as to what else we can do. Perhaps we can use a different technique and employ the use of some mechanical devices."
4. "I prefer that" or "It would be helpful to me if . . ."

   Dental professionals should state the alternative action. For example, "I prefer that you use dental floss after every meal."

*Effective Communication Application—
"I" Messages*

Dr. Felix Hertz has a habit of always picking the same person to lead the discussion on office morale, thus arousing feelings of discomfort in that individual. In such a situation the "I" message may take the following form:

1. "Dr. Hertz, When you ask me to get the discussion started on staff morale . . ."
2. "I feel really uncomfortable and anxious . . ."
3. "It puts me in a very difficult spot with everyone else. I feel that they think I have the answer to everything. This makes me very uncomfortable."

"I" statements are helpful in dealings with sensitive issues. Giving positive "I" messages also builds relationships. "I" messages facilitate team cohesiveness, enhance compliance behaviors, and reinforce the behavior. For example, showing appreciation for assistance given by one of the staff members: "Mary, I really appreciate that you were able to fill in for me last week. It made life a lot easier for my family." Or, when a patient has been particularly successful with her oral hygiene: "Jane, I am very excited about the progress you have been making with your plaque control. There is quite a difference in your oral health from a month ago. You are making real progress."

 Case #1 Application

The dental team in the scenario at the beginning of the chapter used "I" messages. The patient, Mr. McPherson, was on time for his scheduled appointment but the hygienist was 30 minutes behind schedule. The entire dental team took time to express their thoughts and feelings with Mr. McPherson to help ensure a positive outcome in what could have been a potentially stressful situation.

Active listening expands the "I" message concept. Active listening involves the taking of positive steps to ensure correct interpretation of the speaker's words. In other words, active listening conveys to the speaker the knowledge that the listener understands what the speaker is saying. Nonverbal cues for effective listening are discussed earlier in the chapter.

Although these aids encourage communication, dental hygienists may find the following two specific behaviors especially helpful:

1. *Paraphrase to reflect understanding.* After patients ask questions or make statements about their health, practitioners can restate them in their own words and ask whether they understood the patients correctly.
2. *Prepare to listen.* A little preparation for active listening helps ensure continuing high-quality communication. Two considerations are suggested: (1) Preparation includes reflection on the agenda for the meeting, review of cases for the day, or thoughts about what to say to a patient. (2) Distractions such as superfluous noise, clutter, and competing thoughts interfere with attention owed to the communication partner. The listener also must be able to see the speaker's nonverbal cues. Examples of reducing distractions include placement of oneself at the eye level of a pediatric patient or movement of the chair back to sufficiently observe the body language of a senior patient.

 *Effective Communication Application—
Paraphrasing*

A patient is concerned about his new dentures becoming loose. He says, "I'm going to a fancy dinner party tonight. I know they are going to have some real special foods there and I really like the way the hostess prepares her meals. I guess I better just stay with the soft foods, huh?" A sincere and knowing response might be, "Mr. Lentz, it sounds like you are worried that you might eat something that will loosen your new dentures. Is this a concern you have?"

Or a mother might ask about a procedure her child is about to undergo: "Danielle, is it common for the doctor to take out healthy teeth before placing braces?" Danielle might respond, "You seem concerned about the need to remove permanent teeth. Let's see whether Dr. Smith has a moment to talk with you about this concern."

Paraphrasing comments made by dental team members also helps keep communication on track. A receptionist said, "Every time I get a new system in place our doctor reverts to the old one. I don't know what I have to do to train him to use the new system." Paraphrasing this statement to express understanding may reduce the tension. For example, the dental hygienist may say, "I hear your frustration in getting us to adopt and manage the new filing system. It's hard for us and particularly for Dr. Fernandez to adapt to these new behaviors. Maybe I can help in the transition."

 RITICAL THINKING ACTIVITIES

1. Using the case study in the beginning of the chapter, identify the effective elements of communication that Andrea used during her interaction with Mr. McPherson.
2. Using personal encounters, reflect on your own communication style. Keep a journal for several days and identify the specific occasions when you demonstrated effective elements of communication. In addition, identify the barriers in the maintenance of effective communication skills.
3. Write a composite of the communication skills that you would look for if you were a dentist hiring a dental hygienist for a full-time position in a private practice dental office.
4. Observe a senior dental hygiene while they are providing services to a patient. List the nonverbal forms of communication used by both the student and the patient.

Continued

CRITICAL THINKING ACTIVITIES—cont'd

5. Conduct an interview with a geriatric patient while a fellow student observes you. The interview should include a thorough medical, dental, and social history. The peer observer should record all verbal and nonverbal elements of communication that enhanced the interview in addition to those that served as a barrier for effective communication.

6. Select a periodontally involved patient and provide oral hygiene instruction while a classmate videotapes this session. Critique your own communication style and identify areas that can be changed to enhance your communication effectiveness.

REVIEW QUESTIONS

1. Dr. Marian Jones, a dentist, is discussing the treatment plan with her patient, Bill Truman. The patient states, "Do I really need the periodontal surgery that you are describing, Dr. Jones?" Which of the following responses made by Dr. Jones would demonstrate *reflective listening?*
   a. "Yes, Mr. Truman, you already know the answer to that question."
   b. "Are you nervous, Mr. Truman?"
   c. "Yes, Mr. Truman, but don't worry, it won't be a painful procedure."
   d. "Mr. Truman, you seem to be concerned about the surgery."

2. Laura Buffington, a patient, is discussing her oral hygiene practices to her dental hygienist, Teresa. Ms. Buffington laments that she has been trying so hard to floss on a regular basis but can't seem to get to it every day as Teresa advised. Which of the following responses made by Teresa would demonstrate *empathy?*
   a. "Two or three times a week? You'll have to do better than that, Ms. Buffington."
   b. "You'll lose your teeth, Ms. Buffington, if you don't start flossing every day."

   c. "Ms. Buffington, that's a great start. I know it's hard to fit it in to the schedule."
   d. "Don't blame me, Ms. Buffington, when Dr. Blank tells you that you'll need surgery."

3. Effective listening is a passive process. Effective communication involves participation by both the sender and receiver of the message.
   a. Both statements are true.
   b. Both statements are false.
   c. The first statement is true; the second statement is false.
   d. The first statement is false; the second statement is true.

4. "Dr. Gonzalez, I am not comfortable charging Mr. Hartrick's insurance company for quadrant scaling when he does not need it. I believe that it is wrong to submit insurance claims for treatment that is not indicated. I would like to schedule Mr. Hartrick for a maintenance 6-month prophylaxis." Kim, the dental hygienist, was demonstrating which communication skill?
   a. Empathy
   b. Providing feedback using "I" statements
   c. Paraphrasing
   d. Genuineness
   e. Both *b* and *d* are correct.

 SUGGESTED AGENCIES AND WEB SITES

Because of the ever-changing nature of the Internet, some of the web sites listed here may have changed since publication. Please refer to Mosby's Evolve web site for the most current information.

American Communication Association: http://www.Americancomm.org

Britannica (key word being *communication;* houses an article on the history of communication): http://www.Britannica.com

 ADDITIONAL READINGS AND RESOURCES

Carkhuff RR: New training for the helping professions: toward a technology for human and community resource development, *Couns Psychol* 3:12-30, 1972.

Egan G: *The skilled helper: a model for systematic helping and interpersonal relating,* Monterey, Calif, 1975, Brooks Cole.

Ekman P, Friesen WV: *Unmasking the face: a guide to recognizing emotions from facial cues,* Englewood Cliffs, NJ, 1975, Prentice Hall.

Goleman D: *Emotional intelligence,* New York, 1995, Bantam.

Hall ET: *The silent language.* Garden City, NY, 1969, Doubleday.

Katzenbach JR, Smith DK: *The wisdom of teams.* New York, 1993, Harper Collins.

Knapp ML: *Nonverbal communication in human interaction,* New York, 1972, Holt, Rinehart & Winston.

Rogers CR: *On becoming a person,* Boston, 1961, Houghton Mifflin.

ADDITIONAL READINGS AND RESOURCES—cont'd

Satir V: *People making,* Palo Alto, Calif, 1972, Science and Behavioral Books.

Tamparo CD, Lindh WQ: *Therapeutic communications for health professionals,* ed 2, Albany, NY, 2000, Delmar.

Tannen D: *You just don't understand,* New York, 1990, Ballantine Books.

REFERENCES

1. Adler R, Towne N: *Looking out/looking in,* ed 2, New York, 1978, Holt, Rinehart & Winston.
2. Ekman P: Facial expression. In Seigman AW, Feldstein S, editors: *Nonverbal behavior and communication,* Hillsdale, NJ, 1978, Erlbaum.
3. Ekman P, Friesen WV: Nonverbal leakage and clues to deception, *Psychiatry* 32:88-106, 1969.
4. Gazda GM et al: *Human relations development: a manual for health sciences,* Boston, 1975, Allyn and Bacon.
5. Gordon T: *Parent effectiveness training,* New York, 1970, Plume.
6. Hall ET: *The hidden dimension,* Garden City, NJ, 1969, Doubleday.
7. Hawkins S: *A brief history of time,* New York, 1988, Bantam.
8. Knapp ML: *Essentials of nonverbal communication,* New York, 1980, Holt, Rinehart & Winston.
9. Luft J: *Of human interaction,* Palo Alto, Calif, 1969, Natural Press Books.
10. Miller GR, Steinberg M: *Between people: a new analysis of interpersonal communication,* Chicago, 1975, SRA.
11. Zunin L: *Contact: the first four minutes,* New York, 1972, Ballantine Books.

PART II

Chapter 5
*Exposure Control and Prevention
of Disease Transmission*

Chapter 6
Workstation Design and Positioning

Chapter 7
*Instrument Design and Principles
of Instrumentation*

Chapter 8
Instrument Sharpening

Competency Statements

The learner is expected to possess knowledge, skills, judgments, values, and attitudes to develop the listed competencies.

Core Competencies
- Adhere to state and federal laws, recommendations, and regulations in the provision of dental hygiene care.
- Provide dental hygiene care to promote patient health and wellness using critical thinking and problem solving in the provision of evidence-based practice.
- Use evidence-based decision making to evaluate and incorporate emerging treatment modalities.
- Assume responsibility for dental hygiene actions and care based on accepted scientific theories and research as well as the accepted standard of care.
- Provide quality assurance mechanisms for health services.
- Provide care to all patients using an individualized approach that is humane, empathetic, and caring.

Courtesy American Dental Education Association, Washington, DC.

Environmental Ergonomics

Health Promotion and Disease Prevention

- Respect the goals, values, beliefs, and preferences of the patient while promoting optimal oral and general health.
- Identify individual and population risk factors and develop strategies that promote health related quality of life.
- Evaluate factors that can be used to promote patient adherence to disease prevention and/or health maintenance strategies.
- Evaluate and utilize methods to ensure the health and safety of the patient and the dental hygienist in the delivery of dental care.

Community Involvement

- Facilitate client access to oral health services by influencing individuals and/or organizations for the provision of oral health care.

Patient Care

- Select, obtain, and interpret diagnostic information recognizing its advantages and limitations.
- Recognize predisposing and etiologic risk factors that require intervention to prevent disease.
- Recognize health conditions and medications that impact overall patient care.
- Identify patient needs and significant findings that impact the delivery of dental hygiene services.
- Obtain consultations as indicated.
- Perform dental hygiene interventions to eliminate and/or control local etiologic factors to prevent and control caries, periodontal disease, and other oral conditions.
- Determine the outcomes of dental hygiene interventions using indices, instruments, examination techniques, and patient self-report.

Professional Growth and Development

- Access professional and social networks and resources to assist entrepreneurial initiatives.

CHAPTER 5

Exposure Control *and* Prevention *of* Disease Transmission*

Kathy B. Bassett

Chapter Outline

Case Studies: Infection Control and Disease
  Prevention
Theory (Literature)
  Factors in disease transmission
  Risk of exposure
  Microbial resistance
  Infectious diseases of concern for dental
    healthcare providers

Government agencies: regulations, standards,
  and guidelines
Regulatory terminology and explanations
Techniques, Procedures, and Supportive Evidence
  Goal of an infection control program
  Putting hazard abatement and standard
    operating procedures to work

Key Terms

Acquired immunodeficiency
  syndrome (AIDS)
Bioburden
Biofilm
Biohazardous materials
Bloodborne pathogens
Centers for Disease Control
  and Prevention (CDC)
Contaminated
Decontamination
Engineering controls (EC)
Environmental Protection
  Agency (EPA)
Exposure control plan (EPC)

Exposure incident
Food and Drug
  Administration (FDA)
Guidelines
Hazard abatement
Host reservoir
Host susceptibility
Human immunodeficiency
  virus (HIV)
Occupational exposure
Occupational Safety and
  Health Administration
  (OSHA)

Other potentially infections
  materials (OPIM)
Parenteral
Pathogenic
Personal protective
  equipment (PPE)
Recommendations
Regulated waste
Regulations
Resident flora
Resource Conservation
  and Recovery Act
  (RCRA)

Routes of transmission
  Aerosol or droplet
  Autogenous
  Direct
  Indirect
  Waterborne
Source individual
Standard operating
  procedures (SOP)
Standard precautions (SP)
Standards
Virulence
Work practice controls (WPC)

 ## *Learning Outcomes*

1. State the basic principles and science of disease
   transmission and common infectious diseases of
   humans, infection control in the dental workplace, and
   safety as applied to biohazards in the dental workplace.
2. Identify the names of state and federal regulatory and
   advisory agencies that concern infection control
   practices and management of biohazardous materials.
3. Integrate basic science, clinical practice, professional
   standards of care, and regulatory standards for infection

   control and work-practice safety to prevent disease
   transmission and the health of both employees and
   patients in the dental workplace.
4. Apply effective principles of infection control and safe
   handling of biohazardous materials to provide a safe
   environment for dental hygienists, co-workers, patients
   in the dental workplace, and household members.
5. Comply with federal, state, and local standards and
   regulations for the dental workplace.

*See Appendix E for information about the Guidelines for Infec-
tion Control in Dental Healthcare Settings—2003.

Infection Control and Disease Prevention

Case 1: Infection Control and Nonclinical Personnel

Ruth Levine is in her early 50s and works as an office manager in a small dental practice; she is a hard-working and supportive member of the staff. Her primary duties are at the front desk.

Ruth has been suffering from significant fatigue, a chronic fever, and swollen glands for several weeks. She has seen her physician and has had multiple tests performed with no significant findings. At her last appointment the physician expressed concerned about Ruth's liver function tests. After additional studies were performed, with no conclusive findings, Ruth was referred to a liver specialist for evaluation. The specialist decided to perform a liver biopsy. However, on the day of the procedure, the physician postponed the biopsy to run one more additional test; Ruth's blood sample was taken.

Case 2: Sterilization Cycle Failure

While cleaning her treatment area after a patient appointment, a second-year dental hygiene student noticed that the cycle integrator on the sterilization bag for the instruments she just had used had not changed color (indicating that the physical parameters for sterilization had not been met).

On further investigation, she discovered that two loads of instruments had been distributed without indication that appropriate sterilization had taken place. The instruments appeared to have been used during a student laboratory (in which students practiced on one another), and some had been used on general clinic patients. At least one patient is confirmed to have been exposed to unsterilized instruments, and no other students are able to confirm whether the instruments they used during that session were from the un-

sterilized load. A few remaining unused instrument packs are located, repackaged, and returned for proper sterilization. The patients on whom the instruments were used (the source of contamination) all appear to be first-year dental hygiene students (all of whom had been patients in second-year clinic the previous day).

Case 3: Safe Handling of Sharps

As the dental hygienist withdrew a curet from a patient's mouth, a significant mass of blood and debris adhered to the blade of the instrument. Without giving it a second thought, the hygienist picked up a 2 × 2 gauze square and wiped the instrument clean with a pinching motion before returning to work.

Case 4: Patient Protection

Jim Birdwell awoke one morning with a sore eye. He complained of a "grainy sort of feeling," as if he had a piece of sand in his eye and rubbed his eyes, thinking that it was just a "sleeper," and thus increased his discomfort. Mr. Birdwell figured that it would eventually wash its way out and ignored the feeling. After a couple of hours the pain increased. His attempts to flush out his eye with water were unsuccessful.

After subsequent evaluation by a physician, Mr. Birdwell was referred to an ophthalmologist. Mr. Birdwell's diagnosis was an infection on the outer surface of his eye, just out of his line of sight. The grainy feeling he experienced was the formation of scar tissue. The ophthalmologist speculated that some type of bacterial matter had worked its way into his eye, causing the infection.

---

*A*s healthcare providers it is the responsibility and duty of dental hygienists to practice professionally and ethically. To this end, dental hygienists must carefully integrate basic science, principles of safety, professional standards of care and policy, along with numerous federal, state, and local regulations applied to infection control in healthcare settings. Once this responsibility is understood, dental hygienists then must provide their patients oral healthcare services in a way that protects the health of both the patients and dental healthcare workers.

The Internet has provided access to a wealth of information, from basic science to federal regulations, enhancing professional education and development. Throughout this chapter, web sites are referenced for further study and more in-depth information on each topic. To help understand and apply the principles and implications of infection control procedures and professional responsibility, four case histories represent four actual events.

THEORY (LITERATURE)

Infectious disease transmission can pose significant problems in the dental workplace. All dental healthcare workers

(DHCP) must understand the basic principles of disease transmission, infection control, and safety to minimize the risks associated with exposure to biohazardous agents. Dental professionals must pay close attention to basic sciences and integrate safety practices to comply with the numerous guidelines, standards of care, and regulations initiated to protect the health of patients and healthcare workers.

To ensure an understanding of the risks presented and implement safe work practices, federal regulations require that all healthcare professionals participate in specific training in infection control practices for exposure to and handling of **biohazardous materials.** Training programs must include the following elements:

- Basics of disease transmission
- Epidemiology of infectious diseases
- Modes of transmission for infectious agents
- Exposure prevention
- Precautionary measures

FACTORS IN DISEASE TRANSMISSION

Disease transmission is influenced by a number of factors (Table 5-1). To fully understand this process, the DHCP

TABLE 5-1

Basic elements of disease transmission

Host source	Escape from host	Entry into new host
Surface skin	Natural oral activity (speech, cough, sneeze)	Inhalation
Oral tissues	Natural oral activity (speech, cough, sneeze)	Ingestion
Saliva	Artificial (hands, instruments, aerosols, spatter)	Contact with mucous membranes
Blood	Artificial (hands, instruments, aerosols, spatter)	Penetration of intact skin

must consider the nature of infectious microorganisms, source of these agents, methods by which these agents escape the source and are transmitted to a new host, and factors that affect infection of the new host. In addition, an understanding of the ways in which these microorganisms vary in their resistance to destruction by the host immune system or destroy by other means is important. To control disease transmission in the dental environment, the DHCP must apply these principles and associated factors appropriately to work situations.[64,94]

Nature of Microorganisms and Infectious Agents

Not all microorganisms found on or in tissues are considered disease producing, or **pathogenic,** by nature. Many microorganisms, referred to as **resident flora,** are found normally in humans and are necessary for routine body functions; these include microorganisms normally found in the oral cavity.[64] The body has adapted to and can even benefit from their presence. Both nonpathogenic and pathogenic organisms are present in the oral environment. However, even resident flora can be pathogenic if they increase in numbers greater than normal or are transferred to sites in the body where these microorganisms are not normally present.

Three basic categories of microorganisms can be found in the oral environment and are easily spread through oral activities and dental procedures. The following definitions are taken from *Mosby's Dictionary of Medicine, Nursing, and Allied Health* (sixth edition).

Virus: a minute parasitic microorganism much smaller than a bacterium that, having no independent metabolic activity, may replicate only within a cell of a living plant or animal host; consists of a core of nucleic acid (DNA [deoxyribonucleic acid] or RNA [ribonucleic acid]) surrounded by a coat of antigenic protein sometimes surrounded by an envelope of lipoprotein; *examples:* common cold viruses, herpes, hepatitis, HIV, measles, rubella

Bacteria: any of the small unicellular microorganisms of the class Schizomycetes; vary morphologically, being sphere-shaped (cocci), rod-shaped (bacilli), spiral (spirochetes), or comma-shaped (vibrios); the nature, severity, and outcome of any infection caused by a bacterium be-

ing characteristic of that species; *examples* of infectious bacteria: tuberculosis, *Staphylococcus* strains, *Streptococcus* strains, *Neisseria gonorrhea,* and *Legionella* strains

Fungi (mushrooms, yeasts, molds, etc.): a general term for a group of eukaryotic, thallus-forming organisms that require an external carbon source; lack both chlorophyll and chemolithotrophic systems; can be saprophytes (organisms living on dead organic material) or parasites; reproduce by budding (simple fungus) or spore formation (multicellular fungus); may invade living organisms, including humans, as well as nonliving organic substances; of 100,000 identified species, 100 common in humans and 10 pathogenic; *examples* of fungal infections: *Pneumocystis carinii* pneumonia, *Cryptococcus neoformans, Candida albicans,* and histoplasmosis

Sources of Microorganisms and Infectious Agents

Common sources of potentially infectious microorganisms, known as **host reservoirs,** in the dental environment include both patients and DHCPs. Microorganisms may be found in a number of host reservoirs—on surface skin and in body tissues and fluids, including blood and saliva.

Methods of Escape, Routes of Transmission, and Entry

Microorganisms can escape the host reservoir and spread through natural occurrences, such as during speaking, coughing, sneezing, or another oral activity; through artificial means, such as carried on hands, instruments, equipment; or through aerosols and spatter.

Transmission to a new host environment may be via direct contact, such as direct deposit, or indirect contact, such as onto an inanimate surface or hands and subsequent transfer from one area to another or one person to another.

Primary Routes of Transmission

Once the microorganisms have escaped one host, they can be spread to a new host by the following primary **routes of transmission:**[9,78,94]

Direct describes transfer from a specific person or host reservoir (source) directly to another person (host). Bloodborne microorganisms are transmitted by direct contact with blood, through blood products, and in blood-contaminated saliva.

Indirect describes transfer from a specific person or host reservoir (source) to an inanimate object, such as a surface or item, and subsequent transfer to another person (host).

Aerosol or droplet transfer is from a person or host reservoir (source), subsequently incorporated into materials that become airborne, and ultimately transferred to a person (host). This method can be both cross-infection or autogenous infection (back to the source). Blood and blood products in saliva are frequently incorporated into droplets, splatter, and aerosols generated during many common dental procedures. Aerosols are considered invisible particles less than 50 microns in size (usually less than 5 microns). Splatter or droplets are considered visible particles greater than 50 microns.[10,23]

Autogenous (self-infection) transfer is a result of the introduction of a microorganism from one area of the body to another. Although the microorganism may be nonpathogenic in one part of the body, it may be pathogenic when introduced to another susceptible site. Examples include the bacteremia induced during subgingival scaling. A bacteremia peaks in approximately 15 minutes and normally is cleared from the body in 20 to 30 minutes; however, infective endocarditis can develop in susceptible individuals.

Waterborne transfer describes a subject of more recent concern—transmission of microorganisms through contaminated dental unit waterlines.[1,4] A film of microorganisms can attach tenaciously to the inner surface of waterline tubing, a formation known as a **biofilm.**

A number of causes and contributing factors are cited for how this phenomena occurs. When portions of this biofilm dislodge, they are carried through the waterline and can be expelled into the patient's mouth during dental procedures. If the organisms are pathogenic and the patient is a susceptible host, then an infection can develop. As many as 40 different microorganisms have been identified in contaminated waterlines.[97] Although several of these can be pathogenic, two are of significant concern for dentistry: *Legionella pneumophila* and *Pseudomonas aeruginosa.*[5,97]

Entry and Transmission to a New Host

Entry into a new host is considered a completed transmission, usually occurring in the dental environment through contact with mucous membranes, through parenteral inoculation, through inhalation, through breaks in the skin, or through ingestion of microorganisms carried in blood, saliva, and oral tissues.

After exposure and transmission of pathogenic microorganisms, a number of factors affect whether infection will occur (Fig. 5-1), including the **virulence** of the pathogen, dose of microorganisms transmitted, and the new host's ability to resist infection.[64] The virulence or nature of a microorganism determines its pathogenicity, its degree of infectiousness, and the conditions necessary for infection to occur. Regarding dose, some highly pathogenic organisms require a very small dose to initiate an infection, whereas others require a large dose exposure before infection is likely. For example, hepatitis B is much more virulent than **human immunodeficiency virus (HIV).** The probability that an infection will occur is demonstrated as an equation shown in Fig. 5-2.

Host Susceptibility

Also of importance in the disease transmission equation are factors not directly related to the microorganism itself. The body has a number of protective barriers and systems to help prevent infection. Intact skin is the primary physical barrier of the body. Physiological characteristics of the respiratory system also function as primary barriers (or filters) to infectious agents. If these physical barriers fail, the body's next line of defense is the immune system.

The integrity of the host's immune system, or its ability

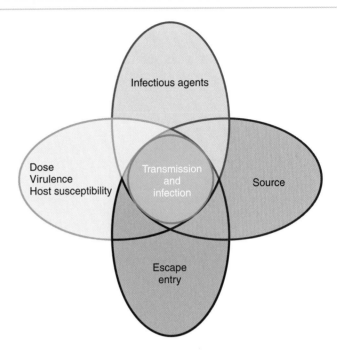

FIG. 5-1 Factors of disease transmission and infection.

$$\text{Infection} = \frac{\text{Virulence} \times \text{Dose of organisms}}{\text{Host resistance}}$$

FIG. 5-2 Transmission equation.

to resist infection, is important in the prevention of infection. **Host susceptibility** is affected by the individual's general state of health and ability to resist infection, including the presence of other conditions, diseases, or infections (co-infection) that can weaken the immune system. In addition to co-infection by a systemic disease, host immunosuppression can be induced by physical defects (such as heart valve damage or prosthetic joints), immunosuppressive drugs (such as chemotherapeutic agents), organ transplants (with associated antirejection drugs), and the natural physiological processes associated with stress, fatigue, and aging.[64]

Host immunity can be increased through natural or acquired immunity (having had the disease) or artificial immunity (immunization). Natural and acquired immunity varies among individuals and is a direct reflection of the person's general health.[85]

RISK OF EXPOSURE

Oral healthcare procedures by nature challenge the body's natural barrier and defense systems, creating an "at risk" environment and situations for patients and DHCPs because of the continual contact with blood, saliva, oral mucous membrane, and tissues; the use of sharp instruments and needles with a danger of injury; and the wide variety of procedures routinely performed.

Infectious agents may be passed from patient to DHCP, from DHCP to patient, to other staff members, and then

TABLE 5-2

Environmental survival of microorganisms

ESTIMATED SURVIVAL AT ROOM TEMPERATURE		
Agent (disease)	**Route(s)**	**Survival**
Bacterial		
Mycobacterium tuberculosis (tuberculosis)	Saliva, sputum	Months
Staphylococcus aureus (staphylococcal infections)	Saliva, skin, exudates	Days
Streptococcus pyogenes (streptococcal endocarditis)	Open wound, blood	Hours to days
Treponema pallidum (syphilis)	Direct contact with lesions	Seconds
Viral		
Respiratory viruses (flu, colds pneumonia)	Salivary secretions	Hours
HAV (hepatitis A)	Blood, feces, saliva	Days
HBV (hepatitis B)	Blood, saliva, other body fluids	Months
HIV (HIV-related diseases, AIDS)	Blood, other body fluids	Days
HSV 1 and 2 (recurrent herpes, herpetic whitlow, herpetic conjunctivitis)	Saliva, secretions	Minutes

Modified from Nisengard RJ, Newman MG: *Applied microbiology and immunology,* ed 2, Philadelphia, 1988, WB Saunders.
HAV, Hepatitis A virus; *HBV,* hepatitis B virus; *HIV,* human immunodeficiency virus; *AIDS,* acquired immunodeficiency syndrome; *HSV,* herpes simplex virus.

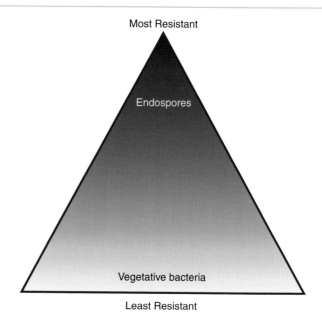

FIG. 5-3 Microbial resistance.

carried home to associates, friends, spouses, children, and other family members. The occurrence of infection after exposure to pathogenic organisms depends on a number of factors with respect to host resistance; microorganisms that exist within one individual without any clinically apparent or significant disease could be quite harmful if transferred to another individual. Although DHCPs may exhibit significant resistance to exposure to pathogenic microorganisms due to the wearing of special protective equipment, frequent immunizations, and a higher level of general health, many patients may be susceptible and at higher risk of infections.

MICROBIAL RESISTANCE

To reduce the risk of infection by pathogenic microorganisms spread in the dental environment, an understanding of the nature of the organism in relationship to environmental survival time, methods of decontamination, and sterilization is necessary. For example, HIV remains viable (capable of transmitting infection) on environmental surfaces (Table 5-2) for merely seconds, whereas hepatitis B virus remains viable for weeks without appropriate decontamination.[64] In addition, some microorganisms are more resistant to decontamination than others; for example, bacterial endospores (such as tuberculosis) are the most resistant to destruction by disinfection and sterilization procedures, whereas vegetative bacteria are the least resistant[64,80] (Fig. 5-3). This knowledge

enables the healthcare worker to apply appropriate measures for disinfection and sterilization of items contaminated by these organisms.

INFECTIOUS DISEASES OF CONCERN FOR DENTAL HEALTHCARE PROVIDERS

Of significant concern in the dental environment are several diseases that can be transmitted by bacteria, viruses, and fungi.* Understanding the nature of the organisms, specific transmission factors, symptoms of infection, and the impact of infection can reinforce the importance for control of exposure to and transmission of infectious agents (Table 5-3; see the suggested agencies and web sites [1-9] at the end of this chapter).

Diseases Caused by Viral Agents

The diseases listed in the following sections are caused by infection with viral agents (see the suggested agencies and web sites [10-11] at the end of this chapter).[9,64,94]

Hepatitis Infection
Hepatitis infection is a viral liver infection that can be caused by a group of viruses. The transmission of hepatitis in healthcare settings is a significant concern. The Occupational Safety and Health Administration (OSHA) has determined that healthcare workers are at great risk of contracting hepatitis B virus because any exposure may result in infection.[76]

To manage exposure to hepatitis, an understanding of the various types of the disease, associated routes of transmission, and prevention strategies is necessary (Table 5-4). To date, seven different hepatitis viruses have been identified: hepatitis A virus (HAV), hepatitis B virus (HBV), hepatitis C virus (HCV), hepatitis D virus (HDV),

---

*References 9, 17, 42, 64, 82, 87, 94.

TABLE 5-3
Summary of significant infectious diseases

Disease	Pathogen	Transmission	Related manifestations	Serious complications
Caused by Viral Agents				
Human immunodeficiency disease	HIV	B, OBF, SC	Secondary oral infections (viral, bacterial, fungal, neoplasms)	AIDS, opportunistic infections, death
Chickenpox	VZV	S, B, AD	Oral lesions, latent shingles	Conjunctivitis, shingles, encephalitis
Common cold	Rhinoviruses (others)	S, B, AD	Sore throat, respiratory infection	Temporary disability
Cytomegalovirus	CMV	S, B	Adults—mononucleosis-like syndrome	Birth defects with immunosuppression, death
Hepatitis A, E	HAV, HEV	Oral, fecal	*	*
Hepatitis B	HBV	S, B, AD	Jaundice	Chronic disability, carrier state,
Hepatitis C	HCV	S, B, AD	Liver inflammation	hepatocellular carcinoma, co-infection, death
Hepatitis D	HDV	B	*	*
Herpes, ocular	HSV 1	S, B, AD	Herpes conjunctivitis	Potential blindness
Herpes, simplex (1 or 2)	HSV 1 or HSV 2	S, B, SC	Primary gingivostomatitis, oral herpes, herpetic whitlow	Painful lesions, disability
Infectious mononucleosis	EBV	S, B, AD	Sore throat, oral ulcers	Temporary disability, latent disease
Influenza	Influenza viruses	S, AD	Sore throat, respiratory infection	Pneumonia, death
Measles, rubella	Rubella virus	S, NR, AD	Vascular rash	Congenital defects, infant death
Measles, rubeola	Rubeola virus	S, NR, AD	Vascular rash	Temporary disability, encephalitis
Mumps	Mumps virus	NR	Parotitis	Temporary disability, male sterility
Pneumonia, viral	Cold and influenza viruses	B	Respiratory infection	Death
†Severe acute respiratory syndrome	SARS-CoV	S, AD, NR, direct contact	Cough, difficulty breathing, hypoxia and radiographic evidence of pneumonia	Death
†West Nile	WNV	mosquito	Fever, headache, skin rash, swollen lymph nodes, neck stiffness, stupor, disorientation, coma, tremors, muscle weakness and paralysis	Encephalitis, meningitis, death
Caused by Bacterial Agents				
Gonorrhea	*Neisseria gonorrhea*	SC	Gonococcal pharyngitis	Arthritis, female sterility, infant blindness
Legionnaire's disease	*Legionella pneumophila*	NR	Respiratory infection	Death
Pneumonia, bacterial	*Staphylococcus aureus, Streptococcus pyogenes*	NR, B	Respiratory infection	Death
Staphylococcal infections	*S. aureus*	S, AD, nosocomial, direct	Skin lesions	Skin lesions, bacteremia, endocarditis, death
Streptococcal infections	*S. pyogenes*	S, B, AD	Streptococcal pharyngitis, "strep throat," skin lesions	Rheumatic heart disease, pneumonia, endocarditis, kidney problems, death
Syphilis	*Treponema pallidum*	SC, congenital	Primary chancre, oral ulcers	Central nervous system damage, death
Tuberculosis	*Mycobacterium tuberculosis*	S, AD	Productive cough more than 3 weeks	Disability, death
Caused by Fungal Agents				
Candidiasis	*Candida albicans*	S, AD, direct	Oral thrush, cutaneous infection	Opportunistic infection

S, Saliva, *B,* blood, *OBF,* other body fluids; *AD,* aerosol/droplets; *SC,* sexual contact; *NR,* nasal/respiratory; *HIV,* human immunodeficiency virus; *AIDS,* acquired immunodeficiency virus; *VZV,* varicella-zoster virus; *CMV,* cytomegalovirus; *HAV,* hepatitis A virus; *HEV,* hepatitis E virus; *HBV,* hepatitis B virus; *HCV,* hepatitis C virus; *HDV,* hepatitis D virus; *HSV,* herpes simplex virus; *EBV,* Epstein-Barr virus.
*Content between symbols applies to all forms of hepatitis.
†See Appendix B for more information.

TABLE 5-4

Summary comparison of human hepatitis viruses

					HEPATITIS VIRUSES—BASIC FACTORS			
Viral agent	Incubation period	Host reservoir	Primary transmission	Chronic carrier state	Serum markers	Terminology	Significance in diagnosis
HAV	2 to 7 weeks	Feces, saliva, blood	Oral–fecal	No	Anti-HAV	Antibody to HAV	Detectable at onset of symptoms; persists for lifetime
					IgM anti-HAV	IgM class antibody to HAV	Indicates recent infection; detectable for 4 to 6 months after infection
HBV	6 weeks to 6 months	Blood, other body fluids (serum-derived, such as saliva)	Parenteral, sexual, perinatal	Yes	HBsAG	HB surface antigen	Surface antigen HBV; detectable in large quantity in serum
					HBeAg	HBe antigen	Soluble antigen of HBV; correlates with viral replication and infectivity
					Anti-HBs	Antibodies to HBsAg	Indicates past infection, inmunity, passive immunity, or immunization
					Anti-HBe	Antibodies to HBeAg	Presence in serum of carrier; indicates low titer
					Anti-HBc	Antibodies to HBcAg	Indicates past infection; undetermined time period
					IgM anti-HBc	IgM antibodies to HBsAg	Indicates recent infection; detectable for 4 to 6 months after infection
HCV	2 weeks to 6 months	Blood	Parenteral	Yes	Anti-HCV	Antibodies to HCV	Delayed detection; no distinction between acute and chronic infection; persists for lifetime; does not indicate immunity
							Present in early infection, during viremia intermittently; does not indicate degree of infectivity
							Indicates liver damage; may increase with HCV infection; may indicate effectiveness of treatment
HDV	3 to 7 weeks	Blood	Parenteral	Yes	HDAg	HD antigen	Detectable in early acute delta infection
			Sexual		Anti-HDV	Antibodies to HDV	Indicates past or present infection
HEV	2 to 9 weeks	Feces	Oral–fecal	No	Anti-HEV	Antibodies to HEV	Clinical tests for HEV unavailable; diagnosis by exclusion
HGV	2 to 7 weeks	Blood	Parenteral Perinatal	Unknown	Anti-HGV	Antibodies to HGV	Detectable in infection
					HGV RNA	Hepatitis G RNA	Present in early infection; persistent at least 1 year
						Alanine aminotransferase	Indicates liver damage; may increase with HGV infection; possible correlation to early infection

Modified from Centers for Disease Control (ACIP), Protection against viral hepatitis *MMWR* 39 (RR-2):6-7, 1990.
HAV, Hepatitis A virus; *IgM*, immunoglobulin M, *HBV*, hepatitis B virus; *HBsAg*, hepatitis B virus surface antigen; *HBeAg*, hepatitis B e antigen, *HBCAg*, hepatitis B core antigen; *HCV*, hepatitis C virus; *HDV*, hepatitis D virus; *HEV*, hepatitis E virus; *HGV*, hepatitis G virus; *HDAg*, hepatitis D antigen; *RNA*, ribonucleic acid.

hepatitis E virus (HEV), and hepatitis G virus (HGV).* Hepatitis F virus (HFV) has been reported but not confirmed, and little is known about it. The most common symptoms of hepatitis infection are flulike symptoms that include fatigue, diarrhea, fever, muscle and joint pain, nausea, abdominal discomfort, and classic to hepatitis infection, jaundice. Persistent and chronic infection can lead to severe liver damage and death (see the suggested agencies and web sites [12-13] at the end of this chapter).

Hepatitis A virus

HAV[9,47,48,87] is the most prevalent hepatitis infection. It is transmitted through oral–fecal cross-contamination, ingestion of foods or water contaminated by an infected person, or close person-to-person contact. Incubation is typically 30 days after exposure but can occur between 15 and 50 days. Proper hand-washing techniques are the most effective means to prevent transmission.

*References 9, 11, 43, 48, 64, 88, 94.

Body Piercing and Tattooing

Body piercing and tattooing have become popular fashion trends in Western industrialized nations within recent years. Risks involved with such trends include chronic infection, prolonged bleeding, scarring, chipped teeth, abscesses or boils, and speech impediments. More serious risks include the transmission of HBV and HCV, tetanus, and even HIV.* Currently 26% of the United States have regulatory authority over body-piercing establishments, whereas only 4 states exercise such authority.† With little or no regulation and little incentive for employees in such facilities to take precautions against infections or health hazards, dental hygiene services must include prevention and education of such risks. Body-piercing and tattoo education can be implemented into any disease prevention discussion and/or protocol.

Certain practices can make body piercing and tattooing more safe, including the cleanliness of the shop and the equipment used for the procedure. Are the same universal precautions (UP) followed in dental hygiene care implemented? Practices such as wearing of disposable masks and gloves, single use of needles and subsequent proper disposal, and sterilization of every item that comes near the customer are important disease-prevention and transmission standards that should be followed in body-piercing and tattoo establishments. Follow-up instructions and care also should be emphasized. The treated area should be kept clean with soap, not alcohol, and the individual should not pick or tug at the area. If oral piercing has been done, an antibacterial mouthwash should be used after eating to reduce infection. Care should be taken to ensure healing, with close observation of any signs of infection or complication. A physician should be contacted immediately if the area becomes sore, irritated, or infected.

*Folz BJ et al: Hazards of piercing and facial body art: a report of three patients and literature review, *Ann Plast Surg* 45(4):374-81, 2000.
†Braithwaite RL, et al: Risks associated with tattooing and body piercing, *J Public Health Policy* 20(4):459-70, 1999.

Testing for HAV is done by screening for the antibody to HAV. Vaccination to prevent HAV infection is available and can provide long-term protection against the disease. An immune globulin injection can help prevent HAV infection if it is administered within 14 days of exposure for persons who have not been vaccinated or previously infected. Not all symptoms are experienced by infected persons, and in many cases children may not experience symptoms at all; adult infection usually causes severe illness that can last several months.

Hepatitis E virus

Infection with HEV shares some of the characteristics of HAV, such as a lack of a chronic phase.[48,87] Incubation is typically 2 to 9 weeks after exposure, with mild symptoms. Testing for HEV is done by laboratory screening. Immune globulin injection has not been shown to be useful in the prevention of infection after exposure, and no vaccination is currently available. HEV is seen primarily in underdeveloped countries with contaminated water supplies; outbreaks have not been observed in the United States.

Hepatitis B virus

Infection with HBV[9,27,45,87] is transmitted through blood, blood products, and/or body fluids (including saliva). HBV is the most significant hepatitis of concern in healthcare settings. Its viral life span on inanimate objects can be from 7 to 14 days, with virulence remaining high. Incubation can be from 1 to 6 months after initial exposure. Testing for HBV is done by a number of laboratory tests to detect antibodies against the HBV surface antigen (HBsAg); antibodies often appear before symptoms develop and may remain 6 months after recovery. As many as 90% of infections are subclinical cases, and a high number of these cases develop into a carrier state, with the host being contagious but not showing any clinical symptoms of disease. HBV infection and its sequela continue to be a major cause of death.

The greatest concentration of HBV intraorally is in the gingival sulcus, a common site of bleeding during many dental procedures. Past studies have shown nearly twice the prevalence of HBV among dental healthcare workers when compared with the general public.[27]

The Centers for Disease Control and Prevention (CDC) recommends that all healthcare professionals who may be exposed to bloodborne pathogens receive the HBV immunization.[21,22] This vaccine has been proven to provide effective immunity to HBV infection. OSHA requires that all workers be offered the immunization by employers before being assigned to work-related tasks that put them at risk of exposure. Studies done in the 1980s identified a decrease in the number of dental professionals naturally infected with HBV from 15% to 8% over an 8-year period, demonstrating effective protection with HBV immunization.[27]

Hepatitis C virus

Infection with HCV* is transmitted through blood, blood products, and/or body fluids. Incubation can be from 2 to 6 months after initial exposure, and many people show no symptoms at all. HCV also has become a significant concern in healthcare settings. Currently no vaccine exists.

As with HBV, subclinical cases can establish a carrier state, with the host being contagious without showing any clinical symptoms of disease. Approximately 95% of infected people show no symptoms at all.

HCV has been treated with the drug Interferon, and recently an additional combination therapy of REBERTRON,[53] containing REBETROL (Ribavirin, USP) and INTRON A (interferon alfa-2b, recombinant), injections is showing promise for treatment of chronic HCV.

Hepatitis D virus

Infection with HDV[9,47,49,87] is transmitted through blood, blood products, and/or body fluids. HDV infection is the severest form of viral hepatitis and is only acquired as a co-infection to HBV. The host first must be infected with acute or chronic HBV for HDV infection to occur.

Hepatitis G virus

Infection with HGV (also known as *HGBV-C*)[47,50] is transmitted through blood, blood products, and/or body fluids. HGV is considered a distant relative of HCV. At this

---

*References 9, 28, 46, 51, 52, 55, 88.

time HGV can be identified only through sophisticated laboratory testing. The nature or frequency of HGV infection is unclear, and uncertainty persists about risk factors and means of prevention. Transmission through blood transfusion has been documented, as has perinatal infection; other modes of transmission are possible but have not been well documented. An increased prevalence of HGV exists among people with frequent exposure to blood or blood products, and co-infection with HBV and/or HCV is common (representing similar modes of transmission). The disease state caused by HGV infection remains unclear, and no significant evidence exists that HGV infection has any important sequela; it does not seem to worsen with co-infection. No proven treatment or commercial screening tests are currently available.

In addition, a large number of other viral agents can be responsible for acute inflammatory diseases of the liver that can appear to be a hepatitis infection. The most prominent include viral agents in the herpes family, such as herpes simplex virus, cytomegalovirus, and Epstein-Barr virus.

Herpes Viruses

The eight identified types of human herpes viruses (HHV)* are (1) HHV-1 and (2) HHV-2, the herpes simplex viruses (HSV-1 and HSV-2); (3) HHV-3, varicella-zoster virus (VZV); (4) HHV-4, Epstein-Barr virus (EBV); (5) HHV-5, cytomegalovirus (CMV); (6) HHV-6, which has been associated with roseola; (7) HHV-7, the sequela for which is unknown; and (8) HHV-8, which has been associated with Kaposi's sarcoma.[61,88] HHV-1 through HHV-5 are discussed further in this chapter.

Herpetic diseases are carried by viral agents transmitted in saliva, blood, droplets, and through sexual contact; some can be acquired through respiratory exposure. The incubation period varies for each type of infection. Herpetic infections often cause recurrent diseases that are manifested by vesicular skin lesions found in the oral cavity, on the genitalia, and on surface skin.

A characteristic of viruses of this family is the ability to establish a latent state (dormant with a potential for recurrent infection) in the host cells they infect. Each such virus has been implicated in central nervous system infection, specifically meningitis and meningoencephalitis.

Herpes lesions are observed frequently in HIV-infected individuals and manifest as significant infections with painful, persistent oral lesions or asymptomatic shaggy white plaques on the tongue known as *hairy leukoplakia*. CMV and EBV have been associated with oral malignancies related to *acquired immunodeficiency syndrome (AIDS)*, CMV with Kaposi's sarcoma, and EBV with AIDS-associated lymphoma.[42]

Herpes simplex virus

HSV[9,64,94] has an affinity for epithelial cells and commonly attacks mucous membranes, skin, eyes, and the nervous system. Transmission is through contact with contaminated saliva, and the incubation period is 2 to 12 days. Transient shedding of the virus, even with a lack of symptoms, is common. Primary infection may or may not be clinically evident; 80% to 90% of primary infections are asymptomatic.

After primary infection takes place, the virus persists in the neural ganglia that innovate the site as a latent infection, with symptoms reoccurring at a later time. Between episodes of infection, HSV remains dormant in sensory ganglia. In response to stimuli, recurrent lesions appear in the initially infected area, causing a wide variety of chronically occurring diseases (see the suggested agencies and web sites [14] later in this chapter).

Infection with HSV type 1 and type 2 (HSV-1 and HSV-2) is most easily differentiated by the body sites of infection and method of transmission. Type 1 infections are most commonly noted in the oral cavity, whereas type 2 infections are generally transmitted sexually and noted on the genitalia. Both types can manifest as skin infections, such as recurrent perioral infections and herpes labialis, the most frequent manifestation.

Other manifestations of herpes infection include herpetic whitlow (most frequently developing around finger nail beds); ocular herpes/herpetic keratitis, which can be primary or recurrent (causing corneal ulcerations and/or lesions of the conjunctiva); genital infections; and neonatal infections.

Herpes simplex type 1 virus. HSV-1 is the most significant viral disease affecting the oral mucosa. Only an estimated 10% of patients infected with HSV-1 show symptoms. Primary infection of HSV-1 most commonly occurs in the mouth, usually in children between ages 6 months and 6 years. Specific caution should be exercised around children with broken skin or lesions because they are highly susceptible to infection. The majority of primary infections are subclinical, but some develop as severe gingivostomatitis. Fever and lymphadenopathy may accompany this infection. The lesions generally heal spontaneously in 1 to 2 weeks.

Herpes labialis is characterized by recurrent lesions on the lips, occasionally occurring within the oral cavity. In younger patients, lesions can be seen on the buccal mucosa, tongue, soft palate, lips, and gingiva. Lymphadenopathy in cervical and submandibular nodes is frequent with primary infection.

Herpes gingivostomatitis is characterized by the presence of vesicles and ulcerations on oral mucosa that is attached to the periosteum, such as the gingiva.

Herpetic conjunctivitis (keratitis) and ocular herpes infection are the leading cause of blindness due to corneal infections in the United States. This infection can occur alone or simultaneously with oral infection; it almost always manifests unilaterally and begins as conjunctivitis, with vesicles on the eyelids.

Herpetic whitlow is characterized by swelling, redness, and tenderness, with subsequent vesicle formation on the fingers. This infection is often seen around the cuticles and nailbeds, occurring where small breaks in the skin are present. Herpetic whitlow was more commonly documented in dental personnel (and subsequently transmitted to patients) before the universal use of gloves.

Herpes encephalitis manifests most commonly during periods of nonepidemic viral encephalitis and is caused by HSV.

Herpes simplex type 2 virus. HSV-2 manifests as herpes genitalia and is the most common genital disease in women, second only to syphilis in men. Oral lesions also

---

*References 9, 42, 59, 64, 88, 94.

can occur from HSV-2 infection (see the suggested agencies and web sites [15] later in this chapter).

Cytomegalovirus. CMV is transmitted through blood, saliva and crevicular fluids, sexual transmission, congenital means, and possibly through respiratory exposure. Incubation can range from 3 to 12 weeks. CMV has a propensity for salivary glands. The majority of the adult population has been infected with CMV, resulting in lifelong latent association in the host. Reactivation can result in severe infection in hosts with immunosuppression.

Infection may involve multiple organ systems, and acute infection may mimic infectious mononucleosis or hepatitis. The most common clinical presentation of CMV infection in the compromised individual is that of a mononucleosis-like syndrome, with the next most common syndrome being pneumonia. No effective therapy exists for the treatment of CMV pneumonitis. CMV infection can be severe in neonatal transmissions (see the suggested agencies and web sites [16] later in this chapter).

Epstein-Barr virus. EBV may be excreted into saliva during the infectious stage of mononucleosis and for weeks after infection. It is acquired primarily by oral contact, through contact with saliva, and less commonly through blood transfusion. During the incubation period, the virus can replicate in the oropharynx for 4 to 7 weeks while the individual continues to be infectious. EBV may persist in blood lymphocytes for years after infection and manifest in latent disease. Clinical symptoms include fever, pharyngitis, and cervical lymphadenopathy. EBV also has been found in the white hairy plaque on the tongue of HIV-infected persons, known as *hairy leukoplakia.*

Infectious mononucleosis is the primary EBV infection in young adults. More than 90% of adults have been exposed to EBV, and differentiation from other causes of mononucleosis is made through antibody testing (see the suggested agencies and web sites [17] later in this chapter).

Varicella-zoster virus. VZV enters the body via the respiratory tract and is transmitted by airborne water particles through sneezing and coughing and by direct contact with skin lesions. After a 2-week incubation period, cutaneous vesicles develop, a primary infection known as *chickenpox.* During primary infection, VZV migrates to the dorsal root ganglia and along sensory nerves, establishing a latent infection known as *shingles.*

Chickenpox is a viral exanthematous disease (manifested by cutaneous lesions). The incubation period is 10 to 21 days. Chickenpox is usually benign in healthy children, but in immunocompromised children the disease can be deadly. The most obvious clinical symptom is the small vesicles on the skin that go through three distinctive phases—from fluid-filled vesicles, to pustules, to dry crusted lesions—and can be found anywhere on the body, including the oral cavity (see the suggested agencies and web sites [18] later in this chapter).

Shingles is the result of latent or persistent VZV infection, established in spinal cord ganglia similar to other herpes virus infections. This recurrent infection, herpes zoster (shingles), is painful and can be severe or life-threatening (see the suggested agencies and web sites [19] later in this chapter).

Human Immunodeficiency Virus Infection and Acquired Immunodeficiency Syndrome

The HIV virus [9,14,64,94] establishes primary infection, the subsequent latent disease state is known as *acquired immunodeficiency syndrome (AIDS).*

HIV infection is transmitted by a viral agent present in the blood and body fluids of an infected host. The incubation period for HIV varies; the clinical onset of symptoms has been noted from a few weeks to several months. The severity of HIV-related diseases and the development of AIDS is directly related to the degree of immune system dysfunction. Numerous opportunistic infections and cancers can develop in the HIV-infected host; the five primary types of HIV-associated lesions are: (1) fungal (e.g., candidiasis, histoplasmosis), (2) viral (hairy leukoplakia, HSV), (3) bacterial (gingival, periodontal), (4) neoplastic (Kaposi's sarcoma, lymphoma), and (5) others (Parotitis). Co-infections may pose a greater hazard than HIV itself.

With the use of protease inhibitors in the treatment of HIV infection, a decline has been noted in the most common oral lesions associated with HIV, such as hairy leukoplakia and oral candidiasis. However, at the same time a significant increase has been noted in oral warts linked directly to the use of protease inhibitors.[66]

HIV-related diseases and AIDS include a vast number of associated opportunistic infections, and the course of disease identifies its classification. The CDC has established a classification system for HIV infection (Box 5-1; see the suggested agencies and web sites later in this chapter). This system lists the vast, clinically identified secondary infections and laboratory test factors involved in the diagnosis and management of HIV disease.

HIV disease is not considered a high-risk hazard in dentistry with appropriate use of universal precautions (UP), but it is a concern if an exposure incident does occur. Appropriate follow-up is critical (see the discussion on post-exposure management later in this chapter). Because of the extensive information on HIV and AIDS, the suggested agencies and web sites (20-22) later in this chapter should be consulted for study on HIV, AIDS, and related infections.

Measles

Rubeola[9,64,28] (hard measles) is a viral infection that was once widespread and highly communicable in children before the introduction of a vaccination. A second form of measles known as *rubella*[9,64,94] (German measles) manifests with much milder symptoms than rubeola. Transmission is airborne, through water droplets, or via direct contact with nasal and throat secretions of infected hosts. The incubation period for rubeola is 7 to 18 days and for rubella, 14 to 23 days. Symptoms include fever, conjunctivitis, cough, and Koplik's spots on the buccal mucosa, followed by a red, blotchy rash on the face that spreads to the body.

Congenital defects and death in infants both are serious complication of measles infection in pregnant women and infants. Vaccination is required in the United States for all infants, with booster shots administered to school-aged children (see the suggested agencies and web sites later in this chapter).

Respiratory Diseases

A number of respiratory diseases are acquired primarily through respiratory transmission.[9,64,94] The common cold

BOX 5-1

CDC Definitions of AIDS

CLINICAL CATEGORIES OF HIV INFECTION

CD4+ T-lymphocyte categories	Category A	Category B	Category C
Category 1 (≥500 cells/μL)	A1	B1	C1*
Category 2 (200 to 499 cells/μL)	A2	B2	C2*
Category 3 (<200 cells/μL)	A3*	B3*	C3*

Category A

One or more of the following conditions is present in an adolescent or adult† with documented HIV infection:

Asymptomatic HIV infection

Persistent generalized lymphadenopathy

Acute (primary) HIV infection with accompanying illness or history of acute HIV infection

Conditions listed in Categories B and C must not have occurred.

Category B

Symptomatic conditions in an HIV-infected adolescent or adult are present that are not included among conditions listed in clinical Category C and that meet at least one of the following criteria:

The conditions are attributed to HIV infection or indicate a defect in cell-mediated immunity.

The conditions are considered by physicians to have a clinical course or to require management complicated by HIV infection.

Examples of conditions in clinical Category B include but are not limited to the following:

Bacillary angiomatosis

Candidiasis, oropharyngeal (thrush)

Candidiasis, vulvovaginal, that is persistent, frequent, or poorly responsive to therapy

Cervical dysplasia (moderate or severe)/cervical carcinoma *in situ*

Constitutional symptoms, such as fever (38.5° C) or diarrhea lasting more than 1 month

Hairy leukoplakia, oral

Herpes zoster (shingles) involving at least two distinct episodes or more than one dermatome

Idiopathic thrombocytopenic purpura

Listeriosis

Pelvic inflammatory disease, particularly if complicated by tubo-ovarian abscess

Peripheral neuropathy

For classification purposes, Category B conditions take precedence over those in Category A. For example, an individual previously treated for oral or persistent vaginal candidiasis (and who has not developed a Category C disease) but who is now asymptomatic should be classified in clinical Category B.

Category C

The clinical conditions listed in the 1993 AIDS surveillance case definition are present.† For classification purposes, once a Category C condition has occurred, the person will remain in Category C.

Conditions include the following:

Candidiasis of bronchi, trachea, or lungs

Candidiasis, esophageal

Cervical cancer, invasive†

Coccidioidomycosis, disseminated or extrapulmonary

Cryptococcosis, extrapulmonary

Cryptosporidiosis, chronic intestinal (greater than 1 month duration)

Cytomegalovirus disease (other than liver, spleen, or nodes)

Cytomegalovirus retinitis (with loss of vision)

Encephalopathy, HIV-related

Herpes simplex: chronic ulcer(s) (greater than 1 month's duration) or bronchitis, pneumonitis, or esophagitis

Histoplasmosis, disseminated or extrapulmonary

Isosporiasis, chronic intestinal (greater than 1 month duration)

Kaposi's sarcoma

Lymphoma, Burkitt's (or equivalent term)

Lymphoma, immunoblastic (or equivalent term)

Lymphoma, primary, of brain

Mycobacterium avium complex or *M. kansasii,* disseminated or extrapulmonary

Mycobacterium tuberculosis, any site (pulmonary† or extrapulmonary)

Mycobacterium, other species or unidentified species, disseminated or extrapulmonary

Pneumocystis carinii pneumonia

Pneumonia, recurrent†

Progressive multifocal leukoencephalopathy

Salmonella septicemia, recurrent

Toxoplasmosis of brain

Wasting syndrome due to HIV

CDC, Centers for Disease Control and Prevention; *AIDS,* acquired immunodeficiency virus.

*Indicates criteria for AIDS diagnosis.

†An adolescent or adult is defined as greater than or equal to 13 years of age.

is the most frequently occurring infection worldwide. As many as 200 viruses have been linked casually to the common cold, with the most common being rhinovirus, coronavirus, myxoviruses, and adenovirus. The incubation period is 48 to 72 hours. The three primary routes of transmission are by virions suspended in droplets that are sneezed or coughed directly onto a new host; by aerosols that can remain airborne for long periods of time, being inhaled and then inoculated onto the nasal mucosa; and by direct contact and transfer through contaminated hands, with inoculation into the nose or mucosa of the eye. Colds are cited as the most common reason for absenteeism in the workplace, and transmission is promoted in crowded conditions such as school classrooms. In the United States, adults typically experience two to four colds per year, whereas children experience six per year. If acute oropharyngitis is present, a secondary infection by *Streptococcus pyogenes* can lead to rheumatic heart diseases. Pneumonia is another secondary infection with serious complications (see the suggested agencies and web sites [23] later in this chapter).

Influenza[19,20] infection (commonly known as *the flu*) is generally attributed to exposure to two primary types of viruses: influenza types A and B. Type A virus infections are the most common worldwide. The predominant mode of transmission is direct contact through airborne water droplet exposure. The virus can survive for hours in dried mucus. Incubation is short, generally 1 to 5 days. A vaccine is valuable for high-risk groups, such as the elderly, individuals with immunosuppressive diseases, and healthcare workers (see the suggested agencies and web sites [24-25] later in this chapter).

Mumps infection occurs when its virus enters through the upper respiratory tract via saliva or other secretions. The incubation period is 16 to 18 days, and the virus may be present in saliva for 6 to 7 days before clinical symptoms appear. The main clinical manifestation of mumps is inflammation of the salivary glands and clinical swelling of the parotid glands, although the virus spreads throughout the body. Mumps virus infection can be prevented by immunization (see the suggested agencies and web sites later in this chapter).

Viral pneumonia can develop as a secondary complication to any viral infection, such as colds, the flu, and lower respiratory tract infections, as well as a sequela to measles and chickenpox. Transmission factors primarily include person-to-person contact via droplet aerosols and on contaminated hands. A pneumonia vaccine is available.

Diseases Caused by Bacterial Agents

The diseases discussed in the following sections are caused by infection with bacterial agents (see the suggested agencies and web sites [26] later in this chapter). [9,64,94]

Gonorrhea
Gonorrhea is an infection caused by the species *Neisseria gonorrhea*. Transmission is through contact with exudates from mucous membranes of infected persons and almost always results from sexual activity with an infected individual. Gonorrhea can be infectious for months in untreated asymptomatic individuals, with an incubation period of 2 to 7 days (see the suggested agencies and web sites [27] later in this chapter).

Legionella
Legionella species[5,9,24] manifest as two distinct acute bacterial infections: legionnaires' disease and Pontiac fever. Several strains of the causative agent, *Legionella* species, have been identified. Transmission is usually airborne from aerosol-producing devices and air-conditioning units. Person-to-person transmission has not been documented. The incubation period is 2 to 10 days for legionnaires' disease and 24 to 48 hours for Pontiac fever (see the suggested agencies and web sites [28] later in this chapter).

Bacterial Pneumonia
Bacterial pneumonia can follow acute lower respiratory tract infection with *Streptococcus pneumoniae*. Several other bacterial agents (including oral bacteria) also have been implicated in pneumonia infections. The most common types of infection vary between adults and children. Transmission is spread through airborne water droplet or direct oral contact, or indirectly from articles freshly soiled with respiratory discharges. Incubation for bacterial pneumonia may be as short as 1 to 3 days. Infection is characterized by a sudden onset of chills and fever. Pneumonia is a serious secondary illness and a noted cause of death in infants, the elderly, and immunocompromised persons.

Staphylococcus *Infections*
Staphylococcus microorganisms[80], such as *S. aureus* and *S. epidermidis*, are part of the normal resident flora of the body for many individuals. As much as 50% of the population harbors the organisms in the nose, with higher percentages noted for hospital personnel. *S. aureus* is a major cause of nosocomial and community-acquired infections and manifests in a number of ways, including skin infections such as impetigo and gastrointestinal tract infection that cause vomiting and diarrhea; *S. aureus* also is responsible for the acute febrile disease infection known as *toxic shock syndrome*.

Autoinfection is responsible for at least one third of infections, with draining lesions and purulent discharge being the most common sources of epidemic spread. Transmission is by contact with a person who either has lesions or is asymptomatic (harboring pathogenic strains in the anterior nasal passages). The hands are the most important vehicle of transmission. The incubation period is most commonly is 4 to 10 days but varies and can be indefinite. Staphylococcus is communicable as long as lesions continue to drain or a carrier state persists, and autoinfection may continue during the period of nasal colonization or throughout the duration of active lesions.

Many *S. aureus* infections today do not respond to common antibiotic treatment due to the emergence of resistant strains. As many as 80% of *S. aureus* strains are resistant to penicillin. Such resistant strains have developed to most aggressive types of antibiotics available, such as methicillin and vancomycin. These strains pose serious challenge for healthcare providers (see the suggested agencies and web sites [29-30] later in this chapter).

Streptococcus *Infections*
Streptococcus infections are caused by bacterial agents: group A (*S. pyogenes*) and group B (*S. agalactiae*) streptococcus. Group A is the causative agent for a variety of diseases (such as sore throat, scarlet fever, and impetigo), whereas group B is responsible for two distinct and serious forms of infections in newborn infants. The primary mode of transmission is via direct or intimate contact with carriers. Microorganisms harbored in the nasal passage are particularly likely to transmit infection. *Streptococcus* infections are rarely transmitted by indirect contact with objects or hands, and casual contact rarely leads to infection. The incubation period is short, usually 1 to 3 days, whereas the infectious period lasts for 10 to 21 days in simple cases. More aggressive cases that include purulent discharge can remain infectious for weeks. Bacteria may be present on the skin 1 to 2 weeks before the development of impetigo lesions (see the suggested agencies and web sites [31-32] later in this chapter).

Syphilis

Syphilis is caused by the bacterial agent *Treponema pallidum*. Transmission is through direct contact with infectious exudates from obvious or concealed moist lesions of skin and mucous membranes, body fluids, and secretions (saliva, semen, blood, vaginal discharge) of infected persons during sexual contact. Transmission can occur through blood transfusion if the donor is in the early stages of infection. The incubation period is 10 days to 3 months, with the individual being infectious indefinitely; latent infection is expected (see the suggested agencies and web sites [33-34] later in this chapter).

Tetanus

Tetanus is an infection at the site of an open wound injury induced by the tetanus bacillus *(Clostridium tetani)*. Tetanus is usually transmitted through puncture wounds contaminated by soil, dust, or feces. The presence of necrotic tissue or foreign bodies supports the growth of this anaerobic pathogen. The incubation period for tetanus is 3 to 21 days. Highly contaminated wounds may develop infection more rapidly, with more severe symptoms and a very poor prognosis. Tetanus infection can be prevented with a tetanus immunization, the effects of which last about 10 years. Booster shots are recommended at 10-year intervals or after a contaminated injury.

Tuberculosis

Tuberculosis (TB)* is an infection acquired by respiratory exposure to *Mycobacterium tuberculosis*. TB is spread through airborne droplet nuclei, escaping the source during oropharyngeal activities such as coughing, sneezing, and singing and can remain airborne for some time. The incubation period for TB is 4 to 12 weeks from infection to primary lesions or a significant tuberculin test reaction. Clinical illness most commonly develops within 6 to 12 months of infection. Symptoms of pulmonary tuberculosis include a persistent cough, fever, night sweats, fatigue, and loss of appetite. Pulmonary tuberculosis is much more common than extrapulmonary disease, affecting structures such as the lymph nodes, skin, kidney, bones, and joints.

Healthcare employees exposed to acute cases of infection or having repeated, long-term exposure through day-to-day, close contact with an active carrier are at particular risk for developing TB. Over time, TB is walled off in the body and considered inactive. During latent disease, if the host immune system is compromised, TB can reactivate and shed the infectious agent again. A positive skin test does not indicate that the host is infectious but rather that the individual has been infected at some time. A positive TB skin test can result even with inactive, latent infection.

Strict guidelines to reduce exposure to and infection from TB are required by the CDC and OSHA. These guidelines and requirements are applied as indicated based on the frequency of exposure and the number of cases present geographically. They are more commonly applied in medical healthcare facilities but may be applied in dental facilities if the risk of significant exposure is present. Most dental facilities fall into the "minimal" to "very low" risk categories (see the suggested agencies and web sites [35-39] later in this chapter).

Diseases Caused by Fungal Agents

Other diseases are caused by infection with fungal agents, one of which is described in the following section (see the suggested agencies and web sites later in this chapter).[9,64,94]

Candidiasis

The fungal agent *Candida albicans*, which is often part of the normal oral flora, causes candidiasis. Transmission is through contact with secretions of the mouth, skin, and feces of an infected host and from mother to infant during childbirth. Candidiasis, also known as *thrush*, is a common oral condition in newborns. The incubation period is 2 to 5 days in infants but otherwise varies. Candidiasis is communicable while lesions are present. Clinical infection usually occurs when host immune defenses are low, such as in immunocompromised states. Infection usually is confined to superficial layers of the skin and mucous membranes, manifesting clinically as oral thrush. Candidiasis also may present as ulcerations or pseudomembranes in the esophagus and gastrointestinal tract (see the suggested agencies and web sites later in this chapter).

GOVERNMENT AGENCIES: REGULATIONS, STANDARDS, AND GUIDELINES

Due to the diverse nature of the practice of dentistry, several federal, state, and local agencies contribute to the regulations, standards, guidelines, and practices that affect the dental workplace. To integrate the recommendations and requirements of each with the concepts of basic science and microbiology, an understanding of the individual focus of these agencies is important.

Regulatory Terminology

Defining the nature of the authority and impact of each agency or organization is important to compliance with the expectations of each. The following terminology should help explain the intent of the documents and authority of each agency:

Regulations are governmental orders carrying the force of law.

Standards indicate an expectation of compliance with a level of requirement.

Guidelines are policies or rules intended to give practical guidance.

Recommendations are intended to give advice or counsel.

(NOTE: The terms *regulations* and *standards* are often interchanged, as are *guidelines* and *recommendations*, in discussions of the provisions of governing agencies.)

Centers for Disease Control and Prevention

The *Centers for Disease Control and Prevention (CDC)* is a federal agency that studies and monitors the etiology and epidemiology of diseases worldwide. The CDC issues guidelines recommending procedures for the control of

---

*References 6, 8, 15, 16, 19, 29, 30, 31, 32, 33, 34, 93.

disease transmission for public health,[22] including immunization recommendations, infection control and injury prevention, and postinjury or postexposure (PE) protocols (see the suggested agencies and web sites [53-54] later in the chapter). The CDC only issues guidelines; it is not considered an enforcement agency but is the primary source of scientific evidence on which specific standards for healthcare issues are based (see the suggested agencies and web sites [40] later in the chapter).

Occupational Safety and Health Administration

The *Occupational Safety and Health Administration (OSHA)* is a division of the U.S. Department of Labor. OSHA's purpose is to ensure the protection of employee safety through the enforcement of standards or regulations. It exercises federal regulatory authority for compliance by employers. The development and enforcement of standards for healthcare employees are based on CDC recommendations and guidelines.

OSHA standards[76] protect each employee's right to a safe workplace, including practices that help reduce exposure to bloodborne pathogens, provision and maintenance of proper personal protection, rules for the handling of any item contaminated with body fluids and potentially infectious agents, instruction in the proper use and storage of chemical products, and the requirement that an employee be informed of the hazardous nature and all risks inherent to a work assignment. Each employer must ensure that infection control and workplace safety is implemented and monitored (see the suggested agencies and web sites [41] later in the chapter).

DHCPs must remain current with proposed OSHA regulations and revisions that may affect dentistry. Of significant concern are upcoming revisions and final standards in the areas of indoor air quality, use of new engineering controls (stressing the use of devices for the management of contaminated needles and other sharp instruments), and ergonomics. Directives in each of these areas will have a direct impact in dentistry (see the suggested agencies and web sites [41: *Directives*] later in the chapter).

Environmental Protection Agency

The *Environmental Protection Agency (EPA)* is a federal organization responsible for regulating the use and disposal of products and waste that may adversely affect the environment. The EPA can provide information on the classification of chemical agents used in dentistry to help DHCPs select appropriate products for each specific task, such as when to use high- or intermediate-level disinfectants. It can also help interpret manufacturer labeling and label claims for the proper use and handling of a product. All chemical products used for disinfection, sterilization, and/or decontamination must be registered with the EPA. (NOTE: Some products require EPA and/or FDA [Food and Drug Administration] registrations, considerations that should be noted in product selection.)

For many states the EPA is the primary authority on acceptable disposal of medical, infectious, hazardous, and toxic wastes. Each state and/or local government may have primary jurisdiction over waste disposal. Knowing all the agencies with regulatory authority in the area in which a workplace is located is necessary. The most stringent regulations must be applied. Even in states with their own regulations on hazardous waste, the EPA can take precedence if its regulations are more stringent or if the waste causes environmental contamination.

The *Resource Conservation and Recovery Act (RCRA)* designates the generator of the waste as ultimately responsible, no matter where the waste ends up (with or without knowledge). This party must pay for the cleanup costs for any improper disposal of hazardous waste, a concept known as *cradle to grave liability* that is meant to ensure the appropriate disposal of the waste generated (see the suggested agencies and web sites [41] later in the chapter).

Food and Drug Administration

The U.S. *Food and Drug Administration (FDA)* regulates products and equipment that affect living tissue—by ingestion, contact, inhalation, or exposure—including chemical products, drugs, food, medical devices, and accessories to medical devices (e.g., sterilizers, radiology equipment, gloves used for medical care). The FDA has established an infection control devices branch to deal specifically with the numerous infection control items at use in the healthcare industry. The FDA reviews all safety and efficacy data submitted by the manufacturer before granting permission to market a product. The FDA has consumer, radiation safety and hygiene, and quality assurance information available upon request.

The Safe Medical Devices Act of 1990 (SMDA) is a law that places significant reporting requirements on the medical device industry and users of such devices. SMDA requires that device user facilities and distributors, as well as manufacturers of medical devices, report certain device-related problems to the FDA (see the suggested agencies and web sites [43] later in the chapter).

State Agencies

Individual state agencies may mandate aspects of infection control policy and practices in dentistry, such as state-based OSHA plans, licensing boards, dental quality assurance commissions, and/or state public health departments. An even greater number of states regulate the disposal of infectious and/or hazardous medical waste through state EPA offices, local boards of health, and public health departments. In some cases such guidelines may be more stringent than the federal regulations and current professional standards or guidelines.

Local authorities also may place limits on the disposal of medical waste and waste water, particularly if the town is served by septic systems or if the current municipal facilities are affected. Any and all agencies concerned with medical waste should be contacted and their regulations reviewed before any decision on a waste hauling and disposal is made.

Professional Associations

A number of professional associations representing medicine, dentistry, science, health care, and education help set of standards of care, regulations, education, and training in infection control. They serve as resources for healthcare professionals and include but are not limited to the following:

- *Organization for Safety and Asepsis Procedures (OSAP)* is dedicated to the establishment, implementation, and maintenance of scientifically valid and reliable standards for infection control. OSAP is a unique organization of practitioners, educators, and industry members who come together on many levels to share ideas and information promoting sound policies, practices, and technology for infection control (see the suggested agencies and web sites [44] later in the chapter).
- *Association for Professionals in Infection Control and Epidemiology (APIC)* is a multidisciplinary voluntary international organization designed to influence, support, and improve the quality of health care through the practice and management of infection control and the application of epidemiology in all healthcare settings (see the suggested agencies and web sites [45] later in the chapter).
- *American Dental Association (ADA)* takes an active role in setting standards of care and interpreting external regulations for dentistry. Although the ADA affects professional guidelines regarding the prudent and safe practice of dentistry, it does not have any direct regulatory authority. However, DHCPs are expected to follow these basic standards for patient care based on CDC-published guidelines and OSHA standards (see the suggested agencies and web sites [46] later in the chapter).
- *American Dental Education Association (ADEA)* is the leading national organization for dental education. Members include all U.S. and Canadian dental schools, advanced dental education programs, hospital dental education programs, allied dental education programs, corporations, faculty, and students. ADEA's mission is to lead the dental education community in addressing the contemporary issues influencing education, research, and public health. Included in this commitment is the development of curriculum guidelines for dental education regarding infection control[37,79] (see the suggested agencies and web sites [47] later in the chapter).

State and Local Professional Associations and Societies

Local professional associations for dental hygiene, dental, dental assisting, dental laboratory technology, and denturist professionals can be excellent resources for specific state and local regulations. These organizations have affiliations with many of the national associations previously discussed.

REGULATORY TERMINOLOGY AND EXPLANATIONS

Over the past decade new terminology has been applied in the field of infection control. This terminology is defined in federal standards set by OSHA for occupational exposure to bloodborne pathogens. The primary concept, *exposure control,* incorporates the basic science and concepts of infection control, with a focus on prevention of initial exposure to bloodborne pathogens and the transmission of infectious disease. The term *exposure control* is com-

monly interchanged with *infection control,* but readers should understand that exposure control is a primary goal of infection control.

Glossary of OSHA Terms

To help integrate OSHA's standard for exposure control with the basic principles of dental infection control, the following OSHA definitions from the *OSHA Bloodborne Pathogens Standard, Section 29 CFR 1910.1030*[76] are applied (see the suggested agencies and web sites [41] later in the chapter):

Blood means human blood, human blood components, and products made from human blood.

Bloodborne pathogens refers pathogenic microorganisms present in human blood and capable of causing disease in humans. These pathogens include but are not limited to HBV and HIV.

Contaminated is the presence or the reasonably anticipated presence of blood or other potentially infectious material on an item or surface.

Contaminated sharps are any contaminated objects that can penetrate the skin, including but not limited to needles, scalpels, broken glass, broken capillary tubes, and exposed ends of dental wires.

Decontamination refers to the use of physical or chemical means to remove, inactivate, or destroy bloodborne pathogens on a surface or item to the point at which they are no longer capable of transmitting infectious particles and the surface or item is rendered safe for handling, use, or disposal.

Exposure incident is a specific eye, mouth, other mucous membrane, nonintact skin, or parenteral contact with blood or another potentially infectious material that results from the performance of an employee's duties.

Hand-washing facilities are those places providing an adequate supply of running potable water, soap, and single-use towels or hot–air-drying machines.

Hazard abatement involves those policies, procedures, and pieces of equipment that reduce the risk of occupational exposures to bloodborne disease. OSHA's standard to reduce employee exposure to bloodborne pathogens includes the following eight primary categories of control:

1. *Universal precautions (UP)* is an approach to infection control that treats all human blood and certain human body fluids as if they are known to be infectious for HIV, HBV, and other bloodborne pathogens and all material as if it is potentially infectious with a bloodborne pathogen.

2. *Personal protective equipment (PPE)* describes specialized clothing or equipment worn by an employee for protection against a hazard. General work clothes, not intended to function as protection against a hazard, are not considered PPE. In oral health care, PPE refers to those barriers that protect the employee from exposure to infectious/potentially infectious or hazardous materials.

3. *Work practice controls (WPC)* are those controls that reduce the likelihood of exposure by altering the manner in which a task is performed. Methods of performing a task (actions and behaviors) that reduce the chance of an exposure incident are WPCs. They ensure that a task is performed in the safest way possible.

4. *Engineering controls (EC)* are controls that isolate or remove the bloodborne pathogens hazard from the workplace and may involve an actual device or the method of use of the available technology. The purpose of ECs is to reduce the risk by confining or isolating infectious materials, and they must be examined and maintained or replaced regularly to ensure effectiveness.

5. *Housekeeping* ensures that the workplace is maintained in a clean and sanitary condition. The employer shall determine and implement a written schedule for cleaning, including the methods/procedures/tasks to be performed and the materials/products to be used.

6. *Signs and labels* are those symbols used to identify an immediate or recognized hazard, such as the universal biohazard label/symbol, chemical hazard information, fire hazard and evacuation signs, and others.

7. *Record keeping* includes a number of documents that must be kept to verify employment practices and training, such as employee medical records kept for the duration of employment plus 30 years, including immunization records and injury and incident records; training records kept for 3 years; informed refusal/declination records of HBV immunization/ vaccination and other specified/indicated immunizations; postexposure evaluation and follow-up records, including the informed refusal/declination of postexposure follow-up; and material safety data sheets (MSDS), which are part of the OSHA hazards communication standard, not the bloodborne pathogen standard.

8. *Information and training* refers to the requirement that all employees with occupational exposure participate in a training program provided at no cost to the employee during working hours.

Occupational exposure describes reasonably anticipated skin, eye, mucous membrane, or parenteral contact with blood or other potentially infectious material that may result from the performance of an employee's duties.

Other potentially infectious materials (OPIM) refers to the following:

1. Semen, vaginal secretions, cerebrospinal fluid, synovial fluid, pleural fluid, pericardial fluid, peritoneal fluid, amniotic fluid, saliva in dental procedures, any fluid visibly contaminated with blood, and all body fluids in situations in which differentiation among body fluids is difficult or impossible

2. Any unfixed tissue or organ (other than intact skin) from a human (living or dead)

3. HIV-containing cell or tissue cultures, organ cultures, and HIV- or HBV-containing culture medium or other solutions, as well as blood, organs, or other tissues from experimental animals infected with HIV or HBV

Parenteral refers to piercing of mucous membranes or the skin barrier through needle sticks, human bites, cuts, and abrasions.

Regulated waste is liquid or semiliquid blood or other potentially infectious materials; contaminated items that would release blood or other potentially infectious materials in a liquid or semiliquid state if compressed, items caked with dried blood or other potentially infectious materials that are capable of releasing these materials during handling, contaminated sharps, and pathological and microbiological wastes containing blood or other potentially infectious materials.

Source individual means any individual, living or dead, whose blood or other potentially infectious materials may be a source of occupational exposure.

Other Related Terminology

To further understand the application of basic infection control language, the following terminology is applied:

Infection control policy (ICP) describes the written directive for infection control efforts and implementation of individual exposure control procedures to reduce or eliminate hazards to which students, employees, and patients may be exposed by direct or indirect contact with infectious body fluids.

Exposure control plan (ECP) is the written statement of specific procedures and tasks to be performed for the prevention of initial exposure to biohazardous materials and substances. The ultimate goal of exposure control is to prevent any exposure, therefore eliminating the *initial* transmission of infectious agents that can lead to subsequent infection.

Standard operating procedures (SOP) are the documented practices to be followed during the performance of any risk-related task or procedure.

Performance-based (or procedural-based) involves consideration of the actions and consequences involved in the performance of a task or procedure, in contrast to choices based on beliefs or presumptions about patient risk factors related to disease transmission.

TECHNIQUES, PROCEDURES, AND SUPPORTIVE EVIDENCE

The basis of a good infection control program is effective implementation of appropriate SOP, which integrates a number of safety concepts recommended by governing agencies such as the CDC[22] and OSHA.[76] These concepts include the eight (previously defined) OSHA primary hazard abatement strategies to reduce the risk of occupational exposures to bloodborne disease: (1) UP, (2) PPE, (3) WPCs, (4) ECs, (5) Housekeeping, (6) Signs and labels, (7) Record keeping, and (8) Information and training.

GOAL OF AN INFECTION CONTROL PROGRAM

The ultimate goal of an ECP is to eliminate cross-contamination and potential exposure to pathogenic microorganisms for patients and DHCPs during the provision of dental care. Infection control is an outcome of exposure control; through the reduction of exposure to infectious agents few infections should occur. To achieve this goal, both the DHCP and the patient must be aware of the potential risks associated with delivery and receipt of oral healthcare services and accompanying procedures used to significantly reduce these risks.

The primary focus of all exposure control procedures is to prevent or reduce the risk of exposure to infectious agents and minimize the risk of infection from any exposure that does occur during routine tasks. Box 5-2 outlines the steps used to accomplish prevention and reduction.

PUTTING HAZARD ABATEMENT AND STANDARD OPERATING PROCEDURES TO WORK

Integrating science with regulatory demands is necessary for effective implementation of safe work practices and SOP, requiring careful consideration of basic science, disease transmission and infection, and the actual risks for infection.[22,65,76] Many infection control measures protect the health of both patients and DHCPs, including the use of PPE (e.g., protective eyewear, gloves, face masks for the DHCP and protective eyewear for patients), WPC, and EC (e.g., environmental surface decontamination and/or barriers to prevent cross-contamination), and the use of disposable and/or sterilizable reusable items for all procedures in the oral cavity. All these SOP address the various OSHA hazard abatement strategies (see the suggested agencies and web sites later in the chapter).

Assessing the potential for disease transmission throughout the workplace is essential and should be followed by the development of SOP to meet the needs of each workplace. Examples of SOP for dentistry can be acquired from sources such as the CDC *(Recommended Infection Control Practices for Dentistry*[21] and *Practical Infection Control in the Dental Office: A Workbook for the Dental Team*[92]*)* and OSAP *(OSAP Infection Control In Dentistry Guidelines*[65]*)*. (See the suggested agencies and web sites [40, 44, 45] later in the chapter.)

 Universal or Standard Precautions

5-A Given the limitations of routine health history information, the DHCP cannot be certain of the health status of each patient. The DHCP cannot assume that a lack of disease history and clinical findings indicates that the patient is presently free of infectious disease or will remain so on subsequent clinical visits. Many individuals are unaware that they are infected with a disease and that their blood or saliva may be capable of transmitting certain infectious diseases. The infection currently may be subclinical while the individual is contagious, even when that person is asymptomatic (without symptoms), as with chronic carriers of HBV or HCV. Individuals may be unaware of their exposure and may transmit disease or withhold information about the existence of a transmissible disease or condition due to embarrassment, privacy, or discrimination concerns.

Ultimately the DHCP is responsible for the delivery of services in a manner that ensures appropriate care is rendered in the safest way possible, regardless of the health status of the patient. This standard applies not only to direct patient care procedures, but also to those procedures performed as support and routine maintenance for patient care.

In applying SP, the DHCP must assume that every direct contact with body fluids or items that may be potentially infectious is capable of transmitting infection and requires protection and procedures as though such body fluids were infected with HBV or HIV. As previously stated, the goal is to approach each situation as if a risk is known and routinely and comprehensively apply each hazard abatement strategy. This philosophy or approach should be applied to all aspects of dental care and should serve as an example of WPCs intended to meet OSHA requirements (Fig. 5-4).

Host Immunity and Immunizations

One approach to UP is not only to protect the individual from exposure but also to actually increase host resistance to infectious diseases in case an exposure occurs,[9] as in the following examples:
* *Natural immunity.* This type of immunity occurs when an individual is exposed to a disease-producing pathogen that stimulates the immune system to produce

---

BOX 5-2

Steps to Reduce Risk of Exposure and Minimize Risk of Infection

Strive to reduce the number of pathogenic microorganisms present, eliminate cross-contamination, and stop the spread of infection. When primary exposure levels are reduced, the body's normal resistance mechanisms should prevent infection.

Help increase host resistance. Following published immunization protocols for healthcare employees is important.

Treat each potential exposure situation as though disease transmission can occur and take appropriate measures to alter the situation to reduce the risk of exposure. Treat all patients as if they were carriers of an infectious disease, applying universal precautions.

Implement and follow practices that are intended to protect patients, DHCPs, and their families from infection and the subsequent impact of income loss and possible liability.

DHCP, Dental healthcare professional.

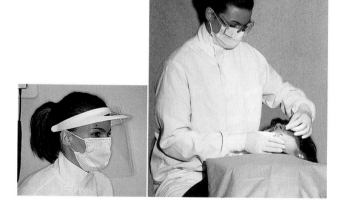

A   **B**

FIG. 5-4 Examples of good personal protective equipment (PPE) and environmental barriers. Well-fitting mask **(A)** and operator with safety glasses, gloves over cuffs, mask, and protective laboratory coat **(B).**

specific antibodies to that pathogen. If this process is successful, the pathogen is destroyed by the host immune system or suppressed to a minor or subclinical state. Once the infection resolves, antibodies remain present in the body and continue to suppress or destroy dormant organisms in the host system. If the individual is exposed to or infected by the same pathogen again, these antibodies are again stimulated. Numerous childhood diseases stimulate natural immunity to the invading pathogen, such as rubella (German measles), mumps, rubeola, and chickenpox.

Another pathogen that stimulates natural immunity is HAV. However, HBV infection may produce natural immunity, or the immune system response may be unsuccessful in destroying the virus, in which case a chronic carrier state may develop. In this state the host continues to be infectious. Natural immunity may last a lifetime, provided the immune system is not injured or suppressed.

- *Artificial or active immunity.* This type of immunity is produced by the introduction of vaccines and immunizations that exogenously stimulate the immune system to produce specific antibodies without the individual actually having the disease. Artificially stimulated immunity may last a lifetime, or a booster dose of the vaccine may be necessary to maintain ongoing protection (such as with childhood immunizations for measles, mumps, and rubella).
- *Passive immunity.* This type of immunity develops in infants from the antibodies passed from the mother. The protection is temporary, and when the antibodies are shed from the infant's system, immunization is required to stimulate artificial immunity.

Recommendations for Immunizations
All DHCP who have contact with patients or materials that are potentially infectious should receive HBV immunization or show evidence of immunity from previous a vaccination or actual infection. OSHA requires that this immunization be offered for free to each "at-risk" employee. Additionally, DHCPs should remain current on immunizations and health screenings as recommenced by the CDC (Box 5-3; see the suggested agencies and web sites [48] later in the chapter), including vaccination for HBV, tetanus and diphtheria (DPT); measles (rubeola), mumps, and rubella (MMR); poliomyelitis, pneumonia, and annual influenza, as well as testing for exposure to TB with a purified protein derivative (PPD) tuberculin skin test.[13,21]

Restricting Healthcare Employee Duties during Illness
Taking care of their own health while reducing the risk of exposure to the patient is also an important aspect of the DHCP's exposure control. Healthcare professionals at times should withdraw from direct patient contact and indirect-contact activities when exhibiting symptoms of some infectious diseases (see Box 5-5 and the suggested agencies and web sites later in the chapter). This concept involves but is not limited to the following conditions: chickenpox, conjunctivitis, CMV, diarrhea diseases (acute stage), HAV, HBV, HCV, herpes simplex (orofacial, whitlow), measles, meningococcal infections, rubella, shingles, *S. aureus* infections, active streptococcal group A infections, TB (active), and viral respiratory infections.

Each situation should be assessed to determine the nature of contact for activities such as direct patient procedures, tasks in treatment areas, instruments and/or cleaning procedures, and avoidance or modification of work assignments to meet the best interests of all parties.

Patient Health History
The first step in any dental appointment is a review of the patient health history (HHx), an important tool used to determine any conditions that may require modifications in infection control products or procedures. Patients with health problems such as iodine allergies, alcohol sensitivity, and latex allergies require modifications to standard infection control procedures that use products containing iodine, alcohol, or latex materials, such as iodophor disinfectants, preprocedural mouthrinses containing alcohol, and the use of any items made from latex (including but *not* limited to rubber dams, rubber polishing cups, nitrous nose hoods, and gloves).

Important to note is that the HHx is *not* a tool for use to screen patients as "infectious disease risks" or to justify increases in infection control measures; such practices are both unethical and illegal. Screening patients as possible infectious disease carriers is acceptable only as it relates to the prescription of appropriate treatment, when necessary during postexposure management (if an exposure incident does occur involving that patient), and in the identification of concerns for modification of procedures.

The HHx, combined with a thorough oral assessment, may indicate the need for referral to another appropriate healthcare provider for differential diagnosis of an infectious disease. Such a referral does not mean that the individual is referred for oral health care elsewhere because that individual is "infected" but that the person's present state of health must be determined so that appropriate treatment can be administered.

A critical note is that HHx information is a confidential document requiring informed consent of the patient before the disclosure of any information to other parties. Specific state laws on patient/medical confidentiality should be consulted.

Extraoral and Intraoral Examination
A comprehensive patient examination often identifies lesions associated with systemic disease; such information is important for appropriate treatment and management of overall patient health.

Personal Hygiene and Appearance
All individuals with patient contact should adhere to high standards of personal hygiene, dressing in a clean, professional manner appropriate for the tasks performed. These expectations may vary among different workplaces, but some basic principles should be followed universally. Although these issues may seem obvious, attention to the basics of healthcare delivery is necessary as a foundation for the appropriate use of required personal protective equipment and sound infection control practices.

Hair
Hair should be kept off the face and should not touch the patient, instruments, or work surfaces. Decorative hair

---

BOX 5-3

Recommendations for Immunizations for Children, Adults, and Healthcare Workers

The following agencies endorse and contribute to recommendations:

Recommendations of the Immunization Practices Advisory Committee (ACIP)

Centers for Disease Control and Prevention (CDC)

United States Public Health Service (USPH)

U.S. Department of Health and Human Services

Immunization and booster dose recommendations for both children and adults are available from the Centers for Disease Control and Prevention (CDC), national Advisory Council for Recommended Immunization Practices (ACIP), and are included in the following list.

Basic Immunizations

Childhood

Measles (rubeola), mumps, and rubella (German measles) (MMR)

Oral polio vaccine (OPV)

Tetanus-diphtheria (Td)

Hepatitis B (HBV)

Adult

Update of childhood immunizations

Influenza

Healthcare employee

Update of childhood immunizations

HBV immunization

PPD/Mantoux screening for tuberculosis

Further Explanations

Childhood immunizations

MMR is provided during childhood and may require booster doses based on periodic titer tests of the antibody levels. Current booster doses are recommended at 10-year intervals or more often when medically indicated.

OPV provides immunization against polio viruses 1, 2, and 3.

Td is a childhood immunization with a recommended 10-year booster.

HBV immunization should begin within 2 months of birth. It is one of the most recent childhood recommendations, and booster dose recommendations will be determined over time by the CDC.

Adult immunizations

Update of childhood immunizations: as recommended by the CDC and as medically indicated

Influenza: annual influenza-type immunization (based on current strain of concern)

Healthcare worker

Update of childhood immunizations and booster doses as necessary; inactivated polio vaccine (IV) for adults older than 18 years who did not receive the OPT as children. This immunization should be provided with the consultation of a physician.

HBV immunization is recommended by the CDC and required by the Occupational Safety and Health Administration (OSHA). OSHA requires that HBV immunization be offered to all employees with occupational exposure to blood or other body fluids that may harbor bloodborne pathogens within 10 working days of the initial assignment unless the individual is already immune due to natural immunity or through previous immunization. The employee may decline the immunization/vaccine once educated about the risks associated with HBV and the efficacy, safety, and risks of the vaccine. In such cases the employee must sign a standardized HBV vaccine declination form but may opt to have the vaccine later, at which time the vaccine must be offered by the employer at no charge to the employee. The declination form is available from OSHA.

Titer testing 1 to 6 months after the last dose of vaccine is not universally recommended by the United States Public Health Service (USPHS), nor is it currently required by OSHA because the vaccine is so successful in producing immunity and the titer test is not considered cost-effective. However, the postvaccine titer test provides evidence that immunity has been achieved, which may be important to the individual who may wish to assume responsibility for the laboratory costs of the titer test.

The titer test is required in the event of postexposure follow-up. In addition, it may be of individual value to confirm that immunity has developed. If an individual does not respond to the vaccine series, another dose or entire series of the vaccine may be required to achieve immunity. If after a second series immunity has not been achieved, the individual should seek the advice of an infectious disease specialist.

PPD/Mantoux screening for tuberculosis bacterium should be performed annually or more often for individuals who work with an at-risk population. The screening is *not* an immunization.

For special modifications in certain circumstances, consult the following source:

Guideline for infection control in healthcare personnel, 1998, *Am J Infect Control* 26(3):289-354, 1998.

or

http://www.us.elsevierhealth.com (Select *periodicals,* then *find journal by name,* then *American Journal of Infection Control,* then *browse,* then *June 1998, v.26. No 3,* then *special article,* and finally type in the title of the previous citation.)

IV, Inactive vaccine; *OPT,* oral polio immunization.

---

accessories can become contaminated by aerosols from procedures and considered inappropriate. Facial hair also is easily contaminated by aerosols from procedures and should be covered by a face mask or shield.

Personal jewelry

Personal jewelry (e.g., rings, watches, earrings, decorative pins) should not be worn during work. Such pieces are contaminated easily by direct contact and aerosols, harbor higher levels of bacteria than does skin, and are difficult to clean.[58] Total bacterial counts are higher when rings are worn, and such jewelry can cause damage to gloves, leaving small breaks in the barrier protection. In addition, microorganisms can be carried home on these items.

Hand care

Hand care is important for healthcare workers.[58,65,70] The skin of the hands and surrounding tissue should be healthy and free of inflammation. The skin is the primary physical barrier against entry of microorganisms into the body and at the same time can be a primary vehicle for

TABLE 5-5

Suggested work restrictions for healthcare personnel*

Disease/infection	Suggested restriction	Duration of restriction
Conjunctivitis	From patient contact and patient environment	Until lesions dry and crust
Cytomegalovirus	None	—
Diarrhea diseases, acute stage	From patient contact and patient environment	Until symptoms resolve
Hepatitis A	From patient contact and patient environment	Until 7 days after onset of jaundice
Hepatitis B (surface antigenemia)	None; refer to state regulations	
Hepatitis C	None[1]	Unresolved
Herpes simplex, orofacial	Evaluate need to restrict from care of patients at high risk.	
Herpes simplex, whitlow	From patient contact and patient environment	Until lesions heal
Measles (active)	Exclusion from duty	Until 7 days after rash appears
Meningococcal infection	Exclusion from duty	Until 24 hours after start of effective therapy
Rubella (active)	Exclusion from duty	Until 5 days after rash appears
Staphylococcus aureus, active	From patient contact and patient environment	Until lesions have resolved
Streptococci group A	From patient contact and patient environment	Until 24 hours after adequate treatment started
Tuberculosis (active)	Exclusion from duty	Until proved noninfectious
Varicella (active)	Exclusion from duty	Until lesions dry and crust
Viral respiratory infection, acute febrile	Consider excluding from the care of patients with high risk and patient environment[2]	Until acute symptoms resolve
Zoster (shingles)		
Localized	Restrict from patients at high risk; cover lesions[3]	Until all lesions dry and crust
Generalized	Restrict from patient contact	

Adapted from Kohn WG, Collins AS, Cleveland JL, et al: Guidelines for infection control in dental healthcare settings, *MMWR,* Dec. 19, 2003, 52 (RR-17); and Bolyard EA: Hospital infection control practices advisory committee. Guidelines for infection control in health care personnel, *Am J Infect Control* 26:289-354, 1998.
*Modified from recommendations of the Advisory Committee on Immunization Practices (ACIP).
1. Unless epidemiologically linked to transmission of infection.
2. Patients at high risk as defined by ACIP.
3. Those susceptible to and at increased risk of varicella.

transmission of infections acquired from microorganisms on the hands. DHCPs *must* take care of their hands and skin to maintain the natural protective function for the health of both themselves and their patients.

Nails. Nails should be kept clean and short, making cleaning of the hands easier. Nails are known to harbor higher levels of bacteria than skin, and long nails are more difficult to clean and may penetrate gloves, creating small tears that reduce the level of protection.

Studies are mixed as to the effects of nail polish and artificial nails on the microbial load on hands. However, studies consistently note the importance of keeping nails short because the majority of flora on the hand is found under the nails.[58,70] Other research has indicated possible adverse reactions between chemicals in nail polish and glove materials, increasing irritation to the fingers and nail beds, and potentially damaging glove materials, thus reducing protection.[58]

Broken skin. Broken skin resulting from dry, chapped, and cracked skin; injury; skin erosions; eczema; or dermatitis should be a concern for DHCPs. In particular, caution should be exercised in patient treatment to reduce the risk that either party may acquire or transmit a secondary infection. This issue should be considered along with other conditions that may limit patient contact (Table 5-5) and other duties.

Hand lotions. Hand lotions often are suggested to reduce the effects on the skin from repeated hand washing, but lotion can become contaminated and act as a reservoir

for microorganisms. Concern also has risen regarding the use of petroleum-based lotions due to their potential to weaken the protective ability of latex gloves by increasing surface permeability and allowing microorganisms to enter. In addition, some question remains as to the compatibility of lotion and antiseptic products; some lotions reduce the antiseptic's ability to disperse bacteria from the skin.

Soaps. Soaps used for hand washing are a basic component infection control, and a number of antiseptic agents are available for use in healthcare facilities. The benefits and limitations of each product should be considered before one is selected. Some products can cause skin irritation over time and are not suitable for repeated use, whereas certain DHCPs may be sensitive to other products. Irritation to the skin can reduce that organ's integrity. If an irritation continues or becomes serious, a dermatologist should be consulted for recommendations. Table 5-6 lists the active ingredients of the most commonly used agents. One significant benefit of several products is the ability to provide continued or "residual" antiseptic protection on the skin to extend throughout the day, known as *substantivity.*

Storage and dispensing of hand-care products. Storage and dispensing must be performed to prevent contamination. Liquid products should be stored in closed containers; disposable containers are best, but if they cannot be used, routine maintenance schedules should be followed. Reusable containers can become contaminated and serve as reservoirs for microorganisms and should be thoroughly washed and dried before refilling.

TABLE 5-6

Hand-hygiene methods and indications

Method	Agent	Purpose	Duration (minimum)	Indication*
Routine handwash	Water and non-antimicrobial soap (e.g., plain soap)†	Remove soil and transient micro-organisms	15 seconds‡	Before and after treating each patient (e.g., before glove placement and after glove removal). After barehanded touching of inanimate objects likely to be contaminated by blood or saliva.
Antiseptic handwash	Water and antimicrobial soap (e.g., chlorhexidine, iodine and iodophors, chloroxylenol [PCMX], triclosan)	Remove or destroy transient micro-organisms and reduce resident flora	15 seconds‡	
Antiseptic hand rub	Alcohol-based hand rub§	Remove or destroy transient micro-organisms and reduce resident flora	Rub hand until the agent is dry§	Before leaving the dental operatory or the dental laboratory. When visibly soiled.§ Before regloving after removing gloves that are torn, cut, or punctured.
Surgical antisepsis	Water and antimicrobial soap (e.g., chlorhexidine, iodine and iodophors, chloroxylenol [PCMX], triclosan) Water and non-antimicrobial soap (e.g., plain soap†) followed by an alcohol-based surgical hand-scrub product with persistent activity	Remove or destroy transient micro-organisms and reduce resident flora (persistent effect)	2-6 minutes Follow manufacturer instructions for surgical hand-scrub product with persistent activity‖	Before donning sterile surgeon's gloves for surgical procedures¶

Reference numbering corresponds to the complete document: Guidelines for Infection Control in Dental Health-Care Settings—2003. *MMWR*, December 19, 2003, 52 (RR-17).

*(7, 9, 11, 13, 113, 120-123, 125, 126, 136-138).

†Pathogenic organisms have been found on or around bar soap during and after use (139). Use of liquid soap with hands-free dispensing controls is preferable.

‡Time reported as effective in removing most transient flora from the skin. For most procedures, a vigorous rubbing together of all surfaces of premoistened lathered hands and fingers for ≥15 seconds, followed by rinsing under a stream of cool or tepid water is recommended (9, 120, 123, 140, 141). Hands should always be dried thoroughly before donning gloves.

§Alcohol-based hand rubs should contain 60%-95% ethanol or isopropanol and should not be used in the presence of visible soil or organic material. If using an alcohol-based hand rub, apply adequate amount palm of one hand and rub hands together, covering all surfaces of the hands and fingers unitl hands are dry. Follow manufacturer's recommendations regarding the volume of product to use. If hands feel dry after rubbing them together for 10-15 seconds, an insufficient volume of product was likely applied. The drying effect of alcohol can be reduced or eliminated by adding 1%-3% glycerol or other skin-conditioning agents (123).

‖After application of alcohol-based surgical hand scrub product with persistent activity as recommended, allow hands and forearms to dry thoroughly and immediately don sterile surgeon's gloves (144, 145). Follow manufacturer instructions (122, 123, 137, 146).

¶Before beginning surgical hand scrub, remove all arm jewelry and any hand jewelry that may make donning gloves more difficult, causes gloves to tear more readily (142, 143), or interfere with glove usage (e.g., ability to wear the correct-sized glove or altered glove integrity).

Hand washing. Hand washing is the most important and extremely effective procedure for the prevention of many infections transmitted by organisms on the hands. Contamination can occur when the hands touch any object not designated as clean, thus causing cross-contamination. Such objects include the DHCP's own hair, work clothing, glasses, and masks contaminated during routine patient procedures.

Hand washing is mandatory before and after patient contact, after any contact with potential sources of microorganisms (such as body fluids and substances, mucous membranes, nonintact skin, and inanimate objects that are likely to be contaminated), after removal of gloves, and before and after treatment room setup and cleanup after treatment. When in doubt about any kind of contamination, the DHCP should wash the hands. The three basic levels of hand-washing protocol for health care are shown in Table 5-6.

Hand-washing procedures in health care vary relative to the tasks to be performed. The recommended basic hand-washing procedure for routine dental procedures begins with the wetting of hands under cool to warm running water, followed by the application of an appropriate hand-washing agent distributed thoroughly over the hands. The hands then should be rubbed together vigorously for 10 to 15 seconds, with all surfaces of the hands and fingers covered, and rinsed well from fingertips to elbows. The combined mechanical action and thorough rinsing are critical for removal, with special attention provided to the fingertip area, not just the palms.

Hand antisepsis is achieved by hand washing or surgical scrub with an antimicrobial-containing soap or detergent and is recommended before the performance of invasive procedures when persistent antimicrobial activity on the hands is desired. The goal is to reduce the numbers of resident skin flora, in addition to the removal of transient microorganisms. The use of an alcohol-based hand rub is approved (October 2002) when soap and water are unavailable.

Products used for hand washing, surgical scrubs, and hand care should be chosen with consideration given to the purpose for use, advantages and disadvantages of the agent, overall cost, and acceptance (biocompatibility) of the product by users. Reusable cloth towels are not recommended for use in hand drying in healthcare facilities. Single-use paper towels or hand blowers are preferred.

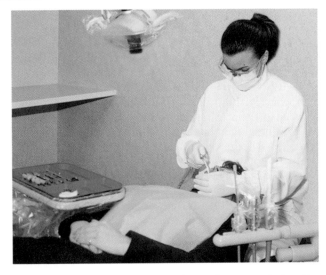

FIG. 5-5 Example of good work practice controls (WPC).

Personal Protective Equipment

5-B   The intent of PPE is to provide protection to the skin, eyes, nose, mucous membranes, and clothing from exposure to biological, physical, (or parenteral) and/or chemical hazards in the workplace. [65,76,77,78] This protection includes contact with blood or other potentially infectious materials (including saliva) that can be reasonably anticipated during the performance of normal work tasks. The selection of PPE is based on the procedures and tasks expected to be performed.

Other individuals, such as the receptionist, may be exposed indirectly to these risks or occasionally have direct contact and also must be trained to use appropriate PPE. For routine procedures in dentistry, this equipment includes but is not limited to the use of gloves, masks, face shields, and protective eyewear, as well as attire, clinic gowns, or uniforms as indicated by the tasks the employee is required to perform (Figs. 5-5 and 5-6).

The use and care of procedurally indicated PPE also integrates in the concepts of WPCs and ECs recommended by OSHA. For example, use of antimicrobial soap to wash contaminated eyewear is an action (WPC) meant to decontaminate protective equipment (PPE) while at the same time the use of a special antimicrobial agent in the soap enhances such effects (EC). Together, this process responds to three OSHA strategies for safety.

Throughout the following paragraphs the reader should look for ways that man and science work together to create the safest work situation possible, reflecting the link between WPC and EC. Individual actions are combined with scientific developments working hand-in-hand to achieve safe working practices.

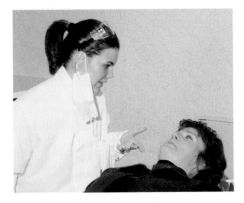

FIG. 5-6 Example of poor work practice controls (WPC)—mask hanging from ear and gloves stuffed into exposed pocket.

Gloves

Gloves are the single most effective element of PPE for the reduction of disease transmission in density. They should be used in addition to, not as a substitute for, hand washing and are required for contact with oral mucous membranes, saliva, blood, or other potentially infectious materials. Most oral health services involve direct contact with the oral cavity (posing biological hazards), whereas infection control practices require routine use of disinfectant agents (posing chemical hazards) and handling of sharp instruments (posing physical hazards). Although not all procedures are done in a blood-contaminated field, saliva in dentistry is also defined as a fluid for which SP apply.

Types

The type of gloves used should be selected based on the tasks to be performed and the individual needs of the person wearing them. Employers must provide gloves in appropriate materials and sizes for each employee. A number of different types of gloves are indicated and available for protection against biological, chemical, and physical hazards anticipated in the work place (see Appendix F).

First the procedures and inherent hazards should be considered. For biological hazards, nonsterile or sterile exam gloves are indicated; for chemical hazards, nitrile rubber utility gloves are needed. In handling of hot trays, equipment, or instruments after sterilization, heat-resistant mitts provide the needed physical protection, and puncture-resistant gloves may be indicated during cleanup of contaminated instruments after patient procedures.

Exam or procedure gloves. Exam gloves are available in several types, including sterile and nonsterile latex or vinyl, latex-free synthetic, powdered and nonpowdered, nitrile rubber exam and utility gloves, and right-left paired or ambidextrous versions.

Nonsterile gloves are dispensed in bulk and should be obtained with clean hands, then rinsed before placement in the patient's mouth. Exam gloves should *not* be washed and reused, even for the same patient.

Surgical gloves are packaged for use when sterile conditions are necessary. Gloves come from the manufacturer in pairs, sealed in sterile packs. A sterile technique is required to don the gloves so as to not contaminate them before use. After the wrapper is opened, only the outside of the wrapper should be touched before the gloves are removed; only the inner surface of the gloves should be touched as the fingers slide between the cuff and palm or back of the gloved hand. Care must be taken to prevent contact with the outer surface of the gloves with the hands or the inner surface of the gloves with the outer surface of the gloves to avoid contamination before use.

Overgloves. Overgloves are thin vinyl or copolymer gloves (like food handlers' gloves) placed over exam glove to prevent cross-contamination. The use of overgloves, worn over treatment gloves, can reduce cross-contamination when the DHCP touches any surface out of the direct treatment area—for example, to retrieve additional supplies from a drawer, use a pen to make a treatment notation, or press an activation button during x-ray taking. Overgloves should be included as a standard part of the treatment room setup.

Utility gloves. Utility gloves are heavy unlined gloves worn during handling of any chemicals or infectious waste; cleaning of contaminated surfaces, instruments, or materials; and environmental surface cleaning and disinfection. Gloves made of nitrile rubber have an increased resistance to instrument punctures and can be autoclaved. Alternatives include reusable utility gloves that can be disinfected after each use (like dishwashing gloves), but such gloves become highly contaminated during clean-up procedures. Procedures used to store these gloves must include washing and disinfection after each use.

Factors for appropriate use

Disposable gloves must be worn whenever contact with blood, saliva, or mucous membranes is present and when materials, substances, or surfaces are potentially contaminated. A new pair of exam gloves must be used for each patient. Gloves should be removed and hands washed when tasks are completed, before the employee leaves the treatment room, and between patients. If damage to the gloves is suspected, the DHCP should remove the gloves and wash the hands. Contaminated gloves should not be washed between patients or removed and reused later on the same patient. Removing the gloves and washing them can damage the integrity of the material, leaving microtears or pin holes that may permit the passage of infectious agents. To prevent contamination of gloves during the donning of PPE, the face mask should come first and the glasses adjusted before the hands are washed and gloves are worn.

Case #1 Application

Ruth's primary duties involve the front desk. She is a valued team member and known to be helpful when the back office is running behind. The other staff members appreciate that she comes into the back and helps clean up the treatment room for the next patient to help them get back on schedule. However, Ruth has not had training in back-office SOP. She admits that she does not always wear gloves when she helps clean.

Only items that are to be sterilized, have surface covers, or are to be disinfected after use are to be touched

with contaminated gloves. Gloves are to be removed when supplies are obtained, materials are removed from the cart, or the chart is handled.

Gloves made of alternative materials should be available for personnel with sensitivity to usual glove materials (such as latex). Individuals with dermatitis related to use of gloves should seek medical attention to determine appropriate modifications to the use of gloves and handwashing procedures.

Experience tells which size glove fits best. The glove selected should fit tightly all around, with no excess, folds, or wrinkling at the fingertips or webs of the hand. However, the glove should not be so tight as to "pull in" on the palm.

Double gloving (two pairs worn at once) may be indicated under certain circumstances, such as if the DHCP has a cut or lesion on the hand. Double gloving provides an in/out barrier for potentially infectious agents.

State recommendations specifically state that gloves should cover the cuffs of long-sleeved gowns. Procedure gloves sold in the United States are quality controlled by the FDA. Recent studies have shown that the use of right- or left-hand ambidextrous gloves may be linked to the development of neuromuscular injures to the hands of dental professionals.[81] Trying several type of gloves is the best way to meet individual needs.

Latex allergy

Exam and surgical gloves made for health care are predominantly made from latex products.* As UP have been implemented, the use of gloves has increased and the incidence of latex allergy appears to be increasing. Surveys have reported that approximately 40% of DHCPs demonstrate sensitivity to latex.[41] A number of conditions can predispose an individual to latex allergy, such as multiple allergic conditions, multiple surgeries, and food allergies to banana, kiwi, and avocado, to name a few. A thorough medical history is critical to help identify high-risk patients and employees.

Type I latex allergy symptoms (immediate hypersensitivity) usually manifest first as localized skin reactions; more serous reactions can manifest as severe respiratory and systemic symptoms as well. Latex allergies can progress from a simple localized dermatitis into a life-threatening allergy, with anaphylaxis.

If any reaction occurs, the individual should have the condition assessed by an allergy specialist to define the specific nature of the reaction and appropriate treatment. Differentiating among reactions to other irritants (such as the powders inside the glove) from actual latex-specific allergies can be quite difficult. An accurate diagnosis of the problem is critical to the selection of appropriate alternatives and, if necessary, the creation of a latex-free environment for the protection of the affected employee.

Several alternatives to latex gloves are available, as are latex gloves without powders. Any problem with latex products should be monitored closely due to the potential severe health problems that may result. No cure exists for latex allergy, and the reactions can increase in severity and even be delayed (type IV hypersensitivity) after the contact is no longer present. Reducing or eliminating

---

*References 12, 13, 38, 41, 71, 74, 90.

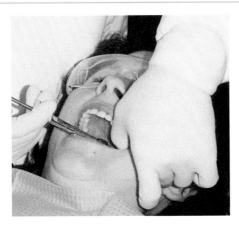

FIG. 5-7 Patient wearing safety lenses.

latex products in the environment is critical when latex-allergic patients or DHCPs are present (see the suggested agencies and web sites [49-52] later in the chapter).

Protective Eyewear

Protective eyewear is required for all procedures that have the potential to create aerosols or spatter. Protective eyewear should provide protection for trauma injuries resulting from flying debris, aerosols/spatter of potentially infectious materials, and/or chemicals.

Types of protective eyewear

Numerous styles of protective eyewear are available, and the user should select the most comfortable version for extended wear. Several styles can even be worn over prescription glasses. Personal prescription glasses must be placed in safety frames to provide adequate protection.

Safety glasses. Safety glasses, or goggles, with top and side coverage provide the highest degree of protection. Standard eyewear models lack protection to the side and top and may not meet the impact requirements for safety glasses (see Figs. 5-5 and 5-6).

Face shields. Face shields may be used in place of safety glasses, particularly for procedures in which significant spatter is anticipated, such as with ultrasonic and air/powder polishing procedures. Reusable shields should be decontaminated between patients. Masks always must be used in combination with face shields, which offer little protection from inhalation for aerosols and are not considered an alterative for masks.

Patient eye protection. Protection for the patient should be provided also, as the same eye hazards exist for the patient during procedures as those for the DHCP (Fig. 5-7).

Case #4 Application

At Mr. Birdwell's last appointment, the ophthalmologist speculated that bacterial matter had gotten in his eye, causing the infection. Questioning by his doctor traced the most probable cause of his eye infection to treatment Mr. Birdwell received for his periodontal disease during his last dental appointment. During the treatment, Mr. Birdwell was not provided safety glasses to wear to protect his eyes from potential spatter from his mouth.

Laser and high-intensity lights. Laser and high-intensity lights used to cure dental materials may cause injury to the eye with repeated exposure. Special light filter glasses and shields should be used during operation of these light sources. The manufacturer's instructions should be consulted for safety specifications.

Factors for appropriate use and care

Protective eyewear and face shields should be put on and adjusted before gloves are donned. Protective eyewear must meet guidelines of the American National Standards Institute (ANSI; see the suggested agencies and web sites [53] later in the chapter) as shatter resistant. Approved eyewear features the ANSI symbol printed on the frame. Other required elements for OSHA approval require that the eyewear has solid side shields (with top and bottom rims also recommended).

Proper size and fit for each individual is important to minimize the need to adjust eyewear during use, taking care not to push eyewear up with contaminated gloves. Pushing up glasses, adjusting masks, or touching the face and hair can promote cross-contamination to or from gloves and should be avoided.

Routine maintenance should include decontamination with soap and water at a minimum. Caution should be taken if chemical disinfectants are used because many of these chemicals may cause irritation to the skin and/or eyes. Use of an antimicrobial soap to wash eyewear between patients reduces both surface contamination and the risk of chemical irritation. Spraying the eyewear with an accepted disinfectant and allowing it to remain wet for at least 10 minutes is recommended for individuals who have *not* demonstrated eye sensitivity to the chemicals. After the 10-minute period, the glasses may be rinsed thoroughly, dried, and reused. When possible, two pairs of protective glasses can help allow time for proper care.

Face Masks

Disposable face masks are to be worn for all procedures in which spatter or aerosols are produced or when a DHCP provider or patient has a respiratory infection. Oral fluids and spatter are routinely generated during dental procedures and can remain airborne for hours after a procedure, eventually settling on environmental surfaces. This type of contamination poses a number of risks from direct inhalation to indirect cross-contamination between PPE and environmental surfaces. The size of these particles vary from visible debris on the DHCP's glasses, hands, arms, or other location to particles so small that they cannot be seen but can be inhaled. Masks also are to be worn in the laboratory when procedures create dust, shavings, or aerosols.

Types and fit

Masks provide two-way protection for possible exposures to and from the patient. They come in several sizes and styles, including molded dome, flat, pleated paper, and variations on both with elastic straps, ear loops, or ties. Masks have a number of different types of surface treatment to prevent or reduce passage of moisture and microorganisms.

To maximize protection the mask must cover the nose, mouth, and facial hair, fitting snugly with no gaps. Properly fitting face masks create a seal for the nose and mouth, reducing the risk of exposure to the respiratory system. For example, if the mask is worn only over the mouth but not the nose, no protection is provided. Gaps along the side of the mask also can allow airborne contamination to seep in and be inhaled through the mouth or nose.

Factors for appropriate selection and use

The DHCP must use science and logic to determine which mask is appropriate for the tasks to be performed. The mask must be able to provide protection to extremely small microorganisms and particles and still function in a moist environment.

Some masks are made of materials or contain dyes that may irritate the skin and/or eyes. Others may be comfortable to wear but are thin and do not provide appropriate protection in a wet environment.

To maintain the integrity of the mask surface, the DHCP should avoid touching the mask with contaminated hands or gloves and remove the mask before leaving the treatment area. The employee should not leave the immediate treatment area with the mask hanging around the neck or from the ear.

Bacterial filtration. One criterion for mask selection is the ability to filter small enough particles to filter out bacterial contaminants. A mask with a filtration level of 95% to 98% of 1- to 3-micron particles provides the DHCP with a high level protection for most exposures.

Duration of wear. Masks must be changed for each patient when contaminated by touch, visibly soiled, or become damp. An estimated 20-minute duration per mask can be expected in a moist/wet environment, but no definitive data exist at this time. Much of the duration expectation depends on the procedures performed, the amount of aerosolization, and the degree of moisture from the DHCP's breath inside the mask. A good practice is to change the mask if it becomes moist on the exterior or inside surfaces.

Protective Garments

Appropriate clinical attire always should be used for dental procedures to protect the skin and underlying clothing from contamination.[54] These garments are to be changed daily or when visibly soiled. As with other PPE, a number of protective garments are available. Selection should be based on the tasks to be performed and the level of protection needed. Moisture-resistant garments are designed to provide additional protection to skin and clothing from potentially saturating contamination.

Garments that are long enough to cover the lap area during sitting, with long sleeves, high necks, tight cuffs, and simple styling are usually best. Often surgical scrubs are worn, in which case the jacket and pants are considered part of the PPE and must be handled accordingly. Protective garments are for use during exposure-prone tasks and should not be worn out of the general treatment area, a practice that allows for cross-contamination of areas not normally decontaminated between patients.

Protective garments are to be provided by the employer, including appropriate laundering and maintenance. These garments are not to be taken home as personal laundry items.

Implementation of Work Practice and Engineering Controls

Numerous WPC and EC are aimed at reducing exposure to hazards during dental procedures and are tailored to the individual workplace. EC available for use in dentistry when properly used (WPC) can reduce the risks of cross-contamination and injury. Combining these practices with the use of appropriately designed products and equipment is the goal of WPC and EC—where science and practice meet.[2,7,21,65,91]

Controls that can be routinely applied by the DHCP to reduce cross-contamination and support the concept of UP[21] include but are not limited to the practices discussed in the following sections.

Barrier Protection

The use of barriers has become a universal practice in dentistry to prevent contact with infectious agents and contamination of environmental surfaces. This practice reduces the risk of transmission to and from these surfaces, while reducing the need to manually clean the treatment room surfaces between patients.

PPE is essentially the use of individual (personal) barrier protection to prevent exposure to the skin, mucous membranes, and clothing of the DHCP and to reduce the risk of inhalation of infectious agents. Both surface barriers and personal barriers, such as gloves and masks (PPE), are designed to be disposed of after each patient and replaced with fresh ones.

Another effective barrier used during exposure-prone procedures is a rubber dam.[10,23,26,91] Although environmental barriers protect surfaces from contamination, a rubber dam is a "reverse" barrier to reduce spattering and aerosolization of oral fluids and blood and should be used whenever possible (Fig. 5-8).

High-Velocity Evacuation

High-velocity evacuation (HVE) should be used whenever procedures generating aerosols and/or spatter are performed, such as the use of high-speed handpieces, ultrasonic or sonic scalers (Fig 5-9), or water spray from the air/water syringe.

Reduction of Microbial Load

One means to reduce the number of microorganisms is to have the patient brush the teeth before the appointment is begun. This practice mechanically reduces the available microorganisms in the oral cavity significantly.

A second approach is to ask the patient to rinse with an antimicrobial mouthrinse before treatment, again the goal being to reduce the volume of available microorganisms. Several mouthrinses are available for patient use before dental treatment, all of which primarily reduce by mechanical means the number of oral microbes in the patient's mouth. Rinsing with a chemical agent that has substantivity, such as chlorhexidine, extends the duration of residual antimicrobial activity and may be a good choice for use before treatment.

X-Ray Equipment

Most often, x-rays are taken in the same room in which the treatment is provided. Therefore the basic treatment room set-up includes the use of protective coverings and/or disinfection procedures for the x-ray equipment, including the x-ray tube head and activation button. Care should be taken to touch only the covered surfaces of the x-ray tube head during alignment. After exposure, film packets must be handled to prevent cross-contamination. Although the contamination during exposure of x-rays

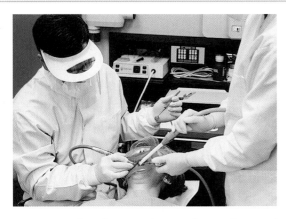

FIG. 5-8 Examples of personal protective equipment (PPE) and environmental barriers—safety glasses on the operator, gloves over the cuffs, well-fitted mask, protective laboratory coat, surface barriers on slow-speed handpiece, use of a rubber dam.

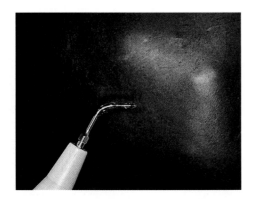

FIG. 5-9 Ultrasonic scaler with spray/aerosol.

usually involves "only" saliva, this potentially infectious body fluid commands the same level of infection control as blood.

Each office's SOP must address WPC aimed at management of contaminated film packets during transportation, opening for development, and disposal of waste. Once the x-rays have been exposed, they are taken to a darkroom or other area for developing; caution is needed so as not to cross-contaminate this area. Gloves must be worn at all times during handling of contaminated packets, and film packets must be disposed of as potentially infectious waste due to saliva contamination.

Disposable Items
The use of disposable items can greatly reduce difficulties associated with surface disinfection, sterilization, and treatment room management. Disposable items should be discarded immediately after use to avoid contamination of other items. Items dispensed for single use must not be reused—ever. Reuse of such items is a violation of FDA regulation for approved devices.

Chairside Safety
Every time the DHCP is present at chairside for patient treatment, the risk of exposure and/or injury exists.

Considering carefully available EC and WPC can minimize these risks. Examples of WPC include the presence of overgloves for reaching into drawers for supplies or writing on charts and the inclusion of an extra pair of cotton pliers with each setup to retrieve extra supplies from clean areas.

Supply-dispensing techniques should prevent contamination of bulk supplies. The DHCP should plan ahead for supplies rather than contaminating supply containers. The goal is to minimize the number of surfaces and items that may be touched with contaminated hands during the patient's appointment.

Needle Stick Safety
The Needlestick Safety and Prevention Act of 2000 supports that employers must consider appropriate and effective safer sharps devices as they become available. Employees are to become involved in the identification and selection of such devices for use in practice, and those decisions must be reviewed annually and noted in office records. When using traditional dental syringe and needle, used needles must never be recapped or otherwise manipulated using both hands: either the one-handed scoop technique or a mechanical device designed for holding the needle sheath must be used.

Use of Transfer Forceps
Some instruments or supplies are not protected by wrapping but may be stored in sterile jars or immersed in liquid disinfectants. These items should be taken from storage with transfer forceps.

Dental Unit Waterline Management

Over the past decade, DHCPs have been made aware of the presence of "biofilm" accumulation in dental unit waterlines (DUWL).* Although limited evidence is available to demonstrate a significant risk to all patients, compelling evidence indicates that the problems related to this microbial accumulation on the inner surface of DUWL can be a problem for immunocompromised individuals.

Biofilm
Biofilm describes colonies of cell growth that attach to the wet inner surfaces of small tubing (Fig. 5-10).[95,97] This tangled matrix of organisms may form up to 400 mm thick. In simple terms biofilm forms "slime," which becomes a microenvironment that can sustain microbial growth of both aerobic and anaerobic organisms and may serve as a reservoir for the transmission of pathogens. This formation of biofilm appears rapidly and adheres to the wet surface by an extracellular polysaccharide fiber matrix, and is highly bound to the surface of the DUWL tubing.

Biofilm can become highly resistant to chemical disinfection and poses a significant challenge to waterline management in dental equipment.

Risk
Exposure to the majority of microorganisms recovered from contaminated DUWL, such as various strains of *Pseudomonas* species, can be managed by a healthy im-

---

*References 1, 3, 4, 6, 18, 24, 39, 56, 61, 63, 73, 95-97.

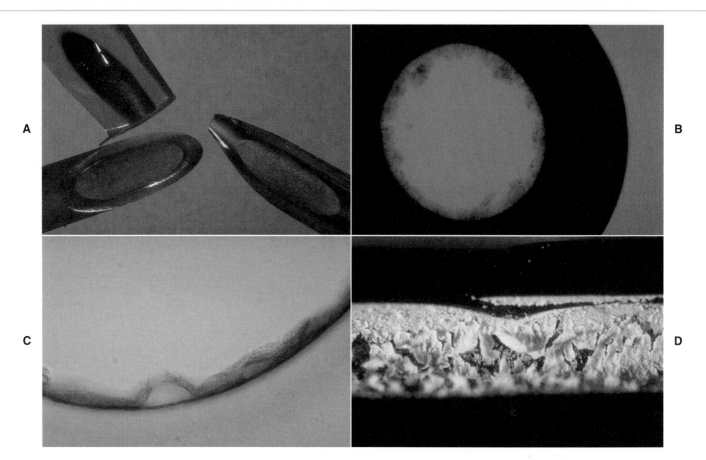

FIG. 5-10 Dental unit biofilms. **A,** Tubing diagonal cut of lumen. **B,** Tubing crosscut with biofilm. **C,** Close-up view of biofilm on inner surface. **D,** Dried biofilm from tubing.

mune system. Of greater concern has been the isolation of *Legionella* species.[24] If conditions are altered in the transmission equation, documentation exists that an infection can follow exposure to the organisms expelled from the waterline during dental procedures.

Management
The challenge for waterline management includes the implementation of both EC and WPC to best control biofilm formation. The ADA has set a goal of 200 CFU/ml (*c*olony-*f*orming *u*nits) or less as the standard for safe water in dental care, termed *potable water,* or water of drinking quality.[4] Some states require that the level of CFUs be 0, requiring the use of sterile water for some invasive procedures. No universal treatment can eliminate the problem, but proper management includes proper equipment, such as antiretraction valves and backflow prevention devices; integration of "point-of-use" waterline filters in the dental unit; use of controlled water sources, such as external water delivery systems that can be cleaned and/or removed or sterilized water delivery systems; and strict adherence to chemical treatment routines by the dental staff members.

Regular maintenance of waterline systems is critical and must include well-managed EC and WPC to be successful. Monitoring the water quality at the point of use, where the water is delivered into the patient's mouth, is one component. Water testing procedures must be integrated into the general office routine.[56,92]

Future OSHA regulations for indoor air quality may further affect the EC and WPC implemented to control DUWL contamination and the management of aerosols generated from those water sources. To stay compliant, the DHCP must monitor local and federal regulations related to health and safety (see the suggested agencies and web sites [44,46] later in the chapter).

General Environmental and Equipment Procedures

Comprehensive infection control practices include preprocedure and postprocedure, as well as direct patient procedures management. Any surface, nonsterilizable equipment, or material that may potentially become contaminated during the course of dental care must be considered.

Work Zones
Defining work areas or *zones* (Fig. 5-11) based on expected levels of exposure can help prevent cross-contamination through the establishment of ground rules for the placement of instruments, procedure items, and materials and can help control their flow during dental procedures. Removing unnecessary items from the treatment area reduces clean-up time. The best place to store equipment and supplies to reduce contamination is in closed cupboards and drawers.

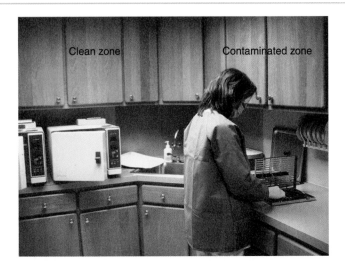

FIG. 5-11 Example of instrument reprocessing area. Work zones *(left)*. Tray break-down and sharps box *(right)*.

Basic WPC and EC for items in the contamination zone range from the use of disposable treatment items and surface barriers to surface cleaning and disinfection to heat sterilization of instruments. Individualizing the needs of each workplace is necessary.

Daily Preparation

Daily preparation of the treatment area and dental unit is another good example of WPC. To ensure that the treatment area is ready to go at the start of the day, SOP should be followed to prepare the treatment room.

Setting up the treatment room for patient care includes tasks such as daily setup of clean water delivery systems, general sanitization of surfaces that may have been contaminated as aerosols settled during the night, and placement of appropriate barrier covers on surfaces that may become contaminated (but are not routinely cleaned and disinfected) between patients.

After washing the hands the DHCP should don utility gloves appropriate to handle chemicals and start with a general sanitization and disinfection of the dental chair, dental unit, and treatment area. A good rule is to cover any surface within 3 feet of the patient's mouth for any treatment that may produce spatter.[10] Cabinet doors and drawers should be closed during treatment.

Although not all surfaces require disposable barriers, their use can simplify treatment room turnover and improve surface asepsis. Research has shown that manual cleaning is not as effective in contamination removal on surfaces as the use of barriers is at preventing it. Changing a barrier appears to be more effective and takes less time than an attempt to adequately decontaminate and disinfect most surfaces manually. Many surfaces have irregular areas that are difficult or impossible to clean adequately, making barriers an effective option.

In place of surface barriers, the use of surface disinfectants is also an accepted practice. In this case, an understanding of the different types of disinfecting agents available and the ways in which their use is intended is important (see the section of this chapter that discusses disinfectants and sterilants). Care should be taken to select an appropriate disinfecting agent and adequately preclean the surface before the agent is applied for disinfection.

The basic procedure begins when an appropriate chemical agent is applied to wet the area (initial contact) and all surfaces are sprayed. Next, the surface is scrubbed and wiped clean (mechanical cleaning/removal) with a gauze square to remove any surface debris and/or residue *(bioburden).* Then the chemical is applied again and allowed to remain moist for the length of time *specified by the manufacturer* to destroy any remaining microorganisms on the surface (disinfection). After the recommended contact time, the chemical is wiped as needed and the surfaces are allowed to dry, an approach referred to as *spray-wipe-spray.*

Environmental Surface Protection

The following surfaces are considered potential areas of contamination and should be cleaned and sanitized at the start of each day: all smooth surfaces in the treatment area (i.e., countertops, tops of cubicle unit partitions); operator, assistant, and patient chairs (including the base of the patient chair and the height adjustment handles); light pole, arm, handles, switch, and light cover (cleaning the cover *only* according to manufacturer's instructions); mobile carts (all switches, hoses, attachments, and nozzles on the power cart), x-ray view box, sink unit, x-ray tube head, and any other items or surfaces that may be touched during patient care.[2,21,65] This SOP helps eliminate all but the most virulent microorganisms and serves as an example of the general housekeeping component of the office procedures.

Once these surfaces have been prepared for the day, disposable barriers are placed on difficult-to-clean items and those best managed with barriers, including the headrest and upper back of the dental chair; light adjustment handles; the power cart with necessary switches, handpieces, and tubing; evacuation tips; air/water syringe; and patient tray (Fig. 5-12).

Preparing the Treatment Room for Patient Treatment

To prepare the for patient treatment, the DHCP should gather the necessary supplies and organize them in the treatment room according to the work zones defined for that work space. The following items are generally considered part of the basic initial preparation: tray and cover; patient bib; disposables, including gauze squares and cotton swabs; treatment supplies (i.e., prophy paste, cups, floss, etc.); patient home-care supplies; chairside biohazard segregation bag and/or chairside waste bag (see Fig. 5-12). In addition, gloves, masks, safety glasses (operator and patient), overgloves, and the patient chart should be easily available.

Clinical DHCPs must ensure that patient charts are managed safely and not contaminated by handling with contaminated hands and subsequently circulated to front-office employees. If possible, charts should be left outside the treatment area. A "no glove" policy for handling charts can reduce the risk of contamination. Some microorganisms can remain virulent on environmental surfaces for some time (see Table 5-2), potentially transmitting infectious agents to any individual who handles a

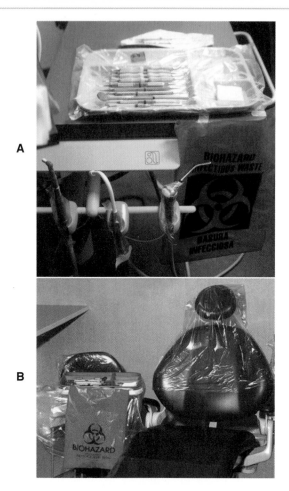

FIG. 5-12 Environmental surface barriers. **A,** Power cart and tubing, instrument tray, and cassette. **B,** Patient and assistant chair backs and biohazard waste bag.

contaminated chart. This caution also applies to the use of pens or pencils that may have been handled with contaminated hands.

Case #1 Application
Ruth regularly handles patient charts, filing, and billing and insurance matters. Often she is the first person to receive the patient chart immediately after the appointment is completed. Ruth has missed several weeks of work, showing lingering signs of a systemic illness. She is extremely fatigued, running a chronic fever, and appears to have some liver dysfunction.

Once all necessary items are set up chairside and barrier covers placed, the patient chair and other equipment should be positioned to enable the patient to sit down easily. The operator's stool should be adjusted to prevent contact with the height and back support adjustment handles during the appointment. Mobile and power carts must be carefully prepared to cover all surfaces that may be touched during treatment, including handpieces, the air/water syringe, suction tubes, and switches (see Fig. 5-13). Inserting suction tips, burs, prophy cups, saliva ejector, and other like items after barriers are placed on tubes and handpieces is a good practice. Although the instrument

tray is a flat, smooth surface and easy to clean, disposable covers also may be used on trays to reduce clean-up time between patients (see Fig. 5-12). When work zones are defined (see Fig. 5-11), a section of the counter area should be designated *clean* and should contain items that are not to be touched with contaminated hands. The treatment area should be double-checked to ensure that the x-ray view box is set up with the patient's x-rays ready to go.

Treatment Room Cleanup
Treatment room cleanup routinely involves the handling of sharp instruments and contaminated waste and the use of chemicals. The DHCP should pay close attention when handling contaminated items; wearing nitrile rubber utility gloves can reduce exposure to contaminated items and injury from sharp objects and provide protection from contact with chemical agents. A systematic approach ensures that all contaminated surfaces are cleaned, instruments and equipment are safely transported for processing, and waste is properly disposed.

Any surfaces visibly contaminated with blood, those that have been touched, or those that may have been contaminated during treatment must be cleaned, disinfected, and/or have their disposable covers changed between patients (see Fig. 5-12).

End of Day
The DHCP should remove all surface barriers at the end of the day and clean and disinfect the treatment room, including any surfaces that may have been contaminated. The manufacturer's instructions should dictate cleanup for all chemicals being used; the spray-wipe-spray procedure should be followed.

Daily equipment routines include flushing of the evacuation system to reduce debris accumulation in the lines and performance of end-of-day procedures for clean water delivery systems. An appropriate cleaning solution always should be used, and manufacturer's instructions should be followed *exactly* for both systems.

Decontamination, Disinfection, and Sterilization Procedures

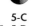

5-C
5-D

Decontamination of contaminated surfaces and instruments after patient treatment requires a variety of procedures.[35,66,68,80,89,94] These procedures vary based on the surface area and/or size of the item, the type of equipment or instruments, the materials from which those instruments are manufactured, and the intended use. The determination about which procedures are required to ensure that the surface or item is safe to touch and reuse becomes one of risk versus benefit.

The risk of cross-contamination (Table 5-7) during reuse of the item or contact with the surface must be determined to be either noncritical (e.g., the seat of the dental chair), semicritical (e.g., working surfaces or suction devices), or critical (e.g., instruments used in the oral cavity, known to be contaminated by blood and/or saliva). Appropriate measures then must be taken to treat the item in a way that renders it safe for use.[80,85,89]

Understanding that both chemical and physical decontamination activities take time and that the microorganisms do not all die at the same time is an im-

TABLE 5-7

Spaulding classifications and chemical agents use

Spaulding risk category	Expected contact	Exposure risk	Level of decontamination	Method of decontamination
Critical	Direct contact Invasive procedures, penetration of mucous membranes, contact with bone Example: Periodontal scalers	Mucous membranes, oral fluids, blood, saliva	Sterilization	Heat sterilization preferred Chemical sterilant (glutaraldehydes)
Semicritical	Direct or indirect contact Contact with mucous membranes, penetration of mucous membranes not anticipated Examples: Dental mouth mirror, dental handpieces†	Mucous membranes, oral fluids, blood, saliva	Sterilization High-level disinfection	Heat Sterilization Chemical sterilant High-level disinfectant (alcohols, chlorines, iodophors, synthetic phenolics, synergized quaternaries,* sodium bromide, and chlorine)
Noncritical	Direct or indirect contact Contact with intact skin, mucous membranes and/or penetration not anticipated Example: Radiograph head/cone	Indirect exposure to oral fluids, blood, saliva	Sanitization Low-level disinfection Barriers	Surface cleaner Intermediate-level disinfectant High-level disinfectant (alcohols, chlorines, iodophors, synthetic phenolics, synergized quaternaries,* sodium bromide, and chlorine)

*Indicates newer generation products; previous formulations were not acceptable surface disinfectants.
†Although considered a semicritical item, dental handpieces should always be sterilized between uses and not high-level disinfected.

portant point.[80] Complete destruction of the target microorganisms requires a series of events over a period of time. Precleaning surfaces to be treated reduces the bioburden (the "load" volume of microorganisms present) that delays this process. Organic matter is capable of neutralizing some agents and sheltering microbes from the agent. Physical cleaning may be adequate for some situations, whereas heat sterilization is required for others. The three most common processes for decontamination in the dental setting are sanitization, disinfection, and sterilization.

Sanitization
Sanitization is the process by which the number of microorganisms is reduced to a relatively safe level, with the focus being on reduction of the "microbial load." This process provides the lowest level of safety and does not destroy any particular microorganism. Sanitization is intended for general housekeeping of noncritical surfaces or for devices made of materials that may deteriorate with the use of stronger agents.

Chemical agents designed for sanitization are considered low-level disinfectants capable of inactivating vegetative bacteria but *not* spores, TB, or nonlipid viruses. Low-level cleaners and disinfectants are not used to decontaminate potentially infectious agents because they are not EPA-registered as effective against TB and therefore not suitable for use in postprocedure cleanup of semicritical or critical surfaces.

Disinfection
Disinfection is the process by which all pathogenic microorganisms are eliminated, with the exception of spore-forming organisms. Disinfection is intended to effectively destroy groups of vegetative bacteria, pathogenic fungi, and some viruses, generally through the use of specific chemicals. However, some thermal disinfection processes also are available.

Chemicals designed for intermediate- and high-level disinfection destroy microorganisms by causing protein denaturation, damaging cell membranes, inhibiting enzymes, or altering nucleic material, most with a combination of these actions.

Intermediate-level disinfectants inactivate all organisms except spores and kill most vegetative bacteria (TB) and viruses (polio II, SA-rotavirus). These chemicals are used for surface decontamination, where a breach in a surface barrier may have occurred, and to treat surfaces not covered with barriers.

High-level disinfectants designed for use in dentistry are capable of inactivating spores when specific contact time recommendations are followed. These products are often referred to as *hospital level disinfectants*. The EPA has set a minimum standard for disinfectants, requiring they be effective against *Pseudomonas* species, lipophilic microorganisms, *S. aureus*, hydrophilic microorganisms, salmonella, and tuberculosis.[83,84]

These chemicals are used to treat heat-sensitive items, such as plastics, and the process often is referred to as *cold sterilization*, terminology that is important to understand. Many of these products, when used for different lengths of time, may be either disinfectants or cold chemical immersion sterilants. Manufacturer's directions are different for disinfection and sterilization, a vital concept, and immersion for longer times is required for sterilization; in addition, for some products the dilution ratios are different. The DHCP *always* should read instructions *carefully*.

Thermal decontamination
Thermal decontamination is a very effective method used to eliminate heat-sensitive microorganisms and on

items that require only an intermediate- or low-level decontamination.[80] The effectiveness of thermal decontamination is due to the use of heat in the form of either steam or hot water, a concept that must not be confused with steam heat sterilization under pressure; the processes are not interchangeable. Thermal decontamination units appear similar to industrial dishwashers.

For the success of any method of disinfection, the bioburden first must be adequately reduced. The spray-wipe-spray method is used for surfaces in the treatment areas. The most important step is precleaning to remove any bioburden. In the case of instruments and equipment used in treatment the same principle applies; the bioburden must be reduced to a level at which disinfection or sterilization can penetrate to completely destroy the microorganisms (see the section on instrument processing).

Chemical classifications

Appropriate disinfection and sterilization chemicals used in dentistry are grouped by the following general chemical classifications: glutaraldehydes, combination phenolics, iodophors, and chlorines (see Table 5-7).[69,83,84]

A suggested ideal disinfectant agent would be effective against a broad spectrum of organisms with a very short contact time, not be inhibited by physical factors such as bioburden, not damage materials on repeated contact, have a residual effect on treated surfaces, and be easy to use, odorless, and economical.[35,61,62] Unfortunately, no products are currently available that meet all these criteria. Products available must be compared by risk versus benefit and the intended use. Science and practice again must join for a safe and effective outcome.

When choosing a disinfection and immersion chemical sterilant product, the DHCP always must read the entire label, the most important step in the use of any chemical in the workplace. To be effective, agents must be used consistently with the manufacturer's specifications. Identifying and understanding the following information is necessary for the appropriate use of any chemical agent: storage and shelf life, mixing and concentration necessary for proper use, special activation, effects of temperature and time on effective use, shelf life after mixing or dispensing, requirements for precleaning (e.g., agent also a cleaner? separate precleaning agent needed?), whether the product is intended for surface or immersion use, and the contact time for tuberculocidal action. In addition, consideration must be given to any label's warnings.

The DHCP always should take the time to determine whether any potential toxic effects or precautions or special handling instructions are necessary for the disposal of used solutions. For the safety of the DHCP, nitrile gloves should be used to handle chemicals because standard latex or vinyl exam gloves do not provide adequate skin protection.

Appropriate products must have an EPA registration number on each, verifying that the product meets the minimum use standards. For intermediate- and high-level disinfection agents, these products feature a label statement that product is effective against *Mycobacterium tuberculosis*. When selecting an agent for operatory cleanup, the DHCP should check the required contact time factor to ensure its effectiveness within in a reasonable time period for treatment room turnaround. OSHA requires that products used for disinfection are registered with the EPA as effective against *M. tuberculosis* and HIV (see the suggested agencies and web sites [42] later in the chapter).

Chemical disinfection

Chemical disinfection is used for both environmental surfaces and some heat-sensitive semicritical instruments.[68,69,80] Surface disinfection in dentistry is accomplished most frequently with the use of alcohols, chlorine compounds, iodine compounds, phenolics, and hydrogen peroxide.[80,83,84] Agents always should be selected based on their intended use; for example, glutaraldehyde solutions should not be used on environmental surfaces because they are extremely toxic to the skin and respiratory system.

Instrument disinfection is accomplished most frequently by immersion in 2% glutaraldehyde solutions. All specific manufacturer's directions *must* be followed, and items to be disinfected must be clean of debris before immersion or surface treatment. Although these chemicals are a good choice for use with heat-sensitive semicritical items, they are limited in comparison to heat sterilization because biological monitoring is not possible; nothing confirms that effective disinfection has occurred. Immersion disinfection is not appropriate for critical items.

Sterilization

Sterilization is the process by which microorganisms, including spore-forming organisms, are destroyed.[80,94] **5-E** Heat sterilization has long been considered the most effective method of sterilization and is particularly effective when combined with steam or chemical vapor pressure (Fig. 5-13). Ethylene oxide also is an accepted and reliable method, and with new technologies on the horizon, other methods may be as effective or even more effective in the future. Because sterilization equipment and chemical sterilants are considered medical devices, they are regulated by the FDA. All equipment and chemicals used for sterilization should be registered and approved as medical devices by that organization.

Each practice setting must examine the type of equipment used, the available space and ventilation needs of

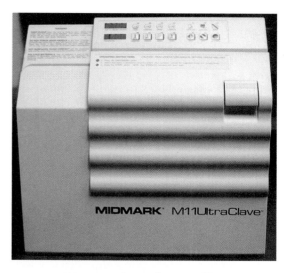

FIG. 5-13 Steam heat sterilizer.

that equipment, and the time management issues of instrument reprocessing. No one method can meet all the needs of every practice setting.

Consequently, the following criteria should be considered in the selection of appropriate method(s) and equipment:

- That materials and items to be sterilized are compatible with each method of sterilization
- That the volume of items to be processed at any one time is limited by the chamber capacity of the equipment
- Time considerations for reprocessing and the cycle time needed for each method
- Packaging materials and their compatibility with the method and equipment
- The availability of process indicators and biological monitors for each method

The most common methods of sterilization[80,85] in dentistry implement four primary types of heat sterilizers.

Autoclaves

Autoclaves heat water in the chamber, creating steam under pressure. The penetration of this steam sterilizes instruments by causing coagulation and inactivation of the cellular proteins of microorganisms. These units operate at temperatures of about 250° F at 15 to 40 pounds per square inch (psi) of pressure for about 30 minutes in a standard cycle. Distilled water is used in the reservoir. The units are highly compatible with many types of materials and feature good penetration of steam into packaged items. One major disadvantage is the corrosion that may occur on unprotected carbon steel instruments. Surgical and stainless steel items are highly compatible with this method of sterilization.

Chemical vapor

Chemical vapor sterilizers produce an unsaturated chemical vapor, and microbial destruction occurs when heat and pressure enhance the penetration of formaldehyde and alcohol vapors. A standard cycle for this type of unit is approximately 260° to 270° F at 20 to 40 psi for about 20 minutes. A proprietary solution with active ingredients of formaldehyde and alcohol is used in the reservoir. Some advantage may be gained from a shorter cycle time, with less corrosion to metals, including carbon steel. Distinct disadvantages are that items must be completely dry before packaging and processing and that the chemical vapor requires special ventilation.

Dri-Clave

Dri-clave sterilizers rely on heat alone to oxidize cellular material of organisms. Dry heat ovens operate at temperatures of 320° F for 2 hours to 340° F for 1 hour, respectively. A significant advantage to dry heat is that it does not rust or corrode metal, a quality that becomes especially important for hinged instruments. Dry heat is not recommended for handpieces or plastic materials.

Ethylene oxide

Ethylene oxide sterilizers operate at room temperature (about 75° F) for 2 to 12 hours, depending on the load. Ethylene oxide features good penetration to surfaces and does not damage heat- or moisture-sensitive materials, including rubber, plastics, and handpieces; it also evaporates without a residue. Because heat is not used, metal instruments may be used immediately after processing.

Disadvantages to ethylene oxide sterilizers, however, include a long cycle time, retained gas in some rubber and plastics, extra safety precautions necessary for toxic gases, and the necessary 24 hours to aerate plastics and rubber items before reuse.

Chemical sterilization

Chemical sterilization is another accepted alternative for heat-sensitive items. The process involves total immersion of the instrument in a glutaraldehyde product for the time specified by the manufacturer (often 8 to 10 hours). When instruments are removed, handled, and exposed to the air, they are no longer sterile. This practice is accepted for semicritical items but should not be used for critical items (see Table 5-7). Items removed from the agent can be bagged and labeled to protect them during storage (e.g., photographic mirrors).

Sterilization Monitors

An essential part of instrument sterilization is monitoring, which is done at a variety of levels to ensure proper operation of sterilization equipment and instruments.

Physical cycle monitor

The first level of monitoring includes physical checks of equipment during processing, such as confirmation that cycle indicators come on at appropriate times to signal that the equipment is operating properly. Sterilizers have a number of "read out" methods depending on the age of the equipment that range from dials and gauges, to lights, to LCD panels and printers. The goal of this level of monitoring is to allow the operator to determine that the equipment is running at appropriate temperature, pressure, and time parameters. For each load, monitors for fluid levels, temperature, pressure, and time should be checked. Physical controls, such as pressure gauges and thermometers, are used widely but should be considered secondary methods used to monitor the efficacy of sterilization.

Cycle integrators

The next level of monitoring involves cycle integrators, which are chemical sensors integrated into packaging materials and/or tape that appear as small dots, squares, or strips. When exposed to the correct parameters of heat and pressure, the indicators change color dramatically, indicating that the packages have been run through a sterilization cycle and all physical conditions have been met. Some less sophisticated sensors are sensitive only to heat and can be misleading; they can change with moderate heat when instrument packs are stored in a warm sterilizer before a cycle. Using true integrators that measure two or more parameters is an important concept.

Case #2 Application

The first indication of a problem was when the student noticed that the cycle integrator on the sterilization bag for the instruments she had just used had not changed color (indicating that the physical parameters for sterilization had not been met). Without this monitor, she would not be able to determine whether a pack had been exposed to a sterilization cycle.

Further checking of processing records identified the persons who had operated the sterilizer for the two batches in question, and an interview revealed that they had not been present to monitor each initial physical check when the sterilizing unit had been started. They were unable to confirm that the equipment appeared to be operating properly. At this point, two levels of monitoring indicated a potential problem.

Biological indicators

The third and most reliable level of monitoring is the use of biological indicators (BIs) that are placed throughout the load before it is subjected to the sterilization process. These test strips or vials are treated with microorganisms that require high levels of heat to kill. The biological indicator to be used for steam sterilization is *Bacillus stearothermophilus* spores and the proper organism used to test dry-heat sterilization processes is *Bacillus subtilis*.

Test protocol. To assess sterilization, test strips are placed into the sterilization chamber during a normal cycle. After the complete cycle, the BIs are incubated with a control and monitored for microbial growth. If the load contains wrapped items, a test pack should be prepared containing a spore strip and should be positioned in the center of the sterilizer load. Then the sterilizer should be operated in accordance with manufacturer's instructions. This test is usually sent to a laboratory, but some in office kits are available.

If complete sterilization has occurred, the processed test will show no growth, whereas the unsterilized control indicates microbial growth. Failure of a sterilizer to successfully sterilize the biological indicator should initiate a recall of all materials processed in that machine. Follow-up through verification (a repeat of the BI testing) should be performed. Before an assumption is made that the error is mechanical, the WPC should be reviewed to determine whether the error was "operator-based," such as through overloading of the sterilizer, a common cause of sterilization failure.

This test does not guarantee the sterility of instruments but does confirm that the equipment is operating properly to achieve sterilization. BI testing is required as a part of routine equipment maintenance and office infection control practices. The interval of BI testing is set by a variety of agencies and may vary for each jurisdiction. Following the regulations for each workplace location is critical to ensure safety.

Case #2 Application
Records on the sterilizer used indicated that the unit routinely passed a weekly BI test, so it was presumed that the error may be with operator, not the equipment.

Instrument Management
After all dental procedures are performed, instruments and equipment must be reprocessed for future use.* At this point, items have been contaminated and must be handled safely until they are disinfected and/or sterilized.

Transporting contaminated items
The first step in contaminated transfer is to gather all items and use appropriate EC and WPC to prevent exposure or injury during the transfer of items to the reprocessing area. WPC may include the use of utility gloves (PPE), hard-sided transport bins, and instrument cassettes (EC). Care must be taken not to create further cross-contamination and prevent injury from any sharp items (WPC).

Cleaning instruments to reduce bioburden
As previously noted, all organic debris and bioburden *must* be removed from surfaces and instruments prior to disinfection and sterilization processes.[80,94] Bioburden

inhibits the ability of the chemical to penetrate to the surface and completely destroy infectious microorganisms.

For environmental surfaces, use of the spray-wipe-spray approach to precleaning is a good example of the manual reduction of bioburden before a disinfection chemical is applied. During the cleaning of sharp instruments for sterilization, the safest WPCs include a hands-off approach. The most effective means to reduce bioburden on contaminated instruments without extensive hand scrubbing is with the use of an ultrasonic cleaner, which creates a physical vibration and utilized energy wave to disperse the bioburden. After the instruments and cassettes are inspected for residual debris, items should be rinsed according to the type of ultrasonic solution used (some are designated as *no rinse*) and then dried and packaged for the method of sterilization implemented. If instruments must sit for a period of time prior to ultrasonic cleaning, the use of a presoak agent can help keep the debris moist so that an ultrasonic cleaner can remove it easily. To help reduce debris from collections on the tips of hand instruments during procedures, instrument tips may be dipped into hydrogen peroxide at chairside to remove debris immediately.

Packaging instruments for sterilization

Selecting appropriate packaging for the method of sterilization used is another important step. [80,94] A number of pouches, wrapping types, and cassettes are available to manage dental instruments; these may be constructed of paper and/or plastic, and some of cloth. Cassettes are an excellent means to reduce possible injury during the handling of sharp instruments throughout the reprocessing cycle. Pouches and wrapping material large enough to contain a variety of cassettes also are available. Reviewing the manufacturer's instructions for each sterilization unit is necessary to ensure that appropriate wrapping materials are used. Selecting packaging materials that integrate sterilization monitoring processes can assist in an overall monitoring program.

To help monitor and retrieve packs, if sterilization is in question, every pack that is sterilized should be labeled with a control number to indicate the sterilizer used, the cycle or load number, the date of sterilization, and an expiration date (if time limits are placed).

Case #3 Application
In following up on this pack, the student discovered that the batch number was used to determine which group of instruments were processed together. This number describes another level of monitoring and tracking. The information was used to determine that two groups of instruments had been distributed without indication that appropriate sterilization had taken place.

Sterilization

All items that can be sterilized should be.[40,44,57,80,91] Heat sterilization is the most effective method available. The critical factors[80] used to develop SOP may include the method of sterilization to be used, appropriate packaging materials and methods, appropriate storage and appropriate handling of the package, appropriate environmental controls, cleanliness, appropriate sterilization methods, and appropriate inventory control. The goal is to achieve sterilization of instruments and critical items used in a safe and effective manner for the patient and the DHCP.

---

*References 2, 21, 57, 74, 75, 80, 91.

Loading the sterilizer in a way that allows for the appropriate physical criteria to be met and maintained throughout the cycle is critical to load sterilization. Instruments should be loosely packed to allow penetration throughout the pack, to avoid excess packing material, and to refrain from overloading of the sterilizer chamber. Room must be available for the heat, steam, and/or chemicals to circulate around and through the packs with maximal penetration to the instruments.

As to a specific type of sterilizer, no one universal standard for sterilization is recommended because of the enormous variations found from facility to facility. However, any sterilizer used in health care must be FDA-approved as a medical device for this purpose. Therefore each DHCP facility is responsible for its own assessment of the needs and the environment for sterilization at the point of use and for the proper operation of the unit selected.

Storage of sterilized items

Sterilized packs of instruments should be positioned so that packaging is not crushed or punctured by items in the bags, which can compromise sterility.[80] All items should be stored in clean, dry areas that allow the oldest packs to be used first. Both open and closed shelving systems are used, and ideally items should be protected from dust. Instruments may be stored as sterile tray set-ups, as groups, or individually wrapped. Evidence must appear on the wrapping, such as autoclave tape or color indicator, that the correct temperature was achieved in the sterilization cycle.

Care should be taken in the storage of sterilized items because the integrity of the package can be compromised by improper handling and storage. If any packaging is damaged, the contents should be considered contaminated or nonsterile. Instruments must be repackaged and resterilized if any sign of damage to the wrapping is apparent.

Research has defined the length of time sterile goods can be stored and still be considered sterile to range from as short as 1 week to indefinitely. A number of factors can affect this determination, including the wrapping material used, the manner of handling, use of cassettes for sharp instruments, and the conditions for storage. Time limits should be determined for each work environment.

The results of the use of nonsterile items can be disastrous for the patient. Therefore proper sterilization and monitoring are critical, as is the maintenance of the sterility of the items after processing. Any breach in the integrity of the packaging or outer wrapping can compromise the barrier of the packaging material. Proper storage and evaluation of package integrity is more important than a time reference; if a hole in the package is discovered, for example, 10 minutes is not long enough to maintain sterility.

Managing Sharps and Related Injury

Numerous opportunities occur for the DHCP to become injured by a sharp object. All DHCPs *must* routinely apply WPC and EC to reduce the handling of contaminated sharps, including reusable items (instruments) and disposable items (needles, burs, wires, matrix bands). Careful transport, cleaning, and disposal practices are required. All sharp items should be handled with the utmost care. Using utility gloves, transport bins and instrument cassettes provides protection when the DHCP recycles instruments.

Recapping needles should be performed only with the use of a recapping device (EC) or a one-handed scoop technique (WPC). Two-handed needle recapping without a protective device is not permitted. The recapping device should be prepared before the needle is unsheathed.

After use the needle is removed from the syringe with the sheath in place, the exposed sharp end is placed over the opening of the sharps container, and the sheath-covered needle is placed into the container. Needles should *never* be bent or broken in any way after use (the no-handling approach). Current revisions to OSHA regulations include an increased focus and emphasis on the use of EC to prevent sharps-related injuries for healthcare employees. Due to the potential serious outcome of percutaneous injury, WPC and EC should be strictly followed. As soon after use as possible, the sharps must be removed from the treatment area and disposable items placed into an appropriate puncture-proof, leak-proof container. Items to be placed in the sharps container are shown in Box 5-4. Sharps must never be forced into an overfilled container (Fig. 5-14).

If an injury involves a potential exposure to human body fluid or materials contaminated with body substances (as would occur with a needle-stick, splash to mucous membranes, or nonintact skin) it should be reported as soon as possible to a staff member.

Case #3 Application

What is the risk to the dental hygienist in wiping a contaminated instrument free of visible debris with a gauze sponge (via a pinching motion) during a procedure, then returning directly to the mouth? This process could be repeated numerous times during a scaling appointment without the hygienist giving it a second thought.

BOX 5-4

Items to be Placed in Sharps Container

Used and unused anesthetic carpules (unless other containers are designated for glass carpules)
Anesthetic needles
Other syringe needles
Worn-out burs
Broken instruments
Instrument tips
Any other sharp items that may injure individuals handling waste

---

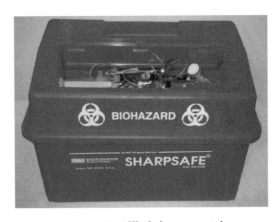

FIG. 5-14 Overfilled sharps container.

TABLE 5-8

CDC recommendations for management of persons exposed to blood*

HUMAN IMMUNODEFICIENCY VIRUS POSTEXPOSURE MANAGEMENT

Source has AIDS *or* is positive for HIV *or* refuses to be tested	Source tested and found seronegative with no clinical manifestations of AIDS or HIV infection	Source cannot be identified
1. The exposed employee should be counseled about the risk of infection. 2. The exposed employee should be evaluated clinically and serologically for evidence of HIV infection as soon as possible after the exposure. 3. The exposed worker should be advised to report and seek medical evaluation for any febrile illness that occurs within 12 weeks after the exposure. 4. The exposed employee should be advised to refrain from blood donation and to use appropriate protection during sexual intercourse during the follow-up period, especially the first 6 to 12 weeks after exposure. An exposed employee who tests negative initially should be retested 6 weeks, 12 weeks, and a minimum of 6 months after exposure to determine whether transmission has occurred.	No further follow-up is necessary unless one or both of the following is true: 1. Evidence suggests that the source may have been recently exposed. 2. Follow-up is requested by the employee or recommended by a healthcare provider. If testing is done, the guidelines in the left column may be followed.	Decisions regarding appropriate follow-up should be individualized. Serologic testing should be performed if the employee is concerned that HIV transmission may have occurred.

HEPATITIS B VIRUS POSTEXPOSURE MANAGEMENT

Employee	Source HBsAg positive	Source HBsAg negative	Source unknown or not tested
Unvaccinated	1. Hepatitis B vaccine should be initiated. *and* 2. Employee should receive a single dose of hepatitis B immune globulin (HBIG) as soon as possible (within 24 hours, if possible).	Hepatitis B vaccine should be initiated.	Hepatitis B vaccine should be initiated.
Previously vaccinated Known responder	Employee should be tested for anti-HBs: 1. If adequate, no treatment is necessary. 2. If inadequate, a hepatitis B vaccine booster dose is necessary.	No treatment	No treatment
Known nonresponder	1. Employee should receive two doses HBIG (second dose 1 month after the first dose). *or* 2. Employee should receive 1 dose HBIG plus 1 dose hepatitis B vaccine.	No treatment	If source is known to be high risk, employee may be treated as if source were HBsAg positive. Employee should be treated for anti-HBs: 1. If inadequate, a hepatitis B vaccine booster dose should be administered.
Response unknown	Employee should be tested for anti-HBs: 1. If inadequate, 1 dose HBIG plus a vaccine booster dose should be administered. 2. If adequate, no treatment is necessary.	No treatment	2. If adequate, no treatment is necessary.

Data from Centers for Disease Control and Prevention (CDC): *Practical infection control in the dental office,* Atlanta, 1993, CDC. Data based on recommendation from Hepatitis B virus: a comprehensive strategy for eliminating transmission in the United States through universal childhood vaccination—recommendations of the Immunization Practices Advisory Committee (ACIP), *MMWR CDC Surveill Summ* 40(RR-13):1-25, 1991.
*Once an exposure has occurred, the blood of the source individual should be tested for hepatitis B surface antigen (HBsAg) and antibody to human immunodeficiency virus (HIV antibody). Local laws regarding consent to test source individuals should be followed. Testing of the source individuals should be done at a location where appropriate counseling is available; posttest counseling and referral for treatment should be provided.

Although this practice is common, it is not safe. If the instrument is both sharp and contaminated with a significant mass of blood and debris (adhered to the blade of the curet), a puncture or small tear to the glove that could possibly break the skin, would potentially expose the DHCP to infectious agents. Simply developing a one-handed debriding technique, such as moist cotton rolls taped to the tray edge, eliminates this risk.

Postexposure management

Postexposure evaluation and follow-up is determined by a designated staff member and/or attending healthcare provider.[13,21,25,72,76] Postexposure follow-up may include testing of the source and recipient blood, medically indicated prophylaxis, counseling, and evaluation of subsequent reported illnesses.

Preparation for the possible event of an injury is important for its timely management. Guidelines and protocols are available from the CDC,[21] OSHA,[76] and the ADA (Table 5-8; see the suggested agencies and web sites [53-54] later in the chapter).

Laboratory Procedures

As with instrument processing and handling of x-rays, items that are removed from the immediate treatment area also must be handled to prevent cross-contamination,[2] including all materials and appliances that require handling for laboratory work, cleaning, or repair. These items must be disinfected before they are transported from the office. In addition, all appliances and materials coming from the laboratory phase of care must be disinfected and rinsed before they are tried or inserted into the patient's mouth, including removable prostheses and appliances and any instruments contaminated during the laboratory phase of treatment (such as spatulas, lab knives, acrylic burs and stones, carvers). All impression/treatment trays must be disinfected after each use.

Impression and bite registration materials vary in their compatibility to disinfection agents. The manufacturer's information always must be consulted to ensure that the impression isn't damaged. Both biohazardous and chemical risks are present in the management of impressions, and the DHCP should use appropriate PPE.

When removable appliances are polished with an office dental lathe, WPC again should be used to eliminate cross-contamination from the pumice and/or rag wheel. PPE to protect the eyes also is indicated.

Waste Management

Waste generated in the dental environment is classified in a variety of ways based on the potential risk to humans and/or the environment during the disposal, transport, and/or treatment of the waste.[2,21,40,60,67] These categories include physical, biohazardous, and chemical wastes. General waste does not pose any significant risk; infectious (biohazardous) waste and toxic (chemical) waste pose possible or definite risks. Biohazardous waste is identified as either sharps or saturated absorbent material that is "dripping" with blood and/or saliva.

Relevant waste categories that are regulated include items referred to as *sharps,* including used and unused needles, local anesthetic needles and carpules, instruments and broken glass; human tissues and foreign bodies, including teeth removed during surgery; blood-contaminated material or items that would release blood; or other potentially infectious materials, including saliva, if compressed. Sharps removed from their original packaging should be disposed of in the biohazard-labeled, puncture-resistant, leak-proof containers found near the site or use of disposable sharps.

All waste generated during treatment should be considered contaminated and therefore potentially infectious. Biohazardous waste from the patient's mouth is to be segregated at the point of generation during treatment in designated containers in the treatment room and in the facility's main waste receptacle after completion of treatment. Materials placed in this bag include but are not limited to soaked or blood-contaminated cotton rolls, gauze, cotton pellets, and similar items.

Each facility should consult its local governing agency for rules and regulation about collection, storage, transport, and treatment of biohazardous and toxic waste from a healthcare facility. The regulations vary widely, and strict adherence to local regulations is required.

The overall health and safety of each patient and DHCP is in the hands of each employee. A commitment to sound practices based on inherent risk and science are necessary for the health of all involved.

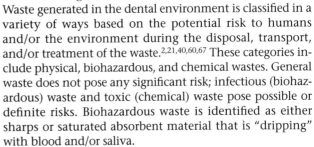

RITICAL THINKING ACTIVITIES

1. Review the first case study about Ruth, the dental office manager. Remember that Ruth's primary duties are at the front desk, although she occasionally helps when the back office is running behind schedule. Ruth's duties require that she regularly handles patient charts, filing, and billing and insurance papers. Often, she is the first person to receive the patient chart immediately after completion of the appointment.

   Considering that Ruth has missed several weeks of work and is showing lingering signs of a systemic illness, it is possible that she has contracted an illness at work. Using this knowledge, address the following issues:

   a. Review her work responsibilities and determine whether she is considered high risk for occupational transmission.

   b. Which tasks would put her at risk?

   c. Is she at risk from the work practices of others in the office?

   d. Which OSHA abatement strategies would reduce the previously stated risks?

2. Review the second case study about the dental hygiene student in her second (final) year. If you had

Continued

CRITICAL THINKING ACTIVITIES—cont'd

been the student who noticed that the cycle integrator on the sterilization bag had not changed for the instruments you had used, which steps would you need to take to identify which load(s) of instruments had been distributed without indication that appropriate sterilization had taken place?

You have determined that the instruments appear to have been used during a student laboratory, and some have been used on general clinic patients. At least one patient is confirmed to have been exposed to unsterilized instruments, but no other students are able to confirm whether the instruments they used that session were from the same load. Review the SOP for your sterilization area, given the same incident, and answer the following questions:

a. Could you determine the following?
1. How many packs must be found; how many were sterilized in the batch(es) in question?
2. How many packs had been opened and used?
3. For which patients or activities were the packs used?
4. Which procedures would assist you in determining on whom the instruments in question were used?

b. If you are unable to follow up on tasks 1 through 4, develop a SOP that would allow you to track the loads in question.

3. Review the third case study about the dental hygienist wiping an instrument tip clean. Think about times in which you have observed a dental hygienist withdraw an instrument from a patient's mouth with a significant mass of blood and debris adhered to the working end. Without thought, many hygienists reach over with a pinching motion and wipe the instrument clean with a piece of gauze. Consider the following issues:
a. Discuss the risks involved in wiping instruments in your fingers.
b. Examine resources in your clinic and develop a hands-free method to debride your instrument during patient treatment.
c. Present an argument in favor of the implementation of safer work practice controls.

4. Review the fourth case study about Mr. Lightfoot and reflect on his activities before he developed the eye infection:
a. Do you agree with the probable cause of his infection?
b. Which OSHA WPCs would provide protection from this incident in the future?
c. Are safeguards in place in your clinic to prevent such an incident?
d. Which SOPs could be implemented to prevent a repeat occurrence?

REVIEW QUESTIONS

1. An infection resulting from the introduction of microorganisms from one area of the body to another occurs by which of the following methods?
   a. Autogenous transmission
   b. Aerosol transmission
   c. Direct transmission
   d. Indirect transmission

2. Which is the most important factor in the development of an infection within a host?
   a. The dose of the pathogenic microorganisms transmitted
   b. The integrity of the host's immune system
   c. The virulence of the microorganisms transmitted
   d. All the above have significance impact on the development of disease; one factor cannot be singled out.

3. Which of the following diseases are caused by bacterial agents?
   a. Candidiasis, hepatitis, legionella
   b. Legionella, pneumonia, tuberculosis
   c. Influenza, pneumonia, tuberculosis
   d. Candidiasis, legionella, tuberculosis

4. You have purchased some instrument trays for use in the office that are made of heat-sensitive plastic, and the following label was included in the package:

Dental Set-Up Tray
To Sterilize: Use alcohol or other approved disinfectants.

Which of the following statements is correct?
   a. The instructions provided are correct; sterilization of the tray would be accomplished.
   b. The instructions provided are partially correct; sterilization of the tray would be accomplished with the use of alcohol but not with other approved disinfectants.
   c. The instructions provided are partially correct; sterilization of the tray would be accomplished with other approved disinfectants but not with alcohol.

REVIEW QUESTIONS—cont'd

   d. The instructions provided are incorrect; sterilization of the tray would be not be accomplished by either method listed.

5. OSHA has defined which of the following as primary hazard abatement strategies to reduce the risk of occupational exposures to bloodborne diseases?
   a. Universal controls (UC), housekeeping, and engineering precautions (EP)
   b. Universal precautions (UP), personal protective engineering (PPE), and labels
   c. Universal precautions (UP), work practice controls (WPC), and record keeping
   d. Universal controls (UC), personal protective equipment (PPE), and training

SUGGESTED AGENCIES AND WEB SITES

Because of the ever-changing nature of the Internet, some of the web sites listed here may have changed since publication. Please refer to Mosby's Evolve web site for the most current information.

Infectious Diseases of Concern for Dental Healthcare Providers
1. National Center for Infectious Diseases: http://www.cdc.gov
2. The Lightning Hypertext of Disease, Pathology Informatics, Inc.: http://www.pathinfo.com
3. CDC, National Center for Infectious Diseases: http://www.cdc.gov
4. CDC ("Health topics A to Z"): http://www.cdc.gov/health
5. CDC *(Emerging Infectious Diseases)*: http://www.cdc.gov
6. Infectious Disease News: http://www.infectiousdiseasenews.com
7. *MMWR*: http://www2.cdc.gov
8. CDC ("Emerging infectious diseases resource links"): http://www.cdc.gov
9. National Institutes of Health: http://www.nih.gov

Diseases Caused by Viral Agents
10. David M. Sander, PhD ("All the Virology on the World Wide Web"): http://www.tulane.edu
11. Division of Viral and Rickettsial Diseases: http://www.cdc

Hepatitis Infection
12. HepNet (the Hepatitis Information Network): http://www.hepnet.com
13. CDC ("Viral hepatitis"): http://www.cdc.gov

Herpes Viruses
14. International Herpes Management Forum: http://www.ihmf.org

Herpes Simplex 2
15. CDC ("Genital herpes"): http://www.cdc.gov

Cytomegalovirus
16. CDC ("Cytomegalovirus [CMV] infection"): http://www.cdc.gov

Epstein-Barr and Infectious Mononucleosis
17. National Center for Infectious Diseases ("Epstein-Barr virus and infectious mononucleosis"): http://www.cdc.gov

Varicella-Zoster Virus
18. CDC ("Varicella-zoster virus [chickenpox]"): http://www.cdc.gov
19. CDC ("Herpes zoster [shingles]"): http://www.cdc.gov

HIV Infection and AIDS
20. AEGIS (pronounced *ee-jis*): http://www.aegis.com
21. HIVDENT: http://www.hivdent.org
22. CDC ("HIV infection and AIDS"): http://www.cdc.gov

Common Cold
23. CDC ("Adenoviruses"): http://www.cdc.gov

Influenza
24. CDC ("Influenza prevention and control"): http://www.cdc.gov
25. CDC ("Human parainfluenza viruses"): http://www.cdc.gov

Diseases Caused by Bacterial Agents
26. CDC, Division of Bacterial and Mycotic Diseases: http://www.cdc.gov

Gonorrhea
27. CDC ("*Neisseria gonorrhea*"): http://www.cdc.gov

Legionella
28. CDC (Legionellosis: legionnaires' disease and Pontiac fever"): http://www.cdc.gov

Staphylococcus Infections
29. CDC ("Toxic shock syndrome"): http://www.cdc.gov
30. CDC ("Preventing emerging infectious diseases: a strategy for the 21st century"): http://www.cdc.gov

Streptococcus Infections
31. CDC ("Group A streptococcal [GAS] disease"): http://www.cdc.gov
32. CDC ("Group B streptococcal [GBS] disease"): http://www.cdc.gov

Syphilis
33. AEGIS: http://www.aegis.com
34. Encarta ("Syphilis"): http://encarta.msn.com

Tuberculosis
35. CDC ("Tuberculosis"): http://www.cdc.gov
36. National Tuberculosis Center: http://www.umdnj.edu
37. Columbia University Medical Informatics: http://www.cpmc.columbia.edu
38. *TB and Outbreaks Weekly*: http://www.newsrx.net
39. Encarta ("Tuberculosis"): http://encarta.msn.com

Continued

SUGGESTED AGENCIES AND WEB SITES—cont'd

Government Agencies: Regulations, Standards, and Guidelines

40. Centers for Disease Control and Prevention (CDC): http://www.cdc.gov
41. Occupational Safety and Health Administration (OSHA): http://www.osha.gov
42. Environmental Protection Agency (EPA): http://www.epa.gov
43. Food and Drug Administration (FDA): http://www.fda.gov

Professional Associations

44. Organization for Safety and Asepsis Procedures (OSAP): http://www.osap.org
45. Association for Professionals in Infection Control and Epidemiology (APIC): http://www.apic.org
46. American Dental Association (ADA): http://www.ada.org
47. American Dental Education Association (ADEA): http://www. adea.org

Recommendations for Immunizations for Children, Adults, and Healthcare Workers

48. CDC, National Immunization Program: http://www.cdc.gov

Latex Allergy

49. CETRA Latex-Free: http://www.latexfree.com
50. The Latex Allergy Information Resource: http://www.anesth.com
51. Allergy Internet Resources (AIR): http://www.immune.com
52. Spina Bifida Association ("Latex in the hospital environment"): http://www.sbaa.org

Other

53. American National Standards Institute: http://www.ansi.org
54. CDC ("Public health service guidelines for the management of healthcare worker exposures to HIV and recommendations for postexposure prophylaxis"): http://www.cdc.gov
55. Northwest Fisheries Science Center ("MSDS sheets"): http://research.nwfsc.noaa.gov

 ADDITIONAL READINGS AND RESOURCES

Centers for Disease Control and Prevention: *CDC year-end HIV/ AIDS surveillance report,* Atlanta, 2000, CDC.

Miller CH, Palenik CJ: *Infection control and management of hazardous materials for the dental team,* St Louis, 1998, Mosby.

Occupational Safety and Health Administration: *Revisions to bloodborne pathogens standard.* Federal Register, 29 CFR. Part 1910. Washington, DC, January 18, 2001, OSHA.

OSAP: *Chemical agents for surface disinfection reference chart,* Annapolis, Md, 1998, OSAP.

OSAP: *Infection control guidelines,* Annapolis, Md, 1997, OSAP.

OSAP Monthly Focus: Annapolis, Md, OSAP.

OSAP Position Paper: *Surface/environmental asepsis,* Annapolis, Md, 2001, OSAP.

OSAP Position Paper: *Percutaneous injury prevention,* Annapolis, Md, 1997, OSAP.

OSAP Position Paper: *Instrument processing,* Annapolis, Md, 1997, OSAP.

OSAP Position Paper: *Laboratory asespsis,* Annapolis, Md, 1998, OSAP.

Rhode J: Ambidextrous gloves—can they contribute to carpal tunnel syndrome? *Dent Today* 9(5):1-2, 1990.

 REFERENCES

1. American Dental Association: Dental unit waterlines: approaching the year 2000. *J Am Dent Assoc Association Report* 130:1653-64, 1999.
2. American Dental Association: Infection control recommendations for the dental office and the dental laboratory [CD-ROM], *J Am Dent Assoc* CD-ROM:672-80, 1996.
3. American Dental Association: *Statement on backflow prevention and the dental office.* ADA position statement. Chicago, 1996, The Association.
4. American Dental Association: *Statement on dental unit waterlines,* Chicago, 1995, The Association.
5. Atlas, et al: Legionella contamination of dental-unit waters, *Appl Environ Microbiol* 61:1208-13, 1995.
6. Bednarsh HS, Eklund KJ, Mills S: Check your dental unit water IQ, *Dent Assist* 65(6):9-10, 1996.
7. Bednarsh HS, Eklund KJ: *Dental staff health and safety training,* Brunswick, Me, 1999, InVision.
8. Bednarsh HS, Eklund KJ: CDC issues final TB guidelines, *Access* 10(5):6-13, 1995.
9. Benenson AS: *Control of communicable diseases in man,* ed 15, Washington DC, 1990, American Public Health Association.
10. Bentley CD, Burkhart NW, Crawford JJ: Evaluating spatter and aerosol contamination during dental procedures [CD-ROM], *J Am Dent Assoc* May:579-84, 1994.
11. Bernstein DE, de Medina MD: *Hepatitis viruses,* Deerfield Beach, Fla, 1998, Health Studies Institute, Inc.
12. Blanco C et al: Latex allergy: clinical features and cross-reactivity with fruits, *Ann Allergy* 73:309-14, 1994.
13. Bolyard EA et al: Guideline for infection control in health care personnel 1998. *Am J Infect Control* 26:289-354, 1998.
14. Carmichael CG et al: *HIV/AIDS: what health professionals need to know,* Miami, Fla, 1996, Health Studies Institute, Inc.
15. Centers for Disease Control and Prevention: Guidelines for preventing the transmission of Mycobacterium tuberculosis in health-care facilities, 1994. *MMWR CDC Surveill Summ* 43(RR-13);1-132, 1994.
16. Centers for Disease Control and Prevention: *Infection control in dentistry—airborne* [Internet], Atlanta, 1999, The Centers [http://www.cdc.gov].
17. Centers for Disease Control and Prevention: *Infection control in dentistry—bloodborne* [Internet], Atlanta, 1999, The Centers [http://www.cdc.gov].

18. Centers for Disease Control and Prevention: *Infection control in dentistry—waterborne* [Internet], Atlanta, 1999, The Centers [http://www.cdc.gov].

19. Centers for Disease Control and Prevention: Prevention and control of influenza. Part I. Vaccines, *MMWR CDC Surveill Summ* 43(RR-9):1-13, 1994.

20. Centers for Disease Control and Prevention: Prevention and control of influenza. Part II. Antiviral agents—recommendations of ACIP, *MMWR CDC Surveill Summ* 43(RR-15):1-10, 1994.

21. Centers for Disease Control and Prevention: Guidelines for Infection-control in dental healthcare settings 2003, *MMWR CDC Recommendations and Reports* 52(RR17):1-61, 2003.

22. Centers for Disease Control and Prevention: Recommendations of the Advisory Committee on Immunization Practices: use of vaccines and immune globulins for persons with altered immunocompetence, *MMWR CDC Surveill Summ* 42 (RR-4):1-17, 1993.

23. Ceisel RJ et al: Evaluating chemical inactivation of viral agents in handpiece splatter [CD-ROM], *J Am Dent Assoc* Feb: 197-202, 1995.

24. Challacombe SJ, Fernandes LL: Detecting *Legionella pneumophila* in water systems: a comparison of various dental units [CD-ROM], *J Am Dent Assoc* May:603-8, 1995.

25. Chenoweth CE, Gobetti JP: Postexposure chemoprophylaxis for occupational exposure to HIV in the dental office [CD-ROM], *J Am Dent Assoc* Aug:1135-39, 1997.

26. Christensen GJ: Using rubber dams to boost quality, quantity of restorative services, *J Am Dent Assoc* 125:81-2, 1994.

27. Cleveland JL: Hepatitis B vaccination and infection among U.S. dentists, 1983-1992, *J Am Dent Assoc* Sept:1385-90, September 1996.

28. Cleveland JL et al: Risk and prevention of hepatitis C virus infection: implications for dentistry, *J Am Dent Assoc* 130:641-47, 1999.

29. Cleveland JL et al: TB infection control recommendations from the CDC, 1994: considerations for dentistry [CD-ROM], *J Am Dent Assoc* May:593-600, 1995.

30. Columbia University Department of Medical Informatics, TB resources: *About tuberculosis* [Internet], New York, 1999, The University [http://www.cpmc.edu/tbcpp/abouttb.html].

31. Columbia University Department of Medical Informatics, TB resources: *TB: getting cured* [Internet], New York, 1999, The University [http://www.cpmc.columbia.edu/tbcpp/tbcure. html].

32. Columbia University Department of Medical Informatics, TB resources: *Preventing tuberculosis* [Internet], New York, 1999, The University [http://www.cpmc.columbia.edu/tbcpp/prevent/ html].

33. Columbia University Department of Medical Informatics, TB resources: *The tuberculin skin test* [Internet], New York, 1999, The University [http://www.cpmc.columbia.edu/tbcpp/skintest. html].

34. Columbia University Department of Medical Informatics: Tuberculosis resources [Internet], New York, NY, 1999, The University [http://www.cpmc.columbia.edu/tbcpp/.html].

35. Cottone JA, Terezhalmy GT, Molinari JA: *Practical infection control in dentistry*, ed 2, Media, Pa, Williams & Wilkins, 1996.

36. Cuny EJ, Fredekind R, Budenz AW: Safety needles: new requirements of the Occupational Safety and Health Administration bloodborne pathogens rule, *J Calif Dent Assoc* 26(7):525-30, 1999.

37. Curriculum Guidelines for the dental care management of patients with bloodborne infectious diseases, *J Dent Ed* 55:9: 609-19, 1991.

38. Diagnosis: latex allergy! Now what? *Latex Allergy News* I(1), 1999 (entire issue).

39. Eleazer PD et al: A chemical treatment regimen to reduce bacterial contamination in dental waterlines, *J Am Dent Assoc* 128:617-23, 1997.

40. *Environmental management and pollution prevention: a guide for dental programs*, adapted from Local Hazardous Waste Management Program of King County: *Waste management guidelines for King County dental offices*, King County, Wash, 1993, The Program.

41. Falcons KJ, O'Fee PD: Latex allergy: implications for oral health care professionals, *J Dent Hyg* 72(3):25-32, 1998.

42. Fons MP et al: Multiple herpes viruses in saliva of HIV-infected individuals [CD-ROM], *J Am Dent Assoc* June:713-19, 1994.

43. Gillcrist JA: Hepatitis viruses A, B, C, D, E, and G: implications for dental personnel, *J Am Dent Assoc* 130:509-520, 1999.

44. Goodman HS, Carpenter RD, Cox MR: Sterilization of dental instruments and devices: an update, *Am J Infect Control* 35(2): 323-37, 1992.

45. HepNet—The Hepatitis Information Network: Education Events Featured Articles: *Epidemiology* & *natural history of hepatitis B* [Internet], Schering, Canada, 1998, HepNet [http://www.hepnet.com/boca/seef2.html].

46. HepNet—The Hepatitis Information Network: Education Events Featured Articles: *Epidemiology and natural history of hepatitis C, virus infection, hepatitis C* [Internet], Schering, Canada, 1998, HepNet [http://www.hepnet.com/boca/epiden. html].

47. HepNet—The Hepatitis Information Network: *Hepatitis A: Hepatitis A—what is it?* [Internet], Schering, Canada, 1998, HepNet [http://www.hepnet.com/hepa/hepafact.html].

48. HepNet—The Hepatitis Information Network: *Hep Update: Hepatitis A, D, E, & G* [Internet], Schering, Canada, 1998, HepNet [http://www.hepnet.com/update14.html].

49. HepNet—The Hepatitis Information Network: *Hepatitis D: The hepatitis D virus* [Internet], Schering, Canada, 1998, HepNet [http://www.hepnet.com/hepd/wormhdv.html].

50. HepNet—The Hepatitis Information Network: *Hepatitis G press release: Hepatitis G* [Internet], Schering, Canada, 1998, HepNet [http://www.hepnet.com/hepg/hepg1.html].

51. HepNet—The Hepatitis Information Network: *HepNews press release: hepatitis A deadly in hepatitis C sufferers* [Internet], Schering, Canada, 1998, HepNet [http://www.hepnet.com/ hepc/news12898.html].

52. HepNet—The Hepatitis Information Network: *HepNews press release: new report on hepatitis C epidemic indicates time is now to stop killer disease* [Internet], Schering, Canada, March 16, 1998, HepNet [http://www.hepnet.com/hepc/news31698. html].

53. HepNet—The Hepatitis Information Network: *HepNews press release: Schering-Plough reports results of clinical studies of Rebertron combination therapy for hepatitis C at American Association for the Study of Liver Diseases meeting* [Internet], Schering, Canada, November 9, 1999, HepNet [http://www.hepnet.com/ hepc/news110999.html].

54. Huntley DE, Campbell J: Bacterial contamination of scrub jackets during dental hygiene procedures, *J Dent Hyg* 72:3:19-23, 1998.

55. American Medical Association, JAMA HIV/AIDS Information Center: *Treatment center—secondary prevention recommendations* [Internet], Chicago, 1999, The Association http://www. ama-assn.org/special/hiv/treatmnt/guide/rr4719/rr4719j.html].

56. Karpay RI et al: Validation of an in-office dental unit water monitoring technique, *J Am Dent Assoc* 129:207-11, 1998.

57. Kolstad RA: The emergence of load-oriented sterilization, *J Am Dent Assoc* 125:51-4, 1994.

58. Larson EL: APIC guideline for handwashing and antisepsis in healthcare settings, *Am J Infect Control* 23:251-69, 1995.

59. Merchant VA: An update on herpes viruses, *J Calif Dent Assoc* 24(1):38-46, 1996.

60. Metro King County Hazardous Waste Management Program: *Disinfectants and cleaners* [Internet], Seattle, 1999, King County http://www.metrokc.gov/hazwaste/yb/disinfectant. html].

61. Miller CH, Palenik CJ: *Infection control and management of hazardous materials for the dental team,* St Louis, 1998, Mosby.
62. Molinari JA: Practical infection control for the 1990s: applying science to government regulations [CD-ROM], *J Am Dent Assoc* September:1189-97, 1994.
63. Murdoch-Kinch CA et al: Comparison of dental water quality management procedures [CD-ROM], *J Am Dent Assoc* September:1235-43, 1997.
64. Nisengard RJ, Newman MG: *Oral microbiology and immunology,* Philadelphia, 1994, WB Saunders.
65. Organization for Safety and Asepsis Procedures (OSAP): *Organization for safety and asepsis procedures infection control in dentistry guidelines,* Annapolis, Md, September 1997, OSAP.
66. OSAP Monthly Focus: *1999 in review: Infection control highlights & headlines from the past year. Focus #11.* Annapolis, Md, 1999, OSAP.
67. OSAP Monthly Focus: *Dental office waste management. Focus #10.* Annapolis, Md, 1998, OSAP.
68. OSAP Monthly Focus: *Emerging diseases with an impact on dentistry. Focus #9.* Annapolis, Md, 1999, OSAP.
69. OSAP Monthly Focus: *Environmental surface disinfection. Focus #6.* Annapolis, Md, 1998, OSAP.
70. OSAP Monthly Focus: *Hand asepsis. Focus #3.* Annapolis, Md, 1998, OSAP.
71. OSAP Monthly Focus: *Latex-associated allergies & conditions. Focus #4.* Annapolis, Md, 1998, OSAP.
72. OSAP Monthly Focus: *Postexposure prophylaxis: Focus #5. CDC issues recommendations for healthcare workers exposed to HIV,* Annapolis, Md, 1998, OSAP.
73. OSAP Position Papers: *Dental unit waterlines,* Annapolis, Md, January 1997, OSAP.
74. OSAP Position Papers: Instrument processing, Annapolis, Md, January 1997, OSAP.
75. OSAP Position Papers: Percutaneous injury, Annapolis, Md, January 1997, OSAP.
76. Occupational Safety and Health Administration: *OSHA regulations: bloodborne pathogens.* Final rule. Federal Register, 29 CFR. Part 1910.1030. 56(235):64175-82, Washington, DC, December 6, 1992, OSHA.
77. Occupational Safety and Health Administration: *Personal protective equipment for general industry.* Final rule. Federal Register, 29 CFR. Part 1910.132. 59(66):16334-64, Washington, DC, April 6, 1994, OSHA.
78. Personal protective equipment for protection against exposure to bloodborne organisms, *J Pract Hyg* May/June:48-51, 1999.
79. Recommended clinical guidelines for infection control in dental education institutions, *J Dent Educ* 55:9:621-30, 1991.
80. Reichert M, Young JH: *Sterilization technology for the health care facility,* ed 2, Gaithersburg Md, 1997, Aspen.
81. Rhode J: Ambidextrous gloves—can they contribute to carpal tunnel syndrome? *Dent Today* 9(5)1-2, 1990.
82. Runnells RR: *Infection control in the wet finger environment,* Salt Lake City, Utah, 1984, Publishers Press.
83. Rutala WA: APIC guideline for selection and use of disinfectants, *Am J Infect Control* 24:313-42, 1996.
84. Rutala WA: *Chemical germicides in health care, International Symposium,* Washington, DC, May 1994, Association for Professionals in Infection Control and Epidemiology, Inc.
85. Sanchez E, Macdonald G: Decontaminating dental instruments: testing the effectiveness of selected methods [CD-ROM], *J Am Dent Assoc* March:359-68, 1995.
86. Shulman ST, Phair JP, Sommers HM: *The biologic & clinical basis of infectious diseases,* Philadelphia, 1992, WB Saunders.
87. Slavkin HC: The A, B, C, D, and E of viral hepatitis [CD-ROM], *J Am Dent Assoc* November:1667-70, 1996.
88. Slavkin HC: Infection and Immunity [CD-ROM], *J Am Dent Assoc* December:1792-6, 1996.
89. Spaulding EH: Chemical disinfection of medical and surgical materials. In Lawrence CA, Block SS, editors. *Disinfection, sterilization, and preservation,* Philadelphia, 1968, Lea & Febiger, pp. 517-531.
90. Sussman GL, Beezhold DH: Allergy to latex rubber *Ann Intern Med* 122:43-6, 1995.
91. U.S. Department of Health and Human Services, CDC: *Practical infection control in the dental office,* Atlanta, October 1993, CDC.
92. Using millipore samplers in dental settings, Millipore Technical Brief, TB094 [Internet], Bedford, Mass, 1998, Millipore.
93. Westlund R, Kim HH, Schulman J: *Tuberculosis resurgent,* Miami, Fla, 1995, Health Studies Institute.
94. Willett NP, White RR, Rosen S: *Essential dental microbiology,* Norwalk, Conn, 1991, Appleton & Lange.
95. Williams JF et al: Assessing microbial contamination of dental unit waterlines: prevalence, intensity and microbiological characteristics, *J Am Dent Assoc* 124:59-65, 1993.
96. Williams HN et al: Assessing microbial contamination in clean water dental units and compliance with disinfection protocol [CD-ROM], *J Am Dent Assoc* September:1205-11, 1994.
97. Williams HN, Baer ML, Kelley JI: Contribution of biofilm bacteria to the contamination of the dental unit water supply [CD-ROM], *J Am Dent Assoc* September:1255-60, 1995.

CHAPTER 6

Workstation Design *and* Positioning

Beckie M. Barry, William Woodall

Chapter Outline

Case Study: Musculoskeletal Problems Resulting
  from Equipment
Workstation and Positioning for the Dental
  Hygienist
Musculoskeletal Problems
    Prevalence
    Definitions
    Additional considerations
Normal Anatomy and Anatomical Changes
Positioning
    Operator positioning
    Patient positioning

Operator positioning during instrumentation
  procedures
Positioning for ultrasonic scaling
Position of dental equipment
Recognition of errors in positioning
Reducing Fatigue
    Magnification systems
    Armrests
Treatment and Exercises
    Types of exercises

Key Terms

Biocentric technique
Dioptre magnification
Ergonomics
Eye loupes
Facet joint
Fiber optics
Herniated or
  "slipped" disc

Kyphosis
Ligaments
Lordosis
Musculoskeletal disorders (MSDs)
Neutral position
Nucleus pulposus
Occupational Safety and Health
  Administration (OSHA)

Operator positioning
Patient positioning
Performance Logic (PL)
  positioning
Postural syndrome
Proprioceptive
Repetitive strain injuries (RSIs)

Semisupine position
Supine position
Synovial joints
Telescopic loupes
Thoracic outlet syndrome (TOS)
Work-related musculoskeletal
  disorders (WMSDs)

Learning Outcomes

1. Develop an appreciation for evidence-based knowledge of ergonomics in the dental environment.
2. Understand the relationship among correct operator posture and positioning, patient and equipment positioning, and musculoskeletal problems.
3. Describe the physical changes that occur from repetitive strain injuries (RSIs).
4. Demonstrate correct operator, patient, and equipment positioning for maximal efficiency and minimal risk for development of musculoskeletal problems.
5. Compare, contrast, and evaluate alternative operator and patient positions.

6. Correct improper positioning by recognizing cues that indicate that an aspect of positioning is incorrect.
7. Develop awareness of new technology that may reduce operator stress and fatigue and promote optimal performance.
8. Incorporate preventive exercises into workday activities such as instrumentation and when at home.
9. Apply correct operator, patient, and equipment positioning for maximal efficiency for ultrasonic scaling.
10. Observe and recognize positioning that may cause RSDs.

Musculoskeletal Problems Resulting from Equipment

Juanita Mineke is a dental hygienist who practiced 6 years as a clinician in private practice and for the past 6 years as an educator. As part of her educational employment, she participated in the university's private practice plan. She chose to work one half-day a week for a general dentist and initially worked on a day when the other hygienist was not in the office. This schedule allowed her to use the full-time hygienist's room, which was set up with state-of-the-art equipment. The equipment components facilitated easy access and manageability of the light, bracket tray, handpieces, suction, and air/water (a/w) syringe and offered maximum visibility through proper lighting. In addition, the operator's chair provided adjustable back support with adjustable chair height.

Juanita changed her half-day schedule 8 weeks later to a day when the other hygienist was also working. This placed Juanita in the "extra" treatment room, the one set up for denture try-ons and emergency patient screenings. This smaller room restricted free movement of equipment and personnel; access to the suction and a/w syringe required stretching across the patient; reaching the instrument tray required Juanita to stretch and twist each time she changed instruments, and the operator's chair was the surplus secretarial chair from the front office. After 4 months, Juanita began experiencing tingling and numbness in the little and ring finger of her left hand, followed shortly by the same feeling in her right hand. Pain in right thumb and wrist followed the tingling and numbness.

The situation described in the case study occurred in the middle 1980s before extensive knowledge of *ergonomics,* repetitive strain injuries, and cumulative trauma disorders in the dental hygiene profession was widespread. The case illustrates that this hygienist failed to immediately recognize the consequence of using inadequate equipment placement. Perhaps she held a common belief that her body was immune to musculoskeletal problems.

WORKSTATION AND POSITIONING FOR THE DENTAL HYGIENIST

The practice of dental hygiene requires the operator to perform intricate tasks in a relatively small area with limited visibility. Often this results in the practitioner assuming an uncomfortable posture, such as leaning forward, dropping the head, and rolling the shoulders forward to improve visibility; projecting the arms away from the body; and remaining in a static position for a long time.

Proper positioning is critical for the dental hygienist's physical longevity in the practice of dental hygiene. Mention of *musculoskeletal disorders (MSDs)* associated with dentistry is found in the dental literature of the late 1950s and 1960s. However, musculoskeletal disorders related to the practice of dental hygiene were scarcely documented before the early 1980s. Numerous studies over the past 20 years identify musculoskeletal disorders as a common oc-

cupational complaint of dental hygienists, even temporarily or permanently compromising the hygienist's ability to work.* These complaints range from neck, shoulder, and back problems to carpal tunnel and thoracic outlet syndrome, all of which affect dental hygiene students, recent graduates, and experienced hygienists. Age and the number of years of professional experience do not seem to make a significant difference. Although early recognition of these problems is important, even better is development of postural habits to promote prevention.

Current collective terms for these complaints are *repetitive strain injuries (RSIs)* in the physical therapy literature, cumulative trauma disorders (CTDs) RSI in the dental hygiene literature, and *work-related musculoskeletal disorders (WMSDs)* in government literature.

> This chapter will use the term *repetitive strain injuries (RSIs)* synonymously with *cumulative trauma disorders* and *work-related musculoskeletal disorders.*

This chapter focuses on the following:
- Normal anatomy, anatomical changes, and treatment of RSI
- Proper positioning of the operator, equipment, and patient for treatment procedures
- Cues for identification of improper positioning
- The use of *eye loupes* and arm rests to reduce fatigue
- Treatment and exercises to incorporate into practice
- Proper positioning of the operator, equipment, and patient for ultrasonic scaling treatment procedures

This chapter also briefly defines the various repetitive strain injuries/cumulative trauma disorders and current federal guidelines that address the workplace.

> The clinician in the photographs in this chapter is not wearing personal protection equipment so that posture and positioning examples are more easily visualized.

MUSCULOSKELETAL PROBLEMS

PREVALENCE

In the United States, WMSDs account for 34% of all lost workday injuries and illnesses with business costs exceeding $15 billion in worker's compensation each year.[22] Estimates are that dental practitioners lost more than $41 million of income in 1990 as a result of CTDs.[23] The lost workdays and the rising costs of workers' compensation resulted in the development of an ergonomic standard for workers in general industry by the *Occupational Safety and Health Administration (OSHA).* Individual states are

---

*References 1, 8, 10, 15, 21, 22, 31.

also developing their own form of ergonomic standards designed to prevent MSD. OSHA defines ergonomics as follows:[22]

> . . . *the science of fitting the job to the worker. When there is a mismatch between the physical requirements of the job and the physical capacity of the worker, WMSD can result.*

> Examples of musculoskeletal disorders, according to OSHA, are injuries or disorders to nerves, *ligaments,* muscles, tendons joints, cartilage, and spinal discs.

OSHA also recognizes that individuals who repeatedly perform the same tasks, sustain awkward working positions, use a great deal of force, repeatedly lift heavy objects, or have a combination of these risk factors are most likely to develop WMSDs.

OSHA's ergonomics program standard was issued on November 14, 2000, and took effect January 16, 2001. Congress, acting under the authority of the Congressional Review Act of 1996, filed a joint resolution disapproving of OSHA's ergonomic standard. President George W. Bush on March 20, 2001, signed the joint resolution, stating:

> *The safety and health of our nation's workforce is a priority for my administration. Together we will pursue a comprehensive approach to ergonomics that addresses the concerns surrounding the ergonomics rule repealed today. We will work with the Congress, the business community, and our nation's workers to address this important issue.*

This information is available in its entirety at the following web address: http://www.osha-slc.gov.

In a news release issued on April 26, 2001, Secretary of Labor Elaine L. Chao outlined a number of ergnonomic principles that urge an approach based on prevention. The principles include and/or are based on prevention, sound science, incentives, flexibility, feasibility, and clarity. This information also is available in full at the following web address: http://www.osha.gov/media/oshnews.

Because of the increased awareness and diagnosis of these conditions, the terms *ergonomics, RSI, CTD, carpal tunnel syndrome (CTS),* and **thoracic outlet syndrome (TOS)** are now common in the dental literature. Therefore even though dental hygiene is not specifically identified as a job that will be affected by OSHA's proposed ergonomic standard, dental hygienists are exposed to five of the six risk factors listed.

DEFINITIONS

Repetitive strain injuries (RSIs) are defined as follows:[17]

> . . . *cumulative trauma disorders resulting from prolonged repetitive, forceful, or awkward movements. These movements result in damage to the muscles, tendons, and nerves. RSIs are referred to as* repetitive stress injuries, CTDs, repetitive motion disorders, occupational overuse injuries, *and* work-related musculoskeletal disorders.

The dental professional is at risk for developing RSIs for three main reasons: the repetition of tasks performed,

---

BOX 6-1

Carpal Tunnel Syndrome and Thoracic Outlet Syndrome

6-A
6-B

Carpal Tunnel Syndrome (CTS)
Description: CTS[24] is a form of peripheral neuropathy leading to compression of the median nerve between the forearm flexor muscle tendons and the transverse superficial carpal ligament. This syndrome is more prominent in women and occurs more frequently after 40 years of age.

Symptoms: Pain, numbness, or pins-and-needles sensation in the thumb, index, and middle fingers (may even include ring finger) and on the radial side of the hand may occur. It also may include the wrist, forearm, and shoulder. Pain begins slowly and may progress to a constant sensation. The affected individual may state that the pain is usually worse at night and that daily activities are limited because of the increased weakness and/or clumsiness of the involved hand.

Causes: The condition can result from compression or vascular insufficiency of the median nerve at the carpal tunnel. Possible causes for the compression or vascular insufficiency include cumulative trauma, overuse injury, and physiological disorders or structural changes. In dentistry possible causes result from flexion or overextension of the wrist. Systemic conditions that have been associated with CTS include thyroid disorders and arthritis.

Thoracic Outlet Syndrome (TOS)
Description: This is a combination of symptoms marked with paresthesias and pain that slowly appear in the shoulder, neck, arm, or hand and extend to the anterior portion of the chest wall. Onset occurs between 35 and 55 years and is seen more frequently in women.

Symptoms: The affected individual may experience fatigue after overhead arm activities, pins-and-needles sensation in the affected arm, and muscle spasms in the shoulder and neck areas.

Causes: Cause is undetermined but may be due to compression of the brachial plexus, axillary artery, and the subclavian vessels. In dentistry this can be a result of dropping of the head too far forward (forward flexion) and rounding (slumping) of the shoulders and/or working with the arms above the waist level.

---

awkward postures during work, and high workforce (force needed to perform a task).[34] Other contributing factors include static or sustained positions, insufficient rest breaks, vibrations, high pressures, poor tool/workstation design, poor-fitting equipment, and poor worker fitness level. Whether called *RSI, CTD,* or *WMSD,* musculoskeletal pain/problems (especially in the lower back, neck, and shoulder area), carpal tunnel syndrome, and thoracic outlet syndrome are occupational hazards in the dental hygiene profession.[1,8,10,21,23]

These complaints and injuries do not appear suddenly, nor are they visible conditions that can outwardly or readily be seen. They occur as a result of repetitive (chronic) movements and are noticed only after the nerves and tendons become inflamed and painful.

Box 6-1 briefly describes two common musculoskeletal conditions and their symptoms. The musculoskeletal conditions are addressed in the treatment and exercise section of the chapter.

ADDITIONAL CONSIDERATIONS

Although dental hygiene programs provide fundamental instructions for students on proper **operator positioning** and **patient positioning,** many do not offer additional information on ergonomics.[3] Pain associated with improper positioning is not always met with suggestions for relief.[14] Common solutions are directed toward the improvement and maintenance of appropriate postures and strengthening exercises. Attention to and awareness of new approaches in instrumentation techniques, new technology, and positioning associated with such techniques and technology is needed to reduce stress and fatigue.

Another consideration is the variety of effects of and treatments for RSIs. Each person has a different body structure and a unique threshold to various activities and tasks. Furthermore, systemic diseases, such as diabetes, may mimic or contribute to RSIs.[11] Although information is available in the medical/dental literature and on the Internet, to seek a diagnosis and subsequent treatment for these conditions from the appropriate healthcare provider is critical.

The following sections describe normal anatomy—changes that can occur as a result of improper operator, patient, and equipment positioning; and appropriate operator, patient, and equipment positioning. Dental hygiene students should develop and maintain these good postural habits early in their clinical education.

NORMAL ANATOMY AND ANATOMICAL CHANGES

An understanding of the musculoskeletal RSIs of the neck and back that most often affect dental hygienists requires a familiarity with the anatomy of the area. The spine is a dynamic structure made up of many smaller units. It is not a static structure designed to be a simple rigid post; instead it is designed to move. Joints between each of the 25 vertebrae make up the moveable segments of the spine. These joints have similar characteristics to other **synovial joints** throughout the body and must be treated as such. The vertebrae stack on top of another with an intervertebral disc found between the bodies of adjacent vertebrae. The spine, when in proper static alignment, has three normal curves. In the cervical and lumbar regions, the normal orientation of the curves is called **lordosis.** This means that the convex side of the curve is anterior, whereas the concave side of the curve is posterior. In the thoracic region the curve is oriented exactly opposite the cervical and lumbar curves and is referred to as **kyphosis** (Figs. 6-1 and 6-2). The most common postural abnormalities found at the spine involve decreases in cervical and lumbar lordosis and increases in the thoracic kyphosis, or in common terms, "slouching" (Fig. 6-3). Positioning the spine that maintains the normal curves creates little stress on its soft tissues and joints. However, when the normal curves are lost, either through increase or decrease in the curves, the soft tissues (e.g., muscles and ligaments) have more stress applied to them. Too

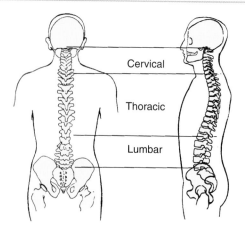

FIG. 6-1 Skeletal view of spine.

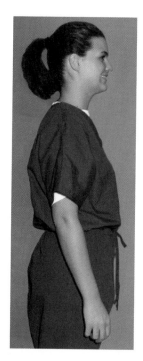

FIG. 6-2 Human view of standing posture.

much stress continually applied to these soft tissues may result in painful conditions.

The intervertebral discs are similar to a jelly donut (Fig. 6-4). The "gelatinous" center is the **nucleus pulposus,** and the outer layer is the annulus fibrosus. These discs are designed to rest between the vertebral bodies of adjacent vertebrae with the spine in its normal alignment. If the curves of the spine are changed significantly, one side of the disc will be compressed and the other side will be stretched (Fig. 6-5). If these forces are placed on the disc for long periods, eventually the disc can become damaged. Although many different classifications of disc injury exist, in general a torn or stretched annulus can allow the nucleus pulposus to move out and compress a spinal nerve root (Fig. 6-6). This **herniated** or **"slipped" disc** can cause radiating pain into the person's arm or leg.

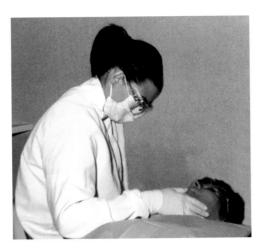

FIG. 6-3 Operator slouching chairside.

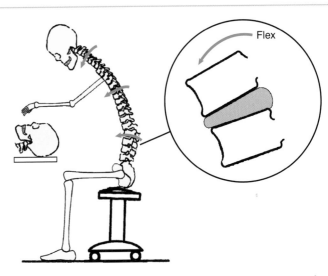

FIG. 6-5 Anteriorly compressed disc with posterior stretch.

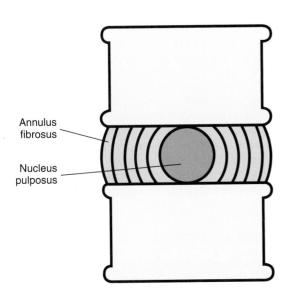

FIG. 6-4 Vertebral disc.

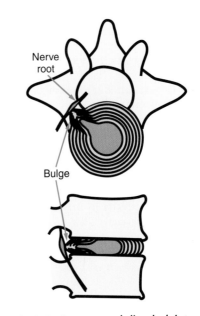

FIG. 6-6 Compressed disc, bulging out.

As previously stated, pain can originate from various soft tissues in the spine. These include ligaments, muscles, intervertebral discs, and the spinal *facet joint* itself. Identifying the cause of the pain is more important than the tissue from which the pain originates.[5] The two most common nontraumatic causes of pain originating from the spine are (1) significant limitation of movement of the joints, as found with immobilization, and (2) abnormal stressing of the structures in and around the spine through overuse in an abnormal pattern.[12,13] The hygienist must understand the cause of pain to prevent or treat the problem.

The first and simplest cause of pain can be from tissue that is of normal length but is maintained in a stretched position for a period of time. *Immobilization* is caused by poor posture. For example, stretching the finger into extreme extension and holding it (Fig. 6-7) may not hurt

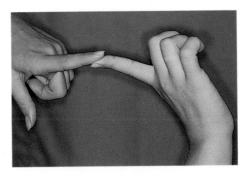

FIG. 6-7 Finger stretched into extreme extension.

immediately, but if that position, or *posture,* is maintained long enough, then pain will occur. In the McKenzie system of classifications, this is referred to as a **postural syndrome.**[12] Slouching forward over a table reading or writing, an almost daily occurrence for most people, eventually results in pain or discomfort in the neck and back (Fig. 6-8). Treatment for this pain involves simply sitting straight and stretching backward. Treatment for postural syndrome is covered in more detail in the treatment section.

The postural syndrome may progress in severity. Complete immobilization, such as that occurring to an extremity that has been placed in a cast, can lead to adaptive shortening of tissues. The tissue does not cause pain when it is left in its shortened state; however, stretching this shortened tissue causes pain. A hygienist who maintains poor posture at work and at home can become immobile due to poor posture. Ultimately this allows tissues around the spine to become shortened and tight. When the individual then attempts movements that stretch the tight structures, as found with an attempt to return to a more normal posture, pain results. In the McKenzie system of classifications, this is referred to as a *dysfunction syndrome.*[12] Because attempts to return to normal postures are painful, individuals with dysfunction syndrome become even less likely to correct their poor postures. The habit of poor posture leads to tissue changes, which makes it even harder to break their bad habits. This vicious circle makes this problem difficult to treat.

When a poor posture becomes typical for an individual, the normal mechanics of the spine become affected. Ligaments and joint capsules are stretched, and muscles have to work overtime to attempt to overcome the poor posture. All these effects may lead to RSI and pain. At this point medical intervention often is necessary to improve the condition, which results in missed time from work and money spent on medical bills.

If left untreated, a dysfunction syndrome can progress to a more severe state, known as a *derangement syndrome.*[15] In this syndrome actual tearing of tissues can occur. For example, the annulus fibrosus tears allow the nucleus pulposus to press against a spinal nerve root. This stage requires medical intervention and may produce chronic effects.

The progressively severe and degenerative continuum from postural to dysfunction to derangement syndromes makes treatment difficult. Early recognition and treatment avoid progression to the next step in the continuum.

POSITIONING

6-C

Risks of musculoskeletal problems are minimized by maximization of the efforts to maintain proper operator, patient, and equipment positions. Good postural habits help prevent these postural syndromes. However, dental hygiene students and even experienced practitioners strive to achieve optimal access to the oral cavity by frequently assuming awkward positions, such as twisting, bending, or leaning over the patient. Fortunately, students' improper postural positions may be corrected by faculty members and clinical instructors. Conversely, practitioners' posture habits usually are unobserved. One pilot study supports the concept that graduates do not practice what is taught. Fewer than one half of the respondents practiced the principles of proper body mechanics as taught during their clinical education, and 63% of the pain reported was attributed to dental hygiene practice.[7]

Students must take the time to develop proper techniques while they are in the educational environment. Breaking bad habits requires approximately 21 days of conscientious effort to correct, so learning and practicing techniques correctly the first time is more efficient and less stressful.[25]

OPERATOR POSITIONING

The positioning of the operator entails two aspects: the operator chair and the working position.

Operator Chair

A critical piece of equipment, if not the most critical for the dental hygienist, is the operator's chair. In the case study, the hygienist began using the front-office secretarial chair rather than a properly designed operator chair. The front-office chair is not appropriate and should not be substituted for a well-balanced chair. According to an authority figure in body ergonomics, ideally the operator's chair should have an adjustable backrest, a reasonable and easily adjustable height range, and a five-wheeled, high-quality base.[25,27] Recent literature also recommends adjustable armrests.[20,25] The use of armrests is discussed later in this chapter.

An easy method used to determine the correct height of the operator chair is for the operator to locate the head of the operator's fibula on the side of the leg (Fig. 6-9). The correct position can be located by placement of a hand on the side of the knee and feeling for the junction between the head of the fibula and the lateral femoral condyle. The head of the fibula is at this joint line. The height of the

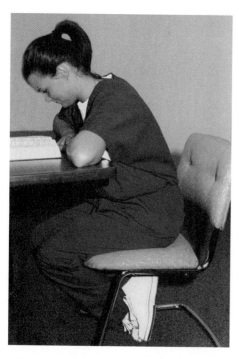

FIG. 6-8 Student slouched while reading.

seat should be adjusted so that the top of the seat cushion is level with the head of the fibula.

The *proprioceptive* self-derivation method is another approach used to determine the operator chair height, assisting the operator in determining a balanced reference posture (Boxes 6-2 and 6-3).

Traditional Working Position

At the correct height the operator should be able to sit tall in the chair with legs separated, thighs parallel to the floor, and feet flat on the floor. The operator's back should be against the chair back so that the lumbar region (small of back) is supported (Fig. 6-10). Operators should be

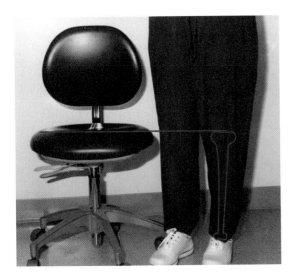

FIG. 6-9 Determining operator chair height.

properly seated in the chair before attempting to correctly position themselves or their patients.

> Incorrect determination of the height of the operator's chair may adversely affect other aspects of correct positioning.

The operator's head should be kept 14 to 16 inches from the patient's oral cavity.[19] The shoulders should be relaxed and not elevated. To help maintain the shoulders at the appropriate height, the elbows should be about even with the occlusal plane and held close to the body. Ideally, the operator's hands should be kept level with the elbows.[32]

Raised arm postures contribute to neck and shoulder complaints. To illustrate this point, readers should raise their elbows to shoulder height and hold the position as the next section is read. Readers will begin to experience neck and shoulder fatigue or strain after a short time. Keeping the elbows out and/or elevated during all-day treatment of patients will eventually contribute to damaging neck and shoulder strain.

Alternative Working Positions

It has been recommended that throughout daily activities the operator should maintain the **neutral position** for optimal musculoskeletal health.[19] The neutral position is the position in which an appendage is not moved away or directed toward the body's midline, including no turning or twisting (Box 6-4). To help maintain this neutral position, suggestions urge the operator imagine a steel pole connecting the hips (pole parallel to floor), with each end

---

BOX 6-2

Proprioceptive Self-Derivation Method of Balanced Reference Posture

This exercise may be conducted in the following two ways:
1. Students work individually as the instructor reads the protocol to the class.
2. Students work in pairs and read the protocol to each other as they progress through the exercise.

Equipment needed: Adjustable operator stool

Protocol
1. Set the *seat* of the stool at the *lowest* possible position.
2. *Sit* on the stool with your *buttocks well supported* and your *feet flat on the floor.* Let your *arms hang freely* at the *sides,* except when adjusting the stool height. Keep your *eyes closed* throughout the exercise and concentrate on how your *body feels.*
3. *Gradually raise the stool* and continue to raise and lower the stool until you reach the height that feels the most stable and comfortable. Readjust if necessary after a few seconds until you are sure this is the best height for you. If you feel that the stool is im-

pinging on your thighs, you may want to slide forward on the stool. Readjust the height again, if necessary. You have now determined your *optimum seating height.*
4. Remember to let your *arms hang loosely at your sides* and *keep your eyes closed.*
5. Take several deep breaths and *relax.* Try to be completely at ease.
6. Move your upper body forward and backward, lean to each side, twist if you wish, and sense the many options available to you for upper body positioning. Finally, decide where you would prefer to *position* your *upper body* to self-maintain a stable, comfortable, and natural upper body posture. Once you have found it, assume and maintain that position.
7. Now do the same with your head and decide where you would prefer to *position* your *head* to self-maintain a stable, comfortable, and natural head position. Once you have found it, assume and maintain that head position.

Continued

From Schoen DH, Dean MC: *Contemporary periodontal instrumentation,* Philadelphia, 1996, WB Saunders.

BOX 6-2

Proprioceptive Self-Derivation Method of Balanced Reference Posture—cont'd

8. Become *proprioceptively aware* of the *body posture you have selected to this point*. If you could, you would probably choose to sit in this manner as you performed a task. It is unlikely that you would choose to alter this *stable, comfortable, and natural posture*.
9. *Think* of the *thumb and index finger* of each hand. With your arms hanging loosely at your sides, *touch* your thumb and index finger together.
10. Making every effort not to alter the posture you have established and keeping your eyes closed, *bring the thumbs and index fingers* of your two hands *together* at a point in front of you, where you would prefer to thread a needle. At this time, you cannot see what you are doing. Once you have found this point, assume and maintain it.
11. Without moving your head or your hands, *open your eyes* and try to see the point at which your two index fingers make contact. At this time, do not concern yourself with the quality of the image you see, only whether you see the point. If you can sit, see, and theoretically thread the needle, maintain this position.
12. If you cannot see the point, or see it only with great and unacceptable discomfort, ask yourself what you would prefer to do to make it possible to see the point, or to see the point with reasonable comfort. If your answer is that you would prefer to *tilt your head* slightly downward, then do so until you can see the point of index finger contact. If your answer is that you would prefer to *move your hands* and relocate the point of index finger contact, do so until you can see the point. If your answer is that you would prefer to *do both,* then do so. Once you have selected your option, maintain this position.
13. This point, where you have decided to thread the needle, is called the *optimum control point.*
14. Once you have satisfied your *natural proprioceptive inclinations,* you may then improve visual acuity problems with the use of corrective eyewear.

Alternative Method to Determine Seat Height

The following method is not as accurate as Steps 1 through 3 of the previous list, but it is an acceptable alternative:

1. Identify the *head of the fibula* on the side of your lower leg. It is the uppermost bone of the lower leg, located approximately at the level of the lower half of the kneecap.
2. *Set* the height of the *seat* of the operator stool to the level of the midpoint of the head of the fibula.

From Schoen DH, Dean MC: *Contemporary periodontal instrumentation,* Philadelphia, 1996, WB Saunders.

BOX 6-3

Characteristics of Balanced Reference Posture

1. *Head* in the least strained position vertically and horizontally
2. *Shoulders* loose, hanging free vertically
3. *Upper arms* loose, hanging free vertically
4. *Lower arms* in the least strained position vertically and horizontally, in line with the palms
5. *Wrists* neither flexed nor extended
6. *Hands* near the level of the apex of the heart, palms vertical, fingers relaxed and flexed, index fingers near the median plane
7. *Back* straight and erect
8. *Buttocks* weight distributed evenly
9. *Thighs* clear and free of distracting contacts, separated and unstrained, front of thighs sloping downward from trunk to knees
10. *Legs* clear and free of distracting contacts
11. *Feet* clear and free of distracting contacts

From Schoen DH, Dean MC: *Contemporary periodontal instrumentation,* Philadelphia, 1996, WB Saunders.

---

bolted to the chair.[19] This position limits or restricts the operator from twisting and helps maintain the pelvic movement forward and backward.

The ***Performance Logic (PL) positioning*** uses proprioceptive self-derivation of balanced reference posture as an alternative method to determine the operator's optimal posture and position described in Boxes 6-2 and 6-3. The **biocentric technique** of positioning also has been suggested and used by clinicians (Box 6-5).[4,6,14,29,33]

The Performance Logic concept developed by Dr. Daryl Beach[6] consists of three basic beliefs: (1) each individual has the "innate capability to self-determine an optimal posture and position for the perception and control of fine motor activity;" (2) this position can be readily reproduced; and (3) this self-determined posture/position is basically the same for each person performing similar tasks.

According to one source, PL:[28]

. . . allows an individual to logically derive the most natural method for the practice of dentistry. Following the principles of performance logic, one can use proprioceptive self-awareness to determine the most effective, stress-free process for performing dental procedures; design an optimal human-centered setting for dental practice; provide the highest quality of oral care; and increase productivity and profitability

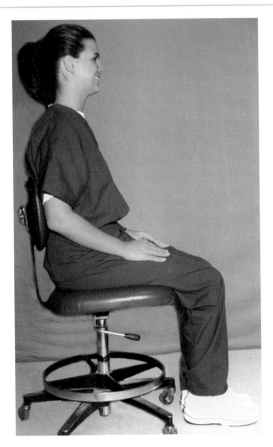

FIG. 6-10 Correct sitting posture.

BOX 6-5

Meador's Biocentric Technique

Harold L. Meador, DDS, BSD, developed the biocentric technique (BT)* in 1960 in response to career-threatening neuromuscular symptoms. "The technique establishes joint neutrality, avoids excessive stress on joints and muscles by having options to shift the work load, and was found effective in coping with neuromuscular pain." The strategy used is based on the maintenance of joints, specifically the wrists, elbows, and shoulders, in a neutral position during instrumentation and shifting of the work load from the smaller muscles to larger muscle groups.

Shifting the workload to different muscle groups is accomplished "through combinations of instrument grasp, attitude of the hands, finger rests, chair positions, and power stokes."

The power stokes, which in this technique include the rocking, pumping, and push-pull strokes, attempts to use the shoulder muscles instead of the hand and forearm. The dynamics of this technique can be self-taught with the use of Power Wheel. The Power Wheel, which was also developed by Meador, provides the guidance necessary for operator positioning, finger rests, grasp, and the type of stroke.

Data from Meador HL: The biocentric technique: a guide to avoiding pain, *J Dent Hyg* 67(1):38-51, 1993.

BOX 6-4

Determining Nunn's Neutral Position

1. The operator should sit tall in the chair, feet flat on the floor, legs slightly apart so that weight is evenly distributed.
2. The stomach muscles should be tightened to help maintain the back against the chair.
3. Allow the hips to slide forward while rotating "the topmost portion of the pelvis in a backward motion (like a cat arching its back)."
4. Allow this portion of the pelvis to rotate forward until the abdomen pushes outward as the back lifts away from the chair back.
5. The neutral position is the most comfortable position midway between the two positions.

From Nunn P: Posture for dental hygiene practice. In Murphy DC, editor: *Ergonomics and the dental care worker*, Washington, DC, 1998, American Public Health Association.

Furthermore, the World Health Organization (WHO) cited the importance of PL, stating the following:[28]

. . . oral health can be improved and the cost of equipment reduced if the workplaces are designed to ensure optimum performance . . . the Performance Logic approach may be considered as a pointer to the future.

The PL approach is a relatively new concept in dental hygiene education. The benefits and limitations of the implementation of PL was studied among students at Vancouver Community College.[33] According to the report:

. . . participants indicated the greatest benefits were increased operator comfort and performance and decreased operator fatigue, muscle strain, and back/neck/shoulder discomfort.

Improved time management, instrument accessibility and control, enhanced intraoral fulcrums, increased patient comfort, less frequent headaches, and augmented indirect vision skills were other benefits reported. Both students and faculty agreed on the major benefits derived from the PL approach. When asked to compare traditional operator and patient positioning with the PL approach, experienced clinicians indicated that PL "definitely" improves the ideal alignment of forces during stroke activation, and decreases operator strain and fatigue. No discernible differences occurred between faculty and student responses, although faculty members provided more detailed information. Limitations were largely focused on equipment features and the patients' acceptance of the **supine position.** Dental hygiene educators should investigate the method described in Boxes 6-2 and 6-3 as an alternative working position.

PATIENT POSITIONING

Dental hygienists should remember that the patient's head is moveable. Although practicing hygienists typically work 8 hours every day, a patient is usually in the dental

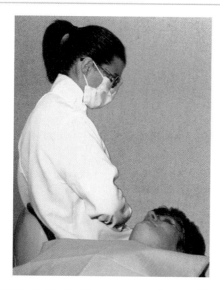

FIG. 6-11 Test for correct patient height.

chair for only 1 to 1½ hours and certainly not every day. Therefore hygienists should place the patient in the correct position and move the patient's head accordingly, rather than constantly assume awkward positions so that the patient is not inconvenienced. However, students frequently become so intent on their work, they forget to move the patient's head and compromise their own positioning to "see better." Assuming awkward positions all day every day leads to musculoskeletal problems.

After the operator is correctly seated in the operator chair, the patient should be positioned. In the traditional and PL working positions, the patient is placed in a supine position, with the dental chair back nearly parallel to the floor. In the supine position, the patient's feet and head are on the same plane. The chair back, however, may be raised approximately 20 degrees *(semisupine position)* to accommodate medically compromised patients. With the traditional working position, the semisupine position may be used to treat the mandibular arch.[19] This use is not recommended with the PL working position. The patient's head should also be at the upper edge of the backrest. The height of the patient's chair off the floor should be determined by the height of the operator's elbows.[18] To test the proper chair height, the operator folds the arms across the waist. The tip of the patient's nose should be lower than the operator's elbow level position (Fig. 6-11). In the PL approach the operator position determines the optimum control point; the patient's mouth is at the height of the optimum control point. This is approximately at the clinician's heart level; thus the operator's hands and elbows form an angle of slightly less than 90 degrees.

As stated, with the PL approach the patient is in the supine position throughout the appointment. The patient's head is moved from a straight position to slightly to the right, further to the right (far right), slightly to the left and further to the left (far left). The patient's maxillary plane should parallel the upper body of the operator. One authority suggests that the relationship of the maxilla to the operator's body posture is usually parallel to the operator's spine.[28] This source further states that this position is true regardless of where the operator is sitting or the site

of treatment and suggests that operators use the maxilla as a gauge to control posture. However, the sources also states the following:

> *. . . conscientious control of the patient's maxillary plane does not guarantee good postural balance for the operator, but lack of control of the patient's maxillary plane is certain to cause poor postures.*

OPERATOR POSITIONING DURING INSTRUMENTATION PROCEDURES

Many different guides can be used to illustrate the various operational positions. Using a clock to establish or guide patient positioning, with the patient's head being at 12 o'clock, is a relatively universal method and is demonstrated in Table 6-1 and Fig. 6-12.[35] These positions are referred to as *zones*, which in location are similar to the clock positions.[18] In the traditional positioning the right-handed operator generally operates from 8 o'clock to 12 o'clock or from the front, middle/back, and back zones on the patient's right side; the left-handed operator performs procedures from the 4 o'clock to 12 o'clock position or front, middle/back, and back zones on the patient's left side.

With the PL approach, the operator works within the range of 10 o'clock to a 12:30 position for the right-handed operator or 2 o'clock to an 11:30 position for the left-handed operator.[29] In Table 6-2, PL operator positions have been translated into the "clock" positions traditionally used by clinicians. The biocentric technique uses the 7 o'clock, 9 o'clock, and 12 o'clock positions.[14]

This author has practiced for years using the traditional approach to positioning for instrumentation. After practicing the PL approach, the author noted that the wrist can maintain a neutral position with this approach more often than with the traditional approach. However, long-term research is needed to determine if this approach eliminates or reduces the musculoskeletal complaints repeatedly experienced and documented by dental hygienists.

POSITIONING FOR ULTRASONIC SCALING

When performing ultrasonic scaling, the operator should be seated in the operator's chair in the same manner as when hand scaling in the 12 o'clock position.[16] In this position, and with the top of the patient's head at the top of the chair, straining of the operator's head and neck is minimized.

Unlike hand scalers, which have single, one-directional cutting edges, any side of the ultrasonic tip is capable of removing calculus or deposits. With this in mind, sextants 2, 3, 4, and 5 and the palatal of sextant 1 and the lingual of sextant 6 can be reached from the 12 o'clock position. From the 9 o'clock position, the facial surfaces of sextants 1 and 6 can be reached and, if it is necessary, reinstrumentation of the palatal of sextant 3 and mandibular anteriors can be accessed. A Hygoformic (Pulpdent Corporation of America, Brookline, Mass.) or a Tipadilly system (Tip-a-dilly, Pelton Crane, Charlotte, N.C.) should be used instead. Water control in sextants 2, 3, 4, and 5 can be obtained by placement of the Hygoformic saliva ejector in the left mandibular vestibule. With the patient's head

TABLE 6-1
Traditional positioning

Area by sextant	Operator position	Patient's head	Chin position
Right-Handed Operator			
Posteriors			
Maxillary right facial	8 to 9 o'clock	Slightly away from operator	Chin up
Maxillary left lingual			
Mandibular right facial			Chin down
Mandibular left lingual			
Maxillary right lingual	11 to 12 o'clock	Slightly toward operator	Chin up
Maxillary left facial			
Mandibular right lingual			Chin down
Mandibular left facial			
Anteriors			
Maxillary facial and lingual surfaces toward operator	8 to 9 o'clock	Straight ahead*	Chin up
Mandibular facial and lingual surfaces toward operator	8 to 9 o'clock	Straight ahead*	Chin down
Maxillary facial and lingual surfaces away from operator	11 to 12 o'clock	Straight ahead*	Chin up
Mandibular facial and lingual surfaces away from operator	11 to 12 o'clock	Straight ahead*	Chin down
Left-Handed Operator			
Posteriors			
Maxillary right facial	3 to 4 o'clock	Slightly toward operator	Chin up
Maxillary left lingual			
Mandibular right facial			Chin down
Mandibular left lingual			
Maxillary right lingual	1 to 2 o'clock	Slightly away from operator	Chin up
Maxillary left facial			
Mandibular right lingual			Chin down
Mandibular left facial			
Anteriors			
Maxillary facial and lingual toward operator	3 to 4 o'clock	Straight ahead*	Chin up
Mandibular facial and lingual surfaces toward operator	3 to 4 o'clock	Straight ahead*	Chin down
Maxillary facial and lingual surfaces away from operator	1 to 2 o'clock	Straight ahead*	Chin up
Mandibular facial and lingual surfaces away from operator	1 to 2 o'clock	Straight ahead*	Chin down
or			
Maxillary facial and lingual surfaces away from operator	1 to 2 o'clock	Straight ahead*	Chin up

*Operator may request that patient move the head away/toward operator as the operator moves from cuspid to cuspid.

turned slightly to the left, the water flows in that direction. For palatal aspects of sextant 1 and lingual aspects of sextant 6, the saliva ejector is placed in the right mandibular vestibule, and the patient's head is turned slightly to the right. This efficient water control requires only one movement of the operator, patient, and saliva ejector.

The sequence described is different from the one traditionally taught for ultrasonic instrumentation and may require practice until the clinician feels competent and confident. The traditional technique has the operator positioned similarly to the position used for hand scaling and thus requires more movement from both the operator and patient.

POSITION OF DENTAL EQUIPMENT

Dental Lighting

Proper lighting is a critical component in patient care. Although the use of *fiber optics* in dentistry has produced advances, its use in dental hygiene is limited. The overhead light still is indispensable, and proper placement is neces-

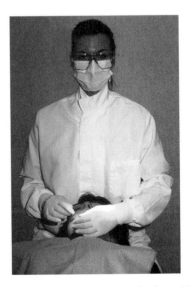

FIG. 6-12 Operator at 12 o'clock position.

TABLE 6-2

Proprioceptive and self–derivation-based Performance Logic instrumentation positions for operator and patient equated to traditional clock positions

Area	Operator positioning	Patient's head position	Patient position
Right-Handed Operator			
Maxillary right facial	10 o'clock	Straight to slightly to patient's left	Patient in supine position for maxillary and mandibular arches
Maxillary anterior facial	11 to 12 o'clock	Slightly to patient's right*	
Maxillary left facial	11 to 12 o'clock	Slightly to patient's right to far right	
Maxillary right facial	11 o'clock	Far right	
Maxillary anterior lingual	11 to 12 o'clock	Slightly to patient's right*	
Maxillary left lingual	12 o'clock	Slightly to patient's right to far right	
Mandibular left facial	11 o'clock	Far right	
Mandibular anterior facial	12 o'clock	Straight to slightly to patient's right*	
Mandibular right facial	10 o'clock†	Slightly to patient's left	
Mandibular left lingual	10 o'clock	Slightly to patient's left	
Mandibular anterior lingual	12 o'clock	Slightly to patient's right*	
Mandibular right lingual	12 o'clock	Far right	
Left-Handed Operator			
Maxillary right facial	1 to 2 o'clock	Slightly to patient's left	Patient in supine position for maxillary and mandibular arches
Maxillary anterior facial	1 to 2 o'clock	Slightly to patient's left*	
Maxillary left facial	2 o'clock	Straight to slightly to patient's right	
Maxillary right lingual	12 o'clock	Slightly to patient's left to far left	
Maxillary anterior lingual	1 o'clock	Far left*	
Maxillary left lingual	12 o'clock	Slightly to patient's right (toward operator) to far right	
Mandibular left facial	Approximately 1 to 2 o'clock	Slightly to patient's right (toward operator)	
Mandibular anterior facial	12 o'clock	Straight to slightly to patient's right (toward operator)*	
Mandibular right facial	1 o'clock	Far left	

*Operator may ask patient to move the head toward/away from operator as operator moves from cuspid to cuspid.
†Clock position changed from that depicted in Schoen and Dean's *Instrumentation* text, which demonstrates the position at approximately 12 o'clock, with patient's head slightly to the right. At this position, reaching the area is extremely difficult.

sary to allow the hygienist to maintain an ergonomically correct position. Two primary dental lighting systems are available: (1) the light fixed in a ceiling-mounted track and (2) the dental light attached to a pole connected to the patient's chair. Regardless of the type system used, the correct light position used to view the mandibular arch is directly above the patient's head, with the beam directed into the oral cavity. To view the maxillary arch, the light should be directly above the patient's chest, with the beam directed into the patient's oral cavity on an angle (slightly tilted upward). To maximize illumination the light should always be at arm's length (approximately 36 inches). Positioning the light closer lessens the illumination.

Equipment Positioning

The instrument tray, handpieces, suction, and air/water syringe should be reasonably accessible and as close to the operator as possible to avoid excessive bending/twisting. Approximately 20 inches is a reasonable working distance for equipment.[25] This distance enhances good posture. Handpiece tubing should be straight, not coiled, and have a smooth outer surface.[26] Straight tubing decreases the force and grasp strength required to pull and detangle the coil. A smooth outer surface is more easily disinfected. In

the case presented at the beginning of this chapter, the use of the front-office chair and the inaccessibility of the dental equipment were the two main causes of the resulting musculoskeletal problems.

RECOGNITION OF ERRORS IN POSITIONING

The following section provides five problems and the cues students should be aware of to help recognize incorrect positioning of operator or patient. Identifying corrections to the following situations may help the student more readily recognize the problem and correct it:

1. *Problem:* An operator has to move the dental light sideways because a shadow is being cast in the oral cavity.
   Solution: The student's position or the patient's head position should be corrected. Rarely, if ever, is movement of the dental light sideways the correct light position.
2. *Problem:* A student knows she is holding the instrument correctly and has the correct working end but finds herself unable to adapt the cutting edge to the surface or activate the working or exploratory stoke.
   Solution: When the student faces this situation, she should stop the procedure and self-assess patient and operator positioning rather than assume an awkward position.

3. *Problem:* The student operator's body is at 9 o'clock, and the chair back is at 11 o'clock. The operator, intent on his work, moves to a different area of the oral cavity without moving the operator chair and consequently adapts his body to reach the area.
Solution: The student needs to move the operator chair as he works to maintain proper posture.

4. *Problem:* The student becomes fatigued and begins to slouch in the chair with legs either extended or crossed.
Solution: When the student realizes this has occurred, she needs to stretch and incorporate the exercises described later in the chapter. Slouching in the chair creates an enormous amount of extra force on the shoulder and neck area, thus exacerbating fatigue.

5. *Problem:* The student never truly learns to use the dental mirror for indirect vision. Failure to use indirect vision results in a student assuming an awkward position to gain visual access and places the operator and patient at unnecessary risk. The operator has compromised posture, and the subsequent poor visibility may result in tissue laceration.
Solution: The student should take every opportunity during the educational process to practice and develop the skills required to master indirect vision. An exercise that may help students develop this skill is to practice tracing an object while looking in a hand mirror. Using a red and a blue pencil highlights how exactly the student is tracing.

REDUCING FATIGUE

For 20 years, musculoskeletal disorders have been reported in the literature, and efforts have been made in the educational setting to instruct the student on proper body mechanics, to correct poor posture when observed in clinic, and, with some schools, to offer additional ergonomic materials.

New equipment and equipment modifications can reduce the occurrence of musculoskeletal problems. An example is the use of magnification systems and armrests for the operator's chair.

MAGNIFICATION SYSTEMS

Two ways to increase visibility are to move closer to the object or to magnify it. Without magnification, students and practitioners typically bend forward to "see better." Bending forward has already been discussed as an improper posture that exacerbates fatigue. The other option is magnification. Although the use of eye loupes (magnification) in dentistry is not equal to that in medicine, the use in dentistry has witnessed a gradual increase. Common use of eye loupes for dental hygienists is likely to follow. A leading manufacturer of magnification systems estimates that 15% to 20% of the dental hygiene programs have already begun requiring the purchase of eye loupes for clinical practice.[2]

Two types of magnification systems are used in dentistry:[9] the single-lens magnifier and the multi-lens magnifier systems. For clinical use, the single-lens magnifier system is probably not the best choice in the selection of a magnification system for clinical practice. The single-lens produces *dioptre magnification,* which restricts the operator's working distance to a set length. With this restricted working distance, maintaining focus is difficult

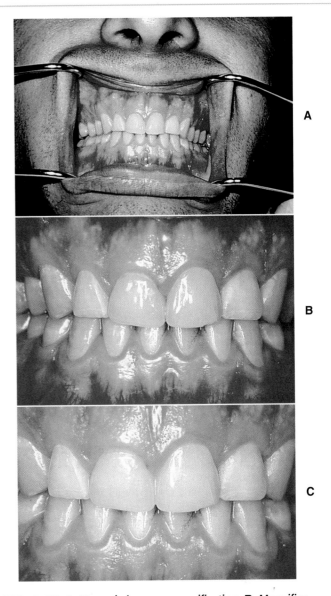

FIG. 6-13 A, Normal view—no magnification. **B,** Magnification 2.0×. **C,** Magnification 2.5×.

because the operator has limited range and opportunity for movement. This places the operator in a restricted position/posture that could increase poor posture and back and neck pain.

The multilens *(telescopic loupes)* is the better choice for magnification. These loupes offer improved posture and optical performance. The models currently available use Galilean optics. These are preferred in dentistry because of the relatively wide field depth, which is maintained as the magnification increases. In dentistry, a magnification power of 2× to 3.5× is recommended.[28] Strassler states that a periodontists may use a 2× to 2.5× magnification power, general dentists and dental hygienists may use 2× for scaling and root-planing procedures.[32] In the previously mentioned study by Sunell completed at Vancouver Community College, the dental hygiene faculty and students used 2.5× magnification.[33] It appears that the range for dental hygienists would be 2× or 2.5×. These power levels offer a greater field depth than those needed by oral surgeons and endodontists (Fig. 6-13).[30]

A 2- to 3-week learning curve is required for the operator to become confident and comfortable using eye loupes. Also an accurate measurement of the operator's working distance must be determined before selection of the proper magnification power. In addition, when the operator requires prescriptive lenses, the same prescription must be added to the magnification system.

To further illustrate the benefits of eye loupes, the Vancouver study, which used the PL approach to positioning, also incorporated the use of eye loupes into the program.[33] Participating faculty members and students reported a decrease in neck, back, and shoulder complaints; an increase in visual acuity; reduced eye strain; and minimal need for exaggerated forward head flexion. An additional benefit to the eye loupes was demonstrated in radiographic interpretation. Cost, the time involved in learning to adapt, and the inability to easily view the patient's facial expressions were identified as drawbacks to their use.

Overall, the use of eye loupes makes it unnecessary to bend or lean forward to "see better." This assistance keeps the operator in a balanced musculoskeletal position, thus reducing the muscle fatigue experienced by numerous practitioners.

ARMRESTS

The use of adjustable armrests is another equipment improvement that is probably used more by dentists than by dental hygienists (Fig. 6-14). However, dental hygienists must consider the benefits of armrests in the reduction of muscle fatigue. The main benefit of an operator armrest is in the increased operator arm stability and the reduction of muscle activity in the upper trapezius (the muscle between the neck and the shoulder). This muscle helps to suspend the shoulder girdle to the trunk and is the muscle that is typically irritated with postural syndromes. When properly used, forearm rest can reduce up to 12% of body weight stress off the spine.[27] Reducing the strain essentially reduces the cumulative fatigue currently experienced by dental hygienists. In addition to the operator chair armrests, one researcher recently devised a horseshoe-shaped cushion that is adapted to patient's headrest.[27] This cushion provides additional support to the operator's wrist and forearm, thus decreasing the strain placed on these areas.

TREATMENT AND EXERCISES

Good posture is key to good health. To both prevent and treat the common musculoskeletal RSIs reported by dental hygienists, good posture habits must be reinforced. Poor posture is actually a bad habit. How can injuries be prevented when the activities of the job potentially require the use of poor posture on a routine basis? Poor posture can't always be avoided during the practice of dental hygiene. However, hygienists should minimize the total time the poor posture is maintained.

What are good posture and poor posture? Generally, good posture includes the head being held back over the shoulders. The shoulders should be back and not rounded forward. When the hands are in use, the elbows should be held as close to the side as possible, for as much of the time as possible. As stated earlier, the dental hygienist should sit squarely on the chair with the lumbar spine in a normal amount of lordosis and touching the backrest of the seat. The thighs should be parallel to the floor and feet should be flat on the floor (see Fig. 6-10). Too many poor postures exist to name them all, but most of them involve some degree of forward flexion. In other words, when the hygienist leans forward and down, the head strains forward, the body moves to the edge of the seat, and the lumbar spine slumps. The list could go on forever. The importance of the maintenance of good, correct posture whenever possible cannot be overstated. But what does a hygienist do when it is impossible to maintain good posture?

Hygienists must break up the time spent in a poor posture position that they are forced to endure in their work. For example, if a hygienist is in a poor posture while performing a procedure, that hygienist can change the poor posture while changing position or reaching for a different instrument (Fig. 6-15). Specific postural exercises that can be performed chairside during these short breaks in treatment are described later in this chapter. This prevents extended periods of the previously described self-imposed immobilization.

The hygienist benefits from periodic breaks from patient treatment, but anyone who has been involved in patient care realizes that this is not always possible. How-

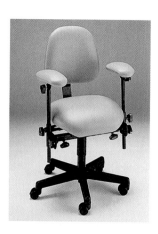

FIG. 6-14 Armrests.

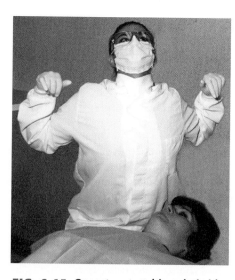

FIG. 6-15 Operator stretching chairside.

ever, discontinuing poor posture at chairside is always possible during a patient treatment.

Because poor postures cannot be completely avoided during the practice of dental hygiene, hygienists must do as much as possible in their personal lifestyles to minimize the possibility of developing an RSI. Keeping good postures and spinal mobility while not at work, taking part in an aerobic/cardiovascular exercise programs, and not smoking helps accomplish this. In addition, limiting those activities that are similar to tasks performed as dental hygienists, such as needlework, helps minimize exposure to continuous poor posture.

The most important aspect of these lifestyle changes is posture and spinal mobility away from work. While at work, every hygienist is going to have some postural syndrome symptoms as previously described; therefore they must limit these poor postures while away from work. If they don't, they will progress to the dysfunction syndrome even more quickly. Good postures while away from work include posture while driving, watching television, reading, and all other activities of daily living (Fig. 6-16). Although good posture cannot be maintained all the time, the hygienist does not want poor posture to become typical.

An exercise program that targets the hygienist's cardiovascular system can be a tremendous help in the prevention of musculoskeletal RSI injuries. The optimal lifestyle includes exercise three to four times a week for 30 to 60 minutes of continuous exercise at a target heart rate of 70% of that person's maximum heart rate. Exercising at a

level lower than this is still beneficial. Exercise just once a week or at heart rates below 70% of an individual's maximum is still better than no exercise.

Although the problems associated with the use of tobacco and nicotine are becoming common knowledge, many people may not be aware of the effect of nicotine on the capillary blood supply to the structures of the spine. Nicotine can inhibit blood flow to tissues, altering tissue response to injury. This is just one more reason not to use tobacco products. Chapter 12 discusses tobacco, chemical dependency, and addictive behavior.

TYPES OF EXERCISES

Exercises used to both treat and prevent musculoskeletal RSIs can be divided into three main groups: postural exercises, stretching exercises, and strengthening exercises. Postural and stretching exercises are by far the most important in the prevention of musculoskeletal RSIs.

Postural Exercises

The four main postural exercises are neck retraction, neck extension, shoulder retraction, and low back extension. Neck retraction is performed by an attempt to slide the head back over the shoulders without extending the face upward. If performed correctly, the head doesn't tilt; it just slides straight back, correcting the forward head posture (Fig. 6-17).

Neck extension involves a simple upward look as far as the head can reach (Fig. 6-18). Neck retraction must be done before neck extension is attempted. If neck extension is done before the forward head is corrected the person ends up with the "turtle" posture in the cervical spine (Fig. 6-19). This hyperextension is not healthy for the cervical spine.

Shoulder retraction is performed when the shoulders are brought back and an attempt is made to pinch the shoulder blades together (Fig. 6-20). This is a simple exercise that breaks the habit of forward shoulders. A combination of neck retraction and shoulder retraction can be performed when the individual lies supine on the floor with a small towel roll placed at the base of the skull (Fig. 6-21). The person can lie in this position for 10 to

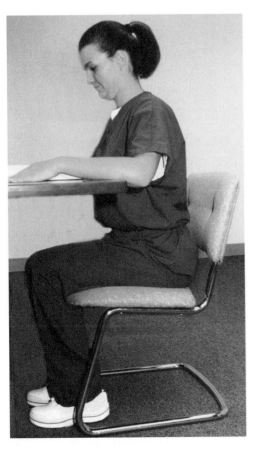

FIG. 6-16 Student reading with good posture.

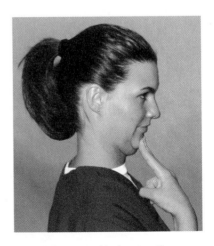

FIG. 6-17 Neck retraction.

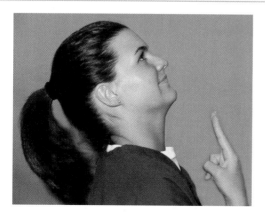

FIG. 6-18 Neck retraction and extension. Retraction occurs first, followed by extension from a retracted position.

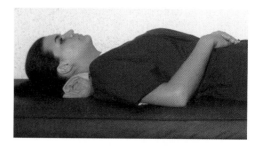

FIG. 6-21 Operator lying on table with towel roll.

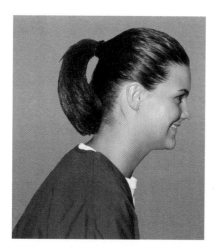

FIG. 6-19 "Turtle" posture.

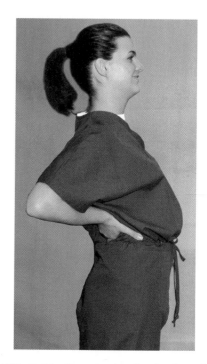

FIG. 6-22 Operator leaning backward.

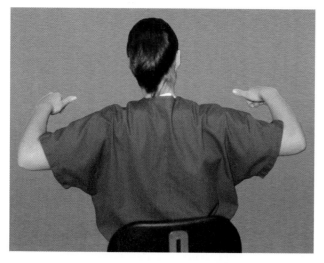

FIG. 6-20 Shoulders back.

leaning (Fig. 6-22); this exercise can be performed standing or sitting. It helps reverse the affects of the forward slumped posture.

These simple postural exercises can be incorporated into daily activities. They easily can be performed chairside during patient care during movement from one position to another or during changing of instruments. Many individuals do some of these movements periodically throughout the day without even thinking about it. These descriptions just allow the hygienist to do the exercises in the most correct manner possible.

Stretching Exercises

Specific stretching exercises should be performed to address muscles that can become tight if poor postures are maintained. With any stretching exercises, all stretches should be done slowly and held for at least 10 seconds. Stretching when the tissues are warm is ideal, such as after

15 minutes and let gravity pull the neck and shoulders into retraction. This is a good exercise to do after a long day of patient care.

Low back extension can be accomplished by placement of the hands on the low back, followed by a backward

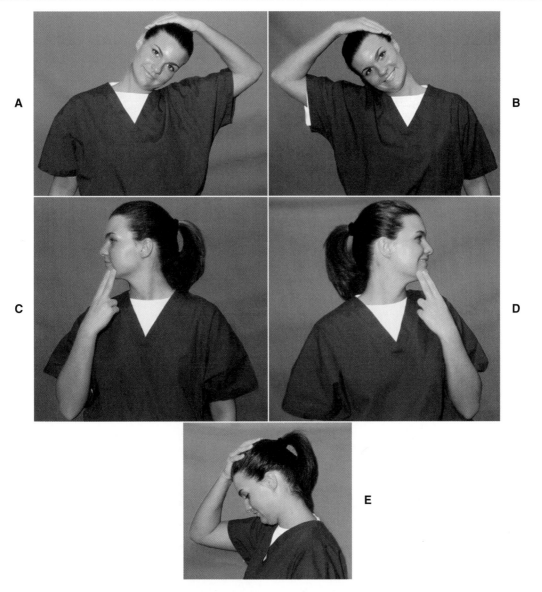

FIG. 6-23 A, Left lateral flexion. **B,** Right lateral flexion. **C,** Right lateral rotation. **D,** Left lateral rotation. **E,** Forward flexion.

exercise or a hot shower. The first area to address is the neck. It should be stretched into lateral flexion to both sides, rotation to both sides, and forward flexion (Fig. 6-23). The stretching exercises should not cause a lasting increase in symptoms of pain. If stretching causes pain to increase or become more persistent, the exercise should be discontinued and medical evaluation should be sought.

The anterior aspect of the shoulder is the next area to stretch. A corner stretch (Fig. 6-24) is the simplest, most effective exercise for this region. The stretch should be felt across the front of the shoulders into the chest. This is an important exercise that helps stretch out muscles that have become tight during the maintenance of a rounded shoulders posture.

Strengthening Exercises

Developing strength in neck, back, and shoulder musculature does not *automatically* cause better posture. It will,

however, help place that person in a better posture. As stated previously, posture is a habit. Developing strength in certain muscles helps a person develop good habits.

Strengthening exercises begin with isometric exercises for the neck, performed by the person pushing the head into the hands without letting the head move. This movement should be held for a count of five, and five repetitions of each exercise should be performed (Fig. 6-25). The next exercise involves extension of the shoulder and retraction of the scapulae. It can be accomplished with resistance from an outside source, such as weights or elastic band (Fig. 6-26), or with resistance from the person's body weight (Fig. 6-27). In a gym these exercises might be described as bar pull-downs, rowing exercises, or shoulder extension. A key to this exercise involves pinching of the shoulder blades together (scapular retraction) as the shoulders are extended. Other shoulder exercises include military press, bench press, and shoulder depression. The lower back can be addressed by exercises that strengthen

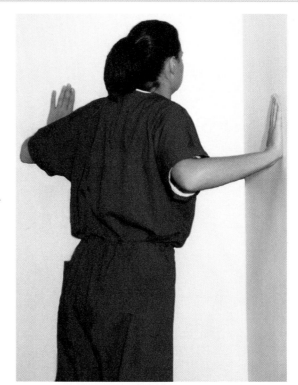

FIG. 6-24 Corner stretch.

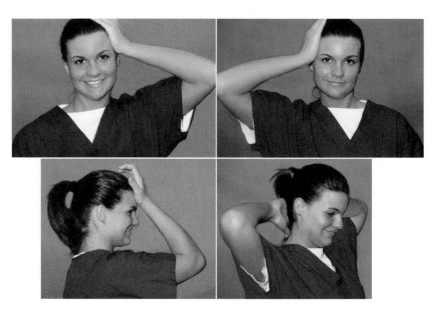

FIG. 6-25 Isometric exercises.

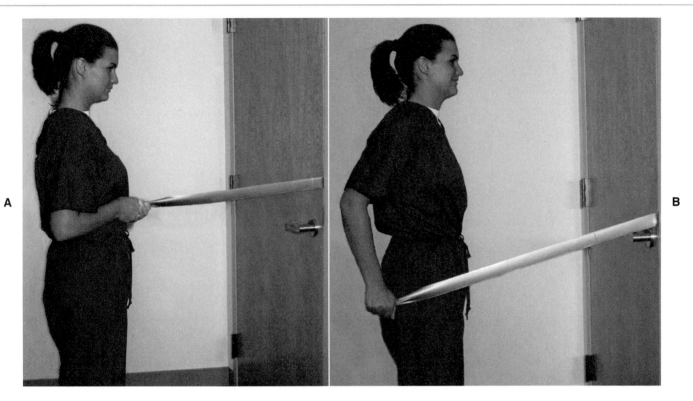

FIG. 6-26 Clinician pulling elastic band. **A,** Bilateral shoulder extension and scapular retraction. **B,** Single-shoulder extension.

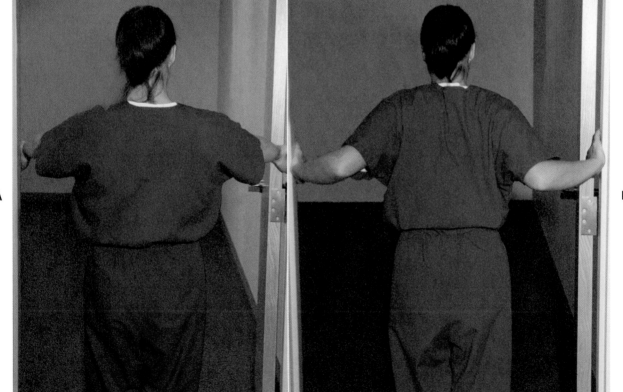

FIG. 6-27 Clinician pulling in the door frame. **A,** Beginning position. **B,** Ending position.

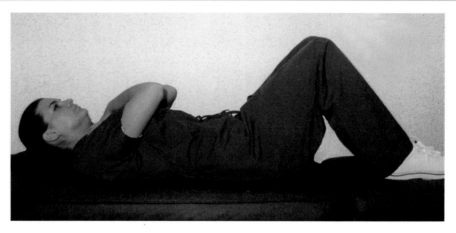

FIG. 6-28 Clinician performing crunches.

the abdominals. Sit-ups or crunches (Fig. 6-28) accomplish this, but care must be taken with these exercises. The person doing the exercise should not pull on the neck while performing the exercise. This unnecessarily stresses the neck and makes the exercise less efficient. Also the exercise should be done without the feet being held down by someone or something else. Readers may benefit from joining a gym or fitness center and receiving instruction in the proper performance of all of the exercises. A trained professional can help determine appropriate weights/resistance and number of repetitions to perform so that the exercise program can be performed in the safest and most efficient manner possible.

RITICAL THINKING ACTIVITIES

1. Practice the exercises described in the section on postural exercises beginning on p. 129.
2. Find the head of the fibula and determine the correct operator chair height.
3. Using the traditional working position, correctly position the following:
   a. Position yourself in the operator chair
   b. Position a student partner in the dental chair
   c. Adjust the equipment to work on the mandibular arch and have the student partner's head turned toward the operator

      Attempt to activate an exploratory stroke on the mandibular left lingual. Can you as the operator see? Does this feel correct? Does a shadow in the oral cavity limit visibility? Next, have the student partner turn the head slightly away from you. Can you see? Does it feel correct? Is there a shadow cast on the arch? Is it possible to activate a stroke without struggling? What positions were incorrect? How was it improved?

4. Determine your own balanced reference point as described in Boxes 6-2 and 6-3.
5. Practice the PL approach to positioning described in Boxes 6-2 and 6-3.
6. Observe another dental hygiene student's posture and positioning and identify correct and incorrect postures/positions.

REVIEW QUESTIONS

Question 1 refers to the case study presented at the beginning of the chapter.

1. Which of the following is the most likely cause for the development of Juanita's musculoskeletal problems?
   a. Improper instrumentation positioning
   b. Improper patient positioning
   c. Improper positioning of the dental equipment
   d. Improper chair height

2. In McKenzie's classification system, which of the following syndromes is the most difficult to treat?
   a. Derangement syndrome
   b. Postural syndrome
   c. Dysfunction syndrome

REVIEW QUESTIONS—cont'd

3. Physiologically, which of the following describes the number of normal curves in the human spine?
   a. Two
   b. Three
   c. One
   d. Four

4. The human spine has *two normal lordosis curves* and *two normal kyphosis curves.*
   a. The first part of the sentence is true, and the second part is false.
   b. Both parts of the sentence are true.
   c. Both parts of the sentence are false.
   d. The first part of the sentence is false, and the second is true.

5. Which of the following describes the recommended distance of the operator's head to the patient's oral cavity?
   a. 6 to 8 inches
   b. 8 to 10 inches
   c. 14 to 16 inches
   d. It does not matter as long as the operator is comfortable.

6. The dental light should be approximately _____ from the oral cavity.
   a. 12 inches
   b. 18 inches
   c. 24 inches
   d. 36 inches

 SUGGESTED AGENCIES AND WEB SITES

Because of the ever-changing nature of the Internet, some of the web sites listed here may have changed since publication. Please refer to Mosby's Evolve web site for the most current information.

Computer-Related Repetitive Strain Injury:
http://www.engr.unl.edu

Occupational Safety and Health Administration:
http://www.osha.gov

 ADDITIONAL READINGS AND RESOURCES

Agur AMR: *Grant's atlas of anatomy,* Baltimore, 1991, Williams and Wilkins.

Anderson, KN, ed: *Mosby's medical, nursing, and allied health dictionary,* ed 5, St Louis, 1998, Mosby.

Kendall FP, McCreary EK, Provance PG: *Muscles, testing and function,* Baltimore, 1993, Williams and Wilkins.

Moore KL, Dalley AF: *Clinically oriented anatomy,* Philadelphia, 1999, Lippincott Williams & Wilkins.

Murphy DC: *Ergonomics and the dental care worker,* Washington DC, 1998, American Public Health Association.

Nordin M, Ortengren R, Anderson GBJ: Measurement of trunk movements during work, *Spine* 9:465-9, 1984.

Norkin CC, Levangie PK: *Joint structure and function,* Philadelphia, 1993, FA Davis.

Palm N: Ergonomics, *J Mich Dent Assoc,* 76(5):28-30, 1994.

Pollack R: Dental office ergonomics: how to reduce stress factors and increase efficiency, *J Can Dent Assoc* 62(6):508-10, 1996.

Ylippa V et al: Physical and psychosocial work environments among Swedish dental hygienists: risk indicators for musculoskeletal complaints, *Swedish Dent J* 21(3):111-20, 1997.

 REFERENCES

1. Barry RM, Woodall WR, Mahan JM: Postural changes in dental hygienists: four year longitudinal study, *J Dent Hyg* 65(3): 147-50, 1992.
2. Baudo TV: Personal communication, March 2000, Surgitel Systems.
3. Beach JC, DeBiase CB: Assessment of ergonomic education in dental hygiene curricula, *J Dent Educ* 62(6):421-25, 1998.
4. Belenky MM: Human-centered ergonomics: proprioceptive pathway to occupational health and peak performance in dental practice. In Murphy DC, editor: *Ergonomics and the dental care worker,* Washington, DC, 1998, American Public Health Association.
5. Caillet R: *Soft tissue pain and disability,* ed 2, Philadelphia, 1988, FA Davis.
6. Colangelo G, Belenky MM: Performance logic: a key to improving dental practice, *J Dent Prac Adm* 7(4):173-7, 1990.
7. Dean MC, Romberg E, Fletcher J, Rogers S: Back, neck, and shoulder pain: results of a pilot study, *J Dent Educ* 61(2):229, 1997.
8. Gravois S, Stringer RB: Survey of occupational health hazards in dental hygiene, *Dent Hyg* 54:518-23, 1980.
9. Kanca J, Jordan PG: Magnification systems in clinical dentistry, *J Can Dent Assoc* 61(10):851-6, 1995.
10. Macdonald G: Hazards in dental workplace, *Dent Hyg* 61:212-8, 1987.
11. Marxhausen P: *Computer related repetitive strain injuries* [Internet], 2000, [http://www.engr.unl.edu].
12. McKenzie R: *The lumbar spine: mechanical diagnosis and treatment,* Waikanae, New Zealand, 1981, Spinal Publications New Zealand Ltd.
13. McKenzie R: *Treat your own back,* Waikanae, New Zealand, 1997, Spinal Publications New Zealand Ltd.

14. Meador HL: The biocentric technique: a guide to avoiding occupational pain, *J Dent Hyg* 67(1):38-51, 1993.

15. Miller DL: An investigation into attrition of dental hygienists from the work force, *J Dent Hyg* 65:25-31, 1991.

16. Miller N: Ultrasonic instrumentation and debridement: current application in dental hygiene therapy, *J Pract Hyg* 4(1): 25-31, 1991.

17. Nainzadeh N, Malantic-Lin A, Alvarez M, Loeser AC: Repetitive strain injury (cumulative trauma disorder): causes and treatment, *Mt Sinai J Med* 66(3):192-6, 1999.

18. Nield-Gehrig JS, Houseman GA: *Fundamentals of periodontal instrumentation,* ed 3, Baltimore, 1996, Williams and Wilkins.

19. Nunn P: Posture for dental hygiene practice. In Murphy DC, editor: *Ergonomics and the dental care worker,* Washington, DC, 1998, American Public Health Association.

20. Oberg T: Ergonomic evaluation and construction of a reference workplace in dental hygiene: a case study, *J Dent Hyg* 67(5):262-7, 1993.

21. Oberg T, Oberg U: Musculoskeletal complaints in dental hygiene: a survey study from a Swedish county, *J Dent Hyg* 67(5):257-61, 1993.

22. Occupational Safety and Health Administration: *Ergonomics* [Internet], 1999, OSHA [http://www.osha-sla.gov].

23. Osborn JB et al: Musculoskeletal pain among Minnesota dental hygienists, *J Dent Hyg* 64:132-8, 1989.

24. Pauls JA, Reed KL: *Quick reference to physical therapy,* Gaithersburg, Md, 1996, Aspen.

25. Pollack R: Dento-ergonomics: the key to energy-saving performance, *Calif Dent Assoc J* 24(4):63-8, 1996.

26. Pollack R: The ergo factor: the most common equipment and design flaws and how to avoid them, *Dent Today* 15(1):112-3, 120-1, 1996.

27. Pollack-Simon R: Beware of your chair: sitting down is not enough!, *Dent Today* 15(9): 78, 80-1, 1996.

28. Rucker LM, Boyd MA: Optimizing dental operatory working environments. In Murphy DC, editor: *Ergonomics and the dental care worker,* Washington, DC, 1998, American Public Health Association.

29. Schoen D, Dean MC: *Contemporary periodontal instrumentation,* Philadelphia, 1996, WB Saunders.

30. Shugars D et al: Musculoskeletal pain among general dentists, *Gen Dentistry* 35(4):272-6, 1987.

31. Stockstill JW, Harn SD, Strickland D, Hruska R: Prevalence of upper extremity neuropathy in a clinical dentist population, *J Am Dent Assoc* 124:67-72, 1993.

32. Strassler HE et al: Enhanced visualization during dental practice using magnification systems, *Compendium* 19(6):595-6, 600, 602, 604, 606, 608, 610, 1998.

33. Sunell S, Maschak L: Positioning for clinical dental hygiene care preventing back, neck, and shoulder pain, *Probe* 30(6): 216-9, 1996.

34. Wolny K, Shaw L, Verougstraete S: Repetitive strain injuries in dentistry, *Ontario Dent* 76(2):13-9, 1999.

35. Woodall I: *Comprehensive dental hygiene,* ed 4, St Louis, 1993, Mosby.

CHAPTER 7

Instrument Design *and* Principles *of* Instrumentation

Mary Kaye Scaramucci

Chapter Outline

Evolution of Instruments
Parts of the Instrument
    Handle
    Shank
    Working end
Instrument Identification
    Classification
    Design name
    Design number
    Design features of specific instruments

Case Study: Instrument Selection Evaluation
Fundamentals of Instrumentation
    Instrument grasp
    Fulcrum
    Adaptation
    Angulation for insertion and activation
    Activation
    Types of strokes

Key Terms

Area-specific curet
Calculus
Circumferential
Cross-section
Curet
Cutting edge
Explorer
Face

File
Fulcrum
Handle
Knurled
Lateral pressure
Lateral sides
Long axis

Oblique
Parallel
Periodontal debridement
Perpendicular
Shank
Sickle
Tactile sensitivity

Terminal shank
Tip
Toe
Ultrasonic instruments
Universal
Vertical
Working end

Learning Outcomes

1. Categorize instruments by design features as to ideal location for use and type of deposit removal.
2. Describe the function of each part of any instrument.
3. Analyze each principle step by step as it relates to instrumentation.
4. Select the appropriate instrument by design based on the periodontal condition.

5. Demonstrate correct principles of instrumentation in preclinical and clinical sessions.
6. Compare and contrast the ultrasonic scaler design and principles of use with hand instruments in periodontal debridement.
7. Recognize the appropriate order of the principles of instrumentation.
8. Determine through observation the type of instrumentation stroke being applied.

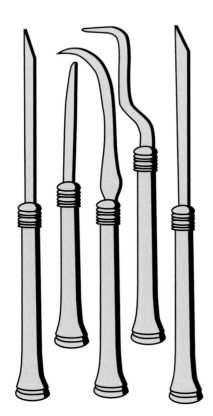

FIG. 7-1 Pierre Fauchard's calculus-removing instruments (1728).

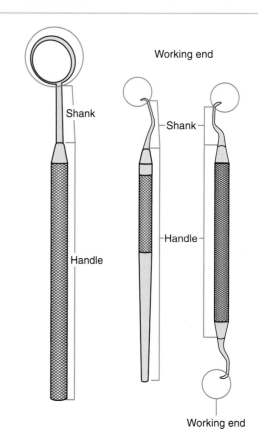

FIG. 7-2 Instrument parts. *Handle* is used to grasp instrument. *Shank* connects the handle and the working end and permits adaptation of the working end to the tooth surface. *Working end* does the work of the instrument.

EVOLUTION OF INSTRUMENTS

Instruments for *calculus* removal have been in existence as early as the twelfth century. An Arabian physician wrote about the formation of calculus and described and illustrated various instruments that would remove it. He invented 14 scalers and recommended a thorough cleaning of the teeth.[1]

In 1728 Pierre Fauchard of France was compelled to invent his own set of instruments because "most of the instruments used for cleaning the teeth seem to me very unsuitable and even clumsy."[1] His instruments shown in Fig. 7-1, consisted of a rebbet chisel, parrot's bill, graver with three *faces,* small knife, and z-shaped hook.

James Snell of London published a guide to scaling in 1832, which unequivocally recommended instruments with special design features for specific tooth surfaces. Snell was noted for his belief that use of a different instrument for the right and left side of the mouth was a "new method" for calculus removal.

From that point, instruments designed for the detection and removal of calculus deposits have evolved into various modern-day instruments: *curets, sickles, files,* hoes, *explorers,* periodontal probes, and ultrasonic scalers. Instrument design is dependent on the type of deposit to be removed and specific tooth surfaces. Designers of instruments over the years strove to develop those that are easy to use, conform well to the tooth surface, and function effectively. The goal of instrumentation, however, has

changed significantly. No longer is the goal to have glassy, smooth root surfaces but rather a removal of endotoxin from the root surface, which can be accomplished with either hand or *ultrasonic instruments.*

The novice clinician benefits from understanding the relationship of instrument design to *periodontal debridement* techniques. Understanding the specific design features of contemporary instruments affords the clinician the critical thinking skills necessary to appropriately adapt and successfully use any instrument. This chapter identifies the parts of hand-activated instruments, their design features, and methods of use.

PARTS OF THE INSTRUMENT

To follow the principles of instrumentation in an effective manner, the clinician must be thoroughly familiar with specific terminology that identifies the standard parts of the instrument. All dental instruments consist of three parts: the *handle, shank,* and *working end* (Fig. 7-2). Each has specific design features that help the clinician determine the proper use of each instrument.

HANDLE

Handles on hand instruments vary in weight, diameter, and texture. The handles shown in Fig. 7-3 can be nar-

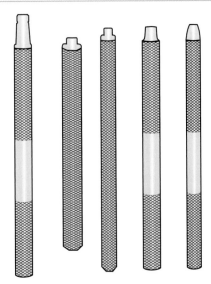

FIG. 7-3 Instrument handles. Handles are available in a variety of shapes and styles. The following factors should be considered in the selection of instrument handles: *Weight*: Hollow handles increase tactile sensitivity and minimize operator fatigue. *Diameter*: Large handles maximize control and encourage a lighter grasp. *Serration*: Knurled handles enhance control by providing a positive gripping surface.

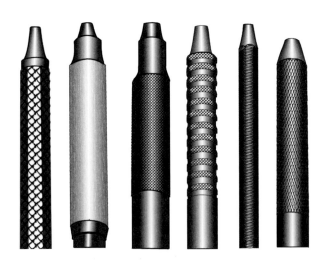

FIG. 7-4 Handle serration (knurling). Handle serrations vary from manufacturer to manufacturer. Some designs offer better control than others.

row and solid or wide and hollow. Narrow handles are normally heavier in weight, whereas wide handles are lighter in weight. To prevent finger fatigue and to ease the instrumentation skills of the novice clinician, wide, hollow handles are the instruments of choice. First graders learning to write use pencils as round and large as a pretzel rod. The size of the pencil makes it easier to hold and use. The writing skills do not change as the pencil size shrinks. The same occurs with perfection of dental hygiene skills.

Hollow handles offer the additional advantage of being more efficient at transmitting tactile sensations. Because much of the instrumentation is below the gingival margin and therefore is not visible, the clinician must rely on vibrations transmitted from the instrument to discern the topography of the root surface. When an instrument is drawn over a calculus deposit, varying degrees of vibrations are transmitted to the instrument handle, which in turn, are felt in the hand of the clinician. It is similar to the sensations felt in the steering wheel when a car drives over a speed bump or a gravel road. This sensation is known as **tactile sensitivity** and is a critical component of instrumentation.

The surface texture of the handle can be **knurled** or smooth (Fig. 7-4). The amount and type of texture helps provide a firm grasp of the instrument and prevents slipping, particularly in a wet environment. Knurling can vary from manufacturer to manufacturer. However, the "waffle iron" pattern provides the best grasp and control.[2]

The handle of an ultrasonic **tip** is actually the round receptacle (handpiece) into which the tip or insert slides. Water to cool the tip flows through the handpiece. Tac-

tile sensitivity is not a design feature of the ultrasonic handle.

SHANK

The shank is located at the end of the handle, between the handle and the working end, and varies in diameter, curvature, and length. The design features of the instrument shank reflect its intended use. Shanks with a thick diameter are considered rigid in nature and therefore are capable of removing heavy calculus deposits. If the diameter of a shank is thin, it is considered a flexible design for removal of light calculus. Thin, flexible shanks also increase tactile sensitivity for the clinician. The curvature of the shank is defined as the bends that deviate from the **long axis** of the handle (Fig. 7-5). The curvature of the shank determines the area where the instrument can be used. Shanks containing many deviations from the long axis are used in treatment areas with restricted access, such as posterior teeth. Shanks with few or no deviations are used in treatment areas with easy access, such as anterior teeth.

The length of the shank is measured by the first bend away from the handle to the beginning of the working end; this measurement determines the area of use (Fig. 7-6). Short shanks (Fig. 7-7, *B*) are used in unrestricted treatment areas, whereas long shanks (see Fig. 7-7, *A*) are used in restricted areas. The **terminal shank** is that portion of the shank closest to the working end, as illustrated in Fig. 7-6. The terminal shank serves as an important visual cue for the clinician to determine if the correct working end has been chosen. The general rule is the terminal shank is **parallel** to the long axis of the tooth. The functional shank can be short, long, or moderate in length. Moderate to long functional shanks are needed to reach the tooth or root surfaces of difficult access, such as posterior teeth. Short functional shanks are used to reach the tooth or root surfaces of easy access, such as anterior teeth.

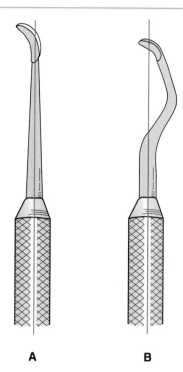

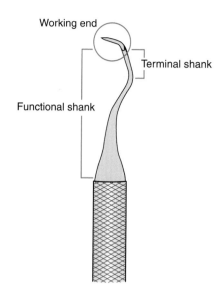

FIG. 7-5 To determine whether an instrument shank is straight or curved, the reader should hold the instrument so that the tip or the toe of the working end is facing the reader. A straight shank is one that has no bends that deviate from the long axis of the shank. A curved shank has one or more bends that deviate from the long axis of the shank. **A,** Straight shank. **B,** Curved shank.

FIG. 7-6 The instrument shank. Terminal shank extends between the blade and the first bend. Functional shank extends from the working end to the handle.

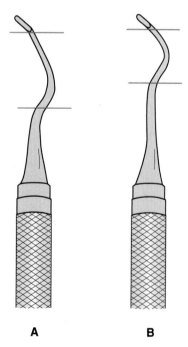

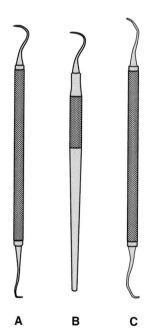

FIG. 7-7 The functional shank length extends from the working end to the shank bend closest to the instrument handle. **A,** A long functional shank. **B,** A short functional shank.

FIG. 7-8 **A** and **C,** Double-ended instrument. **B,** Single-ended instrument. The working ends in **A** are unpaired, whereas the working ends in **C** are paired.

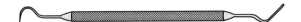

FIG. 7-9 Unpaired double-ended instrument. One working end is a probe, whereas the other is an explorer. Collectively this instrument is considered an instrument of examination.

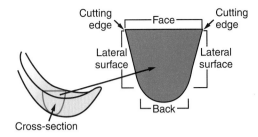

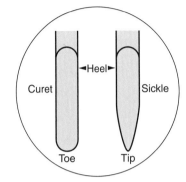

FIG. 7-10 The working end (blade) is made of several components: the face, lateral surfaces, cutting edge, and back. A blade that ends with a rounded toe is classified as a curet. A blade that ends with a pointed tip is classified as a sickle.

The shank on an ultrasonic insert/tip is specific to each manufacturer. Because the power to remove the deposit is the converted electrical energy, the shank on a tip is comparatively rigid. Tips are either straight for anterior teeth and posterior teeth, where adaptable, or contraangled for posterior teeth.

WORKING END

The working end of the instrument is that portion of the instrument that comes in contact with the tooth and performs the intended task. The working end can be wirelike or rod-shaped or a blade. Instruments can have one working end, termed *single-ended instruments,* or two working ends, termed *double-ended instruments* (Fig. 7-8). Double-ended instruments can be paired or unpaired. Paired working ends, as seen in Fig. 7-8, *C,* are mirror images of each other and perform the same function in opposite areas of the mouth. For example, one working end can be used on the facial surfaces of the maxillary right quadrant, and the same end can be used on the lingual surfaces of the left quadrant. Double-ended instruments provide the best efficiency and motion economy because for every double-ended instrument used, the clinician would need two single-ended instruments to complete the same task. Unpaired working ends as seen in Fig. 7-10, *A,* are not mirror images and do not always perform the same function. However, unpaired working ends are useful, depending on the type of instrument at each end. Many unpaired instruments are double-ended based on their function. Instruments such as explorers and probes, as seen in Fig. 7-9, may be combined because they are considered instruments of examination.

The actual parts of the working end vary with each instrument. Some working ends are wirelike or rod-shaped with a sharp or blunt point, as illustrated in Fig. 7-9, whereas others have a blade, face, *lateral sides,* back, and *toe* as shown in Fig. 7-10. Explorers and probes are wirelike or rod-shaped, forming a sharp or blunt point at the end. The side or tip of these instruments is adapted to the tooth surface during instrumentation. The working ends of scaling instruments are slightly more integral. The face and lateral sides join to form a blade or *cutting edge.* Some instruments have two cutting edges, whereas others have only one. The toe of the working end can be rounded or pointed. The back of the working end is opposite the face and may be rounded or pointed depending on the instrument classification (Fig. 7-10). Identifying and understanding the intricate working ends of instruments is vital to proper instrumentation skills and preservation of the original shape and design of each instrument during sharpening. The working end of an ultrasonic instrument is shaped similarly to a hand instrument except that the ultrasonic instrument has no true cutting edges.

BOX 7-1

Instrument Classification

Scaling		*Examination*
Sickles	Chisels	Explorers
Curets	Ultrasonics	Probes
Files	Implant maintenance	
Hoes	instruments	

INSTRUMENT IDENTIFICATION

CLASSIFICATION

Instrument identification is divided into three components: classification, design name, and design number. The shape of the working end of the instrument determines instrument classification. Scaling instruments are classified as sickles, curets, files, hoes, chisels, and ultrasonics, whereas examination instruments are classified as explorers and probes (Box 7-1).

Sickle scalers are designed to remove heavy supragingival calculus deposits and consist of a pointed toe and pointed back. These instruments are triangular in cross-section (Fig. 7-11).

Curets may be used supragingivally and subgingivally to remove fine calculus deposits, particularly in root planing. Curets are designed with rounded toes and backs, and the working end is semicircular in cross-section (Fig. 7-12).

Files are excellent for crushing large tenacious calculus deposits and consist of a rounded or rectangular working end with multiple cutting edges (Fig. 7-13). Hoes and

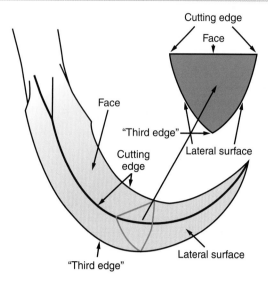

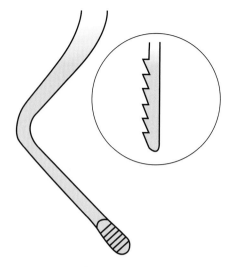

FIG. 7-11 The sickle scaler has two cutting edges. Lateral surfaces join to form a pointed back (sharp third edge) that should be dulled to reduce possible tissue trauma. The face of the instrument is the surface between the two blades that converges to form a point.

FIG. 7-13 Files are composed of a series of parallel blades on a flat working head. Heavy files have a few large blades, whereas fine files have many small blades.

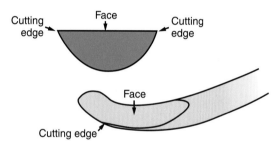

FIG. 7-12 The universal curet has a rounded back and rounded toe that enhances its use in subgingival areas. This back and toe are less likely to cause inadvertent trauma than the sharp-edged back and pointed toe of the sickle.

chisels are designed to remove supragingival calculus. Both instruments have a beveled working end (Fig. 7-14).

Ultrasonic instruments are *universal;* they can be used supragingivally or subgingivally to remove any type of deposit.

Explorers are designed for maximum tactile sensitivity and consist of a fine wirelike working end with a sharp point. Explorers vary in shape and size, and all are circular in cross-section (Fig. 7-15). Probes are considered instruments of measurement, consisting of a rodlike, blunted working end. The working end is also delineated in millimeter markings. Probes are either circular or rectangular in cross-section (Fig. 7-16).

DESIGN NAME

The design name usually is located on the instrument handle and typically is based on the name of the inventor or the academic institution for/from which the instru-

ment is designed. For example, Gracey curets are named for Clayton Gracey, a dentist who invented the original series of 14 single-ended, area-specific instruments in the late 1940s. A team of educators from the University of North Carolina developed the UNC-15 probe, and the EXD 11/12 was developed by Old Dominion University. The design name may provide information about the instrument's origins or design elements to assist in its classification (Fig. 7-17).

DESIGN NUMBER

The design number, also located on the handle, helps describe specific instruments of choice. The Gracey series consists of numerous instruments, and specific numbers identify each instrument (Fig. 7-18). The series consists of the Gracey 1/2, 3/4, 5/6, and so forth up to the 17/18. As a general rule, lower-number instruments are designed for easy access areas, such as anterior teeth, and higher-number instruments are for difficult-to-reach areas or posterior teeth.

On the other hand, probes are identified by a design number that represents the millimeter markings. The earlier reference of the UNC-15 probe indicates that the millimeter markings of this probe are incremented to 15 mm. Other probes, such as the PCP-10 or PCP-12, indicate a 10- and 12-mm increment, respectively.

DESIGN FEATURES OF SPECIFIC INSTRUMENTS

Dental Mirrors

The dental mirror is used as a supplement to enhance access to instrumentation. Dental mirrors have four uses: indirect vision, retraction, indirect illumination, and transillumination. The primary purpose of the mirror is to see oral structures that cannot be seen directly without compromising operator positioning. This technique is known

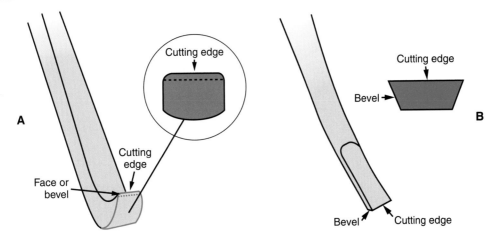

FIG. 7-14 A, The hoe has one blade with a firm shank. When placed beneath a ledge of calculus, a vertical stroke is usually successful in removing deposits. As shown, the corners of the blades should be dulled with a sharpening stone. **B,** Like the hoe, the chisel has a single blade with a firm shank. The cutting edge is at the end of the instrument so that when it is pushed against a deposit, the leading edge engages the calculus.

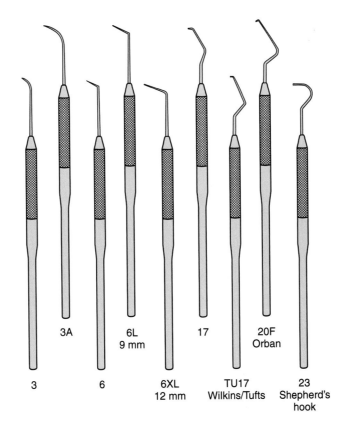

FIG. 7-15 Explorers used to detect caries and examine teeth for calculus and other irregularities are available in a variety of shapes and sizes.

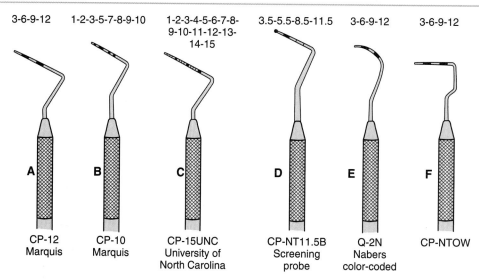

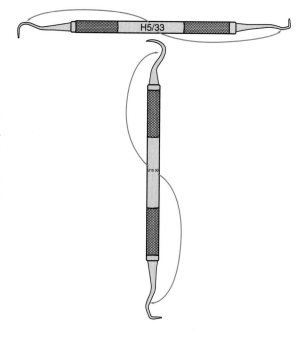

FIG. 7-17 Instrument markings. When the design name and number are labeled along the length of the handle, each working end is identified by the number closest to it. If the design name and number are labeled around the instrument handle, the first number (on the left) identifies the working end at the top and the second number identifies the working end at the bottom of the handle.

as *indirect vision,* and the reflected image is reversed in the mirror. Indirect vision is essential for instrumentation in the maxillary right palatal aspect (left palatal for left-handed) and the palatal aspects of anterior teeth. Constant practice is required to become competent in the viewing of oral structures through the mirror.

The mirror is also used to retract tissue to enhance visibility with direct vision. The cheeks and tongue can be gently moved by the face of the mirror to enhance visibility. Il-

lumination allows the clinician to use the mirror as a spotlight to reflect light from the dental light unto a specific area of the mouth. This technique works best in the maxillary left palatal aspect (right palatal for left-handed).

Transillumination seemingly makes the tooth transparent. This technique is useful in the anterior sextants and consists of placement of the mirror behind the teeth and direction of the dental light *perpendicular* to the long axis of the teeth. Variations in density from the pres-

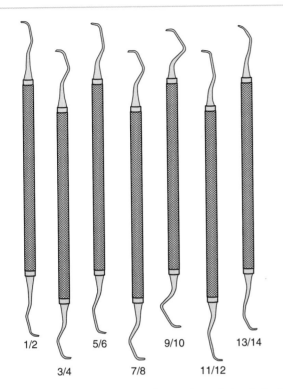

1/2   5/6   9/10   13/14

3/4   7/8   11/12

FIG. 7-18 Gracey curets provide a variety of shank designs to facilitate access to all areas of the dentition. Each instrument is specific to the area. The design of the working end is well suited for removal of fine deposits in subgingival areas. The original series consisted of 14 instruments.

ence of calculus and dental caries become apparent (see Chapter 16).

Mirrors can be one sided or two sided. A two-sided mirror permits the clinician to observe a visible image on either side. The two-sided mirror is preferred because the clinician can retract and use for indirect vision simultaneously. Three types of mirror faces exist. The plane or flat surface mirror has a reflecting surface on the back of the mirror lens and may produce a double image. The concave surface produces a magnified image that may be distorted. The front surface mirror has the reflecting surface on the front of the lens that eliminates the double image, producing a clear image. The front surface mirror is the mirror of choice for dental hygiene procedures. However, this mirror can be easily scratched, and care should be taken to protect the mirror during the bioburden removal and sterilization process. Mirrors should not be placed in the ultrasonic, where other instruments can bump against the face of the mirror, causing scratching. The mirror face should also be wrapped in gauze before sterilization to prevent scratching.

Explorers

Explorers are considered instruments of evaluation. They are used to examine the tooth and root surface for the presence of caries, calculus, and surface irregularities such as the cementoenamel junction and deficient or overhanging margins of restorations. The design features in-

clude a fine, wirelike working end, sharp point, and circular in **cross-section**. The shape of the explorer can vary from a shepherd hook, right angle, pigtail, or contra-angled (see Fig. 7-15).

Periodontal Probes

Like the explorer, the periodontal probe is an instrument of evaluation and cannot be used to remove calculus. Probes are used to measure sulcus depth, determine sulcus topography, measure the amount of attached gingiva, identify gingival bleeding, measure the size of lesions, and aid in calculus detection and identification of root morphology. The design features include a rod-shaped working end and a smooth, blunted point. The probe is round or rectangular in cross-section and marked in millimeters (see Fig. 7-16). The millimeter markings can be color-coded with black markings that will not chip, flake, or fade with sterilizing.

Clinicians should know how the probe is calibrated because the millimeter markings may vary. Some probes are calibrated in increments of 3 mm (see Fig. 7-16, *A*), whereas others are calibrated as 1-2-3-5-7-8-9-10 (see Fig. 7-16, *B*). The UNC-15 is calibrated to 15 mm. This probe is calibrated as 1-2-3-4-5-6-7-8-9-10-11-12-13-14-15 (see Fig. 7-16, *C*). A new screening-type probe has been developed with markings of 3.5-5.5-8.5-11.5 (see Fig. 7-16, *D*). Two types of probes that vary in shape include the Nabers probe (see Fig. 7-16, *E*) used to provide an accurate root furcation measurement, and the Novatech right-angle probe (see Fig. 7-16, *F*) designed for easier adaptation in the posterior regions. Table 7-1 is a quick reference for use of examination instruments.

Sickle Scalers

Sickle scalers are designed for removal of supragingival calculus deposits. The shank of these instruments can be straight, for anterior teeth, or contraangled for posterior teeth. The working end consists of two parallel cutting edges that join to form a pointed toe. The face of the blade may be flame-shaped or triangular, whereas the back is pointed or blunted (see Fig. 7-11). The pointed back and two straight cutting edges limit its use subgingivally because the gingival tissue may be traumatized.

Area-Specific Curets

Curets are used for subgingival calculus removal and root debridement. The original Gracey series consisted of 14 single-ended instruments referred to as **area-specific curets**. Fig. 7-18 shows all 14 as double-ended instruments designed for specific teeth and/or tooth surfaces (Table 7-2). Although two visible cutting edges are curved and join to form a rounded toe, only one edge is used for debridement. The unique feature of the Gracey curet is the offset face of the blade. The face of the blade is at a 60- to 70-degree angle to the shank, rendering one cutting edge lower than the other. When viewing the face of the working end with the terminal shank perpendicular to the floor, the clinician can see a lower and higher cutting edge (Fig. 7-19). The lower cutting edge is the blade that removes calculus. The purpose of this offset angulation is to permit easy insertion

TABLE 7-1

Areas for examination instrument use

Instrument	Area of use	Surfaces	Terminal shank	Description of use
Probe	Anteriors	All	Parallel with tooth surface	Insertion at distal line angle; light walking stroke into interproximal; light walking stroke from distal across straight facial or lingual; light walking stroke from mesial line angle into interproximal
	Premolars	All	Parallel with tooth surface	Insertion at distal line angle; light walking stroke into interproximal; light walking stroke from distal across straight buccal or lingual; light walking stroke from mesial line angle into interproximal
	Molars	All	Parallel with tooth surface	Insertion at distal line angle; light walking stroke into interproximal; light walking stroke from distal across straight buccal or lingual; light walking stroke from mesial line angle into interproximal
11/12 Explorer*	Anteriors	All	Parallel with long axis	Insertion at midline; light walking stroke into interproximal
	Premolars	Distal	Parallel with long axis	Insertion at distal line angle; light walking stroke into interproximal
		Straight buccal and lingual	Oblique	Insertion at distal line angle; light walking stroke to mesial line angle
		Mesial	Parallel with long axis	Mesial line angle; light walking stroke into interproximal
	Molars	Distal	Parallel with long axis	Insertion at distal line angle; light walking stroke into interproximal
		Straight buccal and lingual	Oblique	Insertion at distal line angle; light walking stroke to mesial line angle
		Mesial	Parallel with long axis	Mesial line angle; light walking stroke into interproximal

*During insertion and activation the instrument tip or toe is pointed in the direction of the proximal surface toward which the instrument is moving.

TABLE 7-2

Areas for Gracey curet use

Gracey/area-specific curet	Area of use	Surfaces	Terminal shank	Description of use
1/2	Anteriors	All	Parallel with long axis	Insertion at midline; scaling into interproximal
3/4	Anteriors	All	Parallel with long axis	Insertion at midline; scaling into interproximal
5/6	Anteriors	All	Parallel with long axis	Insertion at midline; scaling into interproximal
7/8	Premolars	All	Parallel with long axis	Insertion at midline; scaling into interproximal
	Molars	Straight buccal and lingual	Oblique	Insertion at distal line angle; scaling to mesial line angle
9/10	Premolars	All	Parallel with long axis	Insertion at midline; scaling into interproximal
	Molars	Straight buccal and lingual	Oblique	Insertion at distal line angle; scaling to mesial line angle
11/12	Premolars	Straight buccal and lingual	Oblique	Insertion at distal line angle; scaling to mesial line angle
		Mesial	Parallel with long axis	Mesial line angle; scaling into interproximal
	Molars	Straight buccal and lingual	Oblique	Insertion at distal line angle; scaling to mesial line angle
		Mesial	Parallel with long axis	Mesial line angle; scaling into interproximal
13/14	Premolars	Distal	Parallel with long axis	Insertion at distal line angle; scaling into interproximal
	Molars	Distal	Parallel with long axis	Insertion at distal line angle; scaling into interproximal
15/16	Premolars	Straight buccal and lingual	Oblique	Insertion at distal line angle; scaling to mesial line angle
		Mesial	Parallel with long axis	Mesial line angle; scaling into interproximal
	Molars	Straight buccal and lingual	Oblique	Insertion at distal line angle; scaling to mesial line angle
		Mesial	Parallel with long axis	Mesial line angle; scaling into interproximal
17/18	Premolars	Distal	Parallel with long axis	Insertion at distal line angle; scaling into interproximal
	Molars	Distal	Parallel with long axis	Insertion at distal line angle; scaling into interproximal

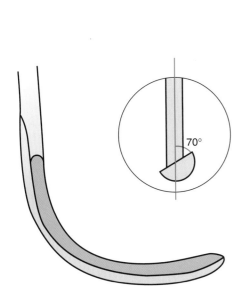

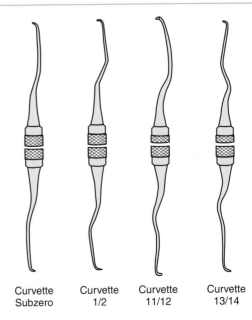

FIG. 7-19 Note the offset relationship of the cutting edge of this Gracey. One blade is lower than the other.

FIG. 7-21 Vision curvettes. Curvette Subzero: Long shank reaches deep into the sulcus, adapting to the facial and lingual root surface. Curvette 1/2: For anterior and premolar surfaces as well as interproximal areas. Curvette 11/12: For mesial surfaces of molars with improved adaptation into furcations. Curvette 13/14: For distal surfaces of molars with improved adaptation into furcations.

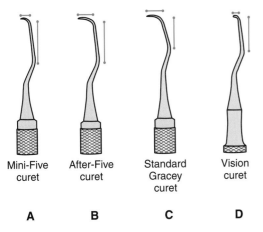

| Mini-Five curet | After-Five curet | Standard Gracey curet | Vision curet |
| A | B | C | D |

FIG. 7-20 Comparison of area-specific curets. **A,** The Mini-Five curet has a long terminal shank and small working end. **B,** The After-Five curet has a long terminal shank and standard working end. **C,** The standard Gracey curet. Compare the terminal shank and working end with the Mini and After-Five. **D,** Vision curvette has a long shank with 5-mm and 10-mm markings and a 50% curved working end.

below the gingival margin and adaptation to the tooth surface. The working end of the Gracey may be styled smaller in overall size, known as the *mini Gracey curet.* The overall working end is approximately half the length of the standard Gracey. The mini is designed to adapt to narrow pockets or furcations (Fig. 7-20, *A*).

The Gracey curets used in the anterior region consist of slight contraangled shanks, whereas those instruments used in the posterior region have multiple contraangled shanks. The long, flexible shanks are designed for superior access in difficult-to-reach areas with an increase in tactile conduction. Because of the limited ability of these Graceys

to remove moderate to tenacious calculus deposits, the Gracey series has been designed with rigid shanks. Graceys with rigid shanks are stronger and can remove more tenacious deposits; however, a slight reduction in tactile sensitivity results.

The After-Five Gracey offers yet another unique style. The After-Five curet has a terminal shank that has been redesigned to be 3 mm longer than the standard curet (Fig. 7-20, *B*). This design feature affords access to deep periodontal pockets and root surfaces of 5 mm and beyond. Many times the After-Five feature is coupled with the mini–working end to create an instrument that can reach the base of a deep, narrow periodontal pocket.

Various innovations have resulted in several contemporary redesigns by the Hu-Friedy Company of the original Gracey series. The Gracey mesial-distal curets (11/14 and 12/13) are a combination of the instrument used on the facial/mesial surfaces and distal surfaces of posterior teeth. This feature allows the clinician to complete a posterior sextant with one instrument as opposed to the combination of the 13/14 and 11/12. Another pattern design mimics the 11/12, in which the shank has accentuated contraangled bends and the cutting edge is positioned to reach the mesial surfaces of posterior teeth and is known as the Gracey 15/16. The Gracey 17/18 is an accentuated version of the 13/14, improving access to the distal posterior surfaces.

The vision curvette series (Fig. 7-21) instruments have long shanks with 5- and 10-mm shank markings, and a 50% shorter, curved working end. These instruments exhibit improved adaptation into furcations and deep periodontal pockets. Finally, the Turgeon Modified Gracey

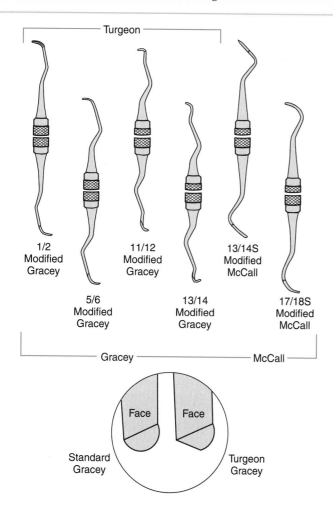

FIG. 7-22 Turgeon Modified Gracey Curets. Note the angulation of a standard Gracey versus the Turgeon Gracey.

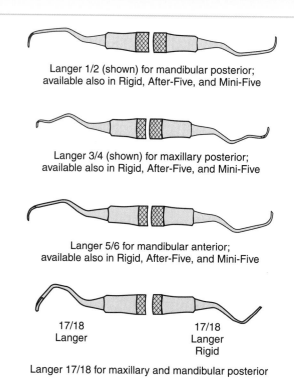

FIG. 7-23 Langer curets combine the features of the Gracey and universal curet. The Langer has two cutting edges like the universal and the shank design of the Gracey. The Langer series consist of the 1/2, 3/4, 5/6, and 17/18. The series can be modified as rigid, After-Five, or Mini-Five.

series is designed with a different cross-section of the blade angulation (Fig. 7-22), providing a sharper cutting edge that is easier to sharpen. The blades are also narrow for easy insertion subgingivally.

Universal Curets

Universal curets have a variety of styles and patterns. However, they all possess basic design features representative of all universals. The universal design permits adaptation to all tooth surfaces of the anterior and posterior regions alike, without the changing of instruments. The working end consists of two parallel and straight cutting edges that join to form a rounded toe (see Fig. 7-12). Both cutting edges are used for calculus removal and root debridement. The face of the blade is at a 90-degree angle to the shank. Universal curets require great care to ensure the opposite cutting edge is not engaged to remove the pocket lining adjacent to the root surface. The Langer curets are unique types of universal instruments (Fig. 7-23). These instruments have the shank design of a Gracey curet with a universal cutting edge design. They feature a series of working ends such as L1/2 for mandibular posterior teeth, L3/4 for maxillary posterior teeth, L5/6 for maxillary and mandibular anterior teeth, and the L17/18 for maxillary and mandibular posterior teeth. The Langer series can also be obtained with a rigid or After-Five shank as well as a mini–working end.

Hoes

The hoe scaler shown in Fig. 7-14, *A,* is designed to remove ledges of calculus and heavy stain from the facial, lingual, and palatal surfaces of teeth. The face of the blade joins the beveled toe to form one straight cutting edge. This face of the blade is at a 99- to 100-degree angle to the instrument shank, whereas the toe has a 45-degree bevel. Hoes consist of straight or contraangled shanks. The straight shank is designed for anterior teeth and the contraangled shank is designed for posterior teeth.

Chisels

Chisels, as shown in Fig. 7-14, *B,* are designed to remove supragingival calculus deposits between teeth, particularly in the anterior region. Like hoes, chisels have one straight cutting edge and a beveled toe. The blade is slightly curved to enhance adaptation around tooth surfaces and is positioned at a 45-degree angle to the face of the working end. Chisels have straight or curved shanks.

Files

Periodontal files are used to crush large pieces of tenacious subgingival calculus. The working ends are either oval or rectangular in shape, containing multiple rows of straight cutting edges and are shown in Fig. 7-13. Files have

TABLE 7-3
Areas for scaling instrument use

Instrument	Area of use	Surfaces	Terminal shank	Description of use
Anterior sickle*	Anteriors	All	Parallel with long axis	Placement at midline; scaling into interproximal
Posterior sickle*	Premolars	Distal	Parallel with long axis	Placement at distal line angle; scaling into interproximal
		Mesial	Parallel with long axis	Placement at mesial line angle; scaling into interproximal
	Molars	Distal	Parallel with long axis	Placement at distal line angle; scaling into interproximal
		Mesial	Parallel with long axis	Placement at mesial line angle; scaling into interproximal
Universal curet*	Anteriors	All	Oblique	Insertion at midline; scaling into interproximal
	Premolars	Distal	Parallel with long axis	Insertion at distal line angle; scaling into interproximal
		Straight buccal and lingual	Oblique	Insertion at distal line angle; scaling to mesial line angle
		Mesial	Parallel with long axis	Mesial line angle; scaling into interproximal
	Molars	Distal	Parallel with long axis	Insertion at distal line angle; scaling into interproximal
		Straight buccal and lingual	Oblique	Insertion at distal line angle; scaling to mesial line angle
		Mesial	Parallel with long axis	Mesial line angle; scaling into interproximal
Hoe	Anteriors	Straight buccal and lingual	Parallel with long axis	No insertion; placement is coronal to gingival margin; stroke pulled downward toward incisal
	Premolars	Straight buccal and lingual	Parallel with long axis	No insertion; placement is coronal to gingival margin; stroke pulled toward occlusal
	Molars	Straight buccal and lingual	Parallel with long axis	No insertion; placement is coronal to gingival margin; stroke pulled toward occlusal
Chisel	Anteriors	Interproximal	Perpendicular with long axis	No insertion; stroke pushed from facial to lingual
File	Anteriors	Straight facial and lingual	Parallel with long axis	Insertion apical to deposit; stroke pulled toward incisal
	Premolars	Straight buccal and lingual	Parallel with long axis	Insertion apical to deposit; stroked pulled toward occlusal
	Molars	Straight buccal and lingual	Parallel with long axis	Insertion apical to deposit; stroke pulled toward occlusal

*During insertion and activation the instrument tip or toe is pointed in the direction of the proximal surface toward which the instrument is moving.

straight or contraangled shanks. Table 7-3 identifies areas of use for all scaling instruments.

Ultrasonics

The ultrasonic scaler was introduced to dentistry in the early 1950s for the removal of decay in cavity preparation. With the advent of the high-speed handpiece, the ultrasonic scaler was no longer needed for its originally designed purpose. In the late 1950s the ultrasonic scaler was used for heavy supragingival calculus removal. Along with the evolution in design, additional benefits soon were realized, and today the most common use by far of this instrument is in periodontal debridement and calculus and plaque removal.

Each unit consists of a control box, a handpiece, insert tips, associated hoses, and a foot-activated pedal. The handpiece is filled with water through depression of the foot pedal, and the selected tip is inserted. The tip is then "tuned" by manipulation of the power setting and water flow until a fine, mistlike spray is achieved when the tip is activated.

The ultrasonic unit uses electrical energy to convert to mechanical energy, and the cycles per second depends on the type of mechanical energy conversion and the specific equipment. The tip in most units vibrates at 28,000 times

Case Study

Instrument Selection Evaluation

A recent dental hygiene graduate, Shanele Jackson, agreed to substitute in a dental practice for 1 day. Her first patient had a slight amount of supragingival calculus and a moderate amount of plaque. The tray set-up brought by the dental assistant included the following instruments:
- Periodontal probe
- Pig-tail ("cow horn") explorer
- Anterior sickle scaler
- Prophy angle-disposable
- Gracey curet, 1-2

Is this an adequate tray set-up given the clinical presentation?

per second. When the tip is placed on a deposit, it virtually implodes as the vibrating force destroys the crystal structure of calculus. Use of the ultrasonic unit includes specific techniques, cautions, and some (few) contraindications (see Chapter 31).

FUNDAMENTALS OF INSTRUMENTATION

7-A
7-B   *INSTRUMENT GRASP*

Understanding the design features of the basic instruments is necessary to apply the principles of instrumentation. These principles describe the relationship of the instrument to the hand and to the tooth or root surface. The fundamentals of instrumentation include grasp, *fulcrum,* adaptation, insertion, angulation, and activation (Box 7-2). Instrument grasp describes how the clinician holds the instrument. The two grasps used during dental hygiene care are (1) the modified pen grasp and (2) the palm grasp. The palm grasp has limited usage: to hold and use the air/water syringe or tuck the mirror away when not in use. With this grasp the syringe/instrument is held in the palm of the dominant hand, and the fingers are wrapped around the handle. The thumb is free to activate the air and water buttons or to provide leverage on the shank of an instrument (Fig. 7-24).

The modified pen grasp is a variation of the pen grasp. Whereas a pen grasp varies from person to person, the modified pen grasp requires all clinicians hold the instrument in a similar manner. Fig. 7-25 shows a typical pen grasp. Students should notice placement of thumb, index, and middle finger.

Three advantages of the modified pen grasp are control of the instrument, prevention of finger fatigue, and increase in tactile sensitivity. The instrument is held in the dominant hand with the pads of the index finger and thumb opposite each other on the handle closest to the working end. The thumb and index finger are not touching, therefore creating a tripod effect with the middle finger placed along the shank of the instrument. This tripod effect balances the instrument in the clinician's hand to provide stability and control. By keeping the index finger and thumb separated, the clinician can roll the instrument between these digits with ease and control. The thumb is either straight or slightly bent in a c-shape, whereas the index finger is straight from the fingertip to the second joint. The index finger bends at the second joint, and the instrument handle rests somewhere between the second and third joint. If the index finger bends at the first joint, it will result in loss of wrist motion and power for scaling. The side pad near the fingernail of the middle finger is against the shank and serves to guide the instrument. The middle finger also bends at the second joint and should not be used to apply pressure to the instrument. The middle and ring finger always should remain in contact somewhere along the length of either finger. This contact ensures proper wrist motion and limits the amount of finger motion to activate the instrument (Fig. 7-26).

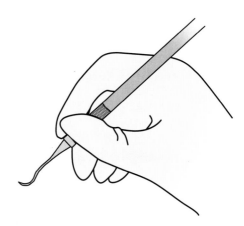

FIG. 7-25 Typical pen grasp, with the thumb and index finger grasping handle. The middle finger supports the instrument from underneath. The pen grasp varies from person to person.

BOX 7-2		
Fundamentals of Instrumentation		
1. Grasp	3. Adaptation	5. Angulation
2. Fulcrum	4. Insertion	6. Activation

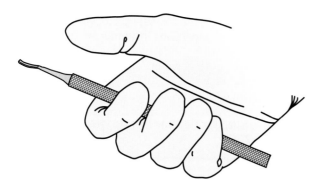

FIG. 7-24 Palm grasp. The instrument handle is held in the palm grasp by cupped index, middle, ring, and pinky fingers.

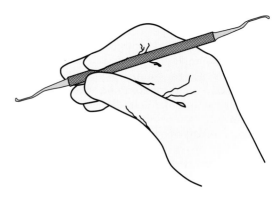

FIG. 7-26 The modified pen grasp with both first and second fingers holding the handle, opposed by the thumb. The third finger is in position to rest on the tooth to create stability and to act as a finger rest to move the instrument and hand as a unit.

FULCRUM

The fulcrum or finger rest serves as a stabilizing point for the instrument, prevents injury to the patient and operator, and enables the hand and instrument to move as a single unit. The pad, specifically the tip of the ring finger of the dominant hand, serves as the fulcrum finger (Fig. 7-27). When activating the instrument, the clinician exerts downward pressure on the fulcrum finger and slightly squeezes the instrument with the index finger and thumb to increase stability and control during scaling while not causing patient discomfort. A lazy fulcrum in which the clinician uses the middle of the pad can hinder the maneuverability or pivot of the fulcrum finger, thereby limiting the ability to adapt, angle, and activate the instrument properly. General guidelines for an appropriate fulcrum include the placement of the ring finger on solid tooth surface, in the same arch, and close to the work area.

The fulcrum finger serves as a pivot point for instrument adaptation and activation. This action of the fulcrum finger and wrist is what is needed to activate the instrument. The hand, wrist, and forearm should be in a straight line to lessen the strain on the carpal nerve, preventing carpal tunnel syndrome.

Auxiliary or Advanced Fulcrums

Although the conventional intraoral fulcrum may be the only fulcrum permitted during skill development, a variety of advanced types of fulcrums deviate from the general intraoral fulcrums. Advanced fulcrums are necessary during certain circumstances that may prohibit following the intraoral guidelines. The advantages include enhanced access to the treatment area, improved instrument to tooth angulation, and an increase in power because of the wider range of motion in the wrist, hand, and arm. Serious disadvantages include lack of stability and control that the traditional intraoral fulcrum offers, as well as a possibility for client/operator injury. These fulcrums should be practiced and used only once the traditional intraoral fulcrum has been mastered. Advanced fulcrums build on the skills learned with the intraoral fulcrum.

Four variations of the traditional intraoral fulcrum include cross-arch, opposite-arch, finger on finger, and reinforced. The cross-arch fulcrum in Fig. 7-28 requires a finger placement on solid tooth structure. Although the placement is in the same arch, it is in the opposite quadrant of instrumentation. Opposite arch fulcrum shown in Fig. 7-29 is placement of the finger rest in the opposite arch of instrumentation. For example, the clinician is instrumenting the mandibular anterior sextant while a finger rest is on the maxillary anterior sextant. Finger-on-finger

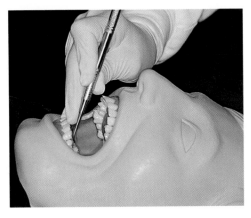

FIG. 7-28 Intraoral cross-arch fulcrum. The clinician fulcrums in quadrant four to instrument in quadrant three. A cross-arch fulcrum permits greater movement of the hand and instrument as a unit, thereby increasing lateral pressure.

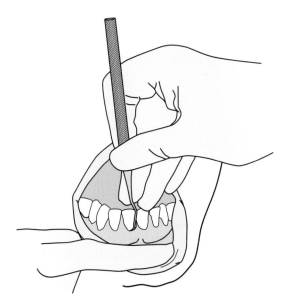

FIG. 7-27 The finger rest in the modified pen grasp is intraorally on a solid tooth surface, in the same arch and as close as possible to the working area.

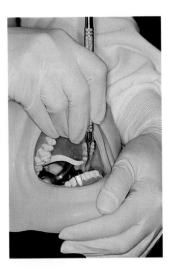

FIG. 7-29 Intraoral opposite-arch fulcrum. The clinician fulcrums in the maxillary arch to instrument in the mandibular arch. Like the cross-arch fulcrum, this alternative fulcrum provides greater movement and pressure.

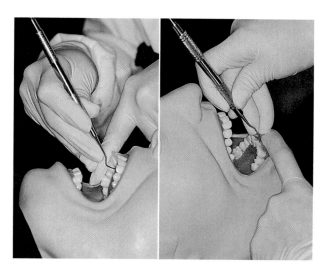

FIG. 7-30 Intraoral finger-on-finger fulcrum, also referred to as the *built-up fulcrum.* It can be used in the maxillary posterior area or the mandibular anterior area. This fulcrum permits superior instrument-to-tooth angulation.

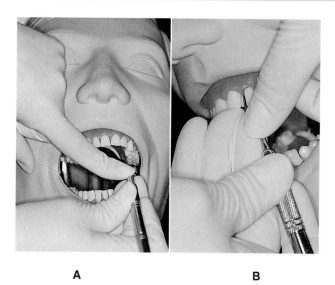

A   B

FIG. 7-31 Intraoral reinforced fulcrum. By placement of a finger **(A)** or thumb **(B)** near the end of the shank closest to the handle, lateral pressure is increased.

fulcrum follows the general principles of a finger rest in the same arch and close to the working area, but the actual placement of the fulcrum finger is on the finger of the nondominant hand. This type of fulcrum (Fig. 7-30, *A*) works in the maxillary right quadrant (left quadrant for the left-handed clinician) during instrumentation of the buccal and palatal surfaces and in the mandibular anterior facial sextant (Fig. 7-30, *B*). For the maxillary right quadrant, the index finger of the nondominant hand serves to retract the check and is placed in the occlusal surfaces of the posterior teeth. The index finger also serves as a finger rest for instrumentation. In the mandibular region, the index finger of the nondominant hand is placed in the vestibule and retracts the lower lip. Again the clinician uses the index finger as a rest for the fulcrum finger, as shown in Fig. 7-30, *B*. A reinforced fulcrum allows the clinician to exert more pressure on scaling. This variation requires caution to prevent the instrument from breaking or injury to the patient. The reinforced fulcrum follows all principles of a finger rest in the same arch, on solid tooth surface, and as close to the working area as possible. The caveat is the addition of the thumb or index finger of the nondominant hand placed on the shank of the instrument. Pressure is gently exerted by the index finger (Fig. 7-31, *A*) or thumb (Fig. 7-31, *B*) to increase **lateral pressure** on the instrument to remove the deposit. Fig. 7-31 illustrates this technique as ideal in the maxillary left lingual quadrant (right lingual for left-handed clinicians). This technique works best with rigid instruments.

Extraoral fulcrums can help the clinician establish the correct instrument for tooth angulation. The extraoral fulcrum shown in Fig. 7-32 is ideal in the maxillary posterior region, where instrument angulation may be challenging. When using an extraoral fulcrum on the maxillary right facial quadrant (left facial for the left-handed clinician), the

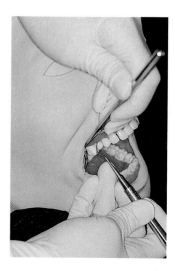

FIG. 7-32 Extraoral fulcrum. By using an extraoral fulcrum, the clinician is afforded the opportunity to increase motion and stroke power. The fulcrum on the maxillary right requires a palm-up approach.

clinician places the back of the hand against the client's chin, with the nail side of the middle and ring fingers gently pressing against the face. The clinician's palm is facing up. Instrumentation on the left maxillary facial quadrant (right facial for the left-handed operator) requires a modified palm-down approach. This time, the pads of the middle and ring fingers are placed against the chin while light pressure is exerted against the face (Fig. 7-33).

The use of ultrasonic instruments can require auxiliary finger rests to control water flow, especially for the maxillary arch.

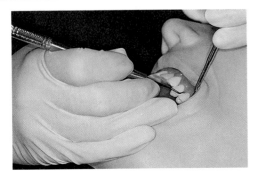

FIG. 7-33 The extraoral fulcrum on the maxillary left is approached with a modified palm-down approach.

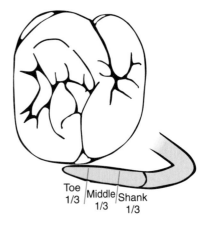

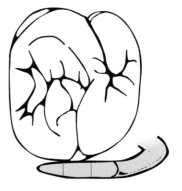

FIG. 7-34 The toe third of the cutting edge should be adapted to the tooth surface. When adapting the toe third, notice the middle and heel thirds are not touching the tooth surface. Notice how these surfaces are rotated away from the tooth. When the middle or heel third is adapted to the tooth surface, then the toe third is not against the tooth, resulting in trauma to the gingiva.

ADAPTATION

Adaptation is the third principle of instrument. It is defined as the relationship between the instrument and the tooth surface that is maintained during instrumentation. A well-adapted instrument prevents damage to the tooth and surrounding tissue and allows for efficient calculus removal. Proper adaptation of the instrument to the tooth surface means placement of the lower one third to two thirds of the instrument working end (Fig. 7-34), specifically the lower third the cutting edge of scaling instruments or the side tip of the explorer and probe, against the tooth. The goal is to keep the side tip or lower one third of the cutting edge or working end against the tooth surface at all times, while the terminal shank is maintained parallel to the long axis of the tooth.

Adaptation of the instrument varies as the instrument is activated around the tooth. The size and shape of individual tooth surfaces dictate how much of the working end is adapted to the tooth surface. Line angles, proximal surfaces, and anterior teeth have the lower one third adapted to those surfaces, whereas facial/lingual surfaces of molars may be able to accommodate the lower two thirds. Clinicians can adapt the instrument by rolling the handle between the index finger and thumb and pivoting on the fulcrum finger. Another aspect of appropriate adaptation is initial placement of the lower one third of the instrument on a specific area of the tooth. The tooth surface location varies from instrument to instrument but is usually at the mesial or distal line angles of posterior teeth and the midline of anterior teeth.

The ultrasonic instrument is adapted in much the same way as hand instruments. The point of the instrument is never adapted directly on the tooth surface, and the side one-third end of the tip is used in debridement.

ANGULATION FOR INSERTION AND ACTIVATION

Angulation is the fourth principle of instrumentation. Angulation is defined as the angle formed by the face of the instrument's working end with the surface to which the instrument is applied (Fig. 7-35). The angle varies, depending on whether the instrument is being inserted before activation or activated for scaling or root planing. Instruments used subgingivally must be inserted before activation. Initial angulation to insert an instrument to the base of the sulcus should be as close as possible to 0 degrees.

This angulation requires the face of the blade to be against the tooth surface. To achieve this position, the clinician tilts the instrument handle as close to the tooth surface as possible, permitting easy insertion with the toe third of the working end beneath the gingival margin and preventing injury to the hard and soft tissue. Once the insertion angle is accomplished, various angles are established depending on the type of stroke applied. If the clinician is beginning an exploratory or examination stroke, the angle should be approximately 5 degrees so that the cutting edge of scaling instruments is not engaged against the tooth surface.

If the working stroke is a scaling stroke for calculus removal, the angulation will be closer to but less than 90 degrees. This angulation affords the clinician with the greatest opportunity to engage the hard deposit. If the work stroke is a root-planing stroke, the angulation will lessen to 60 to 80 degrees. A smaller angulation smoothes the root surface and does not cut or gouge the root, which is the goal of root planing. As a general rule, proper angulation is established when the terminal shank of the instrument is parallel to the long axis of the tooth. This

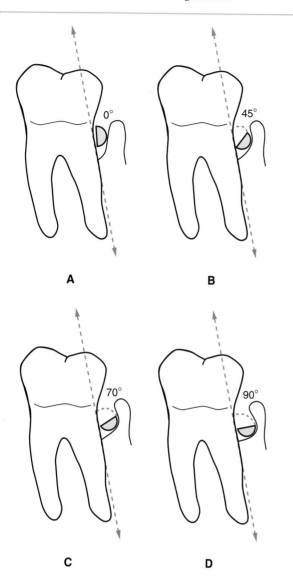

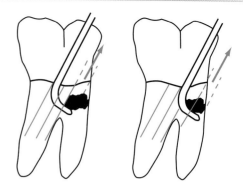

FIG. 7-36 Once the cutting edge is engaged at the proper angle to the tooth, vertical or oblique overlapping strokes can be used for debridement.

FIG. 7-35 Angulation. **A,** Insertion angle of close to zero degrees is ideal for initial blade placement prior to activation. **B,** A 45-degree cutting edge to tooth angulation is too close to effectively remove calculus (with burnishing most likely to occur). **C,** A 70-degree cutting edge to tooth angulation that is ideal for debridement. **D,** A 90-degree cutting edge to tooth angulation that is too open with the potential to damage the adjacent tissue. Observe the terminal shank as the cutting edge to tooth angle is increased.

position is accomplished by tilting of the instrument handle slightly from the tooth after the instrument is inserted. Special care should be taken around line angles and proximal surfaces when instruments have two cutting edges. Care must be taken to disengage the cutting edge adjacent to the gingival sulcus. To disengage this cutting edge, the terminal shank should be tilted toward the proximal tooth surface that is being scaled.

The tip of the ultrasonic instrument is inserted gently beneath the gingiva, adapted to the tooth surface, and activated. The tip also can be placed supragingivally, then gently guided subgingivally as the tip is activated. The tip never remains for more than a second in any given location because energy from the number of vibrations or cycles per second generated by the tip may cause heat and resultant tooth sensitivity.

ACTIVATION

Instrument activation is defined as a single unbroken movement made by an instrument. Activation is divided into exploratory strokes and working strokes. Exploratory strokes are used to detect calculus and root irregularities. These strokes are used intermittently with scaling instruments or continuously with explorers and probes. Exploratory strokes are light and long, covering the entire root surface. Work/scaling strokes for calculus removal are firm, short, and controlled, whereas root-planing strokes are not as firm and longer. Scaling strokes are used on the enamel and root surface for plaque and calculus removal, and root-planing strokes are used only on the root surface for debridement of residual calculus deposits and removal of endotoxins.

Root-planing strokes are designed to smooth the root surface and follow scaling strokes. The instrument grasp is light when exploratory strokes are used, a bit firmer for root-planing strokes, and very firm for scaling strokes. The pressure the clinician exerts on the instrument with the thumb and index finger while pushing with the fulcrum finger determines the firmness of the instrument grasp, known as *lateral pressure,* which varies with the type of stroke used.

Proper pressure is necessary to ensure that calculus is removed efficiently without removal of an excess amount of cementum and dentin. If too much pressure is used, the root surface can become gouged. If too little pressure is used, the instrument will slide over the calculus deposit. Calculus should not be removed in layers because it burnishes the deposit into the root surface. Burnished calculus is difficult to remove and can prevent complete tissue healing.

Stroke direction in relationship to the long axis of the tooth can be **vertical, oblique,** or horizontal. Vertical and oblique strokes are predominantly used on the proximal surfaces of the tooth or root, and horizontal strokes are used mainly on facial and lingual surfaces of the tooth or root

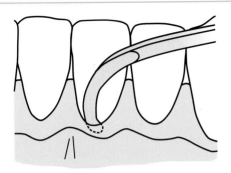

FIG. 7-37 Debridement strokes in a horizontal (circumferential) direction are used in areas where vertical or oblique strokes are not effective. Horizontal strokes work well on the facial and lingual surfaces of mandibular anterior teeth because of their narrow shape.

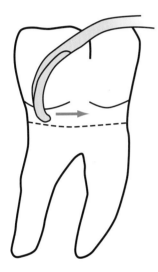

FIG. 7-38 Strokes in a horizontal direction also are used on line angles of posterior teeth.

(Fig. 7-36). The toe third of the instrument is adapted to the tooth surface, and the instrument is pulled by the action of the lateral movement of the wrist and forearm rock. Certain circumstances require a horizontal *(circumferential)* stroke direction. Some mandibular anterior teeth are extremely narrow, prohibiting proper adaptation of the instrument working end (Fig. 7-37). These strokes also are used on line angles of posterior teeth due to lack of proper adaptability (Fig. 7-38). Circumferential strokes must be used with care to prevent damage to the epithelial attachment. To accomplish this stroke, the toe is inserted into the sulcus at a 90-degree to the epithelium. Short, controlled strokes are used in a horizontal direction. This stroke direction requires more finger motion than wrist and forearm to accomplish this movement and should be used in limited situations.

Various types of strokes are used with different instruments. The common stroke type for scaling instruments to remove calculus is a pull stroke, although some instruments require the push stroke for calculus removal. A combined push/pull stroke that is equally light in pressure is used with the explorer in an exploratory stroke around the tooth. The walking stroke is used with the periodontal probe to walk the instrument along the junctional epithelium.

Stroke, or instrument movement, with the ultrasonic scaler consists of short, rapid instrument movement against the surface being scaled or debrided. Lateral pressure is not needed, and the instrument is never held in one place for more than one second.

TYPES OF STROKES

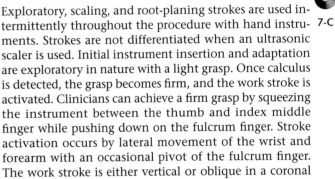

7-C

Exploratory, scaling, and root-planing strokes are used intermittently throughout the procedure with hand instruments. Strokes are not differentiated when an ultrasonic scaler is used. Initial instrument insertion and adaptation are exploratory in nature with a light grasp. Once calculus is detected, the grasp becomes firm, and the work stroke is activated. Clinicians can achieve a firm grasp by squeezing the instrument between the thumb and index middle finger while pushing down on the fulcrum finger. Stroke activation occurs by lateral movement of the wrist and forearm with an occasional pivot of the fulcrum finger. The work stroke is either vertical or oblique in a coronal direction.

Calculus is easier to remove in segments rather than in an attempt to remove the entire deposit at once or to shave it in layers. Once the calculus is identified by location and size, the deposit should be mentally divided into sections. The goal is to remove the entire deposit section at a time, a process known as *channel* or *zone scaling* (see Fig. 7-36).[2,3,4] Channel scaling is critical in the interproximal area. The toe third of the cutting edge is directed beneath the contact area and interdental papilla to provide complete coverage of the proximal tooth surface. Overlapping the scaling strokes in the proximal surfaces occurs from the facial and lingual aspects of instrumentation.

When the work stroke is completed, the clinician uses an exploratory stroke to determine the texture of the root and to ensure complete calculus removal. If the entire deposit is removed and the root surface feels rough, the clinician initiates the root-planing strokes. These strokes require a firm grasp that is not as firm as the scaling grasp. The root-planing stroke is activated by the same means as the scaling stroke; however, the strokes are more numerous, longer, and lighter in nature. Once all zones of the root surface have been instrumented in some manner, and the clinician determines the root is smooth, the next tooth is instrumented.

Certain situations occur when the exploratory stroke is the only necessary stroke on a tooth surface. If the clinician uses a scaling instrument to explore a tooth surface for calculus and finds none, the work stroke is not needed. Subgingival surfaces of all teeth should be instrumented in some way. Scaling instruments should be used with an exploratory stroke or a combination of exploratory, work, and root-planing strokes. When only exploratory strokes are used, the clinician is deplaquing the gingival sulcus to disrupt any bacterial colonies that may have formed between appointments. This instrumentation is the minimal amount required for all patients.

RITICAL THINKING ACTIVITIES

1. A fellow student has a tray set-up of various scaling instruments. She is asking for your assistance in identifying the various instruments by name, use, and location in the oral cavity. The set-up consists of curets, sickles, probes, explorers, and dental mirrors. Several specialty instruments such as files, chisels, and hoes also are included. Using knowledge of the design features for scaling instruments, help your colleague with instrument identification and use.

2. Now that the instruments have been identified, assist the classmate with instrument practice on the typodont. Observe the principles of instrumentation and assist with skill development. Troubleshoot by identifying problems that can be encountered and suggestions to overcome the problem.

3. Examine the instrument grasp in the following illustrations. Determine the possible errors with each grasp and which technique errors could result from an inappropriate grasp.

4. Using two dental mirrors, practice instrument grasp and fulcrum technique in the clinic with a student partner. Remove the mirror from one of the instruments. Holding the handle in the dominant hand, work on grasp, fulcrum, and pivoting in each sextant of the mouth.

5. Create an identification test with instruments from your kit. Cover the design name and number and try to identify the instrument and its location for use.

6. Practice instrumentation in groups of three in the clinic. One student serves as operator, another as patient, and the third as evaluator. Using your instrument evaluation form, the evaluator will examine operator technique for strengths and weaknesses. The patient should evaluate the operator for infection control, ability to communicate effectively, and "bedside" manner. Rotate these positions every hour so that all students have an opportunity to serve in each role.

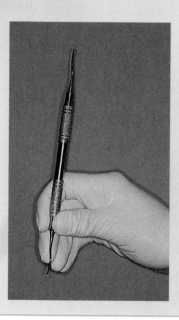
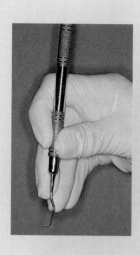
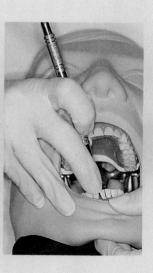

REVIEW QUESTIONS

1. One of the instruments on the tray in the first critical thinking activity has a working end with two straight cutting edges that join to form a point. This instrument is most likely which of the following?
   a. Curet
   b. Sickle
   c. Hoe
   d. File
   e. Explorer

2. Another instrument on the tray has two straight cutting edges that join to form a rounded toe. This instrument is most likely which of the following?
   a. Curet
   b. Sickle
   c. Hoe
   d. File
   e. Explorer

REVIEW QUESTIONS—cont'd

3. Instruments with multiple straight cutting edges parallel to one another are most likely called which of the following?
   a. Curets
   b. Sickles
   c. Hoes
   d. Files
   e. Explorers
4. The advantages of the use of instruments with wide hollow handles include which of the following?
   a. Improves tactile sensitivity
   b. Prevents finger fatigue
   c. Improves instrument control
   d. All the above
   e. None of the above
5. A variation in the thickness of the instrument shank has an effect on the amount of calculus that can be removed. Thin flexible shanks remove fine calculus deposits, whereas thicker, more rigid shanks remove moderate to heavy calculus deposits.
   a. The statement is correct, but the reason is not.
   b. The statement is incorrect, but the reason is correct.
   c. Both statement and reason are correct.
   d. Both statement and reason are incorrect.
6. In a proper modified pen grasp, which of the following is correct?
   a. Index finger, middle finger, and thumb create a tripod on the instrument handle.
   b. Pads of index finger and thumb are opposite each other on the handle, while middle finger rests on the shank.
   c. Middle finger area adjacent to shank rests on ring finger.
   d. Tip of ring finger serves as the fulcrum.
   e. All the above
7. An intraoral fulcrum provides which of the following functions?
   a. Prevents operator fatigue
   b. Prevents injury to the patient

   c. Enables hand and instrument to move as a unit
   d. All the above
   e. None of the above
8. In which of the following ways is proper adaptation of the instrument working end to the tooth surface maintained during activation?
   a. By rotating the instrument between the index finger and thumb
   b. By squeezing the instrument between the index finger and thumb
   c. By pushing down on the fulcrum finger
   d. By moving the instrument handle away from the tooth
   e. None of the above
9. The angle formed by the face of the working end of the instrument to the tooth surface in order to remove calculus should be which of the following?
   a. Less than 45 degrees
   b. Greater than 90 degrees
   c. Less than 90 degrees
   d. Greater than 45 degrees
   e. Both *c* and *d*
10. Which of the following best describe the "channel" scaling strokes?
    a. Short and firm
    b. Overlapping
    c. Vertical or oblique
    d. Engages edge of deposit
    e. All the above
11. The use of an ultrasonic scaler removes which of the following?
    a. Supragingival calculus
    b. Subgingival calculus
    c. Plaque
    d. a only
    e. a, b, and c

ADDITIONAL READINGS AND RESOURCES

Hodges K: *Concepts in nonsurgical periodontal therapy,* Albany, NY, 1998, Delmar.

Hu-Friedy: *Hygiene catalog and reference guide,* ed 2, Albany, NY, 1998, Delmar.

Perry DA et al: *Techniques and theory of periodontal instrumentation,* Philadelphia, 1990, WB Saunders.

Phagan-Schostok PA, Maloney KL: *Contemporary dental hygiene practice,* vol 1, Chicago, 1988, Quintessence Books.

Schaffer EM: Periodontal instrumentation: scaling and root planing, *Int Dent J* 17(2):297-319, 1967.

Woodall IR: *Comprehensive dental hygiene care,* ed 4, St Louis, 1993, Mosby.

REFERENCES

1. Glenner RA: The Scaler, *Bull Hist Dent* 38(1):31-33, 1990.
2. Nield JS, Houseman GA: *Fundamentals of dental hygiene instrumentation,* ed 2, Philadelphia, 1988, Lea & Febiger.
3. Nield-Gehrig JS, Houseman GA: *Fundamentals of periodontal instrumentation,* ed 3, Baltimore, 1998, Williams & Wilkins.
4. Pattison AM, Pattison GL: *Periodontal instrumentation,* ed 2, East Norwalk, Conn, 1992, Appleton & Lange.

CHAPTER 8

Instrument Sharpening

Mary Kaye Scaramucci

Chapter Outline

Case Study: Disadvantages to the Use of Dull
   Instruments
Goals for Maintenance of Sharp Instruments
Sharpening Needs
Testing Sharpness
Sharpening Technique
Devices Used to Sharpen Instruments
   Mechanical
   Mounted stones
   Hand-held stones
Workstation and Equipment
Manual Sharpening Methods
   Stationary instrument/moving stone technique

Specific Instruments
   Sickles
   Area-specific curets
   Universal curets
   Hoes
   Files
   Chisels
   Explorers
Common Technique Errors
Care and Maintenance of a Sharpened Instrument

Key Terms

Acrylic test rod
Angles
Arkansas stone
Beveled edges

Burnished calculus
Cutting edge
Honing machine
India stone

Mandrel-mounted stones
Parallel
Perpendicular
Rounded edges

Slow-speed handpiece
Sludge
Wire edge

Learning Outcomes

1. Value the need for sharp instruments and demonstrate sharpening as indicated by criteria in the chapter.
2. Become knowledgeable of the types of sharpening methods and equipment (stones) to make appropriate selections for sharpening instruments.
3. Select an appropriate sharpening method for instrument design and explain the rationale for this selection.
4. Debate the pros and cons of the sharpening techniques that remove metal from the lateral sides of the working end or from the face of the blade.

5. Explain the rationale used to learn the stationary instrument/moving stone technique over the moving instrument technique/stationary stone.
6. Explain the care and maintenance of all varieties of sharpening stones.
7. Demonstrate the steps used to sharpen each of the following instruments: sickles with flame-shaped cutting edges, sickles with straight cutting edges, Gracey curets, universal curets, hoe scalers, files, explorers.
8. Recognize instrument sharpening errors based on instrument contours.

Disadvantages to the Use of Dull Instruments

A student is debriding quadrant 1 of a patient classified as a periodontal case type II B. She is having difficulty removing calculus deposits from the distal surface of teeth #2 and #3. The student is following the principles of instrumentation accurately, yet the deposits cannot be removed. Further observation of the instrument under a bright light reveals a definite reflection of light along the cutting edge.

*I*n 1908 G. V. Black said:[12]

> *Nothing in the technical procedures of dental practice is more important than the care of the cutting edges of instruments. No man has ever yet become a good and efficient dentist until after he had learned to keep his cutting edges sharp.*

This statement is just as applicable today to the practice of dental hygiene as it was in 1908. It takes the clinician only a few strokes with a dull instrument to appreciate the clinical benefits of a well-maintained, properly sharpened dental instrument. The sharpness of the **cutting edge** must be evaluated with each use, and the maintenance of a sharp cutting edge requires time, practice, and precision.[11]

This chapter discusses the goals of sharpening, with an explanation of the various sharpening devices available and equipment needed. Other objectives include an understanding of the importance of the maintenance of sharp instruments and the original design, in addition to the acquisition of skills necessary to master the sharpening procedure. The sharpening technique requires an understanding of the parts of the instrument, the **angles** of the working end, and precise principles of sharpening.

GOALS FOR MAINTENANCE OF SHARP INSTRUMENTS

Instrument sharpening is a critical component of the periodontal debridement process. Simply stated, periodontal debridement cannot be accomplished with dull instruments. The goals of instrument sharpening are the following:
- To produce a functionally sharp edge
- To preserve the shape (contour) of the instrument
- To maintain the useful life of the instrument

To achieve these goals, the clinician should have a precise understanding of the design features of each instrument before learning the sharpening technique. A review of instrument design in Chapter 7 is essential.

The union of the lateral side and face forms the cutting edge of a scaler and curet (Fig. 8-1, *A*). The sharp cutting edge is the most exact meeting of the lateral side and face. Undesirable **wire edges** are unsupported metal fragments extending beyond the cutting edge from the lateral side

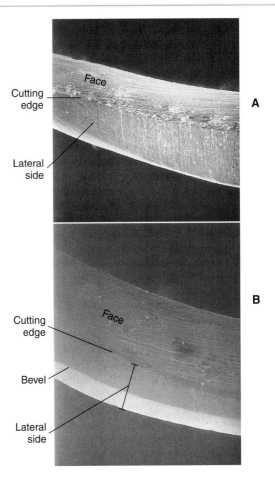

FIG. 8-1 A, Scanning electron micrograph showing the junction of face and lateral side of a curet, which forms the cutting edge. **B,** Scanning electron micrograph showing a bevel on the lateral side of the curet, resulting from incorrect sharpening technique.

or face of the blade. Also undesirable are **rounded edges** that began as sharp edges but are dulled through use or overuse or **beveled edges** that are cutting edges created beneath the original cutting edge by improper stone-to-instrument placement. Therefore the goal of instrument sharpening is to reestablish the sharp edge. Ideally, the internal angle formed by the juncture of the face and lateral sides is 85 degrees and should be maintained throughout the sharpening procedure. A deviation of the stone-to-instrument placement of only 5 degrees can alter the ideal internal angle, which renders the instrument less functional. Little room exists for error in the maintenance of an effective cutting edge.

The outcome of an accurate sharpening technique is to remove a minimum amount of metal from the instrument blade to reestablish the fine cutting edge while maintaining the original shape and texture of the instrument.[17] Maintaining the original shape of the instrument is equally important as the maintenance of a sharp edge. Volumes of research, care, and time are incorporated into the design of instruments to produce effective and safe instruments for debridement. To change the original shape of an instrument by a poor sharpening technique is

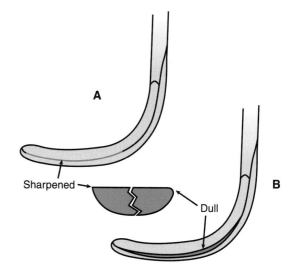

FIG. 8-2   A, A sharp cutting edge does not reflect light. **B,** A dull cutting edge appears as a bright area at the junction of the face and lateral surface.

to create an environment for ineffective treatment and potential harm to the patient.

Maintaining the sharpness of periodontal instruments has many advantages (Box 8-1). Properly sharpened instruments reduce operator fatigue, improve calculus removal, save time, enhance tactile sensitivity, and minimize patient discomfort. Sharp instruments improve the tactile sensations transmitted through the instrument, which improves the clinician's detection skills because the instrument does not need to be held in a tight grasp. Scaling efficiency is increased because sharp instruments remove calculus easier by requiring fewer instrumentation strokes by the clinician. Sharp instruments save time and lessen operator fatigue. Less pressure is required with sharp instruments, which improves control of the instrument and decreases the likelihood of root gouging.

 Case Application
The student was having difficulty removing deposits. What other problems was this student likely experiencing?

In addition, sharp instruments decrease the probability of burnishing calculus by "biting" into the deposit and not shaving over it. ***Burnished calculus*** is calculus that was not completely removed, most often because of a dull or improperly sharpened instrument. When a deposit is smoothed but is not completely removed, it continues to harbor plaque and builds new calculus more readily. Burnished calculus is many times more difficult to detect and remove than nonburnished deposits.

Most importantly, sharp instruments minimize patient discomfort. With dull instruments, the grasp is tighter and more pressure is applied to the tooth surface. This increase in pressure is uncomfortable to the patient and makes the clinician seem heavy-handed. The tighter grasp also makes it easier for the instrument to slip off the tooth surface, increasing the likelihood of trauma to the surrounding tissue.[14] The clinician cannot hope to attain clinical excellence without mastering the skill of instrument sharpening.

SHARPENING NEEDS

Unlike other equipment maintenance procedures, no standard time frame exists for instrument sharpening. The clinician cannot set a specific schedule of instrument sharpening, for example, every Monday morning. Instruments should be sharpened before every scaling and root-planing procedure or whenever the instruments become

dull during treatment. Considerations include the number of patients scheduled for the day, the frequency of use, the degree of patient difficulty, and the type of procedure to be completed. To lessen the chance of contamination with nonsterile instruments, sharpening should occur after sterilization. Dulling of the fine, sharp edge is a normal outcome of scaling and root planing. Approximately 15 working strokes produce a slightly rounded cutting edge, whereas 45 strokes create a very rounded cutting edge.[2,5] Ideally, instruments should be sharpened at the first sign of dullness.[7,18,19,20]

TESTING SHARPNESS

The relative sharpness of an instrument can be determined by a visual or tactile test. A sharp cutting edge appears as a line having no shape or width. A dull cutting edge has a wide, rounded shape. When light is directed on a dull cutting edge, it reflects the light and appears shiny.

 Case Application
The cutting edge of the student's instrument reflected light. A sharp cutting edge having no width cannot reflect light and has a lackluster appearance (Fig. 8-2, *A;* see also Fig. 8-1, *A*).

The tactile test for sharpness uses an ***acrylic test rod.*** The instrument is held in the dominant hand with a modified pen grasp while the test rod is held in the nondominant hand. A fulcrum should be established either on top of the test rod or on the side (Fig. 8-3). Following the principles of instrumentation for activation, the clinician should draw the cutting edge of an instrument across the rod. If the instrument catches or cuts into the acrylic, the instrument is sharp. When the instrument glides over the rod, the instrument is considered dull. Care must be taken to examine or test the entire length of the cutting edge to ensure sharpness of the entire length of the cutting edge.

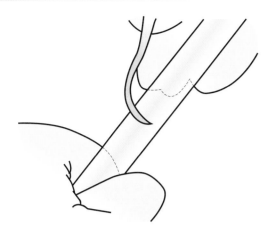

FIG. 8-3 Acrylic test rod is used through application of light pressure against the stick with the instrument at its working angle.

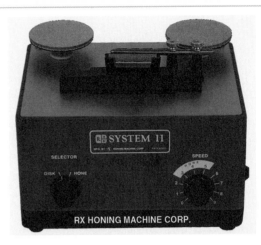

FIG. 8-4 A sharpening honing machine. This method removes metal from the face of the blade.

SHARPENING TECHNIQUE

The sharpening technique uses the grinding of a coarse stone against the instrument to create a sharp edge. Three different hand methods result in sharp instruments. The first advocates grinding the face of the blade. The second method reduces the lateral surface to create a sharp edge through movement of a shaping stone against a stationary cutting edge. In the third, the instrument moves against a stationary shaping stone. The first method, reduction of the face of the blade, creates a weaker instrument that in turn will break more readily.[2,6,7,8,12] Either the stationary stone or stationary instrument method of sharpening produces a wire edge that may interfere with the sharp edge of the blade. Researchers indicate that the direction of the wire edge may have a profound effect on the quality of sharpness.[1,2,4]

Wire edges are unsupported metal fragments that extend beyond the cutting edge from the lateral side or the face of the blade. They are termed *functional* or *nonfunctional*. Studies have indicated that when the wire edge is **parallel** to the scaling direction, the edge is considered functional. A functional wire edge does not gouge into the tooth surface; it "digs in" to the tooth deposit. Therefore it helps remove accretions and does not damage the tooth. Grinding against the lateral sides produces functional wire edges.[1,2,4]

A nonfunctional wire edge is a metal fragment that is **perpendicular** to the scaling direction and is produced when the instrument is sharpened from the face of the blade. Nonfunctional wire edges produce gouging on the root surface and do not aid in the removal of accretions from the tooth,[1,2,4] thus establishing a second reason for sharpening the lateral surfaces of an instrument.

DEVICES USED TO SHARPEN INSTRUMENTS

MECHANICAL

A **honing machine** is an example of a mechanical sharpening device (Fig. 8-4). It is a bench-type piece of equipment that follows the principles of instrument preservation. Specially designed honing disks are mounted on top,

and the instrument is positioned by a sharpening guide according to the instrument classification. The stones are mechanically rotated as the working end is pressed against the stone. The disk rotates up to a powerful 7000 rpm. This device removes metal from the face of the blade, and the clinician controls the pressure.

The honing machine saves time because sharpening occurs rapidly. However, if the clinician is inexperienced and not confident in instrument positioning and application of pressure, the instrument can be ruined quickly. In addition, although sharpening guides assist with proper angulation of instrument to stone, the device sharpens so quickly that the gentle curve of the Gracey or the flame-shape of some sickles is lost.

MOUNTED STONES

Mandrel-mounted stones, as illustrated in Fig. 8-5, are used with a **slow-speed handpiece.** The stones attached are cylindrical in shape with either a flat end or cone-shaped end. Most common mounted stones are Arkansas or Ruby. The rotating stone should be larger than the diameter of the instrument blade. While the handpiece is activated at a slow speed, the stone is passed over the face of the blade to sharpen both cutting edges at once. This method requires stabilization of the instrument in one hand and the handpiece in the other. Again if the clinician is inexperienced with application of pressure, too much of the face of the blade can be removed quickly, rendering the instrument useless.

HAND-HELD STONES

Hand-held stones are a common tool for instrument sharpening. These stones are available in a variety of shapes and materials. Stones can be rectangular and flat, rectangular and wedge-shaped, or cylindrical in shape (Fig. 8-6). Although no one stone shape is superior, the flat stone is ideal for the moving instrument technique and the cylindrical stone is efficient in removing wire edges. The wedge-shaped stone contains a rounded side that can

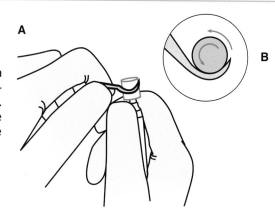

FIG. 8-5 Mandrel-mounted stones. **A,** A mounted stone with a diameter appropriate for the curved blade to be sharpened is positioned across the face for even sharpening of the cutting edges. **B,** With low speed to minimize heat production, the rotating stone is passed along the face of the instrument. Near the toe, the stone is moved upward to prevent flattening of a curved instrument.

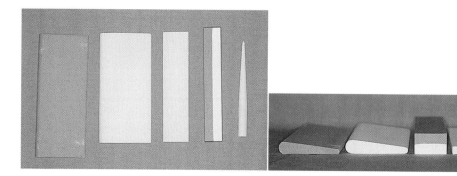

FIG. 8-6 Stones used to sharpen instruments. Stones come in a variety of shapes, sizes, and textures.

TABLE 8-1

Sharpening stone comparison chart

Name	Origin	Method	Lubricant	Texture	Application
Arkansas stone	Natural	Unmounted, mounted, or rotary	Oil	Fine	Routine sharpening and finishing
India stone	Synthetic	Unmounted	Water or oil	Medium	Sharpening of excessively dull instruments or those requiring recontouring
Ceramic stone	Synthetic	Unmounted	Water or dry	Fine	Routine sharpening and finishing
Composition stone	Synthetic	Mounted	Water	Coarse	Reshaping of excessively worn instruments

Courtesy Hu-Friedy Manufacturing Company, Inc., Chicago.

be used like the cylindrical stone to remove wire edges, thus serving as an all-purpose stone.

Stone types vary from natural, quarried from natural mineral deposits *(Arkansas stone),* to synthetic (man-made). Texture varies from fine to medium to coarse. Selection of type and texture are based on the extent to which the cutting edge needs sharpening or recontouring. Sharpening stones are made of abrasive particles that are harder than the surface of the instrument to be sharpened. Coarse stones have larger particles and quickly remove metal from the instrument. Finer stones have smaller particles and remove less material from the instrument. If instruments are excessively dull or require a great deal of recontouring, a coarse stone *(India stone)* is recommended. A fine or medium (Arkansas) stone is preferred for routine sharpening and instrument finishing and has been shown to produce a quality edge.[10] A sharpening stone comparison chart aids in appropriate stone selection (Table 8-1).

Stone Care

Hand-held stones require care to maintain their longevity. First, stones should be lubricated as specified by the manufacturer before use. Stones require either water or oil as a lubricant, and the two lubricants should never be interchanged.[7] The lubricant is used to reduce heat from friction, prevent metal particles from embedding into the stone, and prevent dryness.[3,7] Cleaning the stone also

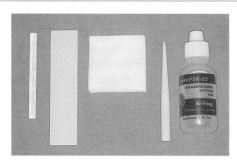

FIG. 8-7 Supplies used for instrument sharpening. From left to right: Acrylic test rod, rectangular Arkansas stone, cotton gauze, cylindrical sharpening stone, and lubricating oil.

BOX 8-2

Sharpening Armamentarium

Light source
Stable work surface
Magnification
Sharpening stones
Test stick/rod
Gauze
Personal protective equipment (PPE): eye protection, exam gloves, mask
Lubricating oil (as needed)

---

should be based on manufacturer's guidelines, especially with the artificial stones. Natural stones can be cleaned with soap and water or abrasive emery paper. Sharpening stones should be cleaned, properly packaged, and sterilized with every use. Stones lubricated with oil before use may bleed oil when sterilized. These stones may be wrapped in a gauze square to absorb the oil. Some manufacturers require lubrication before sterilization. To maintain the useful life of the stone, sharpening should not be limited to one area of the stone. Using the entire stone's surface can prevent grooving of the stone.

WORKSTATION AND EQUIPMENT

Sharpening should be performed at the first sign of dullness, which means a sharpening workstation needs to be incorporated into the dental hygiene treatment room. Ideal conditions include a firm countertop to support the instruments and a light source such as the dental light or a high-intensity lamp. A magnifying glass is helpful to observe wire edges but is not necessary. An armamentarium for instrument sharpening should consist of the following (Fig. 8-7):

- A fine stone
- A medium to coarse stone
- A conical stone
- A sharpening file for sharpening periodontal files
- Gauze for *sludge* (debris created by metal particles and lubricant during sharpening) removal
- Personal protective equipment (PPE), including eye protection, mask, and examination gloves

Ideally, instruments should be sharpened when sterile, before the beginning of the appointment. When sharpen-

ing is necessary during patient treatment, all sharpening armamentaria must be sterile. In addition, sharpening always should be completed with the appropriate work practice controls in place, including PPE, a solid work surface, and an appropriate light source (Box 8-2).

MANUAL SHARPENING METHODS

Two methods of instrument sharpening with hand-held stones can be used. In one method, the sharpening stone is placed in a stationary position and the instrument is moved across the surface of the stone. In the other method, the instrument is held in a stationary position and the sharpening stone is moved against the instrument. Although these techniques vary significantly in visibility and control, both methods require skill, visual acuity, control, and precision to master. Researchers have discovered that when students use the stationary instrument/moving stone method, effective sharpening is accomplished.[8] This method permits the clinician to see the shape of the face of the blade, an important feature because the method reduces the width of the instrument blade. Therefore instruments can be more evenly contoured to provide a better fit subgingivally without significantly reducing the instrument strength.[5] This chapter presents the stationary instrument/moving stone technique.

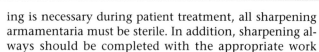
8-A
8-B
8-C
8-D

STATIONARY INSTRUMENT/MOVING STONE TECHNIQUE

The following steps are useful for sharpening:

- *Select* the appropriate stone for the type of instrumennt to be used and the degree of dullness.
- *Lubricate* the stone based on manufacturer's suggestions. Apply small drops of oil or water and rub them into the flat surfaces of the stone.
- *Grasp* the instrument to be sharpened in a palm grasp or modified pen grasp with the nondominant hand placed against the countertop (Fig. 8-8).
- *Rest* the hand holding the instrument on the tabletop and the instrument handle against the edge of the countertop (Fig. 8-9). If the instrument is not stabilized against a hard stationary surface, it may move slightly during the sharpening process and the stone will not be drawn across the blade correctly or consistently.
- *Point* the toe of the instrument toward the clinician and the face of the blade parallel to the floor. The instrument should be held low enough for the clinician to be able to look down on the face to visualize the contour (Fig. 8-10).
- *Hold* the stone in the dominant hand. If a wedge-shaped stone is being used, the wedge should be directed toward the clinician. Two ways exist to hold the stone; both require the stone to be held lengthwise. Method 1 involves grasping of the stone at either end with the thumb on top and fingers on the bottom (Fig. 8-11). Method 2 is similar to a palm grasp where the stone is grasped near the bottom (see Fig. 8-8, *A*). If a rectangular flat stone is used, it can be grasped from the sides as shown in Fig. 8-8, *A*.
- *Position* the stone on the lateral side of the instrument, near the heel of the working end at a 90-degree angle to the face of the blade (Fig. 8-12).

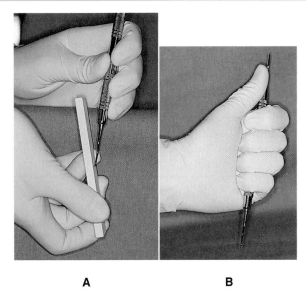

A   **B**

FIG. 8-8 A, Instrument is held in the nondominant hand. This grasp is the modified pen grasp with the bottom of the hand braced against the tabletop. **B,** Instrument is held in the nondominant hand with a palm grasp. Again, the hand should be braced against the tabletop.

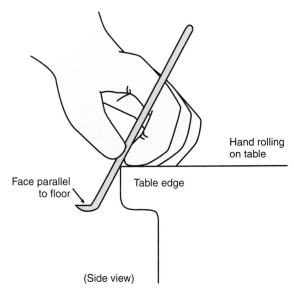

FIG. 8-9 While the hand is braced against the tabletop, the instrument handle is secure against the edge of the tabletop.

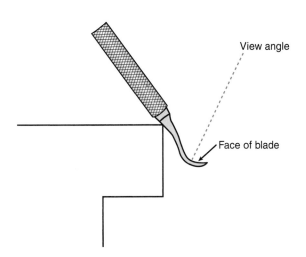

FIG. 8-10 Through bracing of the instrument against the edge of the tabletop, the instrument is positioned for a clear view of the face of the blade.

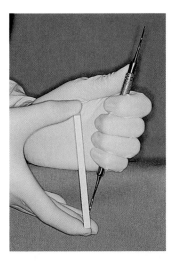

FIG. 8-11 The stone is grasped in the dominant hand in a palm grasp with thumb on top and fingers on bottom.

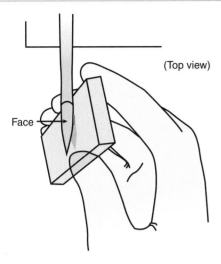

FIG. 8-12 If the stone is not wedge-shaped, it can be grasped in a modified palm grasp with thumb on lateral surface toward clinician and fingers on opposite lateral surface.

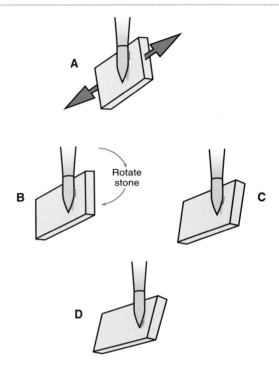

FIG. 8-14 A, Beginning at the heel of the working end, the stone is inched around the cutting edge, following the contour as in **B** and **C. D,** The sharpening stroke is completed on a downstroke when the stone is against the toe of the working end.

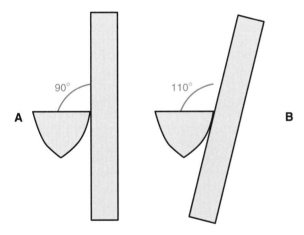

FIG. 8-13 A, Stone at initial placement or "set-up" of 90 degrees to face of blade. **B,** Stone at sharpening activation placement of 110 degrees to face of blade.

- *Move* the stone from the 90-degree position to 100 to 110 degrees (Fig. 8-13).
- *Begin* the sharpening motion on a downstroke, moving the stone down and up while maintaining the 100- to 110-degree angulation. The downstroke should consist of firm pressure, whereas the upstroke should be lighter.
- *Continue* the down/up motion, following the contour of the cutting edge until the toe is reached (Fig. 8-14).
- *Stop* the sharpening procedure on a downstroke to reduce the chance of creating a wire edge.

The entire procedure should include approximately four to five stroke sequences, and the down/up movement of the stone should be ½ to 1 inch in length.

- *Reposition* the stone on the lateral side of the opposite cutting edge of the instrument near the heel at a 90-degree angle (Fig. 8-15).
- *Move* the stone away to a 100- to 110-degree angle from the face of the blade.
- During the sharpening process, *observe* for a layer of sludge. Sludge is a mixture of the lubricant and metal shavings appearing on the face of the blade as the stone is drawn across the cutting edge. Sludge indicates that the correct angle is being maintained.[14]
- *Wipe* the sludge from the instrument, using a gauze square.
- *Test* the instrument for sharpness, using a plastic rod or visual inspection.
- *Follow* the sharpening steps to sharpen the opposite cutting edge as previously described.
- When sharpening is completed, *observe* the cutting edge for wire edges. Because wire edges, whether functional or nonfunctional, do not wholly contribute to the cutting ability of the instrument, they should be removed.
- To remove a wire edge, using a conical shaped stone, *gently stroke* the stone along the face of the blade, maintaining a minimal amount of pressure (Fig. 8-16).

Many students who are beginning to learn the sharpening technique have difficulty visualizing the stone-to-instrument angles necessary for proper sharpening. Because sharpening must be precise to maintain the contour and cutting edge of scaling instruments, an angle guide may be

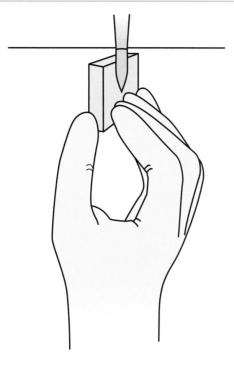

FIG. 8-15 Grasping the stone in the dominant hand, the clinician positions it against the heel of the left side of the working end.

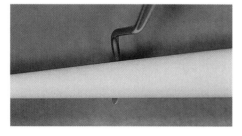

FIG. 8-16 Tapered cylindrical stone is applied to the facial surface of the instrument to help remove wire edges.

helpful to students. Research has indicated that angle guides enhance the clinician's ability for precise sharpening.[9]

Many commercial angle guides are available; however, a guide can be made with a notecard and protractor. A 90-degree vertical line is drawn in the middle of a 3-inch × 5-inch notecard. With a protractor, to the left of the center line another line is drawn that represents 110 degrees and another line to the right of the center representing 110 degrees. The center line is used for instrument placement and initial stone placement, whereas the right and left angle lines represent stone angulation for sharpening. The face of the working end should be perpendicular to the center line. The guide can be placed on the countertop near the edge, or it can be folded over the edge to serve as a guide. A piece of masking tape can be placed on either side of the 110-degree line to further enhance stone positioning (Fig. 8-17).[9] In addition, the guide can be laminated and disinfected for use during patient treatment.

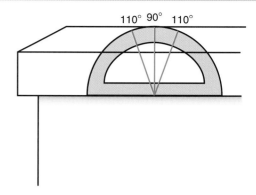

FIG. 8-17 An angle guide can assist the beginner in precise instrument-to-stone placement.

SPECIFIC INSTRUMENTS

SICKLES

Sickle scalers have two cutting edges and a pointed tip. Examine the shape and contour of the face of the blade and cutting edges. The majority of sickles have a flame-shaped contour, which means the cutting edges are not straight but gently curved from heel to toe. However, some sickles, particularly those called *jacquettes*, may be triangular in contour. When sickle scalers are flame-shaped, the entire cutting edge cannot be placed against the sharpening stone. The stone should be positioned at the heel portion of the working end and then rotated along the cutting edge until the stone is flat against the side of the tip as seen in Fig. 8-14. If the sickle is triangular with straight cutting edges, then the entire cutting edge can be sharpened at one time, meaning that the stone can be placed along the entire cutting edge and sharpened at once. Box 8-3 shows the steps necessary to sharpen sickle scalers.

A helpful tip for stone movement along the cutting edge is to place a 1-inch-diameter dot with a pencil in the middle of the stone. When the stone is positioned against the heel of the instrument, the dot should be against the heel. As the stone is moved forward, the dot always should remain in contact with the cutting edge (Fig. 8-18).

See Chapter 7 to review the basic design of each instrument.

AREA-SPECIFIC CURETS

Area-specific curets, such as the Gracey curets, have two edges and a rounded toe; however, only one cutting edge is used for instrumentation. When the terminal shank of a Gracey curet is perpendicular to the floor, the face of the blade is angled or "offset" from the shank to create an upper and lower cutting edge. This offset cutting edge gives the Gracey curets area-specific use. The most important step in sharpening these curets is to determine the correct cutting edge to be sharpened. The cutting edge used in in-

‍‌‍‍

BOX 8-3

Technique Used to Sharpen Sickle Scalers

Flame-Shaped Sickle
1. Position the instrument in the nondominant hand.
2. Place the instrument handle against the countertop with the face of the blade parallel to the floor.
3. Place the sharpening stone in the dominant hand and position it against the heel of the surface.
4. Angle the stone at a 90-degree angle to the face of the blade.
5. Move the stone away from the cutting edge to obtain a 110-degree angle to the face of the blade.
6. Activate the stone in a downward stroke that is ½ to 1 inch in length.
7. Follow the curvature of the blade with the sharpening stroke, while using slight overlapping strokes.
8. Complete sharpening action on a downward stroke when the toe portion is flat against the stone.
9. Sharpen the opposite cutting edge in the same manner.
10. Clear wire edges with conical stone and remove sludge with gauze.
11. Check for instrument sharpness.

Triangular Sickle
1. Position the instrument in the nondominant hand.
2. Place the instrument handle against the countertop, with the face of the blade parallel to the floor.
3. Place the sharpening stone in the dominant hand and position it flat against the entire cutting surface, from heel to toe.
4. Angle the stone at a 90-degree angle to the face of the blade.
5. Move the stone away from the cutting edge to obtain a 110-degree angle to the face of the blade.
6. Activate the stone in a downward stroke that is ½ to 1 inch in length.
7. Complete sharpening action on a downstroke.
8. Sharpen the opposite cutting edge in the same manner.
9. Clear wire edges with conical stone and remove sludge with gauze.
10. Check for instrument sharpness.
11. Complete sharpening action on a downstroke when the side of the toe is flat against the stone.
12. Sharpen the opposite cutting edge in the same manner.
13. Clear wire edges with conical stone and remove sludge with gauze.
14. Check for instrument sharpness.

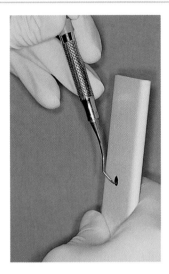

FIG. 8-18 A dot can be applied to the center of the stone as a guide during the rotation of the stone along the cutting edge. As the stone moves forward, the dot is kept against the cutting edge.

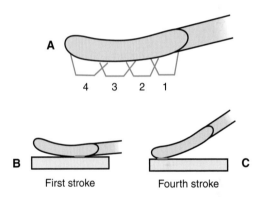

FIG. 8-19 A, Four different adaptations of the stone are necessary to sharpen the entire surface. **B,** First stroke should start at the heel of the blade. **C,** Last stroke should end at the toe.

strumentation is the lower cutting edge. The upper edge is caled the *nonworking edge* or *trailing edge*. To position the instrument correctly for sharpening, the face of the blade must be placed parallel to the floor. The clinician should examine the angle of the face when the terminal shank is perpendicular to the floor, then determine whether the handle should be moved to the right or the left to make the face of the blade parallel to the floor.

The sharpening stone should be placed at the heel of the blade and rotated along the cutting edge until the stone contacts the line angle of the toe (Fig. 8-19). Plac-

ing a dot on the sharpening stone, a helpful tip with sickles, also may be used with the Gracey curet as a guide.

Occasional sharpening of the toe maintains the overall shape of the Gracey curet. Instead of stopping on a downstroke at the line angle of the toe, the clinician should continue the sharpening stroke, increasing the angle of the stone 15 to 25 degrees from the face of the blade as it is moved around the toe. The sharpening process is stopped on a downstroke once the line angle of the opposite side of the toe is reached (Fig. 8-20). Pressure around the toe should be light because only the shape is being maintained; a cutting edge is not being created. Box 8-4 lists the steps used to sharpen area-specific curets.

UNIVERSAL CURETS

Universal curets have two useable and parallel cutting edges and a rounded toe. Unlike the Gracey curets, both

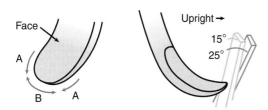

FIG. 8-20 Sharpening the toe. The clinician lightly sharpens by moving the stone around the corner of the toe. As the tip of the toe is reached, the stone-to-face angle is increased by 15 to 25 degrees.

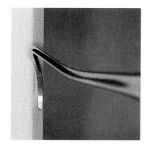

FIG. 8-21 The stone is positioned at a 90-degree angle to face of the blade with complete contact from heel to toe.

BOX 8-4

Technique Used to Sharpen Area-Specific Curets

1. Position the instrument in the nondominant hand.
2. Place the instrument handle against the countertop with face of blade parallel to the floor. (The handle of the instrument must be angled to the right or left.)
3. Place the stone in the dominant hand and position against the heel of the blade at a 90-degree angle to the face of the blade; the anterior portion of the stone will not be in contact with the instrument.
4. Angle the stone away from the cutting edge to obtain a 110-degree angle to the face of the blade.
5. Use light pressure, begin at the heel of the instrument, and activate the stone in a downstroke ½ to 1 inch in length.
6. Rotate stone along its vertical axis as the stone is moved from heel to toe.
7. Follow the curvature of the blade with the sharpening stroke, while using slight overlapping strokes.
8. Complete sharpening action on a downstroke when the stone contacts the line angle of the toe.
9. Round the toe from the cutting edge every fourth or fifth sharpening.
10. Clear wire edges with conical stone and remove sludge with gauze.
11. Check for instrument sharpness.

BOX 8-5

Technique Used to Sharpen Universal Curets

1. Position the instrument in the nondominant hand.
2. Place the instrument handle against the countertop with the face of the blade parallel to the floor.
3. Place the stone in the dominant hand and position against the entire length of the cutting edge of the instrument at a 90-degree angle to the face of the blade.
4. Move the stone away from the cutting edge to obtain a 110-degree angle to the face of the blade.
5. Using light pressure along the entire length of the cutting edge, activate the stone in a downstroke that is ½ to 1 inch in length.
6. Continue with down and up strokes without moving the stone forward.
7. Complete sharpening action on a downstroke.
8. Sharpen the opposite cutting edge in the same manner.
9. Round the toe from both cutting edges once every fourth or fifth sharpening event.
10. Clear wire edges with conical stone and remove sludge with gauze.
11. Check for instrument sharpness.

---

cutting edges of the universal curets must be sharpened. The cutting edges are straight from heel to toe; therefore the entire cutting edge can be placed against the sharpening stone (Fig. 8-21). When rounding the toe, the clinician should lift the stone away from the heel of the blade and begin rotating around the toe, as shown in Fig. 8-20. The toe of the universal curet must be rounded from both cutting edges. Rounding should stop at the toe line angle opposite the cutting edge being sharpened. The steps necessary to sharpen the universal curet are outlined in Box 8-5.

A helpful tip that helps maintain instrument-to-stone contact is to draw a 1-inch vertical line with a pencil down the middle of the stone. The line is placed against the instrument so that it is positioned in the middle of the working end. As the stone is moved up and down against the working end, the line should remain positioned in the center as shown in Fig. 8-22.

HOES

Hoe scalers have one straight cutting edge and a beveled toe. (The toe is flat and angled from the cutting edge.) When a hoe scaler is sharpened, the stone is placed on a countertop and the hoe is pulled across the stone. The instrument is held in the dominant hand with a modified pen grasp and a finger resting on the stone. The beveled working end should be placed flat against the stone with the handle of the instrument at approximately a 70-degree angle to the stone and the working end at approximately 45 degrees to the stone (Fig. 8-23). Gently and evenly, pull the instrument across the length of the stone two to three times. Pressure should be exerted on the pull stroke. The instrument should be lifted from the stone at

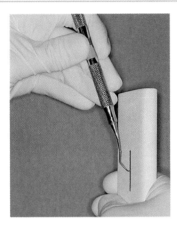

FIG. 8-22 A straight line can be drawn down the center of the stone to serve as a guide for the universal curet. By keeping the line in contact with the cutting edge during sharpening, the clinician maintains correct stone-to-instrument contact.

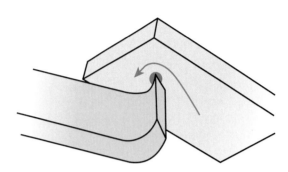

FIG. 8-24 Rounding the corners of the hoe scaler. A flat stone is drawn over each end of the cutting edge with a gentle rolling motion.

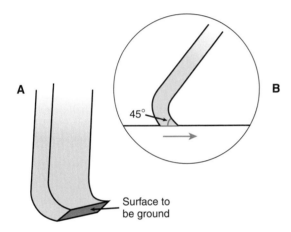

FIG. 8-23 Sharpening hoe. **A,** The beveled toe is the surface to be ground. **B,** The bevel is placed flat against the stone. To maintain the angle of the bevel, the handle-to-stone angle should be approximately 70 degrees.

the conclusion of the pull stroke and placed on the stone again to perform another pull stroke. At the conclusion of the sharpening procedure, the stone is pulled over the corner angles to round the sharp corners (Fig. 8-24). The steps necessary to sharpen a hoe are listed in Box 8-6.

FILES

Periodontal files are unique in that they have several cutting edges, much like the hoe. A special sharpening file is needed to sharpen the rows of cutting edges on the file's working surface.[16] Fig. 8-25 shows the technique used to sharpen a periodontal file. The sharpening file is placed in each of the V-shapes formed by two cutting edges. The sharpening file is drawn back and forth across the edge of each row while the file is maintained within the area between cutting edges. The clincian then moves the sharpening file to the next area and continues the process of sharpening the next cutting edge.

> ### BOX 8-6
>
> **Technique Used to Sharpen Hoes**
>
> 1. Place the stone flat on the countertop.
> 2. Hold the instrument in the dominant hand, using the modified pen grasp with a finger rest on the stone.
> 3. Position the bevel flat against the stone. (The handle should be at approximately a 70-degree angle from the stone.)
> 4. Pull the hoe across the length of the stone two to three times, maintaining the 70-degree angle with the finger rest.
> 5. To round the corners, hold the stone in the dominant hand and the instrument in the nondominant hand with the beveled toe facing away.
> 6. Round the corner closest to the stone by pulling the stone over the corner angles from heel to toe.
> 7. Turn the instrument around so that the bevel is toward the clinician and sharpen the opposite corner in the same manner by pulling the stone over the corner angle from heel to toe.
> 8. Remove sludge with gauze.
> 9. Check for instrument sharpness.
> 10. Check for dullness at the corners by determining whether the corners glide over the test stick.

CHISELS

Although chisels seldom are used in modern instrumentation techniques, sharpening of the chisel is necessary to maintain a sharp cutting edge for the instrument's occasional use. Fig. 8-26 demonstrates the technique used to sharpen a chisel. The stone is stationary, and the chisel bevel is placed on the stone and drawn across the stone to sharpen the cutting edge.

EXPLORERS

Explorers also may be sharpened to produce a sharper point or recontour the working tip. Given the current

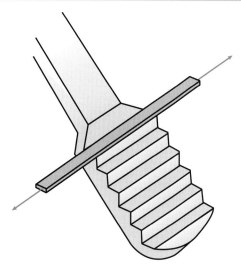

FIG. 8-25 The tang file is positioned parallel along the entire length of the cutting edge. Each edge is individually sharpened.

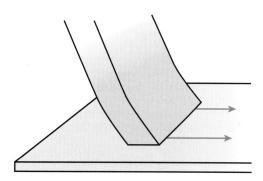

FIG. 8-26 The chisel is adapted to the stone in the same manner as the hoe. Note the increase in angle of the shank to the stone. The handle is positioned at an 80-degree angle to the stone.

recommendations for detection of carious lesions, the need for a pinpoint on an explorer is in question (see Chapter 16). To sharpen explorers the clinician places the side of the tip against the stationary stone, and using light pressure, moves the instrument against the stone, away from the tip. The explorer tip is rotated slightly, and the process is repeated until all sides have been sharpened.

 COMMON TECHNIQUE ERRORS

8-E The goal in instrument sharpening is to maintain the shape and contour of an instrument and at the same time to create a sharp cutting edge. If the exact principles are not followed, then the shape and contour can be destroyed, rendering the instrument unusable. Common technique errors include the following:
- Sharpening beyond the pointed toe of a sickle shortens the overall length of the instrument (Fig. 8-27).
- Flame-shaped or curved cutting edges can be flattened if the stone is *not* rotated along the cutting edge to maintain the correct contour (Fig. 8-28).

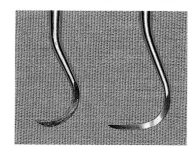

FIG. 8-27 Sickle scalers can be easily shortened by sharpening, which changes the balance of the instrument.

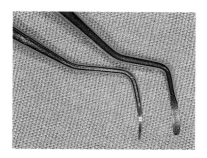

FIG. 8-28 Poor contour of curet blades. The most common error in Gracey curet sharpening is not following the contour of the cutting edge and sharpening a small portion of the edge with each downstroke. The contoured cutting edge loses its shape and becomes a straight cutting edge that no longer adapts to the root surface.

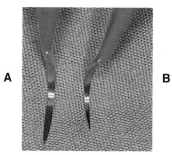

FIG. 8-29 Sharpening was not started at the heel of the blade. Sickle blades must be sharpened entirely from heel to toe to preserve the contoured blade design. **A,** A new sickle with a distinct contour. **B,** A sickle blade that has been thinned at the center. Its contoured shape is lost.

- When the stone is not placed at the heel of the instrument or the last downstroke is made with excess pressure or a longer than normal downstroke, gouging can occur along the cutting edge, creating an uneven edge (Fig. 8-29).
- Rounding the toe of a curet too often or with too much pressure can shorten the overall length of the working end (Fig. 8-30).

All these technique errors can render an instrument ineffective.

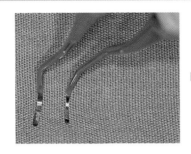

A   **B**

FIG. 8-30 Rounding the toe of curets too often or not often enough. Universal curets can easily be thinned at the working end if the toe of the blade is not rounded. Many curets end up losing the rounded toe and look like sickles with pointed toes. **A,** A brand new universal curet. **B,** A curet that has been thinned with a pointed toe.

CARE AND MAINTENANCE OF A SHARPENED INSTRUMENT

Unnecessary dullness of instruments is preventable. Instruments should not be overly crowded in an ultrasonic before sterilization because they can become dulled when instruments bump against each other in the ultrasonic bath.[18] Stainless steel instruments may be sterilized with saturated steam (250° F), chemical vapor (270° F), or dry heat (340° F) without dulling the cutting edges. However, saturated steam sterilization does have a negative effect on carbon-steel instruments.[13]

When instrumenting around amalgam restorations or fabricated crowns, the clinician should be aware that nicking of the cutting edge or at least a dulling effect easily may occur. Instruments that have become too thin from continuous sharpening and use should be discarded to prevent breakage during debridement (see Figs. 8-29 and 8-30).[15]

Instrument sharpening is an important procedure to maintain the usefulness of instruments and to effectively remove deposits from the teeth. Ideally, sharpening should be performed at the first sign of dullness. If the clinician always is prepared to sharpen instruments by keeping a sterile stone and test stick available with all patient treatment, sharpening can be done quickly and effectively.

RITICAL THINKING ACTIVITIES

1. Obtain a variety of used instruments. Examine the working end of each instrument for design and shape. Determine whether the shape has been altered from sharpening in any way. If it has, identify sharpening errors that could have caused the current shape.
2. View extremely dull instruments under a high-intensity lamp. Observe the shiny line along the cutting edge. Compare a brand new instrument with the dull instrument under a high-intensity lamp. What differences can you detect?
3. Sharpen an extremely dull instrument. Before removing the sludge, observe the cutting edge under a high-intensity lamp with a magnifying glass. Look for the wire edges and/or layer of sludge.
4. Coat the roots of sterilized extracted teeth with nail polish and corn meal. When the coating has dried, scale the root surfaces with dull instruments. Observe the pressure and difficulty during attempts to remove the deposits with dull instruments. Now, sharpen the dull instruments and repeat the process. Observe the ease of deposit removal.
5. Observe a clinician in private practice during an instrumentation procedure. Ask the clinician's opinion on sharpening procedures and observe the technique. What observations can you make? Is the technique the same as what you have been taught? How does it differ? What steps did the clinician follow when sharpening during the appointment? When are instruments sharpened in that practice?

REVIEW QUESTIONS

Question 1 refers to the case study presented at the beginning of the chapter.

1. Which of the following can occur through the use of dull instruments for debridement?
   a. Operator can lose tactile sensitivity for calculus detection.
   b. Calculus can be burnished into the root surface during debridement.
   c. Instrument can slip during debridement, resulting in injury to the patient.
   d. Operator may have to increase pressure to the instrument for calculus removal.
   e. All the above

2. Which of the following would be the ideal procedure to maintain desirable instrument sharpness throughout the debridement process?
   a. Sharpen instruments at the beginning of each day.
   b. Keep sterile sharpening equipment available for all procedures.
   c. Sharpen instruments before placing them in the autoclave.
   d. Use a magnifying glass while sharpening.

Continued

REVIEW QUESTIONS—cont'd

3. When the sharpening stone is correctly applied to a sickle or curet just before activation, which of the following describes the angle formed by the stone to the face of the blade?
   a. 70 to 80 degrees
   b. 60 to 80 degrees
   c. 45 to 90 degrees
   d. 100 to 110 degrees

4. Which of the following procedures is appropriate to sharpen a flame-shaped sickle scaler?
   a. Keep the stone continuously in contact with the entire length of the cutting edge of the instrument.
   b. Hold the instrument in a pen grasp.
   c. Place the stone at the heel of the instrument and follow the contour of the cutting edge to the tip.
   d. Use long strokes with heavy pressure on the downstroke.

5. Which visible cue can the clinician use to assume the cutting edge of the instrument is sharp?
   a. The clinician may observe the wire edge on the blade.
   b. The edge will reflect light and appear bright and shiny.
   c. The edge will not reflect light and appear as a dull line.
   d. The edge will have a layer of sludge.

6. Which of the following is the initial placement of the instrument against the sharpening stone before the sharpening procedure is initiated?
   a. 60 Degrees
   b. 90 Degrees
   c. 100 Degrees
   d. 110 Degrees

7. When the hoe is sharpened, which of the following is true?
   a. The entire cutting edge is against the stone.
   b. The handle is approximately 70 degrees from the stone.
   c. The instrument is held in a modified pen grasp with a finger rest on the stone.
   d. The beveled toe is placed flat on the stone.
   e. All the above

8. When the universal curet is sharpened, which of the following is true?
   a. The stone should contact the entire cutting edge from heel to toe.
   b. The instrument is used in a pen grasp.
   c. The stone is placed at the heel of the instrument and follows the contour of the cutting edge to the toe.
   d. Long strokes with heavy pressure are used.

9. To round the toe of an area-specific curet, which of the following techniques is *not* correct?
   a. Round from both cutting edges of the same working end.
   b. Round from one cutting edge of the working end.
   c. Increase stone-to-face angle by 15 to 25 degrees.
   d. Round the toe every fourth or fifth time the instrument is sharpened.

10. When sharpening an area-specific curet, the clinician should perform which of the following?
   a. Hold the instrument in a pen grasp.
   b. Place the stone at the heel of the instrument and follow the contour of the cutting edge to the toe.
   c. Make sure the stone is in contact with the entire cutting edge of the instrument from heel to toe.
   d. Use long strokes with heavy pressure.

 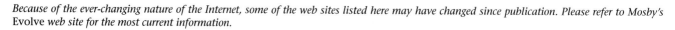

SUGGESTED AGENCIES AND WEB SITES

Because of the ever-changing nature of the Internet, some of the web sites listed here may have changed since publication. Please refer to Mosby's Evolve web site for the most current information.

Edge Dental, Inc.: http://www.Edgedental.com
G. Hartzel & Son, Inc.: http://www.ghartzelandson.com
Hu-Friedy Manufacturing Company, Inc.:
   http://www.Hu-Friedy.com

Premier Dental Products: http://www.premusa.com
Thompson Dental Manufacturing: http://www.tdent.com

REFERENCES

1. Antonini CJ et al: Scanning electron microscope study of scalers, *J Periodontol* 48(1):45-8, 1977.
2. Balevi B: Engineering specifics of the periodontal curet's cutting edge, *J Periodontol* 67(4):374-8, 1996.
3. Claney P: Sharpening hand cutting instruments, *Dent Assist* 55(6):23-4, 1986.
4. Clark SM, Ueno H: An examination of periodontal curettes: an SEM study, *Gen Dent* 38(1):14-6, 1990.
5. Green E: *Sharpening curets and sickle scalers*, ed 2, Berkeley, 1972, Praxis.
6. Huang CC, Tseng CC: Effect of different sharpening stones on periodontal curettes evaluated by scanning electron microscopy, *J Formosan Med Assoc* 90(8):782-7, 1991.
7. Hu-Friedy Department of Education: *Smarten up, sharpen up*, ed 2, Chicago, 1982, Hu-Friedy.
8. Marquam BJ: Strategies to improve instrument sharpening, *Dent Hyg* 62(7):334-8, 1988.
9. Mazzone DM: Quantitative evaluation of scaling instrument contour and sharpening techniques [master's thesis], Ann Arbor, Mich, 1983, University of Michigan.

10. Murray GH et al: The effects of two sharpening methods on the strength of a periodontal scaling instrument, *J Periodontol* 55(7):410-3, 1984.

11. Paquette OE, Levin MP: The sharpening of scaling instruments: I. An examination of principles, *J Periodontol* 48(3):163-8, 1977.

12. Paquette OE, Levin MP: The sharpening of scaling instruments: II. A preferred technique, *J Periodontol* 48(3):169-72, 1977.

13. Parkes RB, Kolstad RA: Effects of sterilization on periodontal instruments, *J Periodontol* 53(7):434-8, 1982.

14. Pattison AM, Pattison GL: *Periodontal instrumentation,* ed 2, East Norwalk, Conn, 1992, Appleton & Lange.

15. Perry DA et al: *Techniques and theory of periodontal instrumentation,* Philadelphia, 1990, WB Saunders.

16. Schoen DH, Dean, MC: *Contemporary periodontal instrumentation,* Philadelphia, 1996, WB Saunders.

17. Smith BA et al: The effect of sharpening stones upon curet surface roughness, *Quint Int* 18(9):603-13, 1987.

18. Wilkins EM: *Clinical practice of the dental hygienist,* ed 8, Philadelphia, 1999, Lippincott Williams & Wilkins.

19. Woodall IR: *Comprehensive dental hygiene care,* ed 4, St Louis, 1993, Mosby.

20. Zimmer SE: Instrument sharpening—sickle scalers and curettes, *Dent Hyg* 52(1):21-4, 1978.

PART III

Chapter 9
Life Stage Changes

Chapter 10
Comprehensive Health History

Chapter 11
Physical and Extraoral Examinations

Chapter 12
Tobacco and Chemical Dependencies

Chapter 13
Intraoral Examination

Chapter 14
Clinical Manifestations of Common Medications

Chapter 15
Periodontal Examination

Chapter 16
Hard Tissue Examination

Chapter 17
Radiographic Evaluation and Utilization

Chapter 18
Nutritional Assessment

Chapter 19
Intraoral Photographic Imaging

Chapter 20
Supplementary Aids

Competency Statements

The learner is expected to possess knowledge, skills, judgments, values, and attitudes to develop the listed competencies.

Core Competencies
- Apply a professional code of ethics in all endeavors.
- Adhere to state and federal laws, recommendations, and regulations in the provision of dental hygiene care.
- Provide dental hygiene care to promote patient health and wellness using critical thinking and problem solving in the provision of evidence-based practice.
- Use evidence-based decision making to evaluate and incorporate emerging treatment modalities.
- Assume responsibility for dental hygiene actions and care based on accepted scientific theories and research as well as the accepted standard of care.
- Provide quality assurance mechanisms for health services.
- Communicate effectively with individuals and groups from diverse populations both verbally and in writing.
- Provide accurate, consistent, and complete documentation for assessment, diagnosis, planning, implementation, and evaluation of dental hygiene services.
- Provide care to all patients using an individualized approach that is humane, empathetic, and caring.

Health Promotion and Disease Prevention
- Promote the values of oral and general health and wellness to the public and organizations within and outside the profession.

Courtesy American Dental Education Association, Washington, DC.

Patient Assessment

- Respect the goals, values, beliefs, and preferences of the patient while promoting optimal oral and general health.
- Refer patients who may have a physiologic, psychological, and/or social problem for comprehensive patient evaluation.
- Identify individual and population risk factors and develop strategies that promote health related quality of life.
- Evaluate factors that can be used to promote patient adherence to disease prevention and/or health maintenance strategies.
- Evaluate and utilize methods to ensure the health and safety of the patient and the dental hygienist in the delivery of dental hygiene.

Community Involvement

- Assess the oral health needs of the community and the quality and availability of resources and services.
- Provide screening, referral, and educational services that allow clients to access the resources of the health care system.

Patient Care

- Select, obtain, and interpret diagnostic information recognizing its advantages and limitations.
- Recognize predisposing and etiologic risk factors that require intervention to prevent disease.
- Obtain, review, and update a complete medical, family, social, and dental history.
- Recognize health conditions and medications that impact overall patient care.
- Identify patients at risk for a medical emergency and manage the patients care in a manner that prevents an emergency.

- Perform a comprehensive examination using clinical, radiographic, periodontal, dental charting, and other data collection procedures to assess the patient's needs.
- Determine a dental hygiene diagnosis.
- Identify patient needs and significant findings that impact the delivery of dental hygiene services.
- Obtain consultations as indicated.
- Prioritize the care plan based on the health status and the actual and potential problems of the individual to facilitate optimal oral health.
- Establish a planned sequence of care (education, clinical, and evaluation) based on the dental hygiene diagnosis; identified oral conditions; potential problems; etiologic and risk factors; and available treatment modalities.
- Establish a collaborative relationship with the patient in the planned care to include etiology, prognosis, and treatment alternatives.
- Make referrals to other healthcare professionals.
- Perform dental hygiene interventions to eliminate and/or control local etiologic factors to prevent and control caries, periodontal disease, and other oral conditions.
- Control pain and anxiety during treatment through the use of accepted clinical and behavioral techniques.
- Determine the outcomes of dental hygiene interventions using indices, instruments, examination techniques, and patient self-report.

Professional Growth and Development

- Access professional and social networks and resources to assist entrepreneurial initiatives.

CHAPTER 9

Life Stage Changes

Kenneth Shay, Victoria C. Vick

Chapter Outline

Case Study: Appreciating Lifestyle Changes to
  Build Rapport and Guide Treatment
Life Stages
  Physical-physiological characteristics
  Psychosocial-behavioral characteristics
  Anticipatory guidance
Early Childhood (Birth to 6 Years)
  Physical-physiological characteristics
  Psychological-behavioral characteristics
Later Childhood (7 to 12 Years)
  Physical-physiological characteristics
  Psychological-behavioral characteristics

Adolescence to Young Adulthood (13 to 20 Years)
  Physical-physiological characteristics
  Psychological-behavioral characteristics
Early Adulthood (21 to 39 Years)
  Physical-physiological characteristics
  Psychological-behavioral characteristics
Mature Adulthood (40 to 60 Years)
  Physical-physiological characteristics
  Psychological-behavioral characteristics
Late Adulthood (61 Years and Older)
  Physiological characteristics
  Psychological-behavioral characteristics

Key Terms

Anticipatory guidance   Intervention
Biopsychosocial   Prevention

 ## *Learning Outcomes*

1. Institute anticipatory guidance principles of health outcomes with patients in each life stage.
2. Identify specific patient needs for each life stage.
3. Develop patient relationships based on the knowledge of issues relative to each life stage of patients.
4. Understand the relationship of biological and psychosocial aspects of patient care.

5. Apply issues specific to the various life stages to the development of preventive and therapeutic interventions.
6. Apply knowledge of anticipatory guidance and patient needs to a variety of patients at different life stages.

Case Study   Appreciating Lifestyle Changes to Build Rapport and Guide Treatment

Yolanda is the hygienist for a suburban general dental practice. Bridgette Tremaile, a patient new to the area and a stylish woman in her mid 40s, is her first patient of the day. Mrs. Tremaile has nicely maintained dentition with a few older amalgams that are starting to look in need of replacement, several small interproximal anterior composites that are beginning to discolor, and a three-unit porcelain bridge replacing tooth #19. Probing interproximally causes some slight bleeding and mild marginal edema, but her mouth is nearly plaque-free. Mrs. Tremaile also has some light intrinsic staining near the cervicals of her incisors, which a review of her health history suggests probably is due to tetracycline prescribed for her as a child. Yolanda focuses much of her patient education time on flossing and then calls the dentist's attention to the deteriorating restorations, the cervical staining, and the gingivitis. The dentist completes the exam; recommends an onlay, two composites, and a computer synthesis of the way in which her anterior teeth would appear with veneers; and makes another appointment for the woman for the next week.

At the second appointment, Mrs. Tremaile brings her 15-year-old daughter, Georgette, for a cleaning and examination. When the mother has been seated, Yolanda stops in to say hello. Mrs. Tremaile confesses that she hasn't really gotten into the habit of flossing yet. With her permission, Yolanda evaluates her gingival tissues and notes a complete absence of inflammation and no bleeding on probing. Puzzled, Yolanda notes these observations in the chart and turns her attention to Mrs. Tremaile and Georgette, who is chewing gum and seems angry. Georgette answers questions in monosyllables and makes no eye contact. When the examination begins, she constantly turns her head away to clear her throat, swallow, or lick her lips. Her hair and clothes are unclean, and she has mild facial acne.

Yolanda notices that Georgette is wearing a pendant of a soccer ball and asks her whether she plays, and if so, which position. She responds that she is a goalkeeper and wants to play but hasn't been able to find an appropriate team since the family moved to "this stupid dump of a town." Yolanda tells her that she was a goalkeeper in college and now referees on weekends and would be glad to put Georgette into contact with several teams in the area. Georgette's affect improves immediately as she and Yolanda discuss their common interest, and the appointment proceeds smoothly. On examination Georgette has a full adult dentition except for the third molars and abundant plaque and significant gingivitis except in the anterior facial areas. Caries is developing in occlusal and buccal pits of all first molars. Her edematous tissues have created some pseudopocketing. After the prophylaxis, which Georgette clearly finds uncomfortable, Yolanda focuses her educational efforts on diet, the importance of oral health to overall health and appearance, and proper brushing technique. (Chapter 42 discusses hormonal imbalances and their effects on dental health.)

Approximately 6 weeks later, Mrs. Tremaile returns for her appointment with the dentist. Yolanda sees that Georgette has accompanied her and chats with the teen briefly in the reception area. She appears radiant and excitedly relates that one of the teams Yolanda suggested selected her as first-string goalkeeper and that the team has won both games in which she has played. She also mentions that she's been trying to put to use some of the dietary tips Yolanda suggested. As Yolanda sets up the treatment room, she sees the girl's mother in the dentist's treatment room. Yolanda greets the woman and inquires about the flossing; she responds that she has been doing it daily, as part of a deal with her daughter to get them both into the habit. Yolanda glances at the woman's mouth and is surprised and a little dismayed that she has a fairly notable marginal gingivitis. As Yolanda leaves the room, the patient asks, "Why do you suppose my mouth always seems more sensitive right before my period?" Yolanda then realizes that much of the soft tissue inflammation you have observed previously was probably due to hormonal factors.

After answering the woman's question, Yolanda proceeds to the treatment room and momentarily thinks that she must be hallucinating; her first impression is that the girl's mother is in the chair now. After a moment of confusion, she realizes that this patient, who although quite youthful looking, is obviously of a more advanced age and is Georgette's *grandmother*, Simone Bouvoir. She is a widow in her 70s who has been invited to live with her daughter's family while she works on a graduate degree in Russian literature at the local university. Despite her extremely youthful appearance, her health history reveals that she is being treated for non–insulin-dependent diabetes (NIDDM), hypertension, glaucoma, and hypothyroidism.

Before the examination, Mrs. Bouvoir removes the remains of a mint from her mouth. She has upper and lower partial dentures that are clean, but they are causing stomatitis in the bearing tissues. She has generalized gingival recession and many open gingival embrasures. Mrs. Bouvoir also has several crowns, and most of her teeth have at least one if not more than one restoration. The large MODBL (amalgam covering most of the tooth's surface) on tooth #14 appears to have a large carious lesion. Although her plaque control in most areas is fairly good, her mouth seems dry; most of the abutment teeth have a thick coating of adherent plaque, and the underlying tooth structure feels sticky. Yolanda focuses her educational efforts on the use of an interproximal brush, acid attacks, and the importance of fluoride and begins periodontal debridement procedures in the upper right quadrant. Later, when the dentist has completed the intraoral examination, Yolanda overhears Mrs. Bouvoir deferring endodontics on #14 in favor of extraction and modification of the upper partial.

LIFE STAGES

9-A   This chapter discusses life stages in terms of the dual role of psychology and physiology on physical well-being. This approach uses a *biopsychosocial* model rather than the biomedical model, acknowledging the complex interaction of biological and individual psychological and social factors that mediate health and illness (Box 9-1).[16,49,56]

PHYSICAL-PHYSIOLOGICAL CHARACTERISTICS

The first of these is the group of "physical-physiological" components, which largely affect the diagnostic and therapeutic role of the dental hygienist. Physical-physiological components include anatomical characteristics (such as the number and condition of teeth, restorations, and prostheses; soft tissue characteristics and bony support; size and condition of the dental pulp; and accessibility of the teeth), pathological findings (oral diseases, systemic conditions that affect oral health, and systemic conditions that might be exacerbated by oral conditions), and physiological factors (tissue response, pulpal response, manual dexterity, sensory abilities, salivary flow, airway protection, and homeostatic mechanisms). Although physical-physiological factors largely influence diagnosis and therapy, they also may affect education and motivation as well, such as when disease (or the medication taken to control disease) plays a significant role in other health conditions of the patient.*

PSYCHOSOCIAL-BEHAVIORAL CHARACTERISTICS

The second group of components is the psychosocial-behavioral factors, which largely influence the educational and motivational efforts of the dental hygienist. Psychological-behavioral factors include the patient's perception of self relative to family and to society, perceived locus of control, learning ability, concentration ability, and life circumstances.† The degree to which dental disease can affect a patient's life often is not broadly considered. Many oral conditions may undermine self-image and self-esteem, discourage social interaction, and be significant

---

*References 18, 20, 23, 40, 43, 52, 63.
†References 5, 12, 13, 19, 24, 26, 39, 41, 54.

> ### BOX 9-1
>
> **Characteristics of the Biopsychosocial Model**
>
> *Physical-Physiological*
> Anatomical characteristics of the teeth, soft and hard tissues, and accessibility of the teeth
> Pathological findings, oral and systemic
> Physiological factors (tissue and pulpal response, manual dexterity, salivary flow, sensory abilities)
> *Psychosocial-Behavioral*
> Patient's perception of self in relation to family and society
> Perceived locus of control
> Learning and concentration ability
> Life circumstances

chronic stressors.[49] They also may lead or contribute to other health issues, such as heart disease, diabetes, and low–birth-weight babies, and interference with vital functions, such as food selection, chewing, and swallowing.* The strong connection between oral health and a person's overall well-being emphasizes the importance of the dental hygienist's interaction with patients on many psychosocial-behavioral levels: attitude, health beliefs, motivating factors, living situation, and previous dental experiences. Just as physical-physiological factors demonstrate some cross-over, psychosocial-behavioral factors may in turn affect diagnosis and therapy. For example, a psychiatric disorder influences oral health (e.g., bulimia, which causes tooth destruction through regurgitation, or depression, which can impair oral hygiene) or fear of dental procedures impairs communication or otherwise interferes with the provision of care.[5,17,19,29,51]

ANTICIPATORY GUIDANCE

The clinician should be adept at anticipation of the best ways to approach a patient and identification of important patient characteristics before initiating care. *Anticipatory guidance* is useful in dentistry to help the clinician predict patient needs and plan an educational approach to best meet those needs.[44,55] For example, characteristic physical and psychological findings are encountered in patients at certain stages of life. Certainly every person is unique, and being a certain age does not guarantee possession of all of the characteristics typically associated with that age. However, familiarity with these characteristics allows recognition of physical findings that are not ordinary. Communication also benefits from an understanding of how different stages of life are likely to feature certain behaviors and attitudes. As the hygienist develops a more informed relationship with a patient, the initial age-indexed approach evolves to accommodate individual differences.

Dental hygiene practice demands application of diagnostic-therapeutic skills and educational-motivational skills. These skills are used in a different manner according to each patient because every patient differs in dentition, manual dexterity, health behaviors and attitudes, learning ability, and language skills. The patient's age helps explain many of these characteristics. In each dental appointment the hygienist is with a patient for only a short time, although the interactions may occur repeatedly over a number of years or even decades. Thus the challenge for the dental hygienist is to discern as much about a patient as quickly as possible—health, habits, and learning ability—to quickly identify what to be alert to, what to provide, what to teach, and how to communicate with that patient most effectively. This is determined partially by a set of factors generally associated with different life stages.

EARLY CHILDHOOD (BIRTH TO 6 YEARS)

This life stage is characterized by profound change and energy. The age segment begins with the unborn baby and encompasses the infant, the toddler, and finally the preschool and school-age child (Table 9-1).

---

*References 4, 18, 22, 23, 38, 40, 47, 49, 53, 62.

The growth rate in the first 6 months of life is faster than it will be at any other time during an individual's life. The human infant's weight doubles during the first 3 months after birth, and it triples within the first year. If growth continued at the rate typical of the first 6 months, the average 10-year-old would be 100 feet tall and weigh approximately 240,000 tons (based on computations for the data at 6 months of life).[27]

PHYSICAL-PHYSIOLOGICAL CHARACTERISTICS

Physiologically, growth is most pronounced during early childhood. Long bones continue to grow and are responsible for energy and stature; the facial features become more defined. Along with skeletal development the child's musculature and motor skills develop equally quickly. Infants and children show remarkable and rapid progress in the development of their motor skills, and by the end of the first year most infants are able to crawl, stand up, and take their first steps.[26,27] Walking, running, and climbing skills develop by the late toddler stage.[26,27] Eye-hand coordination develops and allows them to examine and manipulate objects. Practical skills such as self-dressing and self-feeding are developed during the toddler stage. Improved motor skills and coordination during preschool

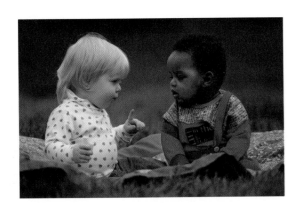

years allow them to become more independent. At this stage children may begin to brush their teeth; however, they still require assistance to ensure they have thoroughly cleaned their teeth.[9]

Numerous texts devoted to the child's physiological development and written in lay terms are particularly useful for parents and caregivers to anticipate the physiological stages from neonatal to age 5 (see the additional readings and resources at the end of the chapter).

Oral Health

Although not immediately apparent, prenatal care is an essential antecedent to a lifetime of dental health. Teeth begin to develop in utero, early in the gestational process. The teeth are affected by environmental factors (e.g., nutrition, maternal health, and medications taken during pregnancy) and lifestyle choices (e.g., alcohol consumption, smoking, and illegal drug use), which can profoundly affect the developing baby.[4,6,30,45,49]

Heavy maternal smoking during pregnancy may lead to delayed tooth formation. Children exposed to cigarette smoke from both parents exhibited up to a 35% reduction in tooth maturation.[42] Another example of such influence is a mother's calcium deficiencies affecting the development of bones and teeth in the fetus. Research has also indicated that low–birth-weight infants are more likely to suffer from developmental disturbances of enamel mineralization.[37] The enamel mineralization of the primary incisors starts at 4 months of gestation, followed in sequence by the other primary teeth and is complete at about 1 year of age. An increased incidence of disturbances in enamel mineralization has been observed in children born preterm, those suffering from severe asphyxia, and in children of mothers with diabetes. The importance of the provision of proper prenatal dental education by the hygienist cannot be overstated.*

*References 4, 6, 30, 37, 42, 44, 45, 49, 55.

TABLE 9-1
Early childhood characteristics

Age	Anatomical	Pathological	Physiological
Prenatal	Primary teeth begin forming in the fourteenth week of pregnancy.	Illness and medications taken during pregnancy can affect tooth formation.	Enamel formation begins in utero.
Birth to 6 months	Eruption of first primary tooth may occur by age 6 months.	Decreased birth weight increases prevalence of enamel defects.	Permanent teeth begin forming 3 to 4 months after baby's birth.
6 months to 1 year	By age 1 year baby may have four to eight primary teeth.	Medication taken for chronic use or periodic use may affect oral health.	Parent-caregiver to infant oral hygiene should begin with eruption of the first tooth.
1 year to 18 months	By age of 18 months child may have 12 primary teeth.	Dental visits should begin. Infants sleeping with bottle are at increased risk for tooth decay.	Weaning to a cup by age 1 year is desirable. Walking begins, as does possibility of trauma.
18 months to 2 years	By age two 16 primary teeth may be present.	Weaning from pacifier or finger sucking habits should begin.	Self-feeding is established, and a great variety of foods are enjoyed.
2 years to 3 years	All 20 primary teeth should be present.	Dental visits should occur every 6 months.	Evaluate fluoride adequacy.
3 years to 6 years	All 20 primary teeth should be present.	Dental visits should occur every 6 months.	Child is given some responsibility for oral hygiene.

During these first developmental years parents play a critical role in setting direction for the child's future oral health. The hygienist must communicate the concept of "keeping teeth for a lifetime" to parents or primary caregivers[9] to ensure a profound effect on the future dental health of that child. Educating children in oral hygiene behaviors must be coordinated with the children's ability both to comprehend the information and to perform the particular task required.[27] Providing education and anticipatory guidance for parents concerning sources of adequate fluoride, normal-abnormal oral development, sucking habits (thumb or pacifier), bottle use, tooth eruption, tooth cleaning, injury *prevention,* and overall dietary habits sets the foundation for a lifetime of good oral health.* The American Academy of Pediatric Dentistry recommends that first dental consultations occur shortly after eruption of the first tooth or no later than 1 year of age.

Dental caries is the most commonly experienced oral disease in children at this life stage. In spite of success with the inclusion of fluoride in many public water systems and the use of fluoridated dentifrice in this country, much progress is yet to be made. The incidence of caries in certain populations still poses a significant public health problem. A hygienist's focused attention to a patient's diet, access to adequate fluoride, oral hygiene habits, and caregiver attitude toward the importance of dental health are essential in the *interventions* for the prevention of dental caries and should be components of every child's dental visits.†

Although many children today remain caries-free because of fluoridated water and dentifrice, one group of children is not so fortunate. Those children have a tremendous amount of decay at an early age. This decay is initiated when a bottle of cariogenic liquid such as milk or sweetened juice is given to a child to encourage sleep or to quiet the child. The liquid simply "pools" around the teeth. This produces a constant acidic assault to the enamel and promotes rampant decay. This condition is referred to as *early childhood caries (ECC).* An estimated 5% to 10% of all children experience some degree of ECC. Some populations, such as Native Americans, are affected to a much larger degree.[17,42,45,49] The dental hygienist may help prevent this condition through patient education and anticipatory guidance with a child's parents or caregiver.

Children are more likely than adults to contract acute diseases such as influenza, measles, colds, and other common childhood conditions. Although chronic conditions are not likely to pose a threat to the development of the dentition, an acute episode of high fever or pharmacological intervention could adversely affect tooth development.[7,17,30,45] An additional challenge for the dental hygienist is to be observant; the clinical signs of some childhood diseases first manifest in the oral environment (e.g., measles).

PSYCHOLOGICAL-BEHAVIORAL CHARACTERISTICS

Much of the psychological and behavioral energy in this life stage is devoted to the concept of self and how the self fits into the world.[27] Each child relates to the environment in a unique way. For example, one 2-year-old is outgoing, cannot wait for a dental visit, is proud of her teeth, and is eager to please. Another child of the same age is fearful, will not leave the safety of his parents' arms, and will not or cannot cooperate during a dental examination. Although generalizations on psychological-behavioral aspects of any age may be misleading, they set the stage for anticipatory guidance in medicine and dentistry.[27,55]

This particular age group of children poses several challenges to both the clinician and the caregiver in terms of oral care. Their personalities, attention spans, and motor skills undergo enormous change. Some children immediately accept having their teeth brushed, whereas others struggle with having someone else brush their teeth. Balancing a toddler's physical ability and emotional maturity during toothbrushing before bedtime may be challenging for any parent.

Nonnutritive Sucking

One of an infant's natural reflexes is sucking. Most young children have an emotional need for sucking beyond what is required to attain nourishment. This instinctual behavior is calming and is an important step in the development of self-regulation and emotional control.

However, at some point nonnutritive sucking may become a problem. Constant and intense sucking may damage the primary and permanent dentition and the jaw. The constant sucking action continuing into the early years creates constant muscular pressure inward that can cause movement of structures medially. Although initial support for the nonnutritive sucking habit and the emotional benefits it provides is appropriate during early childhood, weaning must occur at the appropriate time. Between the ages of 2 and 4 years weaning should begin so that sucking the thumb or pacifier stops completely by the time the first permanent teeth erupt. Parents should be involved in identification of the best approach to help their child discontinue the nonnutritive sucking habit without causing undue stress to the child.[42]

LATER CHILDHOOD (7 TO 12 YEARS)

As children continue to grow physically and mature emotionally, they become more secure in independent activities. Children at this age begin to demonstrate their individuality and general behavior patterns. During this period of change, girls and boys tend to diverge in gender role acceptance and react to the opposite sex with controlled disdain.

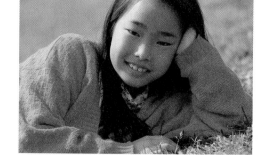

---

*References 1, 9, 17, 34, 42, 45, 49, 55.
†References 9 ,10, 16, 17, 30, 36, 42, 45, 55.

PHYSICAL-PHYSIOLOGICAL CHARACTERISTICS

During the later childhood years, growth and development continues: the human face begins another phase of maturity; jaw growth continues; a child of this life stage has more teeth than at any other stage, considering both the primary and developing permanent dentitions (Table 9-2).

Oral Health

During this developmental stage the hygienist should provide education and anticipatory guidance to the child and parents concerning fluoride supplements, sealants, tooth eruption, oral hygiene, dietary habits, and injury prevention.[1] The child should be included in the discussion of anticipated consequences of good or poor oral care habits because children should become responsible for their own oral health. Although they will certainly still need the influence and guidance of a primary caregiver, they should be developing the coordination and motor skills and motivation to effectively brush and floss their own teeth at this age.[9,10]

Although the majority of United States children enjoy excellent oral health, some experience a high level of disease. The dichotomy of adequate access to dental care, as identified in the surgeon general's *Report on Oral Health in America,* which has found a disproportionate number of economically disadvantaged, minority children receiving inadequate if any dental care.[49] If left untreated, oral diseases frequently lead to serious general health problems and significant pain. These children experience persistent pain, the inability to eat comfortably, and embarrassment in front of their peers.[49] These same children may be turned off by dentistry later in life. When children from families who are socioeconomically challenged gain access to dental care, the hygienist's role as educator and role model becomes even more important. These children do not have the benefit of routine visits, and the time spent with them may influence their dental behaviors for a lifetime.

This life stage also presents with many opportunities for oral trauma.[14,17,25] Whether the child is involved in organized sports or simply riding a bicycle, the risk of orofacial trauma increases. In fact, accidents are the leading cause of death in children aged 1 to 14 years. If a child develops an interest in a contact sport, prevention of orofacial trauma becomes important. The use of a mouthguard in a contact sport is fundamental to the safety of the sport, as is wearing a protective helmet, whether playing baseball, riding a bike, or rollerblading.

PSYCHOLOGICAL-BEHAVIORAL CHARACTERISTICS

This life stage continues the exploration in the understanding of the concept of self. Peers begin to exert a major influence in behaviors and, for the most part, children of this and the next life stage spend more time outside the home than in it. Children begin to understand and use simple logic as they gain an understanding of relational concepts.[24,27] Understanding these constructs is a prerequisite to assume responsibility for their oral care.

A bright, healthy smile at this age often sets the tone for a child's social interaction. During these developmental years a child's social skills evolve. A smile marred by decayed or damaged teeth may lead to ridicule and rejection by peers. Children of this age are seeking approval and guidance; through those needs the hygienist can best provide oral health instruction. A child with even a modest improvement in oral hygiene responds to praise and the acknowledgment of accomplishment by trying to achieve even better results for the next visit. The hygienist may provide positive feedback that enhances self-confidence and the sense of competency that is integral to this developmental stage. The hygienist can support the child's sense of accomplishment and competency by saying, "I am proud of the way have been keeping your back teeth much cleaner since your last visit." Emphasizing even minimal improvement fosters additional progress.

ADOLESCENCE TO YOUNG ADULTHOOD (13 TO 20 YEARS)

Adolescence is clearly a period of transition from the dependence of childhood to the independence of adulthood. It may be characterized in terms of sexual maturity,

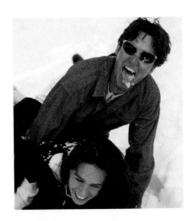

TABLE 9-2			
Later childhood characteristics			
Age	**Anatomical**	**Pathological**	**Physiological**
7 years to 9 years	First permanent teeth begin to erupt around age 6.	Sealants on first molars aid in decay prevention.	Independent and active child is at risk for oral trauma.
10 years to 12 years	This is the "ugly duckling" stage of mixed dentition.	Increased plaque formation may occur in children afraid to brush loose teeth.	Early orthodontic intervention or space retainers may be necessary.

identity development, and a period of social transition into adulthood. This group is often identified as defiant, lazy, and egocentric. However, they are experiencing such significant change that even they do not necessarily understand their behavior.[12,24,27]

PHYSICAL-PHYSIOLOGICAL CHARACTERISTICS

Adolescence can be defined in strictly biological terms (Table 9-3). Puberty and all associated physical changes may occur between the ages of 9 and 17. The pituitary gland is responsible for the control of the production of estrogens (from the ovaries in females) and androgens (from the testes in males). These hormones, responsible for the development of sex organs, incur profound physical and emotional influences during this life stage. Physically, both males and females experience accelerated growth, height, weight, and muscle mass. Because of the pattern in growth spurts adolescents may appear clumsy and awkward. Lack of physical coordination may become an issue and may affect self-esteem. Dermatological changes, including acne, are often evident in this life stage and may cause immense concern in teens.[12,17,24,46]

Oral Health

This age group of patients present clinicians with particular challenges to oral health care.[17,46] A significant number of adolescents are fortunate enough to have benefited from fluoridated water and dentifrice and often have not experienced any caries activity. However, these patients need to understand the importance of good oral hygiene relative to plaque control and their periodontal health regardless of whether they have experienced a caries problem. Some adolescents present with no caries but have poor plaque control. Although age is on their side, over time they will likely experience gingival problems and possibly periodontal deterioration.

The practice of anticipatory guidance with this group of patients is sometimes difficult but rewarding to the clinician. Although education regarding the importance of oral health to overall health may seem to fall on deaf ears,

these patients are usually receptive to a clinician's true interest in their well-being.[35]

One oral condition that becomes more apparent during adolescence is malocclusion. Malocclusion is not considered a disease as much as a condition or variation from proper alignment of the teeth and jaw. Many minor malocclusions have little or no impact on the patient's oral or general health and may not need treatment. However, some malocclusions can be disfiguring and can affect chewing and speaking. Cases involving craniofacial disturbances such as missing or unerupted teeth or severely malformed palates require treatment to maintain health and function. Many malocclusions are treated primarily for aesthetic reasons.

Careful consideration is critical in the making of any decision about orthodontic treatment. Families must consider risk factors and the potential benefits and costs involved in the treatment of malocclusion. One significant psychological benefit often achieved through orthodontic treatment is an enhanced self-image, which may have a profound positive effect on an adolescent's life.

PSYCHOLOGICAL-BEHAVIORAL CHARACTERISTICS

The adolescent focus is once again on the self. They seek, enjoy, and respond well to attention. They are physically maturing but not yet considered adults. Many inflated emotions result from their efforts to seek independence, which are often complicated by the conflicted state of fear of breaking or distancing the parental attachment. The quest for independence is accomplished by the questioning of authority figures, especially parents, and an increase in respect from adults outside the family circle.[27] These years are rarely easy ones for teen or parent. Change is difficult.

These patients require the clinician to be an educator and a good communicator. Each of these patients has priorities, needs, and interests and is trying to establish a unique lifestyle. The clinician must consider each of these variables when deciding what information each patient needs. In the case study at the beginning of this chapter the hygienist's sensitivity to the 15-year-old patient's

TABLE 9-3			
Adolescent and young adult characteristics			
Age	**Anatomical**	**Pathological**	**Physiological**
13 years to 14 years	Period of mixed dentition continues. Most primary teeth are shed.	Beginning of hormonal changes may increase gingival problems. Frequent snacking and unbalanced diet may increase caries risk. Bulimics are at risk for rampant caries because of increased acid.	Patient has physical skills and proper dentition to master flossing. Bulimia and anorexia may manifest.
14 years to 16 years	Dentition consists of permanent teeth.	Hormonal changes may increase gingival problems. Frequent snacking and unbalanced diet may increase caries risk. Bulimics are at risk for rampant caries because of increased acid.	
17 years to 18 years	Wisdom teeth may erupt.	Oral irritation occurs with tobacco use.	Use of tobacco products may begin.

needs and life circumstances provided the basis for a patient-clinician relationship that resulted in improved oral hygiene and overall well-being. The hygienist realized a common interest with the patient, which led to the patient improving her attitude toward and responsibility for her oral hygiene needs. That sensitivity also gave the patient confidence in other aspects of her life. The rewards of clinical practice often extend beyond the clinical setting.

Cognitively the adolescent begins to think less concretely and to understand and use some abstract thought constructs. This higher level of thinking allows adolescents to begin self-assessment and the development of their own identities. Some teenagers experience great experimentation in the determination of their values, beliefs, and attitudes. However, others seem to move quietly into this period, feeling quite comfortable with childhood experiences and having little need to question or change their sense of self. Seeking identification with adult role models is a manner in which many teenagers begin to build their own identities (see case study at the beginning of the chapter).[24,27]

Issues concerning body appearance begin to manifest at this age as concerns over clothing and possessions begin to play a major role in identity and self-esteem. The pressure from peers or parents may produce psychological problems in the form of eating disorders. Bulimic behavior results in a specific form of dental caries, in which the enamel of teeth is dissolved by the acid produced by repeated vomiting. The patient with bulimia often presents with teeth that have a dull, chalky enamel surface. Often the lingual/palatal surfaces appear eroded from the gastric acids produced during vomiting. An oral exam indicating bulimia should result in a frank discussion with the patient and the patient's parents and a referral to the appropriate healthcare professional. This particular psychological problem should be approached from a medical-dental team perspective. The psychiatrist or other mental health professional should be aware of and involved in the progress or deterioration of the patient's oral health as it relates to the patient's recovery from this eating disorder.[2,17,51]

EARLY ADULTHOOD (21 TO 39 YEARS)

The changes that occur during the adult years may not seem as dramatic as those typified in childhood and adolescence, but they are just as real (Table 9-4). The transition from adolescence to adulthood is marked by the independent choices one makes. The sense of identity that one creates as an adolescent is put to use. Psychological and social adjustments must be made for marriage, parenthood, and career choice. Although young adulthood is a season of excitement and opportunity in the identification of a person's place in life, it is also a stressful period as many life-defining choices are made.[27,40]

PHYSICAL-PHYSIOLOGICAL CHARACTERISTICS

In terms of physical status of adulthood, the twenties and thirties usually are seen as the peak of physical health, although the occurrence of chronic diseases later in life is often influenced by lifestyle decisions made during these years. Health, generally taken for granted as a child and adolescent, for the first time may become a concern. The impact of oral health on general health has been the focus of a significant body of research and has identified several

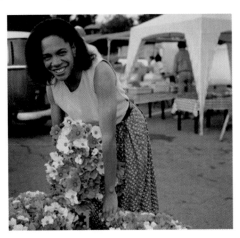

Age	Anatomical	Pathological	Physiological
20 years to 40 years	Natural adult dentition	Gingival inflammation resulting from inadequate plaque control Occurrence of caries because of changes in diet and poor plaque control	Overall health affected by lifestyle choices
	Natural adult dentition	Periodontitis	May be causal factor in low birth weight infants
	Natural adult dentition	For women: pregnancy gingivitis	Hormonal changes resulting from pregnancy
41 years to 60 years	Natural adult dentition	Periodontitis leading to loss of alveolar bone	Onset of menopause and osteoporosis
	Natural adult dentition	Gingival bleeding and periodontitis in response to what might otherwise be acceptable plaque levels (onset of bone loss is often rapid)	Onset of NIDDM
	Natural adult dentition	Periodontitis	Potential increased risk of cardiovascular disease or stroke

TABLE 9-4

Adulthood characteristics

systemic diseases exacerbated by oral disease.* In terms of anticipatory guidance this may be a powerful and important motivator for adults.

Oral Health

Dentally, the focus for these patients is often on the maintenance of a level of oral health acquired through childhood and adolescence.[31,49,54] Some individuals may experience a pronounced increase in dental caries as they leave home and begin making their own decisions in areas affecting oral health, such as nutrition and self-care products or a move to a location without water fluoridation. These people need to make appropriate changes to deal with the onset of potential new caries activity. They may be surprised and perhaps question the presence of cavities.

Although this may be a rude awakening to adulthood, it is better addressed sooner rather than later. The hygienist must be tactful in the presentation of this information to avoid offending the patient and damaging the clinician-patient relationship, which is so important to the long-term receptiveness to oral care by the patient. The clinician may need to ask patients to relate major life changes when taking their histories because that information may be helpful in assessment of changes in the patients' caries activities. Patients cope with their change in health status by learning logical reasons for caries development and actions to reduce or eliminate the caries activity.

During this life stage many individuals will marry and start families, so oral care of expectant mothers and unborn children become relevant issues. The dental hygienist can expect to educate pregnant women about their oral health and the impact certain lifestyle choices can have on the oral health of the baby. Expectant women experience significant hormonal changes, which can often result in oral manifestations such as pregnancy gingivitis, a definite topic for oral care education. Dispelling myths such as "you lose one tooth for every child you have" is another aspect in the education of the patient in this life stage. An expectant woman should not fear damage to her teeth during pregnancy if she maintains adequate care and gets the necessary vitamins and minerals for both herself and her unborn child. Explaining the relationship between gingivitis during pregnancy and its effects on fetal development (e.g., preterm low birth weight) can significantly elevate the importance of oral self-care during this phase of adult life.[47] This is a period of great receptivity to medical-dental knowledge because expectant parents generally seek and appreciate information regarding health changes.

Young adults who needed orthodontic treatment during adolescence but for whatever reason did not receive treatment may have that orthodontic treatment done at this time. Patients of this age are beginning to realize the importance of their teeth from an aesthetic standpoint and as an important element of their health. However, the aesthetic appearance of their teeth is indeed important to their overall oral health.

---

*References 8, 22, 38, 40, 49, 53, 62, 63, 64.

PSYCHOLOGICAL-BEHAVIORAL CHARACTERISTICS

This life stage is one of great transition and personal development.[13,24] People begin to define themselves and build their futures. Interest in oral condition includes a strong interest in presentation in their social environments.

This can be used to the hygienist's advantage as a powerful motivational strategy. Health promotion theory indicates that people often are more willing to comply with health instruction if an aesthetic benefit is involved than they would be to gain only the health benefit.[5,33] For example, an overweight patient with diabetes wants to lose weight. Although a health benefit exists in weight loss, often a change in appearance is the real motivator behind the change in eating and exercise behavior. This knowledge of health promotion theory allows the hygienist to present oral care information or treatment options to the patient in terms that are relevant but beyond immediate apparent oral health benefits.

These young adults are now developing buying habits, even health habits, and are often influenced by advertising and the entertainment industry. In today's commercial environment it is difficult for people to ignore advertisements when purchasing oral care products. These patients look to their dental professional for guidance in the appropriate selection of their oral care regimen and specific products. Counseling provided to these patients strongly influences their current and future oral health habits.

MATURE ADULTHOOD (40 TO 60 YEARS)

As the middle years of adulthood approach many people feel settled. They have chosen their lifestyles and have established their places in the societal framework. However, this is also a time of reexamination of one's accomplishments and life situation. During this period, children generally leave home and start families of their own; for some, careers are winding down. Thus a period of apparent peacefulness is also laden with significant, stressful life changes. During this phase of life the reality of aging and a sense of finality begin to become apparent. Before reaching this age people often have a sense that they are invulnerable and that life and its possibilities are limitless.[24]

A trend in this age group's increasing role as caregiver is becoming apparent. Individuals at this life stage may now have to care for aging parents, adult children who have

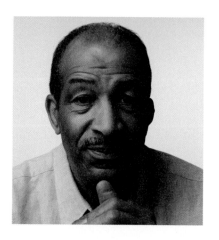

returned home, or grandchildren.[49] They have become known as the "sandwich" generation because they may be caring for children and parents at the same time. As life expectancies continue to increase, it is possible for parents to spend fewer years caring for their children than caring for their aging parents.

PHYSICAL-PHYSIOLOGICAL CHARACTERISTICS

During "middle age" people often begin to notice specific changes about themselves that, until this point, they thought happened only to other people. People begin to notice gray hair, thinning hair, a tendency to gain weight more easily, and physical inability to do the things they had done when they were younger. These physiological changes occur in different time frames for many reasons, such as familial traits, lifestyle choices such as exercise (or lack of), nutrition, stress, smoking, obesity, and alcohol abuse.[24,49] Given the myriad of possible interactions between these multiple factors, each patient must be evaluated individually and not in the context of general health amid an entire pool of patients.[64]

Numerous physiological changes occur during this life stage that have an effect on oral health, or conversely, many oral conditions may affect other aspects of physiological health.[38,49] A patient's understanding of the importance of oral health to overall health is extremely important. Initially the link of periodontal disease to systemic diseases was thought to be unidirectional, but growing evidence shows that the relationship may be bidirectional.[18,53]

Research connecting oral health to cardiovascular disease, stroke, diabetes, and other systemic conditions has begun to emerge.* Case-control and cross-sectional studies indicate that periodontitis may confer a twofold increase in the risk for cardiovascular disease.[22] These interrelationships may prove extremely important in the development of appropriate intervention-prevention strategies from both the dental and the medical outcomes perspectives.[64] This body of knowledge calls for a team approach to patient care between the medical and dental communities.

Oral Health

The oral health of patients in this group increases in complexity. As they age they also begin to experience the onset of various chronic conditions. These conditions or often the therapies used to treat them may have significant effect on the oral tissues. For example, the onset of diabetes in someone with previously excellent plaque control may result in significant bleeding. This occurrence may frighten the patient, and the clinician should consider this in treatment planning and observation.

These patients must be educated (i.e., provided with anticipatory guidance) regarding the etiology of the gingival bleeding and the associated precautions needed. Medications for chronic conditions may cause xerostomia, and root caries may also pose a problem for this age group. As more of these patients present with complex medical and psychological issues, the importance of the use of a biopsychosocial model in assessment of their needs becomes even more important. This group often tries to downplay the importance of their changing health conditions, so thoroughness is critical in updates of the medical-psychological (life status) histories at each visit. Any significant change should be noted. This change may be the onset of diabetes, the addition of medication for hypertension, or a significant psychosocial change such as a divorce, children leaving for school, or older parents no longer able to care for themselves. These changes should be considered as potential factors in oral disease and its treatment and prevention.[31,49]

During this time frame most women experience perimenopause and menopause. With the accompanying decline of estrogen women are more susceptible to osteoporosis (reduced bone density), which also may affect the dental alveolar structure. Loss of dental alveolar bone that often may accompany osteoporosis is usually completely unexpected by the patient. The effect of reduced estrogen levels on bone density must be considered as a potential contributing factor in the onset of periodontal disease.[23,48]

Counseling female patients regarding the role of estrogen in periodontal disease is another example of anticipatory guidance playing an important role.

PSYCHOLOGICAL-BEHAVIORAL CHARACTERISTICS

This life stage is accompanied by a lot of change, some related to growth opportunities and other changes that mark the onset of endings. These patients face the failure or fulfillment of their life's hopes and dreams. Change seems to mark each phase or life stage, and as with the others, change may be difficult. Clinicians should note such changes as divorce, job loss, death of a parent, or other significant events, if possible. The stress that accompanies such change can often bring about depression or anxiety,[24] both of which may affect oral health.[39] These topics are best not solicited from patients directly but rather with open-ended questions such as, "What's new in your life?" Patients are often grateful to have someone to whom they can confide some of life's changes but need to take the lead in initiating that discussion.

People in this group are often self-conscious about their appearance and the fact they are growing older. The physical affects of aging become more and more apparent.[24] Because our culture places such significance on youth and beauty, the aging process may be devastating to their self-esteem. As a person matures the teeth tend to darken with age, which is just another visual sign of aging. Tooth whitening is relatively inexpensive, easy, painless, and quick. It provides patients with a more youthful smile that in turn can boost their self-confidence. Approaching the topic sometimes may be challenging; therefore "cues" in the reception area and operatory are helpful. Patients who view whitening literature in the waiting room may ask about their options, which invites a discussion of available options.

Cosmetic options to restore a more youthful smile range from cosmetic whitening with a peroxide-based product to more significant procedures, including veneers, replacement of amalgam restorations with composite materials, and porcelain crowns. The patient may

---

*References 8, 18, 22, 38, 40, 53, 62.

be more likely to feel comfortable discussing these topics with the hygienist, at least at first, before consultation with the dentist. A patient's bright smile and enhanced self-esteem brought about through appropriate counseling by the dental team may be rewarding to the dental team.

The female patient approaching middle age is faced with hormonal changes inevitably brought about with the onset of menopause. These changes often present as significant alterations in emotions because the hormonal changes often bring about mood swings, depression, anxiety, and a general feeling of malaise.* Clinicians must be alert to these changes in addition to the potential physiological ones mentioned earlier and approach the patient in a calm and courteous manner.

These transitional years are filled with psychological milestones that the clinician must consider in the determination of treatment plans and provision of treatment. Awareness of and sensitivity to the major life changes people face may make a tremendous difference in the relationship that develops between patient and clinician. This relationship may be rewarding and enriching to both patient and clinician.

LATE ADULTHOOD (61 YEARS AND OLDER)

Probably no age group is as encumbered with and affected by popular misconception as is the oldest segment of the population. Most of the popular lore about the last stages of life is based not on personal experience but on a variety of secondhand information, usually derived from and later colored by personal interactions. Through much of the twentieth century, most Americans have learned and shared sets of unrealistic stereotypes about their elders. Some are negative: senile, ineffectual, crabby, deaf, poor, toothless, inflexible, repetitive, self-centered, and helpless. Others are positive but equally inaccurate when used to describe tens of

millions of people: sweet, generous, funny, cute, energetic, wise, helpful, and selfless.[24]

Both positive and negative terms share a fundamental flaw; they do not account for individuality. Just as making sweeping generalizations about a group of children would be incorrect, even more incorrect would be to assert at once that the group of children has lived unique lives for 60 years. They are no longer the diverse, unique individuals that they were 60 years previously. Therefore dental hygienists should deliberately set aside culturally instilled and likely inaccurate beliefs—termed *stereotypes*—about patients over the age of 60. This allows the hygienist to be attuned to the actual mix of physical-physiological and psychological-behavioral characteristics that is truly relevant to that patient (Table 9-5).

PHYSIOLOGICAL CHARACTERISTICS

Chronic Disease

An older person unquestionably is more likely than a younger one to live with one or more chronic diseases and/or disabilities. Unlike acute disease (such as influenza), which has a clearly defined beginning and ending, chronic diseases do not go away. The effects of chronic diseases

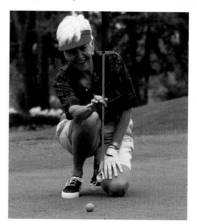

*References 13, 23, 24, 36, 39, 48.

TABLE 9-5

Late adulthood characteristics

Age	Anatomical	Pathological	Physiological
60 years and over	Natural adult dentition or partial to complete edentulism	Root caries Recurrent root caries Gingivitis Periodontitis	More challenging to practice adequate oral hygiene because of changes such as arthritis, dementia, poor eyesight, impaired coordination, and decreased grip strength
		Periodontitis correlated with tooth loss and predisposition to candidiasis	Diabetes
		Recurrent decay Gingivitis Halitosis	Lowered salivary flow because of medications or disease
		Gingival hyperplasia	Calcium channel blockers for cardio-vascular disease and hypertension
		Oral cancer (largely male)	Impaired salivary flow and taste perception; impaired oral intake and ability to chew and swallow

such as hypertension, atherosclerosis, arthritis, and hearing loss are encountered more with advancing age both because their pathophysiologies are cumulative (i.e., the physiological changes that bring them about gradually accumulate over time) and because the changes are essentially irreversible.[21]

Oral Health

The effects of chronic disease on oral health and oral care are diverse. Arthritic changes may have significant effects on oral hygiene care: grasping and manipulation of oral hygiene devices can become painful, cumbersome, or impossible.[52] Declining visual acuity (particularly close-up and in dim light) and hearing loss may impair the efficacy of patient instructions that are given verbally or in writing. Diabetes, which affects nearly 10% of older Americans, interferes with the management of periodontal disease, is strongly correlated with tooth loss, and predisposes to candidiasis.[63] Individuals with congestive heart failure may need to remain in an upright position during care to avoid experiencing pulmonary distress. Cognitive impairment resulting from past cerebrovascular disease or progressive dementia (most commonly Alzheimer's disease) often interferes with the provision and quality of daily care and may affect patient cooperation during dental appointments.[57,61]

Increasing prevalence of chronic disease customarily leads to increasing use of medications to slow disease progression and/or to minimize the effect of disease on function and comfort.[21] Most medications commonly prescribed to older patients have the capacity to bring about significant oral health consequences.* Salivary hypofunction is a potential consequence of nearly 80% of the 200 most commonly prescribed medications. Absence of an adequate supply of properly constituted saliva increases intraoral acidity and raises bacterial counts, thereby fostering gingivitis, caries, and halitosis. Several of the calcium channel blockers, prescribed for cardiovascular disease and hypertension, cause a gingival hyperplasia in a quarter to a third of those ingesting the drugs. Cyclosporin, indispensable to prevent graft rejection in patients who have received an organ transplant (such as a kidney, heart, or liver), causes similar challenging periodontal effects. A wide variety of medications, including diuretics, beta blockers (for hypertension), and antineoplastic chemotherapy agents, are known to cause painful oral ulcerations.

Oral diseases in advanced age are the same as the maladies of younger adults, although their presentations may be distinctive. With advancing age dental caries is more likely to be recurrent, and root areas of the teeth are more intensely affected. Tooth loss affects individuals at all ages, but in older individuals, it is more likely to result in multitooth edentulous spans and even fully edentulous arches.[30,58,59]

Periodontal disease in older adults generally presents as loss of attachment, recession, and exposed root areas, rather than as deep and suppurating pockets. The reason for the different clinical presentations is because teeth susceptible to the more destructive forms of the disease are more likely to have been lost by advanced age. Teeth still present in late life are more likely to show signs of prior attachment loss that has fallen short of causing exfoliation. Oral cancer is most prevalent in individuals (mostly men) in their 50s and 60s but actually declines in prevalence by age 70 and beyond.[57]

Although chronic diseases are more common in elderly persons, aging must not be confused with disease. Everyone ages, but not everyone is afflicted with a particular disease—true even when the disease is common, such as arthritis in elderly individuals or gingivitis is those with one or more natural teeth. Most commonly held (but inaccurate) expectations about older individuals are in fact disease changes rather than changes due to the aging process itself. Deafness, confusion, dry mouth, tooth loss, stiffness, and curvature of the spine are physiological states that, although more common in older persons, are in fact due to identifiable causes that are independent of the aging process.

The aging process is universal, progressive (the changes are additive over time), and irreversible (the causative agent, time, cannot be modified or eliminated, unlike in the case of disease). The exact mechanisms of aging are still being identified, but their effects are expressed at all levels in the organism.

The summary significance of the various age-related changes is frailty: impairment to withstand stress. Persons of advanced age often display high levels of function and health within the circumstances in which they customarily function, but their apparent robustness must not be confused with the resiliency of youth. People of advanced age and excellent health may slip on the ice or trip over a rug in the home. When they do, their slower reflexes are more likely to result in a fall, and the fall more likely to result in a fracture, and the fracture more likely to result in extended hospitalization and isolation than would occur in a younger person.

Oral health in young adults is generally not thought to be a critical factor in overall wellness, except in extreme cases of neglect or immunocompromise. But in an older individual, who may remain healthy only as long as his or her diet remains undisturbed, social relationships are not impaired, and one or more implanted prosthetic devices remain uninfected, oral health may be a genuinely life-or-death matter. Preventive dentistry in advanced age is not merely cosmetic or discretionary but a rational and cost-effective method for ensuring that a problem-prone yet essential body system remains healthy and functional.[57,61]

Aging in the Oral Cavity

Age-related changes in the oral cavity are difficult to separate from changes resulting from disease and environment, but they may have significant effect on oral health care behaviors. The most familiar age change concerns the gradual but steady deposition of secondary dentin on the walls of pulp chambers. Caries or prior restoration of a tooth stimulates a similar change, as do severe intraoral temperature swings. But whatever the cause, pulps of older teeth are smaller, resulting in a diminished need for blood supply and a consequent decline in nerve supply.

---

*References 7, 11, 20, 21, 28, 50, 57, 60.

Patients become less aware of unexpected sensitivity to sweets or other helpful reminders for dental attention and are more tolerant of fractured but asymptomatic teeth. Thus patients who are accustomed to waiting until they perceive need for dental care before they arrange for appointments may become infrequent but high-need consumers of dental care. Because of pulpal insensitivity older patients tend to be more tolerant of oral care that would be intolerable without local anesthetic in younger patients, although diversity of psychological overlays of the dental experience and of pain perception makes this generalization far from universal.[19,24,43]

PSYCHOLOGICAL-BEHAVIORAL CHARACTERISTICS

Diversity within the aged population is not limited to physical characteristics. Socioeconomic differences throughout life, educational and vocational opportunities, early experiences with healthcare providers, cultural beliefs about health and the dentition, and exposure to societal attitudes about the role of the aged are different for each older person and have combined in each case to result in the emergence of a unique—and ever-changing—individual. Yet through all this diversity are some generalizations that can be made and should be kept in mind when working with persons of advanced age.

The first generalization concerns changes in the perceived importance and ultimate fate of the natural dentition. Persons born around the beginning of the twentieth century most likely went through childhood and the appearance of the permanent dentition without having ever received dental care other than possibly extractions. Restorations and preventive care were unknown to the vast majority of Americans until later in the twentieth century. Total tooth loss among persons ages 90 years and older, which often had occurred by a person's 20s or 30s or even earlier, is much higher than it is among Americans who matured after World War I. In this next-oldest group, including persons aged between their mid-70s to mid-80s, are a large number of individuals who benefited in early adulthood from the growing number of better-trained and more accessible dentists. These improvements in dental care resulted in a higher degree of tooth retention in early adulthood. Those born in the 1920s and 1930s were the first Americans for whom dental care was generally available from childhood. The children born in the 1940s, 1950s, and early 1960s, known in popular culture as the "Baby Boomers," include millions of Americans who have been exposed to fluoridated drinking water and dentifrice since birth.

Exposure to growing levels of oral health awareness, rising sophistication, and improvement of dental materials have raised most older Americans' expectations of their dentitions and of the dental professions. Members of the two oldest groups of Americans (years 70 to 80 to 90 and above) who retain some teeth may believe their dentition has lasted longer than they'd ever thought possible; therefore they are somewhat resigned to deterioration to the edentulous state. In contrast, older individuals who have been exposed to preventive and restorative dental care throughout their lifetimes are more likely to continue such habits and practices into seniority and to take efforts to preserve their dentitions.

A second generalization concerns the relationship between a health provider and an older person. Until the later 1960s, most adults deferred to their physicians' and dentists' opinions. Patients believed, or behaved as if they believed, that clinicians knew what was in each patient's best interests and would act accordingly. Most patients knew little about their conditions or treatments other than what they were told. Today the public generally knows, or wants to know, all about health care.

Persons of advanced age are far more likely than their younger counterparts to maintain an unshakable faith in their providers and to give less legitimacy to their own concerns and questions. Dentists and dental hygienists are trained to empower patients by listening to and addressing their concerns and remaining open to alternatives that the patients suggest. They may inadvertently offend patients who habitually have no desire to be part of the clinical decision process and are disinterested or even frankly annoyed to hear details about their health or treatment. In addition clinicians who expect older patients to be perfectly open with them because the patients have been given ample opportunities to voice concerns or ask for clarifications may be puzzled when home-care instructions are not followed, to the point of compromising care. Dentists and dental hygienists caring for older patients must be mindful of this disparity in expectations and should take extra efforts to elicit information or repeat important instructions in patients who may not accept their right to be part of the clinical process.

A third generalization relates to the earlier discussion concerning aging and disease and to the immediately preceding point about communication. Older persons—particularly males—are notorious underreporters of symptoms. The customary explanation is that believing that old age is, for example, accompanied by pain, poor vision, or loose teeth reduces the likelihood of raising these issues with a physician, optometrist, or dentist and increases the likelihood of accepting and trying to adjust to these conditions. Oral healthcare providers must be alert for clues that the older patient is just accepting something that represents a treatable, unhealthful oral state, such as a new crown that is "just a little high" or an endodontically treated tooth that continues to hurt. This may be avoided by educating the patient about what sensations should be expected from a treatment and in particular which sensations mandate professional attention.

A fourth generalization deals with the respect accorded a patient of advanced age.[3] Healthcare providers display two characteristic habits when confronted with a debilitated older person in the company of a relative or caregiver who is younger or otherwise somewhat more robust.[15] The first habit is to become engaged with the other person in a dialog regarding the patient. This individual may be more prompt or appropriate in responding or may initiate responses even when questions are directed toward the patient. However, unless the patient indicates a preference otherwise, the healthcare provider should not allow discussion with the third party to supersede interaction with the patient. To do otherwise is to indicate that the patient is inadequate, incompetent, or otherwise diminished relative to the others present.

The second habit a healthcare professional may display is to call patients by their first names. When older individuals become dependent, a tendency exists to begin to treat them like children, such as speaking for them, reinterpreting their statements, and minimizing their complaints. Addressing a total stranger, who may be the retired president of a Fortune 500 company or the chairperson of the board of a foundation, by first name can unconsciously but effectively deprive them of identity and self-respect. Until a patient of advanced age has specifically requested to be called by first name, that person should be addressed as *Mr., Mrs., Ms.,* or *Miss.*

The fifth important generalization is that patients of any age are still capable of learning new tasks, as long as their cognitive abilities are not impaired by disease. Abundant research published in the educational and psychological literature has demonstrated repeatedly that learning ability is not impaired by age alone. Older learners may require a greater number of repeated exposures to the new material, may have visual or auditory impairments that require special efforts on the part of the instructor, or may need to have their own knowledge on an issue validated before incorporating new material. But they will learn, and once having learned may actually retain and apply the new material to a greater degree than they could when they were younger. "You can't teach an old dog new tricks" is an untrue adage. Teachers of "new tricks" must realize the shortcoming of delivering a message in a particular, set fashion that fails to adjust for learner style. When the particular needs of the cognitively unimpaired older person are identified and addressed, learning proceeds with excellent results.

CRITICAL THINKING ACTIVITIES

1. Develop a training activity-program to take into a nursing home to present to the residents. Keep in mind what physical, psychological, and medical issues they may be experiencing as you develop your program.
2. Develop a series of educational brochures, one for each life stage, and submit them to various organizations or corporations to seek support for broad distribution, especially to underserved populations.
3. Think of interactive educational activities for preschool children that would provide them useful yet entertaining and engaging oral health education.
4. Investigate the various cultural differences that may accompany each "life stage" and develop a short educational module for one or more of them. Try to obtain funding for distribution to the particular group you have chosen to develop your module around.
5. Investigate the various systemic diseases that are influenced by oral health/disease and develop a short article that can be released to the local media.

REVIEW QUESTIONS

Questions 1 and 9 refer to the case study presented at the beginning of the chapter.

1. In which of the following statements is anticipatory guidance used appropriately with Georgette, the 15-year-old patient introduced in this chapter?
   a. "I see that you are beginning to accumulate a lot of plaque around the gums. It will be best if you can start to pay more attention to that and remove it on a daily basis."
   b. "You need to floss your teeth more often! You already have a significant amount of gingival bleeding."
   c. "Your teeth are so beautiful. To keep them looking that way you should floss them every day, especially because you are going into a period of development during which you will experience a significant change in your hormones. Amazingly, that increase in hormones can lead to periodontal disease if you aren't aware of how to prevent it."
   d. "I know that your parents are concerned about the health of your teeth and have invested a lot of time and expense so that you can have a healthy mouth. You should pay more attention to how you take care of them so that you won't disappoint your parents."

2. The method of assessment and treatment planning presented in this chapter can best be described as which of the following?
   a. Medical model
   b. Biopsychosocial model
   c. Prevention model
   d. None of the above

3. Which aspects of someone's life could be affected by serious and visible dental caries?
   a. Perception of self
   b. Perceived locus of control
   c. Amount of social interaction
   d. All the above

4. To effectively use anticipatory guidance in your work with your patients, which of the following is (are) important?
   a. Anticipation of patient needs
   b. Understanding of the patients' particular life circumstances
   c. Knowledge of life stages and the general health-related events that accompany those stages
   d. All the above

Continued

REVIEW QUESTIONS—cont'd

5. The condition known as *early childhood caries* is *not* initiated with which of the following when the infant is put to bed?
   a. Giving an infant a bottle with fluoridated water
   b. Giving an infant a bottle with fortified milk
   c. Giving an infant a bottle with a fruit drink
   d. Giving an infant a bottle with soda pop

6. The nonnutritive sucking habit does not provide which of the following benefits?
   a. Calming effect
   b. Self-regulation
   c. Control of emotions
   d. Improved coordination

7. The outcome faced by children who experience a high level of oral disease includes which of the following?
   a. Persistent dental pain
   b. Inability to eat comfortably
   c. Embarrassment with peers
   d. Potential for poor nutrition
   e. All the above

8. The tooth development in the fetus can be affected by which of the following?
   a. Alcohol consumption
   b. Poor posture
   c. Illegal drug use
   d. Poor nutrition
   e. *a, c,* and *d*

9. All the following behaviors can result in successful therapy with adolescent patients, such as Georgette from the case study. Which one is the *exception*?
   a. Listening to their concerns
   b. Demanding that they change their oral care habits
   c. Showing an interest in who they are outside of the dental office
   d. Complimenting them on some aspect of their oral health care regimen

SUGGESTED AGENCIES AND WEB SITES

Because of the ever-changing nature of the Internet, some of the web sites listed here may have changed since publication. Please refer to Mosby's Evolve web site for the most current information.

Administration on Aging: 330 Independence Avenue, SW; Washington, DC 20201: http://www.aoa.dhhs.gov

American Academy of Pediatric Dentistry: 211 East Chicago Avenue, #700; Chicago, IL 60611-2663, (312) 337-2169; FAX (312) 337-6329: http://www.aapd.org

American Association of Retired Persons (AARP): http://www.aarp.org

American Society for Geriatric Dentistry: Suite 948, 211 East Chicago Avenue, Chicago, IL 60611, (312) 440-2660: http://www.aoa.dhhs.gov

National Institutes of Health: Bethesda, MD 20892: http://www.nih.gov

National Institute on Aging: Building 31, Room 5C27, 31 Center Drive, MSC 2292, Bethesda, MD 20892, (301) 496-1752: http://www.nia.nih.gov

ADDITIONAL READINGS AND RESOURCES

Chauncey HH: *Clinical geriatric dentistry: biomedical and psychosocial aspects,* Chicago, 1985, American Dental Association.

Eli I: *Oral psychophysiology: stress, pain, and behavior in dental care,* 1992, CRC Press.

Little JW, Falace DA, Miller CS, Rhodus NL: Dental management of the medically compromised patient, ed 6, St Louis, Mosby (in press).

McDonald RE, Avery DR: *Dentistry for the child and adolescent,* ed 7, St Louis, 1999, Mosby.

Pinkham JR, Fields HW Jr, McTigue DJ: *Pediatric dentistry: infancy through adolescence,* ed 3, Philadelphia, 1999, WB Saunders.

REFERENCES

1. Adair SM: Overview of the history and current status of fluoride supplementation schedules, *J Public Health Dent* 59(4): 252-8, 1999.

2. Altshuler B: Anorexia nervosa and bulimia—a review for the dental hygienist, *J Dent Hyg,* 10:466-71, 1986.

3. Atchison KA, Anderson RM: Demonstrating successful aging using the international collaborative study for oral health outcomes. *J Public Health Dent* 60(4):282-8, 2000.

4. Barnett R, Shusterman S: Fetal alcohol syndrome: review of literature and report of cases, *J Am Dent Assoc* 111(10): 591-3,1985.

5. Ben-Sira Z: Eclectic incentives for health behavior: an additional perspective on health-oriented behavior change, *Health Educ Res* 6:211-29, 1991.

6. Bergner L, Susser MW: Low birth weight and prenatal nutrition: an interpretive review, *Pediatrics,* 46(6):946-66, 1970.

7. *Burket's oral medicine diagnosis and treatment,* ed 9, Philadelphia, 1994, JB Lippincott.

8. Casamassimo PS: Relationships between oral and systemic health, *Pediatr Clin North Am* 47(5):1149-57, 2000.

9. Charonko CV, BeBiase CB: Dental health for children: an adult responsibility, *J Pract Nurs* 34:45-54, 1984.

10. Christen JA, Christen AG: Behavioral considerations in preventive dentistry: six lessons learned from the past, *J Indiana Dent Assoc* 66(4):17-21, 1987.

11. Ciancio S: *American dental association guide to dental therapeutics,* Chicago, 1998, ADA Publishing.

12. Copas BE et al: Coping with stress during childhood and adolescence: problem progress, and potential in theory and research, *Psychol Bull* 127(1):87-127, 2001.

13. Donahue EM et al: The divided self: concurrent and longitudinal effects of psychological adjustment and social roles on self-concept differentiation, *J Pers Soc Psychol* 64(5):834-46, 1993.

14. Everett MS: Mouth protectors, *J Dent Hyg* 56:27-33,1982.

15. Eyison J et al: A comparative study of the attitude of dental students towards the elderly, *Eur J Prosthodont Restor Dent* 1(2):87-90,1992.

16. Feldman RS: *Understanding psychology,* ed 4, New York, 1996, McGraw-Hill.

17. Finkbeiner BL, Johnson CS: *Mosby's comprehensive dental assisting—a clinical approach,* St Louis, 1995, Mosby.

18. Fowler EB, Breault LG, Cuenin MF: Periodontal disease and its association with systemic disease, *Mil Med* 166(1):85-9, 2001.

19. Friedlander AH et al: Dental management of the geriatric patient with major depression, *Spec Care Dentist* 13(6):249-53, 1993.

20. Gage TW, Pickett FA: *Mosby's dental drug reference,* ed 5, St Louis, 2001, Mosby.

21. Ganong WF: *Review of medical physiology,* ed 13, East Norwalk, Conn, 1987, Appleton & Lange.

22. Genco RJ: Periodontal disease and the risk for myocardial infarction and cardiovascular disease, *Cardiovasc Rev Rep* 19(3):34-40, 1998.

23. Genco RJ, Grossi SG: Is estrogen deficiency a risk factor for periodontal disease? *Compend Contin Educ Dent* 19(suppl 22) 23-30, 1998.

24. Gerow JR: *Psychology: an introduction,* ed 3, New York, 1992, Harper Collins.

25. Going RE, Loehman RE, Chan MS: Mouthguard materials: their physical and mechanical properties, *J Am Dent Assoc* 89:132-8, 1974.

26. Health and Human Services: *Health United States report,* ed 20, Washington, DC, 1995, HHS [http://www.os.dhhs.gov].

27. Hetherington EM, Parke RD: *Child psychology: a contemporary viewpoint,* ed 4, New York, 1993, McGraw-Hill.

28. Jenkins GM: *The physiology and biochemistry of the mouth,* ed 4, Oxford, England, 1978, Blackwell Scientific Publications.

29. Johnson DL, Rue VM: The bulimic dental patient: recognition and recommendations, *J Dent Hyg* 8:372-7,1985.

30. Johnson NW: *Dental caries markers of high and low risk groups and individuals,* Cambridge, 1991, Cambridge University Press.

31. Kiyak HA: Successful aging: implications for oral health, *J Public Health Dent* 60(4):276-81, 2000.

32. Lawrence L, McLeroy KR: Self-efficacy and health education, *J School Health,* 56(8):317-21,1986.

33. Levine RA, Shanaman RH: Translating clinical outcomes to patient value: an evidence-based treatment approach, *Int J Periodont Restor Dent* 15(2):187-200, 1995.

34. Levy GF: A survey of preschool oral health education programs, *J Public Health* 44(1):10-8, 1984.

35. Linn EL: Teenagers' attitudes, knowledge, and behaviors related to oral health, *J Am Dent Assoc,* 92:946-51,1976.

36. Martin FJ: New age dentistry for children, *Dent Teamwork,* Sept:220-223, 1988.

37. Mellander M et al: Mineralization defects in deciduous teeth of low birthweight infants, *Acta Paediatr Scand* 71:727-33, 1982.

38. Meurman JH: Dental infections and general health, *Quint Internat* 28(12):807-11, 1997.

39. Miller L: Depression in middle age patient, *Encephale,* 18(4):507-10,1992.

40. Miller LS et al: The relationship between reduction in periodontal inflammation and diabetes control: a report of 9 cases, *J Periodontol* 63(10):843-8, 1992.

41. Moss ME et al: Exploratory case-control analysis of psychosocial factors and adult periodontitis, *J Periodontol* 67:1060-9, 1996.

42. Moss SJ: Preventive techniques in infant dental care, *Nurse Pract* 7:37-48, 1988.

43. Niessen LC, Gibson G: Aging and oral health for the 21st century, *Gen Dent,* 48(5):544-9, 2000.

44. Nowak AJ, Casamassimo PS: Using anticipatory guidance to provide early dental intervention, *J Am Dent Assoc* 126(8):1156-63, 1995.

45. Nowak AJ, Warren JJ: Infant oral health and oral habits, *Pediatr Clin North Am* 47(5):1043-66, 2000.

46. O'Rourke T, Smith BJ, Nolte AE: Health risk attitudes, beliefs and behaviors of students grades 7-12, *J Student Health* 54(5):210-4, 1984.

47. Offenbacher S, Katz V, Fertik G: Periodontal infection as a possible risk factor for preterm low birth weight, *J Periodontol* 67(suppl):1103-13, 1996.

48. *Oral health for women,* 2001, Aboutsmiles.com: http://www.aboutsmiles.com

49. *Oral health in America: a report of the surgeon general,* Washington, DC, 2000, Department of Health and Human Services.

50. Remick RA, Blashberg B: Clinical aspects of xerostomia, *J Clin Psychiatry* 44(2):63-5, 1983.

51. Renshaw DC: Dentists and bulimia-anorexia nervosa, *Pa Dent J* 52(4):20-1, 1985.

52. Risheim H, Kjarheim V, Arneberg P: Improvement of oral hygiene in patients with rheumatoid arthritis, *Scand J Dent Res* 100:172-5, 1992.

53. Rose LF, Steinberg BJ, Minsk L: The relationship between periodontal disease and systemic conditions, *Compend Contin Ed Dent* 21(10A):870-7, 2000.

54. Ruel-Kellerman M: What are the psychosocial factors involved in motivating individuals to retain their teeth? dreams and facts, *Inter Dent J* 34:105-9, 1984.

55. Sanchez OM, Childers NK: Anticipatory guidance in infant oral health: rationale and recommendations, *Am Fam Physician* 61(1):115-20, 2000.

56. Saunders RP: What is health promotion? *Health Educ* 19(5):14-8,1998.

57. Shay K: Identifying the needs of the elderly dental patient. the geriatric dental assessment, *Dent Clin North Am* 38(3):499-523, 1994.

58. Shay K: Root caries in the elderly: an update for the next century, *J Indiana Dent Assoc* 76(4):37,39-43, 1998.

59. Shay K: Restorative considerations in the dental treatment of the older patient, *Gen Dent* 48(5):550-4, 2000.

60. Shay K, Reuhlar MR, Renner RP: Oropharyngeal candidosis in the older patient, *J Am Geriatr Soc* 45(7):863-70, 1997.

61. Shay K, Ship JA: The importance of oral health in the older patient, *J Am Geriatr Soc* 43(12):1414-22,1995.

62. Shlossman M et al: Type 2 diabetes mellitus and periodontal disease, *J Am Dent Assoc* 121(4):532-6, 1990.

63. Taylor GW, Loesche WJ, Terpenning MS: Impact of oral diseases on systemic health in the elderly: diabetes mellitus and aspiration pneumonia, *J Public Health Dent* 60(4):313-20, 2000.

64. Vick VC, Harfst SA: The oral risk assessment and early intervention system—a clinician's tool for integrating the biopsycho-social risk into oral disease interventions, *Compend Contin Educ Dent,* 21(30suppl):57-62, 2000.

CHAPTER 10

Comprehensive Health History

Mary R. Pfeifer, George M. Taybos

Chapter Outline

Case Study: Significance of a Thorough Health History
Essential Elements of a Health History
    Patient identification (biographical data)
    History of present oral condition
    History of illness
    Family history
    Social history
Review of Organ Systems
    Skin
    Extremities (musculoskeletal system)

Eyes
Ear, nose, and throat
Respiratory system
Cardiovascular system
Gastrointestinal system
Genitourinary system
Endocrine system
Hematopoietic system
Neurological system
Psychiatry
Dental History

Key Terms

Addison's disease
Adrenocorticotropic hormone (ACTH)
Angina pectoris
Angular cheilosis
Atrial dysrhythmia
Chancre
Chronic obstructive pulmonary disease (COPD)
Comprehensive dental history
Comprehensive health history
Congestive heart failure (CHF)
Crohn's disease
Cushing's disease (primary aldosteronism)
Diabetes mellitus (DM)
Dyspnea

Dysuria
Edema
Endogenous
Epistaxis
Exogenous
Fainting (syncope)
Family history
Fibromyalgia
Hematuria
Hepatitis
History of illness
History of present oral condition
Hypertension
Hyperthyroidism
Hypothyroidism

International normalized ratio (INR)
Ketoacidosis
Lupus
Myasthenia gravis
Myocardial infarction (MI)
Nicotinic stomatitis
Parathyroid hormone (PTH)
Paresis
Pellagra
Pernicious anemia
Polycythemia
Polydipsia
Polyuria
Ptosis

Rheumatic heart disease (RHD)
Scleroderma
Sjögren's syndrome
Social history
Teratogens
Thrombocytopenia
Tinnitus
Transient ischemic attacks (TIAs)
Trigeminal neuralgia (cranial nerve V)
Tuberculosis
Type 2 herpes
Upper respiratory infections (URIs)
Vasovagal syncope
Ventricular fibrillation

 ## Learning Outcomes

1. Recognize the health history components and the importance of each to the acquisition of an accurate health database by exploring appropriate follow-up questions.

2. Explore uses, side effects, and other characteristics of medications.

3. Analyze verbal and written patient responses to the health questionnaire to anticipate and/or initiate treatment plan modifications and medical or dental consultation.

*M*edicine has progressed to the point at which conditions once considered debilitating or pernicious are routinely treated and/or managed effectively.[15] These afflicted individuals are now leading longer and more productive lives with the assistance of medications that control their disorders.[8] Advances in medical technology make it possible to replace a variety of body tissues and organs with both donated organs and prosthetic devices. The combination of medical advances and the cultural belief that "pills" can cure any and all aches, pains, and maladies creates a challenge for the dental healthcare team in treating an older, often medically compromised patient population who may be taking a myriad of both prescription and over-the-counter drugs.

The aging (geriatric) population in the United States is the most rapidly growing segment of the population. Presently 12% of the population is 65 years of age or older, and this number will increase to 23% by 2040.[12] Miller and colleagues state that the use of medications is on the rise and the patterns of use vary according to age, gender, race, health, and access to health care.[5] They report that the group of individuals age 80 years or older take four times as many drugs at the group ages 18 to 33 years. More than 48% of the people over age 80 took multiple drugs. The same study also noted that females took more than two thirds (68.9%) of all the drugs reported.[8]

Therefore the dental healthcare team members are treating the following: (1) an older population, (2) patients with medically compromising conditions, and (3) a dental population in which more than 40% of patients are taking a prescribed medication or multiple medications. Thus the overall health status of the dental patient must become as much the concern of the dentist and dental hygienist as the thorough and accurate diagnosis and treatment of oral disease.[4,6,14]

The success of the dental treatment depends on both the dentist's and dental hygienist's clinical expertise and the patient's ability to tolerate and positively respond to the treatment. Halpern, in 1979, reported that 13.6% of an adult patient population at a U.S. dental school required a formal medical consultation because of a medical problem.[6] A study by Nery and colleagues[9] found that 46.3% of the patients at a dental school presented with compromising medical conditions. Sonis and colleagues[14] reviewed a group of patients in 1983 and reported medical problems present in more than 50% of that study population. Rhodus and colleagues evaluated dental school patient populations in 1976 and 1986 and found an increase in the percentage of patients with identifiable medical problems from 7.3% in 1976 to 24.6% in 1986 (Fig. 10-1).[10] A 1995 review of a dental school population revealed that 45% of the patients reported medical problems on their health history questionnaires (see Fig. 10-1).

The dental healthcare team members must be aware of this changing profile in their dental patient population. The team has the following goals:
- Ensure proper patient management
- Modify, if necessary, the dental treatment to minimize or prevent any interference with the patient's medical management for their systemic medical disorder(s)
- Manage patients with life-threatening medical disorders
- Recognize medical disorders and be able to monitor their physical status to ensure stability of their medical condition(s)

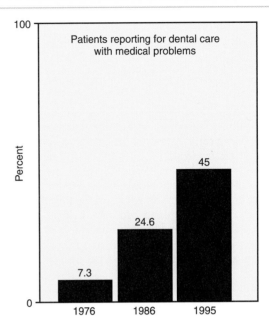

FIG. 10-1 Increase in the number of dental patients with medical problems.

- Be aware of the patient's medications, the drug actions, and the potential drug interactions
- Promote and enhance communication and rapport between the treating dentist, the patient and the patient's physician
- Prevent the possibility of litigation[10,13]

Chapter 3 provides more information on this topic. Ultimately, the dental healthcare clinician is legally and professionally responsible for the health and welfare of a patient during a dental treatment. This responsibility includes an appreciation of both the recognition and management of medical disorders when present.[9]

ESSENTIAL ELEMENTS OF A HEALTH HISTORY

The phrase "Never treat a stranger" is attributed to Sir William Oster. His point was that the healthcare provider should know as much about the patient as possible. This ensures a thorough and proper diagnosis and the patient's ability to tolerate the proposed dental procedures. The patient's health history therefore becomes an important vector in both gathering critical medical-dental information and establishing clinician to patient rapport. The current trend among dental healthcare providers is to combine the printed *comprehensive health history* (composed of subjective responses from the patient) with a verbal review of the patient's responses by the dentist and dental hygienist. The essential elements of a medical history are listed in Box 10-1.

PATIENT IDENTIFICATION (BIOGRAPHICAL DATA)

Gender

While taking the patient's history, the dental hygienist should begin formulating thoughts about the patient's health status. Certain medical conditions have a gender prevalence. Thyroid dysfunction, thyroid carcinoma,

Significance of a Thorough Health History

You greet a 58-year-old African-American male patient, Stanley Belzak, in the reception room. He is obese and is seated on the edge of the chair and leaning forward, resting on his walking cane. When you call his name, you notice that Mr. Belzak strains to stand and is unsteady. After a few seconds he begins to stand upright and walk toward you. His gait is slow and unsteady despite the use of a cane.

Once in the dental treatment room, his transition into the dental chair is slow and labored. After being seated in the dental chair, he requires a few moments to "catch his breath." To sit back in the chair, Mr. Belzak requires your assistance in elevating his lower legs onto the dental chair.

The dental hygienist should mentally review the office emergency protocol.

A review of Mr. Belzak's health history reveals the following:

- *Age 42:* Mr. Belzak was diagnosed with non–insulin-dependent diabetes mellitus, treated with Glucotrol 15 mg once/day and Glucophage 1000 mg twice/day. He states that he checks his blood sugar daily with a Dextrostix and that his fasting blood sugar is usually about 180+.
- *Age 45:* He was diagnosed with **chronic obstructive pulmonary disease (COPD),** high blood pressure, and **atrial dysrhythmia.** Mr. Belzak states that his initial blood pressure before medication was 190/112. The **hypertension** is being treated with an angiotensin-converting enzyme (ACE) inhibitor (Accupril 40 mg twice/day), a diuretic (furosemide 60 mg/day), and a potassium supplement (K-Dur–8 mEq Extencaps: two Extencaps twice/day). Mr. Belzak's atrial dysrhythmia resulted in multiple **transient ischemic attacks (TIAs),** and he is presently being managed with Lanoxin (0.125 mg/day) and Coumadin (alternating doses of 5 mg and 2.5 mg). His last **international normalized ratio (INR)** was 2.5.
- *Age 55:* A physical examination revealed an enlarged prostate gland. The prostate-specific antigen (PSA) was within the normal range. His physicians decided to evaluate annually; no medications were prescribed at this time.
- *Age 56:* Mr. Belzak was diagnosed with **angina pectoris.** This condition is being managed with Adalat (20 mg three times/day). At the time of diagnosis, the physician detected a heart murmur (HM). An echocardiogram revealed a stenotic aortic valve. In addition to the existing COPD, Mr. Belzak is now experiencing **congestive heart failure (CHF).**
- *Allergies:* Mr. Belzak states that he is allergic to penicillin and sulfonamides.
- *Social history:* Mr. Belzak is a widower. (His wife died 2 years ago.) He has two grown children, a son and daugh-

ter, and he lives at home alone. He smokes two packs of cigarettes per day now (one pack per day until his spouse died). He has smoked for at least 40 years (40+ pack years). He states that he has tried to quit on numerous occasions using the gum and patch, but they didn't work. His alcohol consumption is minimal (less than three drinks per week). The chance of this patient experiencing a mild to moderate form of depression should be considered.

- *General:* Mr. Belzak states that he is supposed to see his physician every 3 months, but he has not seen her regularly since his spouse died. His medications have been refilled by a telephone call to the physician's office.

The dental hygienist must encourage this patient to see his physician and perhaps make a follow-up phone call a week or so later to determine whether he has done so. This attempted phone call should be noted in the patient's dental chart.

Mr. Belzak's dental status consists of the following findings:

- *Caries:* Interproximal enamel lesions, root caries, and Class V lesions in every sextant
- *Periodontal disease:* Gingival recession, increased probing depths with spontaneous bleeding, overt marginal inflammation, generalized edematous gingival tissue, with the mandibular buccal area exhibiting a pronounced hypertrophy
- *Missing teeth:* Numerous teeth are missing in the maxilla and mandible. To replace the missing teeth in the maxilla, Mr. Belzak wears a removable partial denture. He states that he has a partial denture for the bottom teeth, but because it doesn't fit well, he doesn't wear it.
- *Oral soft tissues:*
  Palate: A generalized whitish appearance is present, with numerous elevated areas with a red center **(nicotinic stomatitis).** The palatal tissue below the framework of the partial denture is bright red.
  Buccal mucosa: Generalized atrophic appearance, with the presence of ulcerative lesions, with a white, lace-like pattern in the posterior mandibular regions
  Lips: The patient complains that the lips feel swollen. **Angular cheilosis** is present.
- *General comments:* Mr. Belzak states that he brushes his teeth twice a day. He uses whatever toothpaste is on sale. He does not use a mouthrinse; he does not floss or scrape his tongue. He states that his mouth feels dry and he has to drink fluids often during the day to keep his mouth moist. A clinical assessment determines that no saliva is pooling in the floor of the mouth, and the buccal mucosa does not appear to have a saliva layer.

cerebrovascular disease, rheumatoid arthritis, Sjögren's syndrome, *fibromyalgia,* systemic *lupus* erythematosus, and temporomandibular joint dysfunction are more commonly found in female patients. Conditions with a male predominance are oral and pharyngeal carcinoma, laryngeal carcinoma, genital carcinoma, and human immunodeficiency virus infection.[5]

Age

Age has a direct bearing on the presence of and morbidity and mortality caused by medical problems. Increasing age typically increases a person's tendency to develop medical conditions. The most prevalent causes of death (in order of prevalence) by age bracket are as follows (Table 10-1):[5]

- Ages 1 to 19 years: accidents (cancer a distant second for females; homicide for males)
- Ages 20 to 39 years
  Males: (1) accidents, (2) suicide, and (3) homicide
  Females: (1) accidents, (2) cancer, and (3) heart disease
- Ages 40 to 59 years
  Males: (1) heart disease, (2) cancer, and (3) accidents
  Females: (1) cancer, (2) heart disease, and (3) accidents
- Ages 60 to 79 years
  Males: (1) heart disease, (2) cancer, and (3) COPD
  Females: (1) cancer, (2) heart disease, and (3) COPD
- Age 80 years or older
  Males: (1) heart disease, (2) cancer, and (3) cerebrovascular accident (CVA)
  Females: (1) heart disease, (2) cancer, and (3) CVA

> **BOX 10-1**
>
> **Elements of a Health History**
>
> Patient identification (biographical data)
> History of present oral condition (chief complaint)
> History of illness (medical history)
> Family history
> Social history
> Vital signs (see Chapter 11)
> Review of organ systems

Another consideration with age is the onset of ***diabetes mellitus (DM).*** When DM occurs at a young age, the individual generally is insulin-dependent (no secretion of insulin from the beta cells of the pancreas) and prone to ***ketoacidosis*** (diabetic coma). When DM occurs in later years (after age 40), the pancreas can still secrete insulin and the treatment is focused on increasing the secretion of insulin and/or increasing the insulin receptor activity.

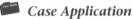 *Case Application*

Mr. Belzak is 58 years old. This age group is prone to heart disease, cancer, non–insulin-dependent diabetes, and COPD.

Race

A greater percentage of African Americans are affected with hypertension than other ethnic groups. The disease presents itself at an earlier age than for Caucasians. The 5-year survival rate for oral and pharyngeal carcinomas in African Americans is dramatically less than for Caucasians—34% versus 55%.[5]

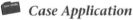 *Case Application*

Mr. Belzak is African American.

HISTORY OF PRESENT ORAL CONDITION

Complaint

The dental hygienist should record accurately the patient's descriptions of oral symptoms. The chief complaint should be stated in the patient's words. The most common complaint for a person seeking dental treatment is pain. After determining the chief complaint, the hygienist should begin to document the chronology of the patient's dental problem *(history of present oral condition)*. The complaint should be documented with the following information: duration/progression, domain, character, and relation to physiological function.

Case Application

Mr. Belzak states that he has a lower partial denture, but he doesn't wear it because it doesn't fit. He also states that his lips feel swollen and his mouth is always dry.

> **TABLE 10-1**
>
> Leading causes of death

Age	Accidents	Homicide	Suicide	Heart disease	Cancer	COPD	CVA
1 to 19	1 M/F	2 M			2 F		
20 to 39	1 M/F	3 M	2 M	3 F	2 F		
40 to 59	3 M/F			1 M	1 F		
				2 F	2 M		
60 to 79				1 M	1 F	3 M/F	
				2 F	2 M		
80+				1 M/F	2 M/F		3 M/F

Modified from Greenlee RT et al: Cancer statistics, 2001, *Cancer J Clin* 51(1):15-36, 2001.
M, Male; *F,* female; *COPD,* chronic obstructive pulmonary disease; *CVA,* cerebrovascular accident.

Duration and Progression

Questions for consideration include the following: How long has this symptom been present? Has this problem developed quickly or was it a slow and progressive process? Have the oral symptoms become more intense, or are they better? Do the symptoms change in character during the day?

Domain

Is the pain/discomfort localized, diffuse, or does it radiate to other sites in the head and neck region? When documenting an oral lesion, the exact location must be noted: for example, anterior floor of the mouth adjacent to teeth #22 to #24.

Character

What is the character of the symptoms? Is the pain sharp or dull? Do the symptoms appear suddenly and disappear, or are the symptoms present all the time? Notation regarding an oral lesion should include the following information: color (white, red), pigmentation, ulcerative, exophytic (elevated, growing outward), or a combination of these clinical features.

Relation to Physiological Function

How does the patient's chief complaint affect normal function? Can this individual chew on the affected side? Does mastication increase or decrease the intensity of the symptoms?

 Case Application
Mr. Belzak reports that he can't chew well because he can't wear his lower partial denture and he has to drink fluids all day to keep his mouth wet.

HISTORY OF ILLNESS

The medical history is important to a thorough understanding of a patient's health status. This document helps to ensure the patients' safety, health, and well-being. It also is a powerful legal document. Serious systemic diseases may have a direct impact on the diagnosis, treatment, and progression of disease associated with the oral cavity and dentition. The dental hygienist must be aware of the implications of systemic diseases and illness, not just on the condition of the oral cavity.[4,9,10,13,15]

The present health history illustrates the chief complaints and gives a full, clear, and chronological summary of how each of the signs and symptoms develop and what events are related.

The past history explores prior illnesses, hospitalizations, operations, drug reactions, injuries, anesthesia, congenital or development problems, and/or other medical interventions.

Obtaining the health history and talking with the patient is often the most important part of establishing a professional relationship. Establishing a safe environment promotes trust and confidence. This provides further information on the effect of an illness on patients' lives.

The dental hygienist must understand the differences between a sign and a symptom. A sign is something observable. For example, the patient is sweating, or the skin color is pale. A symptom is something the patient feels and reports, such as nausea or dizziness.

Collecting medical information regarding the **history of illness** involves collecting information about symptoms. Generally, the easiest method is to have the patient provide an outline of the present problems and then, together with the dental hygienist, go back to fill in all the pertinent details.[15] The dental hygienist must learn the appropriate questions. Positive findings on a completed health history require follow-up questions in the form of a personal interview. The OPQRST–MEDICATIONS format is helpful in asking focused questions to positive findings.[11]

10-A

O: Onset or Other Episodes
When did it start (time/date)? Have you had other episodes like this one? When? What follow-up occurred?

 Case Application
Mr. Belzak states that he was diagnosed with non–insulin-dependent DM at age 42; COPD, hypertension, and atrial dysrhythmia at age 45; benign prostate hypertrophy at age 55; angina pectoris and a stenotic aortic valve at age 56.

P: Provocation or Problems Associated with the Event
What were you doing when the event occurred? Did anything make it better or worse? Are any residual problems due to this event? What are you currently doing for it?

Q: Quality or Quantity
Describe what the pain, pressure, ache felt like. Is any amount of lasting damage or injury due to the event?

R: Radiation or Reaction
Did the pain radiate or did you have any other reaction to the event?

S: Severity, Symptoms, or Surgery
Grade the severity of pain on a scale of 1 (insignificant) to 10 (worst ever experienced). Were there other associated symptoms related to the episode? Did surgery result due to this event? What is your current status? Were there any complications?

 Case Application
Mr. Belzak's fasting blood sugar is in excess of 180. This documents poor control of the DM. The patient's obvious limited mobility is a result of the progression of the COPD and CHF.

T: Time or Tests
When did it start? How long did it last (minutes, hours, days)? Were there any tests conducted at the hospital for this event?

 Case Application
Mr. Belzak checks his blood sugar daily with a Dextrostix, and the fasting blood sugar level is usually about 180+. The patient's latest INR was 2.5.

Medications
The dental hygienist should record the patient's past and current medications, dosage, and compliance in taking

the medication. This includes home remedies, vitamins, birth-control pills, over-the-counter medication (aspirin, sleeping pills, cough syrup, antacids, antihistamines), and prescription medication (including borrowed from friends and family members). The hygienist should list all the names of the medications (a drug manual may be helpful for difficult names to spell) and understand the possible side effects that may relate to dental hygiene care.

 Case Application

Mr. Belzak's medications would be listed as follows:
DM: Glucotrol 5 mg/day, Glucophage 1000 mg bid
Hypertension: Accupril 40 mg bid, furosemide 60 mg/day, and K-Dur 8 mEq Extencaps bid
Atrial dysrhythmia: Lanoxin 0.125 mg/day and Coumadin alternating doses of 5 mg and 2.5 mg/day
Angina pectoris: Adalat 20 mg tid

The OPQRST–MEDICATIONS format may not always apply to all positive responses in the health history. However, it provides a simple template in the initiation of follow-up questions to positive responses. For example, a patient circles *yes* to having a heart attack on the health history. Focused questions may include but are not limited to the following:

O: Onset or Other Episodes
When (month/year) did you have a heart attack? Have you ever had other episodes like this? Does heart disease run in your *family history?*

P: Provocation or Problems Associated with the Event
What were you doing when this happened? Are any current problems in your activities of daily living associated with this event?

Q: Quality or Quantity
Describe the pain that was involved. Did any damage to the heart muscle occur?

R: Radiation or Reaction
Did the pain radiate to other areas or stay in the chest area? Did a more serious illness result from this episode, such as CHF?

S: Severity, Symptoms, or Surgery
On a scale of 1 to 10, how bad was the episode? (Some people have heart attacks and do not even realize it.) Did this require surgery? Do you have chest pains now?

T: Time or Tests
What period of time passed before you went to the hospital for medical care? (Some people are in denial and may wait 2 to 3 days.) What tests did the physician perform, such as a cardiac catheterization, electrocardiogram (ECG), or echocardiogram?"

Medications
What medications are you currently taking for this condition, dosage and frequency?

Other information to elicit from each patient includes the following:
- The name, address, and phone number of all physicians who have treated/are treating the patient
- If surgeries have occurred, the date and year, the hospital and doctors' names, the diagnosis, any complications, follow-up treatment, and current status
- Allergies to anesthetics, medications, penicillin, food, iodine, latex, or bees or seasonal allergies

- A history of childhood illnesses such as polio, rheumatic fever, whooping cough, measles, rubella, mumps, and chicken pox (it can no longer be assumed that all adults have had common communicable childhood diseases, such as chicken pox)

FAMILY HISTORY

The family history helps determine the following:
- Predisposition to certain diseases
- History of diseases that occur in the family
- Cultural beliefs about health care and medicine

The family history helps assess a patient's risk for developing certain diseases. A pattern of familial illnesses may prove useful in the care of and development of a treatment plan for patients. It also may suggest what health concerns the patient might have. This is a good time for patient education.

The diseases that tend to have a strong familial and hereditary factors include diabetes, high blood pressure, allergies, cancer, asthma, stroke, epilepsy, arthritis, heart disease, hemophilia, sickle cell anemia, and chronic myelogenous leukemia (CML). If the patient has diabetes, ask the patient whether any family members have diabetes (including aunts, uncles, siblings, cousins, and grandparents).

At the conclusion of obtaining the family history, the clinician should ask the patient, "Is there anything else that you think is important for us to know?" In certain situations, such as vague, complicated, or contradictory histories, it may be helpful to ask, "What do you think is wrong with you?" and "Have you discussed this with your physician recently?"

 Case Application

Mr. Belzak did not provide any history of his parents or siblings; however, he does have a son and daughter who may be at increased risk for developing DM and hypertension.

SOCIAL HISTORY

The patient's personal history may alert the dental team to possible environmental and cultural factors that can significantly influence the patient's overall health. Each patient should be viewed as a multiple dimensional person, having emotional, physical, spiritual, social, and intellectual needs. Recording the patient's *social history* is helpful in the determination and assessment of the personality and overall well-being of the patient.

Emotional

Emotional well-being factors include a recent death, divorce, relocation to a new area, new job, or a recent marriage. Any of these emotional issues may result in positive or negative stress for the patient and provide the clinician with a better understanding of the patient's present "state of mind."

Psychosocial

Psychosocial history occasionally may suggest factors contributing to the patient's illness and helps the clinician evaluate the patient's source of support, likely reactions to illness, coping mechanisms, strengths, and concerns. It also helps the clinician become more closely acquainted with the patient.

Personal

Personal information includes the patient's birthplace, place raised, cultural background, education, marital status, general life satisfaction, source(s) of stress, and interests.

Habits

Habits include nutrition and diet; patterns of eating and sleep; exercise; quantity of coffee, tea, alcohol, tobacco, and illicit drugs; or overuse of prescription medications. When recording the use of tobacco, the clinician should determine the type, amount used per day, and the duration of years.

Asking about the use of alcohol and drugs is often difficult for dental healthcare workers. However, alcohol and drugs are often directly related to the patient's health and dental symptoms. Tolerance and dependence on a substance may significantly affect the management of the patient. Patients who routinely smoke cigarettes and drink alcohol have a higher incidence of oral cancer. Thus gathering the necessary information is important to the creation of a correct assessment and treatment plan. Questions about alcohol and drugs follow questions about coffee and cigarettes. The clinician should ask specifically about the type of alcohol consumed, such as beer, wine, or liquor, and prescription medications, such as nerve pills, sleep pills, or diet pills.

Addictions

If a patient is a recovering alcoholic, the clinician must avoid suggesting alcohol-containing preparations, such as commercial mouthwashes. Special considerations when treating a patient with addictions are important on the use and effects of anesthesia and pain management, decreased wound healing time, poor nutritional state, and lack of oral care.

Occupation

The clinician should record the patient's usual type of work, present work if different, types of physical and mental strains, and exposure to toxins, gases, and other carcinogens or *teratogens.*

Environmental

Does the patient travel extensively for a living? Is the patient exposed to contagious diseases and other sources of infection?

Cost of Care Resources

What cost of care resources are available to the patient? Does the patient have concerns in this regard? A candid discussion about these issues may alter the treatment plan extensively.

REVIEW OF ORGAN SYSTEMS

The review of organ systems[15] is important to both the clinician and the patient because it documents existing medical conditions, the medical management of the patient's problem(s), and the physical status of the patient. The review of organ systems also may suggest the presence of undiagnosed medical problems and/or may give a direct relationship of the oral signs and symptoms to a medical condition, such as severe oral ulcerations with *Crohn's disease,* glossodynia with anemias, increased caries incidence, and candidiasis with head and neck radiation therapy patients. A medical compendium and a drug reference book in the treatment room provide appropriate references when needed to understand diseases, disorders, treatments, drug therapies, and oral sequelae.

SKIN

The clinician should ask patients whether they have or have ever had any of the following:
- Itching (pruritis), dermatitis (contact or atopic [skin rash]), and/or eczema
- Psoriasis or seborrhea
- Pigmentations
- Skin cancer(s), appearance of moles, and/or melanoma
- Allergies or adverse reactions to latex, medications, and/or metals

Itching, Dermatitis, and Eczema

A common cause of itching (pruritis) is psychogenic (i.e., a reaction to stress). Itching in the scalp area is often associated with a bitter taste and glossodynia. Itching without a visible rash may be due to drug reaction and may be caused by over-the-counter (OTC) drugs such as aspirin, or by prescribed drugs such as opiates, quinidine, penicillin, or other antibiotics. The clinician should ask patients exactly what their reactions were (adverse reaction versus anaphylaxis) and to describe the symptoms associated with the incident.

Itching may be localized (e.g., dermatitis). The most common inflammatory skin disease is eczematous dermatitis. The various types include primary contact dermatitis, allergic contact dermatitis, and atopic dermatitis. All three share the common presentation of a breakdown of the epidermis.

 Case Application
Mr. Belzak probably developed a rash because of the past use of penicillin and sulfate medications and most likely developed a sensitivity rather than a true allergy.

Psoriasis and Seborrhea

Psoriasis is a common chronic disease characterized by dry, silvery, well-circumscribed plaques of various locations and sizes. A strong association exists with family history of psoriasis and reflects an autosomal dominant inheritance. Seborrhea is an inflammatory scaling and involves the scalp and face. It is apparent as a dry or greasy diffuse scaling of the scalp with variable degrees of itching.

Pigmentations

Genetic Factors

Vitiligo is an autosomal dominant trait characterized by a localized or generalized hypomelanosis of the skin and hair. Vitiligo has a strong association with **Addison's disease, hyperthyroidism, hypothyroidism, pernicious anemia,** and alopecia areata.

Neurofibromatosis is a dominant trait characterized by *café au lait* spots. The presence of six or more spots with diameters of greater than 1.5 cm is a strong indicator of the diagnosis of neurofibromatosis.

Peutz-Jegher's syndrome is a dominant trait characterized by the presence of mucocutaneous hypermelanosis on the lips and in the oral cavity. The importance of the oral finding is that this entity is associated with polyposis of the jejunum and ileum. The polyps are most often benign.

Metabolic and Endocrine Factors

Hypermelanosis or hemochromatosis are familial disorders of iron metabolism that produces liver damage resulting in cirrhosis. Iron deposition in the pancreas and adrenal glands results in DM and hypoadrenalism. The skin becomes hyperpigmented (bronze).

Adrenal gland disorders resulting in the overproduction of **adrenocorticotropic hormone (ACTH)** and melanin-stimulating hormone (MSH) cause Addisonian hyperpigmentation.

Nutritional Factors

Kwashiorkor, decreased protein in the diet, causes the hair to change color to a brownish-red, then to gray. Sprue, or malabsorption in the small intestine, produces a brown pigmentation that can occur anywhere on the body. **Pellagra,** deficiency of niacin, has a cutaneous component that begins as erythematous appearing skin and then progresses to a darker keratotic skin.

Chemical and Physical Factors

Progesterone, whether **endogenous** (resulting from pregnancy) or **exogenous** (resulting from birth control pills), may cause hyperpigmentation on the abdomen and forehead. This is known as *melasma* or *chloasma*.

Skin Cancer(s) and Malignant Melanoma

Moles may be small or large; flat or raised; smooth or hairy; flesh-color, yellow-brown, or black. If a mole enlarges suddenly or becomes spotty in color, has an irregular border, or becomes painful and bleeds, it must be excised. Approximately 40% to 50% of malignant melanomas arise from ordinary moles. The presence of color changes may be caused by actinic damage, a melanoma, basal cell carcinoma, keratoacanthoma, and squamous cell carcinoma.

Allergies and Adverse Reactions to Latex, Medications, and Metals

Many allergies to medications, metals, and latex are due to the body developing antibodies or sensitized lymphocytes that develop during a sensitization period after an initial exposure to a specific agent. A later exposure to the same agent (penicillin) may result in a severe sensitive reaction (itching, hives, vomiting) or a life-threatening reaction (anaphylaxis).

 Case Application

Mr. Belzak complains that his lips feel swollen. On the medical history form, the patient lists that he is taking Accupril 40 mg twice/day. Angioedema (swollen lips) is a reported side effect in patients taking ACE-inhibitors (Accupril, Monopril, Prinivil, Zestril, and Altace).

EXTREMITIES (MUSCULOSKELETAL SYSTEM)

The patient should be asked whether he or she has ever had any of the following:

- Stiff and swollen joints, arthritis (rheumatoid or osteoarthritis [degenerative joint disease, or DJD]), and/or osteoporosis
- Lupus, polymyositis, *scleroderma*, and/or **Sjögren's syndrome**
- Muscle weakness and/or pain and fibromyalgia
- Bone deformity and/or fracture
- Prosthetic joints
- Conditions requiring cortisone therapy

Stiff and Swollen Joints, Arthritis, and Osteoporosis

Swollen and painful joints may be caused by trauma, infection, metabolic disturbances, immunological disturbances, and/or neoplasms. The patient experiences pain, swelling, stiffness, and decreased or limited motion in addition to redness and a feeling of warmth.

Rheumatoid arthritis (RA) is a chronic, systemic inflammatory disease of the joints. The deformities of RA are due to the inflammatory destruction of the articular surfaces. RA appears to have a 3:1 female predilection. Osteoarthritis (DJD) is a noninflammatory disorder of the joints that results in the deterioration of the bone and cartilage. The incidence of DJD increases with age. DJD affects almost every individual age 70 and older.[4] Osteoporosis is an increased porosity of the bone that places individuals at an increased risk of hip and/or spinal vertebrae fractures.

Dental Considerations

Oral self-care strategies must be evaluated carefully to accommodate any lack of manual dexterity.

Lupus, Polymyositis, Scleroderma, and Sjögren's Syndrome

Lupus is a chronic, progressive disease often presented as a butterfly face rash. Symptoms include photosensitivity, arthritis without deformities, oral and nasal ulcerations, and pericarditis. Polymyositis is a connective tissue disease characterized by dermatitis and **edema,** inflammation, and degeneration of the muscles. Scleroderma varies in progression and severity. It is seen more in women than in men, causing diffuse fibrosis, degenerative changes, and vascular abnormalities in the skin, articular structures, and internal organs. Sjögren's syndrome occurs most frequently in post-menopausal women, causing severe dry mouth and keratoconjunctivitis; it is often related to rheumatoid arthritis (see Chapter 40).

Muscle Weakness/Pain and Fibromyalgia

Ocular palsies are manifested by double vision (diplopia). Drooping of the eyelid *(ptosis)* may be an early sign of *myasthenia gravis.* Facial palsy (known as Bell's Palsy) is the paralysis of the facial nerve. This condition is usually unilateral, and the patient is unable to smile, expose teeth, or close the eye on the affected side. Fibromyalgia is a nonspecific illness characterized by overall fatigue, muscle and joint pain, tenderness, and stiffness.

Bone Deformity/Fracture

Bone is a dynamic tissue that is constantly being repaired and remodeled throughout an individual's life. The calcium-to-phosphorus ratio is important in bone health. Any condition that alters the calcium-to-phosphorus ratio affects the integrity of the bone. *Parathyroid hormone (PTH),* calcitonin, vitamin D, and serum protein all affect the calcium-to-phosphorus ratio. Vitamin D affects the calcium and phosphorus absorption from the gastrointestinal tract. Serum protein is directly related to the amount of calcium and phosphorus bound to the albumen. Thus liver and GI tract problems may have a direct effect on the health of the skeletal tissue.

Prosthetic Joints

More than 400,000 total joint prostheses are placed annually. The prostheses replace both the hip and the knee. Pain is the main reason that the surgery is performed, and osteoarthritis is the major medical condition causing the joint pain. The question has been answered regarding whether the patient with a total joint prosthesis should receive antimicrobial prophylaxis before invasive dental procedures. American Dental Association guidelines state that the majority of total joint prostheses are not at risk for developing a late joint infection caused by a dental procedure.[1] However, patients who have a total joint prosthesis and also have an immunocompromising disease (i.e., uncontrolled insulin-dependent DM, systemic lupus erythematosus, or severe and symptomatic rheumatoid arthritis) may benefit from antimicrobial prophylaxis (antibiotic premedication). The trend today, however, is to sharply curtail the use of antimicrobial agents in clinical situations in which no proven benefit exists.

EYES

The clinician should ask whether patients have or have ever had any of the following:
- Double vision
- Drooping eyelid
- Glaucoma
- Cataracts

Double Vision

Double vision (diplopia) occurs when the points of the visual receptors are far apart and two images are formed. Other causes of double vision may occur in the cerebrum: trauma, cerebrovascular accident, or vascular abnormalities. Damage to the optic nerve also may cause double vision.

Drooping Eyelids

Drooping of the eyelid may be an early manifestation of myasthenia gravis. This also may occur with *paresis* of the third cranial nerve.

Glaucoma

Glaucoma is an elevation of the intraocular pressure and is the most common cause of blindness in many regions of the world. Chronic primary open-angle glaucoma is the most common type of glaucoma.[7] The canal of Schlemm is the site of the resistance to outflow of the aqueous material. An estimated 2% of the population have this type of glaucoma.

Cataracts

A cataract is a developmental or degenerative opacity of the lens. The classic symptom is a progressive painless loss of vision. The degree of vision loss depends on the location and the extent of the opacity. Pain may occur if the cataract swells and produces secondary glaucoma.

The dental hygienist must carefully evaluate oral self-care strategies to accommodate vision impairment.

EAR, NOSE, AND THROAT

The hygienist should ask patients whether they have or have ever had any of the following:
- Hearing loss, *tinnitus,* hearing aid, and/or vertigo
- Frequent nosebleeds
- Frequent sore throats and/or tonsillitis
- Sinusitis and/or rhinitis
- Hoarseness
- Mouth ulcers, canker sores, fever blisters, and/or cold sores
- Tobacco and/or smokeless tobacco use

Hearing Loss, Tinnitus, Hearing Aid, and Vertigo

Transient hearing loss may be caused by an acute or chronic external otitis. Hearing loss also may be due to a malformed auditory organ anatomy and/or impaired transmission of the sound waves via the eighth cranial nerve.

Tinnitus is a ringing in the ears and is a subjective phenomenon. Approximately 90% of the population has reported tinnitus at one time or another. Salicylates and quinine drugs are notorious for causing tinnitus.

Patients with hearing deficits, regardless of whether they use hearing aids, may require the dental hygienist to speak louder and face the patient during interactions.

Patients with vertigo may feel they are moving in space with a loss of equilibrium.

Frequent Nosebleeds (Epistaxis)

The most common cause of *epistaxis* (nosebleed) is the tearing of Kiesselbach's plexus as a result of nosepicking. Epistaxis also may occur as a normal finding during an upper respiratory infection (URI) or may be a sign of hypertension, a bleeding diathesis (clotting deficiency, *throm-*

bocytopenia or *polycythemia)*, nasal tumors, or Osler-Rendu-Weber disease (hereditary hemorrhagic telangiectasia, HHT).

Frequent Sore Throat (Pharyngitis) and Tonsillitis

Sore throat is the most common manifestation of pharyngitis. Two thirds of all cases of pharyngitis are due to viral *upper respiratory infections (URIs).* Serious complications of a bacterial pharyngitis are peritonsillar cellulitis or abscess. Carcinoma of the tonsillar tissue, although rare, is the second most common tumor of the superior airway. Signs of a tonsillar carcinoma include reports of pain in one enlarged tonsil with no signs or symptoms of an infection.

Tonsillitis is an infection of the tonsils, usually resulting from viral or streptococcal infections.

Sinusitis and Rhinitis

The most common predisposing factor for acute sinusitis is a viral URI. This leads to blockage of draining of the paranasal sinuses and the development of pain, tenderness, and low-grade fever. The maxillary sinus is the most common sinus infection, characterized by pain, swelling, and tenderness in the anterior portions of the maxilla and infraorbital regions; infection in the frontal sinus is characterized by pain over the forehead; ethmoid sinus infection is characterized by pain in the upper lateral areas of the nose; and sphenoid sinus infection is characterized by pain and tenderness over the vertex of the skull, mastoid bones, and the occipital portion of the head.

Rhinitis (runny nose), the most frequent URI, is characterized by edema and nasal discharge and obstruction and vasodilation of the nasal mucous membrane.

Hoarseness

Hoarseness is a change in the character of the voice most commonly resulting from a local laryngeal infection. Hoarseness may be caused by exophytic lesions such as papillomas and tumors and disorders of the structures around the upper airway (such as edema or tumors of the esophagus). Uncomplicated hoarseness resulting from benign local factors is of short duration; however, persistence of symptoms of hoarseness longer than 2 to 3 weeks warrants a direct examination by an otolaryngologist.

Mouth Ulcers, Canker Sores, Fever Blisters, and Cold Sores

Oral ulcers associated with pain are a common reason the patient seeks dental treatment. These ulcers may be due to trauma, viral/bacterial, or autoimmune reactions.

Tobacco and Smokeless Tobacco Use

Tobacco use (all forms) is a major cause of illness and death. A movement in the healthcare profession is trying to establish tobacco assessment as the fifth vital sign (after blood pressure, pulse, temperature, and respiration). Dental hygienists may have a significant impact in education and cessation of tobacco with patients (Chapter 12).

RESPIRATORY SYSTEM

The dental hygienist should ask the patients whether they have or have ever had any of the following:
- Cough
- Blood in the sputum
- Wheezing and asthma
- Bronchitis and emphysema (COPD)
- Exposure to *tuberculosis*
- Pneumonia

Cough

A cough is an explosive expiration of air that clears the tracheobronchial tree of secretions and foreign bodies. Inflammatory, chemical, or thermal stimulation of the cough may cause coughing receptors. Most commonly acute episodes of coughing are due to viral or bacterial infections, whereas chronic cough is due to bronchitis (usually caused by cigarette smoking), pulmonary tuberculosis, or pulmonary neoplasms.

Blood in Sputum

Blood in the sputum is known as hemoptysis. Many diseases, such as lung carcinoma, a bronchial tumor or bronchiectasis, lobar pneumonia, lung infarction, and pulmonary edema, may cause hemoptysis.

Wheezing and Asthma

The classic triad of symptoms for asthma is coughing, wheezing, and *dyspnea.* Viral URIs, physical exertion, emotional excitement, and exposure to allergens can precipitate asthmatic attacks. Asthma is a reversible lung disorder characterized by narrowing of the airways, resulting from bronchial constriction, edema, and inflammation of the bronchial mucosa. Have inhaler available during appointment.

Bronchitis and Emphysema (COPD)

Bronchitis usually is associated with cigarette smoking, which results in bronchial irritation with increased production of mucous and structural changes in the bronchi that results in significant airway obstruction.

Emphysema is an enlargement and destruction of the alveolar tissues in the lungs. This is generally a predictable sequela of long-term cigarette use. COPD consists of both bronchitis and emphysema. Both of these conditions are preventable by not smoking or cessation of smoking.

Exposure to Tuberculosis

In the past decade, the incidence of tuberculosis has increased. This is due to many factors, which include the influx of infected foreigners to this country and the increased rate of infection in immunocompromised chronic diseases, such as acquired immunodeficiency syndrome (AIDS). A distinction must be made between the individual who has the disease and the individual who has the infection. The individual who has the infection has been exposed to the organism and exhibits a positive purified protein derivative (PPD) or Mantoux test. They do not have any active lung lesions nor do they have any organisms in their sputum. If treated, they give a history of taking INH (isoniazid) for about a year. These individuals cannot transfer the organism to another person; they are not infectious.

The individual who has the disease has a positive PPD or Mantoux test, positive lung findings, and organisms in the sputum. These individuals can transfer the disease to other individuals up to the time that they have a negative sputum culture (generally 2 to 3 weeks on multiple drug therapy; see Chapter 5).

Pneumonia

In the elderly population, pneumonia may be fatal. This population must have a current pneumonia vaccination. Another population at risk is individuals who have had a splenectomy (removal of the spleen).

CARDIOVASCULAR SYSTEM

The hygienist should ask whether patients have or have ever had any of the following:
- Shortness of breath (SOB)
- *Fainting (syncope)*
- Pain or pressure in the chest and/or angina
- Swelling of the ankles
- High or low blood pressure and/or orthostatic hypotension
- Rheumatic fever (RF)
- Congenital heart disorder
- HM
- Cardiac dysrhythmia, abnormal heartbeat, and/or flutter
- Pacemaker, defibrillator
- CHF
- History of endocarditis
- Prosthetic heart valve
- Heart attack *(myocardial infarction [MI])*
- Arteriosclerosis and/or atherosclerosis
- Stroke and/or TIA

> Certain conditions in this organ system may place a patient at risk for endocarditis.

Shortness of Breath

Shortness of breath (SOB) or abnormal awareness of breathing is a cardinal sign of disease of both the respiratory and cardiovascular systems. An early manifestation of left ventricular heart failure is dyspnea (difficulty in breathing) at rest or during the performance of a menial task. The dyspnea related to heart disease develops and progresses relatively quickly in comparison to dyspnea resulting from respiratory disease (COPD).

Fainting (Syncope)

Fainting, or syncope, is a momentary loss of consciousness that may be due to cardiovascular problems, dysrhythmias, hyperventilation, neurological, or metabolic problems. *Vasovagal syncope* is usually precipitated by a physical or an emotional event. Have vasoconstrictor available.

Pain or Pressure in the Chest and Angina

Myocardial ischemia results in an increase in the oxygen supply in relation to the need of oxygen in the heart muscles caused by atherosclerosis of the coronary arteries. Symptomatic myocardial ischemia is known as angina pectoris. The pain from an MI may be distinguished from angina pain in that the MI pain is more severe, of longer duration, and unresponsive to nitroglycerin (NTG). Have nitroglycerine available.

Swelling of the Ankles

Swelling of the ankles may be a sign of right ventricular failure that results in systemic venous congestion and edema.

High or Low Blood Pressure and Orthostatic Hypotension

Arterial blood pressure must be maintained at adequate levels to provide perfusion of the capillary system. The blood pressure depends on the level of the preload (venous return), the afterload, and the myocardial contractile force.

Essential hypertension is the most common cause of elevated blood pressure, and this form of hypertension has a familial tendency. The elevated blood pressure may be manifested with an increase in the systolic pressure. An increased preload resulting from anemias, hyperthyroidism, and/or aortic insufficiency may cause this. A normal stroke volume that is pumped out into a noncompliant arteriosclerotic aorta also results in an elevated systolic pressure. The diastolic blood pressure is elevated when the afterload is increased as a result of an increased arteriolar resistance.

Hypertension, if untreated or poorly managed, results in secondary end-organ damage to the heart, kidney, and central nervous system. This significantly shortens the lifespan of the individual by 10 to 20 years.

Hypotension results from a decrease in the cardiac output or a decrease in the peripheral resistance. A fall in the blood pressure upon standing is known as orthostatic hypotension and is a common finding in older adults with atherosclerosis. (See Chapter 11, Physical and Extraoral Examination, p. 225.)

Rheumatic Fever

Rheumatic fever (RF) is an inflammatory disease that occurs as a delayed sequel to a pharyngeal infection with a group A streptococci. The infection may affect the heart, joints, skin (erythema marginatum), central nervous system (chorea), and subcutaneous tissues. Rheumatic fever can be fatal in the acute stage and can result in *rheumatic heart disease (RHD),* which is characterized by a deformity of the heart valves and the presence of an audible HM. Rheumatic heart disease applies only to those situations in which the individual had rheumatic fever and the rheumatic fever infection directly caused the heart valve deformity and HM.

Dental Considerations

An individual with a damaged heart valve caused by rheumatic fever should be managed in accordance with the American Heart Association guidelines (Boxes 10-2 through 10-4). However, a patient with a history of rheumatic fever who does not have heart valve damage is not at increased risk for developing infectious endocarditis and thus should not receive an antimicrobial prophylaxis regimen.

Congenital Heart Disorder

The list of congenital heart disorders is lengthy. It includes aortic valve (stenosis and bicuspid), ventricular septal defects, coarctation of aorta, patent ductus arteriosus, and tetralogy of Fallot. Untreated tetralogy of Fallot is considered a risk category for infective endocarditis (IE). The others are in the moderate risk category.

Heart Murmur

An HM results from vibrations of the heart valve leaflets as a result of turbulent blood flow through valves and chambers of the heart.[2] HMs may be classified by intensity of the sound ranging from grade I (barely audible) to a grade VI (very loud and audible with the stethoscope not on the chest).

The discovery of HM requires careful assessment and diagnosis by the physician. HMs may be classified as ei-

---

BOX 10-2

American Heart Association Guidelines for the Prevention of Endocarditis

High-Risk Category
Prosthetic cardiac valves, including bioprosthetic and homograft valves
Previous bacterial endocarditis
Complex cyanotic congenital heart disease
    Single ventricle states
    Transposition of the great arteries
    Tetralogy of Fallot
Surgically constructed systemic-pulmonary shunts or conduits
Moderate-Risk Category
Most other congenital cardiac malformations (other than those listed above)
Acquired valvular dysfunction
    Rheumatic heart disease
Hypertrophic cardiomyopathy
Mitral valve prolapse (MVP) with valvular regurgitation and/or thickened leaflets
Negligible-Risk Category
(no greater risk than general population)
Endocarditis prophylaxis is *not recommended* for the following conditions:
Isolated secundum atrial septal defect
Surgical repair of atrial septal defect, ventricular septal defect, or patent ductus arteriosus (without residue beyond 6 months)
Previous coronary artery bypass graft (CABG) surgery
Mitral valve prolapse without valvular regurgitation
Physiological, functional, or innocent heart murmurs
Previous Kawasaki disease without valvular dysfunction
Previous rheumatic fever without valvular dysfunction
Cardiac pacemakers (intravascular and epicardial) and implanted defibrillators
Dental procedures
Antibiotic prophylaxis recommended
Extractions
Periodontal procedures
    Surgery
    Scaling
    Root planing
    Probing and recall maintenance
    Subgingival placement of antibiotic fibers/strips
Prophylactic cleaning (when bleeding is anticipated)
    Teeth
    Implants

Endodontic procedures
    Instrumentation beyond the apex
Orthodontic procedures
    Initial placement of bands
Local anesthesia
    Intraligamentary injections
Other procedures
    Dental implants
    Reimplantation of avulsed teeth
Dental procedures
Antibiotic prophylaxis not recommended
Restorative dentistry
    Operative procedures
        Includes restoration of carious teeth
    Prosthetic procedures
        With or without retraction cord
        Clinical judgment may indicate antibiotic use in selected circumstances that may create significant bleeding
        Includes replacement of missing teeth
Local Anesthesia
    Block injections
    Infiltration injections
Endodontic procedures
    Intracanal treatment
    Post placement
    Coronal build-up
Other procedures
    Placement of rubber dam
    Taking of impressions
    Taking of oral radiographs
    Fluoride treatments
    Postoperative suture removal
Orthodontic procedures
    Appliance adjustment
    Placement of brackets
Placement of removable appliances
    Prosthodontic
    Orthodontic
Shedding of deciduous/primary teeth

Modified from American Heart Association: *Prevention of bacterial endocarditis* (Tables 1 and 2), Dallas, 1997, The Association.

Prophylactic Regimens for Dental, Oral, Respiratory Tract, or Esophageal Procedures

Standard Prophylactic Regimen
Amoxicillin
    Adults: 2.0 g
    Children: 50 mg/kg
    Oral route: 1 hour before the dental procedure
Patients Unable to Take Oral Medications
Ampicillin
    Adults: 2.0 g IM or IV
    Children: 50 mg/kg IM or IV within 30 minutes before the dental procedure
Patients Allergic to Penicillin
Clindamycin
    Adults: 600 mg
    Children: 20 mg/kg
    Oral route: 1 hour before the dental procedure
Cephalexin* or Cefadroxil*
    Adults: 2.0 g
    Children: 50 mg/kg
    Oral route: 1 hour before the dental procedure
Azithromycin or clarithromycin
    Adults: 500 mg
    Children: 15 mg/kg
    Oral route: 1 hour before the dental procedure
Patients Allergic to Penicillin and Unable to Take Oral Medications
Clindamycin
    Adults: 600 mg
    Children: 20 mg/kg IV within 30 minutes before the dental procedure
Cefazolin*
    Adults: 1.0 g
    Children: 25 mg/kg IM or IV within 30 minutes before the dental procedure

Modified from American Heart Association: *Prevention of bacterial endocarditis* (Table 4), Dallas, 1997, The Association.
IM, intramuscularly; *IV,* intravenously.
*Use of cephalosporins: Avoid in patients with a history of a type I hypersensitivity reaction (urticaria, angioedema, or anaphylaxis) to penicillin.
Total children's dose should not exceed adult dose.

Antimicrobial Prophylaxis Review

Determine the medical risk factor.
    Cardiovascular
        Prosthetic heart valves
        History of infective endocarditis (IE)
        MVP with regurgitation
    Total joint replacement
        Few patients are premedicated
Establish optimal oral health.
Maintain optimal oral health.
Complete periodic dental examinations.
Prevent or treat acute oral infections.
Provide antimicrobial mouthrinse before treatment.
Prescribe and monitor antimicrobial prophylaxis for invasive procedures.

ther innocent/benign functional or the result of valvular abnormality. It is not unusual for a child, adolescent, or active young person to be told that he or she has an HM. Most of the time this finding is due to strenuous myocardial contraction, which results in a stronger blood flow during systole and the movement of the blood from the large ventricle into the smaller sized aorta and blood vessels. In thin-chested young persons, the sound of the movement of the blood is easier to hear. These findings are termed *innocent heart murmurs* and are not a risk factor for the development of IE. Thus antimicrobial prophylaxis is not recommended for this type of HM.

HMs resulting from diseased heart valves may increase the patient's risk to develop IE. Anatomical disorders of the heart valves that result in a pathological murmur are as follows:
- Mitral valve stenosis
- Mitral valve prolapse with regurgitation
- Aortic stenosis
- Subaortic stenosis
- Pulmonic stenosis
- Tricuspid valve stenosis

Aortic stenosis was identified in the case study. According to the American Heart Association, this condition is a risk factor for the development of IE.[3] Because this patient is unable to take penicillin (which includes amoxicillin), he would require premedication for invasive dental and dental hygiene procedures with clindamycin.[3]

The previously listed valvular defects result in turbulent blood flow that creates the audible murmur heard with the stethoscope. In accordance with the American Heart Association, a patient with an HM resulting from these valvular disorders should receive antimicrobial prophylaxis for certain high-risk dental procedures (i.e., invasive dental procedures such as oral surgical procedures and endodontic or periodontal surgery; see Boxes 10-2 through 10-4).

Cardiac Dysrhythmia, Abnormal Heartbeat, and Flutter

Normal heartbeats originate in the sinoatrial node. The impulse then enters the atrioventricular node. From there is a pass through the bundle of His into the left and right bundles. Any electrical deviations may result in abnormal heartbeats.

Pacemaker and Defibrillator

If the heart rate decreases significantly, a pacemaker is inserted in the chest to restore a normal heart rate. Severe dysthymias that result in disorganized ventricular contractions *(ventricular fibrillation)* may result in death if intervention (i.e., cardiopulmonary resuscitation [CPR]) is not implemented immediately. To prevent this life-threatening form of dysrhythmia, defibrillators are implanted to "shock" the person back into a more stable heart rhythm.

Congestive Heart Failure

With CHF the ventricle cannot adequately pump blood to the critical organs and periphery. This results in left ventricular hypertrophy, left ventricular failure, pulmonary edema, and peripheral edema.

History of Endocarditis

Endocarditis is an infection of the endocardium characterized by an elevated temperature, presence of HMs, petechiae, anemia, emboli, and vegetations on the endocardium that result in heart valve damage, myocardial abscess, or aneurysm. Males are affected with IE almost twice as often as females. The median age for the infection is in the 50s. Endocarditis of the right side of the heart is associated with cardiac diagnostic procedures and intravenous (IV) drug abuse. Cardiac surgeries have resulted in an increase of nosocomial endocarditis. An increase in the elderly population with calcific changes on the valve leaflets is another subset of IE patients.[7] IE, if untreated, is almost always fatal, and when treated, the morbidity and mortality varies according to the patient's age, severity of the disease, site of infection, microorganism, and complications.

Dental Considerations

IE is considered a high-risk factor for the development of another infection of the endocardium. Therefore the American Heart Association recommends antimicrobial prophylaxis for these patients when undergoing invasive dental procedures[3] (see Boxes 10-2 through 10-4).

Prosthetic Heart Valves and Inserts

Heart valves that become nonfunctional and result in serious cardiovascular problems are surgically replaced with prosthetic devices. The heart valve that most commonly has prosthetic replacement is the mitral valve, followed by the aortic valve. The presence of a prosthetic heart valve is a high-risk factor for developing IE and *must* be premedicated with an antimicrobial agent before high-risk dental procedures. Prosthetic devices such as stents in the coronary vessels, Dacron graft material, and synthetic tube material placed in the major vessels do not place the individual at increased risk for developing IE. Therefore antimicrobial prophylaxis for dental procedures is not recommended[3] (see Boxes 10-2 through 10-4).

Heart Attack (Myocardial Infarction)

A heart attack (myocardial infarction [MI]) may result in permanent damage to the myocardium and thus a decreased capability of the heart to pump blood to the periphery. If a patient gives a history of a heart attack, the clinician must determine (1) the date of the MI and not treat within 6 months time (2) degree of damage, (3) present medications, (4) lifestyle modifications resulting from the MI, and (5) patient health status. (See Boxes 10-2 through 10-4 for premedication guidelines.)

Arteriosclerosis and Atherosclerosis

Arteriosclerosis is a generic term for a number of diseases in which the arterial wall becomes thickened and losses elasticity (such as in aging). Atherosclerosis begins with fat and plaque deposits in the smooth muscle of the arterial wall. If the deposits continue, complete occlusion prevents blood flow in the arteries.

Stroke and Transient Ischemic Attack

Cerebral vascular accident or stroke is the most common cause of neurological disability in developed countries. Most strokes are due to atherosclerosis and hypertension.

TIAs usually are due to cerebral emboli arising from plaques or atherosclerotic ulcers involving the carotid or ventricle arteries. TIAs are often recurrent and at times presage a stroke. Often TIAs are referred to as "mini-strokes." The plaques in the carotid may be visualized in a dental panoramic radiograph.

GASTROINTESTINAL SYSTEM

The hygienist should ask patients whether they have or have ever had any of the following:
- Difficulty in swallowing (dysphasia)
- Abdominal pain and/or ulcers
- Gastroesophageal reflux
- *Hepatitis* and/or jaundice

Difficulty in Swallowing (Dysphagia)

Difficulty in swallowing (dysphagia) is a subjective symptom. This may be due to an emotional disturbance or a disease/dysfunction condition. Dysphagia is caused by a transport dysfunction of the musculature of the esophagus. Swallowing disorders may be due to neuromuscular disorders (e.g., myasthenia gravis or bulbar palsy) or lesions (e.g., esophageal carcinoma, the strictures associated with progressive systemic sclerosis [scleroderma], or Plummer-Vinson syndrome, and the disseminating candidiasis that can be found in AIDS). Patients who have xerostomia or who have had head and neck radiation therapy also have difficulty with swallowing.

Abdominal Pain and Ulcer

The area of pain in the abdomen is important in determining the cause of the pain. Pain in the right upper quadrant (RUQ) may be a sign of hepatitis (liver), cholecystitis (gall bladder), or carcinoma of the head of the pancreas. Pain in the left upper quadrant (LUQ) may be a sign of an enlarged spleen or inflammation or carcinoma of the tail of the pancreas. Pain in the lower right quadrant (LRQ) may be a sign of acute appendicitis or pneumonia in the lower right lung; pain in the lower left quadrant (LLQ) may be a sign of diverticulitis; and pain in the epigastric area may be a sign of acute pancreatitis.

Patients with a history of ulcers also have a distinct location and character of pain. Gastric ulcers produce a diffuse pain on the left side, whereas duodenal ulcers have pain localized to the right side with a focal area of tenderness. The cycle of pain for the duodenal ulcer is as follows:

Pain → Food → Relief → Pain

For the gastric ulcer the pain cycle is as follows:

Pain → Food → Increased pain

Gastroesophageal Reflux

Gastroesophageal reflux disease (GERD) is a reflux or regurgitation of gastric contents into the esophagus. Patients should stay in a semi-sitting position during treatment.

Hepatitis and Jaundice

Jaundice means a greenish-yellow color. A jaundiced condition manifested by a yellow discoloration of the skin, mucous membranes, and sclera is due to an increase in the bilirubin level in the blood. Bilirubin increases with an increased rate of destruction of red blood cells, a decreased conjugation of the lipid soluble bilirubin in the liver, and/or a decreased rate of removal of the conjugated bilirubin via the bile duct into the small intestine. Newborn infants may have jaundice.

Thus a history of jaundice is not necessarily synonymous with a history of hepatitis, an inflammation of the hepatocyte, or cells in the liver. Some causes are medications/drugs, toxic chemicals, alcohol, and viruses.

Causes of Viral Hepatitis
Causes of viral hepatitis are as follows:
- Hepatitis A: waterborne/foodborne; fecal-oral route; no carrier state; vaccine available
- Hepatitis B: bloodborne; carrier state; vaccine available
- Hepatitis C: bloodborne; carrier state; no vaccine; variable clinical progression
- Hepatitis D: bloodborne; occurs only in presence of HBV infections; HBV vaccine effective
- Hepatitis E: waterborne/foodborne; fecal-oral route; no vaccine
- Mononucleosis: Epstein-Barr virus (EBV) transmitted in saliva; no carrier state

Dental Considerations
The concern in dentistry is the transmission of viral hepatitis from a patient to the dental healthcare worker (DHCW) or other patient. With the acceptance of universal precautions and the hepatitis B vaccine, the threat to the DHCW has been decreased significantly. However, clinicians should still thoroughly review the patient's medical history and attempt to identify the cause of jaundice or hepatitis (see Chapter 5).

GENITOURINARY SYSTEM

The hygienist should ask patients whether they have or have ever had any of the following:
- Difficulty and/or pain on urination
- Blood in the urine
- Excessive urination
- Kidney infections and/or urinary calculi
- Renal or kidney dialysis
- Sexually transmitted disease and/or venereal disease
- Pregnancy and/or breast cancer
- Prostate cancer

Difficulty and Pain on Urination (Dysuria)

Dysuria may be a sign of prostate enlargement (hypertrophy or carcinoma), streptococcal glomerulonephritis, cystitis (bladder infection/inflammation), urethritis, pyelonephritis, and/or gonorrhea.

Blood in the Urine (Hematuria)

Hematuria, whether microscopic or overt, is a serious sign. Hematuria may be caused by severe hypertension (end organ damage to the kidneys), acute glomerulonephritis, trauma, cystitis, gonorrhea, bladder carcinoma, or a toxic reaction to drugs.

Excessive Urination (Polyuria)

Four major medical disorders could cause *polyuria:*
- DM
- Diabetes insipidus
- Acquired renal lesions
- Psychogenic *polydipsia*

Kidney Infections and Urinary Calculi

Kidney infections may occur anywhere in the urinary tract. Infections in the lower urinary tract are known as *cystitis* and *urethritis* and are caused by colonic flora or gonococci. Infections of the upper urinary tract are known as *pyelitis* and *pyelonephritis.* Kidney infections are not to be confused with glomerulonephritis, which is an autoimmune response to a streptococcal infection.

Urinary calculi (stones) may occur anywhere in the urinary tract. They can cause pain, obstruction, and secondary infections. Approximately 1 in every 1000 adults requires hospitalization for kidney stones.

Renal or Kidney Dialysis

When the kidneys are no longer able to maintain body homeostasis because of kidney failure, the patient is treated by hemodialysis. Dialysis is a process during which the blood is removed from the patient, passed through membranes and filters to remove impurities, restored with electrolyte concentration, and then returned to the patient. For patients on a regular dialysis program, blood pressures should not be taken on the arm where the shunt or fistula has been placed. This population tends to be at an increased risk for IE.

Sexually Transmitted Diseases and Venereal Disease

Sexually transmitted diseases (STDs), such as gonorrhea and syphilis, remain a concern. Syphilis may present with classic oral lesions. In the primary stage, a *chancre* may be present (teeming with infectious organisms); in the secondary stage, mucous patches and split papules may be present; and in the tertiary stage, a gumma and interstitial glossitis may be present. Genital herpes *(type 2 herpes)* and genital warts (*Condyloma acuminatum*) may be present in the oral cavity and in the genital mucosa (see Chapter 5).

Pregnancy and Breast Cancer

In the unstable pregnant woman, oral self-care education should be stressed, and planned definitive dental procedures should be discussed with her physician. With a stable pregnant female, any trimester is suitable for dental hygiene procedures.

Breast cancer, the most common malignancy with women, occurs more commonly after menopause. All women should be encouraged to have routine mammograms and to perform monthly self-breast exams.

Dental Considerations

Patient education should include current concepts in the link between gingivitis and preterm, low-birth-weight infants.

Prostate

More than 198,000 cases of prostate cancer occur annually. Prostate cancer is a common malignancy in men over age 50, and the incidence increases with each decade of life.[5]

ENDOCRINE SYSTEM

The hygienist should ask patients whether they have or have ever had any of the following:
- Thyroid gland problems
- Weight change
- DM
- Excessive thirst
- Adrenal hyperfunction (Cushing's syndrome) and adrenal hypofunction (Addison's disease)

Thyroid Gland Problems

When patients state they have or have had thyroid problems, the clinician must ascertain the nature of the problem and how it is being managed. Is the patient taking levothyroxine (Synthroid), what is the dose, and how often is the thyroid function evaluated? A patient who is obese or gaining weight and relates symptoms of fatigue, drowsiness, cold intolerance, and poor memory and who presents with physical signs including dry, coarse skin and hair, decreased heart rate, loss of the lateral one third of the eyebrow, and prolonged reflexes may have decreased thyroid gland activity (hypothyroidism). However, a patient who relates symptoms of headaches, diarrhea, increased appetite, weight loss, and heat intolerance, and whose physical signs include exophthalmia, increased heart rate, and dyspnea, may have increased thyroid gland activity (hyperthyroidism).

Dental Considerations

An undiagnosed hyperthyroid patient or a known hyperthyroid patient whose medical management has not been stabilized should not be given a dental local anesthetic agent with a vasoconstrictor (see Chapters 35 and 36).

Weight Change

In an adult, an increase in body weight may reflect an increase in adipose tissue or an accumulation of fluid. Obesity is the single most prevalent metabolic disorder in countries with an abundance of food. Obesity occurs when the caloric intake is greater than the energy requirement of the body for normal physical growth and maintenance. Increased fluid retention may be due to excessive salt intake, fluid intake, or a decreased sodium and water excretion. A decreased sodium and water excretion may indicate a cardiovascular, renal, hepatic or adrenal problem. Weight gain resulting from increased fluid retention occurs in a short period of time (hours to days). Excessive loss of weight may be the first indication of a wasting disease such as HIV infection. Weight loss also is an ominous prognostic indicator of the progression of a malignancy (see Chapters 44 and 45).

Diabetes Mellitus

DM is the most prevalent of all endocrine disorders. The two major types of DM are insulin-dependent diabetes mellitus (IDDM; type I) and non–insulin-dependent diabetes mellitus (NIDDM; type II). IDDM is acquired at younger ages, in people with a thinner physique. Those with type I are prone to develop ketoacidosis and do not produce any insulin. NIDDM is typically acquired by obese individuals (60% to 90% of individuals with NIDDM are obese), those more than 40 years of age, and those who are ketosis-resistant and produce insulin. The problem is in the amount of insulin produced and/or the insulin receptor activity.[12] (See Chapter 20, Supplementary Aids, p. 373).

Dental Considerations

For the dental clinician, the most common problem for this patient is insulin shock. Common oral findings in the patient with diabetes are xerostomia, resulting in an increased caries rate, candidiasis, and periodontal disease. The patient with diabetes who is well-managed with hypoglycemic agents does not appear to have any compromise in healing or combating infections.

Excessive Thirst (Polydipsia)

Increased thirst (polydipsia) and increased urination (polyuria) should alert the clinician to the possibility of the presence of diabetes. This finding also may be present in the patient with *Cushing's disease (primary aldosteronism)*.

Adrenal Hyperfunction (Cushing's Syndrome) and Adrenal Hypofunction (Addison's Disease)

Cushing's syndrome is a myriad of clinical signs resulting from long-term exposure to excessive levels of cortisol, whether from hypersecretion of the adrenal gland or high-dose steroid therapy.

Addison's disease is the opposite of Cushing's; it is a severe adrenal hypofunction.

Dental Considerations

The patient with Addison's disease may require additional steroid supplement during stressful events, including some dental procedures (i.e., periodontal surgery or multiple extractions).

HEMATOPOIETIC SYSTEM

The hygienist should ask patients whether they have or have ever had any of the following:
- Easy bruising
- Excessive bleeding
- Anemia and/or sickle cell anemia
- Hemophilia
- Leukemia
- Radiation and/or chemotherapy
- HIV/AIDS

Easy Bruising

The presence of a bruise may be explained by eliciting a history of trauma, or it may be the sign of a vascular or platelet abnormality.

Excessive Bleeding

Bleeding is one of the most serious manifestations of a disease process. The presence of blood, whether from the gingival sulcus representing periodontal disease or in the form of hematuria or hemoptysis, should alert the clinician to pursue this concern. Excessive bleeding may be due to the patient taking medications such as Coumadin, aspirin, or nonsteroidal antiinflammatory drugs (NSAIDs), or it may represent a defect in that patient's hemostatic system.

Anemia and Sickle Cell Anemia

Anemia is a manifestation of an underlying disease process. Approximately 20% of females in the United States have iron-deficiency anemia. Anemia is a decrease in the oxygen-carrying capacity of the red blood cells (RBCs) and may be manifested as a decrease in the hemoglobin content or a decrease in the number of RBCs. The anemic patient is tired, weak, and faint and has headaches and is intolerant of cold. Oral findings in the anemic patient may range from no obvious changes in the oral tissues to the classic beefy red, bald tongue, and the subjective complaint of altered taste or glossodynia. These findings should alert the clinician to the possible presence of an anemic condition.

Taking dietary replacement of either iron or folic acid can reverse iron- and folate-deficiency anemia. If vitamin B_{12} is the deficient factor, B_{12} injections are required to treat this condition. An undiagnosed or untreated vitamin B_{12} deficiency (pernicious anemia) may result in irreversible degeneration of the spinal cord.

Sickle cell anemia is a chronic anemia in African Americans, affecting 0.3% of African Americans in the United States.[7] The sickle cell trait affects 8% to 13% of African Americans and doesn't result in any signs or symptoms.[7] The anemia in sickle disease is severe. The red blood cell (RBC) sickles or loses its shape and plugs up small vessels, causing swelling of the spleen and liver, thus severely compromising the immune system and placing the patient at risk for infection. A sickle cell event is extremely painful.

Dental Considerations
Radiographically, the molar region may present with a decreased trabecular pattern, characterized by a "stepladder" pattern.

Hemophilia

This hereditary disorder results in a deficiency of clotting of blood. Hemophilia A (factor VIII deficiency) is the most common form. Genetically, hemophilia is transmitted to males and carried by females. Patients with hemophilia have factor VIII ranging from 1% to 25% of the norm. Regardless of the range, dental surgical procedures result in severe bleeding.[7]

Dental Considerations
Before invasive dental procedures, patients with hemophilia should have factor VIII replacement, and their factor VIII level should be 30% of normal or greater at the time of the dental procedure.

Leukemia

Leukemia is an increase in the number of immature cells of the white blood cell line. Leukemia may arise in either the granulocytic or lymphocytic line. The acute forms of leukemia may have oral signs such as bleeding around the gingiva, leukemic infiltrates in the oral tissues, candidiasis, serious fungal infections (aspergillosis or mucormycoses), and debilitating viral infections. The patient's hematologist may ask the dental clinician for assistance in his or her efforts to control intraoral hemorrhage or to determine the cause of oral lesions: fungal, viral, or graft-versus-host.

Radiation and Chemotherapy

See Chapters 44 and 45.

HIV/AIDS

See Chapters 5 and 44.

NEUROLOGICAL SYSTEM

The hygienist should ask patients whether they have or have ever had any of the following:
- Frequent headaches
- Dizziness and/or fainting
- Epilepsy and/or seizure disorder
- Neuritis and/or neuralgia
- Paralysis
- Alzheimer's disease
- Muscular dystrophy
- Multiple sclerosis and/or demyelinating disease
- Lyme disease
- Parkinson's disease

> See Chapter 41 for detailed neurological system information.

Frequent Headaches

Headaches along with fatigue, hunger, and thirst represent an individual's most frequent complaints of discomfort. A headache most often is the expression of minor tension or fatigue associated with the events of the day. However, if the individual is incapacitated by the headache and the headache is of a long duration, the individual may have migraine headaches, or some underlying organic disease state may exist.

Dizziness and Fainting

Dizziness may be related to a hypoglycemic state, anemias, and disturbances in the vestibular component of the auditory nerve.

Fainting refers to a lack of strength with the sensation of impending loss of consciousness. Dizziness and fainting rarely appear when the patient is in the recumbent position (see also the section on the cardiovascular system).

Epilepsy (Seizure Disorders)

Epileptic attacks may occur at any time, day or night, and occur regardless of the patient's position. The onset is sudden; an aura is present; the patient becomes unconscious; and tonic-clonic contractions begin. After the seizure terminates, the patient is confused, may have a headache, and is physically exhausted.

Patients with seizure disorders must take their medication(s) as prescribed. If they do have seizures during treatment, the clinician must ensure that they do not injure themselves. If they are standing, the clinician should ease them to the floor and make sure that the head does not strike the floor.

Patients with seizure disorders who are treated with phenytoin (Dilantin) may exhibit gingival enlargement.

Neuritis and Neuralgia

Neuralgias that affect the head and neck region are ***trigeminal neuralgia (cranial nerve V)*** and glossopharyngeal neuralgia (cranial nerve IX).

Paralysis

The most common head and neck paralysis is Bell's palsy. This is due to an inflammatory reaction in or around the nerve in the area of the stylomastoid foramen. Bell's palsy may be associated with DM, the postsequelae of a viral infection, or a recurrent herpes infection.

Alzheimer's Disease

Alzheimer's disease is a degenerative process with loss of cells in the cerebral cortex, resulting in memory loss. Behavior may be variable from childlike to angry and aggressive. A caretaker typically escorts the patient to the dental office. The clinician should maintain a close watch of these patients.

Muscular Dystrophy

This is an inherited progressive muscle disorder, characterized by wasting and atrophy of muscle.

Multiple Sclerosis and Demyelinating Disease

Multiple sclerosis is a slowly progressive CNS disorder. In the brain and spinal cord patches of demyelination occur, resulting in multiple and varied neurological symptoms and signs, usually with remissions and exacerbations.

Lyme Disease

Lyme disease is a tick-transmitted disorder that results in neurological, cardiac, and joint problems.

Parkinson's Disease

Parkinson's disease is a degenerative central nervous system disorder characterized by slow movement, rigid muscles, and tremors at rest and inability to remain upright.

PSYCHIATRY

The hygienist should ask patients whether they have or have ever had any of the following:
1. Nervousness
2. Depression and/or bipolar disorder

Nervousness

Many patients admit to being nervous or anxious about dental treatment. If this is in direct relation to a stressful event, this is accepted as a normal response. However, if the nervousness is uncontrollable and accompanied by physical effects, then further evaluation may be necessary before any dental procedures are performed (see Chapters 34 and 43).

Depression and Bipolar Disorder

Depression is a recognized medical illness and a myriad of pharmacotherapeutic agents exist to treat this disorder. Clinicians should accurately document the antidepressant medication. The tricyclic agents are notorious for causing xerostomia. An increased rate of caries, recurrent caries, presence of candidiasis, and inflamed tissues may reflect this in the oral cavity.

 Case Application

You suspect that Mr. Belzak may suffer depression. He will have a much more difficult time in tobacco and substance cessation than someone who has not experienced depression.

Bipolar disorder is having depression and elevated "manic" periods. Bipolar disorder has a younger age of onset between episodes and a higher rate of social dysfunction (see Chapter 43).

DENTAL HISTORY

The patient's past ***comprehensive dental history*** provides the dental hygienist with insight into the patient's dental intelligence and the patient's priority for dental health and dental treatment. A review of the patient's dental history includes an assessment of the following:

The frequency of dental visits: Did the patient return on a regularly scheduled frequency or use dental services infrequently? Were special circumstances affecting this behavior? This information reveals the patient's attitude toward dental health and the importance of preventive dental procedures.

The reason for the past dental visits: Were previous dental visits for emergency treatment only, or were they part of the patient's regular healthcare maintenance schedule? This information reveals the patient's knowledge about dental health and the importance of regular examinations. When patients participate in a regular dental health program, their appreciation of the importance of good oral health and regular dental examinations are greater than for the patients who seek oral care only when they are in pain.

Type of dental care provided in the past:

Extractions: Were the extractions part of orthodontic therapy, the result of unrestorable caries due to an orofacial trauma, or due to of bone loss resulting from periodontal disease? Were the extractions performed because the patient could not afford the recommended treatment?

Periodontal therapy: Does the patient have a past history of periodontal disease? Has the patient had periodontal surgery? Did the patient participate in a periodontal therapy maintenance regimen? How has the patient responded to the periodontal treatment? All of these questions help the clinician determine the prognosis of treatment for this patient.

Restorative dentistry: Were the restorations placed as part of a comprehensive dental program, or were they placed as part of managing a dental emergency?

Prosthodontic dentistry: Was the reason for the dental prostheses aesthetic to replace missing teeth? How well is the patient maintaining the dental prosthesis?

Temporomandibular joint: Does the patient have a history of TMD? How has the TMD been treated in the past? How successful was the past treatment?

Parafunctional habits: Does the patient give a history of clenching or bruxism; mouth breathing; or biting objects (pencils, pipestems, fingernails)? How were the parafunctional habits managed, and what was the success of the treatment?

Oral hygiene behavior: What is included in the patient's current oral self-care regimen? Were these procedures recommended by the dental health professional? Were any self-care recommendations made in the past but not followed? This information helps the clinician focus future oral care strategies.

Dental radiographic examination(s): Information relative to a radiographic exam provides two important facts. One is the patient's understanding of the need and use of dental radiographs in the diagnosis and treatment of their dental needs. Second, the information provides background on the thoroughness of the patient's previous dental examinations.

Family dental history: What is the dental status of the patient's parents? This response can reveal the patient's attitude about the importance of "saving" the teeth. It can help identify behaviors and beliefs likely to affect compliance.

Fluoride history: Has the patient lived in a community with optimally fluoridated water? If so, for how long? What about during childhood? Depending on the age of the patient, current information, and past history of the use of fluorides, this can provide additional information regarding risk of dental caries.

 CRITICAL THINKING ACTIVITIES

1. The dental hygienist often refers to a medical reference textbook (e.g., *The Merck Manual*, Merck, Sharpe, and Delmar Laboratories, Rockway, N.J.). In the index area in the back of *The Merck Manual*, become familiar with looking up specific diseases and locating the disease in the main text area. For example, look up sickle cell anemia, bradycardia, cataracts, and eclampsia.

2. Refer to a drug reference textbook (e.g., *Mosby's Dental Drug Reference*). In the index area in the back of the reference book, become familiar with looking up specific medications and locating the medication in the main text area. Focus on the actions/pharmacodynamics, the route and dosage, the contraindications and precautions, the adverse/side effects, and the relationship to dental hygiene care.

3. Review a completed health history on a clinic patient and do the following:
   a. Compare the medications the patient is taking by looking up each medication in a drug reference manual.
   b. Look up the diseases or disorders listed on the medical history in a medical reference manual.

   c. Assess the relationship between the patient's medication(s) and the identified medical problems.

4. Review three to five health/dental histories of clinic patients in each of the following age ranges and determine where they fall in the grid for disease incidence/death, as presented in this chapter:
   a. 1 to 19 years: men and women
   b. 20 to 39 years: men and women
   c. 40 to 59 years: men and women
   d. 60 to 79 years: men and women
   e. 80+ years: men and women
   What conclusions can you draw, based on your observations? Might any personal habits have changed their health profile, such as smoking, diabetes, exercise?

5. Review your clinic medical/dental history forms. Are there any additions/deletions you would make based on this chapter?

6. Role-play with a peer partner, explaining the importance of a thorough medical/dental history. The "patient" should be unwilling to fill out such a "long" form and should want to know why all this "stuff" is necessary. "After all," the patient may say, "I am just having my teeth cleaned."

CRITICAL THINKING ACTIVITIES—cont'd

7. Identify which portions of the organ systems review, when answered positively, place a patient at increased risk for dental disease.

8. Identify which portions of the dental history review, when answered positive, place a patient at increased risk for systemic disease.

 REVIEW QUESTIONS

1. The essential elements of a health history include all *except* which of the following?
   a. Full mouth radiographic survey
   b. Vital signs
   c. Patient identification
   d. History of present oral condition (chief complaint)
   e. Social history

2. The history of a patient's present oral condition would include which of the following examples?
   a. Glucotrol by mouth for diabetes
   b. Blood pressure of 180/98
   c. Dull, constant pain in upper right molar
   d. 40-year history of cigarette smoking

3. All *except* which of the following are components of the social history?
   a. Alcohol use
   b. Emotional status
   c. Occupation
   d. Age
   e. Level of education

4. The American Heart Association recommends that certain dental patients receive antimicrobial premedications before a dental prophylaxis. For which of the following conditions would premedication be recommended?
   a. History of rheumatic fever
   b. Functional heart murmur
   c. Prosthetic aortic valve
   d. Myocardial infarction 3 years ago

5. During the past 10 years, the incidence of tuberculosis (TB) has increased. Which of the following would indicate active (infectious) TB in a dental patient?
   a. Positive PPD test
   b. Negative PPD test
   c. History of taking INH for 6 months
   d. Positive sputum
   e. Negative chest (x-ray) films

6. Common oral findings in the patient with diabetes include all *except* which of the following?
   a. Xerostomia
   b. Candidiasis
   c. Progressive periodontal disease
   d. Caries
   e. Fluorosis

 SUGGESTED AGENCIES AND WEB SITES

Because of the ever-changing nature of the Internet, some of the web sites listed here may have changed since publication. Please refer to Mosby's Evolve web site for the most current information.

American Association for Retired Persons: 601 E Street, NW, Washington, DC 20024; (800) 424-9046: http://www.wellweb.com

American Diabetes Association: 1660 Duke Street, Alexandria, VA 22314; (703) 232-3472 or (800) ADA-DISC: http://www.diabetes.org

Arthritis Foundation (of which Sjögren's syndrome is a subcomponent), 1330 West Peach Street, Atlanta, GA 30309; (404) 872-7100 or (800) 283-7800: http://www.arthritis.org

American Cancer Society: 1599 Clifton Road NE; Atlanta, GA 30329; (404) 325-2217 or (800) ACS-2345: http://www.cancer.org

American Dental Association: 211 Chicago Avenue, Chicago, IL 60611; (312) 440-2500: http://www.ada.org

American Dental Hygienists' Association: 444 N. Michigan Avenue, Suite 3400, Chicago, IL 60611; (312) 440-8900; (800) 243-2342; FAX 312-440-8929: http://www.adha.org

American Lung Association: 1740 Broadway, New York, NY 10019; (212) 315-8700: http://www.lungusa.org

American Heart Association: 77320 Greenville Avenue, Dallas, TX 75231; (800) AHA-USA1 or (214) 373-6300: http://www.amhrt.org

American Journal of Nursing: http://www.nursingcenter.com/

American Medical Association: 515 North State Street, Chicago, IL 60610; (312) 464-5000: http://www.ama-assn.org

American Nursing Association: 600 Maryland Avenue, SW, Suite 100 West, Washington, DC 20024; (800) 274-4262: http://www.nursingworld.org

American Pharmaceutical Association: 2215 Constitution Avenue, NW, Washington, DC 20037; (202) 628-4410 or (800) 237-APHA: http://www.aphanet.org

American Red Cross: 17th and D Sts. NW, Washington, DC 20006; (202) 737-8300: http://www.redcross.org

Center for Disease and Prevention (CDC): Division of STD Prevention, 1600 Clifton Road NE, Atlanta, GA 30333; (404) 639-3311: http://www.cdc.gov

CDC National AIDS Hotline: (800) 227-8922

Food and Drug Administration: 8800 Rockville Pike, Bethesda, MD 20852; (301) 295-8228: http://www.fda.gov

International Federations of the Red Cross: http://www.ifrc.org

National Health Information Center: (800) 336-4797

Continued

SUGGESTED AGENCIES AND WEB SITES—cont'd

National Institutes of Health (including National Institute of Aging, Diabetes, Child Health, Alternative Medicine, Women's Health, Heart, Lung and Blood & Neurological Disorders and Stroke): 900 Rockville Pike, Bethesda, MD 20892: http://www.nih.gov

National Institute of Mental Health: 4500 Fishers Lane, Room 15C-05, Rockville, MD 20857; (301) 443-4513: http://www.nimh.nih.gov

National Osteoporosis Foundation: 1232 22nd Street NW, Washington, DC 20037-1292; (202) 223-2226: http://www.nof.org

National Stroke Association: 300 East Hampden Avenue, Englewood, CO 80110; (303) 649-9299: http://www.stroke.org

The Dental Record, Inc.; 111 E. Wisconsin Avenue, Suite 1300, Milwaukee, WI 53202; (800) 243-4675; (414)-276-3954

Breast Cancer
Women's Health Weekly: http://www.newsfile.com
National Breast Cancer Coalition: http://www.natlbcc.org

Cancer
Lymphoma Research Foundation of America: http://www.lymphoma.org
National Cancer Institute: http://www.nci.nih.gov

General Interest/Wellness
National Institute of Occupational Safety and Health: http://www.cdc.gov/niosh
World Health Organization: http://www.who.org
Health *(USA Today)*: http://www.usatoday.com/life/front.htm
Medscape: http://www.medscape.com

Medications
Drug InfoNet: http://www.druginfonet.com

Men's Health Issues
Prostate.com: http://www.prostate.com

Mental Health
American Psychiatric Association: http://www.psych.org
American Psychological Association: http://www.apa.org

Nutrition
American Dietetic Association: http://www.eatright.org

Stroke
National Institute of Neurological Disorders and Stroke: http://www.ninds.nih.gov

Substance Use/Misuse
National Clearinghouse for Alcohol and Drug Information: http://www.health.org

Tobacco Cessation
QuitNet: http://www.quitnet.org
Tobaccofreekids.org (tobacco use cessation): http://www.tobaccofreekids.org
Americans for Nonsmokers: http://www.no-smoke.org

 ## ADDITIONAL READINGS AND RESOURCES

Gage TW, Pickett FA: *Mosby's dental drug reference,* ed 6, St Louis, (in press), Mosby.

Samples of other medical history forms may be obtained by calling or writing University of Mississippi Medical Center, School of Dentistry, 2500 North State Street, Jackson, MS 39216-4505; Thomas J. Smith, DDS, MS, JD–Associate Dean for Clinical Programs, (601) 984-6025

University of Mississippi Medical Center, School of Health-Related Professions, Department of Dental Hygiene, 2500 North State Street; Jackson, MS 39216-4505; (601) 984-6310.

 ## REFERENCES

1. Advisory statement: Antibiotic prophylaxis for dental patients with total joint replacements, *J Am Dent Assoc* 128:1004-8, 1997.
2. American Hearth Association: *Cardiovascular disease in dental practice,* Pub. No. 71-0009. Dallas, 1991, The Association.
3. Dajani AS et al: Prevention of bacterial endocarditis: recommendations by the American Heart Association, *J Am Dent Assoc* 128:1142-51, 1997.
4. Epstein IA: Blood examination in the practice of dentistry, *J Am Dent Assoc* 16:1808-20, 1929.
5. Greenlee RT et al: Cancer statistics, 2001, *Cancer J Clin,* 51(1):15-36, 2001.
6. Halpern IL: Medical consultation: essential in today's dental practice, *Dent Surv* 2:26-9, 1979.
7. *Merck Manual,* ed 16, Rahway, NJ, 1992, Merck Sharp and Dohme Research Laboratories.
8. Miller CS et al: Documenting medication use in adult dental patients: 1987-1991, *J Am Dent Assoc* 123:41-8, 1992.
9. Nery EB et al: Prevalence of medical problems in periodontal patients obtained from three different populations, *J Periodontol* 58:564-8, 1987.
10. Rhodus NL, Bakdash MB, Little JW, Haider ML: Implications of the changing medical profile of a dental school patient population, *J Am Dent Assoc* 119:414-6, 1989.

11. Seidel HM, Ball JW, Dains JE: *Mosby's guide to physical examination,* ed 4, St Louis, 1998, Mosby.

12. Ship JA, Mohammed AR: *Clinician's guide to oral health in geriatric patients,* Baltimore, 1999, American Academy of Oral Medicine.

13. Simpson TH, Halpern IL: Health appraisal of apparently well persons in oral diagnosis, *J Dent Educ* 37:27-30, 1973.

14. Sonis ST, Fazio R, Setkowicz A: A comparison of the nature and frequency of medical problems among patients in general practice and hospital dental practice, *J Oral Med* 38:58-61, 1983.

15. Taybos GM, Terezhalmy GT, Pelleu GB: Assessing patients' health status with the navy dental health questionnaire, *US Navy Med* 2:24-31, 1983.

CHAPTER 11

Physical *and* Extraoral Examinations

Nelson L. Rhodus, George M. Taybos

Chapter Outline

Case Study: The Examination Process
Physical Evaluation
Principles and Techniques of Physical Evaluation
  General physical observations
  Principles of clinical examination for the head
    and neck
  Components of the HEENT
  Supplemental diagnostic aids

Vital Signs
  Temperature
  Pulse
  Respiration
  Blood pressure
  Tobacco assessment
Referrals and Consultations

Key Terms

Aspiration
Auscultation
Crepitus
External auditory meatus

Inspection
Lymph nodes
Muscles
Palpation

Parotid glands
Percussion
Salivary glands
Submandibular glands

Sublingual glands
Temporomandibular joint (TMJ)
Thyroid gland

 ## Learning Outcomes

1. Perform a thorough extraoral examination, identifying structures and abnormalities during the examination.
2. Perform vital signs on patients according to techniques presented in the chapter.

3. Evaluate readings obtained when taking vital signs and identify whether precautions or consults are needed before the performance of dental hygiene care.
4. Evaluate the TMJ and facial symmetry on a patient.

This chapter provides information to the dental hygiene student to enable proficient performance of the head and neck (head, eyes, ears, nose, and throat [HEENT]) examination and an in-depth assessment of the dental patient's vital signs. This information is limited to the extraoral portion of the HEENT examination. The intraoral examination is discussed in Chapter 13.

The techniques used to perform the HEENT examination include *inspection, palpation, auscultation,* and *percussion.* The structures to be examined include the facial and neck skeleton, *muscles,* glands, blood vessels, and skin. The vital signs to be reviewed include blood pressure, pulse rate, temperature, respiration, and an assessment of tobacco use.

The thorough HEENT examination and assessment of

the vital signs reveal any deviations from normal. The most important concept is that the dental hygienist must be comprehensive in evaluating *all* the essential information and findings and must recognize *any* variations from normal. Follow-up monitoring, additional diagnostic evaluations, consultations, or referrals must then be planned accordingly. Regular performance of these techniques makes the comprehensive examination an efficient process. This process leads to an accurate determination of any pathological or infectious process in the head and neck region. A thorough evaluation of the patient's vital signs may reflect disease beyond the head and neck region.

This chapter also presents a review of the vital signs and the anatomical structures in the head and neck and the techniques by which to examine them.

Case Study

The Examination Process

Fadi Jabir has returned for his supportive-care appointment. He has not been to the dental office in 18 months. While you review his health history, Mr. Jabir reports having been diagnosed with prostate cancer shortly after his last visit and that he has had surgery and chemotherapy. He states that his physician gave him a clean bill of health at his last medical visit 4 months ago. While performing the extraoral exam, you note enlarged lymph nodes in the supraclavicular area.

> **BOX 11-1**
>
> **General Physical Observations**
>
> | | |
> |---|---|
> | Stature | Hair |
> | Body type | Extremities |
> | Symmetry | Sexual characteristics |
> | Gait | Responses |
> | Mobility | Function |
> | Posture | Cleanliness, personal hygiene, |
> | Color | dress |
> | Skin | Odor |

From Halstead C et al: *Physical evaluation of the dental patient,* St Louis, 1982, Mosby.

PHYSICAL EVALUATION

The dental hygienist is in an excellent position to assist in the diagnosis of systemic pathology. Recognition of normal anatomy and physiology, normal variations, and the early signs and symptoms of disease is important. These observations lead to a diagnosis and proper treatment.

The recognition of variations from a normal health status is crucial for two major reasons. First, this observation may identify medical or dental conditions that are undiagnosed. Second, the observation may determine the status of the identified conditions. Patients may have a more serious status for their medical condition, and this may place them at risk for serious complications from the dental treatment.

The thorough, comprehensive examination facilitates recognition of medical problems; the need to modify or defer treatment; or the need for referral to the appropriate healthcare provider. The clinician should not discount the importance of the comprehensive exam for every patient lest something significant, serious, or even disastrous go unrecognized.

The dental health of the patient is the primary focus of the dental hygienist's attention. However, before the examination of the oral cavity, the clinician must see the dental patient as a whole human being. Medical diseases may present a serious threat to the patient's life. Attention to serious medical conditions supersedes any routine dental treatment. Recognizing the patient with a serious medical condition such as hypertension or diabetes mellitus and making the proper referral may save a life. Modifying dental treatment to prevent a medical emergency (stroke, heart attack) or serious medical condition (infective endocarditis, bleeding) is the responsibility of everyone in the healthcare field.

PRINCIPLES AND TECHNIQUES OF PHYSICAL EVALUATION

Illness is the interaction of a particular disease process with an individual patient. Subjective sensations resulting from the disease that are reported by the patient are called *symptoms. Signs* of illness are objective findings that are observed by the clinician (see Chapter 10). The comprehensive examination must be performed in a systematic, standardized manner to avoid missing any signs or symptoms of an infection or medical problem. Detection of illness depends on the determination and accurate interpretation of the symptoms and signs and therefore relies principally on the knowledge, training, and skill of the clinician. To paraphrase Sir William Osler, what the mind does not know, the eyes cannot see. The examination process begins the moment the dental hygienist meets the patient and continues throughout the appointment.

GENERAL PHYSICAL OBSERVATIONS

General physical observations begin the minute the dental hygienist encounters the patient. By carefully observing the patient in the reception room and in the treatment room and at all times during the appointment, the dental hygienist may detect variations from normal or a disease process in the patient. General physical observations are shown in Box 11-1.

Body type, stature, and symmetry are related to hereditary characteristics. These characteristics also may reflect endocrine or metabolic problems. Variations from normal gait, mobility, and posture may reflect a musculoskeletal or inflammatory connective tissue disorder or a central nervous system (CNS) disturbance. The patient's responses and personal hygiene may be related to CNS or psychological problems or general physical debilitation. Color of the skin may reveal liver disease (jaundice), cardiovascular disease (cyanosis), bleeding disorders (petechiae-red, anemia-pallor), or infections. Characteristics of the distribution of body hair, such as alopecia (sparse or loss of hair) or hirsutism (excessive body hair), or hyperpigmentation of the skin and excessive secondary sexual characteristics (gynecomastia) may indicate endocrine (hormonal—hyperthyroidism, pituitary, or adrenal), CNS, or drug problems.

Examination of the extremities may reveal changes in the color of the skin, presence of bleeding or bruising, arthritic changes in the wrist and fingers, clubbing of the fingertips, or cyanosis of the nail beds. All of these findings may indicate a serious medical problem. Odors may indicate metabolic disorders such as diabetes mellitus (ketoacidosis) or renal disease (uremia).

PRINCIPLES OF CLINICAL EXAMINATION FOR THE HEAD AND NECK

The basic techniques of diagnosis are inspection, palpation, auscultation, percussion, diascopy, and **aspiration.** These techniques are used every time an examination is performed.

Inspection

Inspection is a systematic, standardized observation of a set of criteria performed in an orderly manner to ensure completeness and accuracy of the examination. Inspection includes evaluation of bilateral symmetry, the comparison of the anatomy on one side of the head, face, and neck to the opposite side. Most normal anatomical structures are bilaterally symmetrical. If a structure of the head, face, or neck appears different on one side than the other, this may indicate some pathological process. For example, the clinician performs an inspection of the head (skull), the skin, mucosa, eyes, ears, and other anatomical structures in the head and neck.[1,3]

Palpation

11-A Palpation is used to determine the size, texture, consis-
11-B tency, symmetry, firmness, fluctuant, and other qualities evaluated by the sense of touch. Often a structure cannot be adequately evaluated simply by inspection. The structure must be palpated to determine its true nature. Palpation may be accomplished by using both hands, comparing one side of the head, face, and neck with the other in terms of texture, size, and consistency. This is called *bimanual palpation* (see Fig. 11-6).

In certain cases unilateral palpation may be used to assess anatomical structures. With unilateral palpation, one anatomical structure is pressed against another to assess the contents of that area. In some areas, bidigital palpation (two fingers) may be necessary, as in the floor of the mouth. Bidigital compressions are used when examining lymph nodes. These round nodes may be detected much more easily with a circular motion performed during compression. For example, the clinician may palpate the structures of the neck, lymph nodes, **thyroid gland, salivary glands,** tongue, and the muscles of mastication.[1,3] Students should note the method of palpation used for examination of each structure.

Auscultation

Auscultation is listening to sounds. This may indicate to the dental hygienist whether the structure being evaluated is normal. Auscultation may be performed by listening with the unaided ear or with the assistance of a stethoscope. For example, the clinician may use auscultation to listen to the TMJ for **crepitus** or popping, to measure the blood pressure, and to assess for the presence of bruits in the carotid artery.[1,3]

Percussion

Percussion is performed by tapping on a structure usually with the fingers, hand, or instrument. This evaluation may help the dental hygienist determine whether a structure is sensitive and the relative density of the structure (solid, hollow, or fluid filled). Examples for which percussion are used include the examination of muscles, bones, and teeth.[1,3]

Although not used frequently, the following are diagnostic techniques used to assist in the diagnosis of certain problems.

Diascopy

Diascopy is the examination technique in which the dental hygienist compresses tissue with a glass slide. This examination technique is used to determine whether a lesion is vascular. The glass slide is pressed evenly over the lesion. If the lesion is vascular, it blanches on diascopy and returns to its original color when the pressure is released.

Aspiration

Aspiration is the removal of fluid from a body cavity. The area aspirated may be a soft tissue lesion or a lesion central in bone. A purulent aspirate indicates an inflammatory or infectious process; yellow, straw-colored fluid is consistent with a cyst; a predominance of blood indicates a vascular lesion such as hemangioma; little or no aspirate may indicate a traumatic bone cyst or air embolism.

COMPONENTS OF THE HEENT

Components of the HEENT evaluation include the following:
- Skeletal (bones and cartilage)
- Muscles
- Lymph nodes
- Glands
- **Temporomandibular joint (TMJ)**
- Blood vessels

The head and neck examination begins with the first contact with the patient. When the dental hygienist meets and interviews the patient, the general physical characteristics of habitus, such as body symmetry, posture, stature, and skin color and texture, are evaluated by inspection. This begins the diagnostic process. Palpation follows inspection because it is *only* by palpation that the proper head and neck evaluation can be completed.

Head and Face

The skeletal structure of the head and face develops through a complex series of events. The growth process depends on many factors that must occur properly for normal anatomy and physiology. Variations in skull size and shape may be due to developmental defects, endocrine or metabolic problems, nutritional disorders, or systemic disease. Enlargements of the skull or facial bones may indicate an acquired disease such as pituitary dysfunction (e.g., acromegaly; Fig. 11-1) or an autoimmune connective tissue disease (e.g., Paget's disease). Malignant or benign conditions may affect the size, shape, and symmetry of the head and face; therefore any swellings in the facial structures must be evaluated. Anatomical landmarks are important to every clinical examination. The

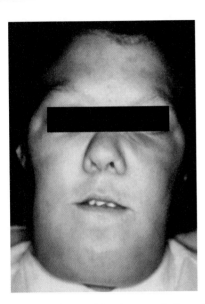

FIG. 11-1 Acromegaly resulting from a pituitary dysfunction.

landmarks in the head and face area are the malar or zygomatic areas, temporal portions of the skull, tragus of the ears, ala of the nose, philtrum of the lip, forehead, and orbits. An evaluation of the patient's skin is an important component of the examination. Any presence of erythema (redness), hyperkeratinization (thickened, white scaly skin), petechiae (ruptured capillaries), ecchymosis or purpura (bruises), angiomas, icteric (yellow, jaundice), or cyanosis (blue, hypoxia) should be noted and evaluated. The above examples are indications of systemic conditions, which may indicate serious medical problems, such as bleeding, infections, rheumatic disease, liver dysfunction, and cardiovascular problems. Hair thickness and distribution may indicate hormonal alterations. Alopecia (hair loss) may be a sign of hyperthyroidism, syphilis, or neurological or psychological problems. Hirsutism (excessive hair growth) may indicate endocrine or other systemic problems.[1,3]

Eyes, Ears, and Nose

The eyes may be the main indicator of systemic disease, such as hyperthyroidism, diabetes, liver disease, CNS disturbances, or infectious diseases. The eyes must be inspected to determine whether they are normal in size, shape, and position. Deviations from normal, such as ptosis (drooping eyelids), nystagmus (rapid, involuntary eyeball movements), hypertelorism, unusually dilated pupils (cranial nerve II or III damage), blue sclera (scleroderma), jaundice (yellow conjunctiva-liver disease), bacterial/viral infections (conjunctivitis), blepharitis (inflamed eyelids), keratoconjunctivitis sicca (dry eyes), retinopathy (diabetes), or exophthalmus (hyperthyroidism) may indicate an underlying medical problem. The examination of the dental patient's ear is limited to the **external auditory meatus** and the preauricular and postauricular areas. The examination of the skin of the ear and nose is performed with the same examination criteria as discussed under the discussion of the head and face.[1,3,7]

Lymph Nodes

Among the most important structures in the head and **11-C** neck are the lymph nodes. Within the boundaries of the head and neck lie hundreds of **lymph nodes** (Table 11-1 and Fig. 11-2). The lymphatic system's major function is to monitor the body's immune system. If infectious organisms or foreign material enter the body and pose a threat of disease, the lymph system activates to remove them. Macrophages engulf bacteria, viruses, and other pathogenic agents. The cellular immune system activates the lymphocytes to neutralize the pathogens. The lymph system removes the pathogens from the body.

During infections the lymph nodes become engorged with immune components, dead cells, and pathogens. The lymph nodes become enlarged and can be palpated. If infections or malignancies are anywhere in the head and neck, the lymph nodes in that anatomical location become enlarged. Lymph nodes may become enlarged during viral infections as influenza, herpes, mononucleosis, human immunodeficiency virus (HIV), chicken pox, colds, and upper respiratory tract infections (URIs). They may also signal bacterial infections, tuberculosis, sinusitis, and fungal infections. Chronic conditions and malignancies also cause lymph node enlargements. Cancer may invade the lymphatic system, in which case the prognosis for survival becomes much more grave. The enlargement of lymph nodes in the head and neck signal important changes that must be recognized by the astute health professional.[1,3,7]

Case Application

You noted enlarged supraclavicular lymph nodes. Given Mr. Jabir's history, what questions might you ask?

Neck (Thyroid)

The thorough examination of the neck is vital. In the mid-line of the neck lies the thyroid gland. The thyroid gland produces hormones that regulate the body's metabolic activities. When abnormalities in tissue development, growth, or hormonal (pituitary) regulation are present, the thyroid tissue may become enlarged. Clinically, this enlargement may be detectable as a goiter (Fig. 11-3). Enlarged thyroid gland tissue may be clinically significant in identifying the patient with hyper- or hypothyroidism. The patient with hyperthyroidism may be at risk for cardiovascular problems (hypertension and arrhythmia).

Adenoma is a neoplasia of the thyroid gland, and early detection of this malignant neoplasm is critical.[1,3,7]

Other abnormalities that appear in the neck are cysts (thyroglossal duct cyst, brachial cleft cysts dermoid cyst, sebaceous cyst, epidermal cyst), muscle problems, tumors, and blood vessel abnormalities such as bruits from atherosclerosis of the carotid arteries. The thorough neck examination reveals these potentially serious conditions.

Salivary Glands

Salivary glands that are infected or obstructed or undergo **11-D** neoplastic changes may become firm and enlarged. The major salivary glands are the paired **submandibular glands** and **parotid glands** (Fig. 11-4). These glands produce more than 90% of all saliva.

The **sublingual glands** and minor salivary glands are small and contribute only about 7% to 8% of saliva. The submandibular glands are located in the posterior part of the mandible and below the floor of the mouth (mylohyoid muscle). These glands are easily palpated even when normal. The ducts of the submandibular glands (Wharton's) exit lingual to the anterior mandibular incisors. The parotid glands are the largest glands and are located on the side of the face anterior to the ear. The ducts of the parotid glands (Stenson's) are located on the superior portion of the buccal mucosa adjacent to the second maxillary molars.[7] The salivary glands or their ducts may become enlarged and painful as a result of a bacterial (*Staphylococcus* or *Streptococcus* organisms) or viral infection. Chronic enlargement of salivary glands may also signal the presence of a neoplasm. Lymphoma, leukemia, adenoid cystic carcinoma, mucoepidermoid carcinoma, and other malignancies may affect the salivary glands. The salivary glands may undergo inflammatory changes as a result of systemic diseases such as Sjögren's syndrome, sicca syndrome, systemic lupus erythematosus, diabetes mellitus, liver disease, and HIV. Salivary gland enlargement may be the result of nutritional deficiencies, chronic alcoholism, or therapy with certain drugs. Sialoliths (calculi or stones) may develop in the ductal system of the salivary glands and cause obstruction. Often the sialoliths can be palpated in the duct, and the gland is enlarged and painful. Any pronounced, prolonged abnormalities of the salivary glands require close monitoring, follow-up, or referral.[1,3]

Muscles

Several muscle groups, including the muscles of mastication, are found in the head and neck region. The muscles in the neck include the sternocleidomastoid, digastrics, omohyoid, and trapezius. These muscles function in mastication, swallowing, positioning, and turning the head. The temporalis, buccinator, masseter, and pterygoid muscles are responsible for mastication and facial expression. Muscle abnormalities are most commonly detected by observing pain upon palpation, changes in the muscle texture or consistency, or a change in head position or facial

TABLE 11-1 Lymph nodes of the head and neck	
Lymph node group	**Areas of drainage**
1. Submental	Tip of tongue, anterior floor of mouth, lower incisors, anterior lower gingiva, mid-lower lip
2. Submandibular	Salivary glands, lips, anterior nose, frontal, maxillary and ethmoid sinuses, buccal mucosa, gingival, teeth (except lower incisors), anterior palate, soft palate, anterior two-thirds of tongue
3. Infrahyoid	Thyroid, larynx, trachea, and part of the pharynx
4. Pretracheal	Thyroid, larynx, trachea, and part of the pharynx
5., 6. Medial and lateral lower deep cervical	Receive lymph drainage from the submental and submandibular lymph nodes. Drainage for the base of the tongue and sublingual region.
7., 8. Medial and lateral upper deep cervical	Receive lymph drainage from the submental and submandibular lymph nodes.
9. Occipital	Skin of posterior scalp
10. Inferior upper deep cervical	Receive lymph drainage from the submental and submandibular lymph nodes. Drainage for the base of the tongue and sublingual region.
11. Nuchal	Skin of back of neck, other nodes
12. Posterior auricular	Skin of scalp and neck, ear
13. Anterior auricular	Ear, skin of face and neck
Not shown on Figure 11-2	
Superficial parotid	Lateral and frontal scalp, ears, eyelids
Deep parotid	Parotid gland, orbit, eyes, conjunctiva
Buccal	Median eyelids, mucous membranes of nose and cheek
Mandibular	Mucous membranes of nose and cheek
Jugulodigastric	Tongue, floor of mouth, lips
Internal jugular	Pharynx, larynx, tonsils, soft palate, tongue
Superficial cervical	Parotid and ear region, angle of the mandible
Spinal accessory	Occipital, nuchal, retroauricular nodes
Supraclavicular	Posterior triangle of neck, spinal accessory nodes, most other nodes

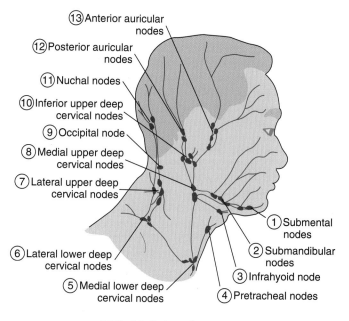

13 Anterior auricular nodes
12 Posterior auricular nodes
11 Nuchal nodes
10 Inferior upper deep cervical nodes
9 Occipital node
8 Medial upper deep cervical nodes
7 Lateral upper deep cervical nodes
6 Lateral lower deep cervical nodes
5 Medial lower deep cervical nodes
1 Submental nodes
2 Submandibular nodes
3 Infrahyoid node
4 Pretracheal nodes

FIG. 11-2 Lymph system.

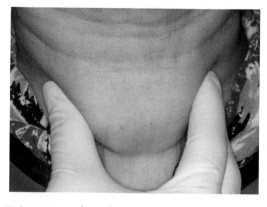

FIG. 11-3 Enlarged thyroid gland tissue (goiter).

expression. Muscles that are enlarged, painful, tender, firm and/or cramping may indicate infection, neoplasia, dysfunction, autoimmune inflammatory connective tissue diseases, metabolic or endocrine disorders, or emotional-psychological disturbances.[1,3]

Bones and Cartilage

Thyroid cartilage, cricoid cartilage, and the tracheal rings are found in the anterior median part of the neck. The cartilage structures provide support and protection to critical structures in the neck. They protect the thyroid gland, the major blood vessels, and the trachea. The hyoid (free-floating bone) is responsible for swallowing.[7]

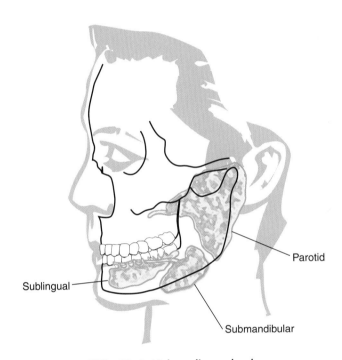

FIG. 11-4 Major salivary glands.

Labels: Sublingual, Parotid, Submandibular

Blood Vessels

The head and neck region has an extensive blood vessel network. The major blood vessels in the neck are the common carotid artery, which branches into the internal and external carotid arteries, and the jugular vein. With advancing atherosclerosis and cardiovascular disease, edema and engorgement of these blood vessels may occur. Many blood vessels are in the face, paraoral structures, eyes, nose, and skin. The blood vessels may become dilated, ruptured, or aneurysmal, resulting in the clinical appearance of petechiae, telangiectasias, angiomas, purpura, hematomas, and ecchymoses. This may indicate the presence of a serious hematologic abnormality and/or bleeding problem.[1,3,7]

Temporomandibular Joint

The temporomandibular joint (TMJ) is found just in front of the ear. The TMJ may be examined by palpation and auscultation (Fig. 11-5). Palpating with the index finger, index and middle finger over the head of the condyle, or a finger just inside the external auditory meatus, allows the dental hygienist to evaluate the function of the TMJ. Auscultation for joint sounds may be accomplished by listening with the unaided ear or with a stethoscope placed over the TMJ (Fig. 11-5). With TMJ dysfunction the dental hygienist may observe obvious deviations in movement as the mandible is opened and closed or moves laterally and/or tenderness, pain, crepitus, cracking, and/or popping during the mandibular movements. Subluxation (locking in the open mandibular position) may occur in advanced TMJ dysfunction.[1,3]

Head and Neck Examination

The HEENT examination begins with the initial encounter with patients: meeting them in the reception area, reviewing their medical history, continuous observing, and then performing the clinical examination. Figs. 11-6 through 11-12 illustrate a sequence and examination of structures in the head and neck. Box 11-2 lists common abnormal findings in the examination of the head and neck.

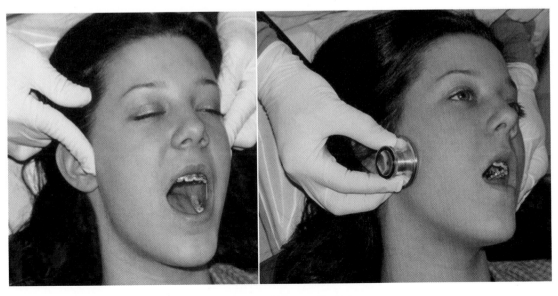

FIG. 11-5 TMJ examination.

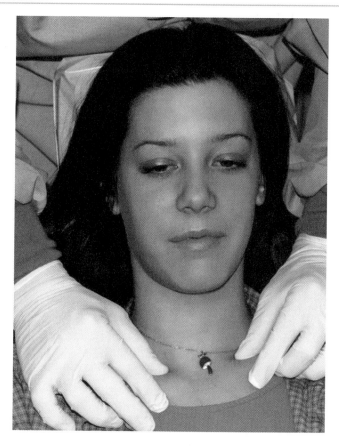

FIG. 11-6 Inspection and bimanual, bidigital palpation. *Anatomical landmarks*: sternum, clavicles. *Structures*: supraclavicular lymph nodes. *Instructions*: The clinician proceeds laterally along the clavicles, pressing down into the supraclavicular triangle and the top of the clavicles, using bidigital circular compression until the trapezius muscle is reached.

FIG. 11-7 Palpation. *Anatomical landmarks*: tracheal rings, cricoid cartilage, thyroid cartilage, hyoid bone, mental protuberance. *Structures*: thyroid gland, submental lymph nodes. *Instructions*: The clinician returns to the sternum and palpates upward in the midline of the neck. The thyroid gland is palpated with the use of bidigital compression. The clinician proceeds upward and palpates the cricoid cartilage and submental lymph nodes.

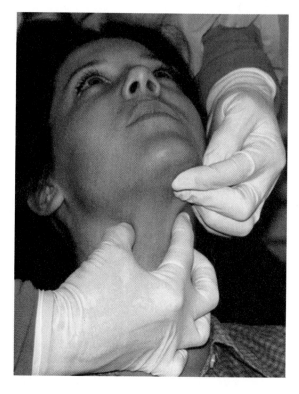

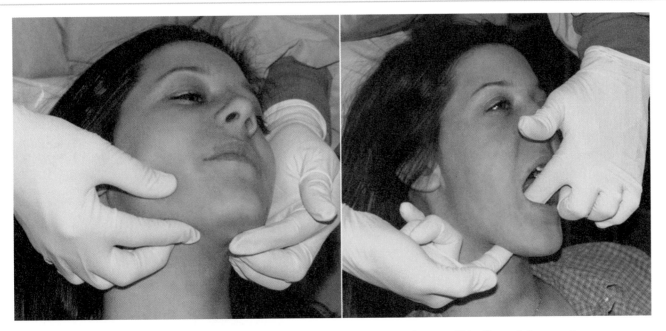

FIG. 11-8 Bimanual, bidigital palpation. *Anatomical landmarks*: mandible, floor of the mouth. *Structures*: mylohyoid muscle, submandibular salivary gland, submandibular lymph nodes. *Instructions*: The clinician palpates under the chin and along the mandible. With one digit compressing the floor of the mouth and another digit placed medially to the inferior border of the mandible, the clinician palpates the submandibular gland and the submandibular lymph nodes.

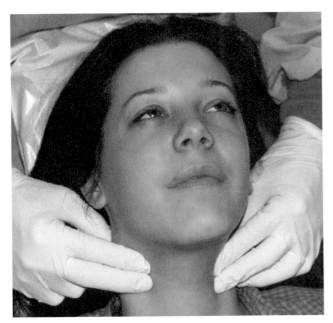

FIG. 11-9 Bimanual, bidigital, circular compression for nodes. *Anatomical landmarks:* sternocleidomastoid muscle, trachea. *Structures:* lymph nodes (jugulodigastric, anterior cervical, accessory, posterior (cervical), carotid artery, jugular vein, skin. *Instructions:* The clinician palpates the anterior aspect of the sternocleidomastoid muscle. The cervical and jugular lymph nodes and the vessels may be detected by palpating the tissue medial to the sternocleidomastoid muscle. The carotid artery (pulse) is palpated here. The clinician palpates the posterior aspect of the sternocleidomastoid muscle (accessory and posterior cervical lymph nodes) down to the insertion of the trapezius muscle and then moves posterior to the cervical spine.

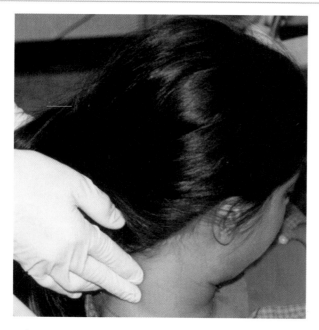

FIG. 11-10 Bimanual palpation. *Anatomical landmarks:* cervical vertebrae, base of skull. *Structures:* lymph nodes (nuchal, occipital), trapezius muscle, skin. *Instructions:* The clinician proceeds bilaterally up the cervical spine, palpating for lymph nodes.

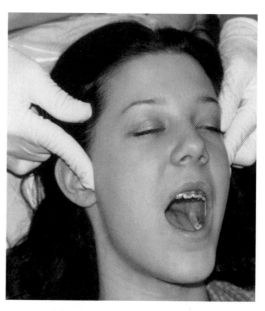

FIG. 11-12 Palpation, bimanual auscultation. *Anatomical landmarks:* TMJ. *Structures:* TMJ. *Instructions:* The examination of the TMJ may be performed by palpation during mandibular excursions. This evaluation may be performed more accurately by using a stethoscope. The masseter muscles, parotid gland, and the facial lymph nodes are examined by movement of the fingers over the lateral aspect of the ramus of the mandible and palpation of the facial tissues (cheek).

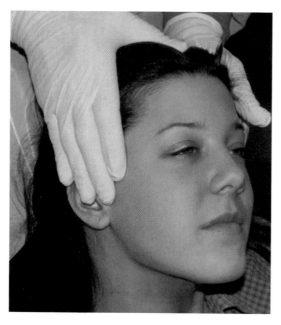

FIG. 11-11 Bimanual palpation. *Anatomical landmarks:* ear, TMJ. *Structures:* lymph nodes, parotid gland, TMJ, skin. *Instructions:* The clinician moves anteriorly to the ears and palpates the posterior auricular lymph nodes and the anterior auricular nodes. The hands are moved upward, and the temporalis muscles are palpated while the patient goes through mandibular excursions. The masseter muscle also may be palpated by movement of the hands down to the cheek and request that the patient clench the teeth.

BOX 11-2

Common Abnormal Findings: Head and Neck

Lymphadenopathy
Hypertrophy of the salivary glands
Thyroid hyperplasia or neoplasia (including adenoma, carcinoma, or goiter)
Dermoid cyst
Sebaceous cyst
Epidermal cyst
Sialadenitis, sialadenopathy
Lipoma

Data from Bricker S, Langlais R, Miller C: *Oral Diagnosis, oral medicine and treatment planning,* Philadelphia, 1994, Lea and Febiger; and Coleman G, Nelson J: *Principles of oral diagnosis,* St Louis, 1992, Mosby.

SUPPLEMENTAL DIAGNOSTIC AIDS

The HEENT examination is primarily one of screening for deviations from normal anatomy and physiology. The dental hygienist may not determine the definitive diagnosis based on the clinical examination; therefore additional diagnostic techniques and evaluations are required to obtain further diagnostic information. These adjunctive diagnostic aids are shown in Table 11-2.

TABLE 11-2

Adjunctive diagnostic aids

Diagnostic aid	Description
Radiographic imaging	Additional radiographs (Waters projection, lateral skull, etc.), CT scans, MRIs, videofluoroscopy, other tomograms, arthrograms, sialograms, etc.
Laboratory tests	Blood tests, microbiological cultures, antibody tests, biopsy, and histologic examination
Special tests	Exfoliative cytology, DNA–PCR, ELISA, salivary function tests, and electromyography

DNA–PCR, Deoxyribonucleic acid–polymerase chain reaction; *ELISA,* enzyme-linked immunosorbent assay; *CT,* computed tomography; *MRI,* magnetic resonance imaging.

VITAL SIGNS

The measurement of the vital signs is an essential component of the patient's database. Physicians use the vital signs to evaluate, diagnose, and to treat their patients. In the early 1900s the leading cause of death was infectious diseases.[10] The medical community developed a standardized assessment to help diagnose the leading medical problem at that time, infections. The standardized assessment became known as the "vital signs" and consisted of the temperature, pulse rate, and respiratory rate.

Blood pressure became a later addition to the vital signs. Today the healthcare professional is faced with a different leading cause of illness and death: tobacco use. Cigarettes are responsible for more than 430,000 deaths annually.[2] As in the past, the vital signs should assess the leading cause of morbidity and mortality of patients.[1,3,7,8] A strong movement in the healthcare professions is underway to make tobacco assessment the "new vital sign." To actually do so would place the healthcare provider at the forefront in embracing the guidelines of the United States Preventive Services Task Force and the National Health Promotion and Disease Prevention Objectives for the Year 2000. As part of the healthcare delivery team, the dental hygienist must take the lead in the promotion and implementation of tobacco assessment as the "new vital sign."[4]

 ## *TEMPERATURE*

11-E An elevated temperature is not an illness. It is how the body stimulates the immune system to defend against infection. To get an accurate temperature, the patient should not have smoked or consumed hot or cold beverages or food for at least 10 minutes before the placement of the oral thermometer. The patient should be resting, either sitting or lying down. Knowledge of the patient's medications is important.[1,3,8]

Normal Temperature

Normal temperature is 98.6° F, or 37° C. The human body has a circadian rhythm with regard to body temperature. The temperature changes during the day with lower readings in the morning and higher readings in the evening.

Hyperthermia

Body temperatures above normal are as follows:
- Slight = normal to 101° F
- Moderate = 101° to 103° F
- High = 103° F or greater

The causes of elevation of body temperature are the following:
- Excessive exercise: increased metabolism
- Infection
- Inflammatory diseases
- Hyperthyroidism: increased metabolic demand
- Factitious causes (purposeful elevation of thermometer reading)

Hypothermia

Causes of hypothermia are the following:
- Hypothyroidism
- Certain viral infections
- Chronic debilitating diseases
- Excessive alcohol intake

PULSE

When taking the pulse, the clinician should ensure **11-F** the patient is seated comfortably. The count should be for 60 seconds. In addition to the rate, the dental hygienist should also assess the rhythm and the force. The most commonly used site for taking the pulse is the radial artery; however, the facial artery and the carotid artery also may be used. The clinician should palpate with the pads of the fingers rather than the thumb.[1,3,8]

Pulse Rate

Normal

The rate varies with the activity, age, and the body's demand for oxygen. The pulse rate varies from 60 to 90 beats/minute in the normal adult and 80 to 120 beats/minute in the normal child. Well-trained athletes may have rates as low as 45 to 60 beats/minute. A rate of 100 beats/minute in the adult is considered to be the upper limit of normal in the relaxed, nonanxious state. Loss of consciousness may occur below 40 beats/minute. A rate of less than 60 beats/minute or more than 110 beats/minute in the adult dental patient with an unremarkable medical history should be investigated/referred.

Sinus Rhythm

Sinus rhythm is the beat of the normal heart with ventricular systoles equally separated in the series and with normal cardiac conduction originating in the sinoatrial node.

Sinus Bradycardia

Sinus bradycardia is a pulse rate less than 60 beats/minute. This rate may be normal for some individuals or secondary to either (1) reduced metabolic from hypothermia, hypothyroidism, or hypoadrenalism or (2) cardiotonic agents or beta blockers.

Sinus Tachycardia

Sinus tachycardia defines a pulse rate greater than 100 beats/minute. It may occur with the

- exercise
- anxiety
- hyperthyroidism
- anemia
- decreased blood volume
- elevated temperature (5 to 10 beats/minute increase for every degree Fahrenheit increase in temperature)
- heart disease

Pulse Rhythm

An even, regular force and rate is what is interpreted as "normal." Regular rate and rhythm may be abbreviated as *rrr*.

Atrial fibrillation describes a total/complete irregularity of the pulse. In atrial fibrillation, the atria do not contract as units; different segments contract separately. Numerous stimuli arrive in complete disorder at the atrioventricular (AV) node. A small number of stimuli are transmitted to the ventricles at irregular intervals.

A 60-second examination of the pulse is mandatory to check for atrial fibrillation. Atrial fibrillation can result from the following: coronary heart disease, mitral stenosis, or hyperthyroidism.

Premature ventricular contractions (PVCs) are ectopic beats or systoles recognized as a pronounced pause in an otherwise normal rhythm. These are caused by an abnormal focus of electrical activity in the ventricles that triggers ventricular contraction. When the next normal impulse arising at the sinoatrial (SA) node arrives at the atrioventricular (AV) node, the ventricles are refractory and do not contract until the next impulse from the SA node.

Although PVCs are not significant in the healthy adult, they are significant when found in a patient with cardiovascular disease, such as coronary heart disease, congestive heart failure, valvular disease, or hypertension. Five PVCs during a 60-second pulse examination in a patient with a history of myocardial infarction (MI) should be urged to seek medical consultation.

RESPIRATION

11-G The type, rate, and depth of breathing should be observed in the patient at rest. The patient has some control over respiration; therefore the rate should be determined without the patient's conscious knowledge, possibly while taking the pulse.[1,3,8]

Normal Respiration

The normal rate of respiration is 12 to 20 breaths/minute for the healthy adult, 24 to 28 for children, and 44 for infants. The rate should be equal and the rhythm regular. The rate, however, is affected by several factors, including the following:

- Age (the rate increases with an increase in age)
- Gender
- High altitudes
- Exercise
- Elevated temperature (increases by 4 breaths/minute for each degree Fahrenheit elevation)
- Metabolic acidosis/alkalosis
- Emotional stress
- Odors

Abnormalities in Respiratory Rate

Respiration in males is diaphragmatic, and the use of chest muscles indicates air hunger. In females, respiration is costal, and the use of the diaphragm could indicate air hunger (dyspnea or SOB). Use of the accessory muscles (neck and shoulder) could indicate dyspnea associated with congestive heart failure, bronchial asthma, or emphysema. Expiration is prolonged in emphysema; pursing of the lips during expiration may be observed, which helps hold the collapsing smaller bronchi and bronchioles open.

Tachypnea, or rapid breathing, can be observed during excitement, stress, exercise, elevated temperature, or metabolic acidosis.

Dyspnea, or difficulty in breathing, can occur in congestive heart failure, congenital heart anomalies, emphysema, pneumonia, or tuberculosis. When dyspnea occurs when the patient is in the supine position, termed *orthopnea,* it is best to perform dental procedures with the patient in an upright position.

Hyperventilation, or deep and rapid breathing, may be observed under emotional stress or diabetic ketoacidosis.

BLOOD PRESSURE

In 1896 Riva-Rocci introduced a sphygmomanometer. In **11-H** 1905 Korotkoff, with the use of the Riva-Rocci sphygmomanometer, introduced the auscultatory method for measuring systolic and diastolic blood pressures.[1,3,5,8] Taking and recording blood pressure is an important part of the examination procedure in dentistry. Opportunity to screen for hypertension is great because patients seek dental care five times more often than medical care. Undiagnosed cases of hypertension may easily be referred for treatment.

Guidelines for High Blood Pressure

In general, it is considered high if an individual's blood pressure is consistently 140/90 mm Hg or higher. For healthy people age 18 or older, Table 11-3 recommends actions to take based on initial blood pressure checks.

Prehypertension

Prehypertension is a systolic pressure ranging from 120 to 139 or a diastolic pressure ranging from 80 to 89. This category underscores the increase health risks as blood pressure rises and underscores the need for better education of healthcare professionals and the public to prevent the development of hypertension. As with all categories, only one of the numbers, either systolic or diastolic needs to be high for the reading to meet these criteria.

Hypertension

Common causes for secondary hypertension include renal artery stenosis/thrombosis; hyperaldosteronism; Cushing's disease; or coarctation of the aorta.

Hypotension

Conversely, hypotension may be the result of syncope, hypoadrenalism (Addison's disease), hypothyroidism, heart failure, anemias, or systemic lupus erythematosus.

TABLE 11-3
What blood pressure means*

Systolic		Diastolic	Group	What to do*
Below 120	and	Below 80	Normal blood pressure	Maintain a healthy lifestyle
120-139	or	180-190	Prehypertension	Adopt a healthy lifestyle
140-159	or	90-99	Stage 1 hypertension	Adopt a healthy lifestyle; take medication
160 or more	or	100 or more	Stage 2 hypertension	Adopt a healthy lifestyle; take medication

* If heart disease, diabetes or kidney disease are present, blood pressure needs to be managed more aggressively. This table recognizes high blood pressure as a single condition.
Source: *Seventh Report of the Joint National Committee on Prevention, Detection, Evaluation and Treatment of High Blood Pressure, 2003.* Numbers expressed in millimeters of mercury (mm Hg).

Orthostatic Hypotension

Orthostatic hypotension is syncope brought on by a sudden change from the horizontal position to the upright position or by prolonged standing (peripheral pooling). Occasionally, patients who stand up quickly after being reclined in a dental chair for a prolonged period of time experience orthostatic hypotension. The clinician should advise all patients to sit for just a minute, before standing, after a dental procedure.

Patients at risk for orthostatic hypotension are those who take narcotics, tranquilizers, or antihypertensive agents or who suffer from diabetic neuropathy or Addison's disease.

Determination of Blood Pressure

The following procedure determines blood pressure:
1. The deflated cuff of the sphygmomanometer is placed on the patient's arm, which is held at heart level. The inflatable bladder of the cuff should be placed over the brachial artery; the lower edge of the cuff should be about 1 inch above the antecubital fossa.
2. The cuff is fastened evenly and snugly.
3. The stethoscope endpiece is placed over the brachial artery. The clinician locates and holds fingers on the radial pulse.
4. With the needle valve closed (air lock), the cuff is inflated until the radial pulse stops. The clinician notes the level of mercury. The dial is pumped 20 to 30 mm Hg beyond the point at which the radial pulse stopped. This is the MIL, maximum inflation level.
5. Using the endpiece of the stethoscope, the clinician listens for the first sound or tap as the air lock is slowly and gradually released. This is the systolic reading.
6. As air is continuously released from the cuff, the sound becomes louder, then gradually muffled, and disappears.
7. The number on the dial at the last distinct sound is the diastolic pressure reading.

FIG. 11-13 Tobacco assessment form.

BOX 11-3
Five *A*'s of Tobacco Treatment

Ask the patient about tobacco use.
Advise the patient as to the effects of tobacco use on overall health.
Assess the patient's level of interest in stopping tobacco use.
Assist the patient by providing nicotine and nonnicotine replacement products.
Arrange for periodic assessments to evaluate progress.

TOBACCO ASSESSMENT

The impetus to make tobacco assessment the fifth vital sign is based on the devastating impact that tobacco use has on overall health (see Chapter 12).[4]

A tobacco assessment might appear as in Fig. 11-13.

Box 11-3 outlines the five *A*'s of tobacco treatment. If the patient gives a positive present history of tobacco use *(ask)*, the dental healthcare worker should *advise* the patient to quit. The patient may not be able to quit using tobacco *(assess)* without help *(assist)*.

The dental clinician should be knowledgeable in counseling the patient in tobacco treatment and developing treatment strategies that may include nicotine replacement (gum, patch, inhaler, nasal spray, and/or the nonnicotine replacement approach [Zyban]). Nicotine is an addictive compound, and tobacco products are the recognized nicotine delivery systems. Stopping the use of an addicting substance may be difficult. The tobacco user should be contacted during treatment at regular intervals to assess progress *(arrange)*. The clinician should expect a modest success rate among patients who attempt to stop their tobacco use. A high relapse rate exists for these patients.[6,9]

REFERRALS AND CONSULTATIONS

Often the knowledge and experience of the dental hygienist is not sufficient to allow for the determination of all possible definitive diagnoses or differential diagnoses.

This is the point in which the astute professional realizes that additional expertise is needed and a consultation is in order. Consultation with a dental specialist (oral medicine, oral pathology, oral surgery) or physician (otolaryngologist, oncologist, dermatologist, or internist) is man- dated when the dental healthcare professional is uncertain of the significance of clinical findings. After the referral, the clinician should always follow up with the patient and/or the consultant to determine the outcome and results of the referral.

RITICAL THINKING ACTIVITIES

1. Take your blood pressure before and after a lab examination. Note which number increased. Why do you think this number increased?
2. Take your blood pressure and then drink 16 oz. of water. Wait 20 minutes without urinating, retake your blood pressure, and compare the readings. Explain the difference noted in the readings.
3. Select three to five patient records. Record vital signs on a sheet of paper. Identify whether these are within normal ranges. Review the medical history and correlate your findings with the vital signs.
4. Evaluate the temporomandibular joint (TMJ) of a minimum of six classmates, family members, or others. Record your findings identifying the number of individuals who had a problem with the TMJ based on your examination. Compare this with the individual's subjective appraisal of problems with this joint.
5. Take a photograph of your face or that of a classmate's. Make sure the eyes are wide open. Draw a line through the midsagittal plane. Draw another line through the pupils. Assess for symmetry.

REVIEW QUESTIONS

1. An examination of the lymph nodes of the head and neck region uses which examination technique?
   a. Palpation
   b. Percussion
   c. Auscultation
   d. Probing
2. Examination of the temporomandibular joint uses which of the following examination techniques?
   a. Probing and percussion
   b. Palpation and percussion
   c. Auscultation and palpation
   d. Auscultation and probing
3. A neoplastic lesion located on the ventrolateral surface of the tongue in the middle third of the tongue may result in an enlargement of which node?
   a. Submental node
   b. Submandibular node
   c. Jugulodigastric node
   d. Mandibular (facial) node
4. Periapical abscesses and/or severe, active periodontal disease may result in an enlargement of which lymph node?
   a. Submental node
   b. Submandibular node
   c. Jugulodigastric node
   d. Mandibular (facial) node
5. Which of the following statements is false?
   a. The thyroid gland is located in the midline of the neck.
   b. A decrease in the size of the thyroid gland is consistent with a hypothyroid condition.
   c. Thyroid hormones regulate metabolic activities.
   d. An enlarged thyroid gland is a significant clinical finding.

6. Which of the following statements is false?
   a. The parotid and submandibular salivary glands produce more than 90% of all saliva.
   b. The parotid gland located anterior to the ear secretes its saliva into the oral cavity via Stenson's duct.
   c. Salivary glands may become inflamed as a result of diabetes mellitus, lupus erythematosus, and/or Sjögren's syndrome.
   d. The submandibular gland is located in the posterior mandible and thus cannot be palpated.
7. Which vital signs are elevated/increased or changed during an infection?
   a. Blood pressure, pulse, and respiration
   b. Pulse, respiration, and temperature
   c. Blood pressure and temperature
   d. Respirations and blood pressure
8. Tobacco assessment is being promoted as the fifth vital sign because tobacco use is the leading cause of morbidity and mortality today. The five A's are used in tobacco treatment (cessation). Which is the correct sequence of the five A's?
   a. Ask, answer, advise, arrange, assist
   b. Advise, answer, assist, arrange, ask
   c. Ask, advise, assess, assist, arrange
   d. Ask, answer, advise, arrange, assist
9. Elective medical and dental procedures should not be performed when the patient's blood pressure is which of the following?
   a. 140/90
   b. 180/110
   c. 140/100
   d. 160/100

REVIEW QUESTIONS—cont'd

10. **Which of the following statements is false?**
    a. The hypertensive patient can be treated by the dental healthcare worker in the horizontal (reclined) position without any potential for an adverse occurrence.
    b. Infection is the leading cause for an elevated temperature.
    c. The dental healthcare worker may detect an undiagnosed hyperthyroid patient by assessing the pulse rate (extremely elevated, 110+).
    d. The hypertensive patient whose blood pressure is maintained in the normal range is not expected to develop end organ damage.

SUGGESTED AGENCIES AND WEB SITES

Because of the ever-changing nature of the Internet, some of the web sites listed here may have changed since publication. Please refer to Mosby's Evolve web site for the most current information.

American Cancer Society: http://www.cancer.org
American Heart Association ("High blood pressure: AHA recommendation"): http://www.americanheart.org
Baylor College of Dentistry ("Detecting cancer through the extraoral examination"): http://www.tambcd.edu
Cansearch (a guide to cancer resources on the Internet): http://www.cansearch.org
Centers for Disease Control and Prevention, National Center for Chronic Disease Prevention and Health Promotion ("Oral health resources"): http://www.cdc.gov
Homestead Schools, Inc. ("Oral examination"): http://www.homesteadschools.com
National Heart, Lung, and Blood Institute, National High Blood Pressure Education Program: http://hin.nhlbi.nih.gov
National Institute of Dental and Craniofacial Research ("Oral cancer: confronting the enemy"); National Institutes of Health, 31 Center Drive MSC 2290, Bethesda, MD 20892: http://www.nidr.nih.gov

National Institutes of Health: U.S. Department of Health and Human Services, 31 Center Drive MSC 2290, Bethesda, MD 20892: http://www.nih.gov
National Institute on Aging ("High blood pressure: a common but controllable disorder"): http://www.nih.gov
National Oral Health Information Clearinghouse: http://www.nohic.nidcr.nih.gov/
NOAH (New York Online Access to Health): http://www.noahhealth.org
National Institutes of Health ("Surgeon general's report on oral health"): http://www.nidcr.nih.gov

ADDITIONAL READINGS AND RESOURCES

American Heart Association: National Center, 7272 Greenville Avenue, Dallas, TX 75231; (214) 373-6300.
Centers for Disease Control and Prevention: National Center for Chronic Disease Prevention and Health Promotion: Division of Oral Health, 1600 Clifton Road, Atlanta, GA 30333; (404) 639-3311.
National Institute of Dental Research: Building 31, Room 2C35, 31 Center Drive MSC 2290, Bethesda, MD 20892-2290.

The National Institute on Aging Information Center: P.O. Box 8057, Gaithersburg, MD 20898-8057; (800) 222-2225; TTY (800) 222-4225.
U.S. Department of Health and Human Services, Public Health Service, National Institutes of Health.

REFERENCES

1. Bricker S, Langlais R, Miller C: *Oral Diagnosis, oral medicine, and treatment planning,* Philadelphia, 1994, Lea and Febiger.
2. Centers for Disease Control and Prevention: Smoking attributable mortality and years of potential life lost (United States, 1988), *MMWR* 266(3):139-44, 1991.
3. Coleman G, Nelson J: *Principles of oral diagnosis,* St Louis, 1992, Mosby.
4. Fiore MC: The new vital sign: assessing and documenting smoking status, *J Am Med Assoc* 266(22):3183-4, 1991.
5. Glick M: New guidelines for prevention, detection, evaluation, and treatment of high blood pressure, *J Am Dent Assoc* 129:1588-94, 1998.
6. Glynn TJ, Manley MW: *How to help your patients stop smoking,* NIH Publication No. 98-3064, June 1998.
7. Halstead C et al: *Physical evaluation of the dental patient,* St Louis, 1982, Mosby.
8. Little JW et al: *Dental management of the medically compromised patient,* ed 6, St Louis, (in press), Mosby.
9. Mecklenburg RE et al: *How to help your patients stop using tobacco,* NIH Publication No. 98-3191, August 1998.
10. Musker DM, Dominquiez EA, Boro-Sela A: Edward Seguin and the social powers of thermometry, *N Engl J Med* 316(2):115-7, 1987.

CHAPTER 12

Tobacco *and* Chemical Dependencies

Robert E. Mecklenburg, Cathy L. Backinger

Chapter Outline

Seduction
Addiction
Intended Consequences
Case Study: Helping a Patient Quit Tobacco Use
Results
Costs of Tobacco Habit
Smokeless/Spit Tobacco
Other Tobacco Products
Essential Elements of Patient History
 Risks
 Initiation
 Progression
Dependence
Relapse
Diagnosis of nicotine dependency and
 addiction
Rituals
Environmental stimuli
Quitting
Techniques, Procedures, and Supportive Evidence
 Helpful methods
 First visit
 Follow-up visits
The Team Approach

Key Terms

Acetylcholine
Addiction
Bidis

Dopamine
Kretek
Neurotransmitters

Nicotine dependence
Norepinephrine
Quid

Serotonin
Tobacco
Tobacco cessation

Learning Outcomes

1. Recognize various ways that tobacco use undermines oral health and dental practice.
2. Recognize that nicotine and other chemical dependencies are chronic, progressive, relapsing conditions of the brain, which alter vital neural functions.
3. Recognize common symptoms of nicotine and other drug dependencies and withdrawal.
4. Recognize that nicotine dependency can be effectively treated with modest, scientifically established methods and periodic reinforcement.

5. Use basic behavioral and pharmacotherapeutic intervention services in clinical practice.
6. Establish clinic policies and practices that ensure routine identification of patient tobacco use status and appropriate methods for care and follow-up.
7. Refer selected patients for specialized treatment of their nicotine and other drug dependencies.
8. Develop an appropriate tobacco cessation program for a patient.
9. Become familiar with forms of tobacco sold in your locale.

Contrary to the thinking presented by Aesop, Hans Christian Andersen, Rudyard Kipling, Walt Disney, and other animators, animals are not anthropomorphic. Living in the thin moment of the present, animals do not share the human abilities of assigning meaning to observations or possess foresight, abstract thought, or self-consciousness. Yet people, beneath these human attributes, do share with animals many basic drives essential to individual well-being and species continuity—drives such as drinking, eating, reproducing, socializing, and avoiding harm.

These basic survival attributes are finely developed in the central nervous system (CNS), especially the brain, as a result of eons of complex, continuing interaction between genetic architecture and environmental stimuli.[2] Early in a person's life, billions of dendritic connections form between neurons, as many as 10,000 per neuron. Many such pathways atrophy if they are not used during growth or if they fall into disuse later. Other pathways assume key roles in human interactions with the environment. Constant interplay between nature and nurture (between genetic makeup and experience) makes people who they are—unique but within limits.

At the chemical level, neurons communicate using *neurotransmitters.* These are monoamines such as *acetylcholine, norepinephrine, serotonin,* and *dopamine.* The release of neurotransmitters at neural clefts stimulates, inhibits, and modulates neural function, hormone production, and other processes through an unimaginably complex system. This system regulates automatic functions and willed behaviors needed to maintain life and one's sense of well-being. Millions of monoamines are carefully metered out by neurons and then, within microseconds of transmitting their signals though synaptic clefts, are cleared away by reuptake into the producing neurons or destroyed by catalysts such as monoamine oxidase. In this symphony of interactions between neurons in the core structures of the brain and neocortex, the brain and mind merge. Other systems throughout the body exist primarily to provide the oxygen, food, and sensory stimuli that nurture the dynamic processes of being, which are expressed in the brain.

SEDUCTION

The human brain is in constant danger of being devastated by psychoactive chemicals. These subvert an individual's perceptions, feelings, personality, and judgment so that the mind gradually changes forever in both subtle and gross ways. Trauma, toxins, and infectious agents only threaten cell viability, but nicotine, alcohol, heroin, opium, cocaine, marijuana, hallucinogens, and other stimulants, depressants, and perception-altering chemicals transform neural cells themselves by altering neurotransmitter functions. They create "liking" feelings that reinforce repetitive use. Neural pathways, neural receptors, and other cell and chemical structures change to compensate for the artificially produced stimuli. As neurons adjust to repeated exposure, the individual gradually increases exposure to "once more" achieve the desired mood-altering effect. The disease is progressive. It erodes basic animal drives and higher human satisfactions as life gradually becomes centered on drug seeking, using, and recovery.

ADDICTION

Once neurons adjust so that their functions are "normal" only in the presence of a psychoactive substance, the sudden absence of the substance creates a neurotransmitter signal deficiency and hormone imbalances that clinically produce impaired emotions, motor skills, and thought processes. Without the artificial stimulus, brain and body react to a sudden plunge in monoamine levels. Feelings of acute anxiety and stress and an inability to concentrate and perform replace the sense of well-being that existed in the presence of the substance. Other conditions commonly occur, such as insomnia, irritability, decreased heart rate, increased appetite, and weight gain.

Long-term psychoactive drug users receive little "pleasure" from their drugs. Rather, use is driven by a compelling need to prevent withdrawal symptoms. What users interpret as "pleasure" is merely relief from the symptoms of withdrawal. Users are trapped when the brain's delicate signal system has been altered, sometimes long before use has even become a daily preoccupation. By definition, individuals who use *tobacco,* alcohol, or other psychoactive substances are at risk of developing a substance-specific chronic, progressive, relapsing disease.[18]

Environmental conditions are often as important as the substance's action. Environments associated with use trigger craving and anticipation. Certain times, places, or events act as cues that stimulate craving for the substance. These social and psychological stimuli become part of the *addiction.* Ritual preparations for use heighten anticipation and concentrate perceptions. Motor pathways that develop with repetitive use become deeply imbedded in patterns of daily living.

Drug seeking, using, and recovery behaviors may overtake important basic motives and behaviors necessary for survival and fundamental to a sense of well-being. The subtle joys people experience from non–drug-related activities become dulled. They often experience diminished intellectual curiosity, lack of interest in accomplishment, inability to effectively organize, altered appetites and sexual desire, impaired social interaction, increased risk-taking behaviors, and limited concern for personal integrity. Indeed, drug-dependent individuals often engage in risky and illegal behaviors to sustain their drug use. Dependency on nicotine, the most prevalent of the drugs that alter brain function, seldom leads to the ethical and legal compromises typically encountered when other drugs are used because tobacco is relatively inexpensive, easily obtained, and still socially acceptable in some environments.[20]

INTENDED CONSEQUENCES

Most adverse mental and physical conditions are inadvertent, perhaps a result of injury, infection, aging, or a genetic glitch. The tragedy of most chemical dependencies, including *nicotine dependence,* is that they occur because of willful exploitation by industries willing to sacrifice a drug user's dignity, health, well-being, and even life itself, for self-serving motives.[35] During the twentieth century, the tobacco industry has produced persuasive campaigns directed at girls and women.[7,28,29] Also, this industry has secured many exemptions from government oversight,

Case Study **Helping a Patient Quit Tobacco Use**

The Patient as a Person

Paula Evans is a 22-year-old who plans to begin a new job in 2 weeks. She wants to start with a good impression, so she is requesting dental hygiene services and a dental checkup before she enters her new position. She says, "I need this job to begin to pay off my school debts and become more independent."

When you inquire about her general health, Ms. Evans states that she tries to take care of herself. She says, "I exercise twice a week." On reviewing her health history forms you verify that she is not aware of any illnesses, not taking any drugs, and is not pregnant. She volunteers, "One day I want to settle down and have a family, but for now I enjoy being single." Her health history form discloses that she smokes, on average, about a pack of cigarettes a day and has for about 5 years. She has her first cigarette within a half hour of waking and smokes about 15 cigarettes a day. Inquiring about this, you learn that she smokes the most during social occasions, which are frequent. You learn that Ms. Evans began smoking when she was 13 and never intended to be smoking after she graduated from high school. She tried to quit twice. About 4 years ago she quit for a couple of weeks but then relapsed when drinking "maybe a little too much at a party." She tried to quit again 2 years ago but began again after a week because she was feeling irritable and "blue" and noticed that she had gained 4 pounds.

Diagnosis and Treatment Plan

Ms. Evan's vital signs are normal. An oral examination shows that she is caries-free and that the few restorations present are sound. Although her oral hygiene was good, the upper anterior gingival area was fibrous and the mesiopalatal probe depths of 3 molars measure 4 to 5 mm.

Ms. Evans is not aware that she has become nicotine dependent, nor that, as young as she is, her smoking is beginning to compromise her desire to be healthy and attractive. The peripheral vasoconstriction properties of nicotine inhibit gingival bleeding and are masking her early-stage periodontal disease.

such as the Consumer Products Safety Act, and insulated itself from liability for tobacco-related injuries, such as by the 1998 settlement with state attorneys general.[21] Huge profits have helped tobacco companies secure a position of power and influence.

RESULTS

- Approximately 46 million adults smoke cigarettes, and millions use other forms of tobacco.
- More than 80% of daily users become dependent before they are legally old enough to buy tobacco, that is, ready to make a rational choice.[38]
- Of those individuals who experiment with cigarette smoking, alcohol, cocaine, heroin, and other drugs, a higher proportion become dependent using cigarettes.[3]
- Those individuals who are dependent on multiple substances report that quitting tobacco use is more difficult than quitting use of other substances.[3]
- In addition to cigarette use, tobacco use involves smokeless tobacco (also called *spit tobacco,* including both oral snuff and chewing tobacco), cigars, pipe tobacco, and newer forms of tobacco such as *bidis* and *kretek*
- More than a third of high school students use one or more of these forms of tobacco, as do 13% of middle school youths.[9]
- All forms of tobacco are harmful, for example, accounting for 30% of all cancers.

COSTS OF TOBACCO HABIT

Each drug has its own constellation of adverse health consequences. Tobacco dependence is responsible for more than one in every six deaths in the United States.[37] Individual differences in susceptibility lead to vulnerability for varying chronic diseases, different losses in quality of life, and different causes of death. Some tobacco users survive a long time. However, half die of a tobacco-related disease. Who would fly if half of all individuals who do so would die in an aircraft accident; perhaps not this flight, but one day? On average, cigarette smokers lose about 12 to 15 years of life, compared with similar groups of nonsmokers.[31]

In addition to the toll on tobacco users and their families, the social cost of tobacco use is high. Tobacco industry gross sales of $46 billion annually are not even half of the estimated direct and indirect annual social costs of $130 billion.[17,34] Such costs do not include intangible costs such as impaired sexual function, pain, disfigurement, lost opportunities, and costs to families and close associates when users are disabled or die prematurely as a consequence of tobacco use. Stated simply, it costs society nearly $3 for every $1 of tobacco sold.

Many oral diseases are caused or aggravated by tobacco use (Box 12-1). For example, the prevalence and severity of adult periodontal diseases are directly related to the intensity and duration of smoking.[14,15,23] In addition, patient tobacco use adds a preventable burden on practice (Box 12-2). For example, oral hygiene services among smokers are more difficult and less enduring. Postsurgical wound healing is poorer. Smokers have twice the risk of experiencing dry socket. Prognoses are poorer after periodontal therapy, implant insertion, and other dental services that depend on healing and resistance to infection.[16] Extra clinic time often is required during the treatment of patients who are ill with tobacco-related diseases for medical consultation and provision of pretreatment medication. Medical emergencies may occur more among smokers. Because tobacco use adversely affects oral health, some treatment options, treatment, and prognoses may be precluded.[26] Because tobacco use is life-threatening, it is ethically and morally sound to routinely use scientifically established, brief, effective tobacco prevention and cessation services with every patient.

BOX 12-1

Tobacco-Induced and Tobacco-Associated Oral Conditions

Oral cancer
Leukoplakia
 Homogenous leukoplakia
 Nonhomogenous leukoplakia (precancer)
  Verrucous leukoplakia
  Nodular leukoplakia
  Erythroleukoplakia
Other tobacco-induced oral mucosal conditions
 Snuff dipper's lesion
 Smoker's palate (nicotine stomatitis)
 Smoker's melanosis
Tobacco-associated effects on the teeth and supporting tissues
 Tooth loss (premature mortality)
 Staining
 Abrasion
 Periodontal disease
  Destructive periodontitis
  Focal recession
  Acute necrotizing ulcerative gingivitis

Other tobacco-associated oral conditions
 Gingival bleeding
 Calculus
 Halitosis
 Leukoedema
 Chronic hyperplastic candidiasis
 Median rhomboid glossitis
 Hairy tongue
Possible association with tobacco use
 Oral clefts
 Dental caries
 Dental plaque
 Lichen planus
 Salivary changes
 Taste and smell

From Mecklenburg RE et al: *Tobacco effects in the mouth,* Bethesda, Md, 1994, U.S. Department of Health and Human Services, Public Health Service, National Institutes of Health. NIH Publication No. 94-3330.

BOX 12-2

Tobacco Effects on Clinical Care

Effects on Oral Health Care
Periodontal therapy
Dry socket
Delayed wound healing
Implant prognosis
Sinusitis
Cosmetic dentistry
Effects of Fitness for Care
Immune system
Medical crises
Medications
Frequent illness
Disabilities
Effects on Family Health and Well-Being
Premature death
Involuntary tobacco smoke

From Mecklenburg RE et al: *Tobacco effects in the mouth,* Bethesda, Md, 1994, US Department of Health and Human Services, Public Health Service, National Institutes of Health. NIH Publication No. 94-3330.

Nicotine is the psychoactive drug in tobacco but not the substance that is most harmful.[5] Combinations of hundreds of tars, particulates, and gases produce carcinogenic, cardiovascular, reproductive, sensory, and other adverse effects. Risks of developing these effects are generally a function of duration and intensity (often expressed in pack years). Most non–diabetes-related adult periodontal disease may be attributed to smoking.[8,36] Withholding of or noncompliance with cessation services as a component of periodontal therapy dramatically lowers a favorable long-term outcome because a major contributor continues. Helping a patient quit is an essential component of his or her dental care.

SMOKELESS/SPIT TOBACCO

Boys and men are nearly eight times more likely to use spit tobacco than girls.[7] About half of users show tobacco-induced white lesions where they hold the **quid.** The juices are rich in tobacco nitrosamines that are powerful carcinogens. Oral cancer risks are even greater, especially when smokeless tobacco is combined with alcohol. One report demonstrates that spit tobacco users double their risk of cardiovascular death.[6] Nicotine from spit tobacco is absorbed through the oral mucosa in a basic environment. Youths begin the smokeless tobacco habit with near neutral pH forms that release little nicotine and are highly flavored to mask the bitter tobacco taste. As tolerance grows, users switch to products with higher pH levels to help transfer larger quantities of nicotine into the blood. Highly dependent users choose forms that are higher than pH 8 and have few, if any, masking flavors. Some spit tobacco users are so dependent that they sleep with a quid in their mouths for continuous nicotine absorption.

OTHER TOBACCO PRODUCTS

Like spit tobacco juices, smoke from cigars, pipes, and bidis has a basic pH (above pH 7.0) and is harsh. Thus most nicotine is absorbed through the oral mucosa and upper brachial tree. Little nicotine reaches the lung alveoli. Cigarette smoke is acidic, having on average a 6.1 pH, and must be inhaled deeply into the lung for nicotine absorption. Some cigarettes are treated with ammonia and other chemicals to increase absorption throughout the brachial tree, and with other chemicals to open and anesthetize the airway, permitting a deeper draw and greater nicotine absorption. The addition of sugars in cigarettes also increases the psychoactive "hit."[4]

ESSENTIAL ELEMENTS OF PATIENT HISTORY

RISKS

The average age of smoking onset is 14.5 years.[38] The younger people begin smoking, the more likely they are to become long-term users, that is, become nicotine dependent. Early tobacco use is often associated with early alcohol use. Children and youths who are users are at greatest risk of experimenting and becoming regular users of other psychoactive substances. Thus tobacco use, especially smoking, is considered a "gateway drug."[38]

INITIATION

The onset of tobacco use usually begins for social or psychological reasons. Other youths offer the product, and it is taken because of curiosity, a desire to fit in, as an act of rebelliousness against authority, to mimic an admired celebrity, or for no obvious reason. Intermittent use extends, on average, for about 4 years before regular (almost daily) use begins.[38]

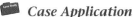 *Case Application*

Ms. Evans' history is typical. She began smoking during her early teens. Youths who have smoked as few as 100 cigarettes are likely to become daily smokers. She is past that point. She also drinks and may occasionally drink more than she intended. Alcohol use is both a common risk factor for relapse and a strong cofactor for oral cancer and other serious chronic health problems. Her routine use of two psychoactive drugs and her remark that she "likes socializing" may suggest that she is in a cluster of individuals who engage in multiple high-risk activities.

PROGRESSION

Nicotine mimics acetylcholine by binding to acetylcholine receptors at the autonomic ganglia, in the adrenal medulla at neuromuscular junctions, and in the brain. At low doses, nicotine stimulates the brain, primarily the cortex via the locus ceruleus. This produces increased alertness and cognition. At higher doses, nicotine tends to stimulate the production of dopamine, providing a "pleasure" effect and sense of well-being (Fig. 12-1). The nicotine promotes a more intense signal, and because the signal is not cleared normally, a lingering effect. In time, the CNS adjusts to this repeated stimuli by increasing the number of neuron receptor sites, returning signals to "normal" function, but now only in the presence of nicotine. Thus to achieve the altered mood desired, higher doses are required over time (Box 12-3). Withdrawal from nicotine use creates a rebound effect that may extend for several weeks or longer, depressing cognitive ability, brain metabolism, emotional stability, and sense of well-being.

DEPENDENCE

The conversion from voluntary to involuntary use is gradual and seldom recognized by the user. The search for re-

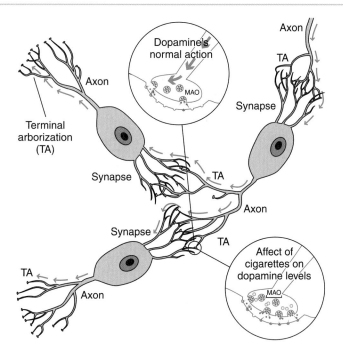

FIG. 12-1 The addictive process. Nicotine is shown replacing the neurotransmitter acetylcholine at the receptor site. This replacement results in increased alertness and cognition. With increased doses of nicotine at the receptor site, dopamine is produced, resulting in a feeling of pleasure and well-being. Because nicotine produced a large discharge of dopamine and this neurotransmitter does not clear from the receptor site as quickly as it would during normal functioning, the signal has an intense, lingering effect. Over time, more receptor sites are produced, returning signals to "normal" intensity and duration, but only in the presence of nicotine.

ward through nicotine use and the avoidance of the penalties of stopping are embedded in the social and environmental context of use. Although synonymous with *nicotine dependence, nicotine addiction* is often used in a broader context. Many behaviors are characterized as addictive. Compulsive eating, gambling, sexual activity, and acquisition of money and goods have been called addictive when they risk and/or compromise inherently advantageous fundamental behaviors.

Drug use is often differentiated as a "dependency," connoting that chemicals directly alter the neurotransmitting functions of the brain. Like purely behavioral addictions, drug-taking behaviors are conditioned by the environment in which a drug is used and the reinforcement of learned, repetitive motor skills. Motor neuron pathways develop memory so that motions used to prepare and use tobacco products become refined and so ingrained within the individual that the user perceives them as efficient, "normal" motions.

RELAPSE

Women more than men state that they smoke to relieve anxiety, overcome depression, and manage weight gain. Unfortunately, it is the interruption of nicotine's action on neurotransmitters that trigger much of such feelings

---

BOX 12-3

American Psychiatric Association: Diagnostic Criteria for Substance Dependency

The American Psychiatric Association (APA) diagnostic criteria applicable to nicotine dependency outline a maladaptive pattern of substance use, leading to clinically significant impairment of stress as manifested by three or more of the following criteria, occurring at the same time in the same 12-month period.

A. Tolerance, as defined by one of the following:
  1. A need for markedly increased amounts of the substance to achieve intoxication or desired effects
  2. Markedly diminished effects with continued use of the same amount of the substance
B. Withdrawal, as manifested by one of the following:
  1. The characteristic withdrawal syndrome for the substance
  2. Using the substance to relieve or avoid withdrawal symptoms
  3. Taking the substance in larger amounts and over a longer period than intended
  4. Persistent desire or unsuccessful effort to cut down substance use
  5. Spending a great deal of time in activities necessary to obtain the substance, use it, or recover from its effects
  6. Reducing or discontinuing important social, occupational, or recreational activities because of substance use
  7. Continued substance use despite knowledge of having a persistent or recurrent physical or psychological problem that is likely to have been caused or exacerbated by the substance

From Hughes JR et al: Practice guideline for the treatment of patients with nicotine dependence, *Am J Psychiatry* 153(suppl):1-31, 1996.

BOX 12-4

American Psychiatric Association: Diagnostic Criteria for Nicotine Withdrawal

A. The individual uses nicotine daily for at least several weeks.
B. The individual abruptly ceases nicotine use or the amount of nicotine used, followed within 24 hours by four or more of the following signs:
  1. Dysphoric or depressed mood
  2. Insomnia
  3. Irritability, frustration, or anger
  4. Anxiety
  5. Difficulty concentrating
  6. Restlessness
  7. Decreased heart rate
  8. Increased appetite or weight gain
C. The symptoms in Criterion B cause clinically significant degrees of impairment in social, occupational, or other important areas of functioning.
D. The symptoms are not due to a general medical condition and are not better accounted for by another mental disorder.

From Hughes JR et al: Practice guideline for the treatment of patients with nicotine dependence, *Am J Psychiatry* 153(suppl):1-31, 1996.

---

she experiences and the decreased metabolism associated with her weight gain.

Case Application

In Ms. Evans' case, social situations may be strongly reinforcing, as suggested by her remark that she smokes most heavily during such occasions. Whereas her first relapse was due to a social situation, Ms. Evans' second relapse was due to her nicotine dependency. She described typical withdrawal symptoms (Box 12-4).

DIAGNOSIS OF NICOTINE DEPENDENCY AND ADDICTION

Nicotine is rapidly metabolized so that the positive effects achieved through the use of a single cigarette may deteriorate within a half hour. Nicotine depletes when sleeping, so withdrawal symptoms are often most intense on waking. Smokers commonly report that the most "satisfying" or "enjoyable" cigarette is the one taken on waking. Without realizing it, they are reporting on their relief from withdrawal. Highly dependent smokeless/spit tobacco users may sleep with a chew so that some nicotine absorption occurs during sleep. Other indicators[10] that an individual is nicotine-dependent are presented in Fig. 12-2.

RITUALS

Individuals who use tobacco or other substances develop rituals around use. For example, a pattern exists involving opening of the pack, tapping and removal of the cigarette, placement of the cigarette into position, lighting, extinguishing of the flame, and storage of the pack and lighter, followed by a set means of holding and drawing on the cigarette and use of the smoke in accord with the dose needed. Fine, often unconscious regulation of each dose occurs to adjust the amount of nicotine absorbed to maximize the effect without its reaching an unpleasant state of nicotine intoxication or overdose. On average, a cigarettes smoker repeats puffing about 10 times per cigarette, receiving a dose that sustains comfort and avoids the onset of withdrawal symptoms for 20 to 40 minutes. A pack-a-day smoker might repeat the puffing act 73,000 times per year. The ritual provides an illusion of control and becomes a source of comfort.

ENVIRONMENTAL STIMULI

Nicotine dependency occurs in a social environment. Anticipation of use can trigger craving, and a social context in which the substance is used heightens desire for it. Cigarette smoking has been socially acceptable in a wide variety of environments, easily triggering a desire to use tobacco. This, coupled with the low cost, easy access, and seemingly ubiquitous encouragement by the tobacco industry has made cigarette smoking easy to develop and continue. An increasing number of policies to make public places smoke-free are incentives for nicotine-dependent individuals to reduce use or quit, in spite of the physical withdrawal symptoms that occur while the brain readjusts to functioning without the presence of nicotine.

Questions		Answers	Points
1. How soon after you wake up do you smoke your first cigarette?		Within 5 minutes	3
		6 to 30 Minutes	2
		31 to 60 Minutes	1
		After 60 minutes	0
2. Do you find it difficult to refrain from smoking in places where it is forbidden?		Yes	1
		No	0
3. Which cigarette would you hate most to give up?		The first one in the morning	1
		All others	0
4. How many cigarettes per day do you smoke?		10 or less	0
		11 to 20	1
		21 to 30	2
		31 or more	3
5. Do you smoke more frequently during the first hours of being awake than during the rest of the day?		Yes	1
		No	2
6. Do you smoke if you are so ill that you are in bed most of the day?		Yes	1
		No	0

Dependence score:

0 to 2	Very low
3 to 4	Low
5	Moderate
6 to 7	High
8 to 10	Very high

FIG. 12-2 Items and scoring for Fagerstrom Test for Nicotine Dependence. (Modified from Fagerstrom K, Schneider NG: Measuring nicotine dependence: a review of the Fagerstrom tolerance questionnaire, *J Behav Med* 12:59-182, 1989.)

QUITTING

Nearly half of high school seniors and 60% to 70% of adults who smoke want to quit.[38] Most individuals who want to quit think about it for years before making a first quit attempt. Most who attempt to quit require several attempts. Less than 10% of individuals who make a self-help quit attempt are capable of achieving long-term abstinence, that is, being free of tobacco for 6 months or longer. Thus only about 2% to 3% of smokers become abstinent each year.[11] Clinical and extra-treatment social support can double to triple long-term abstinence, and, with the use of a Food and Drug Administration (FDA)-approved pharmacological agent, success rates can rise to 20% or more for a single quit attempt. Such rates are not as common among individuals who have low self-efficacy, multiple drug dependencies, or a psychiatric comorbidity, such as clinical depression.

Depressed neuron function during the quitting process should be expected. Reduction in electroencephalographic (EEG) waves, brain metabolism, and other functions become progressively more intense after quitting and peak within a few days. Most relapses occur within the first week.[19] Impaired neuron function may extend more than a month, with recovery of neuronal function taking much longer. Learned, conditioned patterns of behavior exist indefinitely, requiring continued reinforcement of each ex-user coping strategies to counter them.

 Case Application

Ms. Evans is beginning to exhibit oral symptoms from her smoking. Stained teeth and restorations, fibrous gingiva, and the initial formation of pockets spell trouble ahead should she continue to smoke. Fortunately, scientifically sound **tobacco-cessation** services are a natural component of twenty-first century oral hygiene and periodontal dental services. Ms. Evans needs help and wants help, as signaled by her history of attempting to quit.

TECHNIQUES, PROCEDURES, AND SUPPORTIVE EVIDENCE

Who should help Ms. Evans, whose story was outlined in the case study at the beginning of the chapter? All health-care providers can be effective in helping patients quit.

Treatment delivered by a variety of clinician types increases cessation rates. Assistance by dentists and dental hygienists reinforces each other. Help in dental offices complements help provided in medical environments, so individuals who quit with the help of one discipline may have been prepared to do so earlier by someone of another discipline. The consistency and skill involved is more important than discipline. Of course, any patient who quits gains both dental and medical benefits simultaneously, which is not surprising because oral health is completely integrated with general health and well-being.

Dental hygienists are especially appropriate to provide tobacco-cessation services and to reinforce abstinence. Hygienist time is often long enough to integrate the discussion into the service. Hygiene services are quickly reversed by continued tobacco use. Tobacco-related conditions and the results of care are readily visible. Patients are willing to learn in a nonthreatening clinic environment. Evidence exists that dental hygienists can be effective.[22,30]

 ## HELPFUL METHODS

12-A Treatment of disease follows understanding the disease. Unfortunately, threatening or castigating patients or recommending actions or prescribing or recommending smoking-cessation drugs without knowing how they work is ineffective. Uncertain results and frustration in the attempt are likely outcomes. Dental staff members should choose methods proven to be effective and know how each act helps each patient manage dependency. To keep the service effective and brief, clinic teams should follow a simple routine to identify tobacco use and respond appropriately.

The most widely used system for such identification and treatment uses the five *A*'s: *a*sk, *a*dvise, *a*ssess, *a*ssist, and *a*rrange. The steps involving the clinician first were advanced by the National Cancer Institute[24] and then organized into a clinical practice guideline by the Agency for Health Care Quality and Research[12]; these steps were refined further to become the 2000 Public Health Service guideline entitled "Treating Tobacco Use and Dependence."[13] The current guideline is the global standard inasmuch as it is based on more than 6000 clinical tobacco-use intervention studies.

FIRST VISIT

Ask

All patients are asked to fill out a health history that specifically asks questions to discern which patients are tobacco users, as well as the type and frequency of use. The receptionist routinely notes each patient's tobacco use status on the chart so that all team members are aware of it, often along with other vital signs.

 Case Application
Ms. Evans was identified as a tobacco user before she spoke to anyone in the clinic. The patient history form given to her on her visit included routine questions such as "Do you use tobacco?" and "How interested are you in quitting?" If Ms. Evans had not been a user, she could have been commended for being tobacco-free. This commendation is especially important to reinforce ex-user abstinence.

But Ms. Evans is a user, so you should learn the extent of her problem and her interest in solving it. Clues that Ms. Evans is dependent on nicotine include the following:

- She has been smoking for several years and started when she was young.
- She is smoking daily, averaging three fourths of a pack to more than a pack of cigarettes a day.
- She begins smoking within the first hour of awakening.
- She tried to quit twice. Her second relapse was due to withdrawal symptoms, anxiety, and depressed mood and her concern for weight gain.

In addition, Ms. Evans may have a tendency toward multiple dependencies. Her first relapse followed drinking more than she intended. She likes socializing, so she may be frequently in an environment where alcohol is used.

Advise

The clinician should advise the patient to stop. A powerful motivator for an individual to stop smoking is a tobacco-related symptom or condition. The clinician should listen to the patient's reasons and reinforce them. This step is motivational. The clinician is reinforcing the tobacco user's determination to quit. About a third of smokers are content with their use or at least have more reasons to continue use than to quit.

 Case Application
If Ms. Evans had been in this group, possible caring, positive advice is as follows:

"I think you would be doing yourself a huge favor by quitting. Even though you are only 22, I can see where smoking is damaging your gums. Most adult gum disease occurs among tobacco users, and it is hard to treat successfully when a person keeps using it. What are your reasons for wanting to stop?"

Whatever reasons she might have you should reinforce to help quicken her decision to quit.

Assess

This step highlights the critical point when tobacco-using patients decide to make a quit attempt or not. It is a triage step in which a subset of patients who were routinely *asked* and *advised* agree to make a quit attempt. Some might have special problems, addressed later, which suggest that referral would be an option. However, the health-care team can help most patients.

The majority of tobacco users are not be ready to make a quit attempt. The clinician should offer motivational remarks. Of assistance are the five *R*'s: *r*elevance, *r*isks, *r*ewards, *r*oadblocks, and *r*epetition.

Relevance
The importance of quitting should be made real to each patient. The clinician should observe how patients' personal relations, career, hobbies, sports activities, or anything else might be better without tobacco.

Risks
Patients must understand the risks against quality-of-life issues such as threats to their oral health, life-threatening diseases, and to others they care about.

Rewards

The clinician should remind patients about the benefits of quitting in terms of health, money, protection of family, and positive feelings of being tobacco-free.

Roadblocks

The clinician should help them identify obstacles to quitting and suggest that means to overcome each.

Repetition

Few individuals react positively to a new idea. People need time to think about advantages and disadvantages of doing something different. Periodic reminders are taken more seriously.

Case Application

At the very least you should say to Ms. Evans, "I'll be ready to help you *when* you are ready," implying that she will want to quit sometime. To underscore the message, you could provide her with a pamphlet tailored to her interests and situation.

Ms. Evans is already highly motivated. She has tried to quit twice, and she is on her way to a new job where smoking might not be permitted. She wants to make a good impression. The same three parts to *advise* are important: First, you should tell Ms. Evans clearly, but with compassion, that she should quit. Second, you should relate her smoking to a tobacco-related health condition (e.g., her halitosis, stained teeth, and most poignantly the early signs of periodontal disease). A mirror is a helpful visual argument. You should tell Ms. Evans about the cost and problem of these teeth becoming loose and perhaps being lost and the difficulty of successful treatment in smokers. Third, you should solicit Ms. Evans' reasons for wanting to quit so, as she speaks, they become stronger in her mind by having expressed them. Reinforcement of Ms. Evans' reasons, which may have little to do with health, is persuasive; you should expand on them when possible.

Because this patient is interested in her appearance, a powerful argument is how most people do not think smoking is attractive and that it leaves odors in hair, cloths, and breath. Users are not aware of this odor because the tobacco suppresses senses of taste and smell. Also, attractiveness is defined primarily by a healthy appearance, and smoking promotes premature aging, pallor, and leads to conditions that damage the body long before they become clinically evident. The tobacco companies have promoted being thin as an attribute, but it is not the same as attractiveness. Indeed, tobacco company advertising promotes appearance, wealth, popularity, cleanliness, and other features, which the use of their products destroys or with which it has no relationship. If she develops intractable periodontal disease, loss of teeth is going to make Ms. Evans appear older, whereas a healthy dentition would help preserve her attractiveness indefinitely.

Other potential motivation for Ms. Evans to quit smoking includes wanting to protect her body for motherhood. Women who smoke have a harder time conceiving and carrying their babies to term than do women who do not.[33] The unborn baby who is exposed to toxins in tobacco and tobacco smoke experiences a tobacco-induced restricted oxygen flow. Therefore women who smoke during pregnancy are at higher risk of having babies with physical problems and greater learning and behavioral problems as they grow.[32]

Ms. Evans may not be aware of special health risks for women. For the same amount of smoking, women are at a much higher risk than men for developing lung cancer. In addition to chronic, fatal diseases, smoking leads to more days of illness throughout life, especially respiratory illnesses. You may say to Ms. Evans:

> *"Better you should enjoy life tobacco-free and accumulate earned sick leave. Or, if you need sick leave for colds and flu, their symptoms will not be intensified by the burden that smoking places on the respiratory system."*

Another useful argument in this patient's case is that by becoming tobacco-free before beginning her new job, Ms. Evans may find it easier to develop new friends among employees if she is not a smoker among a majority of nonsmoking colleagues. You may remind Ms. Evans that nearly four of every five adults are now tobacco-free, and that the trend is toward being tobacco-free because many are quitting every day.

Assist

This step moves beyond the first three steps (ask, advise, and assess), which are routinely used with all patients. The clinician should offer to help the patient. Successful quitting, defined as 6 months or longer for this chronic disease, is much more likely with help than when attempted alone. The *assist* step focuses on a subset of tobacco users who decide to quit and may address the following topics:

1. *Setting a quit date.* The patient should select the date and take ownership of the attempt.
2. *Coping with stress.* Because quitting smoking is a stressful time for the patient, that individual should not try to add unnecessary stress to the situation, which may jeopardize the effort's success.

Case Application

Ideally, Ms. Evans should select a quit date in the next few days so that she can be smoke-free for a week or more when she begins her new job. You may phrase this information in the following way:

> *"You are much more likely to succeed if you only have one stress to manage at a time. Beginning a new job is stressful, no matter how much people might welcome you, so the quit date should not be at the same time."*

Second, Ms. Evans is concerned about her weight, but she should not try to diet at the same time. She should recognize that her metabolism likely may fall during the first few weeks after quitting, so she will not require as many calories as she usually consumes. She should eat well but avoid sweets and fats. This information is important because her periodic craving for nicotine may be interpreted as hunger. She should know that women usually find it less stressful to quit during their follicular, rather than luteal, phase. The stress of withdrawal also may be dampened by the use of a nicotine replacement agent or bupropion. Last, you may suggest that she increase her exercise program because exercise is a healthy way to manage both stress and weight. The moment she stops smoking, her blood oxygen will improve because she will no longer have the peripheral vasoconstriction of nicotine and the oxygen binding from carbon monoxide and cyanide from the smoke. Nicotine artificially increases heart rate but restricts blood flow to heart muscles, a dangerous condition.

3. *Coping with physical withdrawal, including possible depression.* Both nicotine replacement agents (patch, gum, nasal spray and oral inhaler) and bupropion (Zyban) reduce the duration and intensity of withdrawal from smoking. Both types counter the depression that may occur during the quitting process. Both nicotine gum and bupropion temporarily postpone weight gain. The use of at least one of these products is recommended during withdrawal, and sometimes a combination of nicotine replacement with bupropion is recommended for individuals who have difficulty maintaining abstinence using only one. Some nicotine-replacement agents are purchased by the patient over-the-counter (OTC), whereas others are available only by prescription (Box 12-5). The *American Dental Association Guide to Dental Therapeutics* describes individual attributes, indications, and precautions for each drug.[25]

Two other drugs may be helpful in special circumstances: nortriptyline, a tricyclic antidepressant, and clonidine, an antihypertensive agent. However, neither is approved by the Food and Drug Administration for smoking cessation. Thus they should not be used in dental practice because the treatment of clinical depression and hypertension is commonly considered to be ruled beyond the scope of dental practice. Herbal products such as mint leaf preparations that are commercially promoted for spit tobacco users, although harmless, have not been shown to be effective and are not recommended. Popular behavioral smoking-cessation methods such as the use of hypnosis, acu-puncture, and laser therapy have not been shown to be effective and are not recommended.[38]

4. *Coping with environmental cues to smoke.* Because social events prompt urges to smoke, the dental hygienist should ask the patient whether he or she would stop going to events where smoking is likely or at least suspend going during the first weeks when it will be most difficult to resist. If the patient is involved in a significant relationship with a smoker or is sure to be in situations in

---

BOX 12-5

Food and Drug Administration: Approved Tobacco-Cessation Pharmaceutical Agents

General Information

All smokers who try to quit should receive pharmacotherapy as part of the quitting process except in the presence of contraindications (for example, pregnancy). None of the FDA-approved products for smoking cessation is known to create a cardiovascular risk. Clonidine has been shown to be effective but is not listed as a drug of choice because it has not received FDA approval for tobacco-cessation treatment. Both bupropion and nicotine gum have been shown to delay, but not prevent, weight gain. Bupropion may be the drug of choice if the patient exhibits symptoms of depression. However, no drug has been shown to have a clear advantage in achieving long-term abstinence. All FDA-approved drugs may be used longer than recommended treatment by patients who desire long-term therapy. Combining the nicotine patch with nicotine gum or nicotine nasal spray is more efficacious than a single form of nicotine replacement, and patients should be encouraged to use such combined treatment if they are unable to quit using a single type of nicotine replacement. In addition, bupropion in combination with an FDA-approved nicotine replacement may be more effective than either drug alone. Higher doses than recommended of nicotine-replacement products have not been shown to significantly increase long-term quit rates.

Nonnicotine Tobacco-Cessation Drugs
Bupropion SR (Zyban)
Precautions: No cardiovascular risks are known. The most common side effects are dry mouth and insomnia.
Contraindications: Bupropion SR is contraindicated in individuals with a history of seizure disorder, a history of eating disorder, who use another form of bupropion (Wellbutrin or Wellbutrin SR), or who have used an MAO inhibitor in the past 14 days.

Dosage: Patients should begin with a dose of 150 mg qAM for 3 days, then increase to 150 mg bid. This dose should continue for 3 months after the quit date. Unlike with nicotine replacement products, patients should begin bupropion SR treatment 1 to 2 weeks before their quit date.
Instructions:
Spontaneous quitting: Some patients lose their desire to smoke before their quit date or spontaneously reduce the amount they smoke.
Scheduling of dose: If insomnia is marked, taking the PM dose earlier (in the afternoon, at least 8 hours after the first dose) may provide the individual some relief.
Alcohol: The patient should use alcohol only in moderation.

Nicotine Replacement Tobacco-Cessation Drugs
General Precautions for Nicotine Replacement Therapy
Not an independent risk factor for acute myocardial events. Nicotine replacement therapy (NRT) should be used with caution among particular cardiovascular patient groups; those in the immediate (within 2 weeks) postmyocardial infarction period, those with serious arrhythmias, and those with serious or worsening angina pectoris.
Nicotine Patch
Precautions: Up to 50% of patients using the nicotine patch have a local skin reaction. Skin reactions are usually mild and self-limiting but may worsen over the course of therapy. Local treatment with hydrocortisone cream (1% or 0.5%) and rotating patch sites may ameliorate such local reactions. In less than 5% of patients, such reactions require the discontinuation of nicotine patch treatment.

Modified from Fiore MC et al: *Treating tobacco use and dependence: clinical practice guideline,* Rockville, Md, 2000, Department of Health and Human Services, Public Health Service.
Continued

BOX 12-5

Food and Drug Administration: Approved Tobacco-Cessation Pharmaceutical Agents—cont'd

Dosage: Treatment of 8 weeks or less has been shown to be as efficacious as longer treatment periods. Based on this finding, the following treatment schedules are suggested as reasonable for most patients. Clinicians should consider individualizing treatment based on specific patient characteristics, such as previous experience with the patch, amount smoked, and degree of nicotine dependence. Finally, clinicians should consider starting treatment on a lower patch dose in patients smoking 10 or fewer cigarettes per day or weighing 100 pounds or less.

Drug	Duration	Dosage
Nicoderm CQ*	4 weeks	21 mg/24 hours
Habitrol	then 2 weeks	14 mg/24 hours
	then 2 weeks	7 mg/24 hours
ProStep	4 weeks	22 mg/24 hours
	then 4 weeks	11 mg/24 hours
Nicotrol*	8 weeks	15 mg/16 hours

Instructions:

Location: At the start of each day, the patient should place a new patch on a relatively hairless location between the neck and waist.

Activities: No restriction while using the patch

Time: Patches should be applied as soon as the patient wakes on quit day. With Nicotrol patches, or in patients experiencing sleep disruption, consider removing the patch before bedtime.

Nicotine Gum

Side effects: Common side effects include mouth soreness, hiccups, dyspepsia, and jaw ache. These effects are generally mild and transient and often may be alleviated by correcting the patient's chewing technique.

Dosage: Nicotine gum is available in 2-mg and 4-mg (per piece) doses. Generally the gum should be used for up to 12 weeks, with no more than 24 pieces per day. The gum is most commonly used for the first few months of a quit attempt. Clinicians should tailor the duration of therapy to fit the needs of each patient. Patients using the 2-mg strength should not use more than 30 pieces per day, whereas those using the 4-mg strength should not exceed 20 pieces per day.

Nicorette, Nicorette Mint (OTC only)
Instructions:

Chewing technique: Gum should be chewed slowly until a "peppery" or "minty" taste emerges, then "parked" between the cheek and gum to facilitate nicotine absorption through the oral mucosa. Gum should be slowly and intermittently "chewed and parked" for about 30 minutes or until the taste dissipates.

Absorption: Acidic beverages (e.g., coffee, juices, soft drinks) interfere with the buccal absorption of nicotine, so eating and drinking anything except water should be avoided for 15 minutes before and during chewing.

Scheduling of dose: Patients often do not use enough gum to get the maximum benefit: they chew too few pieces per day and they do not use the gum for a sufficient number of weeks. Instructions to chew the gum on a fixed schedule (at least one piece every 1 to 2 hours) for at least 1 to 3 months may be more beneficial than ad lib use.

Nicotine Inhaler

Local irritation reactions: Local irritation in the mouth and throat was observed in 40% of patients using nicotine inhalers. Coughing (32%) and rhinitis (23%) were also common. Severity generally was rated as mild, and the frequency of such symptoms declined with continued use.

Dosage: A dose from the nicotine inhaler consists of a puff or inhalation. Each cartridge delivers 4 mg of nicotine over 80 inhalations, of which approximately 2 mg is absorbed. Recommended treatment is at least 6 cartridges/day, with a maximum limit of 16 cartridges/day.

Nicotine Inhaler (Prescription only)
Instructions:

Ambient temperature: Delivery of nicotine from the inhaler declines significantly at temperatures below 40° F. In cold weather, the inhaler and cartridges should be kept in an inside pocket or warm area.

Dose reduction: Use is recommended for up to 6 months with gradual reduction in frequency or use over the last 6 to 12 weeks of treatment.

Nicotine Nasal Spray

Nasal/airway reactions: Some 94% of users report moderate to severe nasal irritation in the first 2 days of use; 81% still reported nasal irritation after 3 weeks, although rated severity was mild to moderate. Nasal congestion and transient changes in sense of smell and taste were also reported. Nicotine nasal spray should not be used in persons with severe reactive airway disease.

Nicotrol NS (Prescription only)
Instructions:

Dose delivery: Patients should not sniff, swallow, or inhale through the nose while administering doses. The spray is best delivered with the head tilted slightly back.

Modified from Fiore MC et al: *Treating tobacco use and dependence: clinical practice guideline,* Rockville, Md, 2000, Department of Health and Human Services, Public Health Service.
*Over-the-counter (OTC) drugs.

which smoking occurs, he or she should prepare and repeatedly practice in advance how to refuse offers to smoke. Indeed, individuals whose friendship the patient regards highly should be specifically solicited to help by not smoking in the patient's presence and to help encourage others not to do so.

5. *Coping with deeply ingrained habits.* The clinician should remind the patient that all the rituals of smoking that he or she has repeated thousands of times over the years are well developed and can't be expected to simply disappear. New rituals need to be established to override old ones. The clinician should ask about habits that involve smoking (e.g., driving or eating). In addition, the patient must consider alternative actions to carrying, taking out, lighting, and puffing on a cigarette. The patient may practice fun or distracting alternative behaviors to break the mold.

6. *Coping with other common relapse risks.* The clinician may try to identify those behaviors that have led that patient to break the resolve to quit and begin smoking again and suggest ways the patient can avoid such situations or substitute more healthy alternatives.

Case Application

Ms. Evans may not be alcohol-dependent but must be aware that her resolve may be easily undermined when she drinks, as experience has taught her. She should avoid alcohol during the quitting process, especially because drinking is one of the most common reasons people relapse. You should suggest substituting alcohol-like drinks, such as straight tonic water, that have low sugar. If she uses nicotine gum, she should know that acidic beverages (carbonated drinks, fruit juices, coffee and tea) prevent absorption of the nicotine that suppresses her withdrawal symptoms. She should avoid drinking acidic beverages 15 minutes before and during nicotine gum use.

7. *Providing the patient with (1) a reminder about the chosen quit date and (2) a booklet the patient can use to prepare for that date.* Booklets such as the Public Health Service booklet *You Can Quit Smoking Consumer Guide*[1] (or in Spanish, *Usted Puede Dejar de Fumar Guia del Consumidor*) and the National Cancer Institute booklet *Clearing the Air: How to Quit Smoking . . . and Quit for Keeps.*[27] These sources are written in simple language and contain many tips to prepare individuals to quit and to manage the quitting process.

Arrange

Quitting tobacco use is a process. Typically, developing nicotine dependence takes several months to a few years. Once nicotine dependence is firmly established, quitting may require months before the brain has readjusted to normal function in the absence of nicotine. Even so, learned patterns of behavior and environmental cues continue in memory so that even a single use of tobacco years later may quickly precipitate a return to the previous pattern of use. As for other chronic diseases and conditions, nicotine dependence has a long recovery period and requires a lifetime of patient monitoring and reinforcement.

Case Application

Ms. Evans' first visit should conclude with arrangements for follow-up contacts, ideally face-to-face but at least by telephone. Timing, duration, and frequency of these contacts are important.

FOLLOW-UP VISITS

Timing

The first follow-up contact with a patient is usually conducted by telephone. This brief contact should occur a day or two before the scheduled quit date to accomplish the following:

- To determine whether the patient still plans to quit on that date
- To remind the patient to stop using and discard all tobacco products the evening before

- To ask the patient whether he or she has questions or wants to discuss anything after reading the booklet
- To ask the patient whether he or she is prepared

Case Application

Ms. Evans should be seen within the first week after she quits, perhaps in the third or fourth day because physical withdrawal appears to be a major problem. During this visit, you should continue to provide encouragement, determine what problems she is experiencing, suggest means to overcome each, and ensure that the pharmacological agent selected is being used properly. Are persons around her being helpful? You should reinforce the importance of her avoiding taking even a single puff from a cigarette and reassure her that physical symptoms of withdrawal are normal, part of the healing process, and will start to subside in frequency and intensity as time passes.

Interventions as brief as 3 minutes may help, but longer visits are more effective. Most contact lasts from 3 to 10 minutes.

Any follow-up visit increases the likelihood of long-term success, but four or more person-to-person sessions appear especially effective in increasing long-term abstinence.[13] Visits should occur at least once a month while pharmacotherapy is being used and during the month after it is discontinued. After that, follow-up at regular intervals for routine hygiene services should be adequate. Because nicotine dependency is chronic and relapsing, reinforcement of her abstinence should be provided at every dental visit as enthusiastically as possible. Simply being delighted with her being tobacco-free is a life-saving service.

Relapse

If the patient has relapsed, as most patients who quit will, the clinician should congratulate her on making the attempt. The following techniques are helpful:

- Recognize any period of abstinence as a personal accomplishment—a victory
- Make the session a learning experience
- Determine what led to the relapse: a social situation, physical withdrawal symptoms, an emotional state
- Ascertain where the tobacco came from
- Review the reasons why the patient wanted to quit and ask whether he or she is willing to try again
- Encourage the patient to set a new quit date
- Repeat the key steps: building the patient's determination to quit, helping manage the quitting process, using pharmacotherapy, and encouraging the patient that other individuals who are important to him or her also help in important ways

Repeated quit attempts are important, with an aim to extend the duration of time she is tobacco-free each time. Some patients want to continue using a nicotine replacement for an extended time to dampen their craving.

Common causes for relapse are drinking alcohol, having a significant other who smokes, or failure to use the pharmacological agent properly. As stated, common causes for women include anxiety, depression, and weight gain. The clinician should help the patient develop a coping strategy for each. Repeated quit attempts are the norm; on average, about one in five individuals who quit using clinical assistance and guideline-recommended methods achieve abstinence of 6 months or longer. Success rates increase as the duration and intensity of the help provided increases. Such continued care is similar to the strategy used to treat other chronic conditions.

Referral

The clinician should consider referring the patient if he or she is not willing to try again, not receptive to the suggestion to reconsider quitting in a few weeks, or needs more intensive help than the clinician can provide. Perhaps one in three to one in five to 10 patients is a good candidate for referral, which can take several forms:

- Patients who require more intensive help than the clinician can provide should be referred to a specialist in nicotine dependence or to a group program.
- Patients who have low self-efficacy or self-esteem, have overwhelming personal problems, or are mentally or emotionally disadvantaged, should be referred to an appropriate counselor.
- Patients who have multiple drug dependencies should be referred to a drug treatment program.
- Patients who have psychiatric comorbidities, such as acute depression, should be referred for assessment for psychiatric assistance.

Avoiding the provision of additional assistance to the patient through referral is unethical. Tobacco use presents a clear threat to oral health and life. Abandoning the service is also not good business practice because tobacco use is a long-term liability to the practice. It could present a risk management problem if a tobacco-related oral condition progressed in the absence of continued advice and encouragement to quit.

THE TEAM APPROACH

A few simple management steps permit tobacco intervention services to be integrated into any clinic routine. First, the clinic should have a tobacco intervention coordinator. This individual, usually not the primary care provider, ensures that all new employees are oriented to the system, that a mechanism is in place to identify and follow through with patients, and that appropriate motivational and quit method literature is available. Second, the clinic should have a tobacco-free policy so that signs are posted, tobacco-using staff members are offered help to quit, reception magazines and other materials are free of tobacco advertising, and other steps to convey that tobacco use is not encouraged. Third, patient records and the record-keeping system should facilitate clinical tobacco intervention services. Each chart should have a simple chart reminder, obvious to all staff, that identifies each patient's tobacco use status. The patient history form should determine whether tobacco is used. For example, the American Dental Association history form does this. Tobacco intervention services should be coded. (The ADA code for "Tobacco counseling for the control and prevention of oral disease" is #01320.) Records should provide for progress notes from follow-up visits.

Patients expect and respond to tobacco intervention advice from respected clinicians. Dental teams enjoy providing this service for its ability to draw from an understanding of each patient's physical and mental status and social environment. Helping an individual become tobacco-free, thereby reducing their risks to health and well-being, is extremely rewarding.

Nicotine dependence is a chronic, progressive, relapsing brain condition reinforced by certain social conditions, environmental cues, ingrained repetitive behavior, and tobacco industry strategies that attempt to give reasons to continue or start again. The action of nicotine in the CNS is similar to that of other psychoactive drugs, all of which deprive users of a degree of control over their capacity to think, do, and feel. Tobacco use adversely affects patients' oral health and the dental team's practice.

Although adult cigarette use declined during the 1970s and 1980s, it has remained fairly stable in the 1990s with about 25% of adults smoking cigarettes. Tobacco use by youth increased during the 1990s but may be declining recently. Approximately 35% of high school students use tobacco products: 28% use cigarettes, 15% use cigars, and almost 7% use smokeless tobacco. Youths experiment with any tobacco product that comes to market, most recently 5% using bidis and 6% using kretek.[9]

In recent years, much has been learned about how the brain and mind work and how function is altered by psychoactive substances. In the future, a richer understanding of the underlying molecular and cellular neurological processes should aid patient management in many ways. Although each psychoactive chemical has its own specific actions and effects, all act on the same system and in related ways. Clinicians who become competent in managing nicotine dependence are able to better diagnose and manage patients who have other drug-related and other neurological conditions.

During the 1990s remarkable progress has been made in understanding how the tobacco industry conducts business and the social costs of tobacco use. Public awareness may convert to public outrage as more is learned. The global mortality for tobacco-caused disease is projected to rise from the current annual toll of 4 million deaths a year to 8.4 million per year by 2020.[39] However, the tobacco industry continues to market lethal products and to resist public health measures. A bright future depends on a well-informed, concerned public.

Clinically, brief, practical, scientifically sound tobacco intervention methods exist that should be routinely used in dental practice. Dental hygiene services are easily defeated by tobacco use. Dental hygienists have excellent opportunities to encourage their tobacco-using patients to quit and help them do so. Long-term abstinence is much easier to achieve when a caring person is encouraging and educates patients on how to manage the quitting process. Such help is ethically and morally sound and satisfying with every success.

CRITICAL THINKING ACTIVITIES

1. Develop a presentation for elementary-school students on the brain functions that occur to develop a chemical dependency.

2. Review a group of 10 clinic patient records at random. Identify the number using tobacco and the type of product. Look for any notation as to whether quitting was discussed with the patient and what the outcome or decision was at that time. Keep notes of this activity.

3. Go to a grocery store, convenience mart, and another type of store that sells tobacco products. Identify where tobacco products are kept and whether there is signage about age restrictions on purchasing tobacco products. Record the amount of time you spend in the store and the number of tobacco products purchased while there and the approximate age of the purchaser.

4. Interview three people: someone who has quit smoking over 3 years ago, someone who has recently quit, and someone who has committed to quitting. Ask questions of each about concerns over quitting, successes for those who have quit, support needed to quit, and what got them through the desire to continue use. For the person who has committed to quit, ask about expectations of behavior and means of coping during this time.

5. Answer the following multipart question.

   a. Ask friends who use tobacco why they do it and their thoughts and intentions about doing so in the future. Do not be judgmental. Use your listening skills. Develop a list that shows responses under headings by type, for example as follows:

   Liking tobacco
   Taste, smell, feel, color of container
   Image: helps to appear to be like someone else
   Ability to manage mood: relief of stress, thinking
   Help in weight control
   Help in social situations
   No reasons for using

   Not liking tobacco
   Cost
   Image
   Taste, smell, feel, etc.
   Feeling of not being in control
   Health concerns
   Other reasons

   Interest in quitting
   Not interested at all
   Somewhat interested
   Interested a lot
   Interested and have tried to quit before

   Experience in trying to quit
   How long they were abstinent
   How the quitting process felt
   How many used a nicotine replacement product or other pharmacological aid? Did it make a difference?
   What caused relapses: physical, social, other

   b. Ask individuals whether they would like you to help them quit. Keep track what percentage of those you ask agree to quit with your help.

   c. Help interested friends quit. Help them identify as many reasons as possible for wanting to quit. Talk with them about concerns while quitting, such as experiencing physical withdrawal, stress, weight gain, and other common side effects during the recovery process. Help them identify social situations, places and conditions that are most likely to tempt them to relapse, and offer suggestions about how they might deal with these temptations. Try the different methods suggested in this chapter and think of others. (The chapter cannot cover all common possibilities or anticipate every situation that people confront.) Of course, if a prescription drug is desired, the tobacco user's physician or dentist would have to be consulted. If possible, try to be supportive and positive over at least the first 3 months after your friend quits.

   d. Encourage friends who relapse to try again.

   e. Check to see how the tobacco use status of each clinic patient is determined and learn the system used to encourage users and help them to quit.

These experiences help you learn in an informal, systematic way about the ways tobacco influences people and the obstacles they face when they are trying to quit. Few acts of friendship or professionalism can be stronger than helping someone break free from tobacco use. Success, even limited abstinence, reduces their chances of experiencing tobacco-related health problems, including oral health problems, and the possibility of an entirely avoidable premature death.

REVIEW QUESTIONS

1. On which of the following does nicotine act directly?
   a. The sympathetic nervous system
   b. The neuromuscular junction
   c. The medulla of the adrenal cortex
   d. The brain
   e. All the above

2. Which of the following best describes nicotine?
   a. Not addictive
   b. Not as addictive as heroin and cocaine
   c. As addictive as heroin and cocaine
   d. More addictive than heroin and cocaine
   e. Addictive and the most harmful substance in tobacco

Continued

REVIEW QUESTIONS—cont'd

3. Tobacco use is a strong risk factor for all *except* which of the following conditions?
   a. Periodontal diseases
   b. Tooth loss
   c. Oral cancer
   d. Gingival bleeding
   e. Halitosis

4. Which of the following best describes the effect of tobacco use on dental practices compared with tobacco-free patients?
   a. Greater loss of patients as users succumb to tobacco-related diseases
   b. Greater number of appointment cancellations
   c. Greater need to consult with patients' physicians
   d. Greater risk of in-treatment emergency care
   e. All the above

5. Which of the following describes the oral health team's role in helping patients quit using tobacco?
   a. Is not as effective as medical teams
   b. Is about equally effective as medical teams
   c. Is more effective than medical teams
   d. Is ineffective
   e. Of unknown effectiveness

6. All *except* which of the following describe routine clinical steps in helping patients quit using tobacco?
   a. Asking patients about tobacco use and experience with quitting
   b. Advising patients, showing them examples of tobacco-related oral conditions, and reinforcing their reasons to quit
   c. Attacking patients' misperceptions
   d. Assisting with coping skills and planning strategies
   e. Arranging follow-up in support of the quitting and recovery process

7. Which of the following drugs have been helpful during the quitting process?
   a. Nicotine gum, nasal spray, suppository, and inhaler

   b. Nicotine gum, patch, nasal spray, and Wellbutrin
   c. Nicotine gum, patch, nasal spray, inhaler, and buspirone
   d. Nicotine gum, patch, inhaler, and bupropion
   e. Smokeless tobacco

8. All of the following are predictors of relapse while trying to quit except one. Which one is the *exception*?
   a. A spouse who uses tobacco
   b. Taking a single puff from a cigarette
   c. Moderate alcohol use
   d. Feelings of depression
   e. Having quit before but relapsed

9. Follow-up contacts with the patient should occur just before the quit date and at another time. Which of the following is the other time one should contact the patient?
   a. At least at the end of each of the first 3 months
   b. During the first few days, and monthly during pharmacotherapy
   c. On the quit date and at monthly intervals
   d. Whenever the patient requests it
   e. Every 6 months for life

10. The American Dental Association does all of the following to encourage the oral health team to help patients avoid and discontinue tobacco use except one. Which one is the *exception*?
    a. Adopting policies that encourage clinical tobacco intervention services
    b. Including tobacco counseling in its standard procedure codes
    c. Publishing tobacco company advertising in its journals and newsletters
    d. Describing approved drugs for tobacco cessation in its *Guide to Dental Therapeutics*
    e. Including a tobacco question in the American Dental Association (ADA) health history form

SUGGESTED AGENCIES AND WEB SITES

Because of the ever-changing nature of the Internet, some of the web sites listed here may have changed since publication. Please refer to Mosby's Evolve web site for the most current information.

Agency for Healthcare Research and Quality: Center for Practice and Technology Assessment, Agency for Healthcare Research and Policy, 6010 Executive Boulevard, Suite 300, Rockville, MD 20852; (800) 353-9295; http://www.surgeongeneral.gov

American Dental Association: Council on Access, Prevention and Interprofessional Relations, 211 East Chicago Avenue, Chicago, IL 60611-2678; (312) 440-7494: http://www.ada.org (Click "Research" or "Clinical Issues" and find topic index "Tobacco and Nicotine.")

National Cancer Institute: Tobacco Control Research Branch, Division of Cancer Control and Population Sciences, Executive Plaza North, Room 4039, 6130 Executive Boulevard, Rockville, MD 20892-7337; (301) 496-8584: http://www.cancer.gov and http://www.tobaccofree.gov

National Institutes of Health: publications *Clearing the Air: How to Quit Smoking . . . and Quit for Keeps* (NIH publication No. 95-1647) and *Tobacco Effects in the Mouth* (NIH Publication No 94-3330): (800) 4-CANCER

National Oral Health Clearing House: 1 NOHIC Way, Bethesda, MD 20892-3500; (301) 402-7364: http://www.aerie.com

Office on Smoking and Health, CDC: Office on Smoking and Health, Center for Chronic Disease Prevention and Health Promotion, Centers for Disease Control and Prevention, 4770 Buford Highway, N.E., MS-K67, Chamblee, GA 30342; (770) 488-5703: http://www.cdc.gov/tobacco

ADDITIONAL READINGS AND RESOURCES

Fiore MC et al: *Treating tobacco use and dependence: a clinical practice guideline.* Rockville, Md, US Department of Health and Human Services, Public Health Service, Agency for Healthcare Research and Quality, 2000.

Mealey BL, editors: *Periodontal medicine,* Hamilton, Ontario, 2000, BC Decker, pp 99-119.

The Tobacco Use and Dependence Clinical Practice Guideline Panel, Staff, and Consortium Representatives: A clinical practice guideline for treating tobacco use and dependence: a U.S. Public Health Service report, *JAMA* 283:3244-54, 2000.

US Department of Health and Human Services: *Treating tobacco use and dependence: quick reference guide for clinicians,* ISSN-1530-6402, Washington, DC, HHS.

REFERENCES

1. Agency for Healthcare Research and Quality: *You can quit smoking consumer guide,* Rockville, Md, 2000, U.S. Department of Health and Human Services [Publications Clearinghouse (800) 358-9295].
2. Allman JM: *Evolving brains,* New York, 1999, Scientific American Library.
3. Anthony JC, Warner LA, Kessler RC: Comparative epidemiology of dependence on tobacco, alcohol, controlled substances and inhalants: basic findings from the National Comorbidity Survey, *Exp Clin Psychopharm* 2:244-68, 1994.
4. Bates C, Jarvis M, Connolly G: *Tobacco additives: cigarette engineering and nicotine addiction,* Atlanta, July 14, 1999 (accessed), US Centers for Disease Control and Prevention Tobacco Industry Document site [http://www.cdc.gov/tobacco/industry documents/index.htm].
5. Benowitz NL, editor: *Nicotine safety and toxicity,* New York, 1998, Oxford University Press.
6. Bolinder G et al: Smokeless tobacco use and increased cardiovascular mortality among Swedish construction workers, *Am J Public Health* 84:399-404, 1994.
7. Brandt AM: Recruiting women smokers: the engineering of consent, *J Am Med Wom Assoc* 51:63-6, 1996.
8. Burgan SW: The role of tobacco use in periodontal diseases: a literature review, *Gen Dent* 45:449-60, 1997.
9. Centers for Disease Control and Prevention: Tobacco use among middle and high school students—United States, 1999. *MMWR* 49(03):49-53, 2000.
10. Fagerstrom K, Schneider NG: Measuring nicotine dependence: a review of the Fagerstrom tolerance questionnaire, *J Behav Med* 12:159-82, 1989.
11. Fiore MC: Trends in cigarette smoking in the United States: the epidemiology of tobacco use, *Med Clin North Am* 76:289-303, 1992.
12. Fiore MC et al: *Clinical practice guideline number 18: smoking cessation,* Rockville, Md, 1996, US Department of Health and Human Services, Public Health Service, Agency for Health Care Policy and Research. AHCPR Publication No. 96-0692.
13. Fiore et al: *Treating tobacco use and dependence: clinical practice guideline,* Rockville, Md, 2000, U.S. Department of Health and Human Services, Public Health Service.
14. Grossi SG et al: Assessment of risk for periodontal disease. I. Risk indicators for attachment loss. *J Periodontol* 65:260-7, 1994.
15. Grossi SG et al: Assessment of risk for periodontal disease. II. Risk indicators for alveolar bone loss, *J Periodontol* 66:23-9, 1995.
16. Grossi SG et al: Response to periodontal therapy in diabetics and smokers, *J Periodontol* 67:1094-102, 1996.
17. Harris JE: American cigarette manufacturers' ability to pay damages: overview and a rough calculation, *Tobacco Control* 5:292-4, 1996.
18. Henningfield JE, Cohen C, Pickworth WB: Psychopharmacology of nicotine. In Orleans CT, Slade J, editors: *Nicotine addiction: principles and management,* New York, 1993, Oxford University Press, pp 25-43.
19. Hughes JR et al: Smoking cessation among self-quitters, *Health Psychol* 11:331-4, 1992.
20. Kaufman NJ, Nichter M: The marketing of tobacco to women: global perspectives. In: *Women and the tobacco epidemic: challenges for the 21st century,* Geneva, Switzerland, 2001, World Health Organization.
21. Kelder G, Davidson P, editors: *The multistate master settlement agreement and the future of state and local tobacco control: an analysis of selected topics and provisions of the multistate master settlement agreement of November 23, 1998.* Boston, Northeastern University School of Law, Tobacco Control Resource Center, March 24, 1999.
22. Krall EA, Garvey AJ, Garcia RI. Alveolar bone loss and tooth loss in male cigar and pipe smokers. *J Am Dental Assoc* 130:57-64, 1999.
23. Little SJ, Stevens VJ: Dental hygiene's role in reducing tobacco use, *J Dent Hygiene* 346-50, 1991.
24. Manley M et al: Clinical interventions in tobacco control, *J Am Med Assoc* 266:3172-3, 1991.
25. Mecklenburg MC, Somermann M: Cessation of tobacco use. In: *ADA guide to dental therapeutics,* ed 2, Chicago, 2000, American Dental Association.
26. Mecklenburg RE et al: *Tobacco effects in the mouth,* Bethesda, Md, 1994, US Department of Health and Human Services, Public Health Service, National Institutes of Health. NIH Publication No. 94-3330.
27. National Cancer Institute: *Clearing the air: how to quit smoking . . . and quit for keeps.* NIH Pub. No. 95-1647, Bethesda, Md, 2001, The Institute.
28. O'Keefe MA, Pollay RW: Deadly targeting of women in promoting cigarettes, *J Am Med Wom Assoc* 51:67-9, 1996.
29. Pierce JP, Lee L, Gilpin EA: Smoking initiation by adolescent girls, 1944 through 1988: an association with targeted advertising, *J Am Med Assoc* 271:608-11, 1994.
30. Severson HH et al: Using the hygienist visit to deliver a tobacco cessation program, *J Am Dent Assoc* 129:993-9, 1998.
31. Shopland DR, Burns DM: Medical and public health implications of tobacco addiction. In Orleans CT, Slade J, editors: *Nicotine addiction: principles and management,* New York, 1993, Oxford University Press, pp 105-28.
32. Slotkin TA: The impact of fetal nicotine exposure on nervous system development and its role in sudden infant death syndrome. In Benowitz NL, editor: *Nicotine safety and toxicity,* New York, 1998, Oxford University Press.
33. Stein Z: Smoking and reproductive health, *J Am Med Wom Assoc* 51:29-30, 1996.

34. Summers LH: The economic case for comprehensive tobacco legislation, *Treasury News*. Department of Treasury. Presentation at George Washington School of Public Health, March 25, 1998.

35. Teague C: Survey of cancer research with emphasis upon possible carcinogens from tobacco, R.J. Reynolds internal report. (Bates No. 501932947-2968) February 2, 1953.

36. Tomar SL, Asma S: Smoking-attributed periodontitis in the United States: findings from NHANES III, *J Periodontol* 71:743-51, 2000.

37. US Department of Health and Human Services: *Reducing the health consequences of smoking: 25 years of progress,* Rockville, Md, 1989, US Department of Health and Human Services, Public Health Service, Centers for Disease Control, Office on Smoking and Health. DHHS Publication No. (CDC) 89-8411.i.

38. US Department of Health and Human Services: *Preventing tobacco use among young people: a report of the Surgeon General.* Atlanta, 1994, US Department of Health and Human Services, Centers for Disease Control and Prevention, National Center for Chronic Disease Prevention and Health Promotion, Office on Smoking and Health, p 67.

39. World Health Organization: *Women and the tobacco epidemic: challenges for the 21st century,* Geneva, Switzerland, 2001, The Organization.

CHAPTER 13

Intraoral Examination

Alan W. Budenz, Douglas A. Young

Chapter Outline

Case Study: Thorough Intraoral and Extraoral
  Examination
Examination of the Lips and Labial Mucosa
  Anatomical landmarks and topography
  Examination technique
Examination of the Buccal Mucosa and Vestibular
  Folds
  Anatomical landmarks and topography
  Examination technique
Examination of the Floor of the Mouth
  Anatomical landmarks and topography
  Examination technique

Examination of the Tongue
  Anatomical landmarks and topography
  Examination technique
Examination of the Hard and Soft Palates
  Anatomical landmarks and topography
  Examination technique
Examination of Oropharynx and Palatine Tonsils
  Anatomical landmarks and topography
  Examination technique

Key Terms

Anterior
Dorsal surface
Inferior

Lateral
Medial
Nodule

Pharyngeal
Posterior
Superior

Ventral surface
Within normal limits (WNL)

Learning Outcomes

1. Identify the essential components of a comprehensive intraoral patient examination.
2. Recognize normal anatomical hard and soft tissue landmarks of the oral cavity.
3. Visually evaluate the integrity of the oral mucosa, noting any breaks that may exist and noting any irregularities in color or general appearance.

4. Use palpation, the sense of touch, to determine tissue consistency (soft, firm, hard, nodular), mobility (fixed or movable), and patient tenderness or discomfort.
5. Assess anatomical bilateral symmetry for possible indications of underlying pathology.
6. Appropriately document both normal and abnormal findings.
7. Recognize and describe intraoral lesions.

A thorough examination of the oral cavity is an integral part of any comprehensive diagnostic sequence. The intraoral examination consists of observation, palpation, and evaluation of the lips and labial mucosa, the buccal mucosa and the vestibular folds, the floor of the mouth, the tongue, the hard and soft palates, the oropharynx and palatine tonsils, the gingiva and periodontium, and the teeth. During the examination, visual emphasis should be on assessment of size, shape, color, and location; the sense of touch, or palpation, should emphasize evaluation of consistency, texture, and patient discomfort. The goal of the intraoral examination is to evaluate the status of the various structures of the oral cavity and to detect any abnormalities apparent by sight and/or feel. This chapter discusses examination and evaluation of each of the above areas with the exceptions of the periodontium and the teeth, which are discussed in separate chapters later in this text.

Although careful inspection of all of the described intraoral regions is essential to a comprehensive intraoral examination, the sequence for this examination may be altered to suit individual preferences. The key is for every dental healthcare provider to develop a routine that is consistent and reproducible for every patient. A comprehensive intraoral examination should be performed at regular intervals for all active patients, seen by either the dentist or the dental hygienist, and for every new patient. The general recommendation is for an intraoral examination to be an integral part of a comprehensive assessment of new patients and at all subsequent supportive care appointments.

Documentation of one's findings from the comprehensive intraoral examination is also essential. All findings, both normal and abnormal, should be recorded in a consistent, clear, and specific manner within the chart record, either as part of the treatment record write-up or with a separate documentation form. Fig. 13-1 is an example of a comprehensive head and neck physical examination documentation form, which includes the comprehensive intraoral examination. Normal findings are usually recorded as **within normal limits (WNL),** which recognizes that anatomical features may vary without being abnormal. Any findings considered outside the range of normal should be carefully noted (Box 13-1). Such information is essential for monitoring of the tissue whenever no immediate action is deemed necessary and the practitioner plans to evaluate the finding at follow-up appointments or for referral to a specialist for consultation. A periodontal probe is a useful tool to measure width and length of lesions. The description also should include the lesion's relationship to adjacent structures. Complete tissue lesion description includes size, color, morphology, location, and history. Each descriptive element should include the following:

- *Size:* length, width, and sometimes height, measured with a periodontal probe
- *Color:* as it appears with either single color (red or white) or multiple colors
- *Morphology:* shape, arrangement, consistency, and surface texture
- *Locations:* description as specific as possible, including a list of structures in close proximity
- *History:* duration of lesion and symptoms, including patient habits such as tobacco use

13-A

13-B
13-C

Thorough Intraoral and Extraoral Examination

Hilda Jorgensen, a 43-year-old Caucasian woman, has recently moved to your town and has come to your office for the first time, requesting a routine check-up and cleaning appointment. She reports that she last visited a dental office approximately 2 years ago, and her last appointment was for a routine dental cleaning. She is currently feeling no dental pain and is aware of no abnormalities. She states that she has received dental treatment on a relatively regular basis since childhood and has received cleanings and a number of fillings without incident.

BOX 13-1

Findings Outside Range of Normal

Noted by the following:
- Color
- Texture
- Shape
- Size
- Mobility
- Location

First the clinician should determine whether the lesion is elevated, flat, or depressed. The appropriate algorithm is used (Figs. 13-2 through 13-6) with indicated terms to describe the lesion.

EXAMINATION OF THE LIPS AND LABIAL MUCOSA

ANATOMICAL LANDMARKS AND TOPOGRAPHY

13-D
13-E

The intraoral examination logically begins at the entrance to the oral cavity, the lips. The exposed red portion of the lips, the vermilion border or zone, forms a transition between the skin of the external lips and the moist mucous membrane of the internal labial mucosa. The vermilion border of the lips is a mucous membrane; however, it contains no mucous glands. Because of the unusual thinness of the mucosa, the underlying vascularity readily shows through to create the characteristic reddish color of the lips.

The mucocutaneous junction of the vermilion border with the skin of the external lips generally is quite distinct in young individuals but may become obscured with increasing age. The mucosa of the vermilion border may become thicker over time because of exposure to sun and other elements, and the normal light fissuring of this mucosa layer may become exaggerated and continuous with fissures and folds developing in the skin of the lips. The lower lip is more prone to these age-related changes than is the upper lip.

The skin surrounding the lips may be creased by several folds, or sulci. The upper lip is divided into two halves by a midline depression, a vertical groove, called the

HEAD AND NECK PHYSICAL EXAMINATION

GENERAL APPEARANCE & VITAL SIGNS: Blood pressure_____ /_____   Pulse/min_____   Date_____ /_____ /_____

Weight_____   Recall blood pressure_____ /_____   Pulse/min_____   Date_____ /_____ /_____

Height_____   Recall blood pressure_____ /_____   Pulse/min_____   Date_____ /_____ /_____

Recall blood pressure_____ /_____   Pulse/min_____   Date_____ /_____ /_____

External Structures	
Scalp	WNL
Facial skin	WNL
Facial symmetry	WNL
Eyes	WNL
Nose	WNL
Lips	WNL
Ears	WNL
Salivary glands	WNL
Neck	WNL
Hands	WNL

Oral Cavity	
Lips (mucosal)	WNL
Buccal mucosa	WNL
Parotid flow	WNL
Gingiva	WNL
Oral floor	WNL
SMG flow	WNL
Tongue: lateral	WNL
ventral	WNL
dorsal	WNL
Palate: hard	WNL
soft	WNL
Oropharynx	WNL
Tonsillar pillar	WNL

Ears, Nose, and Throat	
Tympanic membrane	WNL
Nasal cavity	WNL
Larynx: T cords	WNL
F cords	WNL
AE fold	WNL
pyriform	WNL
Epiglottis	WNL

Cranial Nerves

Subjective		Objective motor	
Smell (olf I)	WNL	Eye movement (III, IV, VI)	WNL
Taste (facial VII, glosso IX)	WNL	Nystagmus	+ −
Hearing (acoustic VIII)	WNL	Facial (VII)	WNL
Vision (optic II)	WNL	Trigem (V)	WNL
		Access (XI)	WNL
Objective sensory		Hypogl (XII)	WNL
Trigen (V)	WNL	Sympathetic (pupil)	WNL
Paresthesia	+ −		

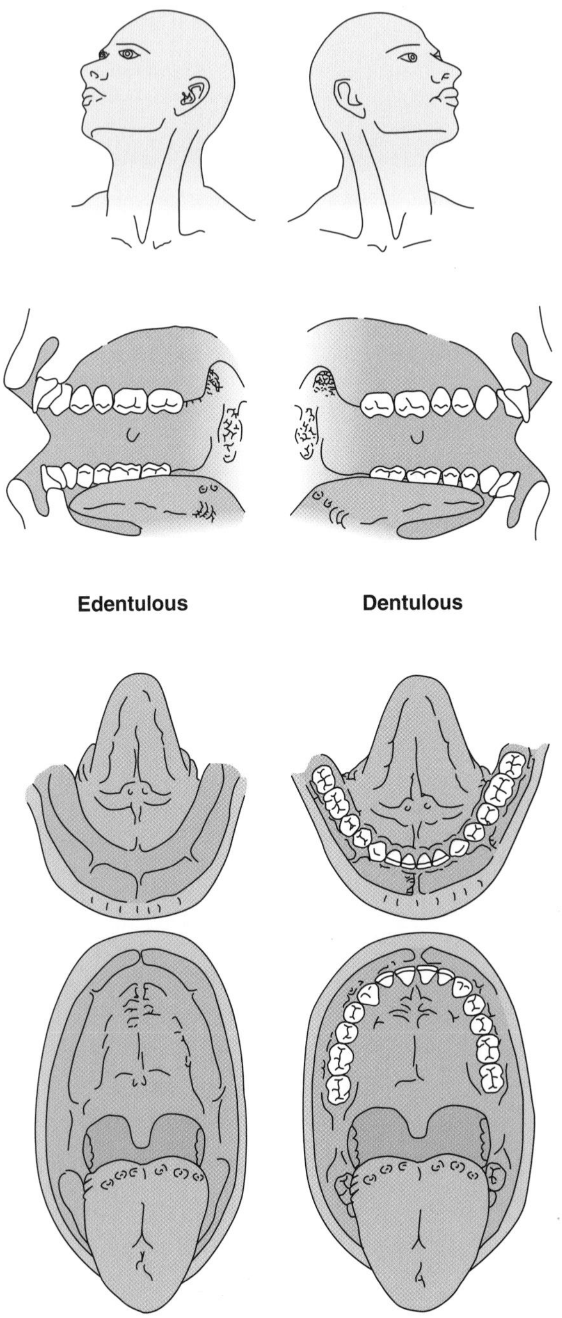

Edentulous   **Dentulous**

FIG. 13-1 Sample of a comprehensive head and neck physical examination documentation form.

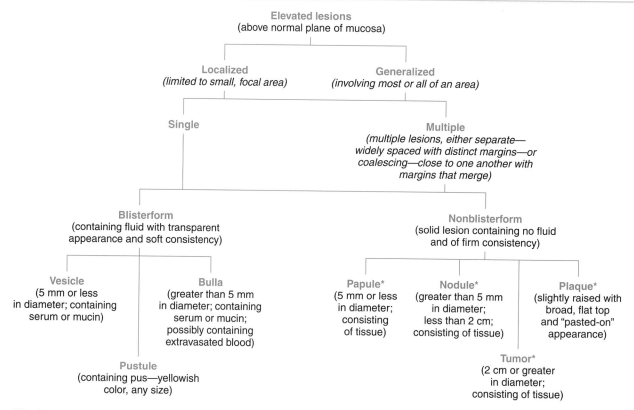

FIG. 13-2 Elevated lesions. (Modified from McCann A: Redi-reference, *Dent Hyg News* 5(2), 1999.)

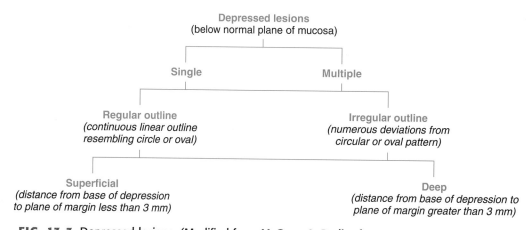

FIG. 13-3 Depressed lesions. (Modified from McCann A: Redi-reference, *Dent Hyg News* 5(2), 1999.)

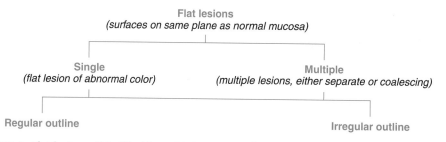

FIG. 13-4 Flat lesions. (Modified from McCann A: Redi-reference, *Dent Hyg News* 5(2), 1999.)

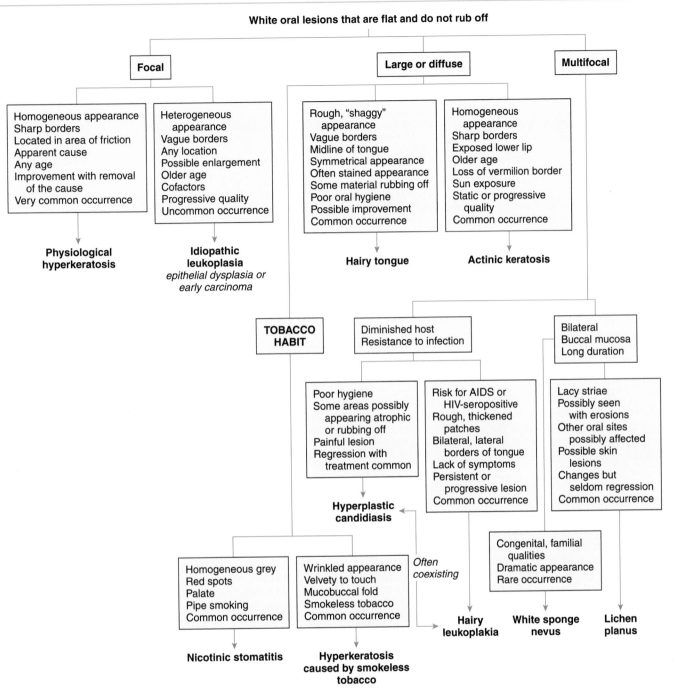

FIG. 13-5 White oral lesions. *AIDS,* Acquired immunodeficiency syndrome; *HIV,* human immunodeficiency virus. (Modified from Coleman GC, Nelson JF: *Principles of oral diagnosis,* St Louis, 1993, Mosby.)

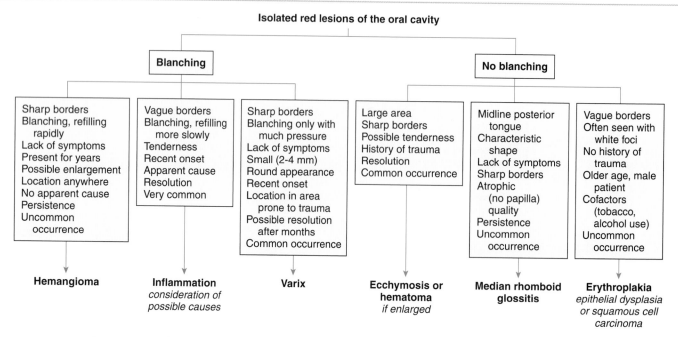

FIG. 13-6 Isolated red lesions. (Modified from Coleman GC, Nelson JF: *Principles of oral diagnosis,* St Louis, 1993, Mosby.)

philtrum. The philtrum extends from the base of the nasal septum superiorly down to the upper lip inferiorly and ends in the center of the lip as a thickened area, called the *tubercle of the lip.* At the corners of the mouth, also known as the *commissures,* the mesial labial fold starts at the junction of the upper and lower lips and extends down and out. Further to the side away from the oral opening, the *lateral* labial fold, or sulcus, runs roughly parallel to the mesial labial fold and extends up to its origin just lateral to the ala, or wing, of the nasal nostril. This fold is also known as the *nasolabial sulcus* or *groove.* The lower lip has a fold running parallel and just **inferior** to the mucocutaneous junction, the mental labial fold.

The thick, pink labial mucosa that lines the internal surfaces of the lips may appear mildly lumpy, or nodular, on visual inspection. This appearance is due to the presence of numerous small mucous glands that keep the labial mucosal surface moist. These are called *accessory salivary glands* and are found just beneath the mucosal surface. In the midline, both the upper and lower lips have a flap of tissue, called a *frenum,* which attaches to the midline mucosa of the maxillary and mandibular alveolar processes. The size and tightness of these frenular attachments vary considerably among individuals, and in some people, the tension exerted by the frenular attachment or its extension up in between the teeth may be a contributing factor to creation of a space, or diastema, between the central incisor teeth. The upper labial frenum frequently may have a small bump or tag of tissue along its free edge. Formation of these fibrous "polyps" on the frenum is thought to result from trauma.

EXAMINATION TECHNIQUE

Evaluation of the lips begins with observation of the patient at rest. The lips are normally in contact or slightly apart. The lip line, the level of the edge of the lip relative to the incisal edge of the teeth, should be observed and noted, both at rest and when the patient smiles. Control of lip movements during speech and smiling also should be observed, and any abnormalities should be noted. Next, the vermilion borders of the lips are carefully examined. This is best done through slight eversion of the lips manually to fully expose them to view. The vermilion border is then evaluated for consistency of color, texture, fissuring, and shape, and again any abnormalities should be precisely noted on the intraoral examination charting form. If the patient is wearing lipstick, this should be thoroughly removed before the examination begins (Fig. 13-7).

Continuing the examination with further eversion of the lips, the clinician gently squeezes the lips between the index finger and the thumb, called *bidigital palpation,* while the mucosal surfaces are carefully viewed. The mucosa should be intact to the view, feel supple to the touch, and the patient should feel no tenderness or discomfort. Any abnormalities to sight or feel should be recorded in detail. Secretion of the mucous glands of the lips may be checked through light drying of the mucous membrane, followed by a close watch for beads of saliva to form on the surface. By gently pulling the lips away from the teeth the clinician may observe the attachments of the labial frena, in addition to the vestibular reflection of the mucous membrane from the lips onto the alveolar processes of the bones, maxilla or mandible, supporting the teeth. The vestibules are the spaces lying between the lips, or cheek, and the gums of the teeth (Fig. 13-8).

Case Application

Mrs. Jorgensen has mildly chapped lips (vermilion border), particularly on the lower lip. The skin around the lips is normal (WNL). The labial mucosa is uniformly moist with apparently normal salivary flow. Palpation of the lips reveals a slightly

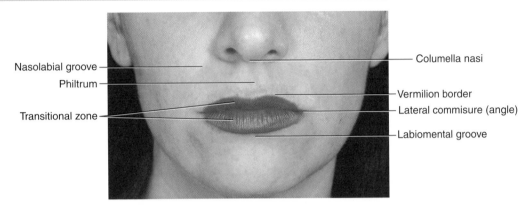

Nasolabial groove

Philtrum

Transitional zone

Columella nasi

Vermilion border

Lateral commisure (angle)

Labiomental groove

FIG. 13-7 Anatomy of the external lip region. The patient's lipstick should be removed before the examination begins. (Modified from Liebgott B: *The anatomical basis of dentistry,* ed 2, St Louis, 2001, Mosby.)

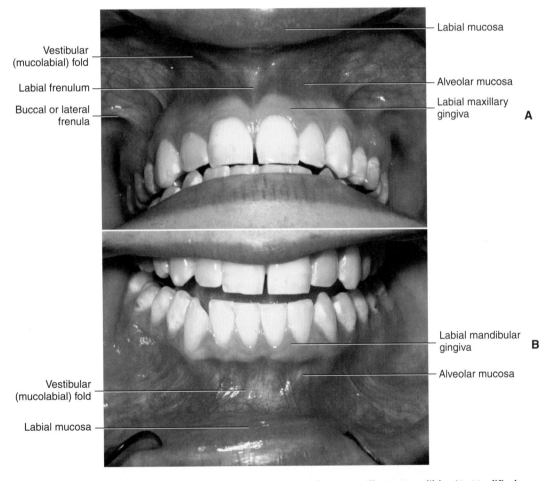

Vestibular (mucolabial) fold

Labial frenulum

Buccal or lateral frenula

Labial mucosa

Alveolar mucosa

Labial maxillary gingiva

A

Labial mandibular gingiva

B

Alveolar mucosa

Vestibular (mucolabial) fold

Labial mucosa

FIG. 13-8 Everted lips exposing the vestibules and frenula. **A,** Maxilla. **B,** Mandible. (**A,** Modified from and **B,** From Liebgott B: *The anatomical basis of dentistry,* ed 2, St Louis, 2001, Mosby.)

External Structures	
Scalp	WNL
Facial skin	WNL
Facial symmetry	WNL
Eyes	WNL
Nose	WNL
Lips	(WNL)	Mildly chapped lips
Ears	WNL
Salivary glands	WNL
Neck	WNL
Hands	WNL

Oral Cavity	
Lips (mucosal)	(WNL)
Buccal mucosa	WNL
Parotid flow	WNL
Gingiva	WNL
Oral floor	WNL
SMG flow	WNL
Tongue: lateral	WNL
ventral	WNL
dorsal	WNL
Palate: hard	WNL
soft	WNL
Oropharynx	WNL
Tonsillar pillar	WNL

Edentulous   **Dentulous**

FIG 13-9 Appropriate chart documentation for examination of the lips and labial mucosa (mildly chapped lips).

lumpy texture produced by the minor salivary glands. The labial frenula and vestibular reflections are WNL. Fig. 13-9 illustrates appropriate charting.

EXAMINATION OF THE BUCCAL MUCOSA AND VESTIBULAR FOLDS

13-F

ANATOMICAL LANDMARKS AND TOPOGRAPHY

The buccal mucosa is the internal lining of the cheek region. This mucous membrane often varies considerably in thickness from one area to another but is generally thick and pink like the labial mucosa with which it is continuous. Frequently, the occlusal plane of the teeth is marked on the mucosa of the cheek by a white line running *anterior* to posterior. This line is produced by the buccal mucosa being pressed between the teeth during chewing by contraction of the buccinator muscle of the cheek. This constant mild abrasion of the cheek mucosa causes an increase in the keratin layer demarking the occlusal plane, forming a hyperkeratotic low ridge called the *linea alba* (Fig. 13-10). The linea alba ends anteriorly at the corner of the mouth, a site often further demarcated by a small, firm *nodule* termed the *caliculus angularis*. An additional raised bump, or papilla, is found on the buccal mucosa opposite the maxillary second molar. A large duct

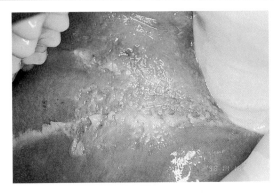

FIG. 13-10 Buccal mucosa with a linea alba and the parotid papilla. (Courtesy Dr. Alice Curran, Jackson, Miss.)

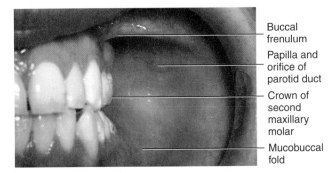

Buccal
frenulum

Papilla and
orifice of
parotid duct

Crown of
second
maxillary
molar

Mucobuccal
fold

FIG. 13-11 Buccal vestibules and frenula. (From Liebgott B: *The anatomical basis of dentistry,* ed 2, St Louis, 2001, Mosby.)

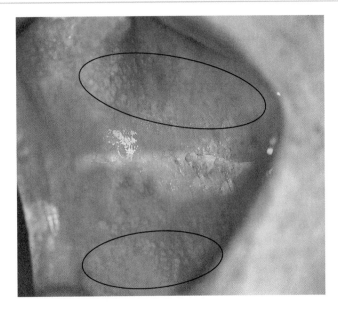

FIG. 13-12 Fordyce granules.

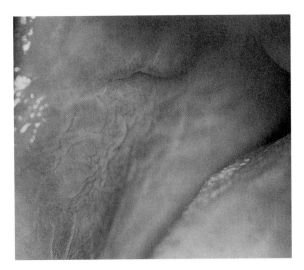

FIG. 13-13 Leukoedema. (Courtesy Dr. Alice Curran, Jackson, Miss.)

draining secretions from the parotid gland into the oral cavity, named the *parotid* or *Stensen's duct,* opens onto the crest of this papilla, and hence it is named the *parotid papilla.* By lightly drying the papilla and the buccal mucosa, the clinician may check secretions from both the minor salivary glands of the cheek and from the parotid gland.

Looking both superiorly and inferiorly into the vestibular folds, or spaces, of the cheek, the clinician observes additional frenular attachments. Called *lateral, labial* or *buccal frenula,* these folds attach the buccal mucosa to the maxillary and mandibular alveolar processes in the area of the first premolar tooth in each quadrant (Fig. 13-11). Frequently small clusters of yellow nodules are found bilaterally in the mucosa of the buccal region and sometimes extending forward into the labial mucosa. These nodules, called *Fordyce granules,* are ectopic sebaceous glands ranging 1 mm or less in diameter, may be flat or slightly elevated, and are found in approximately 80% of adults. Fordyce granules are considered a variation of normal anatomy rather than a pathological change (Fig. 13-12). Another variation commonly seen is leukoedema, which appears as a filmy white, translucent surface of the mucous membrane. In this condition, the mucosa is often highly folded, or wrinkled at rest, but the mucosal lining appears normal when the tissue is gently stretched taut. Leukoedema is most common in people with darkly pigmented skin, and is found in approximately 50% of Caucasian patients and up to 90% of African-American patients (Fig. 13-13). Although this condition is simply a variation of normal, the dentist needs to differentiate leukoedema from a number of other conditions, some pathological, which manifest as white changes of the mucous membrane.

The **posterior** boundary of the buccal mucosa is defined by a low ridge or fold of tissue extending from the crest of the mandible just behind the last molar tooth superiorly up to a point behind and slightly **medial** to the maxillary tuberosity. This ridge is created by a tendinous band of tissue lying deep to the mucosal layer, the pterygomandibular raphe. The pterygomandibular raphe is the common origin for two muscles, the buccinator muscle of the cheek and the **superior** constrictor muscle of the pharynx. This raphe is also an important landmark for administration of local anesthetic injections to the lower jaw (Fig. 13-14). Just distal to the origin of the pterygomandibular fold behind the last mandibular molar tooth is a dense pad of tissue, called the *retromolar pad.*

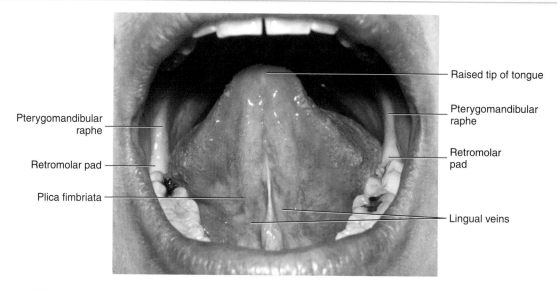

FIG. 13-14 Ventral surface of the tongue showing pterygomandibular raphe, retromolar pad, plica fimbriata, tip of tongue, and lingual veins. (Modified from Liebgott B: *The anatomical basis of dentistry,* ed 2, St Louis, 2001, Mosby.)

EXAMINATION TECHNIQUE

The buccal mucosa can be best visualized when patients open their mouths wide but not completely open. Then a mouth mirror and/or finger may be used to retract the cheek away from the teeth to clearly expose all of the buccal tissue. The patient's head also should be rotated toward and away from the examiner as needed to make both sides of the mouth clearly visible. Alternatively, a finger may be used to retract the cheek, and the mirror may be used to view the buccal tissue indirectly. Gauze should be used to dry the mucosal surface so that secretion of the accessory salivary glands of the cheek may be observed. Flow of saliva from the parotid gland also should be observed and is best done through gentle stroking of the parotid region externally from posterior to anterior to "milk" secretions from the gland. The full extent of the buccal region should be palpated with either bidigital or bimanual palpation, or a combination of the two techniques. Any abnormal findings should be carefully recorded and charted for size, color, shape, texture, mobility, and location.

Case Application

Mrs. Jorgensen's buccal mucosa is marked by bilateral linea alba, raised approximately 1 mm and ending just short of the corner of her mouth. Fordyce granules are present bilaterally, and each group of granules is 10 mm in diameter (see Figs. 13-10 and 13-12). Palpation of the buccal mucosa again reveals a mildly lumpy texture resulting from the minor salivary glands, which are producing a moderately moist mucosal surface. The parotid papilla is bilaterally raised 2 mm and is 4 mm in diameter. After drying, watery (serous) saliva can be readily milked out of both papillae. The buccal frenula and vestibular folds are again within normal limits. Fig. 13-15 illustrates charting of the buccal mucosa findings.

EXAMINATION OF THE FLOOR OF THE MOUTH

13-G
13-H

ANATOMICAL LANDMARKS AND TOPOGRAPHY

Visually, the floor of the mouth is a narrow, horseshoe-shaped depression lying between the base of the tongue and the alveolar processes of the mandible. The mucous membrane covering the floor of the mouth is continuous with that of both the tongue and the mandible, reflecting up off the floor onto these neighboring structures. A prominent landmark in the floor of the mouth is the midline lingual frenulum, connecting from the inferior aspect of the midline medial mandible back into the base and *ventral surface* of the tongue. On either side of the lingual frenulum is a small papilla, the sublingual caruncle, which holds the opening of a duct, called the *submandibular* or *Wharton's duct,* draining from the submandibular salivary gland, located posteriorly in the floor of the mouth and extending into the upper lateral superficial neck just below the inferior border of the mandible, onto the crest of the caruncle, anteriorly. Extending posteriorly from the caruncles, and following the curvature of the mandible, is an elevation of the floor of the mouth formed by the sublingual salivary glands and the pathway of the submandibular duct from the submandibular salivary glands. This elevation is called the *sublingual ridge,* or *sublingual fold.* Along this fold are hairlike projections known as *plica sublingualis.* The sublingual salivary glands drain directly into the oral cavity through a series of short ducts (ducts of Ravinus) that open onto the top of this ridge (Fig. 13-16).

EXAMINATION TECHNIQUE

The clinician may best view the floor of the mouth by asking the patient to lift the tongue up to the roof of the

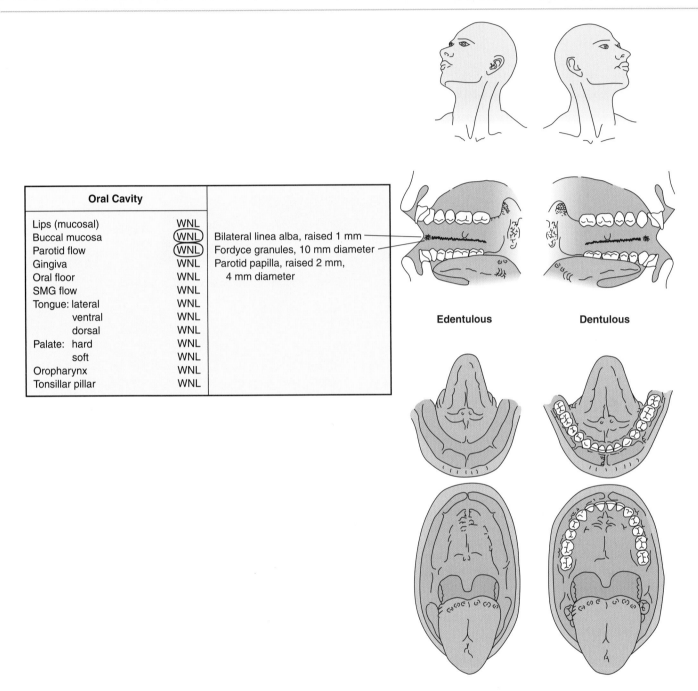

Oral Cavity		
Lips (mucosal)	WNL	
Buccal mucosa	(WNL)	Bilateral linea alba, raised 1 mm
Parotid flow	(WNL)	Fordyce granules, 10 mm diameter
Gingiva	WNL	Parotid papilla, raised 2 mm,
Oral floor	WNL	4 mm diameter
SMG flow	WNL	
Tongue: lateral	WNL	
ventral	WNL	
dorsal	WNL	
Palate: hard	WNL	
soft	WNL	
Oropharynx	WNL	
Tonsillar pillar	WNL	

Edentulous　　　　**Dentulous**

FIG. 13-15 Appropriate chart documentation for examination of the buccal mucosa and the vestibular folds (bilateral linea alba, raised 1 mm; Fordyce granules, grouping 10 mm diameter; parotid papilla, raised 2 mm, 4 mm diameter).

mouth and then using a mouth mirror to further retract the tongue laterally. The mucosa may be gently dried with gauze. The clinician may observe the submandibular and sublingual salivary flow by milking the glands, stroking the skin just below the inferior border of the mandible from posterior to anterior. The floor of the mouth should be palpated with the index finger of one hand in the floor of the mouth and the opposite hand from outside of the mouth gently pressing up from medial to the inferior border of the lower jaw. Palpation is best started posteriorly

from the submandibular region on one side, moving anteriorly through the submental region, and around to the submandibular region of the opposite side. The index finger in the floor of the mouth and is moved gradually around the base of the tongue. Gentle pressure is applied down to palpate structures between the two hands.

The lingual aspect of the mandible also should be palpated carefully. Many patients reveal bony bumps or projections, called *mandibular tori,* particularly in the premolar to cuspid area. These tori are benign bony overgrowths

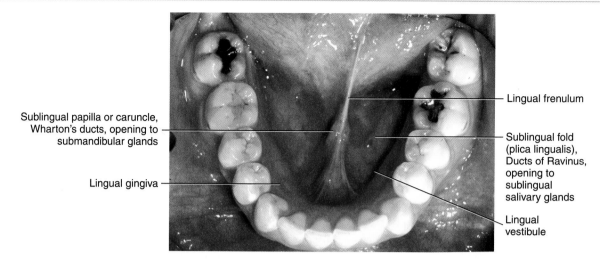

Sublingual papilla or caruncle, Wharton's ducts, opening to submandibular glands

Lingual gingiva

Lingual frenulum

Sublingual fold (plica lingualis), Ducts of Ravinus, opening to sublingual salivary glands

Lingual vestibule

FIG. 13-16 Features of the oral cavity. (Modified from Liebgott B: *The anatomical basis of dentistry,* ed 2, St Louis, 2001, Mosby.)

and should be noted and carefully monitored for any changes over time. Such changes may or may not reflect development of pathological conditions.

Because the base of the tongue sits in the center of the floor of the mouth, it normally is examined in conjunction with the floor of the mouth. However, this portion of the examination is covered in the next section, which considers the tongue as a whole.

Case Application

Mrs. Jorgensen's lingual frenulum has a 1 mm tissue tag just superior to her submandibular caruncles. Milking the submandibular salivary glands produces squirts of fluid from the submandibular ducts. Drying the floor of the mouth before palpation produces rapid flow from the sublingual salivary glands. The lingual vestibule and lingual gingiva appear normal. These findings are shown in Fig. 13-17.

 EXAMINATION OF THE TONGUE

13-I
13-J *ANATOMICAL LANDMARKS AND TOPOGRAPHY*

With the mouth wide open, the tongue fills the floor of the mouth with only the upper, or dorsal, surface of the tongue visible. The dorsum of the tongue is covered by mucous membrane, but unlike the smooth, moist mucosa seen throughout the rest of the oral cavity, the dorsal tongue appears rough. This rough surface is due to the presence of thousands of papillae projecting from the *dorsal surface.*

The most numerous of the papillae are the filiform papillae: small, spikelike projections covering most of the surface of the tongue. These papillae usually appear whitish in color because of an outer covering of keratin, which is constantly being sloughed from the tip of the papillae. The amount of keratin present varies considerably from one individual to another and also varies over time in any given individual because of diet and oral habits. The keratin may become stained by extrinsic factors such as coffee and smoking. Regular brushing of the dorsal surface

of the tongue is recommended as part of proper oral hygiene, particularly to control potential halitosis.

The second most numerous type of papillae found on the dorsum of the tongue is called *fungiform papillae.* As their name suggests, these are small mushroom-shaped projections, which are found scattered amongst the filiform papillae and are most common along the lateral border and tip of the tongue. Fungiform papillae are less keratinized compared with the filiform papillae and are therefore often reddish in color. Also in contrast to the filiform papillae, the fungiform papillae contain taste buds. Posteriorly, at the junction of the horizontal body of the tongue and the vertical root of the tongue is a V-shaped groove with the apex directed posteriorly, termed the *sulcus terminalis.* Running parallel and just anterior to the sulcus terminalis is a row of 7 to 14 large and distinctive circumvallate papillae. Each circumvallate papilla is surrounded by a trough, or crypt, into which numerous taste buds open.

The least prominent type of papillae found on the human tongue are the foliate papillae, sparsely scattered along the lateral borders of the tongue. These papillae are small leaflike projections oriented in vertical ridges. They also contain taste buds.

From the anterior tip, or apex, of the tongue, the dorsum of the tongue is divided in half longitudinally by a midline depression, the median lingual sulcus, which varies in depth from one individual to another. The dorsal surface may be additionally indented by fissures generally oriented perpendicular to the median sulcus. These fissures may again be highly variable in number and depth from one individual to another. A common condition noted on the dorsum of the tongue is termed *wandering glossitis,* or geographical tongue. The epithelium of the papillae is lost, and the dorsal surface becomes smooth in patches, resembling a topographical map. This condition can appear in irregular shapes and can change location, thus the term "wandering" glossitis. One final feature of the dorsum of the tongue is a small pit at the apex of the sulcus terminalis, called the *foramen cecum,* or blind opening, which

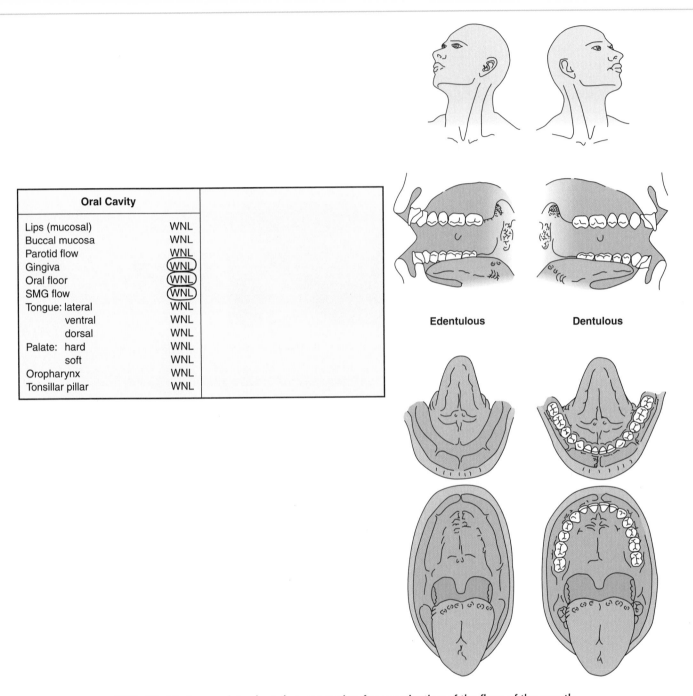

Oral Cavity	
Lips (mucosal)	WNL
Buccal mucosa	WNL
Parotid flow	WNL
Gingiva	(WNL)
Oral floor	(WNL)
SMG flow	(WNL)
Tongue: lateral	WNL
ventral	WNL
dorsal	WNL
Palate: hard	WNL
soft	WNL
Oropharynx	WNL
Tonsillar pillar	WNL

Edentulous   **Dentulous**

FIG. 13-17 Appropriate chart documentation for examination of the floor of the mouth.

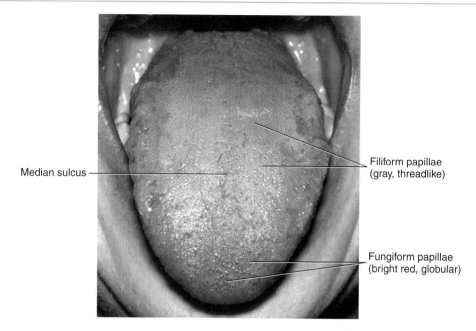

FIG. 13-18 Dorsum of the tongue. (From Liebgott B: *The anatomical basis of dentistry,* ed 2, St Louis, 2001, Mosby.)

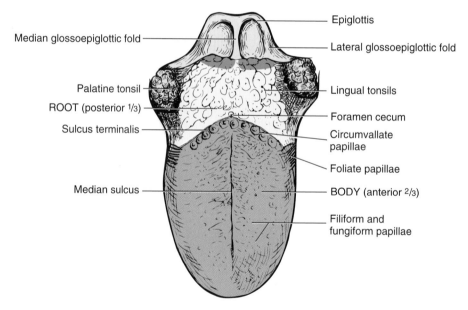

FIG. 13-19 Anatomical landmarks on the dorsum and root of the tongue. (Modified from Liebgott B: *The anatomical basis of dentistry,* ed 2, St Louis, 2001, Mosby.)

marks the site of the former thyroglossal duct. This duct connects the thyroid gland to its site of origin from the base of the tongue (Fig. 13-18).

The vertically oriented root, or base, of the tongue forms the anterior wall of the pharynx, or throat, as it drops away from the back of the oral cavity. This portion of the tongue is composed primarily of lymphoid tissue, called the *lingual tonsils,* which produce a lumpy surface in this region. The lymphoid tissue may at times be mistaken for papillae or pathology when it projects forward into the posterolateral body of the tongue. The body of the tongue

is the anterior two thirds of the tongue and lies fully within the oral cavity (Fig. 13-19).

The ventral surface of the tongue is a thin mucous membrane through which the vasculature is readily visible, particularly the large lingual veins. In older patients, these veins may become varicosed, producing grapelike purplish masses under the tip of the tongue. The lingual frenulum reaches a variable distance up the ventral midline towards the tip of the tongue. Lateral to the lingual veins on each side is a low fold with fingerlike projections, which gives the folds the name *plica fimbriata* (Fig. 13-20).

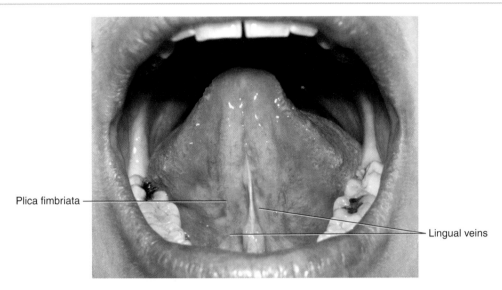

Plica fimbriata

Lingual veins

FIG. 13-20 Ventral surface of the tongue. (Modified from Liebgott B: *The anatomical basis of dentistry,* ed 2, St Louis, 2001, Mosby.)

EXAMINATION TECHNIQUE

The dorsal and lateral surfaces of the tongue are best examined with the patient's mouth wide open and the tongue thrust forward. A piece of gauze either wrapped or draped around the tip of the tongue enables the examiner to gently pull the tongue forward for better visualization. All surfaces of the tongue should be carefully viewed and then palpated as a finger is run firmly over the surfaces. Caution must be used in an examination of the posterior body and the root of the tongue to avoid stimulation of the patient's gag reflex. The clinician may best visualize the root of the tongue by pulling the tongue as far forward as possible and using a mouth mirror to look down at the root surface. Care must be taken not to stimulate the gag reflex of the soft palate or the oropharyngeal wall with the mirror. Use of spray topical anesthetic may be helpful in the visualization of this posterior region and is advised when palpation of the root of the tongue is required for examination of suspected pathologic processes.

The ventral surface of the tongue may be readily viewed when the patient touches the tip of the tongue up to the front of the hard palate. A mouth mirror or fingertip also may be used to push the tongue to first one side and then to the other to view the lateral and posterior ventral surfaces of the tongue.

Case Application

The dorsal surface of the tongue is mildly fissured and is colored a light brown in the central area. On questioning, Mrs. Jorgensen reports that she drinks six to seven cups of coffee per day and does not brush her tongue. Palpation of the tongue is unremarkable, revealing a firm texture and a moist surface. Examination of the ventral surface of the tongue reveals normal lingual veins and a short frenulum. Fig. 13-21 illustrates the findings of this portion of the examination.

EXAMINATION OF THE HARD AND SOFT PALATES

13-K

ANATOMICAL LANDMARKS AND TOPOGRAPHY

The roof of the mouth, the palate, is composed of two subregions, the hard palate and the soft palate. The hard palate forms the anterior two thirds of the palatal region, lying between the alveolar processes of the two maxilla and supported by bony plates projecting horizontally to the midline from the maxilla (Fig. 13-22). The soft palate is the posterior one third of the roof of the mouth and is formed by a group of small palatal muscles covered by a mucous membrane.

Anteriorly, the hard palate begins just lingual to the maxillary central incisor teeth. This area is distinguished by a midline papilla, the incisive papilla, which overlies the incisive, or nasopalatine, canal from the nasal cavity. Extending posteriorly from the incisive papilla is the midline median palatine raphe, which may be marked by a shallow depression or a low ridge created by the direct binding of the palatal mucosa to the underlying bony plates and ending at the posterior extent of the hard palate. The anterior palate is also characterized by the palatine rugae, dense ridges of mucosa radiating roughly perpendicular to the palatine raphe just posterior to the incisive papilla. The mucosal covering of the hard palate is generally thicker than the mucosa seen throughout the rest of the oral cavity due to an increase in the keratin layer, which acts as a protective coating against the abrasive forces of mastication. Such heavily keratinized mucosa is termed *masticatory mucosa* and is a lighter shade of pink than nonmasticatory mucosa because the underlying blood vessels do not show through as clearly. Excessive bony growth at the midline of the palate, termed *torus palatinus* (similar to mandibular tori), is also common.

The junction of the hard palate posteriorly with the

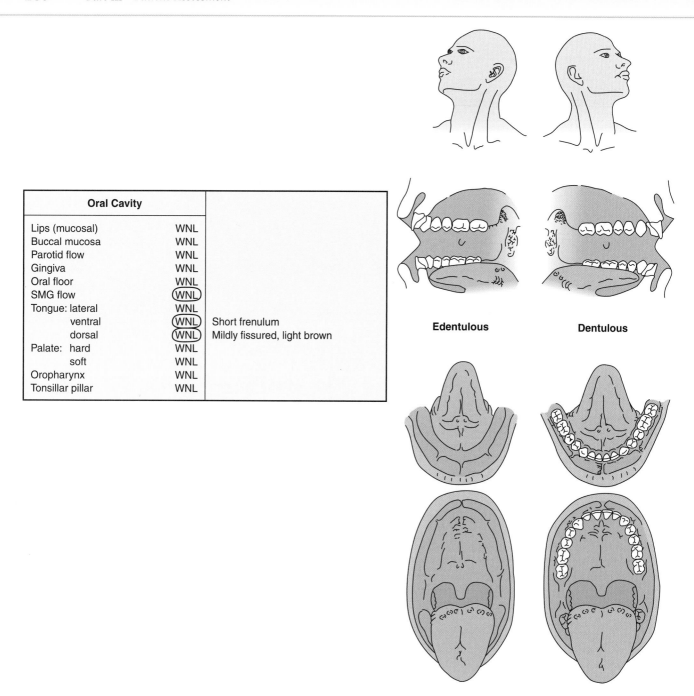

Oral Cavity		
Lips (mucosal)	WNL	
Buccal mucosa	WNL	
Parotid flow	WNL	
Gingiva	WNL	
Oral floor	WNL	
SMG flow	(WNL)	
Tongue: lateral	WNL	
ventral	(WNL)	Short frenulum
dorsal	(WNL)	Mildly fissured, light brown
Palate: hard	WNL	
soft	WNL	
Oropharynx	WNL	
Tonsillar pillar	WNL	

Edentulous   **Dentulous**

FIG. 13-21 Appropriate chart documentation for examination of the tongue (mildly fissured, light brown, short frenulum).

soft palate is indistinct at rest, but can be easily delineated as the appropriately named vibrating line when the patient says "ahh." Just anterior to the vibrating line and on either side of the midline are two small depressions, known as the *palatine fovea,* which are formed by the common openings of two groupings of minor salivary glands. Laterally, the mucosa of the hard palate is continuous with that of the lingual alveolar processes (see Fig. 13-22).

Posteriorly, the soft palate forms a flap hinged off the back edge of the hard palate that separates the oral cavity from the nasal cavity. The flap is generally rounded posteriorly until the midline is approached. At the midline the soft palate has a posterior projection of variable length and width called the *uvula.* The mucosa of the soft palate is thinner than that of the hard palate because of a decrease of the keratin layer and is therefore redder in color than the hard palate (Fig. 13-23). The soft palate may appear inflamed when a patient experiences a cold, cough, or allergy. The mucosa of both the hard and the soft palates has numerous openings of small, accessory salivary glands, which may give the palates a dotted appearance.

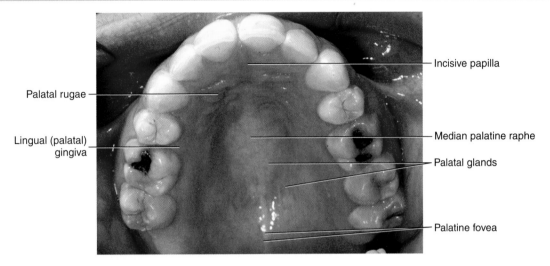

FIG. 13-22 Hard palate. (Modified from Liebgott B: *The anatomical basis of dentistry*, ed 2, St Louis, 2001, Mosby.)

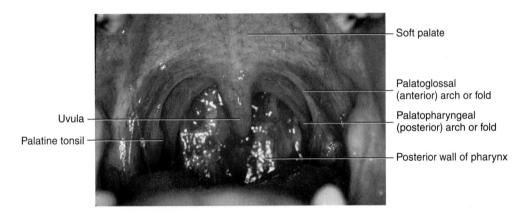

FIG. 13-23 Soft palate. (Modified from Liebgott B: *The anatomical basis of dentistry*, ed 2, St Louis, 2001, Mosby.)

EXAMINATION TECHNIQUE

The hard and soft palates can be best visualized when the patient's head is tilted back as the patient lies in a supine position with the mouth wide open. A mouth mirror is recommended to facilitate complete examination of the entire palatal region. In addition, asking the patient to say "ahh" as the examiner gently depresses the tongue may prove helpful. The hard palate can be easily palpated with a single finger. The mucosa is tightly bound down to bone along the palatine raphe but becomes increasingly resilient as palpation is directed out laterally because of increasing glandular and adipose tissues. Palpation should be continued onto the soft palate cautiously because of the possible stimulation of the patient's gag reflex.

Case Application

Examination of the hard palate reveals a flat, erythematous lesion in the right anterior quadrant measuring 3 mm wide by 5 mm long oriented parallel to the long axis of the palate. Mrs. Jorgensen reports that she burned the roof of her mouth

eating pizza about 4 days ago. The hard palate is firm and moist on palpation. The soft palate is normal on visual examination. Fig. 13-24 illustrates findings for the hard and soft palates.

EXAMINATION OF THE OROPHARYNX AND PALATINE TONSILS

13-L

ANATOMICAL LANDMARKS AND TOPOGRAPHY

The opening from the oral cavity into the posteriorly located oropharynx is termed the *fauces* of the oral cavity, or the *oropharyngeal isthmus*. The oropharynx is demarcated from the oral cavity by a tissue ridge running from the side of the soft palate superiorly down to the posterior lateral edge of the tongue. This ridge is formed by the palatoglossus muscle, and hence its name, the *palatoglossal fold*. The palatoglossal fold also defines the anterior boundary of the palatine tonsillar bed, a depression of the lateral oropharyngeal wall containing the palatine tonsil.

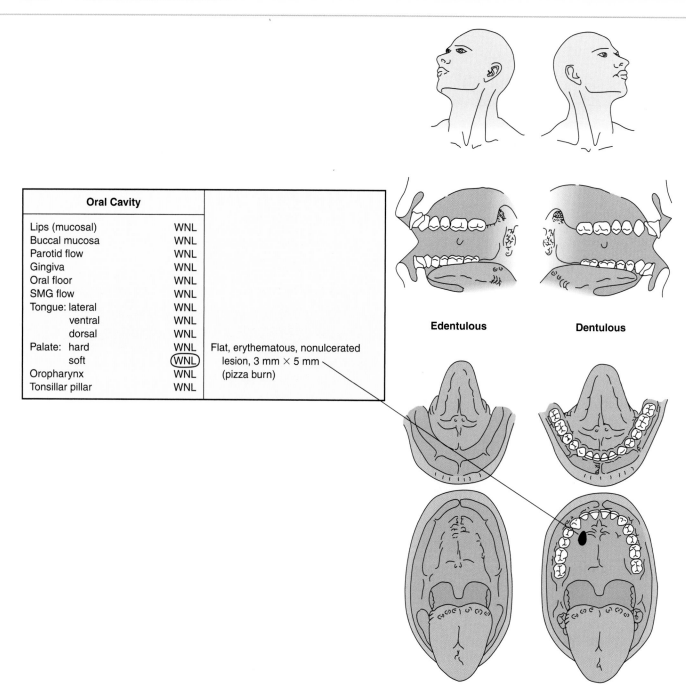

Oral Cavity		
Lips (mucosal)	WNL	
Buccal mucosa	WNL	
Parotid flow	WNL	
Gingiva	WNL	
Oral floor	WNL	
SMG flow	WNL	
Tongue: lateral	WNL	
ventral	WNL	
dorsal	WNL	
Palate: hard	WNL	Flat, erythematous, nonulcerated
soft	(WNL)	lesion, 3 mm × 5 mm
Oropharynx	WNL	(pizza burn)
Tonsillar pillar	WNL	

Edentulous   **Dentulous**

FIG. 13-24 Appropriate chart documentation for examination of the hard and soft palates (flat, erythematous, nonulcerated lesion, 3 mm × 5 mm [pizza burn]).

The posterior boundary of the tonsillar bed is the palatopharyngeal fold, formed by the palatopharyngeal muscle, which extends from the lateral edge of the soft palate down to the larynx. The two folds are also referred to as *the pillars of the fauces.* The anterior pillar is the palatoglossal fold, and the posterior pillar of the fauces is the palatopharyngeal fold.

The palatine tonsillar tissue found lying between the pillars may vary considerably in size, from small, barely discernible lymphoid aggregates to masses large enough to essentially obscure the posterior **pharyngeal** wall, pro-

vided they were not removed by tonsillectomy (see Fig. 13-23). When visible, the posterior pharyngeal wall has a thin mucous membrane and a rich vascular bed, resulting in a deep red coloration. As noted previously, the anterior wall of the pharynx is formed by the lymphoid lingual tonsil of the root of the tongue.

EXAMINATION TECHNIQUE

Examination of this region is largely limited to visual inspection with the exception of cautious palpation of the

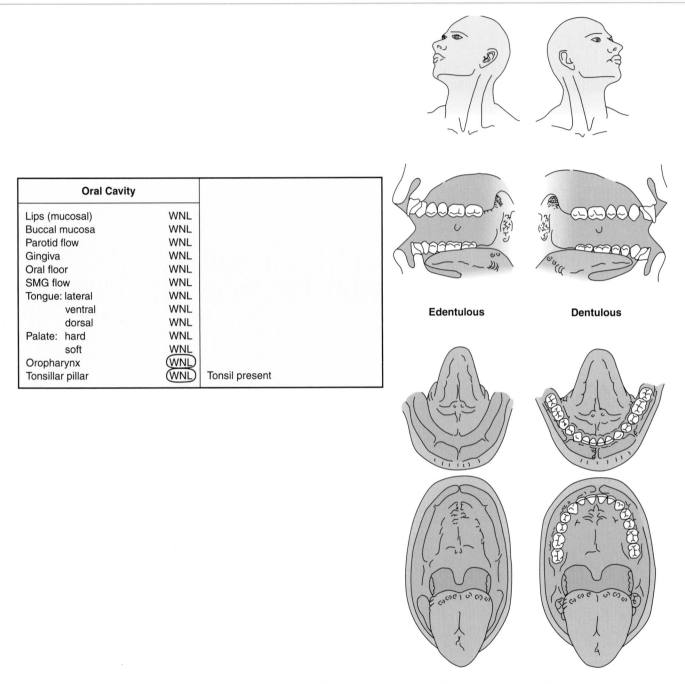

Oral Cavity	
Lips (mucosal)	WNL
Buccal mucosa	WNL
Parotid flow	WNL
Gingiva	WNL
Oral floor	WNL
SMG flow	WNL
Tongue: lateral	WNL
ventral	WNL
dorsal	WNL
Palate: hard	WNL
soft	WNL
Oropharynx	(WNL)
Tonsillar pillar	(WNL) Tonsil present

Edentulous **Dentulous**

FIG. 13-25 Appropriate chart documentation for examination of the oropharynx and the palatine tonsils (tonsil present).

anterior tonsillar pillar and possibly the tonsillar bed. A mouth mirror should be used with care not to stimulate the gag reflex. Spray topical anesthetic may prove helpful with particularly sensitive patients. The clinician usually obtains the best view of the throat by asking the patient to open wide and say *ahh*. Sometimes the clinician may find it helpful to sit the patient in a somewhat upright position so that the patient's tongue falls naturally against the floor of the mouth. This positioning permits the clinician better vision of the oropharynx. Retraction of the tongue forward and/or depression of the tongue of-

ten helps the clinician in visualizing the root of the patient's tongue.

Case Application

The oropharynx appears normal, with a moderately red (vascular), moist mucosa. Mrs. Jorgensen still has her palatine tonsils. They are of normal mucosal coloration and lie low within the tonsillar beds. Fig. 13-25 is an example of appropriate charting of this region, whereas Fig. 13-26 summarizes the findings of the intraoral examination of Mrs. Jorgensen.

HEAD AND NECK PHYSICAL EXAMINATION

GENERAL APPEARANCE & VITAL SIGNS: Blood pressure_____ /_____   Pulse/min_____   Date_____ /_____ /_____

Weight_____   Recall blood pressure_____ /_____   Pulse/min_____   Date_____ /_____ /_____

Height_____   Recall blood pressure_____ /_____   Pulse/min_____   Date_____ /_____ /_____

Recall blood pressure_____ /_____   Pulse/min_____   Date_____ /_____ /_____

External Structures		
Scalp	WNL	
Facial skin	WNL	
Facial symmetry	WNL	
Eyes	WNL	
Nose	WNL	
Lips	(WNL)	Mildly chapped lips
Ears	WNL	
Salivary glands	WNL	
Neck	WNL	
Hands	WNL	

Oral Cavity		
Lips (mucosal)	(WNL)	
Buccal mucosa	(WNL)	Bilateral linea alba, raised 1 mm
Parotid flow	(WNL)	Fordyce granules, 10 mm diameter
Gingiva	(WNL)	Parotid papilla, raised 2 mm,
Oral floor	(WNL)	4 mm diameter
SMG flow	(WNL)	
Tongue: lateral	WNL	
ventral	(WNL)	Short frenulum
dorsal	(WNL)	Mildly fissured, light brown
Palate: hard	WNL	Flat, erythematous, nonulcerated
soft	(WNL)	lesion, 3 mm × 5 mm
Oropharynx	(WNL)	(pizza burn)
Tonsillar pillar	(WNL)	Tonsil present

Ears, Nose, and Throat		
Tympanic membrane	WNL	
Nasal cavity	WNL	
Larynx: T cords	WNL	
F cords	WNL	
AE fold	WNL	
pyriform	WNL	
Epiglottis	WNL	

Edentulous   **Dentulous**

Cranial Nerves			
Subjective		Objective motor	
Smell (olf I)	WNL	Eye movement (III, IV, VI)	WNL
Taste (facial VII, glosso IX)	WNL	Nystagmus	+ −
Hearing (acoustic VIII)	WNL	Facial (VII)	WNL
Vision (optic II)	WNL	Trigem (V)	WNL
		Access (XI)	WNL
Objective sensory		Hypogl (XII)	WNL
Trigen (V)	WNL	Sympathetic (pupil)	WNL
Paresthesia	+ −		

FIG. 13-26 Summary of charted findings for clinical case.

CRITICAL THINKING ACTIVITIES

1. The tongue serves many oral functions. The one we think least about is the task of locating plaque. Place your tongue as far back on the buccal surface of your maxillary teeth as possible. What is the furthest tooth structure you can reach? Survey five classmates; check their response to this question. What problems in patient education could you foresee if tongue placement could not reach the distal of the most distal tooth?

2. Survey five classmates for the following intraoral conditions and tabulate your results:
   a. Leukoedema
   b. Linea alba
   c. Palatine raphe
   d. Salivary caruncles
   e. Fordyce granules
   f. Palatine tonsils

3. Describe the buccal mucosa of a patient with xerostomia. What do you think you would observe?

4. Working with a classmate, determine the best order in which to evaluate intraoral structures. Compare your order of exam with another group. Were there any similarities?

REVIEW QUESTIONS

1. Mucosal tissue that appears wrinkled and filmy white but translucent when gently stretched taut is called which of the following?
   a. Leukoplakia
   b. Candidiasis
   c. Leukoedema
   d. Erythema multiforme

2. Which of the following describes a dense pad of tissue in the area just distal to the pterygomandibular fold behind the last mandibular molar?
   a. Retromolar pad
   b. Raphe
   c. Tuberosity
   d. Buccal mucosa

3. In an examination of the mucosal surface of the cheeks, drying the surface with gauze is best for which of the following reasons?
   a. To increase patient comfort
   b. To gain a true picture of color
   c. To avoid slipping
   d. To observe secretion of accessory salivary glands

4. Fordyce granules can be found on which intraoral structure?
   a. On the hard palate
   b. In the buccal mucosa
   c. In the lip
   d. All the above
   e. All but *a*

5. The sublingual caruncle holds the opening of which of the following ducts?
   a. Palatine fovea
   b. Parotid
   c. Submandibular
   d. None of the above

6. The remnant of the thyroglossal duct, seen as a small pit at the apex of the sulcus terminalis, is termed which of the following?
   a. Mental foramen
   b. Foramen cecum
   c. Sella turcica
   d. Median lingual sulcus

7. The armamentarium necessary to perform the intraoral examination includes which of the following?
   a. Gauze
   b. Mouth mirror
   c. Air
   d. Overhead light
   e. All but *c*
   f. All the above

8. A white line running horizontally on the buccal mucosa is known as which of the following terms?
   a. Leukoedema
   b. Candidiasis
   c. Lichen planus
   d. Linea alba
   e. None of the above

9. The small, spinelike projections covering most of the tongue's surface are which type of papilla?
   a. Filiform
   b. Fungiform
   c. Circumvallate
   d. Foliate

10. Palatine rugae are located on which portion of the palate?
    a. Anterior palate
    b. Palatine fovea
    c. Soft palate
    d. Vibrating line

SUGGESTED AGENCIES AND WEB SITES

Because of the ever-changing nature of the Internet, some of the web sites listed here may have changed since publication. Please refer to Mosby's Evolve web site for the most current information.

American Association of Oral and Maxillofacial Surgery: Consumer Information, 9700 West Bryn Mawr Avenue, Rosemont, IL 60018-5701; (847) 678-6200: http://www.aaoms.org

American Cancer Society: http://www.cancer.org

The American Dental Hygienists' Association ("Oral health information: oral cancer facts"): http://www.adha.org

American Heart Association ("High blood pressure: AHA recommendation"): http://www.americanheart.org

American Heart Association: National Center, 7272 Greenville Avenue, Dallas, TX 75231; (214) 373-6300: http://www.americanheart.org

Baylor School of Dentistry ("Detecting oral cancer: a guide for dentists"): http://www.tambcd.edu

Healthlink USA ("Oral cancer"): http://www.healthlinkusa.com

Homestead Schools, Inc. ("Oral examination"): http://www.homesteadschools.com

Medline Plus ("Health information: oral cancer" [a service of the National Library of Medicine]): http://www.nlm.nih.gov/medlineplus

National Cancer Institute: http://www.nci.nih.gov

National Cancer Institute, News Center: http://rex.nci.nih.gov

National Center for Chronic Disease Prevention and Health Promotion: Oral Health Resources, Division of Oral Health, Centers for Disease Control and Prevention, 4770 Buford Highway, NE, MS F-10, Atlanta, GA 30341; (770) 488-6054: http://www.cdc.gov

National Coalition for Cancer Survivorship: http://www.cansearch.org

National Heart, Lung, and Blood Institute, National High Blood Pressure Education Program: http://hin.nhlbi.nih.gov

National Institute of Dental & Craniofacial Research, National Institutes of Health, Bethesda, MD 20892-2190: http://www.nidcr.nih.gov

National Institute of Dental Research: Building 31, Room 2C35, 31 Center Drive MSC 2290, Bethesda, MD 20892-2290; Telephone (301) 496-4261, Fax (301) 496-9988: http://www.aoa.dhhs.gov

National Institute on Aging: Building 31, Room 5C27, 31 Center Drive, MSC 2292, Bethesda, MD 20892; (301) 496-1752: http://www.nih.gov/nia

National Institutes of Health, U.S. Department of Health and Human Services, 31 Center Drive MSC 2290, Bethesda, MD 20582-2290: http://www.nih.gov

National Institutes of Health ("Oral cancer: confronting the enemy"): http://www.nidr.nih.gov

National Institutes of Health ("Surgeon general's report on oral health"): http://www.nidcr.nih.gov

NOAH (New York Online Access to Health): http://www.noahhealth.org

Northwestern University ("Concepts of intraoral examination") http://faculty-web.at.nwu.edu

Oral Cancer Awareness Initiative: http://www.oral-cancer.org

Oregon Health Sciences University ("Head and neck exam: intraoral examination" [variance of normal buccal mucosa; linea alba]): http://www.teleport.com

University of Minnesota ("Oral cancer self-examination"): http://www.umanitoba.ca

Washington State University ("Dental erosion: case-based learning for dental hygiene treatment"): http://www.wsu.edu

Washington State University ("Tongue piercing: case-based learning for dental hygiene treatment"): http://www.wsu.edu

World Dentistry, Inc. ("Improving the detection and prevention of oral cancer"): http://www.worlddent.com

 ## ADDITIONAL READINGS AND RESOURCES

Avery JK, Steele PF: *Essentials of oral histology and embryology: a clinical approach,* ed 2, St Louis, 1999, Mosby.

Fehrenbach MJ, Herring SW: *Illustrated anatomy of the head and neck,* Philadelphia, 1995, WB Saunders.

Liebgott B: *The anatomical basis of dentistry,* ed 2, St Louis, 2001, Mosby.

Regezi JA, Sciubba JJ: *Oral Pathology: clinical pathologic correlations,* ed 3, Philadelphia, 1998, WB Saunders.

CHAPTER 14

Clinical Manifestations *of* Common Medications

Robert Sherman, George M. Taybos

Chapter Outline

Case Study: Erythema Multiforme
Erythema Multiforme
   History
   Epidemiology
   Signs and symptoms
   Etiological factors
   Associated systemic drugs
   Precipitating factors
   Treatment
Xerostomia
   Signs and symptoms
   Etiology
   Associated systemic drugs
   Management
Lichenoid Drug Reaction
   Signs and symptoms
   Histology
   Associated systemic drugs
   Treatment
Gingival Hyperplasia
   Etiology
   Clinical history
   Mechanism for gingival enlargement

   Histology
   Associated systemic drugs
   Management and treatment
Dysgeusia
   Signs and symptoms
   Anatomy
   Associated systemic drugs
Oral Pigmentation
   Etiology
Hairy Tongue
   Signs and symptoms
   Associated systemic drugs
   Treatment
Angioedema
   Signs and symptoms
   Associated systemic drugs
   Histology
   Treatment
Candidiasis
   Etiology
   Signs and symptoms
   Associated systemic drugs
   Treatment

Key Terms

Angioedema
Candidiasis

Drug interactions
Dysgeusia

Gingival hyperplasia
Lichenoid drug reaction

Xerostomia

Learning Outcomes

1. Identify patients' chief oral complaints as they may relate to their medications.
2. Classify the patients' medication categories.
3. Develop a differential diagnosis of the patient's chief complaint to include a medication as the etiological factor.

4. Confidently discuss the relationship between the patient's chief complaint and medications with the patient's physician and dentist.

267

*M*edications, whether prescription or over the counter (OTC), should obtain the maximal benefit for the individual while producing minimal adverse effects. The dental hygienist must (1) determine all medications that patients are taking, (2) know the desired action of the medication(s), and (3) know the adverse effects of the medication(s). The practice of medicine has progressed to the level that conditions once considered debilitating or fatal are routinely treated and/or managed.[41]

14-A

Approximately 30% of the population is more than 50 years of age. Studies have shown that people 80 years of age and older used four times as many drugs as those in the 18- to 33-year-old age group. Approximately 68.9% of all medications are taken by females.[23] The dental hygienist therefore is treating (1) an older population, (2) a population with medically compromising conditions, and (3) a population in which more than 40% of the patients are taking a prescribed medications or multiple medications.[23] Therefore the overall health status of the patient must become as much the concern of the dental hygienist as the thorough and accurate diagnosis and treatment of oral disease.[13]

Use of medications is increasing. Modern culture promotes the belief that a pill can cure all ailments. However, the medications do not have a narrow range of activity and often cause many unwanted (adverse) effects. The dental hygienist has two concerns when treating patients who are taking medications: Will any adverse *drug interactions* occur from the drug(s) administered or prescribed for the dental hygiene procedure? Do the patients' medications cause oral adverse conditions or symptoms?

Patients are seen by the hygienist for numerous reasons, including an initial oral prophylaxis for a new patient, supportive-care appointment, scheduled or unscheduled posttreatment appointment, or an unscheduled visit for a dental emergency. Most dental emergency appointments are due to pain and/or infection caused by dental caries, periodontal problems, or a postsurgical complication. However, patients are more frequently seeing their dental healthcare providers for concerns not specifically related to caries or periodontal disease. The etiology for these symptoms may be puzzling. The patient reports vague signs and symptoms. The clinical findings may range from normal-appearing tissues to a severe, diffuse ulcerative or erythematous appearance affecting the entire buccal mucosa, dorsum of the tongue, and/or keratinized gingiva. The evaluation of this patient is quite time-consuming; the determination of the etiology of the problem may remain elusive; and the management of the chief complaint, then, is based on addressing of the symptoms and not necessarily the disease process. This patient also may have been seen by a number of both medical and dental professionals without any positive impact in the diagnosis and treatment of the oral condition.

The oral mucosa is an actively dividing tissue and is susceptible to the effects of medications on both its structure and mature appearance. Medications may affect the oral tissues from both local contact and systemic reaction. Thus the dental hygienist must thoroughly review the patient's medical history and accurately determine all prescription and OTC medications the patient is taking.

A review of the 200 most prescribed medications in 1998 reveals that 175 of them are associated with an adverse effect on the oral tissues or structures.[47] Table 14-1

TABLE 14-1

Classification of the 200 most prescribed drugs of 1998

Category	Percentage of prescription
Cardiovascular drugs	27
Hormone replacement	
BCPs, estrogen, progresterone	10
Endocrine—DM, thyroid	6
Antimicrobial agents	12.5
Analgesic agents	8.6
Asthma drugs	5.5
Antianxiety/sedative–hypnotic drugs	5
Antidepressant drugs	4.5
Gastric acid secretion inhibitors	4.5
Antihistamines	3.5
Other classes	13

From Zoeller J: The top 200 drugs, *Am Druggist* Feb:41-8, 1999. *BCPs,* Birth control pills; *DM,* diabetes mellitus.

BOX 14-1

Oral Signs and Symptoms Associated with Adverse Drug Reactions

Angioderma
Candidiasis
Cough
Dysgeusia
Erythema multiforme
Gingival bleeding
Gingival hyperplasia
Glossodynia glossitis
Increased gag reflex
Lichenoid drug reaction
Mouth/jaw discomfort
Mouth ulcerations/ stomatitis
Oral paresthesia
Pharyngitis
Reflux/hyperacidity
Tooth disorder
Vomiting
Xerostomia

---

lists the classes and incidence of prescribed medications causing an oral adverse event, and Box 14-1 lists the identified oral adverse effects from the medications.[47] The more common oral adverse effects are discussed.

ERYTHEMA MULTIFORME

HISTORY

In 1866 Dr. Ferdinand von Hebra in his treatise *On Diseases of the Skin* wrote about "erythema exudativum multiforme."[44] He is credited with originating the term *erythema multiforme (EM)*. The characteristics of EM as described by von Hebra were an acute, self-limiting, mild skin disease characterized by skin lesions, located primarily on the extremities and by a tendency for recurrences. In 1922 Drs. Stevens and Johnson described an acute febrile illness with skin lesions resembling EM, an associated stomatitis, and a severe conjunctivitis with visual impairment.[38] By the early 1940s this severe form of EM was universally known as Stevens-Johnson syndrome. In 1950 Thomas developed the terms *EM minor* to describe the mild cutaneous form that von Hebra discussed and *EM major* to describe the

Case Study **Erythema Multiforme**

A 65-year-old Caucasian man, Harry Liebowitz, is scheduled for his 6-month supportive-care appointment. He states that his mouth is sore and that this soreness has been present for almost the past 6 months.

You review Mr. Liebowitz's medical history and find the following medical problems and medications:

Hypertension	Lopressor
Elevated cholesterol	Lopid
Rheumatoid arthritis	Naprosyn, Darvocet-N100, ASA
GI disturbance	Zantac

Mr. Liebowitz's social history is negative. He states that he has never used any tobacco products and does not consume alcoholic beverages.

Your clinical examination reveals the following:

Buccal mucosa	Bilateral buccal mucosa; diffuse white lacy lesions over erythematous mucosa. On the left side are focal areas of ulcerations 6 mm × 8 mm
Tongue	Left side of the tongue in the middle to posterior third on the ventrolateral surface is a 8 mm × 20 mm area of white lacy lesions over erythematous tissue with ulcerations 6 mm × 10 mm

The overall oral cancer screening examination does not reveal any abnormal findings except the documented lesion on the tongue. This is a high-risk area for oral cancer.

TABLE 14-2

Systemic drugs associated with erythema multiforme

Category	Agents
Antimicrobial agents	Sulfonamides, penicillins, TCN, chloramphenicol, isoniazid, rifampin, clindamycin, dapsone, TMP/SMZ
Oral hypoglycemic agents	Diabinese, Glucotrol
Chemotherapeutic agents	Alkylating agents, MTX
NSAIDs	Aspirin, ibuprofen, fenoprofen, sulindac, Relafen, Daypro
Hormones	Estrogen
Anticonvulsant drugs	Carbamazepine, trimethadione, ethosuximide, Depakote, Dilantin
Opioid analgesic agents	Codeine
Antianxiety agents	Meprobamate
Sedative–hypnotic drugs	Glutethimide (Doriglute)
Muscle relaxants	Quinine
Cardiovascular agents	Diuretics: furosemide Vasodilator: minoxidil ACE inhibitors: Vasotec
Antiinflammatory agents	Glucocorticoids
H$_2$-antagonist agents	Cimetidine
Antihelminth agents	Thiabendazole
Antigout agent	Allopurinol

From Huff JC, Weston WL, Tonnesen MG: Erythema multiforme: a review of characteristics, diagnostic criteria, and causes, *J Am Acad Dermatol* 8(6):763-75, 1983.
TCN, Tetracycline; *TMP/SMZ,* trimethoprine/sulfamethoxazole; *MTX,* methotrexate, *NSAIDs,* nonsteroidal antiinflammatory drugs; *ACE,* angiotensin-converting enzymes.
NOTE: Compare with Table 14-1, listing the incidence of prescriptions by drug category.

---

severe mucocutaneous form that Stevens and Johnson characterized.[21]

EPIDEMIOLOGY

EM occurs in young, healthy individuals, predominantly in males. Most cases occur in the 20-year-old to 40-year-old age group, but about 20% occur in children and adolescents. The annual incidence of EM is estimated to be 0.01% to 1%. The rate of recurring EM cases is 22% to 37%.[21]

SIGNS AND SYMPTOMS

The initial symptoms of EM include the nonspecific complaints of fever, malaise, headache, sore throat, rhinorrhea, and cough. These symptoms appear to be more common in major EM than minor EM. The cutaneous lesion is a round, erythematous macule that becomes papular and progresses to the classic "iris," "target," or "bull's-eye" appearance with the central area of necrosis. The oral mucosa is involved in 25% to 60% of the cases. The oral lesions begin as erythematous areas with edema that quickly progresses to large erosive lesions with a pseudomembranous surface. The oral involvement in EM major is severe and may result in extensive tissue damage and morbidity. EM major has a more prolonged course consistent with the severe mucocutaneous destruction.

EM major has frequent complications. The most common complications involve the eye. Visual impairment resulting from keratitis or conjunctival scarring associated with the disease has been reported in 10% of the cases. Pneumonia has been reported in 30% of the cases and death in 18% of the cases. The gastrointestinal tract may be affected with esophagitis and strictures.

EM minor usually lasts 2 to 4 weeks from onset to healing. EM minor is a benign illness without any complications. The main concern may be difficulty with eating and drinking, which leads to dehydration.[21]

ETIOLOGICAL FACTORS

Etiological factors of EM include the following:
- Infections
- Immunizations
- Neoplasms
- Connective tissue disease
- Physical agent: sunshine, radiation therapy

ASSOCIATED SYSTEMIC DRUGS

Table 14-2 lists systemic drugs associated with erythema multiforme.[21] Compare this table with Table 14-1.

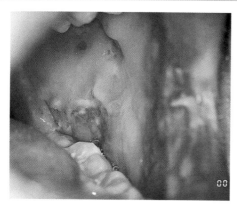

FIG. 14-1 Erythema multiforme. Diffuse ulcerations on the left buccal mucosa and retromolar pad areas.

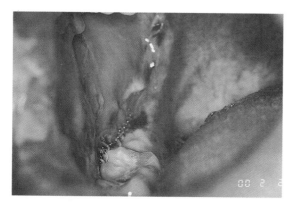

FIG. 14-2 Erythema multiforme. Diffuse ulcerations on the right buccal mucosa and retromolar pad areas.

PRECIPITATING FACTORS

The literature identifies three etiology-related EM syndromes: herpes-associated EM, Mycoplasma-associated EM, and drug-associated EM.

Herpes-Associated Erythema Multiforme

The association of herpes virus infections and EM has been recognized for more than 100 years. The proportion of EM cases ranges from 15% to 63%. This form of EM usually affects young adults and occurs 1 to 3 weeks after the recurrent herpetic infection. Herpes-associated EM generally is in the form of EM minor. The pathogenesis for this form of EM is thought to be either a hypersensitivity reaction to the virus or an inadequate immune response to the recurrent infection (Figs. 14-1 and 14-2).[21]

Mycoplasma-Associated Erythema Multiforme

A clear association exists between EM and *Mycoplasma pneumoniae* infections. This form of EM occurs primarily in children and young adults, follows a severe respiratory infection with *M. pneumoniae,* and resembles EM major.[21]

TABLE 14-3

Drugs linked to minor and major erythema multiforme

Category	Agents
Cardiovascular agents	Vasotec
Anticonvulsant	Dilantin, Depakote
NSAIDs	Relafen, Daypro
Antibiotic agents	TMP/SMZ
Antigout agent	Allopurinol

NSAIDs, Nonsteroidal antiinflammatory drugs; *TMP/SMZ,* trimethoprine/sulfamethoxazole.

Drug-Associated Erythema Multiforme

The best-documented drug-associated EM is related to sulfonamides and more recently trimethoprim-sulfamethoxazole (TMP-SMZ) preparations. The EM occurs usually 7 to 14 days after drug therapy and presents as EM major. Drug-associated EM most likely represents a hypersensitivity reaction to the drug. [21]

A review of the 200 most prescribed drugs in 1998 reveals drugs that have been linked to EM (Table 14-3).[47]

TREATMENT

The treatment by the dental healthcare team is based on the severity of intraoral mucosal lesions, the level of pain, and the degree of difficulty in eating, drinking, and swallowing. The patient with EM major (Stevens-Johnson syndrome) may require hospitalization to ensure adequate hydration and treatment of secondary infections.

The treatment for EM minor remains controversial. For adults, systemic corticosteroid therapy rapidly relieves the oral symptoms, hastens the healing of the intraoral tissues, and has few adverse effects. In addition to the systemic corticosteroid therapy, topical analgesic agents such as diphenhydramine elixir (Benadryl) or 2% viscous lidocaine may be prescribed as rinses to locally decrease the oral pain. Topical steroid rinses such as dexamethasone elixir (0.5 mg/5 ml) may supplement the effects of the systemic corticosteroids.[43]

An important part of treatment is determination of the precipitating factor. If the precipitating factor is a pharmacotherapeutic agent, this agent should not be prescribed for that patient. If the precipitating factor is a recurrent herpetic infection, measures should be employed to minimize reactivation of the latent herpes virus.[43]

Topical Analgesic Agents

Throughout the chapter, *Rx* is the prescription; *Disp* is to dispense; and *Sig* is the direction for the patient on dosing.

Rx: Diphenhydramine hydrochloride (Benadryl) syrup 12.5 mg/5 ml
Disp: 8 oz (240 ml)
Sig: Rinse with 1 tablespoonful (10 ml) for 2 minutes immediately before meals and at bedtime.
or

Rx: Lidocaine hydrochloride viscous 2%
Disp: 100 ml
Sig: Rinse with one teaspoonful (4.9 ml) for 2 minutes before meals and at bedtime; do not swallow.

Topical Steroids

Rx: Dexamethasone elixir (Decadron) 0.5 mg/5 ml
Disp: 8 oz (240 ml)
Sig: Rinse with one tablespoonful (10 ml) for 2 minutes before meals; do not swallow.

XEROSTOMIA

SIGNS AND SYMPTOMS

Xerostomia is a dryness in the mouth from a decrease in the normal salivary secretions; however, xerostomia often is a subjective complaint that is not correlated to an actual decrease in salivary gland activity.

Saliva performs many functions: lubricating and protecting the oral tissues, cleaning the mouth, regulating the oral pH, maintaining the integrity of the teeth, and destroying oral microorganisms. A loss or decrease in saliva production results in many predictable oral changes. The oral mucosa has a dry, atrophic appearance and is more susceptible to trauma (ulcerations) and secondary infections (candidiasis). The teeth are more susceptible to caries activity. In addition to the changes in the mucosa and teeth, the patient may complain of an altered taste, glossodynia or glossitis, and difficulty in mastication and swallowing.[42]

ETIOLOGY

Salivary gland activity is regulated mainly by the parasympathetic nervous system. This salvatory nuclei are stimulated by taste and tactile stimuli from the tongue and other regions in the oral cavity. Another factor that affects salivary gland secretion is the blood supply to the glands. Medications that block or decrease the release of acetylcholine (neurotransmitter) from the neurons result in a decrease in salivary gland secretions; medications that cause an increase in sympathetic activity (adrenaline/epinephrine) result in a decrease of salivary gland activity; and additionally, medications that cause vasoconstriction may result in a decrease in salivary gland secretions.

ASSOCIATED SYSTEMIC DRUGS

The drug categories shown in Table 14-4 can produce xerostomia.

MANAGEMENT

The management of xerostomia is based on the patient's subjective complaints and the clinical findings of the dental hygienist. Patients with xerostomia say their mouth is dry and that they have to sip water all day. The dental hygienist's clinical examination reveals dry oral tissues and a decreased salivary flow (0.1 ml/min or less). This patient

TABLE 14-4	
Systemic drugs associated with xerostomia	
Category	**Agents**
Amphetamines	Adderall
Analgesic agents	
Narcotic agents	Hydrocodone, codeine, oxycodone
NSAIDs	Ibuprofen
Antianxiety/sedative–hypnotic agents	Benzodiazepines
Anticonvulsant agents	Neurontin
Antidepressant agents	
SSRIs	Prozac, Zoloft
Miscellaneous	Serzone, Effexor, Wellbutrin
Tricyclics	Amitriptyline
Antihistamine agents	Claritin, Zyrtec, phenergan, promethazine
Antimicrobial agents	Cipro
Antipsychotic agents	Risperdal
Asthma drugs	Albuterol, Atrovent, Flovent, Rhinocort, Vancenase
Cardiovascular agents	
ACE inhibitors	Zestril, Accupril, Prinivil
Calcium channel blockers	Plendil
Alpha-adrenergic blocker	Hytrin, Cardura, clonidine
Combination agents	Zestoretic
Decongestant agent	Guaifenesin with phenylpropanolamine
Gastric acid secretion inhibitor	Prilosec
Prokinetic GI agent	Propulsid
Skeletal muscle relaxant	Cyclobenzaprine
Tobacco cessation	Zyban

NSAIDs, Nonsteroidal antiinflammatory drugs; *SSRIs,* selective serotonin reuptake inhibitors; *ACE,* angiotensin-converting enzyme; *GI,* gastrointestinal.

may benefit from artificial saliva substitutes (see Chapter 40) to moisten oral tissues and salivary gland stimulators such as Salagen or Evoxac. If the patient exhibits an increased caries rate, the dental hygienist should reinforce oral hygiene procedures and implement a topical fluoride program and antimicrobial rinses.[42]

Salivary Gland Stimulators

Rx: Pilocarpine hydrochloride (Salagen) 5-mg tablets
Disp: 90 tablets
Sig: Take one tablet 30 to 45 minutes before each meal and at bedtime. Maximum of 4 tablets/day
Refills   × _____ (determined by treatment provider)

or

Rx: Evoxac 30-mg capsules
Disp: 90 capsules
Sig: Take one capsule 60 minutes before meals. Maximum of 3 capsules/day.
Refills   × _____ (determined by treatment provider)

Caries Prevention

Rx: Stannous fluoride gel 0.4%
Disp: 4.3 oz
Sig: Place 5 to 10 drops in a custom tray and insert in mouth for 5 minutes daily; do not swallow.

and

Rx: Chlorhexidine gluconate 0.12%
Disp: 480 ml (16 oz)
Sig: Rinse with 0.5 ounces for 30 seconds 2 times a day; do not swallow.

LICHENOID DRUG REACTION

SIGNS AND SYMPTOMS

A *lichenoid drug reaction* results in the appearance of oral lesions that resemble lichen planus. The lesions are located on the posterior buccal mucosa and exhibit a central erythematous area with a surrounding zone of radiating white striae. The patient states the lesion is painful. The designation of a lichenoid drug reaction is based on the temporal relationship by which the individual takes the medication and then subsequently develops the oral lesion. Both lichen planus and lichenoid reactions are thought to represent a delayed hypersensitivity reaction. The cells of the oral mucosa are exposed to an antigenic challenge that initiates interactions that result in both the clinical and histologic appearance of a lichen planus–like lesion (Figs. 14-3 and 14-4).[8,11,37]

HISTOLOGY

The mucosal surface exhibits atrophy and erosion secondary to epithelial cell destruction. The submucosal infiltration consists of T lymphocytes (CD4+ and CD8+) that are located at the basement membrane and parabasilar areas. The lymphocytes adhere to the basal cells in the area where the antigen challenge occurs. This leads to lysis of the basal cells.[8,11,37]

ASSOCIATED SYSTEMIC DRUGS

Table 14-5 provides a list of systemic drugs associated with lichenoid reactions.

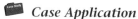 *Case Application*

Mr. Liebowitz is taking a beta blocker (Lopressor), analgesic agents (NSAID: Naprosyn propoxyphene compound), and an H₂ antagonist (Zantac). Each of these drugs has been implicated in causing lichenoid drug reactions.

TREATMENT

The treatment of a lichenoid drug reaction is to eliminate the causative agent, if possible. If the medication cannot be stopped or an adequate substitution cannot be found, the oral signs and symptoms can be managed through initial use of topical corticosteroids (dexamethasone elixir, fluocinonide 0.05%, clobetasol proprionate 0.05%, or triamcinolone 0.1 % ointments in equal parts of Orabase).[43]

The type of corticosteroid therapy is determined by the extent of the lesion. If the lichenoid reaction is localized to a few areas of the oral mucosa, the topical steroid agents placed on the affected mucosa four times a day result in a decrease of the signs and symptoms. If the lichenoid reac-

TABLE 14-5	
Systemic drugs associated with lichenoid drug reactions	
Category	**Agents**
Analgesic agents	NSAIDs, propoxyphene/acetaminophen, acetaminophen/codeine
Antianxiety drugs	Benzodiazepines
Anticonvulsant drugs	Depakote
Cardiovascular agents	Beta-adrenergic blockers, angiotensin II antagonist, calcium channel blockers, cardiac glycoside, diuretics, potassium supplements
Gastric acid secretion inhibitors	H₂-antagonists
Hormone replacement	Thyroid hormone, insulin, sulfonylureas, metformin, oral contraceptives, estrogen, progesterone
Uricosuric agent	Allopurinol

NSAIDs, Nonsteroidal antiinflammatory drugs.

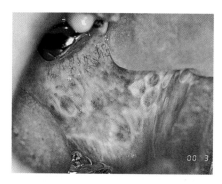

FIG. 14-3 Lichenoid drug reaction. Left buccal mucosa with Wickham's striae on an erythematous tissue and focal areas of ulcerations.

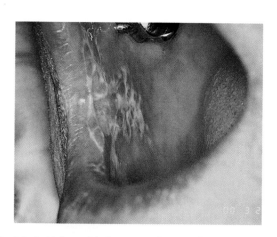

FIG. 14-4 Lichenoid drug reaction. Right buccal mucosa with Wickham's striae on an erythematous tissue.

tion is generalized, rinsing with a tablespoonful (10 ml) of dexamethasone elixir (0.5 mg/5 cc) for 2 minutes four times a day can reduce the erythema and the pain. Systemic corticosteroid therapy is indicated when the lichenoid reaction has not responded to the topical therapy or when the reaction is generalized with severe ulcerations. Oral candidiasis may occur in patients using steroids. These patients should be monitored for the presence of oral candidiasis. Patients with a history of developing candidal infections while using steroids or antibiotics are considered to be candidal carriers and should be prescribed antifungal therapy.[43]

Topical Steroid Agents

Rx:	Fluocinonide ointment (Lidex) 0.05%; mix with equal parts of Orabase
Disp:	10 g
Sig:	Apply a thin film to the lesion after each meal and at bedtime.

or

Rx:	Clobetasol propionate ointment (Temovate) 0.05%; mox with equal parts of Orabase
Disp:	10 g
Sig:	Apply a thin film to the lesion after each meal and at bedtime.

or

Rx:	Triamcinolone acetonide in Orabase 0.1 %
Disp:	5-g tube
Sig:	Apply a thin film to the lesion after each meal and at bedtime.

or

Rx:	Dexamethasone elixir (Decadron) 0.5 mg/5 ml
Disp:	8 ounces (240 ml)
Sig:	Rinse with one tablespoonful (10 ml) for 2 minutes before meals; do not swallow.

GINGIVAL HYPERPLASIA

ETIOLOGY

Anticonvulsant drugs, calcium channel blockers, and cyclosporine are the most common medications associated with *gingival hyperplasia.*[4]

CLINICAL HISTORY

The gingival enlargement usually occurs within 1 to 3 months after initiation of drug therapy. The anterior gingival tissues are the most affected area. Enlargement of the labial gingiva is seen more frequently than the lingual gingiva or edentulous areas. The affected tissues appear normal in color, firm, and lobulated, with a smooth, stippled, or granular surface texture.[4]

MECHANISM FOR GINGIVAL ENLARGEMENT

Many theories have been postulated to explain the gingival enlargement: individual susceptibility, immunological and genetic factors, and a select population of gingival fibroblasts sensitive to the particular medication.[39]

HISTOLOGY

The histologic appearance is similar for phenytoin, calcium channel blockers, and cyclosporine. A chronic inflammatory infiltrate exists with an increased formation of collagen and fibroblasts.

ASSOCIATED SYSTEMIC DRUGS

Phenytoin (Dilantin) is often prescribed for the prevention of seizures (grand mal, status epilepticus, and nonepileptic seizures) and also may be used to manage trigeminal neuralgia. Gingival enlargement is seen in approximately 50% of the patients taking phenytoin and the enlargement is more common in children and adolescents. The severity of the enlargement is directly proportional to the drug dose, the plasma drug level, and the patient's oral hygiene habits.[2] Other anticonvulsant agents that have been reported to cause gingival enlargement are listed in Table 14-6 (Fig. 14-5).[30]

Calcium channel blockers are used to manage hypertension, angina pectoris, cardiac dysrrhythmias, and the prevention of vasospastic angina (Prinzmetal's angina). This class of drugs causes (1) a relaxation and dilatation of the coronary arteries, (2) reduction in the peripheral resistance, (3) decrease in the myocardial oxygen consumption, and (4) decreases in the atrioventricular conduction, heart rate, and blood pressure. Most calcium channel blockers have been reported to cause gingival hyperplasia; however, nifedipine is the most common agent reported.[24] No factors exist for

TABLE 14-6

Selected anticonvulsant agents reported to cause gingival enlargement

Generic name	Brand name
Phenytoin	Dilantin
Valproic acid	Depakote
Phenobarbitol	Barbitol
Mephobarbitol	Mebaral
Primidone	Mysoline
Ethosuximide	Zarontin
Methsuximide	Celontin
Phensuximide	Milontin

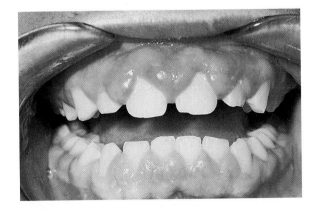

FIG. 14-5 Example of gingival hyperplasia resulting from dilantin therapy for the treatment of seizure disorders.

the prediction of which individuals will develop gingival enlargement.[40] The prevalence rate for gingival enlargement ranges from 6.3% to 43.6% (Fig. 14-6).[12,27]

Selected calcium channel blockers reported to cause gingival enlargement are listed in Table 14-7.[30]

Cyclosporine is an immunosuppressant medication used in the treatment of autoimmune disorders and prevention of rejection of solid organ transplants and bone marrow transplants. Cyclosporine has increased the 5-year survival rate from 50% to 96%, but this medication is not without side effects. Some of the side effects are nephrotoxicity, hepatotoxicity, lymphoma, hypertension, and gingival enlargement. The gingival enlargement occurs in about 25% of the patients taking cyclosporine.[20]

MANAGEMENT AND TREATMENT

Poor oral hygiene is a risk factor directly correlated with the severity of the gingival enlargement. At every dental appointment, the dental hygienist must debride the dentition and reinforce oral hygiene procedures. Ultrasonic debridement with an antimicrobial rinse could be beneficial in reducing bacterial counts. The use of an antimicrobial after-care mouthrinse such as 0.12% chlorhexidine gluconate (Peridex, PerioGard) or an OTC essential oil mouthrinse (e.g., Listerine) may be of benefit by reducing the plaque-forming bacteria and the resultant inflammation. Surgical excision of the enlarged gingiva may be nec-

essary for the most severe cases; however, the enlargement may recur.

The clinical effects of the calcium channel blocker on the gingiva are usually reversible. In consultation with the patient's physician, substitution of the offending drug for a similar drug may reduce or even prevent the gingival enlargement.[45] Discontinuing the offending drug often results in marked improvement within 1 week and a complete resolution within 8 weeks. Patients taking cyclosporine do not have an acceptable alternative immunosuppressive agent. A reduction in the dose of cyclosporine may prove somewhat beneficial in reducing the gingival enlargement in some cases.[7]

Antimicrobial Rinse

Rx:	Chlorhexidine gluconate 0.12%
Disp:	480 ml (16 oz)
Sig:	Rinse with 0.5 oz for 30 seconds 2 times a day; do not swallow.

DYSGEUSIA

SIGNS AND SYMPTOMS

Dysgeusia is a distortion in one's ability to taste. Taste is the perception of salt, bitter, sour, and sweetness by the tongue. Taste may be influenced by the texture of the food and the sense of smell. More than 2 million people in the United States have complaints of taste and smell abnormalities. Taste complaints are more frequently noted in elderly females. These problems may significantly alter individuals' quality of life. Their inability to taste decreases their ability to identify foods, recognize the flavors of foods, and, ultimately, may result in both nutritional and psychological disorders.[5]

ANATOMY

The taste buds are located in the tongue, and taste receptors are located in the soft palate, epiglottis, pharynx, and larynx. Each taste bud is composed of 50 to 150 modified neuroepithelial cells that are renewed every 10 to 14 days.[19] The mushroom-shaped fungiform papillae (200 to 400) appear red and are located on the dorsum of the tongue. Each fungiform papilla contains two to five taste buds. The circumvallate papilla (8 to 12) are located on the dorsum of the tongue in a V-shaped line that separates the anterior two thirds from the posterior one third of the tongue; each papilla contains 250 taste buds. The foliate papillae contain 1300 taste buds and appear as vertical folds on the posterior lateral aspect of the tongue. The soft palate contains 400 taste buds.[6] The chorda tympani branch of the facial nerve (cranial nerve VII) innervates the fungiform papillae, whereas the posterior foliate and circumvallate papillae are innervated by the glossopharyngeal nerve (cranial nerve IX). The superior laryngeal branch of the vagus nerve (cranial nerve X) innervates the epiglottis and esophagus.

An evaluation of the patient who complains of altered taste perception must include a comprehensive medical history that details a complete listing of medications (prescription and OTC). The dental hygienist must question the patient regarding current and past medical conditions,

TABLE 14-7

Selected calcium channel blockers reported to cause gingival enlargement

Generic name	Brand name
Nifedipine	Procardia, Adalat
Verapamil	Calan, Covera, Isoptin, Verelan
Diltiazem	Cardizem, Dilacor XR
Nicardipine	Cardene
Amlodipine	Norvasc
Felodipine	Plendil
Nimodipine	Nimotop
Isradipine	DynaCirc
Nisoldipine	Sular

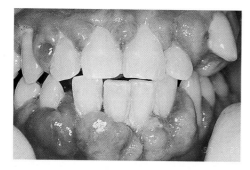

FIG. 14-6 Example of gingival hyperplasia resulting from the patient taking Procardia (nifedipine) for the treatment of hypertension.

such as diabetes mellitus, thyroid gland dysfunction, and radiation therapy. Sinusitis and recent viral upper respiratory infections should be ruled out as possible causes of the altered taste. The onset and duration of the taste disorders should be determined in an attempt to correlate the onset with medications, changes in medications, and medical conditions.

ASSOCIATED SYSTEMIC DRUGS

More than 250 medications have been reported to cause alterations in taste and smell. These drugs may be excreted in the saliva and the gingival crevicular fluid and may modify the taste. Saliva is important in dissolving and transporting tastants to receptors in the taste buds and taste receptors. Drugs that decrease the salivary flow have the potential to cause taste alterations. In addition, drugs that decrease the turnover rate of the taste receptors may result in an altered taste perception (Table 14-8).[1,34,35]

TABLE 14-8
Drugs reported to cause taste alterations

Category	Antimicrobial agents
Antibiotics	Tetracyclines, cephalosporins, fluoroquinolones
Antifungal agents	Griseofulvin, amphotericin
Anticonvulsants	Carbamazepine (Tegretol), Phenytoin (Dilantin)
Antidiabetic agents	Metformin
Antiasthmatic agents	Albuterol, cromolyn sodium, triamcinolone acetonide, Beclometasone
Antiinflammatory agents	NSAIDs, glucocorticoids, acetaminophen, propoxyphene
Antilipid agents	Clofibrate, cholestyramine, gernfibrozil, lovastatin
Antineoplastic agents	5-FU, Imuran 9, cisplatin, carboplatin, bleomycin, tamoxifen
Anti-Parkinson drugs	Levodopa, selegine
Antipsychotic drugs	Lithium carbonate, nortriptyline, lorazepam, triazolam, amitriptyline, sertraline
Antithyroid drugs	Thiamazole, methimazole, carbamizole, methylthiouracil
Arthritis drugs	Penicillamine, allopurinol
Antiviral drugs	Acyclovir
Cardiovascular drugs	Diuretics, ACE inhibitors, beta-adrenergic blockers
Muscle relaxants	Baclofen, cyclobenzaprine
Tranquilizers	Triazolam, flurazepam, chlormezanone
Analgesic agents	Codeine compounds
Gastrointestinal agents	H_2-antagonists, omeprazole

Data from Ackerman BH, Kasbekar N: Disturbances of taste and smell induced by drugs, *Pharmacotherapy* 17(3):482-96, 97; Schiffman SS: Taste and smell disease, *N Eng J Med* 308:1275-9, 1337-43, 1983; and Scott AE: Clinical characteristics of taste and smell disorders, *Ear, Nose Throat J* 68:297-315, 1989.
NSAIDs, Nonsteroidal antiinflammatory drugs; *ACE,* angiotensin-converting enzyme.

ORAL PIGMENTATION

ETIOLOGY

Abnormal pigmentation of the teeth may be caused by tetracycline (TCN) antimicrobial agents. TCN is a broad spectrum, bacteriostatic antibiotic often prescribed for acne vulgaris and ear infections. The systemic ingestion of TCN causes irreversible yellow-brown intrinsic staining in the developing teeth and bones. This type of staining is seen in the gingival third of the affected teeth and results from the deposition of a TCN-calcium orthophosphate complex during tooth development. This staining is directly proportional to the age of drug exposure, the dosage, and the duration of the drug therapy (Figs. 14-7 and 14-8).[29,31]

Minocycline is a semisynthetic TCN with additional antiinflammatory properties. Minocycline is used to treat acne vulgaris and rheumatoid arthritis. Minocycline also is associated with pigmentation of the teeth, bone, sclera, nails, and soft tissues.[22,25] Unlike TCN, which affects the developing teeth and bones, minocycline staining may occur after the teeth are fully developed and erupted. Minocycline is a fat-soluble drug with great penetration into the soft tissues and calcified tissues. It concentrates in the saliva at 30% to 65% of the serum concentration.

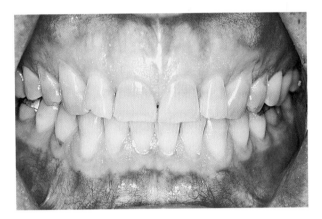

FIG. 14-7 Oral pigmentation. Tetracycline staining of the dentition. This patient was treated with a tetracycline medication during infancy.

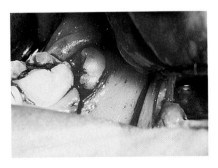

FIG. 14-8 Oral pigmentation. Tetracycline staining of the bone. Because the bone is a dynamic tissue and is constantly remodeling, the uptake of tetracycline in the bone may occur at any age when a peson is exposed to the drug.

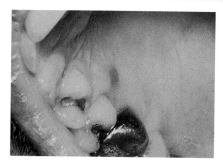

FIG. 14-9 Oral pigmentation. This is a 34-year-old Caucasian female with a medical history of lupus erythematosus. In addition to taking a corticosteroid, she is taking Plaquenil (hydroxychloroquine) to treat the arthritic component of her lupus.

The pigmentation of the developed dentition may be produced by the incorporation of minocycline complexes from the pulp into the dentin and from demineralization of the enamel and the subsequent oxidation of the drug from the saliva and gingival crevicular fluid. The pigmentation is green-gray or blue-gray and is seen in the middle and incisal third of the crown. The gingival third is spared. Minocycline pigmentation is irreversible.[46] The incidence of minocycline-induced pigmentation in the facial bones is reported to be 10% in a study of patients who took oral minocycline for more than 1 year and increased to 20% if the drug was taken for 4 or more years.[10]

Other drugs that have been reported to cause oral pigmentation include the antimalarial agents (chloroquine, hydroxychloroquine, quinacrine [Atabrine]) and the antiretroviral drugs (zidovudine) (Fig. 14-9).[18]

HAIRY TONGUE

SIGNS AND SYMPTOMS

Hairy tongue is a benign condition that results from elongation, hyperkeratinization, and retardation of the normal rate of desquamation of the filiform papillae. Hairy tongue is confined to the middorsal part of the tongue anterior to the circumvallate papillae. The increased length of the filiform papillae produces a matted appearance that may be black, brown, or yellow. The color may be related to chromogenic bacteria or exogenous pigments from food, beverages, or tobacco products.[33]

Predisposing factors for the development of hairy tongue include poor oral hygiene, tobacco use, oxidizing mouthrinses (e.g., hydrogen peroxide), antibiotics, xerostomia, and radiation therapy.[16] Bouquot and Grundlach[3] found the prevalence of hairy tongue to be 0.6 cases per 1000 with a strong male predilection (80%), whereas Farman[15] found a 0.15% prevalence rate in the general population, a 0.72% prevalence in the elderly, and a 22% prevalence in cancer patients (Fig. 14-10).

ASSOCIATED SYSTEMIC DRUGS

Drugs associated with hairy tongue include penicillins, broad spectrum antibiotics, tetracyclines, phenothiazines, griseofulvin, and corticosteroids.[9]

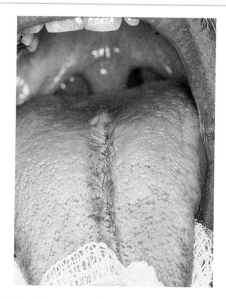

FIG. 14-10 Hairy tongue in a Caucasian male in his late twenties. This patient gives a history of one to two packs of cigarettes per day for the past 8 years and heavy consumption of coffee during the day.

TREATMENT

The conservative management of hairy tongue is for the dental hygienist to instruct patients in the proper technique of scraping the tongue, improving their oral hygiene procedures, and eliminating identifiable predisposing factors. Other more aggressive approaches used to treat hairy tongue include topical applications of podophyllum resin, retinoic acid, or triamcinolone. In severe cases of elongation, surgical removal of the elongated filiform papillae may be performed.

ANGIOEDEMA

SIGNS AND SYMPTOMS

Angioedema is a condition that features an acute onset of swelling in the skin, soft tissues, and subcutaneous and submucosal tissues of the head and neck. Angioedema may present as a painless, nonpitting edema of the face, cheeks, eyelids, lips, tongue, floor of the mouth, soft palate, uvula, and pharynx. The edema is often mild with a quick onset but may progress to laryngeal edema and death. Angioedema may be idiopathic, secondary to foods, food additives, trauma, medications, or a deficiency of the C1 esterase enzyme (Fig. 14-11).[9]

ASSOCIATED SYSTEMIC DRUGS

Drugs that have been implicated in angioedema, are penicillins, aspirin, nonsteroidal antiinflammatory drugs (NSAIDs), propranolol, cimetidine, ACE inhibitors, and angiotensin II receptor antagonists.[9]

HISTOLOGY

The hereditary form is a rare autosomal dominant trait that features the C1 esterase inhibitor deficiency.[9] The

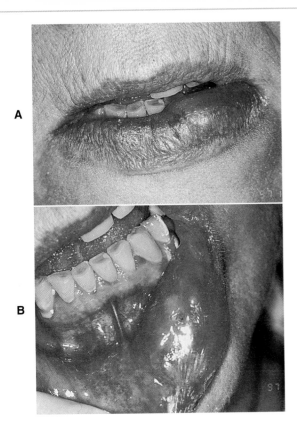

FIG. 14-11 Angioneurotic edema. **A,** Swelling on the lower left lip of a Caucasian female. This swelling occurred shortly after the completion of a dental restorative procedure on tooth #19 performed using the rubber dam. This patient was not sensitive to latex. **B,** Intraoral view of the same individual.

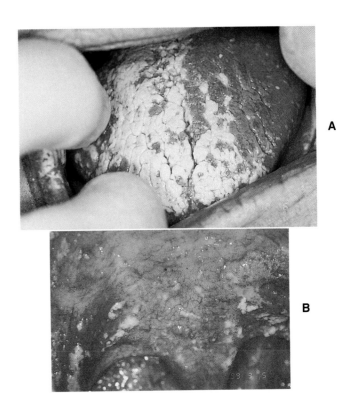

FIG. 14-12 Candidiasis. **A,** 60-year-old female with erosive lichen planus (ELP). Present medications are hormone replacement therapy (estrogen/progesterone) and topical corticosteroids for the treatment of ELP. Pseudomembranous form of candidiasis on the dorsum of the tongue. **B,** Junction of the hard and soft palate.

nonhereditary form features an immunoglobulin E (IgE)-mediated hypersensitivity reaction with mast cell degranulation and the release of histamine. This reaction may occur secondary to the administration of drugs. Angiotensin-converting enzyme (ACE) inhibitors have been reported in the literature to cause angioedema. These drugs are prescribed to treat essential and renovascular hypertension and congestive heart failure. This class of drugs prevents the conversion of angiotensin I to angiotensin II, which is a potent vasoconstrictor. The ACE inhibitors also inhibit an enzyme that degrades bradykinin, a vasoactive substance that promotes vasodilation and fluid accumulation. The overall incidence of angioedema secondary to ACE inhibitors is 0.1% to 0.2%.[36] Most cases occur very shortly after the drug is administered (i.e., within 48 hours).[32]

TREATMENT

Treatment consists of identification of the primary causative factor. If this is a medication, the treatment includes cessation of the suspected drug and administration of diphenhydramine (Benadryl) or hydrocortisone.

Rx:	Diphenhydramine hydrochloride 25-mg capsules
Disp:	Capsules No. 12 (3-day regimen) or 20 (5-day regimen); length determined by treatment provider
Sig:	One capsule every 6 hours for 3 to 5 days.

CANDIDIASIS

ETIOLOGY

Candidiasis is the most common opportunistic fungal infection of the oral cavity and is caused by an overgrowth of the organism *Candida albicans*. The candida organism is a commensal organism found on the skin, gastrointestinal tract, and genitourinary tract. *Candida albicans* exists in a symbiotic relationship with *Lactobacillus acidophilis*. In the healthy patient, the intact epithelium with a competent immune system results in the maintenance of the normal microbial flora and this symbiotic relationship.[14,17,26]

Immunosuppression, endocrinopathies, anemias, nutritional deficiencies, medications, malignancies, dental prostheses, epithelial alterations, age, poor oral hygiene, xerostomia, and a history of smoking are factors that may enable the *C. albicans* to become opportunistic and lead to tissue penetration and infection (Figs. 14-12 and 14-13).[14,17,26]

SIGNS AND SYMPTOMS

The candidal infection may appear as the classic pseudomembranous form, which is characterized by the white plaques that are easily removed, or the atrophic/erythematous form, which is characterized by the loss of filiform

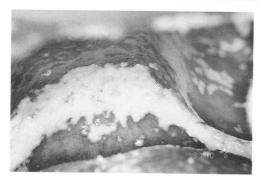

FIG. 14-13 Candidiasis. Combination of pseudomembranous form of candidiasis and the atrophic form. This is an elderly female who has asthma and uses a corticosteroid inhalant three to four times daily.

papillae on the dorsum of the tongue and a thinning and inflammation of the other affected tissues.

ASSOCIATED SYSTEMIC DRUGS

The medications associated with the development of candidiasis are the tetracyclines, glucocorticoids, cytotoxic drugs, and xerostomic agents. The tetracyclines suppress the endogenous microflora that inhibit Candida species growth. The glucocorticoids suppress the nonspecific inflammatory response and cell-mediated immunity. The cytotoxic (methotrexate and cyclophosphamide) and immunosuppressive drugs (azathioprine) cause a decrease in the number of neutrophils and suppress the cell mediated immunity. The xerostomic drugs, such as tricyclic antidepressants and diuretics, decrease the production of saliva and reduce the salivary immunoglobulins (IgA and histidine-rich peptides).[28]

TREATMENT

The treatment is to use an antifungal agent. Topical antifungal treatment is used most frequently in the mild, localized cases in an otherwise healthy individual. The topical agent may include oral suspensions (Nystatin), pastilles, troches, creams or ointments of Nystatin, clotrimazole, or miconazole. Systemic therapy (ketoconazole, fluconazole)

is usually reserved for advanced cases of candidal infections in an immunocompromised patient. The dental hygienist should have the patient return 3 to 7 days after initiation of therapy to assess the effectiveness of the antifungal therapy. The antifungal therapy should be continued for at least twice the time required to produce a resolution of the clinical signs and symptoms.[17,43]

Topical Antifungal Agents

Rx:	Nystatin oral suspension, 100,000 units/ml
Disp:	60 ml
Sig:	Rinse with 5 ml for 2 minutes four times a day and swallow. Continue this regimen for a minimum of 14 days.
Refills	× _____ (determined by treatment provider)

or

Rx:	Nystatin pastilles, 200,000 units
Disp:	70 pastilles
Sig:	Let 1 pastille dissolve in the mouth five times a day until all are gone.

or

Rx:	Clotrimazole troches (Mycelex), 10 mg
Disp:	70 troches
Sig:	Let 1 troche dissolve in the mouth five times a day until all are gone.

or

Rx:	Nystatin ointment
Disp:	15 grams
Sig:	Apply a thin film to the tissue side of your denture base.

Systemic Antifungal Agents

Rx:	Ketoconazole (Nizoral) tablets 200 mg
Disp:	14 tablets
Sig:	Take one tablet daily at a mealtime for 14 days.

or

Rx:	Fluconazole tablets (Diflucan) 100 mg
Disp:	14 tablets
Sig:	Take one tablet daily at mealtime for 14 days.

RITICAL THINKING ACTIVITIES

1. Visit with your local pharmacy. Inquire about the types of instructions given to patients taking antidepressant drugs.
2. Prepare a handout for patient use describing the oral side effects of the following drugs and steps they can take to reduce the side effects:
   Antidepressant
   Phenytoin
   Nifedipine
   Nonsteriodal antiinflammatory agents
3. Select six patient charts. Review the medication history and correlate the history to the dental charting and patient Rx. Can you find any oral symptoms in chart that could be related to the medication listing?
4. You are completing a health history on an elderly patient (age 75) with an extensive medication history. He wants to know why you need to know "all that stuff." How would you reply?

CRITICAL THINKING ACTIVITIES—cont'd

5. Survey a family member. Identify all medications the individual is taking and using a drug reference book, list the potential oral adverse effects of the medications. Inquire as to whether the person currently experiences any of the effects.
6. Role-play discussions with healthcare providers (dentists and physicians) concerning oral manifestations based on the patient's intake of certain medication.

7. Select at random 5 to 10 patient records, list the medications recorded, and review these in a drug reference book for possible oral side effects. Review the same records for oral manifestations that could be related to the given medications.
8. Develop a ready reference for management of specific clinical oral lesions based on specific medications.

REVIEW QUESTIONS

1. Your patient is a 16-year-old boy. His chief complaint is that he has ulcers in his mouth that are causing him pain. This instance has occurred twice before the current visit, but the ulders disappeared in a couple of weeks. On both occasions he reported having had a sinus infection that his physician treated with amoxicillin. Based on the patient's age, gender, and health history, the oral ulcerations most likely are due to which of the following?
   a. Lichenoid drug reaction
   b. Erythema multiforme
   c. Candidiasis
   d. Xerostomia
   e. All the above

2. Which of the following medications has *not* been associated with causing gingival enlargement?
   a. Phenytoin
   b. Calcium channel blockers
   c. Cyclosporin
   d. Prozac

3. All the following medications have been associated with xerostomia *except* which one?
   a. Ibuprofen
   b. Pilocarpine
   c. Prozac
   d. Zestril

4. All the following statements *except* which one are true?
   a. Lichenoid drug reactions produce oral lesions that resemble lichen planus.
   b. The gingival enlargement associated with calcium channel blockers is irreversible.
   c. Minocycline can cause pigmentation in teeth that are completely developed.
   d. Hyperkeratinization of the filiform papillae can result in a "hairy tongue."

5. All the following statements about candidiasis are true *except* which one?
   a. Candidiasis is the most common fungal infection in the oral cavity.
   b. The fungal organism, *Candida albicans,* when found in the oral cavity, is always a pathogenic organism.

   c. Antibiotics and cytotoxic drugs can cause candidiasis.
   d. Two common types of candidiasis are the pseudomembranous and the atrophic forms.

6. Which of the following statements does *not* apply to angioedema?
   a. The soft tissues of the head and neck swell.
   b. Some drugs that have been implicated in angioedema are ACE inhibitors and NSAIDs.
   c. Angioedema is always painful.
   d. One form of angioedema features and immunoglobuline E- (IgE-) mediated hypersensitivity reaction.

7. All the following statements about erythema multiforme are true *except* which one?
   a. Erythema multiforme is most common in young men.
   b. The skin lesions of erythema multiforme are described as *iris, target,* or *bulls-eye* lesions.
   c. Erthema minor is a benign illness without complications and also is known as *Stevens-Johnson syndrome.*
   d. Episodes of erythema multiforme may recur.

8. Which of the following statements is *not* true?
   a. The patient's complain of xerostomia always correlates directly with the amount of saliva that individual produces.
   b. Common drugs that cause xerostomia are NSAIDs, tricyclic antidepressants, and antihistamine agents.
   c. Lichenoid drug reactions are thought to be a delayed hypersensitivity reaction.
   d. One of the mechanisms for dysgeusia is the secretion of drugs in the saliva.

9. Based on a review of Table 14-1, which lists the incidence of prescriptions by drug category, which of the following oral adverse effects would you expect to see most frequently in a general clinical dental practice?
   a. Xerostomia
   b. Angioedema
   c. Dysgeusia
   d. Erythema multiforme

SUGGESTED AGENCIES AND WEB SITES

Because of the ever-changing nature of the Internet, some of the web sites listed here may have changed since publication. Please refer to Mosby's Evolve web site for the most current information.

American Academy of Oral Medicine ("Publications, monographs"): http://www.aaom.com

Canadian Adverse Drug Reaction newsletter: e-mail to webmaster@inet.hwc.ca

Dalhousie University College of Pharmacy ("Useful journals in pharmacy"): http://www.dal.ca

Lexi-Comp (drug information handbook for dentistry): http://www.lexi.com

Mosby's Dental Drug Reference, ed 5 ("Product updates"): http://www.harcourthealth.com

RX List (the Internet drug index): http://www.rxlist.com

ADDITIONAL READINGS AND RESOURCES

American Academy of Oral Medicine: *Clinician's guide to treatment of common oral conditions,* Monograph, AAOM Executive Secretary, 2910 Lightfoot Drive, Baltimore, MD 21209-1452.

Gage TW, Pickett FA: *Mosby's dental drug reference,* ed 6, St Louis, (in press), Mosby.

Terézhalmy GT, Batizy LG: *Urgent care in the dental office: an essential handbook,* Carol Stream, Ill, 1998, Quintessence.

Wynn RL, Meiller TF, Crossley HL: *Drug information handbook for dentistry,* ed 6, Hudson, 2000, Lexi-Comp.

REFERENCES

1. Ackerman BH, Kasbekar N: Disturbances of taste and smell induced by drugs, *Pharmacotherapy* 17(3):482-96, 1997.
2. Addy V et al: Risk factors in phenytoin-induced gingival hyperplasia, *J Periodontol* 54(6):373-7, 1983.
3. Bouquot JE, Gundlach K: Odd tongues: prevalence of common tongue lesions in 23,616 white Americans over 35 years of age, *Quint Intern* 17(l):719-30, 1986.
4. Bradfeldt GW: Phenytoin hyperplasia found in edentulous patients, *J Am Dent Assoc* 123:61-4, 1992.
5. Cowart BJ et al: Clinical disorders of smell and taste, *Occup Med* 12(3):465-81, 1997.
6. Cullen MM, Leopold DA: Disorders of taste and smell, *Med Clin North Am* 83(l):57-74,1999.
7. Daly C: Resolution of Cyclosporine A-induced gingival enlargement following reduction in CsA dosage, *J Clin Periodontol* 19:143-5,1992.
8. Duffey D, Eversole LR, Abemayor E: Oral lichen planus and its association with squamous cell carcinoma: an update on pathogenesis and treatment implications, *Laryngoscope* 106: 357-62, 1996.
9. Eisen DE, Lynch DP: *The mouth: diagnosis and treatment,* St Louis, 1997, Mosby.
10. Eisen DE: Minocycline-induced oral pigmentation, *Lancet* 349:400, 1997.
11. Eisenberg E: Clinicopathologic Patterns of Oral Lichen Planus, *Oral Maxillofac Clin North Am* 6(3):445-63, 1994.
12. Ellis JS et al: Prevalence of gingival overgrowth induced by calcium channel blockers: a community-based study, *J Periodontol* 70(l):63-7, 1999.
13. Epstein IA: Blood examination in the practice of dentistry, *J Am Dent Assoc* 16:1808-20, 1929.
14. Epstein JB, Polsky B: Oropharyngeal candidiasis: a review of its clinical spectrum and current therapies, *Clin Therap* 20(l): 40-57, 1998.
15. Farman AG: Hairy tongue, *J Oral Med* 32(3):85-91, 1977.
16. Flaitz CM: Diseases of the mouth. In *Conn's current therapy 2002,* Philadelphia, (in press), WB Saunders.
17. Fotos PG, Lilly JP: Clinical management of oral and perioral candidiasis, *Dermatol Clin* 14(2):273-80,1996.
18. Giansanti JS et al: Oral mucosal pigmentation resulting from antimalarial therapy, *Oral Surg* 31(l):66-9,1971.
19. Guyton AC, Hall JE: *Textbook of medical physiology,* ed 10, Philadelphia, 2000, WB Saunders.
20. Hassell TM, Hefti AF: Drug-induced gingival overgrowth: old problem, new problem, *Crit Rev Oral Biol Med* 2(l):103-37,1991.
21. Huff JC, Weston WL, Tonnesen MG: Erythema multiforme: a review of characteristics, diagnostic criteria, and causes, *J Am Acad Dermatol* 8(6):763-775, 1883.
22. Hung P, Caldwell JB, James WD: Minocycline-induced hyperpigmentation, *J Fam Pract* 40:183-5,1995.
23. Miller CS, Kaplan AL, Guest GF, Cottone JA: Documenting medication use in adult dental patients: 1987-1991, *J Am Dent Assoc* 123:41-8, 1992.
24. Miller CS, Damm DD: Incidence of verapamil-induced gingival hyperplasia in a dental population, *J Periodontol* 63:453-6, 1992.
25. Morrow GL, Abbott RL: Minocycline-induced scleral, dental, and dermal pigmentation, *Am J Ophthalmol* 125(3):396-7, 1998.
26. Muzyka BC, Glick M: A review of oral fungal infections and appropriate therapy, *J Am Dent Assoc* 126:63-72, 1995.
27. Nery EB et al: Prevalence of nifedipine-induced gingival hyperplasia, *J Periodontol* 66:572-78, 1995.
28. Neville BW et al: *Oral and maxillofacial pathology,* ed 2, Philadelphia, (in press), WB Saunders.
29. Parks ET: Lesions associated with drug reactions, *Dermatol Clin* 14(2):327-37,1996.
30. Rees TD, Levine RA: Systemic drugs as a risk factor for periodontal disease initiation and progression, *Compendium* 16(l):20-42,1995.
31. Regezzi JA, Sciubba JJ: *Oral pathology clinical pathologic correlations,* ed 3, Philadelphia, 1999, WB Saunders.
32. Roberts JR, Wuerz RC: Clinical characteristics of angiotensin-converting enzyme inhibitor-induced angioedema, *Ann Emerg Med* 20(5):555-8, 1991.
33. Sartii GM et al: Black hairy tongue, *Am Fam Physician* 41(6): 1751-5,1990.

34. Schiffman SS: Taste and smell disease, *N Eng J Med* 308:1275-9, 1337-43, 1983.

35. Scott AE: Clinical characteristics of taste and smell disorders, *Ear Nose Throat J* 68:297-315, 1989.

36. Sharma PK, Yium JJ: Angioedema associated with angiotensin II receptor antagonist losartan, *South Med J,* 90(5):552-3, 1997.

37. Shiohara T, Modya N, Nagashima M: The lichenoid tissue reaction, *Int J Dermatol* 27(6):365-73, 1988.

38. Stevens AM, Johnson FC: A new eruptive fever associated with stomatitis and ophthalmia, *Am J Dis Child* 24:526-33, 1922.

39. Stinnett E, Rodu B, Grizzle WE: New developments in understanding phenytoin-induced gingival hyperplasia, *J Am Dent Assoc* 114(6):814-6, 1987.

40. Tam IM, Wandres DL: Calcium channel blockers and gingival hyperplasia, *Ann Pharmacother* 2: 213-4, 1992.

41. Taybos GM, Terézhalmy GT, Pelleu GB: Assessing patients! Health status with the Navy dental health questionnaire, *U.S. Navy Medicine* March-April:24-31, 1983.

42. Taybos GM: Xerostomia—common complaint and challenging dental management problem, *MDA J* 54(3):24-5,1998.

43. Terézhalmy GT, Batizy LG: *Urgent care in the dental office,* Carol Stream, Ill, 1998, Quintessence.

44. von Hebra F (Fagge CH, translator): *On diseases of the skin including the exanthemata,* London, 1866, New Sydenhour Society.

45. Westbrook P et al: Regression of nifedipine-induced gingival hyperplasia following switch to a same class calcium channel blocker, isradipine, *J Periodontol* 68:645-50, 1997.

46. Wolfe ID, Reichmister J: Minocycline hyperpigmentation: skin, tooth, nail, and bone involvement, *Cutis* 33:457-8, 1984.

47. Zoeller J: The top 200 drugs, *American Druggist,* Feb:41-8, 1999.

CHAPTER 15

Periodontal Examination

Francis G. Serio, Katharine R. Stilley

Chapter Outline

Case Study: Completing the Periodontal Examination
Periodontal Anatomy
  Epithelium
Anatomical Landmarks of the Periodontium
  Tooth and gingiva interface
  Gingiva
  Alveolar mucosa
Attachment Mechanisms
  Junctional epithelium
  Gingival connective tissue fibers
Components of the Periodontal Examination
  Visual characteristics of the gingiva
Periodontal Pocket Probing
Location of the Free Gingival Margin in Relation to the CEJ
Calculation of Attachment Loss
Amount of Keratinized or Attached Gingiva
Detection of Marginal and Deep Bleeding on Probing

Detection of Suppuration
Exploration of Furcations
  Classifications
Detection of Mobility
Assessment of Plaque and Calculus
Indices
Dental Factors in Periodontal Disease Risk
  Interproximal contacts
  Restorative materials
  Other contributing factors
Examination and Evaluation of Dental Implants
Technology in the Periodontal Examination
  Identifying inflammation
  Automated probing systems
  Imaging technology
  Laboratory assays of periodontal infections
Classification of Periodontal Disease

Key Terms

Abfraction lesions
Acellular cementum
Acute necrotizing ulcerative gingivitis (ANUG)
Alveolar bone proper
Alveolar crestal fibers
Alveolar mucosa
Anatomic crown
Ankylosed
Apical fibers
Attached gingiva
Attachment apparatus
Basal lamina
Bifurcation
Biologic width
Bone

Bruxism
Buccal mucosa
Calculus
  Subgingival
  Supragingival
Cellular cementum
Cementum
Circular fibers
Clinical crown
Connective tissue
Darkfield microscopy
Dentin
Dentoalveolar (dentoperiosteal) fibers
Dentogingival fibers
Edema
Embrasure

Enamel
Endosteum
Epithelium
Erythema
Free (marginal) gingiva
Free gingival groove
Free gingival margin
Frena
Furcation
Gingiva
Gingival sulcus
Gingivitis
Glycosaminoglycans
Ground substance
Hemidesmosomal attachment
Horizontal fibers
Immunoassays

Indices
Interdental papillae
Interradicular fibers
Junctional epithelium
Koch's postulates
Labial mucosa
Lamina densa
Lamina lucida
Lamina propria
Loss of attachment (LOA)
Materia alba
Melanocytes
Mobility
Mucogingival junction
Nonspecific plaque hypothesis
Nucleic acid probes

Key Terms—cont'd

Oblique fibers
Osteoblasts
Pellicle
Periodontal ligament
Periodontitis
Periodontium
Principal fibers
Proteoglycans

Quiescence
Radiolucent
Radiopaque
Recession
Sharpey's fibers
Specific plaque (or qualitative)
  hypothesis

Stippling
Stratified squamous
  Keratinized
  Nonkeratinized
Stratum basale
Stratum corneum
Stratum granulosum

Stratum spinosum
Sulcular epithelium
Supporting alveolar bone
Suppuration
Transseptal fibers
Trifurcation

 Learning Outcomes

1. Describe the roles of plaque and other local etiological factors in periodontal diseases.
2. Identify the components of a periodontal assessment, their appearance in health and disease, and their significance.
3. Chart an involved periodontal condition, using the correct charting notations.

4. Interpret the periodontal findings from a chart (correctly read a periodontal chart) and discuss the ramifications.
5. Explain the interrelationships and suspected interrelationships between periodontitis and systemic diseases, as presently reported in the scientific literature.
6. Identify those patients who have periodontitis or who are at risk for periodontitis.

The periodontal assessment is the first step in planning a patient's periodontal treatment. The patient must be examined, a list of diagnoses developed, and the treatment plan formulated to address each of the diagnoses. The periodontal assessment is completed after the extraoral and intraoral examination, typically after the dental assessment. In this way, those dental factors that may contribute to the patient's periodontal status have already been identified, such as the following:

- Missing teeth
- Caries
- Open contacts
- Faulty restorations
- Poor restorative margins
- Malpositioned teeth
- Anatomical variations
- Palatogingival grooves
- Cervical enamel projections
- Impacted or supernumerary teeth

Because the appearance of periodontal disease may vary widely, visual inspection of the *periodontium* is not enough. The use of instruments such as the mouth mirror, periodontal probe, explorer, *furcation* probe, fiberoptic wand, compressed air, and study models allows for complete clinical examination of the periodontium. A full-mouth series of radiographs including vertical bitewings (discussed in Chapter 17) provides information about the oral hard tissue: teeth, restorations (if present), and alveolar bone.

The periodontal examination and radiographs provide a "snapshot" of the patient's periodontal health. Although they are not a predictor of future disease activity, they can provide an evaluation of risk factors for developing future disease. Until a reliable predictor of future disease is de-

 Completing the Periodontal Examination

Mollie Bozenski is a well-developed, well-nourished 57-year-old Caucasian woman. She is 5 feet 5 inches tall and weighs 160 pounds. She reports a history of mitral valve prolapse with no regurgitation or audible murmur. She is allergic to penicillin and tetanus toxoid. Her medications include Inderal, Lasix, potassium, and two aspirin per day. She reports eating a balanced diet.

Mrs. Bozenski's clinical examination reveals generalized accumulations of plaque and *calculus.* She has generalized severe marginal *erythema* and *edema.* Plaque or calculus is present on 89% of tooth surfaces. Probings range from 1 to more than 10 mm; 98% of the sites bleed on probing. She has several irregular restorative margins. She has noticed an increase in the spacing between her maxillary right and left central incisors.

Clinical photographs, a complete periodontal charting, and a full-mouth series of radiographs are included (Fig. 15-1; see Fig. 15-13).

veloped, an accurate charting of periodontal findings remains critical to the assessment of effectiveness of therapy and/or the progress of disease. Previous chartings and radiographs are helpful in the evaluation of the rate of periodontal destruction.

This chapter outlines periodontal anatomy and details the various components of the periodontal examination. Classification and descriptions of the periodontal diseases

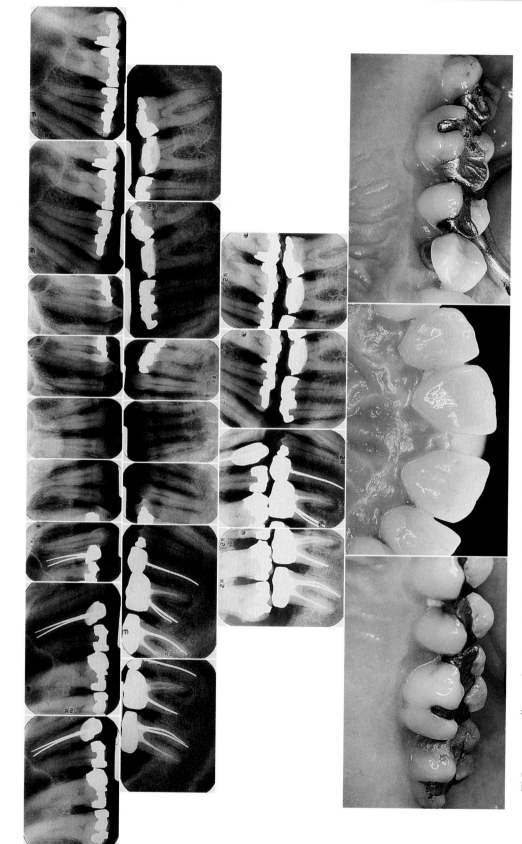

FIG. 15-1 Full-mouth series of radiographs of Mrs. Mollie Bozenski, a well-nourished, well-developed 57-year-old Caucasian woman.

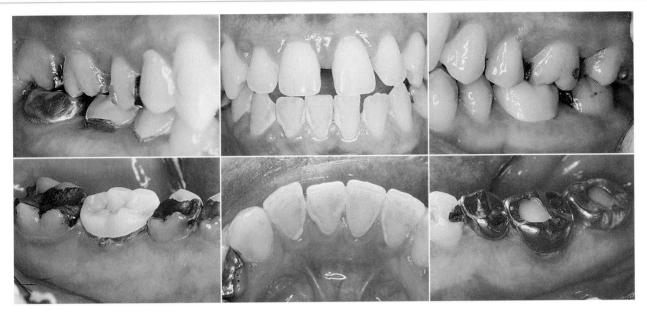

FIG. 15-1, cont'd Full-mouth series of clinical photographs of Mrs. Mollie Bozenski, a well-nourished, well-developed 57-year-old Caucasian woman.

are discussed. Proper rationale, armamentarium, techniques, and clinical findings are presented.

PERIODONTAL ANATOMY

The structures in the mouth are composed of a variety of tissues. The six major dentally related tissue types in the mouth are the following: (1) *epithelium,* (2) *connective tissue,* (3) *bone* (4), *enamel,* (5) *dentin,* and (6) *cementum.* Blood vessels, nerve fibers, and lymphatic channels are also present. Epithelium acts as a protective covering for all of the soft tissues of the body. Connective tissue, with its collection of fibers, blood vessels, and nerves, is found subjacent to the epithelium. Epithelium and connective tissue act as the covering for the jawbones as well as for other bones in the body. The teeth are made of enamel, dentin, and cementum. Enamel, the hardest substance in the body (90% calcified), covers the *anatomic crown.* Dentin constitutes the bulk of both the crown and root of the tooth. Cementum, 45% by volume mineral, covers the surface of the root.

EPITHELIUM

Epithelial tissues differ in structure and function depending on their location. Most oral epithelium is *stratified squamous* and is either *keratinized* or *nonkeratinized.* The epithelium has different layers, or strata. These include the *stratum basale* (basal cell layer), *stratum spinosum, stratum granulosum,* and *stratum corneum* as the outer layer. Keratin is the proteinaceous surface of the epithelium and is either orthokeratin (thicker with few cells), or parakeratin (thinner with some cells and nuclei evident; Fig. 15-2). The keratin gives the *gingiva* its characteristic pink color. The heavier the keratin layer, usually the lighter the color of the tissue as the underlying blood vessels are masked more completely. The gingiva and other masticatory mucosa are covered by keratinized

stratified squamous epithelium, whereas the *alveolar mucosa* and *buccal mucosa* are covered by nonkeratinized stratified squamous epithelium.

ANATOMICAL LANDMARKS OF THE PERIODONTIUM

Several visible intraoral landmarks are associated with the periodontium (Greek *peri,* meaning "around," and *odontos,* meaning "tooth;" Figs. 15-3 and 15-4). These include the tooth crown, *free gingival margin, free gingival groove,* gingiva, *mucogingival junction,* alveolar mucosa, masticatory mucosa, and various frenula.

TOOTH AND GINGIVA INTERFACE

The anatomic crown is that portion of the tooth from the cementoenamel junction (CEJ) to the incisal/occlusal tip of the tooth. The *clinical crown* is that part of the anatomic crown visible in the oral cavity. The free gingival margin is the portion of the gingiva not attached to the tooth. In health, the free gingival margin is typically positioned on the anatomic crown of the tooth at the cervical portion. When *recession* has occurred, the free gingival margin may be located on the tooth root. The free gingival groove is a depression in the gingiva approximately 2 mm apical to the free gingival margin. It is thought to correspond to the base of the sulcus but is an imprecise landmark and most often difficult to observe clinically.

GINGIVA

The gingiva is composed of the *free (marginal) gingiva* and *attached gingiva.*[13,33] The boundaries of the free gingiva are the free gingival margin and the base of the sulcus. The boundaries of the attached gingiva are the base of the sulcus and the mucogingival junction. The mucogingival junction demarcates the gingiva from the alveolar

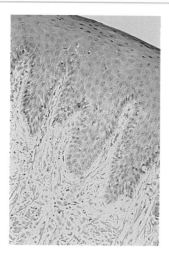

FIG. 15-2 In this histologic section, the darker-stained epithelium is seen at the right. It is covered with parakeratin. The connective tissue is below the rete pegs.

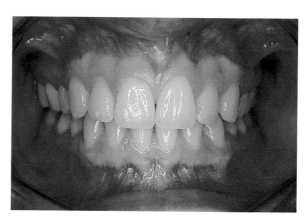

FIG. 15-3 Normal, healthy periodontal tissues and dentition. Anatomical landmarks are identified in Fig. 15-4.

FIG. 15-4 Normal visible landmarks of the periodontal tissues.

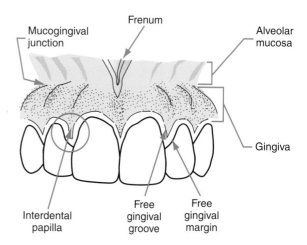

FIG. 15-5 Stippling may be prominent, as shown here, or completely absent. Stippling alone is not a sign of health or disease.

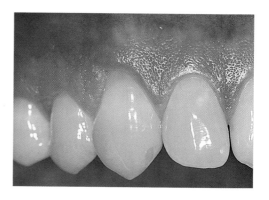

mucosa. On the hard palate, the attached gingiva is continuous with the rest of the masticatory mucosa and is keratinized. The gingiva is covered with keratinized stratified squamous epithelium. This keratinization protects the gingiva from the forces of mastication and toothbrushing. The width of the gingiva varies by location from approximately 1 mm to 9 mm in width. It is generally narrowest on the facial surface of the mandibular canine and first premolar.[6,16]

The surface of the gingiva has a characteristic stippled appearance, similar to the surface of an orange. The intersection of epithelial rete ridges and the interspersing of connective tissue papillae from beneath the surface create this *stippling* effect. The intersecting ridges create the depression; the convexity is caused by the projecting connective tissue papilla[15] (Fig. 15-5). *Melanocytes,* pigment-producing cells, are present in the stratum basale in all gingival epithelium. When melanin pigment is expressed, the gingiva has a brownish color ranging from faint to distinct. Pigmented gingiva is usually normal in dark-skinned individuals, although several diseases and the precipitation of heavy metals such as lead, mercury, and amalgam fillings also may cause gingival pigmentation.

The *interdental papillae* are the pyramidal gingiva found in the interproximal area *(embrasure)* between the teeth. A vertical interdental groove may be evident on the facial surface of the papilla. The col, a saddle-shaped depression in the gingival tissue just apical to the contact of adjacent teeth, connects the facial and lingual or palatal papillae. The col area is generally nonkeratinized and is susceptible to disease. When spaces exist between adjacent teeth, this interproximal tissue is keratinized.

Lamina propria is the connective tissue layer found beneath the epithelium. This layer is composed predominantly of type I collagen fibers, *ground substance,* and cells. In healthy individuals, fibroblasts are the predominant cell type with a small number of monocytes, macrophages, polymorphonuclear leukocytes, lymphocytes, plasma cells, and mast cells present. Some type III and type V collagen is also present. The proportion of the various cell types changes significantly in the presence of inflammation. The ground substance, which serves as a biological glue, consists of protein and carbohydrate complexes called *glycosaminoglycans* and *proteoglycans.*[29] Nerves, lymphatic channels, and blood vessels also are found in this connective tissue.

ALVEOLAR MUCOSA

Alveolar mucosa is covered with nonkeratinized stratified squamous epithelium. The alveolar mucosa is continuous with the *labial mucosa,* which makes up the inside lining of the lips and the buccal mucosa, which lines the inside of the cheeks. The underlying connective tissue is thin with a vascular submucosal layer. The alveolar mucosa has a much redder appearance because of the visibility of these blood vessels through the epithelium. It also contains a significant number of elastic fibers, which allows the alveolar mucosa to regain its shape after being stretched. *Frena* are attachments of the labial mucosa and buccal mucosa to the alveolar mucosa and gingiva.

ATTACHMENT MECHANISMS

JUNCTIONAL EPITHELIUM

The *gingival sulcus* is a space bounded by the free gingival margin, the tooth, and the most coronal attachment of the *junctional epithelium.* The sulcus is lined by nonkeratinized stratified squamous *sulcular epithelium.* The base of the sulcus is formed by the attachment of the junctional epithelium, the most coronal attachment of gingiva to the tooth. The junctional epithelium is stratified with stratum basale and stratum spinosum–type cells; the cells approximating the tooth surface adhere to the tooth by a *hemidesmosomal attachment.* These hemidesmosomes may attach to enamel, cementum, dentin, or to a variety of restorative materials through the *pellicle* and *basal lamina.* The pellicle is a sticky substance composed primarily of proteins high in proline and/or hydroxyproline and mucopolysaccharides. The ultrastructure of the basal lamina includes a *lamina densa* (adherent to the enamel) and *lamina lucida* to which hemidesmosomes attach.[17,36] The junctional epithelium varies in thickness along the tooth. Over time, all epithelial structures undergo constant cell turnover and renewal. The turnover times vary for different types of oral epithelium in experimental animals, as follows:

> 5 to 6 days—palate, tongue, cheek
> 10 to 12 days—gingiva
> 1 to 6 days—junctional epithelium

GINGIVAL CONNECTIVE TISSUE FIBERS

The gingival connective tissue fibers reinforce the epithelial attachment to the tooth and give tissue tone to the gingival papillae. These fibers insert into the cementum and are descriptively termed for their position: *dentogingival fibers, dentoalveolar (dentoperiosteal) fibers, circular fibers,* and *transseptal fibers.* These dense fibers are predominantly type I collagen, although type III and type V collagen are also present. These brace the marginal gingiva firmly against the tooth surface. The transseptal fibers are often also classified as *principal fibers* of the *periodontal ligament.*

Connective Tissue

Numerous types of cells are found in healthy gingival connective tissue. Fibroblasts produce collagen and ground substance and are responsible primarily for the constant turnover of connective tissue fibers and maintaining the stability of this tissue. Small numbers of several types of inflammatory cells, including macrophages, polymorphonuclear leukocytes (neutrophils, PMNs), lymphocytes, plasma cells, and mast cells, are also found. These cells increase dramatically in number when plaque induces the inflammatory response in gingival tissues.

The distance from the most coronal part of the junctional epithelium to the most apical extent of the gingival connective tissue fibers is called the *biologic width* (Fig. 15-6).[11] This biologic width is relatively constant and averages approximately 2.04 mm. The body tries to maintain the biologic width. When the biologic width is compromised or injured by restorative dentistry procedures, the body may induce an inflammatory response to reestablish this dimension. This may result in chronic inflammation even in a site relatively free of plaque.

Alveolar Bone

The *attachment apparatus* of the periodontium consists of the *alveolar bone proper,* which lines the tooth socket of the alveolar bone, the periodontal ligament, and the cementum that covers the tooth root. The alveolar bone proper is dense, lamellated or layered bone into which the *Sharpey's fibers* of the periodontal ligament insert. Sharpey's fibers are connective tissue fibers that insert into any calcified structure, such as bone and cementum. The *supporting alveolar bone* surrounds the alveolar bone proper and supports the tooth sockets.[32] This bone consists of cortical bone on the outer surface covering cancellous

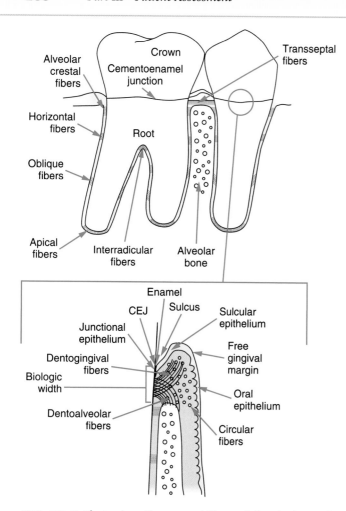

FIG. 15-6 The various tissues and fibers of the gingiva and attachment apparatus.

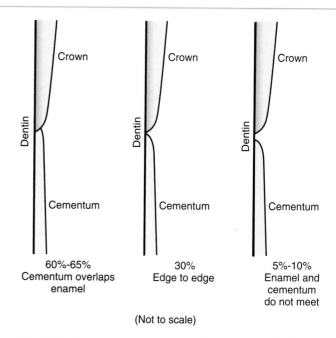

FIG. 15-7 Cementum may overlap the enamel *(left)*, form a butt joint at the cementoenamel junction *(center)*, or leave a gap with the enamel *(right)*.

bone containing yellow or fatty marrow. A layer of tissue called the *periosteum* covers the surface of the bone. The outer layer of the periosteum is composed of dense fibrous connective tissue and the inner (cambium) osteogenic layer contains **osteoblasts.** The lining of the inner surfaces of bone is called the **endosteum.** The endosteum contains both osteoblasts and osteoclasts responsible for the majority of bone remodeling throughout life. The crest of the alveolar bone follows the contours of the cementoenamel junction of each tooth and provides support for the overlying gingiva.

Periodontal Ligament

The periodontal ligament is the connective tissue attachment of the tooth to the alveolar bone proper.[4] The periodontal ligament maintains the biologic activity of cementum and bone, supplies nutrients and removes wastes via the blood and lymphatics, is a source of undifferentiated mesenchymal cells necessary for periodontal regeneration, and provides support for the tooth in the alveolar bone. The periodontal ligament houses a reflex arc that automatically signals the mandible to open when a hard object is accidentally bitten. The principal fibers of the periodontal ligament are arranged into transseptal fibers,

alveolar crestal fibers, horizontal fibers, oblique fibers, apical fibers, and *interradicular fibers.*[20] The transseptal fibers extend interproximally and are embedded in the cementum of adjacent teeth, coronal to the alveolar bone. Intact transseptal fibers may be found even when extensive destruction occurs to the attachment apparatus. The alveolar crestal fibers run from the cementum apical to the junctional epithelium and insert in the periosteum of the crest of the alveolar bone. The horizontal fibers extend from the tooth to the bone at right angles. The oblique fibers, the largest group of principal fibers, runs coronally from the tooth to the alveolar bone proper. These fibers provide the majority of support for the tooth and help the tooth resist displacement from apically applied forces. These forces are transferred from the tooth through the fibers into the alveolar bone proper. The apical fibers surround the apex of the tooth. The interradicular fibers are found extending between the roots of a multirooted tooth.

Cementum

The cementum consists of **acellular cementum,** located on the coronal third of the root surface, and **cellular cementum,** located more apically.[5] Cementum is approximately 45% to 50% inorganic hydroxyapatite; the rest is primarily collagen.

The principal fibers of the periodontal ligament insert into the cemental surfaces. Acellular cementum meets the cementoenamel junction in one of three ways. Approximately 60% to 65% of the time, the cementum extends onto the enamel surface. About 30% of the time the cementum butts against the cementoenamel junction, and in 5% to 10% of the cases, a gap exists between the cementum and the enamel (Fig. 15-7).

Cementum helps to anchor the tooth in the alveolar bone proper by the insertion of Sharpey's fibers of the periodontal ligament. Cementum grows slowly, particularly at the apex of the tooth root, to compensate for tooth wear. This remodeling of cementum also permits continual rearrangement of the inserting fibers of the periodontal ligament. Cementum remodels at a significantly slower rate than does the corresponding alveolar bone proper.

Knowledge of the anatomy of the periodontium provides the necessary foundation for assessment and evaluation of the periodontal status through the periodontal examination.

COMPONENTS OF THE PERIODONTAL EXAMINATION

The components of the periodontal examination are as follows:
- Description of the visual characteristics of the gingiva:
  Color
  Contour
  Consistency
  Texture
- Periodontal pocket probe depths
- Measurement of the location of the free gingival margin/recession
- Calculation of attachment loss
- Measurement of keratinized/attached gingiva
- Detection of marginal and deep bleeding on probing
- Detection of *suppuration*
- Exploration of furcations
- Detection of *mobility*
- Assessment of plaque and calculus accumulations

 Case Application
As you read about the components of a periodontal assessment, refer to Mrs. Bozenski's case. Make notes for each component concerning this patient's condition.

 VISUAL CHARACTERISTICS OF THE GINGIVA

 Cardinal Signs of Inflammation
15-B
15-C

The five clinical signs indicative of the presence of inflammation are shown in Box 15-1. One or more of these signs of inflammation may be present in periodontal disease.

Color

Healthy gingiva has been described as being coral pink. Many individuals have natural melanin pigmentation. When gingival inflammation is present, the gingiva may appear erythematous (red, associated with acute symptoms) and/or cyanotic (purplish, associated with chronic conditions). The erythema is due to the dilation of the capillaries within the gingival tissues. The cyanosis is a result of a decrease in the rate of blood flow through the gingival tissues (venous stasis). This color change may be exaggerated by a decrease in keratinization.

Significant inflammation may exist deep in periodontal pockets while the gingiva maintains a pink color. This is common when the gingiva is thick and fibrotic, such as

---

> **BOX 15-1**
>
> **Signs of Inflammation**
>
> Erythema (redness, *rubor*)
> Edema (swelling, *tumor*)
> Heat (increased tissue temperature, *calor*)
> Pain (*dolor*)
> Loss of function (*functio laesa*)

when the patient is a heavy smoker. Also, severe erythema can exist with both *gingivitis* and *periodontitis*. Therefore color alone is *not* a good indicator of the presence and/or severity of disease.

 Case Application
Note the color of Mrs. Bozenski's tissue.

Contour

Gingival thickness and contours have been classically described as thin and scalloped or thick and flat. In healthy individuals, the gingival margins follow the contours of the underlying alveolar bone and the cementoenamel junctions of the teeth. In cases of disease, these contours change as a result of several factors. In the initial stages of inflammation, up to 70% of the connective tissue that constitutes the gingiva is destroyed. Accompanying edema (accumulation of extracellular fluid within the tissues) may contribute to changes in gingival contour. As the underlying alveolar bone is destroyed, the interproximal gingiva, particularly in the col area, may collapse. As attachment is lost, the gingiva may migrate apically along the root surface, causing recession and exposure of the root surface. In diseases such as *necrotizing ulcerative gingivitis (NUG)*, the tips of the gingival papilla necrose, leaving a "punched out" or cratered appearance to the papilla.

Changes in gingival contour may also manifest in facial indentations called a *Stillman's cleft*. These V-shaped or slitlike areas of localized recession appear at the edge of the marginal gingiva but may extend to a depth of up to 6 mm.

A rimlike enlargement, McCall's festoon, may also be seen. Referred to as *rolled* or *rounded* marginal gingiva, this gingival contour variation, although normal, may lead to plaque accumulation or entrapment, thus fostering inflammation.

The term *festooned gingiva* refers to rolled marginal gingiva on several adjacent teeth, usually noted on facial surfaces (Fig. 15-8).

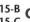 *Case Application*
Note the contour of Mrs. Bozenski's gingiva.

Consistency

As the gingival connective tissue is destroyed during the inflammatory process, gingiva loses its firmness and resiliency. The tissue becomes looser, and the papillae may be retractable, either with an instrument or puff of air. In

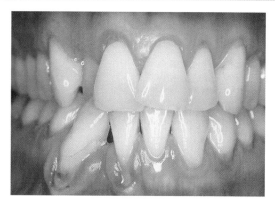

FIG. 15-8 Festooned gingiva and gingival cleft.

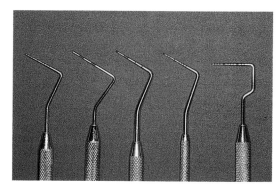

FIG. 15-9 A wide variety of periodontal probes are available. From left to right: Williams, Marquis, PSR Screening, Maryland/Moffitt, and Novatech probes.

healthy individuals, the attached gingiva is firmly bound down to the underlying tooth and bone.

 Case Application
Note the consistency of Mrs. Bozenski's gingiva.

Texture

Stippling is the term used for the orange peel–like appearance to the gingiva. Histologically, stippling is formed by the intersection of epithelial rete ridges and the interspersing penetration of connective tissue papilla. In erythematous tissue, stippling may disappear, although it may be present in thick, fibrotic tissue, which is nonetheless diseased. Stippling is not an absolute sign of health and the absence of stippling is not necessarily a sign of disease.[2]

Case Application
Describe the texture of Mrs. Bozenski's gingiva based on clinical photographs.

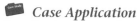 **PERIODONTAL POCKET PROBING**

15-D A periodontal pocket forms as the result of the apical migration of the junctional epithelium in the presence of disease from the cementoenamel junction. A calibrated periodontal probe must be used both to detect the pocket and measure its depth. The periodontal probe consists of a handle connected to a tapered shank and the working end marked in millimeter increments, terminating in a blunt tip. Periodontal probes come in many designs and markings (Fig. 15-9). One of the most common probes, the Michigan "O" probe, has Williams marking at 1-2-3-5-7-8-9-10 mm. The tip of the probe is approximately 0.48 mm in diameter. The World Health Organization (WHO) probe is used in determinations for the Community Periodontal Index of Treatment Needs (CPITN); it is also the probe type used in the Periodontal Screening and Recording (PSR). The WHO/CPITN/PSR probe has a small 0.5-mm ball at the tip and markings at 3.5-5.5-8.5-11.5 mm. This tip is useful for the detection of calculus and measurement of pockets. The WHO design with Williams markings is called the *Moffitt/Maryland probe.* This is perhaps the most versatile manual probe avail-

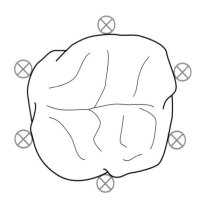

FIG. 15-10 Each tooth should be examined with the periodontal probe at six positions. Bleeding on probing also is checked at these locations.

able. The Novatech probe was designed with a different shaft angulation to facilitate reaching the distal areas of posterior teeth.

Probing measurements are made at six locations circumferentially around a tooth (Fig. 15-10). Measurements are made on the mesiobuccal, mid-buccal, distobuccal, mesiolingual, midlingual, and distolingual surfaces. The probe must be angled at about 10 degrees into the interproximal or col space to ensure an accurate reading. Periodontitis is predominantly an interproximal disease, and this angulation is necessary to place the tip of the probe beneath the contact area and into the col area. Care must be taken not to angle the probe excessively because this results in falsely high readings. Conversely, probing at the transitional line angle of the tooth results in shallow probe readings and missed detection of interproximal disease.

Many factors may influence the accuracy of probe measurements. These factors include probe design, probing force, probe angulation, location of the tooth in the mouth, the presence of coronal and/or radicular calculus, the presence of restorations, tissue sensitivity, and the level of inflammation.

Pockets are measured by *gentle* placement of the tip of

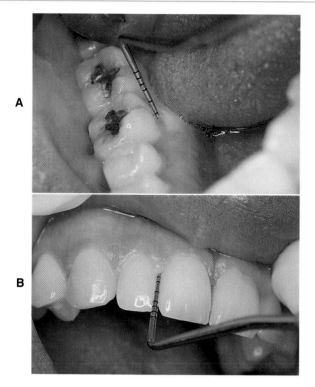

FIG. 15-11 A, The proper position of the periodontal probe is within the sulcus. **B,** Interproximal probing should be as close to the contact as possible with the probe at a 10-degree angle toward the center of the interproximal area.

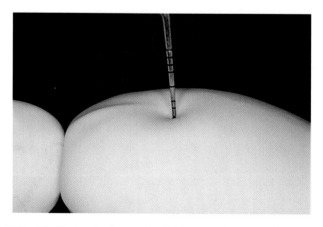

FIG. 15-12 Probe force should be consistent at about 25 grams, similar to the displacement shown on this operator's thumb.

the probe into the sulcus or pocket until resistance is felt (Fig. 15-11). Ideal probing force is approximately 10 to 20 grams pressure, equivalent to pressing of the periodontal probe into the finger pad of the thumb until it depresses approximately 2 mm (Fig. 15-12). Studies have shown that probing force can range from 5 to 105 grams of force.[10] The tendency to probe more gently in the anterior region and more heavily in the molar areas leads to inaccurate measurements and patient discomfort. Obviously, at in-

creased probing forces, the periodontal examination may be uncomfortable for the patient.

When a clinician probes with 25 grams of force, a probe with a tip diameter of 0.5 mm will penetrate into the junctional epithelium in healthy tissue and, in inflamed gingiva, through the junctional epithelium and into the underlying connective tissue.[1,35] Therefore the clinical pocket depth is always greater than the histologic pocket depth (the measurement in a histologic section from the junctional epithelium to the gingival margin).

Development of a consistent probing force and use of the same style probe leads to more reliable measurements. Using the same probe manufacturer also yields a more reliable result because manufacturer variations in probe design and tip diameter cause inconsistencies in probe measurements.

In health, probe depths normally range from 1 to 3 mm. Increased probe depths are an indication of either attachment loss or a coronal proliferation of gingival tissue, which forms a gingival pocket or pseudopocket. Human gingiva always has a probe depth of at least 1 mm, except for the first 10 days of healing after a gingivectomy surgical procedure. A measurement of 0 mm at any location or 1 mm interproximally must be rechecked for accuracy and is usually corrected by proper placement of the probe tip within the sulcus. Probe readings between whole numbers are always rounded up (e.g., 1.5 mm is recorded as 2 mm). Probe depths are recorded on a periodontal chart as a positive number (Fig. 15-13).

 Case Application

Review Mrs. Bozenski's periodontal charting and note areas of probe depths greater than 4 mm.

LOCATION OF THE FREE GINGIVAL MARGIN IN RELATION TO THE CEJ

Recession is defined as the apical migration of the free gingival margin from the CEJ of the tooth, resulting in exposure of the root surface. This recession may be associated with a periodontal pocket or may occur in areas where the probing depths are in the 1 to 3 mm range. The location of recession may be related to tooth anatomy and location in the arch and be caused by inflammatory periodontal disease or as a result of trauma induced by toothbrushing or other mechanical trauma.

Gingival recession may contribute to tooth sensitivity, root caries, or an unpleasant aesthetic appearance. If the previously mentioned conditions are a concern for the patient or if the recession worsens over time, surgical correction of the recession is indicated. Recession in the presence of healthy tissue may be observed without immediate treatment.

Recession is measured in millimeters from the CEJ to the free gingival margin. Recession measurements are made in the same locations as pocket depth measurements. Sometimes it is difficult to detect a CEJ with subtle contours. A free gingival margin apical to the CEJ (recession) is recorded as a positive number. A free gingival margin coronal to the CEJ is recorded as a negative number.

Case Application

Review Mrs. Bozenski's periodontal charting and clinical photographs for areas of gingival recession.

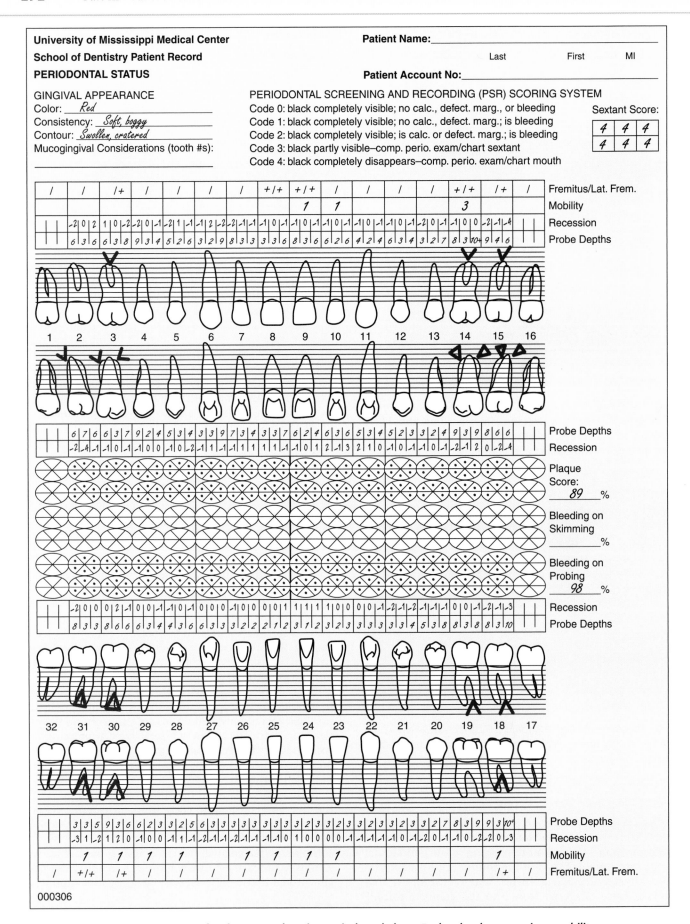

University of Mississippi Medical Center
School of Dentistry Patient Record
PERIODONTAL STATUS

Patient Name:_____
Last   First   MI

Patient Account No:_____

GINGIVAL APPEARANCE
Color: _Red_____
Consistency: _Soft, boggy_____
Contour: _Swollen, cratered_____
Mucogingival Considerations (tooth #s):
_____

PERIODONTAL SCREENING AND RECORDING (PSR) SCORING SYSTEM
Code 0: black completely visible; no calc., defect. marg., or bleeding
Code 1: black completely visible; no calc., defect. marg.; is bleeding
Code 2: black completely visible; is calc. or defect. marg.; is bleeding
Code 3: black partly visible—comp. perio. exam/chart sextant
Code 4: black completely disappears—comp. perio. exam/chart mouth

Sextant Score:

4	4	4
4	4	4

FIG. 15-13 Example of a comprehensive periodontal chart. Probe depths, recession, mobility, furcation involvement, bleeding on probing, bleeding on skimming, the plaque score, PSR score, and other information may be recorded in one place.

000306

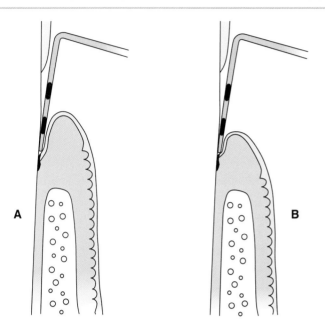

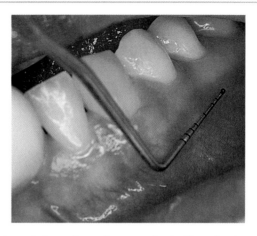

FIG. 15-15 Sometimes the mucogingival junction is not obvious but may be discerned by gentle pushing coronally with the side of the probe. The area of the tissue fold is the clinical mucogingival junction.

FIG. 15-14 Probe depth alone does not tell the whole story. Deeper pockets with less recession may show less attachment loss than shallower pockets with significant recession. **A,** Tooth has a 5-mm pocket and 5-mm attachment loss. **B,** Tooth has only a 2-mm probing but has 7-mm attachment loss.

CALCULATION OF ATTACHMENT LOSS

Probe depth alone does not indicate the amount of periodontal destruction. Attachment loss occurs when the junctional epithelium migrates apically from the CEJ as a result of connective tissue and bone destruction. *Loss of attachment (LOA),* the distance between the CEJ and the base of the pocket, is the true clinical measure of the amount of destruction. LOA, or calculated attachment loss (CAL), is calculated by addition of the probe depth and recession measurement. When the free gingival margin is coronal to the CEJ, the recession measurement is recorded as a negative number. Therefore in this situation the amount of attachment loss is *less than* the depth of the pocket.

The importance in the consideration of attachment loss and not just pocket depth may be illustrated as follows. If only probe depths are considered, it would be logical that a 5-mm pocket would indicate more disease than a tooth with a 2-mm pocket. However, if the 5-mm pocket occurs on a tooth with a recession measurement of 0 mm, the resulting LOA would be 5 mm. If the 2-mm pocket occurs on a tooth with 6 mm of recession, the LOA would calculate to 8 mm (Fig. 15-14).

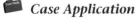 *Case Application*
Note the CAL readings on Mrs. Bozenski's chart and confirm the concept of CAL calculations.

AMOUNT OF KERATINIZED OR ATTACHED GINGIVA

Gingiva is divided into the free gingiva and attached gingiva. Free gingiva is demarcated from the free gingival margin to the base of the sulcus/pocket. The attached gingiva

is that portion from the base of the sulcus/pocket to the mucogingival junction. Below the mucogingival junction is the alveolar mucosa. Often the mucogingival junction is easily distinguished by the color change between the gingiva and alveolar mucosa. In situations in which the mucogingival junction is obscure or significant inflammation is present, the mucogingival junction may be found by placement of a periodontal probe sideways against the alveolar mucosa and gentle pushing in a coronal direction (Fig. 15-15). The clinical mucogingival junction is located where the tissue folds. If the fold occurs at the free gingival margin of the tissue, no keratinized tissue is present. In the absence of inflammation or progressive recession, it is possible for a tooth to have less than 1 mm of attached gingiva and maintain health.

DETECTION OF MARGINAL AND DEEP BLEEDING ON PROBING

Bleeding is the primary sign of gingival inflammation, the importance of which cannot be overemphasized. Although not all gingival inflammation leads to periodontal destruction and LOA, all LOA begins as gingival inflammation. The amount of bleeding may range from sparse to severe. The amount of bleeding may be indicative of the level of inflammation in the tissues but does not necessarily correlate with the amount of attachment loss. Bleeding may be profuse with severe gingivitis or may be scant even though severe attachment loss may occur. Bleeding may occur during gentle probing with a periodontal probe or other instrument while the patient is eating, brushing, or flossing, or it may occur spontaneously. Bleeding, as evidenced by a "pink toothbrush," may be the only indication to patients that anything is wrong with their periodontal health.

During the periodontal assessment, bleeding may be evaluated in two ways. Bleeding on skimming, accomplished by gentle running of the side of the probe between the free gingival margin and the tooth at a 45-degree angle, indicates the presence of marginal inflammation, primarily in the gingiva itself. Bleeding stimulated when the probe is placed to the depth of the pocket indicates the presence of subgingival inflammation and the possibility of ongoing attachment loss. It is not unusual, particularly in smokers, to have minimal bleeding on skimming even in the presence of severe attachment loss with bleeding on probing. The gingiva in smokers is often thick and fibrotic, with a noticeable decrease in marginal inflammation. Clinically, the gingival tissues look healthy. It is only by careful examination that the extent of disease is ascertained. The clinical appearance of gingiva is described as coral pink, but because of varying degrees of pigmentation, keratinization, and vascular blood supply, the gingiva may appear darker or even gray. Thus the gingiva of smokers may actually appear healthy. The detection of bleeding is especially important in the ongoing evaluation of the maintenance patient. More than 30% of the sites that bleed when probed at four consecutive recall appointments were at risk for increased attachment loss.[23,24]

 Case Application
Note areas of bleeding indicated on Mrs. Bozenski's chart. How does this correspond to tissue color, probe depths, and attachment loss?

DETECTION OF SUPPURATION

Suppuration is the formation or secretion of pus. Pus is a fluid product of inflammation consisting of leukocytes and the debris of dead cells and tissue elements liquefied by enzymatic breakdown. It is referred to as *exudate*. The presence of exudate is often, but not always, seen in periodontal inflammation. The presence or absence of exudate does not indicate the severity of disease; it may be present in gingivitis and absent in periodontitis. The amount of exudate is not related to pocket depth. Although the existence of an exudate or suppuration is noted in the periodontal charting, the clinical significance is unclear.

 ## EXPLORATION OF FURCATIONS

15-E
15-F The point at which the root trunk on a multirooted tooth diverges to form more than one root is called a *furcation* or *furca*. In health, furcations are surrounded by alveolar bone and covered by the gingiva. In periodontal diseases, bone loss may progress to the level whereby the furcation is exposed in the oral cavity. Once a furcation becomes involved in the disease process, the possibility of a positive prognosis for that tooth decreases significantly. Furcation measurement is an estimate of the loss of bone support at the areas of root divergence. This reduced bone height is a significant problem for two reasons: (1) the tooth is less stable (possibly mobile), and (2) a furcation is a difficult area to clean for both the patient and clinician. As the extent of furcation involvement increases, the prognosis for that particular tooth decreases.

Furcations between the two roots of the mandibular molars are referred to as **bifurcations** and are accessible from the buccal and lingual surfaces of the tooth. The bifurcation of the maxillary first premolar is accessible from the mesial and distal. **Trifurcations** refer to the three furcations in maxillary molars.

As the name suggests, the buccal furcation is explored directly from the buccal surface of the tooth. Because the

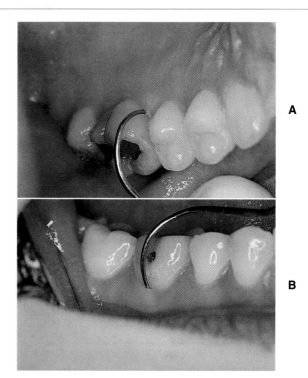

FIG. 15-16 A, The mesial furcation of the maxillary first molar must be examined from a palatal approach due to root anatomy. **B,** Mandibular molar furcations may be examined by direct approach of the furca with the instrument.

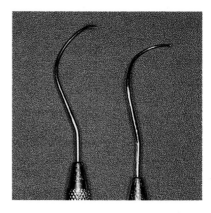

FIG. 15-17 Furcation probes may be found with 3-mm markings (Hamp probe, *right*) or without markings (Nabers probe, *left*).

mesiobuccal root of maxillary molars is broad in the buccopalatal direction, the mesial furcation may be reached only with the use of an approach on the palatal side of the tooth (Fig. 15-16). The distal furcation may be approached either from the buccal or palatal side, depending on the position of the tooth being examined and the adjacent tooth. The Nabers probe, a double-ended curved probe with or without 3-mm band markings, is the instrument used to explore furcations (Fig. 15-17). The tip of the Nabers probe should be held as parallel as possible to the long axis of the tooth and the furcation explored as the probe is moved with a horizontal walking stroke apically and laterally into the furca.

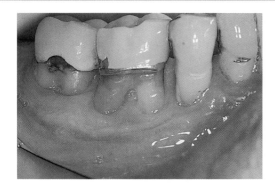

FIG. 15-18 This patient has severe attachment loss resulting in a Class III furcation.

TABLE 15-1

Grades of furcation

Degree	Name	Description	Charting symbol
I	Incipient furcal lesion	Circumferential movement of the probe reveals slight V-shaped indentation (depression) <3 mm horizontally.	∧
II	Patent furcal invasion	Loss of bone extends horizontally underneath roof of furca ≥3 mm horizontally.	∇
III	Communicating furcal invasion	Furcation is open from both facial and lingual approaches (through and through) but covered by gingival tissue.	▲
IV	Clinically visible furcation	Furcation is through and through; loss of bone with furca is visible in the mouth.	◆

Data from Lindhe J, Nyman S: The effect of plaque control and surgical pocket elimination on the establishment and maintenance of periodontal health: a longitudinal study of periodontal therapy in cases of advanced disease, *J Clin Periodontol* 2:67, 1975; and Carranza FA Jr, Takei HH: Treatment of furcation involvement and combined periodontal–endodontic therapy. In Newman MG, Carranza FA Jr, Takei H, editors: *Carranza's clinical periodontology,* ed 9, Philadelphia, 2001, WB Saunders.

 Case Study *Case Application*

Review Mrs. Bozenski's charting and identify which teeth have furcation involvement. Is bleeding indicated in these areas? If yes, why?

CLASSIFICATIONS

Furcations are classified as Class I, II, III, or IV.[8] Class I furcations are incipient, and the Nabers probe penetrates the furcation entrance less than 3 mm. Class II furca can be explored equal to or greater than 3 mm but not all the way through the furca. Class III furca allows the probe tip to pass completely through the furcation opening (Fig. 15-18). A Class IV furca is visible as a result of gingival recession. With the exception of Class I furcation involvement, bone loss in furcations is usually evident on posterior periapical and bitewing radiographs (Table 15-1).

 DETECTION OF MOBILITY

15-G
15-H Because of the soft periodontal ligament between the tooth and alveolar bone proper, teeth are naturally slightly mobile (physiological mobility) unless they are ***ankylosed*** (fused to the bone) in the socket. Therefore tooth mobility is a concern only when it is excessive (2 degrees or greater) or increasing. Possible causes of tooth mobility are listed in Box 15-2. When excessive occlusal or nonocclusal forces are applied to a tooth, the result may be a decrease

BOX 15-2

Possible Causes of Abnormal Tooth Mobility

Attachment loss: Periodontal disease, periodontal surgery, orthodontic correction
Occlusal trauma: Malpositioned teeth, including teeth not in occlusion, clenching, bruxism
Inflammation: Periodontal or periapical, edematous gingival tissues
Diseases of the jaw: Cysts and benign and malignant tumors

in the density of the surrounding bone. Once the excessive force is relieved, the bone density returns to normal. The degree to which excessive or abnormal forces contribute to attachment loss in a periodontium stressed by inflammation is inconclusive.

Measurement of mobility is accomplished by placement of the ends of the handles of two single-ended instruments on the buccal and lingual or palatal middle thirds of the tooth crown, followed by a gentle attempt to rock (move) the tooth in a buccolingual direction (Fig. 15-19).[31] The clinician should observe the contact between the adjacent tooth to observe for tooth movement. Movement is estimated in millimeters from 0 to 3 (Table 15-2). Vertical depressibility of the tooth is also examined

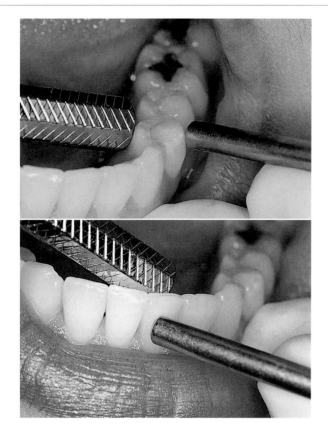

FIG. 15-19 Mobility is detected with the blunt ends of two instruments, not with an instrument and finger.

TABLE 15-2
Tooth mobility

Degree	Description	Charting symbol
1	Tooth moves 0.2 to 1 mm in horizontal direction.	1
2	Tooth moves >1 mm in horizontal direction.	2
3	Tooth is vertically depressible.	3

From Nyman S, Lindhe J: Examination of patients with periodontal disease. In Lindhe J et al, editors: *Clinical periodontology and implant dentistry,* ed 3, Munksgaard, Denmark, 1997, Copenhagen.

by placement of the side of the handle on the incisal or cuspal edge of the tooth with gentle application of pressure in an apical direction. Mobility, particularly implant mobility, also may be evaluated with an electronic device, the Periotest (Siemens AG, Bensheim, Germany). Although it is difficult to get agreement on mobility patterns between two examiners, the relative mobility of one tooth compared with another is the key element in the assessment of mobility patterns.

Case Application
Review Mrs. Bozenski's chart for notations of mobility. What other factors are identifiable with her case to cause mobility?

ASSESSMENT OF PLAQUE AND CALCULUS

Deposits in the oral cavity include plaque, calculus, stain, and *materia alba.* These deposits may be found on the teeth, soft tissues, and on restorative and prosthetic materials.

Plaque is a complex but organized collection of bacterial colonies. Although bacterial plaque is the primary etiology of the periodontal diseases, the type of bacteria, time the bacterial plaque is left undisturbed on the teeth, and host response to the bacteria are all critical factors for the risk of the initiation and progression of periodontal disease.[34,26]

At one time, periodontal diseases were thought to be degenerative in nature. As the general role that plaque plays in inflammation became known, the *nonspecific plaque hypothesis,* or quantitative theory, was proposed. This theory stated that the composition of plaque was not important but that disease depended solely on the accumulation or presence of plaque on the teeth.[27] Current evidence supports the *specific plaque (or qualitative) hypothesis.* This hypothesis states that plaque composition may vary in the types and numbers of microbial organisms and that different periodontal diseases may be caused by different microorganisms. Additionally, periodontal disease activity manifests in bursts of activity causing attachment loss and in periods of *quiescence,* when attachment loss does not progress.

More than 400 species of bacteria have been isolated from human periodontal pockets. Only relatively few of these bacteria are associated with periodontal disease. In health, plaque usually is composed of gram-positive, facultative aerobes that are not motile. The plaque is thin and stains pink with an erythrosin disclosing dye. When plaque is not disturbed, plaque colonies continue to grow and mature and as bacteria die, the bacterial mass becomes thicker. The bacterial types shift to anaerobic cocci, filaments, rods, and spirochetes, and the microbes are generally more gram-negative, motile, and strictly anaerobic. Major components of the cell wall of gram-negative bacteria are lipopolysaccharides, an endotoxin. When a gram-negative bacterial cell dies, the endotoxin is released from the lipopolysaccharides layer, amplifying the inflammation process and promoting tissue damage and bone resorption.

Although several organisms closely associated with the initiation and progression of periodontal disease have been studied, *Koch's postulates* have yet to be satisfied for bacteria associated with either gingivitis or periodontitis. Koch's postulates[12] stipulate that the causative agent of disease must adhere to the following:

- Be routinely isolated from the diseased individual
- Be grown in pure culture in the laboratory
- Produce a similar disease when inoculated into susceptible laboratory animals
- Be recovered from lesions in a diseased laboratory animal

Some researchers have theorized that Koch's postulates will never be satisfied, because of both limitations of the postulates themselves and the nature of the periodontal diseases.[34] In this instance, a potential pathogen must adhere to the following:

- Be associated with disease, as evident by increases in the number of organisms at the diseased site

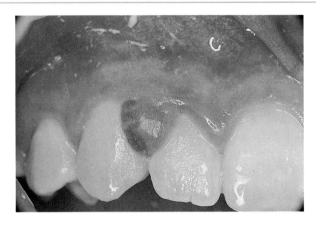

FIG. 15-20 Unstained plaque may often leave a rough appearance on the tooth surface, as seen on the mesial surface of the lateral incisor, resulting in the enlarged gingival tissue.

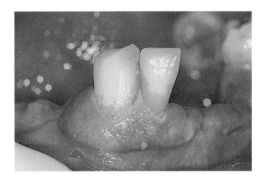

FIG. 15-21 Dyes such as erythrosin allow better visualization of plaque.

BOX 15-3

Suspected Periodontal Pathogens

Actinobacillus actinomycetemcomitans
Bacteroides forsythus
Campylobacter rectus
Eikenella corrodens
Fusobacterium nucleatum
Peptostreptococcus micros
Porphyromonas gingivalis
Prevotella intermedia
Streptococcus intermedius
Treponema species

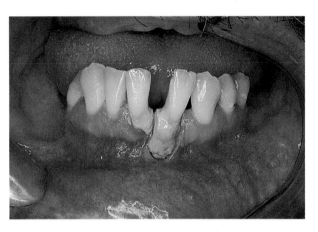

FIG. 15-22 Left undisturbed, calculus may accumulate to a significant size.

- Be eliminated or decreased in sites that demonstrate resolution with treatment
- Demonstrate the stimulation of a host response
- Be capable of causing disease in experimental animal models
- Demonstrate virulence factors responsible for allowing the organism to cause destruction of the periodontal tissues in the host

Many of the microorganisms associated with periodontal disease, or periodontopathogens, are difficult to harvest and successfully culture. A partial list of suspected periodontal pathogens [34,37] is shown in Box 15-3.

How these bacteria relate to one another remains unclear. Is disease initiated by one bacteria and progression caused by another? Because these are mixed infections, does more than one species act together? What is the role of the host in the initiation and progression of disease? These and other research questions are the subject of continuous, ongoing dental research.

Plaque is typically not visible to the untrained eye unless there are significant accumulations. The trained eye can observe plaque by the dullness of the enamel surface and the lack of shine and reflection of light on the teeth (Fig. 15-20). With the application of a disclosing solution or tablet, usually an erythrosin dye, plaque is easy to see (Fig. 15-21). Plaque may be measured in several different ways: quantity, location on the tooth, or age of the plaque. However, of primary importance for periodontal reasons is the location of undisturbed bacterial plaque interproximally and along the gingival margin. Assisting patients in the identification and subsequent removal of these plaque deposits is critical.

Calculus is a calcium and phosphate precipitate that adheres firmly to the tooth surface and dental prostheses (Fig. 15-22). This hard, stonelike material consists of four crystal forms of calcium phosphate: hydroxyapatite (58%), octacalcium phosphate (21%), magnesium whitlockite (21%), and brushite (9%). Microscopically, calculus is a crystalline structure of about 70% to 90% inorganic and organic components. The primary crystalline form is hydroxyapatite with calcium phosphate the principle inorganic portion (75.9%). The variable number of calcium, phosphate, and hydroxyl groups distinguishes these forms of calculus.[7]

Calculus attachment to the tooth surface has been described as one of four mechanisms.[39] The attachment may be by means of (1) an organic pellicle, (2) penetration of calculus into cementum, (3) mechanical locking into surface irregularities, or (4) close adaptation of calculus to unaltered cementum. Often the attachment is tenacious, and the calculus deposits may be difficult to remove with hand instrumentation. Powered instruments may be necessary to assist in removing longstanding calculus deposits.

Although calculus does not cause periodontal disease, it is considered a significant contributing factor to the disease because its surface provides excellent retention for bacterial plaque.[28] Therefore the periodontal assessment must yield an evaluation of the location and quantity of calculus to plan for professional removal and daily control of this deposit. Calculus is detected with the use of a fine-tined explorer or periodontal probe such as the PSR probe or Maryland probe, a good light, and compressed air. The instrument is held with a light grasp and guided along the tooth surface, with the use of tactile sense to feel for irregularities in the smoothness of the crown or root. Radiographs also may be used in calculus detection; heavier interproximal deposits of calculus appear as opaque deposits on the tooth/root surface.

Supragingival (salivary) calculus deposits occur coronal to the gingival margin and are initially whitish or cream-colored until they absorb tobacco and food stains. Supragingival calculus is most frequently found opposite ducts to the major salivary glands, on the lingual surfaces of the mandibular anterior teeth adjacent to ducts from the submandibular glands, and on buccal surfaces of the maxillary posterior teeth adjacent to ducts from the parotid glands. As saliva pools in these areas, minerals from the saliva precipitate onto irregularities in the tooth surface, incorporating plaque contents into the calculus matrix.

As the name suggests, *subgingival* (serumal) calculus forms beneath the gingival margin (Fig. 15-23). Mineral components precipitate from the gingival crevicular fluid to calcify against the root surface, entrapping subgingival plaque as the deposit grows. Subgingival calculus is denser than supragingival calculus and may be located anywhere in the mouth apical to the margin of the gingiva. It can take the form of spicules, solid masses, or sheets of calculus and develops a dark stain from the blood pigment hemosiderin. Occasionally, subgingival calculus is close to the gingival margin and will be visible through the gingival tissue as a darkened spot on the tissue. When recession of the gingival margin occurs so that what was originally subgingival calculus becomes visible, it may be referred to as *supragingival calculus,* even though the derivation and appearance are different from true supragingival calculus.

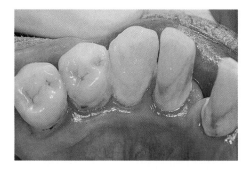

FIG. 15-23 The lighter-appearing calculus is salivary calculus, whereas the darker calculus is serumal calculus. Serumal calculus starts in a subgingival location but may eventually be supragingival as a result of gingival recession.

INDICES

In clinical practice, *indices* are used to evaluate patient oral hygiene proficiency, gingival inflammation, and bleeding changes and to assist in patient education. Indices in periodontal assessment are categorized as bleeding, gingival, plaque, calculus, oral hygiene care, attachment levels, and other measurements of disease severity. As an alternative or addition to the use of an index, clinicians may opt to draw the location of plaque or calculus deposits and record bleeding points on the periodontal chart as documentation and for use as a patient education tool.

When using a bleeding index, the clinician should distinguish whether the bleeding is from a gingival or a periodontal pocket because different procedures may be used to control inflammation in the gingiva and the periodontal pocket. Through appropriate self-care, patients can eliminate marginal gingival bleeding by mechanically controlling the plaque, but patients cannot reach the bacterial masses in deep pockets. To detect marginal bleeding, the periodontal probe is slid or is swept circumferentially at a 45-degree angle, 2 to 3 mm along the inside of the gingival pocket. Bleeding on probing is detected during periodontal probing procedures. Another measurement of interdental gingival bleeding may be obtained by stimulation of the papillary gingival areas with a soft wooden stick such as a STIM-U-DENT, dental floss, or a probe.[30]

Bleeding may be recorded as a dichotomous event (present or absent) or given a score according to how quickly the bleeding appeared, usually waiting 30 seconds or less before recording. Tobacco use has an adverse effect on the periodontium and an effect on bleeding scores. Bleeding scores of smokers have been shown to be both greater and lesser than the scores of nonsmokers. For this reason, bleeding indices should not be compared between smokers and nonsmokers[30] (Table 15-3).

The record of the quantity and location of plaque may serve as patient monitoring and patient education tools. Again, however, clinicians must understand exactly what the index is measuring. Because the quantity of plaque does not equate well to the severity of disease, plaque indices are really a measure of tooth cleaning efficacy. The location of plaque rather than the quantity of plaque is emphasized in other plaque indices. Some indices record plaque only where it is in contact with gingiva; other indices include plaque that occurs on any area of any tooth. Plaque indices may or may not use disclosing agents (Table 15-4).

Gingival indices usually include assessments of color, edema, contour, and bleeding. Clinical signs are generally obtained by inspections for color and contour and by use of the probe to elicit edema or bleeding. Interpretation of color and contour criteria is more subjective than indices that score bleeding (Table 15-5).

Calculus indices are used more frequently in research studies and clinical trials involving anticalculus agents than in clinical practice. In patient care, the quantity and frequency of calculus accumulation is simply one indication of how frequently the patient needs professional debridement. Clinicians may choose to record calculus pictorially by drawing the location and shape of the calculus deposits on the chart rather than obtaining an index (Table 15-6).

TABLE 15-3
Bleeding indices

Name	Year	Authors	Method	Scale
Modified sulcular bleeding index (mSBI)	1987	Mombelli et al[a]	Note bleeding on gentle probing.	Ordinal (0 to 3)
Interdental bleeding index	1985	Caton and Polson[b]	Insert wooden interdental cleaner interproximally facially 1 to 2 mm four times; observe for 15 seconds.	Dichotomous
Eastman interdental bleeding index	1984	Abrams, Caton, and Polson[c]	Insert triangular wooden toothpick midinterproximally.	Dichotomous
Gingival bleeding time index (BTI)	1981	Nowicki et al[d]	Slide probe back and forth against inner margin of gingiva; wait 15 seconds; may repeat once.	Ordinal (0 to 4)
Modified papillary bleeding index (MPBI)	1980	Barnett, Ciancio, and Mather[e]	Add time to PBI.	Ordinal (0 to 4)
Papillary bleeding score (PBS) modified from PBI	1979	Loesche[f]	Insert STIM-U-DENT interproximally.	Ordinal (0 to 5)
Gingival bleeding index	1975	Ainamo and Bay[g]	Perform circumferential stroke at gingival orifice; wait 10 seconds.	Dichotomous
Gingival bleeding index (GBI)	1974	Carter and Barnes[h]	Slide unwaxed dental floss interproximally; wait up to 30 seconds.	Dichotomous
Gingival sulcus index (SBI)	1971	Mühlemann and Son[i]	Perform sulcus probing on dry teeth.	Ordinal (0 to 5; score ≥2 on color if bleeding occurred)

[a]Mombelli A et al: The microbiota associated with successful or failing implants, *Oral Microbiol Immunol* 2:145, 1987.
[b]Caton JG, Polson AM: The interdental bleeding index: a simplified procedure for monitoring oral gingival health, *Comp Contin Edu Dent* 6(2):88, 1985.
[c]Abrams K, Caton J, Polson A: Histologic comparisons of interproximal gingival tissues related to the presence or absence of bleeding, *J Periodontol* 55:629, 1984.
[d]Nowicki D et al: The gingival bleeding time index, *J Periodontol* 52:260, 1981.
[e]Barnett M, Ciancio S, Mather M: The modified papillary bleeding index: comparison with gingival index during the resolution of gingivitis, *J Prev Dent* 6:135, 1980.
[f]Loesche WJ: Clinical and microbiological aspects of chemotherapeutic agents according to the specific plaque hypothesis, *J Dent Res* 58:2404, 1979.
[g]Ainamo J, Bay I: Problems and proposals for recording gingivitis and plaque, *Int Dent J* 25:229, 1975.
[h]Carter HG, Barnes GP: The gingival bleeding index, *J Periodontol* 45:801, 1974.
[i]Mühlemann HR, Son S: Gingival sulcus bleeding—a leading symptom in initial gingivitis, *Helv Odont Acta* 15:107, 1971.

TABLE 15-4
Plaque indices

Name	Year	Authors	Method	Area evaluated
Distal mesial plaque index (DMPI), modified Navy index	1987	Fischman et al[a]	Disclose.	Entire surface with more emphasis at proximals and a measure of quantity
Navy plaque index (modified; MN)	1972	Elliott, Bowers, and Rovelstad[b]	Disclose. Score I (plaque present) for each of nine areas.	Nine divisions of tooth surface with more divisions at gingival margin
Plaque control record	1972	O'Leary, Drake, and Naylor[c]	Record presence of plaque to allow patient to visualize areas.	Four tooth surfaces of all teeth present
Turesky modification of the Quigley-Hein	1970	Turesky, Gilmore, and Glickman[d]	Disclose.	Plaque assessment on facial and lingual surfaces of all teeth

[a]Fischman S et al: Distal mesial plaque index: a technique for assessing dental plaque about the gingiva, *Dent Hyg* 61:404, 1987.
[b]Elliott JR, Bowers GM, Rovelstad GH III: Evaluation of an oral physiotherapy center in the reduction of bacterial plaque and periodontal disease, *J Periodontol* 43:221, 1972.
[c]O'Leary TJ, Drake RB, Naylor JE: The plaque control record, *J Periodontol* 43:38, 1972.
[d]Turesky S, Gilmore ND, Glickman I: Reduced plaque formation by the chloromethyl analogue of vitamin C, *J Periodontol* 41:41, 1970.

Continued

TABLE 15-4

Plaque indices—cont'd

Name	Year	Authors	Method	Area evaluated
Patient hygiene performance (PHP)	1968	Podshadley and Haley[e]	Disclose and record presence or absence of plaque.	#3, #8, #14, #19, #24, #30
Plaque index (PI)	1964	Silness and Löe[f]	Dry teeth; use mouth mirror and explorer.	Gingival one third of tooth surfaces or tooth
Simplified oral hygiene index (OHI-S)	1964	Greene and Vermillion[g]	Perform same as OHI with different teeth selected.	Facial surfaces of #3, #8, #14, #24 and lingual surfaces of #19 and #39
Quigley-Hein plaque index	1962	Quigley and Hein[h]	Disclose.	Surface scored from 0 to 5, with emphasis at gingival margin
Oral hygiene index Debris index Calculus index	1960	Greene and Vermillion[i]	Assess oral cleanliness by estimation of the mouth divided into six segments.	Tooth surface covered with debris and/or calculus

[e]Podshadley AG, Haley JVA: A method for evaluating oral hygiene performance, *Public Health Rep* 83:259, 1968.
[f]Silness J , Löe H: Periodontal disease in pregnancy. II. Correlation between oral hygiene and periodontal condition, *Acta Odont Scand* 22:112, 1964.
[g]Greene JC, Vermillion JR: The simplified oral hygiene index, *J Am Dent Assoc* 68:7, 1964.
[h]Quigley GA, Hein JW: Comparative cleansing efficiency of manual and power brushing, *J Am Dent Assoc* 65:26, 1962.
[i]Greene JC, Vermillion JR: The oral hygiene index: a method for classifying oral hygiene status, *J Am Dent Assoc* 61:172, 1960.

TABLE 15-5

Gingival indices

Name	Year	Authors	Method
Gingival index (GI)	1963	Löe and Silness*	Observe; perform circumferential stroke against soft tissue below gingival margin.
Papillary-marginal-attached index (PMAI)	1947	Schour and Massler†	Observe; press probe against gingiva.

*Löe H, Silness J: Periodontal disease in pregnancy. I. Prevalence and severity, *Acta Odont Scand* 21:533, 1963.
†Schour I, Massler M: Prevalence of gingivitis in various age groups, *J Am Dent Assoc* 35:475, 1947.

TABLE 15-6

Calculus indices

Name	Year	Authors	Method
Marginal line calculus index (MLC-I)	1967	Mühlemann and Villa*	Divide tooth in half (mesial and distal); with air, visualize minute areas of supramarginal calculus next to gingiva on lingual four mandibular incisors.
V-M calculus assessment	1965	Volpe, Manhold, and Hazen†	Measure with probe in three planes.
Calculus surface index	1961	Ennever, Sturzenberger, and Radike§	Use air, mirror, and explorer to detect calculus
Calculus index simplified (CI-S), part of OHI-S	1964	Greene and Vermillion‡	With an explorer, detect calculus on tooth surface or around cervical portion of tooth.

*Mühlemann HR, Villa PR: The marginal line calculus index, *Helv Odont Acta* 11:175, 1967.
†Volpe AR, Manhold JH, Hazen SP: In vivo calculus assessment. Part I. A method and its examiner reproducibility, *J Periodontol* 36:292, 1965.
‡Greene JC, Vermillion JR: The simplified oral hygiene index, *J Am Dent Assoc* 68:7, 1964.
§Ennever J, Sturzenberger OP, Radike AW: The calculus surface index method for scoring clinical calculus studies, *J Periodontol* 32:54, 1961.

TABLE 15-7

Composite periodontal disease indices

Name	Year	Authors	Method
Periodontal scoring and recording index (PSR)	1992	AAP, ADA[a]	This is an individual screening exam. Divide the mouth into six segments; record highest score according to four levels, including bleeding and probe depths.
Extent and severity index	1986	Carlos, Wolfe, and Kingman[b]	This index is for epidemiological purposes. Estimate the attachment level from probe depths—14 sites in each of two contralateral quadrants.
Community periodontal index treatment needs (CPITN)	1982	Ainamo et al[c]	This index is for epidemiological purposes. Use O'Leary's sextants with specified index teeth or worst tooth, WHO probe, and 0 to 4 codes per sextant; evaluate bleeding, deposits, and pocket depth.
Periodontal screening examination	1967	O'Leary[d]	Divide mouth into 6 segments and record highest score; score gingiva by color, contour, and consistency; score periodontium by mesiofacial line angle probe depth; score local irritants.
Periodontal disease index (PDI)	1967	Ramfjord[e]	Select the "Ramfjord" teeth (#3, #9, #12, #19, #25, and #28) and score for gingiva, attachment loss, calculus, and plaque.
Periodontal index (PI)	1956	Russell[f]	Do not use probe; weight scores and combine gingival and periodontal status.

WHO, World Health Organization.

[a]American Academy of Periodontology and American Dental Association: *Periodontal screening and recording* (publication sponsored by Procter & Gamble), Cincinnati, 1992, Procter & Gamble.

[b]Carlos JP, Wolfe MD, Kingman A: The extent and severity index: a simple method for use in epidemiologic studies of periodontal disease, *J Clin Periodontol* 13:500, 1986.

[c]Ainamo J et al: Development of the World Health Organization (WHO) community periodontal index of treatment needs (CPTIN), *Int Dent J* 32:281, 1982.

[d]O'Leary TJ: The periodontal screening examination, *J Periodontol* 38:617, 1967.

[e]Ramfjord SP: The periodontal disease index (PDI), *J Periodontol* 38:602, 1967.

[f]Russell AL: A system of classification and scoring for prevalence surveys of periodontal disease, *J Dent Res* 35(3):350, 1956.

Indices are also available that assess oral cleanliness or oral debris, often combining plaque, materia alba, stain, and calculus into a single score. In patient care, the indices generally include all teeth and all tooth surfaces, unlike epidemiological surveys in which only specified teeth or surfaces may be measured.

Periodontal indices attempt to measure the degree of periodontal destruction. The typical index in periodontal assessment is an historical record, one of past destruction or of current periodontal symptoms that are not predictive of the presence, severity, or future course of the infection (Table 15-7). Currently, evaluating attachment loss or gain is considered one of the most valid measurements of the status of periodontal disease. Although pocket or probe depths are usually obtained in indices of periodontal disease, pocket depth alone does not equate to attachment loss nor necessarily to an unhealthy pocket. Periodontal indices provide only a record of previous destruction, not a prediction of the future course of the disease.

DENTAL FACTORS IN PERIODONTAL DISEASE RISK

Any condition in the patient that enhances the colonization of bacteria, increases the difficulty of plaque control, or alters the initiation or progression of disease should be considered a contributing factor to periodontal disease risk. These factors are listed in Box 15-4.

BOX 15-4

Periodontal Disease Risk Factors

Missing teeth
Caries
Open contacts
Faulty restorations
Malpositioned teeth
Anatomic variations
Palatogingival grooves
Cervical enamel projections
Impacted or supernumerary teeth
Decreased salivary flow

One type of anatomical variation is the palatogingival groove, which commonly appears on the lingual surface of the maxillary lateral incisor. This deep developmental groove extends apically from cingulum on the lingual aspect of the root (Fig. 15-24).

Cervical-enamel projections occur in the furcations of mandibular molars, causing an abnormality in tissue attachment (Fig. 15-25).

Both palatogingival grooves and cervical-enamel projections are considerably more prone to plaque retention and are more difficult to access by normal oral self-care measures.

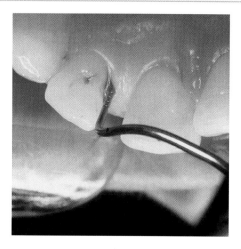

FIG. 15-24 Palatogingival groove.

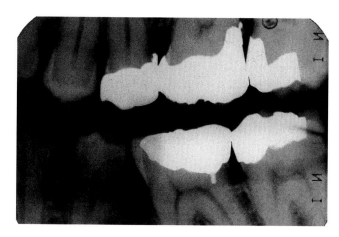

FIG. 15-26 Overhanging restorations are harbingers for plaque accumulation and subsequent inflammation.

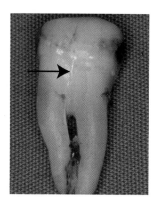

FIG. 15-25 Cervical-enamel projection.

TABLE 15-8

Classifications and descriptions of embrasures

Class	Description
I	Interdental papilla fills space between adjacent teeth in contact.
II	Interdental papilla is partially receded, resulting in small opening under contact.
III	Interdental papilla has completely receded, leaving triangular opening under contact.

Modified from Caranza FA, Newman MG: *Clinical periodontology,* ed 8, Philadelphia, 1996, WB Saunders.

INTERPROXIMAL CONTACTS

Ideally the interproximal surfaces of adjacent teeth contact each other at the heights of contour with the mesial surface of one tooth in contact with the distal surface of the adjacent tooth. The exception is the midline, where two mesial surfaces contact each other and the distal of the last tooth in the arch. The space apical to the contact area forms the gingival embrasure, a roughly pyramidal shaped space filled with gingival papilla. When gingival recession is present, the gingival embrasure may be "open," that is, no tissue filling the space. Table 15-8 classifies and describes gingival embrasure.

Any change in the character of an interproximal contact presents a greater challenge for plaque control. Contact areas that are too broad, too close to the gingiva, or teeth not in contact all contribute to the accumulation of plaque and debris and food impaction. Missing and malpositioned teeth pose additional problems because surrounding teeth in the same arch and the opposing arch move into the space of the missing tooth. Thus over time the interproximal contacts of the teeth may move apart or shift to a position, encouraging food impaction or tissue impingement.

Case Application

What type of embrasure spaces does Mrs. Bozenski have?

RESTORATIVE MATERIALS

Restorations and prostheses must mimic the natural dentition as closely as possible to promote the maintenance of healthy gingiva. Conversely, faulty restorations may present the patient with areas that are exceptionally difficult to clean. Restorative materials with rough surfaces, overhangs, open or worn margins, or poorly contoured interproximal contacts result in plaque retentive areas. Overcontoured or undercontoured restorations provide either too much or too little protection to the gingival embrasure area and may prevent normal physiological cleansing (Fig. 15-26).

OTHER CONTRIBUTING FACTORS

Assessment of saliva, diet, and habits is also important to the quality and health of the periodontal tissues. Salivary flow is a major factor in normal physiological oral cleansing. Individuals with reduced salivary flow, less than 1 ml/minute, are prone to increased plaque retention and increased risk of dental caries. Also, with less saliva available in the oral cavity, the protective mechanisms of the salivary components are reduced. Thus both quantity and quality of saliva should be evaluated with assessment of the periodontal condition.

Attention to the dietary choices of periodontal patients is important so that the periodontal tissue receives adequate nourishment. Coenzymes such as vitamin C are necessary for the proper cross-linking of collagen to occur. Diet also influences plaque growth and retention. Additionally, some oral habits may be damaging to the oral cavity. Clenching and **bruxism** result in abnormal stress on the alveolar bone and may cause flexure of teeth, which results in root concavities called **abfraction lesions**. Incorrect brushing or incorrect use of auxiliary cleaning aids, such as toothpicks, may harm gingival tissues or root surfaces. Tobacco use is damaging to the periodontium. Particularly visible to the patient is the damage to the gingiva when smokeless tobacco quids are held in close proximity to gingival tissue.

EXAMINATION AND EVALUATION OF DENTAL IMPLANTS

For the patient with a dental implant, assessment of the periodontal health around it is an essential part of the periodontal examination. Examination of the surrounding tissue, implant mobility, the presence or absence of bleeding, alveolar bone height, patient satisfaction, and patient care of the implant are part of the implant assessment. Inflammation may develop around an implant, similar to periodontal inflammation. A mobile implant is a failing implant.

The decision of whether to probe around implants is still controversial. Arguments against probing an implant include the possibility of introducing bacteria to the peri-implant area, inadequate data on the relationship between osseointegration and probe depths, and the occasional difficulties encountered when probing around certain prosthetic devices attached to the implant. Modification of assessment procedures is necessary to protect the implant surface[25], usually titanium or hydroxyapatite, and the surrounding tissue. Any instrument used on or around implants must be plastic or graphite, not metal, to avoid alteration of the implant surface or the production of a galvanic reaction (Fig. 15-27). This rule applies to probes, explorers, debridement instruments, rubber cup and air polishers, and personal oral-care devices.

Implant indices for plaque, gingival status, and bleeding have not been validated. The recommendation has been made that any periodontal index used for implants should be separate from the index used on teeth with roots. The appearance of the oral tissue next to the implant may differ, depending on whether the implant is surrounded by gingiva or alveolar mucosa. Careful inspection of the appearance of the implant and its surrounding tissue is necessary to observe cleanliness, deposit accumulation, erythema, bleeding, or the presence of suppuration. Regular intervals of radiographic assessment of alveolar bone level are recommended when monitoring implant health.

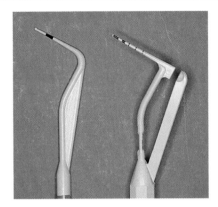

FIG. 15-27 Plastic instruments, such as these probes, must be used around titanium implants.

TECHNOLOGY IN THE PERIODONTAL EXAMINATION

15-I

Traditionally, periodontal examinations have been conducted using manual instruments. However, expanding technology has provided the clinician with automated methods of assessment and with additional diagnostic and monitoring tools. Some of these tests or assays are performed chairside, and some require laboratory analyses.[21,22] Although they are of scientific interest, many of these additional aids have yet to find a place in the everyday diagnosis of periodontal diseases and prediction of disease activity.

IDENTIFYING INFLAMMATION

The PerioTemp (Abiodent, Inc., Danvers, Mass.) measures the sulcus temperature using an electronic probe. It is based on the fact that inflamed tissue has a higher temperature than healthy, uninflamed tissue. An elevated sulcus or pocket temperature may be an early symptom of inflammation. Early gingival inflammation also may be evaluated utilizing the Periotron 8000 (Harco Electronics, Winnipeg, Manitoba, Canada), an instrument that measures the gingival crevicular fluid flow. Crevicular fluid flow increases before either erythema or bleeding is evident in inflamed tissues.[9]

AUTOMATED PROBING SYSTEMS

Several automated probing systems are available that electronically record probe depths and can enter the readings into a computer file. Voice-activated recording systems are now a familiar tool in periodontal assessment. Advantages for these electronic, computerized assessment tools may be efficiency, improved infection control, and consistency in recording measurements. However, the clinician must use the measuring devices properly and understand the limitations of electronic measuring and recording.

IMAGING TECHNOLOGY

Improved methods of assessing bone loss or progression of bone loss have been developed.[14] Using a copying process to provide greater contrast between structures, xeroradiography permits finer visualization of bone quality and density. Subtraction radiography converts radiographic images into digital images that, when superimposed, reveal minimal bone changes (bone loss as *radiolucent,* bone gain as *radiopaque*).

A nuclear medicine method measures bone metabolism through means of a semiconductor radiation probe detector. A radiopharmaceutical is injected into a vein and then read by a semiconductor. A high degree of uptake by the bone may be predictive of future bone loss. Visualizations predictive of bone loss are more valuable than tests or radiographs that show the results of bone loss. As these tools for the evaluation and prediction of bone destruction are improved, they should become part of the armamentarium for the prevention and control of periodontal diseases.

LABORATORY ASSAYS OF PERIODONTAL INFECTIONS

Clinical and radiographic examinations are essential methods of gathering assessment data to aid in the diagnosis of a periodontal condition. However, the ability to gather additional information via laboratory analysis is expanding. One of the earliest chairside procedures analyzing oral flora was the use of phase contrast or *darkfield microscopy* to identify the quantity, shapes, and motility of bacteria in the plaque. Placement of a plaque sample on a slide and examination of it have been used in the office as a patient education and motivational tool and to assist in determining the age of the plaque by its morphology and motility. However, neither types of microscopy can identify specific species of bacteria.[38]

Microbiologists are increasingly able to cultivate the anaerobic oral bacterial species and to associate these bacteria with certain types of periodontal diseases. Culturing permits the microbiologist to recover the widest range of bacterial species. This is an advantage because potential antibiotic use may then be more selective.

However, several problems exist with the cultivation of oral microorganisms. Culturing adequate samples from the diseased periodontal pocket is difficult because the bacteria may not survive the retrieval or transport process to the laboratory. Current culturing techniques do not always foster growth of highly sensitive periodontal pathogens. Culturing is also expensive and time-consuming. Finally, the bacteria that are isolated are only *presumed* to be those initiating or causing disease progression; their absolute role in periodontal disease has not been determined.

In addition to inspection of bacteria through the microscope or the culturing of oral microbes, other microbiological assays are available. These include *immunoassays, nucleic acid probes,* and enzyme assays. Immunoassays employ antibodies to detect bacterial antigens. Some types of immunoassays are available for use by clinicians in the office. The nucleic acid probe uses deoxyribonucleic acid (DNA) and occasionally ribonucleic acid (RNA) to hybridize the organism's genetic code and thus identify some species of oral microorganisms. DNA probes are available for many of the usual periodontopathogens, including *Actinobacillus actinomycetemcomitans, Bacteroides forsythus, Campylobacter rectus, Eikenella corrodens, Fusobacterium nucleatum, Porphyromonas gingivalis, Prevotella intermedia,* and *Treponema denticola.*

Enzyme assays permit detection of enzymes the body may be producing to combat the effects of the periopathogenic organisms. Examples of the enzymes being studied are collagenase, elastase, beta-glucuronidase, and aspartate aminotransferase (AST). Although significant research has been conducted, these assays have yet to find a place in routine periodontal care.[22]

Interleukin-1 (IL-1) is one of the many cytokines involved in the inflammatory process.[19] An association between a specific genotype of IL-1 and severe periodontal disease has been demonstrated.[18] A test has been developed, the PST (Medical Science Systems, Flagstaff, Ariz.), that can determine when a patient has this genotype that can produce as much as four times more IL-1 than other IL-1 genotypes. Although this test does not diagnose disease, it provides information to determine which patients have an increased susceptibility for the initiation and progression of disease. Based on computer models, patients with this specific IL-1 genotype who also smoke significantly increase their odds of developing severe periodontal disease.

CLASSIFICATION OF PERIODONTAL DISEASE

Periodontal disease is the result of predominantly gram-negative anaerobic microorganisms in a gingival pocket and thus stimulating an inflammatory response in the host. In patients susceptible to periodontal disease, this inflammation progresses from gingival inflammation into the attachment apparatus, causing destruction of connective tissue, apical migration of the junctional epithelium, and loss of bone surrounding the tooth. Left untreated, the ultimate fate is loss of a tooth or teeth.

In 1999 the Workshop on Classification of Periodontal Diseases and Conditions developed a new, comprehensive classification system for periodontal disease shown in Box 15-5.[3]

Periodontal classifications are not age-dependent and are not based on the rate of progression. The extent of periodontal disease is classified as *localized* when less than 30% of the existing sites are involved and *generalized* when more than 30% of those sites are involved. The severity of periodontal disease is based on the amount of clinical attachment loss (CAL), with *slight* defined as 1 to 2 mm of CAL, *moderate* as 3 to 4 mm of CAL, and *severe* as 5 mm or more.[3]

Refractory is a term that can be applied to any classification of periodontal disease that is unresponsive to professional therapy and compliant patient self-care. Refractory also is applied to any specific disease category to further clarify the disease.[3]

Categories VI (abscesses of the periodontium), VII (periodontitis associated with endodontic lesions), and VIII (developmental or acquired deformities and conditions) represent specific and special diagnostic and treatment challenges within the scope of periodontics. Of these three categories, category VI is most likely to be used by the dental hygienist.[3]

It is important to understand that knowledge of periodontal diseases is continually changing through research and with the advent of new technology designed to assist in research. As researchers discover more about the etiology and treatment of disease, the current classification system could change.[3]

BOX 15-5

Classification of Periodontal Diseases

I. Gingival Diseases
A. Dental plaque-induced gingival diseases
  i. *Gingivitis associated with dental plaque only*
    1. Without other local contributing factors
    2. With local contributing factors (see VIII.A)
  ii. *Gingival diseases modified by systemic factors*
    1. Associated with the endocrine system
      a. Puberty-associated gingivitis
      b. Menstrual cycle–associated gingivitis
      c. Pregnancy-associated
        1) Gingivitis
        2) Pyogenic granuloma
      d. Diabetes mellitus–associated gingivitis
    2. Associated with blood dyscrasias
      a. Leukemia-associated gingivitis
      b. Other
  iii. *Gingival diseases modified by medications*
    1. Drug-influenced gingival diseases
      a. Drug-induced gingival enlargements
      b. Drug-influenced gingivitis
        1) Oral contraceptive-associated gingivitis
        2) Other
  iv. *Gingival diseases modified by malnutrition*
    1. Ascorbic acid–deficiency gingivitis
    2. Other diseases
B. Non–plaque-induced gingival lesions
  i. *Gingival lesions of specific bacterial origin*
    1. *Neisseria gonorrhea*–associated lesions
    2. *Treponema pallidum*–associated lesions
    3. Streptococcal species–associated lesions
    4. Other
  ii. *Gingival diseases of viral origin*
    1. Herpes virus infections
      a. Primary herpetic gingivostomatitis
      b. Recurrent oral herpes
      c. Varicella-zoster infections
    2. Other diseases
  iii. *Gingival diseases of fungal origin*
    1. *Candida* species infections
      a. Generalized gingival candidiasis
      b. Linear gingival erythema
      c. Histoplasmosis
      d. Other
  iv. *Gingival lesions of genetic origin*
    1. Hereditary gingival fibromatosis
    2. Other lesions
  v. *Gingival manifestations of systemic conditions*
    1. Mucocutaneous disorders
      a. Lichen planus
      b. Pemphigoid
      c. Pemphigus vulgaris
      d. Erythema multiforme
      e. Lupus erythematosus
      f. Drug-induced disorders
      g. Other disorders
    2. Allergic reactions
      a. Dental restorative materials
        1) Mercury
        2) Nickel
        3) Acrylic
        4) Other materials
      b. Reactions attributable to the following:
        1) Toothpastes and dentifrices
        2) Mouthrinses and mouthwashes
        3) Chewing gum additives
        4) Foods and additives
      c. Other allergic responses
  vi. *Traumatic lesions (factitious, iatrogenic, accidental)*
    1. Chemical injury
    2. Physical injury
    3. Thermal injury
  vii. *Foreign body reactions*
  viii. *Not otherwise specified*

II. Chronic Periodontitis
A. Localized
B. Generalized

III. Aggressive Periodontitis
A. Localized
B. Generalized

IV. Periodontitis as a Manifestation of Systemic Diseases
A. Associated with hematological disorders
  i. *Acquired neutropenia*
  ii. *Leukemias*
  iii. *Other*
B. Associated with genetic disorders
  i. *Familial and cyclic neutropenia*
  ii. *Down syndrome*
  iii. *Leukocyte adhesion deficiency syndromes*
  iv. *Papillon-Lefevre syndrome*
  v. *Chediak-Higashi syndrome*
  vi. *Histiocytosis syndromes*
  vii. *Glycogen storage disease*
  viii. *Infantile genetic agranulocytosis*
  ix. *Cohen syndrome*
  x. *Ehlers-Danlos syndrome (Types IV and VIII AD)*
  xi. *Hypophosphatasia*
  xii. *Other genetic disorders*
C. Not otherwise specified

V. Necrotizing Periodontal Diseases
A. Necrotizing ulcerative gingivitis (NUG)
B. Necrotizing ulcerative periodontitis (NUP)

VI. Abscesses of the Periodontium
A. Gingival abscess
B. Periodontal abscess
C. Pericoronal abscess

VII. Periodontitis Associated with Endodontic Lesions
A. Combined periodontal-endodontic lesions

VIII. Developmental or Acquired Deformities or Conditions
A. Localized tooth-related factors that modify or predispose to plaque-induced gingival diseases/periodontitis
  i. *Tooth anatomical factors*
  ii. *Dental restorations and appliances*
  iii. *Root fractures*
  iv. *Cervical root resorption and cemental tears*
B. Mucogingival deformities and conditions around teeth
  i. *Gingival/soft tissue recession*
    1. Facial or lingual surfaces
    2. Interproximal (papillary)

Continued

BOX 15-5

Classification of Periodontal Diseases—cont'd

    ii. Lack of keratinized gingiva
    iii. Decreased vestibular depth
    iv. Aberrant frenum/muscle position
    v. Gingival excess
      1. Pseudopockets
      2. Inconsistent gingival margin
      3. Excessive gingival display
      4. Gingival enlargement (see "Gingival diseases modified by medications" and "Gingival lesions of genetic origin" sections)
    vi. Abnormal color

C. Mucogingival deformities and conditions on edentulous ridges
    i. Vertical and/or horizontal ridge deficiency
    ii. Lack of gingiva/keratinized tissue
    iii. Gingival/soft tissue enlargement
    iv. Aberrant frenum/muscle position
    v. Decreased vestibular depth
    vi. Abnormal color
D. Occlusal trauma
    i. Primary occlusal trauma
    ii. Secondary occlusal trauma

 RITICAL THINKING ACTIVITIES

1. Review clinical photos and describe characteristics of the gingiva.
2. Practice calculating attachment loss using probe depths and recession readings.
3. Complete a comprehensive periodontal charting on a peer or patient.
4. Record periodontal findings for a student clinician.

5. Review patient cases and identify the American Academy of Periodontology's (AAP's) periodontal classification. Provide rationales for your responses.
6. Given sites of bleeding, plaque, and gingival inflammation, calculate an index for each.

 REVIEW QUESTIONS

Questions 1 and 7 refer to the case study presented at the beginning of the chapter.

1. Which of the following is the most appropriate periodontal diagnosis for Mrs. Bozenski?
   a. Aggressive periodontitis and early-onset periodontitis
   b. Chronic periodontitis and adult periodontitis
   c. Periodontitis associated with systemic disease
   d. Refractory periodontitis
   e. Not enough information present to make a diagnosis

2. A secondary diagnosis may include which of the following?
   a. Pregnancy-associated gingivitis
   b. Postmenopausal periodontitis
   c. Occlusal trauma
   d. Aspirin-associated bleeding on probing
   e. Inderal-induced gingival overgrowth

3. During examination of the pocket on the mesiolabial of the maxillary right canine, with 25 gm of probing force, the tip of the probe will *most likely* do which of the following?
   a. Stop at the base of the histologic pocket
   b. Penetrate into but not through the junctional epithelium
   c. Penetrate through the junctional epithelium into the underlying connective tissue
   d. Penetrate through the epithelium and connective tissue and stop when the tip touches the crest of the alveolar bone
   e. None of the above

4. Which of the following is the instrument of choice with which to examine furcations?
   a. Maryland/Moffitt periodontal probe
   b. #23 Shepherd's hook explorer
   c. Pigtail explorer
   d. 2N Nabers probe

5. Which of the following is the furcation involvement on the mesial of the maxillary left first molar?
   a. Class I
   b. Class II
   c. Class III
   d. Class IV

6. Which of the following describes the meaning of the mobility measurement of the maxillary left first molar?
   a. The tooth has three roots.
   b. The tooth is depressible and has lateral mobility.
   c. The tooth is stable in all three dimensions (x, y, and z).
   d. There is nothing to worry about as mobility is measured on a 1 to 10 scale.

7. Based on the medical history presented for Mrs. Bozenski, antibiotic prophylaxis must have been administered before she underwent any type of dental treatment.
   a. True
   b. False

8. Which of the following teeth has the greatest *radiographic* furcation involvement?
   a. Mandibular right first molar
   b. Mandibular left first molar
   c. Maxillary right first molar
   d. Maxillary left first molar

SUGGESTED AGENCIES AND WEB SITES

Because of the ever-changing nature of the Internet, some of the web sites listed here may have changed since publication. Please refer to Mosby's Evolve web site for the most current information.

American Academy of Periodontology: http://www.perio.org
Procter and Gamble, Global Dental Resources: http://www.dentalcare.com (with clicks on *Hygienists' Corner,* then *Dental Hygiene News Online,* and *Periodontics*)

 ## ADDITIONAL READINGS AND RESOURCES

Philstrom BL, editor: Periodontology for the general practitioner, *Periodontol 2000,* 25:7-130, 2001.

Workshop for a classification of periodontal disease and conditions, *Ann Periodontol* 4:1-108, 1999.

 ## REFERENCES

1. Anderson GB et al: Correlation of periodontal probe penetration and degree of inflammation, *Am J Dent* 4:177, 1991.
2. Armitage GC: Clinical evaluation of periodontal diseases, *Periodontol 2000* 7:39, 1995.
3. Armitage GC: Development of a classification system for periodontal diseases and conditions, *Ann Periodontol* 4:1, 1999.
4. Beersten W, McCullouch AG, Sodek J: The periodontal ligament: a unique, multifunctional connective tissue, *Periodontol 2000* 13:20, 1997.
5. Bosshardt DD, Selvig KA: Dental cementum: the dynamic covering of the root, *Periodontol 2000* 13:41, 1997.
6. Bowers GM: A study of the width of the attached gingival, *J Periodontol* 34:201, 1963.
7. Carranza FA Jr: Dental calculus. In Carranza FA Jr, Newman MG, editors: *Clinical periodontology,* ed 8, Philadelphia, 1996, WB Saunders.
8. Carranza FA Jr, Takei HH: Treatment of furcation involvement and combined periodontal-endodontic therapy. In Newman MG, Carranza FA Jr, Takei H, editors: *Carranza's clinical periodontology,* ed 9, Philadelphia, 2002, WB Saunders.
9. Caton J: Periodontal diagnosis and diagnostic aids. In Nevins et al, editors: *Proceedings of the World Workshop in Clinical Periodontics,* Chicago, 1989, American Academy of Periodontology.
10. Freed HK, Gapper RL, Kallwarf KL: Evaluation of periodontal probing forces, *J Periodontol* 54:488, 1983.
11. Gargiulo AW, Wentz FM, Orban B. Dimensions and relations of the dentogingival junction in humans, *J Periodontol* 32:261, 1961.
12. Haake SK: Periodontal microbiology. In Newman MG, Carranza FA Jr, Takei H: *Carranza's clinical periodontology,* ed 9, Philadelphia, 2002, WB Saunders.
13. Hassell T: Tissues and cells of the periodontium, *Periodontol 2000* 3:9, 1993.
14. Jeffcoat MK, Wang I-C, Reddy MS: Radiographic diagnosis in periodontics, *Periodontol 2000* 7:54, 1995.
15. Karring T, Loe H: The three-dimensional concept of the epithelium-connective tissue boundary of gingival, *Acta Odontol Scand* 28:917, 1970.
16. Kennedy J, Bird W, Palcanis K, Dorfman H: A longitudinal evaluation of varying widths of attached gingival, *J Clin Periodontol* 12:667, 1985.
17. Kobayashi K, Rose G, Mahan C: Ultrastructure of the dentoepithelial junction, *J Periodont Res* 11:313, 1976.
18. Kornman KS et al: The interleukin-1 genotype as a severity factor in adult periodontal disease, *J Clin Periodontol* 24:72, 1997.
19. Kornman KS, Page RC, Tonetti MS: The host response to the microbial challenge in periodontitis: assembling the players, *Periodontol 2000* 14:33, 1997.
20. Kvan E: Topography of principal fibers, *Scand J Dent Res* 6:282, 1973.
21. Lamster IB, Grbic JT: Diagnosis of periodontal disease based on analysis of the host response, *Periodontol 2000* 7:83, 1995.
22. Lamster IB: In-office diagnostic tests and their role in supportive periodontal treatment, *Periodontol 2000* 12:49, 1996.
23. Lang NP et al: Bleeding on probing: a predictor for the progression of periodontal disease, *J Clin Periodontol* 13:590, 1986.
24. Lang NP, Joss A, Tonetti MS: Monitoring disease during supportive periodontal treatment by bleeding on probing, *Periodontol 2000* 12:44, 1996.
25. Lang NP, Karring T, editors: *Proceedings of the 1st European workshop on periodontology,* London, 1994, Quintessence.
26. Lindhe J, Nyman S: The effect of plaque control and surgical pocket elimination on the establishment and maintenance of periodontal health. A longitudinal study of periodontal therapy in cases of advanced disease, *J Clin Periodontol* 2:67, 1975.
27. Loesche WJ: Chemotherapy of dental plaque infections, *Oral Sci Rev* 9:65, 1975.
28. Mandel ID, Gaffar A: Calculus revisited, *J Clin Periodontol* 13:249, 1986.
29. Mariotti A: The extracellular matrix of the periodontium: dynamic and interactive tissues, *Periodontol 2000* 3:39, 1993.
30. Newbrun E: Indices to measure gingival bleeding—a leading symptom in initial gingivitis, *Helv Odont Acta* 15:107, 1971.
31. Nyman S, Lindhe J: Examination of patients with periodontal disease. In Lindhe J et al, editors: *Clinical periodontology and implant dentistry,* ed 3, Munksgaard, 1997, Copenhagen.
32. Saffar J-L, Lasfargues J-J, Cherruau M: Alveolar bone and the alveolar process: the socket that is never stable, *Periodontol 2000* 13:76, 1997.
33. Schroeder HE, Listgarten MA: The gingival tissues: the architecture of periodontal protection, *Periodontol 2000* 13:91, 1997.
34. Socransky S: Microbiology of periodontal disease—present status and future considerations, *J Periodontol* 48:497, 1977.

35. Spray JR et al: Microscopic demonstration of the position of periodontal probes, *J Periodontol* 48:148, 1978.
36. Stern I: Current concepts of the dentogingival junction: the epithelial and connective tissue attachment to the tooth, *J Periodontol* 52:465, 1981.
37. Zambon JJ: Periodontal diseases: microbial factors, *Ann Periodontol* 1: 879, 1996.
38. Zambon JJ, Haraszthy VI: The laboratory diagnosis of periodontal infections, *Periodontol 2000* 7:69, 1995.
39. Zander HA: The attachment of calculus to root surfaces, *J Periodontol* 24:16, 1953.

CHAPTER 16

Hard Tissue Examination

Douglas A. Young, Alan W. Budenz

Chapter Outline

Case Study: Examination and Recording of Dental
  Findings
Comprehensive Hard Tissue Charting
Types of Charting Forms
    Anatomical
    Geometrical
    Computer-assisted
Tooth Numbering Systems
    Universal
    Palmer's notation
    International
Infection Control
Caries-Classification Systems and Cavity Design
Charting Existing Conditions
Other Conditions that Modify Teeth
    Erosion
    Abrasion
    Attrition
    Abfraction
Types of Tooth Fracture
    Enamel flaking
    Cracking
    Cusp fracture
    Crown fracture
Charting Caries
Defining Dental Caries and Related Terms

New Caries-Classification Systems
    Mount and Hume
    Computer-based
Current Methods of Caries Detection
    Visual and tactile methods
Recurrent or Secondary Caries
Color Changes in Enamel
Color Changes in Dentin and Cementum
    Affected versus infected dentin
    Active versus inactive caries
Caries-Indicating Dyes
Detection with Dental Radiographs
    New advances in caries detection
    Differing views on surgical restorative
      approaches
Future Caries-Detection Technologies
    Conductance and impedance
    Ultrasound
    Fluorescence
    Optical coherence tomography
Occlusal Analysis
    Angle's classification
    Overbite and overjet
    Maximum incisal opening
    Pathway of opening or closing
    Centric relation–centric occlusion shift
    Initial contacts in excursions
    Traumatic occlusion

Key Terms

Abrasion
Active caries
Angle's classification
Approximal caries
Arrested caries
Attrition
Cavitation
Complete dentures
Cracking
Crown fracture

Cusp fracture
Demineralization
Dental caries
Enamel flaking
Enameloplasty
Erosion
Full gold crown (FGC)
G.V. Black Caries-
    Classification System
Gold foil (GF)

Gold inlay (GI)
Gold onlay (GO)
Inactive caries
Overbite
Overjet
Partial gold crown (¾ GC)
Partially erupted teeth
Periapical radiolucency (PAR)
Porcelain fused to metal
    (PFM)

Porcelain jacket crown (PJC)
Recurrent (secondary) caries
Remineralization
Removable partial dentures
Root canal (RC)
Sealant (SL)
Tooth-colored restorations (TC)
Unerupted teeth
White spot lesion

Learning Outcomes

1. Use a number of different comprehensive charting systems to assess the oral health of new patients and supportive-care patients.
2. Be familiar with the different tooth numbering systems.
3. Use proper infection control during performance of charting procedures.
4. Use the traditional G.V. Black cavity classification and design system to chart existing conditions.
5. Be familiar with new classification systems for carious lesions.

6. Use different charting symbols that represent existing conditions, such as early carious lesions before cavitation, cavities requiring restoration, missing teeth, partially erupted teeth, malposed teeth, existing dental restorations, erosion, abrasion, attrition, abfraction, enamel cracking, and cusp fracture.
7. Become familiar with dental caries and recognize all stages of development of new and recurrent pathology clinically and radiographically.
8. Classify occlusion with Angle's classification system, measuring overbite and overjet and identifying the signs of occlusal trauma.

A proper hard tissue evaluation involves more than just accurate charting of those items visualized during the hard tissue examination. It also involves interpretation of this information and the making of useful clinical decisions. Many conditions may modify teeth. When a dental hard tissue evaluation is performed, a snapshot in time is gained, representing multiple events that could have modified tooth structure in either the recent or distant past. The purpose of hard tissue charting is to capture each snapshot in the chart records for legal, diagnostic, and clerical purposes.

During a hard tissue evaluation, the clinician also must be able to discern between currently active events and the results of history. Accurate dental charts can provide the clinician with a visual representation of every past examination completed on that patient, information that proves invaluable in the comparison and evaluation of many current concerns. In this chapter, comprehensive hard tissue charting of many conditions that modify teeth is reviewed, along with a brief summary of the information currently known about the condition. A brief introduction to occlusal analysis is presented, after which a significant portion of the chapter is dedicated to the detection of **dental caries**. The mechanism of dental caries and its management is covered in further detail in Chapter 22.

Why this emphasis on dental caries in a dental hygiene textbook? Now is an exciting time in the profession, in which knowledge gained in caries research over the past two decades is finally beginning to improve the clinical management of this disease. The information presented in this chapter is a review of the very latest in the field and a source of "new" knowledge for recent graduates. The newly evolving concepts of the way in which dental caries is managed in the United States is still in its infancy; however, a team approach is clearly required, representing a tremendous opportunity for the dental hygiene profession to participate as equally important members of the caries management team.

Examination and Recording of Dental Findings

Case Study

Miguel Cantara, a 37-year-old Hispanic male, has transferred his records to your dental office from his former dentist in another town. He reports that he is overdue for his usual 6-month checkup. His last appointment was for a routine cleaning and replacement of a cracked filling. Mr. Cantara says that he has received a variety of dental treatments since childhood and classifies his dental experiences as quite good. He says that he is unaware of any dental problems.

COMPREHENSIVE HARD TISSUE CHARTING

Comprehensive charting should be an accurate and systematic representation of the dental hard tissues on the day of the clinical exam. The way and order in which this process is accomplished depend on the clinician's preferences. Although no one correct way exists to complete the examination, the method selected should facilitate recording of findings. In that respect, completing the exam logically and consistently each time is important so that all exams are completed, without omissions. Many clinicians prefer to start at tooth #1 and proceed in order to tooth #32 ("universal" system of tooth numbering).

TYPES OF CHARTING FORMS

The manner in which information is recorded in the patient record is a decision that is made by the members of each individual practice. Although many chart formats exist, with countless ways in which to use them, there is no one "right" way; each office team may come up with its own variation of an existing technique. For that reason, only a few of the most commonly used formats—such as anatomical, geometrical, and computer-assisted—are presented in this chapter.

ANATOMICAL

Anatomical charting forms show the anatomy of each tooth in facial, occlusal, and lingual views, usually including the roots of the teeth, as seen in Fig. 16-1. This chart form can record a specific part of the anatomy as it appears in the mouth, such as the distal pit of an upper first molar and specific areas on the roots.

GEOMETRICAL

Geometrical charting forms use a nonanatomical shape to represent each tooth, usually shown from a top or occlusal view only, of the facial, lingual, occlusal, mesial, and distal angles of each tooth, as seen in Fig. 16-2. The same generic shape is used for each tooth and permits charting of primary, adult, or mixed dentition on the same form.

COMPUTER-ASSISTED

Computer-assisted charting uses a computer and a dental software program to help increase the accuracy and speed of the charting procedure (Fig. 16-3). The "charting form" in this case is not a piece of paper but an image seen on the computer monitor. The image format can either be anatomical or geometrical. Although the information is stored in the computer and supports the concept of "paperless" dental records, a neat and professional-looking color form can easily be printed when needed. The information is entered into the computer via a mouse or keyboard and is accomplished instantaneously, saving time. Many software programs offer voice recognition, making charting a one-person operation with improved infection control.

TOOTH NUMBERING SYSTEMS

Just as more than one format exists for charting, different systems are used to designate teeth. The three most common—the universal system, Palmer's notation, and the international system—are summarized in Table 16-1.

UNIVERSAL

The universal system, perhaps the most popular in the United States, numbers the permanent teeth from #1 to #32 and primary teeth from *A* to *T* (Fig. 16-4). Tooth #1 is the maxillary right third molar, tooth #2 is the maxillary right second molar, and so on over to the maxillary left third molar, which is tooth #16. This numbering continues to the mandibular left quadrant, where tooth #17 is the mandibular left third molar and tooth #18 is the mandibular left second molar, continuing to the lower right third molar, tooth #32. The same format is used for the primary dentition.

PALMER'S NOTATION

Palmer's notation numbers the permanent teeth (#1 through #8) and the primary teeth (*A* through *E*), always starting from the midline and working laterally. Therefore the central incisor is designated tooth #1, the lateral incisor tooth #2, the cuspid tooth #3, the first bicuspid tooth #4, and so on to the third molar, which is always tooth #8. When the clinician faces the patient, the quadrant of the mouth is defined by a horizontal line representing the upper arch above and the lower arch below and a vertical line representing the midline. Both the number and the appropriate symbol designating the quadrant are always necessary, as is notation that the left quadrant is on the right and vice versa (Fig. 16-5). For example, the permanent maxillary left central incisor is written as $\underline{|1}$, and the permanent mandibular left first bicuspid is $\overline{|4}$. An example of a primary mandibular right first molar is written as $\overline{D|}$.

INTERNATIONAL

The international system (Fig. 16-6) is numbered the same as Palmer's notation, but instead of designating the quadrants by a symbol, a prefix number is used: 1 for the maxillary right, 2 for the maxillary left, 3 for the mandibular left, and 4 for the mandibular right. For example, the permanent maxillary right central incisor would be 11, and the permanent mandibular left first bicuspid would be 34. However, for the primary dentition the teeth are numbered 1 through 5 instead of with Palmer's notation (*A* through *E*). In addition, the quadrants in the primary dentition are designated by numbers 5 through 8 (5 being the maxillary right, 6 the maxillary left, 7 the mandibular left, and 8 the mandibular right). Thus the primary mandibular right first molar is written as 84.

INFECTION CONTROL

No matter which system is chosen to record the results of a hard tissue examination, proper infection control must be followed. When using paper forms, the clinician must never contaminate the pen or chart by touching them with a contaminated gloved hand. Trying to chart alone, even with overgloves, is extremely inefficient and is not recommended. A chairside assistant who prevents contamination of the operative field is invaluable during charting. As stated previously, the voice-recognition, computer-assisted software can eliminate cross-contamination concerns and in many cases can make charting a single-operator procedure. If single-operator charting is unavoidable and voice-recognition, computer-assisted software is not available, then a voice-activated tape recorder can be used to collect the data, leaving the actual charting to be completed later.

CARIES-CLASSIFICATION SYSTEMS AND CAVITY DESIGN

More than a century ago, Dr. G.V. Black developed a caries-classification system based on location of the carious lesion and cavity preparation designs based on restoration using the materials available in his time (such as amalgam).[31] Although material and preparation technologies have changed significantly in the last 100 years, the G.V. Black classification system and cavity designs still predominate and are discussed in the following section. The

Text continued on p. 316

Baseline Clinical Examination and Re-Evaluation Record

University of the Pacific, School of Dentistry

Patient's Name:_____

Student's Name:_____

Baseline Date:_____   Re-eval Date:_____

Reviewed By (Faculty):_____

	1	2	3	4	5	6	7	8	9	10	11	12	13	14	15	16
Re-eval mobility																
Re-eval Probe																
Baseline Probe																

FACIAL   R   L   **LINGUAL**

| Baseline Probe | | | | | | | | | | | | | | | | |
| Re-eval Probe | | | | | | | | | | | | | | | | |

Re-eval mobility																
Re-eval Probe																
Baseline Probe																

LINGUAL   R   L   **FACIAL**

| Baseline Probe | | | | | | | | | | | | | | | | |
| Re-eval Probe | | | | | | | | | | | | | | | | |

| 32 | 31 | 30 | 29 | 28 | 27 | 26 | 25 | 24 | 23 | 22 | 21 | 20 | 19 | 18 | 17 |

Initial Occlusal and TMJ Findings

CENTRIC RELATION:
Location: ☐ easy   ☐ difficult   ☐ impossible
TMJ discomfort to pressure   ☐ none   ☐ right   ☐ left
Initial tooth contact:_____ vs._____
CENTRIC RELATION-CENTRIC OCCLUSION DISCREPANCY:
Vertical slide _____ mm   Forward slide _____ mm
Lateral slide   ☐ right   ☐ left _____ mm
CENTRIC OCCLUSION:
Canine classification (I,II,III)   right _____: left _____
Right canine vertical overlap _____ mm
Right canine functional horizontal overlap _____ mm
Left canine vertical overlap _____ mm
Left canine horizontal overlap _____ mm
Central incisor vertical overlap _____ mm
Central incisor functional horizontal overlap_____ mm
Wear facets: ☐ minimal   ☐ moderate   ☐ severe

CR TO CO	1	2	3	4	5	6	7	8	9	10	11	12	13	14	15	16
INTERFERENCES	32	31	30	29	28	27	26	25	24	23	22	21	20	19	18	17
RT.	1	2	3	4	5	6	7	8	9	10	11	12	13	14	15	16
LATERAL	32	31	30	29	28	27	26	25	24	23	22	21	20	19	18	17
LT.	1	2	3	4	5	6	7	8	9	10	11	12	13	14	15	16
LATERAL	32	31	30	29	28	27	26	25	24	23	22	21	20	19	18	17
PROTRUSIVE	1	2	3	4	5	6	7	8	9	10	11	12	13	14	15	16
	32	31	30	29	28	27	26	25	24	23	22	21	20	19	18	17

TEMPORO-MANDIBULAR JOINT:
Maximum opening _____ mm
Joint sounds during opening and closing: ☐ none   ☐ right   ☐ left
Joint sounds during excursions: ☐ none   ☐ right   ☐ left
History of TMJ treatment: ☐ yes   ☐ no
Current joint pain: ☐ none   ☐ right   ☐ left

Plaque Index

TOOTH	S C O R E	
SURFACE	Baseline	Re-eval
Facial 3		
Facial 8		
Facial 14		
Lingual 19		
Facial 24		
Lingual 10		
Plaque Index		

FIG. 16-1 Anatomical charting form. (Courtesy University of the Pacific School of Dentistry, San Francisco.)

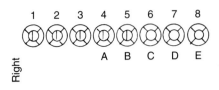

FIG. 16-2 Geometrical charting form, right quadrant only. (Modified from Woodall IR: *Comprehensive dental hygiene care,* ed 4, St Louis, 1993, Mosby.)

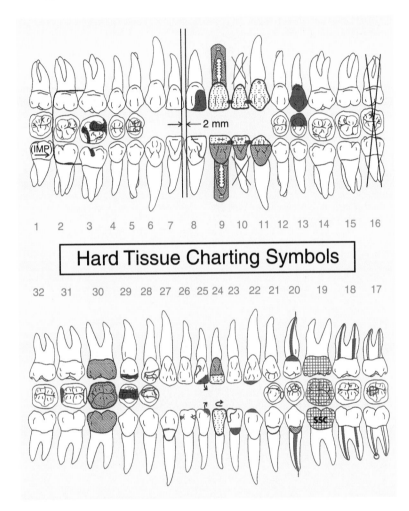

FIG. 16-3 Hard tissue charting symbols. *#1,* Horizontal impaction with tissue line *(black),* IMP on facial view *(black),* and horizontal arrow indicating direction of impaction; *#3,* OL and MO amalgams *(solid blue)* and mesial defect *(red); #5,* DO composite resin *(blue outline)* and O clinical fracture *(sawtooth red); #7-#8,* 2-mm diastema *(black parallel lines and distance in millimeters); #8,* MIFL composite resin *(blue outline)* and F defect *(red); #9,* implant *(slanted blue lines),* transmucosal connector *(opposite blue slanted lines),* PFM crown with visible metal *(slanted blue lines),* and porcelain *(blue stippling)* splinted to #10, *(solid blue); #10,* missing root *(green or black X),* replaced by PFM pontic attached to abutments 9 and 11 *(solid blue bar); #11,* PFM crown; *#13,* MODF portion of tooth fractured *(red); #16,* missing tooth *(black X); #17,* root canal treatment in progress *(green)* with adjacent periapical radiolucency and temporary O filling *(red checkerboard); #18,* occlusal pit defects *(red)* and root canal treated plus post *(green)* [NOTE: situation actually clinically impossible; no access opening present]; *#19,* temporary SCC *(black)* crown *(red checkerboard); #20,* O comp *(blue outline),* F gold foil *(slanted blue lines),* root canal filling *(green)* with overextension *(green); #21,* F comp *(blue outline)* and incipient caries seen only radiographically *(green outline); #22,* I defect—attrition—*(red); #23,* MIF comp *(blue outline)* and F defect—erosion or abfraction—*(red); #24,* PFM as described above; arrow *(black)* showing rotation; *#25,* DL comp resin *(blue outline)* and MIFL fracture *(red and black arrows)* indicating part of tooth missing; *#26,* x-ray findings (unconfirmed clinically) of M caries in enamel only *(green outline),* and D caries into dentin *(solid green); #27,* F comp *(blue outline)* and clinically defective F margin *(red); #28,* MO comp *(blue outline)* [NOTE: outline extended too far on distally occlusal view]; *#29,* MOD alloy—same as amalgam—*(solid blue); #30,* FVC—full veneer crown—*(blue slanted lines);* and *#31,* M enamel caries—seen only radiographically *(green outline)*—and D caries into dentin *(solid green).* Radiographic findings were transferred from radiographic diagnosis worksheet for teeth *#21, #26,* and *#31.*

TABLE 16-1

Summary of tooth numbering systems

System	Primary dentition	Permanent dentition
Universal	Each tooth is designated by a letter (A to T). For example, A is the designation for the maxillary right primary second molar and T is the mandibular right primary second molar. See Figure 16-4.	Each tooth is designated by a number from 1 to 32. For example, #1 is the maxillary right third molar and #32 is the mandibular right third molar. See Figure 16-4.
Palmer's Notation System	Each tooth is lettered (A to E) and positioned within intersecting axes to designate the quadrant. For example, |A‾ would be the notation for the maxillary left primary central and ‾A| would be the notation for the mandibular right primary central. See Figure 16-5.	Each tooth is numbered (1 to 8) and positioned within intersecting axes to designate the quadrant. For example, |1‾ would be the notation for the maxillary left permanent central and ‾1| would be the notation for the mandibular right permanent central. See Figure 16-5.
International System	Each tooth is designated by a quadrant number prefix (5 to 8) and a tooth number suffix (1 to 5). For example, the notation for the maxillary left primary central would be 61 and the mandibular right primary central would be noted as 81. See Figure 16-6.	Each tooth is designated by a quadrant number prefix (1 to 4) and a tooth number suffix (1 to 8). For example, the notation for the maxillary left permanent central would be 21 and the mandibular right permanent central would be noted as 41. See Figure 16-6.

From Woodall IR: *Comprehensive dental hygiene care,* ed 4, St Louis, 1998, Mosby.

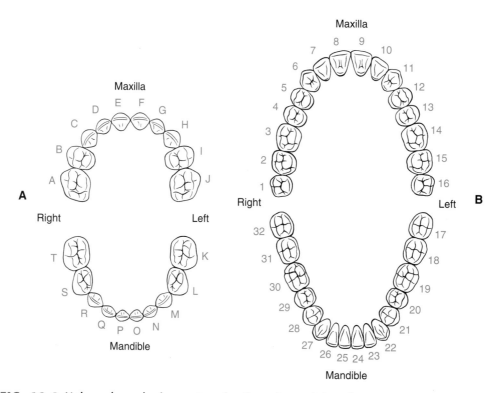

FIG. 16-4 Universal numbering system for the primary **(A)** and permanent **(B)** dentition. (Modified from Finkbeiner BL, Johnson CS: *Mosby's comprehensive dental assisting: a clinical approach,* St Louis, 1995, Mosby.)

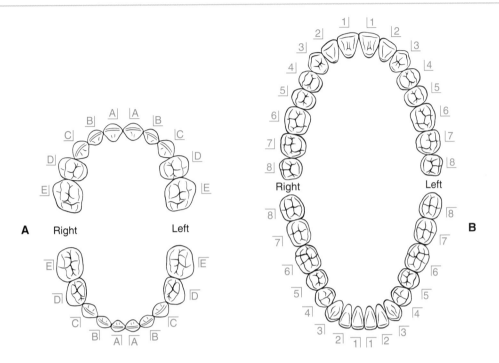

FIG. 16-5 Palmer's notation system assigned to primary **(A)** and permanent **(B)** dentition. (Modified from Finkbeiner BL, Johnson CS: *Mosby's comprehensive dental assisting: a clinical approach,* St Louis, 1995, Mosby.)

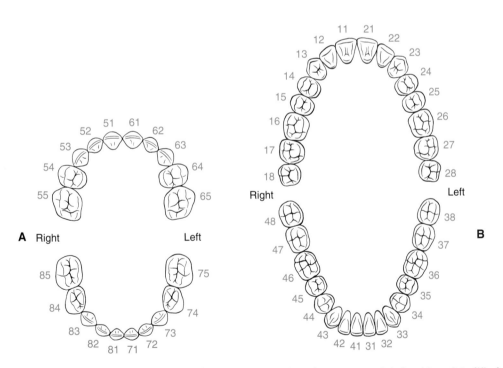

FIG. 16-6 International system assigned to primary **(A)** and permanent **(B)** dentition. (Modified from Finkbeiner BL, Johnson CS: *Mosby's comprehensive dental assisting: a clinical approach,* St Louis, 1995, Mosby.)

G. V. Black classification system (I through VI) based on lesion location is summarized in Table 16-2.

Although not yet in common use, new classification systems have been proposed[30] and will be discussed later in the chapter in the section concerning new caries-classification systems.

TABLE 16-2
G.V. Black Caries-Classification System

Class and description	Illustration
I: All pit and fissure restorations	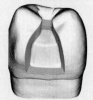
II: Restorations on proximal surfaces of teeth, most often including portion of occlusal surface	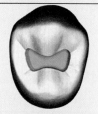
III: Restorations on proximal surfaces of anterior teeth that do not include incisal angle	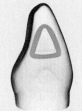
IV: Restorations on proximal surfaces of incisal teeth that *do* include incisal angle	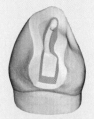
V: Restorations on gingival third of lingual or facial surfaces of all teeth except pit and fissure lesions	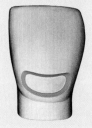
VI: Restorations on incisal edge or occlusal cusp tips	Not shown

Modified from Roberson TM, Heymann HO, Smith EJ: *Sturdevant's art and science of operative dentistry,* ed 4, St Louis, 2002, Mosby.

CHARTING EXISTING CONDITIONS

Accurately charting existing hard tissue conditions is the most important task in charting, regardless of the chart format or numbering system selected. The information and the way in which it is recorded may vary from practice to practice, and room exists for customization depending on office preferences. Therefore the following examples are meant to illustrate the concept rather than to be an all-inclusive formula.

The clinician usually charts missing teeth first by crossing the teeth out with a vertical line or an X in black ink. This method helps to lessen the confusion, especially in mixed dentition. The clinician next depicts *partially erupted teeth* by drawing a line to show the exposed part of the tooth. *Unerupted teeth* are circled. Inclined, drifted, rotated, and supraerupted teeth are illustrated with arrows in the appropriate direction. Diastema are noted as a double line, drawn noticeably between contact areas. *Removable partial dentures* and *complete dentures* are marked with brackets. Restoration outlines are drawn on the appropriate part of the tooth. The type of restorative material is keyed by either blue color, outlined versus filled, or with some kind of letter code. Some examples of a letter-coded system are as follows:

Amalgam (A)
Tooth-colored restoration (TC)
Sealant (SL)
Gold foil (GF)
Gold inlay (GI)
Gold onlay (GO)
Partial gold crown (¾ GC)
Full gold crown (FGC)
Porcelain fused to metal (PFM)
Porcelain jacket crown (PJC)
Acrylic facing (AF)
Root canal (RC)
Periapical radiolucency (PAR)
Stainless steel crown (SSC)
Dental implant (DI)

OTHER CONDITIONS THAT MODIFY TEETH*

EROSION

Erosion (Figs. 16-7 and 16-8) is the superficial loss of dental hard tissue due to a chemical process, usually resulting from nonbacterial acids. The acids that cause erosion may be either extrinsic or intrinsic. Extrinsic acids may include those found in foods and drinks, with examples including low-pH cola drinks, fruit juices, and wine. Some medications and vitamins are also acidic. Gastric acids coming from the stomach are intrinsic acids caused by chronic gastric reflux diseases or bulimia.

Because exposure to acid removes tooth mineral, erosion may very well potentiate *abrasion, attrition,* and abfraction (described in detail in a later section of this

---

*This section was written with significant contributions taken from Mount GJ, Hume WR: *Preservation and restoration of tooth structure,* St Louis, 1998, Mosby.

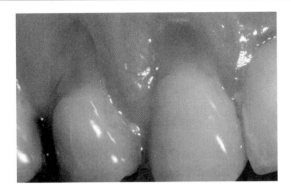

FIG. 16-7 Severe erosion lesions. Teeth #13 and #14 show severe erosion, doubtless exacerbated by toothbrush abrasion. (From Mount GJ, Hume WR: *Preservation and restoration of tooth structure,* St Louis, 1998, Mosby.)

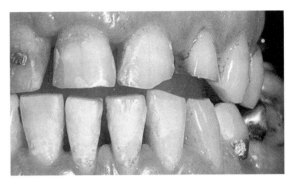

FIG. 16-9 Abrasion on tooth #22 caused by many years of holding a pipe stem in this position. (From Mount GJ, Hume WR: *Preservation and restoration of tooth structure,* St Louis, 1998, Mosby.)

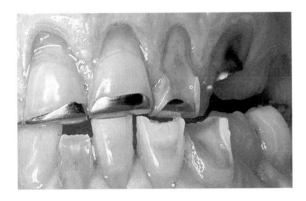

FIG. 16-8 Severe erosion. Quadrant of teeth showing similar erosion to Fig. 16-7 in addition to abrasion. (From Mount GJ, Hume WR: *Preservation and restoration of tooth structure,* St Louis, 1998, Mosby.)

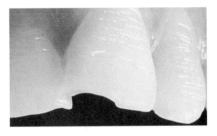

FIG. 16-10 Abrasion on labial of maxillary anterior teeth. The horizontal, parallel scratch marks were caused by toothbrush abrasion. (From Mount GJ, Hume WR: *Preservation and restoration of tooth structure,* St Louis, 1998, Mosby.)

chapter). Partial loss of enamel crystal surfaces or removal of dentin or cementum mineral makes the subsequent removal of mineral easier in the presence of acid. In particular, demineralization of dentin leaves collagen exposed to trauma; if this collagen is then removed or damaged—by toothbrushing, for example—it may no longer be present for remineralization, thus leading to permanent loss of tooth structure. Sources of acids in particular should be investigated when abrasion, attrition, and abfraction are evident.

ABRASION

Abrasion (Figs. 16-9, 16-10, and 16-11) is the wearing of tooth substance by exogenous material forced over the surface by incisive, masticatory, or teeth-cleaning functions. Exogenous material describes anything foreign to the tooth's substance, such as sand, grit, or foreign material found in food and includes the natural abrasive qualities of some foods, as well as any solid material held by or forced against the teeth. Therefore abrasion may occur during mastication or even during teeth cleaning. An abrasion area is generally not well defined and may

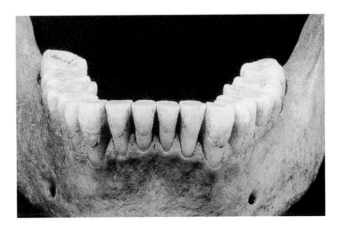

FIG. 16-11 Abrasion pattern on ancient skull specimen. Note the helicoidal wear pattern on posterior teeth, emphasizing the slope toward the tongue in the third molars. (From Mount GJ, Hume WR: *Preservation and restoration of tooth structure,* St Louis, 1998, Mosby.)

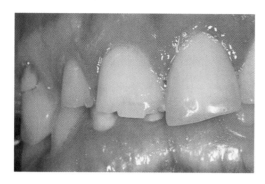

FIG. 16-12 Attrition. Heavy attrition is evident on teeth #6, #7, and #8, as is enamel flaking. (From Mount GJ, Hume WR: *Preservation and restoration of tooth structure,* St Louis, 1998, Mosby.)

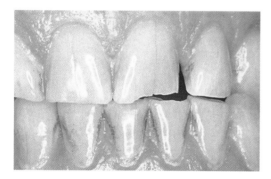

FIG. 16-13 Attrition. Heavy attrition is evident on teeth #21 and #22, largely the result of a deflective incline between the second molars on the right side. (From Mount GJ, Hume WR: *Preservation and restoration of tooth structure,* St Louis, 1998, Mosby.)

manifest as a cusp tip or incisal edge that has been rounded, blunted, or worn flat and often exposes the dentin, causing a "scooped out" appearance that is softer and more porous than enamel. The location and extent of abrasive wear is influenced by such things as occlusion, diet, oral habits, age, loss of posterior teeth, and oral hygiene techniques.

ATTRITION

Attrition (Figs. 16-12 and 16-13) is tooth wear caused by tooth-to-tooth contact without the presence of exogenous material. Persistent tooth grinding is called *bruxism* or *parafunction.* The characteristic feature of occlusal attrition is the development of a wear facet—a flat, often shiny surface and with a well-defined border. The distribution of facets is influenced by the occlusal morphology and the characteristic grinding pattern(s) of the individual. Attrition facets may appear in seemingly impossible locations, such as the facial of a maxillary canine in a patient with

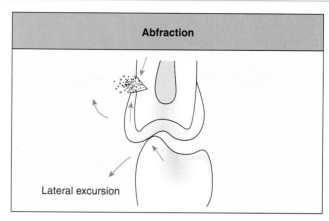

FIG. 16-14 *Abfraction* is a term used to describe possible flexure of a tooth under heavy lateral load, which may lead to displacement or fracture of enamel rods at the cemento-enamel junction (CEJ). The lost enamel exposes more dentin, in which dentin tubules may be crushed by the same stresses and more readily demineralized. These factors may account for isolated "erosion" lesions for which no obvious explanation is evident. (Modified from Mount GJ, Hume WR: *Preservation and restoration of tooth structure,* St Louis, 1998, Mosby.)

Class I occlusion. Careful examination of these uniquely positioned attrition facets can reveal interesting, and occasionally damaging patient habits, which can produce TMJ. In the presence of erosion, the facet may not appear shiny even if the bruxism is active. Facial pain and a stiff jaw (which may also have associated pain and tenderness in the TMJ) are symptoms that may indicate active tooth grinding.

ABFRACTION

Abfraction (Fig. 16-14) is thought to be caused by excessive buccal or lingual occlusal load through either compression or tension in the cervical region of the tooth just above its bony support. The excess load may cause flexure of the tooth, with disintegration of the relatively brittle enamel or dentin in the cervical area. Such disintegration can add to erosion and abrasion, all of which can be contributing factors in so-called toothbrush abrasion.

TYPES OF TOOTH FRACTURE

ENAMEL FLAKING

Small amounts of enamel of various sizes may fracture from the incisal edges of anterior teeth or from the buccal or lingual edges of posterior teeth *(enamel flaking),* possibly the result of unusual incisal or occlusal biting patterns and habits (Fig. 16-15).

CRACKING

Minor **cracking** in enamel is usually asymptomatic and requires no treatment. However, under heavy occlusal load,

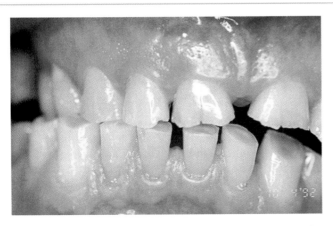

FIG. 16-15 Enamel flaking. Forceful extreme mandibular movement from centric occlusion outward can cause the enamel flaking on the anteriors. (From Mount GJ, Hume WR: *Preservation and restoration of tooth structure*, St Louis, 1998, Mosby.)

more significant cracks can involve the dentin. Cusp movement then is extremely painful due to hydraulic stimulation of odontoblast-sensory nerve receptors.

CUSP FRACTURE

If enough force is exerted against a tooth—either from direct physical trauma or as a result of parafunction—or if the tooth structure is weakened (often by restorative treatment), the tooth may fracture. Cusps most prone to split and fail are the lingual cusps of mandibular molars and the facial or palatal cusps of maxillary first and second premolars. A common *cusp fracture* runs from the pulpal floor of an existing carious lesion downward and outward to the cementoenamel junction (CEJ) and is generally repairable. In contrast, a vertical fracture, which may sometimes involve the root, often is irreparable. Teeth under high occlusal load, such as endodontically treated posterior teeth, are also at increased risk due to loss of tooth structure, and the cusps of these teeth should be protected by a restoration, such as a crown or onlay.

CROWN FRACTURE

The crowns of anterior teeth are most at risk from direct trauma, with the main predisposing factors being the age of the patient and the tooth position. The highest incidence of *crown fracture* occurs in elementary–school-age boys in anterior teeth. Mouthguards are useful in contact sports, but convincing children to use them in playgrounds is often difficult. (Chapter 27 provides more content on the use of mouthguards in athletics.)

CHARTING CARIES

At first glance charting caries sounds very straightforward—simple tracing of the clinical caries on the chart in red as it appears in the mouth. In addition, to encourage a preclinical review of radiographs, some clinicians advocate the outlining of radiographic caries in green before the clinical

---

BOX 16-1

Terms Used to Describe the Results of Dental Caries

Cavitation	Radiographic caries
Demineralization	Histological gold standard
White spot lesion	Polarized light microscopy
Approximal caries	Explorer stick
Root caries	Soft dentin
Pit and fissure caries	Brown spot lesion
Caries dye uptake	Active caries
Clinical caries	Infected dentin

examination begins. These areas (in green) remind the clinician to confirm the radiographic findings clinically, in which case the green outline may be filled in red on the hard tissue chart.

Although this approach sounds simplistic, it contains many inherent pitfalls. Before a carious lesion can be recorded, it first must be detected in the mouth by the clinician. Unfortunately, different clinicians may detect and treat caries, even in the same patient, quite differently. In the last two decades much has been learned about the disease, and as a result, new caries-management techniques are emerging.[1,2,3] However, changing treatment paradigms is far from instantaneous, and thus early adopters and late adopters of new knowledge will always emerge, leading to differing opinions. Therefore dental professionals must review the current understanding of caries. The following sections focus on the definition and detection of dental caries. The mechanism of dental caries and its management is covered in detail in Chapter 22.

DEFINING DENTAL CARIES AND RELATED TERMS

The term *dental caries,* along with its related terms, is often a source of confusion because the same term may be used differently depending on the person using it and the circumstance in which it is used (Box 16-1). Sobering is the realization that not all dental professionals agree on the true meaning of the term *dental caries.* The term is used to describe more than one concept. Understanding this fact can help the clinician and patient communicate.

Dental caries is an infectious disease caused by bacteria. The organisms involved include mutans streptococci and lactobaccili, which produce acid when exposed to dietary fermentable carbohydrates. The acid then diffuses into the tooth and dissolves the tooth mineral, a chemical process known as *demineralization,* and is a result of the disease process. Demineralization can cause many changes in the tooth mineral, not all of which are visible to the naked eye (even with magnification). The term *dental caries* is used rather loosely by dental care workers and is frequently meant to describe the results of the demineralization process—a carious lesion—rather than the disease itself.

Clinicians' use of the term *caries* also may vary. For example, so-called contemporary clinicians who use new caries-management techniques may use the term *caries* differently than so-called traditional clinicians. The traditional clinician uses a surgical approach very similar to the way G.V. Black treated caries more than 100 years ago, in which the focus is on the treatment of carious lesions through removal of decay and placement of restorations. Carious lesions often are detected on a radiograph (radiographic caries) or in the clinical setting with visual and tactile methods (clinical caries). The patient then is periodically recalled, usually based on periodontal criteria, and more restorations are placed if new carious lesions are detected, and so on. Thus when the traditional clinician uses the term *caries,* it usually designates a carious lesion, or "cavity," that needs to be restored rather than a disease that needs to be diagnosed. Detection is not the same as diagnosis because a disease is diagnosed and a carious lesion detected. This seemingly trivial point is the source of much confusion, and when the term *caries* is used, of importance is whether it refers to the disease or the lesion.

Also confusing is the fact that the term *dental caries* may have different meanings depending on whether a clinician or a researcher is using it. Researchers have the luxury of performing experiments *in vitro* (in the laboratory away from the patient's mouth) using specialized equipment and histological techniques such as polarized light microscopy and microradiography, which describe ways to visualize the demineralized mineral in the laboratory. These research terms are sometimes referred to in the literature simply as *the histological gold standard* because they positively identify mineral loss and can be quantitative.

Because such laboratory techniques cannot be used clinically, the histological terms are of little use to the clinician. In addition, mineral loss alone does not mean that the tooth needs restoration. Thus *caries* from a histological or research perspective may not have the same meaning to a clinician. Whenever possible, clinical decisions should be based on scientific knowledge, which requires practitioners to read and understand the appropriate literature. However, if research terms are not defined in a way in which readers outside the field can understand easily, the literature itself can be a source of confusion. Not only must authors carefully define and explain the clinical relevance of the terms they use, but also readers must to be aware of the circumstance or perspective in which terms are being used.

Even clinical terms such as *clinical caries, radiographic caries,* and *carious lesion* are considered vague because they do not define the extent of the lesion in clinically relevant terms. Demineralization is a dynamic process occurring when the tooth is exposed to acid in the absence of protective factors, such as healthy saliva and fluoride. As stated previously, mere mineral loss does not always require surgical intervention. The earliest loss of mineral during the demineralization process is not visible to the naked eye. As more mineral is lost and the enamel becomes more porous, it produces optical changes in the enamel that appear first as a dull *white spot lesion.* The "dull" appearance often suggests that the lesion is in an active state of demineralization and is just one sign of something known as *active caries.* If the demineralization process can be halted or even reversed, the dull appearance often turns shiny, one sign of *inactive caries* or *arrested caries.* This reversal of the demineralization process

is called *remineralization* and will be explained in more detail in Chapter 22.

White spot lesions often discolor with time, causing a brown spot lesion in the enamel (see the later section of this chapter concerning color changes in enamel). The exact mechanism for this occurrence is not yet known and will be discussed in Chapter 22. Again, if the surface of a white or brown spot lesion is smooth (noncavitated) and shiny, the lesion is considered to be arrested or remineralized. On the other hand, if an active carious lesion is allowed to progress, it eventually produces an actual hole, or *cavitation,* into or through the enamel; in the presence of surface cavitation, the control of plaque accumulation is no longer possible, representing a critical point in the process of diagnosis. Once the surface is cavitated, surgical intervention is required to restore a smooth surface that can be maintained free of plaque.

Accurate determination of the type and extent of the carious lesion is clinically important because when carious lesions are detected at an early stage, clinicians may decide to use chemical rather than surgical restorative intervention. Chemical intervention treats the bacterial infection itself and preserves the natural tooth structure by helping the saliva to remineralize the areas of early decay; this process will be discussed in more detail in Chapter 22.

NEW CARIES-CLASSIFICATION SYSTEMS

The *G.V. Black Caries-Classification System* has worked well for the past 100 years where only the standard Black cavity preparations were used. However, new knowledge of caries, coupled with an explosion in restorative material science, now allows nonsurgical treatment modalities and conservative cavity preparation designs. This new knowledge poses problems for the traditional G.V. Black Classification System. For example, no way exists to designate the size of the lesion or describe early lesions that are amenable to conservative treatment with the Black system. Two new classification systems consistent with conservative care are introduced in the following sections; however, neither conservative care nor the proposed classification systems can be considered standard of care at the present time.

MOUNT AND HUME

Recently, a classification system based on two simple parameters, the location and size of a carious lesion, has been suggested.[30,31] The G.V. Black System was designed to classify the cavities that had to be cut to eliminate a carious lesion, and it does not permit recognition of the size of the lesion at all. The system presented here, recently proposed by Mount and Hume, is designed to recognize carious lesions beginning with the very earliest stage, in which remineralization is the indicated treatment rather than surgical intervention. It continues to classify the lesions as they become progressively larger without at any stage specifying a cavity design. This system is quite logical because caries is found typically only in three sites on a tooth—in pits and fissures, at proximal contacts, and on cervical surfaces (sites 1, 2, and 3 respectively). These three sites are consistent with the typical acid challenge patterns created by niches commonly colonized by the pathogens. In other words, plaque accumulates and is

TABLE 16-3

Cavity classification

Site size	Minimal 1	Moderate 2	Enlarged 3	Extensive 4
Pit/fissure (1)	1.1	1.2	1.3	1.4
Contact area (2)	2.1	2.2	2.3	2.4
Cervical (3)	3.1	3.2	3.3	3.4

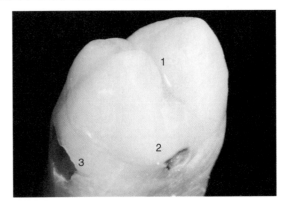

FIG. 16-16 Three sites for caries: *1*, pits and fissures on otherwise smooth surfaces; *2*, contact areas on the proximal surfaces of all teeth; *3*, cervical margins on the crown or exposed root surface of any tooth. (From Mount GJ, Hume WR: *Preservation and restoration of tooth structure*, St Louis, 1998, Mosby.)

difficult to control below the floss contacts, on tooth roots, and in the pits and fissures of teeth. Lesions are treated differently depending on their location (site) and size, explaining the lack of specificity for cavity design.

Size 0 lesions are those early signs of demineralization that may be noted as white spots on visible surfaces or early lesions at the contact areas identified in radiographs. Another example, the occlusal fissures on a newly erupted molar, may fit this classification if they are relatively deep and convoluted.

A size 1 lesion is described as "minimal" but beyond the hope of remineralization treatment. Some cavitation is present, and therefore plaque control cannot be maintained. Some form of surgical intervention is required, but the cavity design should be based on the removal of only sufficient tooth structure to allow access to the dentin lesion, after which the cavity can be sealed with an adhesive restorative material.

Size 2 lesions are described as "moderate." That is, the cavity is beyond minimal, but adequate sound tooth structure remains to support the occlusion. The entire load will be borne by the restoration.

In a size 3 lesion, the cavity needs to be "enlarged" because the tooth structure is seriously weakened. The cavity design must be modified so that the restoration will take the entire occlusal load; otherwise one or more of the cusps is likely to split at the base.

A size 4 lesion is described as "extensive," with bulk failure or major breakdown of a cusp, requiring a cast or bonded final restoration.

Thus a #1.2 lesion in this classification system is really just a numerical way of indicating a medium-sized cavity in the occlusal/incisal surface of tooth relating to the fissure system. By the G.V. Black system this cavity would be a Class I, with a specific cavity preparation design prescribed for its restoration. The cavity design, incidentally, would require the removal of the entire fissure system whether it was carious or not because finishing an amalgam restoration within the fissures is impossible. In contrast with contemporary materials and techniques, a #1.2 lesion can be restored with an adhesive restorative material without the removal of all the fissures because the restorative material can act as a fissure seal and a restoration (Table 16-3 and Fig. 16-16).

COMPUTER-BASED

D.K. Benn and colleagues have suggested a computer-based classification system to help the clinician classify

early and more advanced lesions and also attempts to describe active versus inactive lesions.[4] In this system, several icons represent every possible clinical caries scenario and attempts to classify them by histological lesion depth (as if the clinician could section the tooth in the laboratory to evaluate the depth of the lesion into enamel or dentin). The clinical caries classification is divided into sound, white, and brown spots on the surface, noncavitated pits and fissures, cavitations, noncavitated dentin caries, and cavitated and noncavitated root caries (Fig. 16-17). Radiographic classification is divided into no visible lesion (E0), a lesion in the outer one half of the enamel (E1), and a lesion in the inner half of the enamel (E2). Similarly the dentin is divided into thirds, in which a lesion in the outer third is labeled *D1*, a lesion in the middle third is labeled *D2*, and a lesion in the inner third, including the pulp, is labeled *D3* (Figs. 16-18 and 16-19). The existing tooth condition is recorded on the electronic tooth chart when the appropriate icon is selected, and along with the appropriate clinical and radiographic icons, the computer software automatically suggests a possible treatment for the charted condition (Fig. 16-20).

This suggested classification system has several advantages. First, it reminds the clinician to consider lesion severity and caries activity. Second, it rapidly collects and records data with a simple click of the mouse. Third and finally, the software program automates the decision process, facilitating more consistent interexaminer agreement. Although this system is a step in the right direction, it is not foolproof. One limiting factor is that the system assumes that the clinician can estimate the actual histological lesion depth, which is questionable given today's crude diagnostic tools.

In summary, the preceding sections have presented two proposed classification systems to address the expanding knowledge in modern caries management. Perhaps more important than the discovery of an "ideal" classification system is the challenge to the dental community first to realize the need for new treatment modalities, then to explore new systems, and finally to implement them.

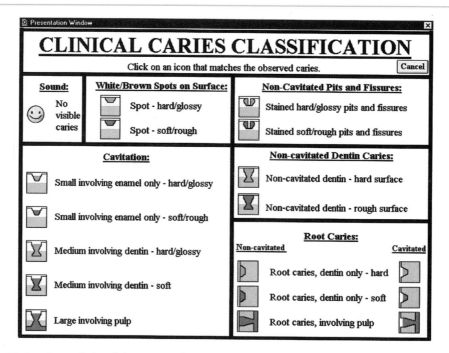

FIG. 16-17 A set of pictorial computer icons represent different stages of lesion severity and activity from various anatomical sites. (From Benn DK et al: Practical approach to evidence-based management of caries, *J Am Coll Dent* 66(1):27-35, 1999.)

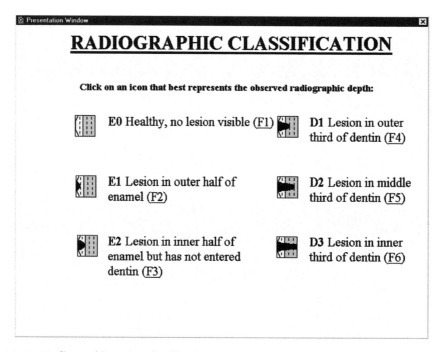

FIG. 16-18 Radiographic caries classification. (From Benn DK et al: Practical approach to evidence-based management of caries, *J Am Coll Dent* 66(1): 27-35, 1999.)

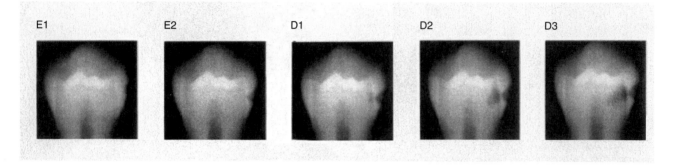

FIG. 16-19 Examples of radiographic lesion classification. *E0,* Healthy, no lesion visible in enamel; *E1,* lesion in outer half of enamel; *E2,* lesion in inner half of enamel; *D1,* lesion in outer third of dentin; *D2,* lesion in middle third of dentin; *D3,* lesion in inner third of dentin. (From Benn DK et al: Practical approach to evidence-based management of caries. *J Am Coll Dent* 66(1):27-35, 1999.)

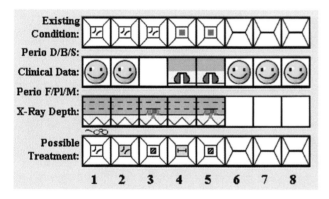

FIG. 16-20 New caries tooth chart. (From Benn DK et al: Practical approach to evidence-based management of caries. *J Am Coll Dent* 66(1):27-35, 1999.)

CURRENT METHODS OF CARIES DETECTION

Any review of the literature on caries detection requires the definition of two commonly used terms—*sensitivity* and *specificity.* Simply put, *sensitivity* is the ability to correctly detect a carious lesion that is truly carious, and *specificity* is the ability to correctly identify health, or an absence of carious lesions. Ideally a caries-detection method would have both high sensitivity and specificity, but in reality the perfect detection tool or method has yet to be found.

VISUAL AND TACTILE METHODS

A typical conventional approach to caries management in the United States often begins with a careful tooth-by-tooth visual and tactile hard tissue exam. The main detection tools consist of a discriminating eye, conventional dental radiographs, and a sharp dental explorer. The clinician examines the tooth surfaces carefully by probing the sharp end of a dental explorer into any suspect areas of the tooth, such as white or brown spot lesions (see the later section of this chapter concerning color changes in enamel), pits and fissures, and marginal discrepancies

(chips or gaps) in existing restorations. The test for caries, as described by Black in 1924 and Sturdevant in 1985,[6] is thought to be positive if the sharp explorer "sticks" when pressure is applied to the tip or has "tug-back" on withdrawal. Because of the narrow tooth morphology in pit and fissure areas, these so-called conventional methods used to detect caries all may be inaccurate.[34] Deep morphology of these areas can cause an explorer to stick or demonstrate tugback not because the area is actually carious but because the sharp explorer has wedged in the narrow pit or fissure (a false-positive result). Conversely, narrow, deep anatomy of these areas may prevent the explorer from actually reaching the base of the pit or fissure, causing the clinician to miss an active carious lesion at the base (a false-negative result). Given these facts, it is not surprising that studies[28] have shown that the use of a dental explorer does not improve detection of pit and fissure caries in comparison to a visual inspection alone. In one study the percentage of correctly diagnosed teeth was only 42%, compared with a histological gold standard method.[28] Such findings are consistent with other studies showing that only 20% to 40% of pit and fissure caries were correctly detected by visual techniques.[43]

Thus the dependence on the dental explorer is not only highly misleading, as in the pit and fissure areas, but also may be potentially harmful to the tooth,[18] especially on partially diminished smooth surfaces. Improper use of a sharp dental explorer during examination can adversely affect teeth[40] by damaging newly erupted teeth,[12] accelerating caries progression,[42] causing cavitations in previously noncavitated lesions,[44] and transmitting pathogens to a tooth not previously infected.[27]

The occlusal surface currently poses the greatest challenge for clinicians. First, most of the incidence of caries today occurs on the occlusal surface.[28] Second, because of deep, narrow morphology the pits and fissures may be impossible to thoroughly clean and thus may act as a niche for bacterial growth.[14] Third, this morphology makes caries detection difficult, especially in early lesions in which a threat of the so-called hidden occlusal lesion exists. A hidden occlusal lesion describes an area in which a seemingly normal-appearing pit or fissure has an undetected lesion underneath that requires surgical intervention. Fourth and

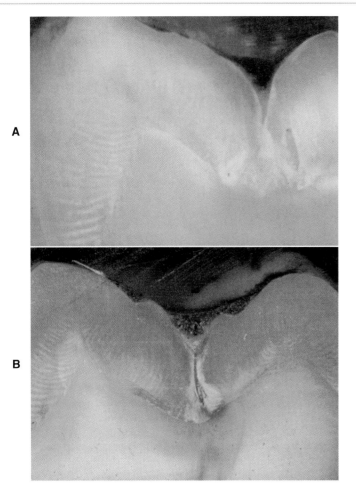

FIG. 16-21 Anatomy of fissures. **A,** A simple, uncomplicated fissure that does not penetrate the full depth of the enamel. **B,** A more common anatomy in which the fissure has demineralized and the dentin is immediately involved. (From Mount GJ, Hume WR: *Preservation and restoration of tooth structure,* St Louis, 1998, Mosby.)

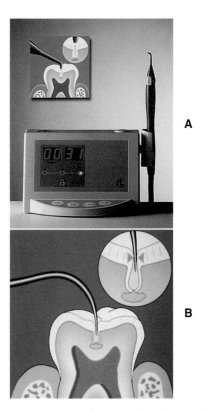

FIG. 16-22 **A,** The DIAGNOdent used to detect subsurface carious lesions. **B,** Shows the inability of the explorer to reach the extent of the subsurface lesion, making the DIAGNOdent preferable for caries detection. (Courtesy KaVo America Corporation, Lake Zurich, Ill.)

last, the deep morphology leaves the enamel layer extremely thin at the base of the fissure (Fig. 16-21).

Pits and fissures now may be examined for visually undetectable caries with the DIAGNOdent (Fig. 16-22), a device that detects and measures pathogenic bacterial byproducts in the subsurface lesion. The next method used to detect subsurface lesions is to perform an ***enameloplasty*** by opening the surface with a small dental bur and evaluating the underlying dental structure (Fig. 16-23). This procedure requires removal of tooth structure and some form of restoration, regardless of whether a carious lesion is present.

RECURRENT OR SECONDARY CARIES

Recurrent, or *secondary,* ***caries*** refers to a new active lesion in relation to the margin of an existing restoration. These terms are always associated with a restoration placed as a result of a previous or primary acid attack. However, many so-called recurrent lesions occur on the tooth surface itself, clearly independent of the restoration, and actually represent a new primary attack called an *outer lesion.* In contrast, if the carious lesion is associ-

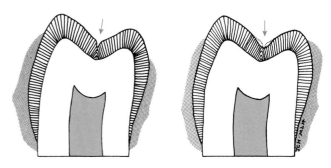

FIG. 16-23 Enameloplasty. (From Roberson TM, Heymann HO, Smith EJ: *Sturdevant's art and science of operative dentistry,* ed 4, St Louis, 2002, Mosby.)

ated with a margin of a restoration between the restoration and the cavity wall, then it is termed a *wall lesion.*[23] Interestingly, secondary caries is more likely to occur at the gingival margins than the occlusal margins (with 94% of amalgams and 62% of composites failing at the gingival floor of the restoration).[29] Thus amalgams rarely fail at occlusal margins, perhaps because of the self-sealing effects of the formed corrosion products. In fact, many experienced clinicians believe that "marginal discrepancies" (or a small explorer "catch" or "ditching" at the margin in the absence of caries) often are falsely being misdiagnosed as secondary caries. Reports are that 75% of operative dentistry is involved in the replacement of existing restorations,[23] many of which may not be secondary caries at all.

Surgical intervention should be undertaken only in the presence of cavitated lesions (because of the inability to control plaque accumulation) and infected dentin, not necessarily ditching or staining. Laboratory and histological studies show a poor correlation between ditching and secondary caries.[22] A color change next to an amalgam restoration should be interpreted with caution because it may simply indicate corrosion products or the physical presence of the silver-colored restoration, rather than caries. Staining around tooth colored restorations, either marginal staining or undermining staining, does not reliably predict soft dentin.[19] Using color change as the only guide would mean that many restorations would be replaced unnecessarily. Microbiological culturing of amalgam restorations shows that intact restorations and "narrow ditches" are minimally infected, requiring no intervention, whereas "wide ditches" are significantly more infected and should be replaced. In addition, findings indicate that color changes alone do not relate to infection and that only frank carious lesions at the margin constitute a reliable diagnosis of secondary caries.[19] Based on previously mentioned studies, one researcher defines a *wide ditch* as one into which the tip of a periodontal probe can fit.[22] Using a dull periodontal probe, a clinician can determine that narrow ditches and color changes alone should not trigger filling replacement, whereas wide ditches or frank carious outer lesions should be restored.[19]

The previous discussion applies to margins in enamel, and extreme caution should be used in any attempt to evaluate the gingival margins in cementum or dentin, where most secondary caries occurs.[29] These margins are often subgingival in cementum or dentin, making the areas both difficult to assess and restore. More precise diagnostic criteria are necessary to help prevent clinical disagreement on secondary caries detection in these areas.

COLOR CHANGES IN ENAMEL

One of the earliest signs of demineralization visible to the naked eye is the white spot lesion. The lesion appears white because the loss of mineral introduces porosities that change the refractive index compared with that of the surrounding translucent enamel. (This type of lesion will be discussed further in Chapter 22; Fig. 16-24). Often the white spot lesion turns brown, thus the term *brown spot lesion* (Fig. 16-25). Dental professionals and researchers do not fully agree on the exact mechanism of this brown change. Many believe that the increased porosity causes exogenous proteins to diffuse and stain the area. One interesting note is that this white-to-brown color shift is most often a sign that the lesion already has remineralized and is resistant to caries. In fact, when remineralized in the presence of topical fluoride, this surface is more than likely fluorapatite and will resist future acid attacks, thus greatly decreasing the probability that a cavitation will occur at that particular site.

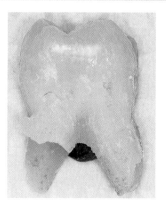

FIG. 16-24   White spot lesion.

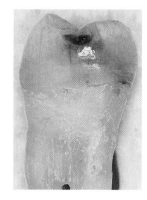

FIG. 16-25   Brown spot lesion.

Perhaps more important than color in enamel is whether the surface is significantly cavitated. Cavitation through the enamel allows bacteria to enter the dentin, whereas an intact enamel surface layer does not allow the bacteria to penetrate the enamel and enter the dentin. The diffusion channels in enamel are too small to let bacteria in but are large enough to allow the entrance of small molecules, such as acid and fluoride. The consequences of failure to remineralize an enamel lesion are usually not as severe as those related to failure to remineralize a dentinal lesion, a fact due to the differences in the rate of caries progression between the two tooth structures. In addition, enamel contains more mineral (85% by volume) than dentin (50% by volume), making remineralization more clinically practical in enamel. The only exception to this concept is that of the pits and fissures, where, because of anatomy and inadequate detection, any color change should be investigated early and met with aggressive preventive strategies when possible.

COLOR CHANGES IN DENTIN AND CEMENTUM

AFFECTED VERSUS INFECTED DENTIN

Why do carious lesions sometimes stain dark or appear brown? This phenomenon may be due to a combination of factors. Many researchers believe that the increase in porosity caused by the demineralization of the dentin allows an ingress of exogenous stain, whereas others in the field believe it is caused by chromogenic bacteria.[17] More recently, the cause for the discoloration of carious dentin has been suggested to be a reaction between demineralized collagen and bacterially derived aldehydes or dietary sugars, or both.[25] Demineralizing acids tend to diffuse ahead of bacteria as they advance through dentin. Usually a demineralized zone called the *affected dentin* lies deeper than the bacteria-filled dentin, known as the *infected dentin.* Only the infected dentin in a carious lesion needs to be removed. The affected layer, because of its increased porosity, is the area that often appears dark brown and can appear broader in rapidly advancing caries than in slowly advancing lesions.

ACTIVE VERSUS INACTIVE CARIES

As stated previously, the use of color alone as an indicator of active caries is risky. Evaluating color changes on root surface cementum and dentin is often challenging and has more severe consequences. Compared with enamel, dentin is much more porous, with less mineral content. Dentin is susceptible to collagenase and is physically closer to the pulp. Many experienced clinicians have noticed that active caries is often normal in color or a very light brown. In contrast, inactive or arrested caries is dark brown to black in color. Microbiological studies have shown that the combination of optical criteria and conventional tactile sense in the clinical removal of caries (until the dentin is firm and hard) results in little to no infected dentin remaining.[20] Therefore the use of hardness and optical appearance as a clinical guide is more reliable than color alone.

The important biological difference between infected and affected dentin is bacteria. The infected dentin feels soft to the touch, is often described as "mushy" or "leathery," and can be removed by careful use of large round bur in a slow-speed handpiece or spoon excavator. Cautious use of a specially formulated caries-indicating dye may help the novice clinician differentiate between affected and infected dentin (as long as the clinician understands that this method is not absolute). Caries-disclosing dyes are used in many dental schools to help students develop the tactile skills necessary to discern infected from affected dentin. Active lesions progress and lead to eventual cavitation, which can be seen radiographically, whereas inactive lesions do not progress and may appear smaller radiographically if remineralized. Again, this information should not encourage unrestrained use of dental radiographs.

CARIES-INDICATING DYES

Recently a number of caries-indicating products have become available on the market. First introduced in the early 1970s, these products consist of a dye in a carrier fluid. Once applied, the dye penetrates partially demineralized dentin because of the increased porosity. When carious dentin underlying carious enamel is exposed during a cavity preparation, the clinician can apply the dye solution to help judge the point at which all the carious dentin has been removed. The clinical goal of caries removal in dentin is to remove only the soft bacterial "infected" dentin, leaving partially demineralized affected dentin be-

hind. Studies conducted in the early 1970s claimed that the dye did not stain noninfected dentin, and to this day the use of caries-indicating dye is met with enthusiasm based on these original studies.[13] However, subsequent studies since have shown that the dye stains demineralized areas of the dentin, not the bacteria itself, and also may stain noninfected dentin. An inherent danger of overremoval of tooth structure is present.[20] Because of this lack of specificity, such dyes are a very crude caries-detecting tool[21] and should not be used as the sole determining factor in clinical caries removal.

DETECTION WITH DENTAL RADIOGRAPHS

Caries just under the floss contact between teeth is called *proximal* or **approximal caries** and is conventionally detected with dental bitewing radiographs. Radiographic detection of caries consists of discerning whether radiolucent (dark) areas on the dental radiograph appear consistent with a carious lesion. Once a carious lesion is detected on the radiograph and preferably confirmed by the visual and tactile examination, the area is treatment-planned for surgical restorative treatment (often amalgam prepared to a G.V. Black outline form). After the restorative treatment is completed, the patient usually is recalled for a periodic oral exam. Ironically, this recall interval is based on the periodontal status of the patient, and recall criteria make little sense given that no direct biological relationship exists between periodontal disease and dental caries. At the recall appointment the patient again is examined for caries and the process repeated if lesions are detected.

Conventional radiographic examination is the accepted standard used to detect proximal lesions and is a fairly crude but objective way to visualize the loss of mineral. Although the radiographic technique may be objective, the interpretation of the resulting image often is not. A common mistake is the assumption that the appropriate treatment for a radiolucent area on a radiograph is to "drill and fill." Studies have shown that demineralization measured in the laboratory with histological techniques is more advanced than the information represented on the radiograph.[24] This one fact is grossly misinterpreted, leading many to believe that clinicians need to be more aggressive at surgically restoring small radiographic proximal lesions because they are actually much deeper than they appear on the radiograph. The interpretation error is in the failure to recognize that early demineralization often can be arrested and remineralized, especially if the surface layer of enamel is intact and noncavitated. In these cases, the loss of mineral is most important to the diagnosis, as is the fact that the intact surface layer prevents bacteria from penetrating through the enamel into dentin. Although small molecules such as acid, calcium, and fluoride can diffuse into and from intact enamel, larger-sized bacteria cannot. Thus when bacteria have not invaded or when little chance exists of invasion into the dentin, nonsurgical treatment modalities should be considered. When the dentin has been invaded by bacteria, it is called *infected dentin,* and all such dentin should be surgically removed. Unfortunately, the conventional radiograph, which may qualitatively show areas where the mineral is less dense, does not show whether the surface is cavitated. Presently, needs exist for better quantitative caries-detection tools and for modification of the drill-and-fill mentality concerning early lesions.

Until such time, dental professionals can apply some common rules of thumb based on laboratory studies and clinical experience. In many states the licensure board generally would reject a proximal lesion if the radiolucency did not "touch" or penetrate the dentinoenamel junction (DEJ). As it turns out, this description is comparable to the E2 or D1 histological lesion described previously. This rule is a good clinical guide used to evaluate proximal lesions on bitewing radiographs until improved methods are perfected. Of course many E2 and D1 lesions may not have cavitated, but the rule of thumb is an acceptable compromise until better quantitative detection methods are available. Clearly E1 lesions should be treated chemically to prevent cavitation.

Used properly, the bitewing radiograph is a valuable tool to evaluate the proximal area but is less reliable in caries detection in the occlusal area, where, as mentioned previously, clinicians often have difficulty discerning pathological processes. Therefore radiographs must be interpreted with great caution to prevent false-positive detections.[34,35] In proximal lesions, minimal sound tissue is in the path of the x-rays, whereas the occlusal surface usually has a thick layer of sound hard tissue on either side, making detection in this area by conventional radiography difficult, unless the lesions are very large. Consequently, occlusal lesions are well advanced by the time they can be detected on a radiograph.[33] In 1995 a group of researchers[11] questioned routine usage of radiographic examination for early occlusal lesions.[35] Computerized digital radiography now is being successfully used in dental practice and subjects patients to less exposure from ionizing radiation; however, it still suffers from the same problems of basic physics and interpretation as described previously.

NEW ADVANCES IN CARIES DETECTION

Recently, two commercial products have shown great promise in improving caries detection—namely DIFOTI (Electro-Sciences, Inc., Irvington, N.Y.) and DIAGNOdent (Diagnodent, Lake Zurich, Ill.). The DIFOTI (digital fiber-optic transillumination) uses computer technology to interpret images captured by shining visible light on the tooth. Instead of ionizing radiation used in a bitewing radiograph, a concentrated beam of visible light is shined on the tooth and an image is captured on the other side of the tooth, where the radiographic film usually is placed. DIFOTI images only detect optical changes at, or near, the surface and it is up to the clinician to discern if the optical changes are from demineralization or from other causes. Although very sensitive at picking up early surface changes, more studies are needed to determine if DIFOTI can be useful in assessing and monitoring lesion depth at all.

The DIAGNOdent is a device that uses laser fluorescence to detect occlusal caries. Sound enamel produces an intrinsic fluorescence, the exact origin of which has yet to be explained. The alteration of sound enamel as the caries process continues leads to changes in fluorescence, enabling observations to be made for potential caries detection.[16,41,42] Specific wavelengths of light can excite fluorescence, and differences between sound and carious tissue can be detected. With the DIAGNOdent a diode laser with a wavelength of 655 nm is used. This technique does not provide a two- or three-dimensional image showing the extent and severity of lesions for later comparison in the determination of a progression or reversal of the lesion.

At the time of this text's publication, both devices are commercially available to clinicians. Although relatively new technologies, these devices represent valuable adjuncts to conventional detection methods. Only time will tell how much impact they will have on early caries detection.

DIFFERING VIEWS ON SURGICAL RESTORATIVE APPROACHES

Traditional G.V. Black cavity preparations are still being taught in U.S. dental schools, used for state licensure examinations, and are the most predominant cavity forms used in private practice today. However, many clinicians believe these conventional treatment philosophies and a lack of aggressive preventive measures have contributed to the overpreparation of tooth structure. Currently, trends are emerging that look for opportunities to preserve tooth structure via prevention and conservative restorative procedures.[31] For example, growing evidence supports the idea that some conservative preparations, which remove much less tooth structure, are at least as retentive as the traditional G.V. Black cavity preparations.[10] The limitations of current detection techniques described previously have lead most traditional clinicians to "watch" questionable areas until they test positive with conventional detection techniques (an explorer "stick" or visible cavitation) or to restore early proximal radiographic lesions. However, some clinicians believe that watching pits and fissures can lead to large subsurface lesion progression, which can go undetected until it is too late for preventive intervention. Still other clinicians believe that using these conventional management strategies, coupled with conventional Black preparation design, results in unnecessary loss of tooth structure. Given current knowledge, preventive sealants and new management protocols require further investigation.

FUTURE CARIES-DETECTION TECHNOLOGIES

Several alternative caries-detection techniques are currently under investigation. Although some are being used clinically in certain countries, most have failed to surface in the United States. Because these methods are appearing in the research literature, each is introduced briefly in the following section.

CONDUCTANCE AND IMPEDANCE

Several approaches have been proposed to take advantage of the ability of water within teeth to conduct electricity.[37] Carious tissue contains more water and therefore conducts electricity more readily. However, experiments using direct current (D.C.) conductance have been disappointing, demonstrating little discrimination between carious tissue and other noncarious porous tissue. Location of the lesion also is difficult to determine.

In contrast, impedance measurements recently have shown considerable promise for lesion detection, demonstrating both high sensitivity and high specificity. This method may prove to be a relatively low-cost approach for the detection of occlusal caries and may help dental professionals decide whether to "open up" the tooth.[26,34,36,37] However, this method lacks two- or three-dimensional images of the lesion and produces no record of position or extent of the lesion.

ULTRASOUND

Potentially, ultrasound may be used to provide images of carious lesions in all tooth surfaces, but, as of yet, this methodology is unavailable specifically for dental use.

FLUORESCENCE

Sound enamel produces an intrinsic fluorescence, the exact origin of which has yet to be explained. As the caries process continues, the alteration of sound enamel leads to changes in fluorescence, enabling observations to be made for potential caries detection.[16,38,39] Specific wavelengths of light can excite fluorescence, permitting detection of differences between sound and carious tissue. Although this technique has shown some promise for smooth surfaces and possibly for occlusal surfaces, it has not yet been perfected and requires more laboratory and clinical validation. This technique also does not provide a two- or three-dimensional image to show the extent and severity of lesions for later comparison to determine progression or reversal of the lesion.

OPTICAL COHERENCE TOMOGRAPHY

A new technique, optical coherence tomography (OCT), produces a tomographic image in two dimensions, showing the extent and potentially the severity of subsurface demineralization.[8,9] Near infrared light is readily transmitted through sound enamel but is scattered by carious enamel. The reflected and back-scattered light can be detected to produce the tomographic image. OCT is in its early research stage and needs more development before it will be ready for clinical use. However, OCT shows great potential because of its ability to produce a permanent image that can record the position and extent of the lesion for future comparison.

OCCLUSAL ANALYSIS

Occlusion is important to all aspects of dentistry at all ages. For example, in the primary dentition the clinician should check for adequate spacing between the deciduous teeth so that enough space remains to allow the permanent teeth to erupt properly. If crowding is present in primary or permanent dentition, an orthodontic evaluation may be indicated. Each time a tooth is restored the dentist must consider the occlusion and the way in which the teeth will function. If such information is not considered, the tooth may be restored with a tooth-to-tooth interference and the patient may later develop headaches and/or jaw pain, which could indicate problems with the TMJ. These examples are just a few of the many demonstrating the important role of occlusion. A comprehensive review of occlusion is beyond the scope of this chapter, but a few basic observations should be recorded during the exam. The extraoral exam in Chapter 11 discusses the way to evaluate the TMJ and the muscles of mastication. The intraoral portion of the occlusal analysis is discussed briefly in the following text.

The basic information to record may include the patient's Angle's classification, overbite, overjet, maximum incisal opening, pathway of opening or closing, amount of movement from centric relation to centric occlusion (CR-CO shift), initial contacts in centric relation (CR), initial contacts in right and left lateral excursions, initial contacts in protrusive movements, and any signs of traumatic occlusion. These terms are defined in the following section, and Fig. 16-26 summarizes one way to chart this information.

ANGLE'S CLASSIFICATION

The *Angle's classification* is the traditional method developed by Dr E. H. Angle in 1899 to identify occlusions that need orthodontic treatment. Originally this system used the position of the mesiobuccal (MB) cusp of the maxillary first molar in relationship to the buccal groove of the mandibular first molar.[41] Later, clinicians added the cuspid relationship as well. The "ideal" occlusion was defined as *Class I*, in which the MB cusp of the maxillary first molar is

Initial Occlusal and TMJ Findings

CENTRIC RELATION:
Location: ☐ easy ☐ difficult ☐ impossible
TMJ discomfort to pressure ☐ none ☐ right ☐ left
Initial tooth contact: _____ vs. _____
CENTRIC RELATION-CENTRIC OCCLUSION DISCREPANCY:
Vertical slide _____ mm Forward slide _____ mm
Lateral slide ☐ right ☐ left _____ mm
CENTRIC OCCLUSION:
Canine classification (I,II,III) right _____ left _____
Right canine vertical overlap _____ mm
Right canine functional horizontal overlap _____ mm
Left canine vertical overlap _____ mm
Left canine horizontal overlap _____ mm
Central incisor vertical overlap _____ mm
Central incisor functional horizontal overlap _____ mm
Wear facets: ☐ minimal ☐ moderate ☐ severe

CR TO CO	1	2	3	4	5	6	7	8	9	10	11	12	13	14	15	16
INTERFERENCES	32	31	30	29	28	27	26	25	24	23	22	21	20	19	18	17
RT.	1	2	3	4	5	6	7	8	9	10	11	12	13	14	15	16
LATERAL	32	31	30	29	28	27	26	25	24	23	22	21	20	19	18	17
LT.	1	2	3	4	5	6	7	8	9	10	11	12	13	14	15	16
LATERAL	32	31	30	29	28	27	26	25	24	23	22	21	20	19	18	17
PROTRUSIVE	1	2	3	4	5	6	7	8	9	10	11	12	13	14	15	16
	32	31	30	29	28	27	26	25	24	23	22	21	20	19	18	17

TEMPORO-MANDIBULAR JOINT:			
Maximum opening _____ mm			
Joint sounds during opening and closing:	☐ none	☐ right	☐ left
Joint sounds during excursions:	☐ none	☐ right	☐ left
History of TMJ treatment:	☐ yes	☐ no	
Current joint pain:	☐ none	☐ right	☐ left

FIG. 16-26 Occlusal charting record. (Courtesy University of the Pacific School of Dentistry, San Francisco.)

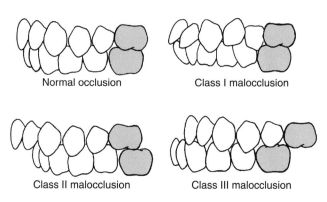

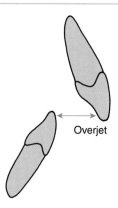

FIG. 16-27 Normal occlusion and malocclusion classes as specified by Angle. This classification was quickly and widely adopted early in the twentieth century. It is incorporated within all contemporary descriptive and classification schemes. (Modified from Proffit WR: *Contemporary orthodontics,* ed 3, St Louis, 2000, Mosby.)

FIG. 16-28 *Overjet* is defined as horizontal overlap of the incisors. (Modified from Proffit WR: *Contemporary orthodontics,* ed 3, St Louis, 2000, Mosby.)

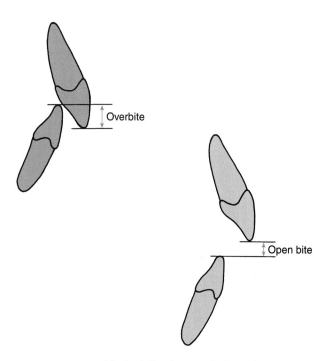

FIG. 16-29 *Overbite* is defined as vertical overlap of the incisors. (Modified from Proffit WR: *Contemporary orthodontics,* ed 3, St Louis, 2000, Mosby.)

in line with the buccal groove of the mandibular first molar, as shown in Fig. 16-27. Class II is defined as having the MB cusp of the maxillary first molar and the maxillary cuspid mesial to the mandibular landmarks. *Class II* can be subdivided further in to division 1 (anterior teeth flared) and division 2 (anterior teeth verted, or inclined, lingually), also illustrated in Fig. 16-27. Lastly, *Class III* is defined as the MB cusp of the maxillary first molar and the maxillary cuspid distal to the mandibular landmarks, as shown in Fig. 16-27. The Angle's classification system does have some drawbacks; however, it only looks at a few teeth to classify the entire mouth and is somewhat subjective in decisions about when the maxillary cusps are not in the ideal Class I relationship. If the cusp is more than a half cusp from an ideal Class I, this cusp is generally accepted as either a Class II or Class III, and even this determination is somewhat subjective.

OVERBITE AND OVERJET

Overbite is the vertical distance that the maxillary anterior teeth overlap the mandibular anterior teeth when the teeth are fully occluded.[41] *Overjet* is the horizontal distance measured from the labial or lingual surface (depending on clinician preference) of the maxillary incisors to the facial surface of the lower incisors when the teeth are fully occluded.[41] Figs. 16-28 and 16-29 demonstrate the ways to measure overbite and overjet.

MAXIMUM INCISAL OPENING

The maximum incisal opening (MIO) is measured from the incisal edges of the anterior teeth when the mandible is opened to its furthest extent (Fig. 16-30).

PATHWAY OF OPENING OR CLOSING

Ideally the midline path of opening and closing of the mandible follows a straight, or linear, path when viewed from the front of the patient. However, this path is not al-

ways the case, and deviations from it should be noted on the chart. Often the path the midline of the mandible takes an S-shape deviation to the right or left.

CENTRIC RELATION–CENTRIC OCCLUSION SHIFT

In its simplest definition, centric relation (CR) is the most retruded position of the mandible, and centric occlusion (CO) is the position of the mandible when the teeth are in maximum intercuspation.[32] The CR and CO are rarely in the same position, and often a shift or slide occurs from the CR to the CO position that can be estimated and recorded in the chart. A CO-CR shift by itself is not necessarily a pathological condition.

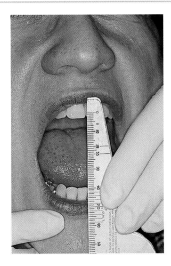

FIG. 16-30 Maximum opening of patient's mandible is measured.

INITIAL CONTACTS IN EXCURSIONS

A protrusive excursion occurs when the mandible moves from the CR or CO position anteriorly until the incisors are in the edge-to-edge position. Ideally when the teeth are in the protrusive position, the posterior teeth should no longer touch. A lateral excursion occurs when the mandible travels from the CO or CR to the right or left until the cuspids on that side are in the cusp-to-cusp position. In that position the teeth on the opposite side should not be in contact. Observing and recording in the chart which teeth touch during the performance of these different excursions can help discern between normal movements and those that may be considered pathological interferences.

TRAUMATIC OCCLUSION

Occlusal trauma is a force capable of producing pathological changes to the supporting periodontium. Two types of occlusal trauma exist—primary and secondary. Primary occlusal trauma occurs when excessive occlusal force is applied to a tooth with normal supporting structures. Secondary occlusal trauma occurs when normal occlusal forces causes trauma to the attachment apparatus of a tooth because of inadequate support structures. Occlusal trauma is not an inflammatory process, is not related to periodontal disease, and does not cause pocket formation.[5,7,15,45] A periodontally involved tooth may, however, be affected adversely by occlusal trauma. Many causes of occlusal trauma exist, including tooth position, oral habits, contacts with foreign objects, and iatrogenic causes.

RITICAL THINKING ACTIVITIES

On a patient charting form, record the following conditions:
- A 2-mm diastema between teeth #9 and #10
- A four-unit bridge between teeth #11 and #14 (abutment teeth: #11 and #14; pontics: #12 and #13)

Tooth #14: all gold extending to the CEJ

Tooth #13: porcelain on the facial extending from the CEJ to the central groove on the occlusal; gold from the central groove to the lingual margin, which is at the CEJ

Tooth #12: porcelain on the facial extending from the CEJ to the central groove on the occlusal; gold from the central groove to the lingual margin, which is at the CEJ

Tooth #11: porcelain on the facial and lingual extending from the CEJ to halfway down the lingual surface; gold on the other half of the lingual surface

- Tooth #2: acrylic temporary crown covering the entire crown to 1 mm below the CEJ
- Tooth #19: occlusal amalgam with an ideal outline form with caries that can be seen clinically along at the margins of the distal pit
- Tooth #5: caries (not to the DEJ) that can be seen radiographically and clinically under the distal contact
- Tooth #7: completed single root endodontics (seen radiographically) with a lingual pit amalgam
- Tooth #30: occlusal composite 2 mm wide along central groove between mesial and distal pits
- Tooth #32: horizontally impacted and completely covered by tissue
- Tooth #8: distal incisal fracture with piece of tooth missing

REVIEW QUESTIONS

1. **All of the following statements are true *except* which one?**
   a. Sensitivity is the ability to correctly identify health or the absence of carious lesions.
   b. A #1.2 lesion is Mount and Hume's classification of a medium-sized cavity in the top of the tooth.
   c. E0 classification means that no lesions are visible.
   d. Secondary caries is more likely to occur at gingival margins than occlusal margins (especially in amalgams).
   e. Bacteria-filled dentin is called *infected dentin.*

2. **All *except* which of the following are limitations involving the use of an explorer to detect occlusal caries?**
   a. It is only 60% accurate.
   b. It can transfer bacteria to other sites.
   c. It can damage intact surfaces.
   d. It can give false-positive results.
   e. It can give false-negative results.

3. **Which of the following statements best describes the process of attrition?**
   a. The wearing of tooth substance by exogenous material forced over the surface by incisive, masticatory, or tooth-cleaning functions
   b. The superficial loss of dental hard tissue due to a chemical process not involving bacteria
   c. Tooth wear caused by tooth-to-tooth contact without the presence of exogenous material
   d. "Flexure" at the cervical region of the tooth, causing loss of mineral
   e. None of the above

4. **Which of the following statements best characterizes abrasion?**
   a. The wearing of the tooth substance by exogenous material forced over the surface incisive, masticatory, or tooth-cleaning functions
   b. The superficial loss of dental hard tissue due to a chemical process not involving bacteria
   c. Tooth wear caused by tooth-to-tooth contact without the presence of exogenous material
   d. "Flexure" at the cervical region of the tooth causing loss of mineral
   e. None of the above

5. **White spot lesions are the result of which of the following occurrences?**
   a. Too much fluoride in water
   b. Too much abrasive in dentifrice
   c. More topical fluoride treatments than warranted
   d. Change in refractive index due to demineralization
   e. Infusion of exogenous proteins into enamel surface

 SUGGESTED AGENCIES AND WEB SITES

Because of the ever-changing nature of the Internet, some of the web sites listed here may have changed since publication. Please refer to Mosby's Evolve web site for the most current information.

Delmar's Online Companion for Dental Charting ("A standard approach"): http://www.delmaralliedhealth.com
Dental Diagnostics: http://www.applied-technologies.com

DHY 104—Preclinical Dental Hygiene Lecture: http://www.dtae.org
Vo-Tech Adult Learning Services ("Dental charting"): http://ae.lisd.k12.mi.us

 ADDITIONAL READINGS AND RESOURCES

Mount GJ, Hume WR: *Preservation and restoration of tooth structure,* St Louis, 1998, Mosby.

Schneiderman A, Elbaum M, Shultz T, Keem S, Greenebaum M, Driller J: Assessment of dental caries with Digital Imaging Fiber-Optic Trans Illumination (DIFOTI): *In vitro* study. Caries Res 1997;31:103-110.

 REFERENCES

1. Anderson MH, Bales DJ, Omnell K-A: Modern management of dental caries: the cutting edge is not the dental bur, *J Amer Dent Assoc* 124:37-44, 1993.
2. Anusavice KJ: Efficacy of nonsurgical management of the initial caries lesion, *J Dent Educ* 61:895-905, 1997.
3. Anusavice KJ: Treatment regimens in preventive and restorative dentistry, *J Am Dent Assoc* 126(6):727-43, 1995.
4. Benn DK et al: Practical approach to evidence-based management of caries, *J Am Coll Dent* 66(1):27-35, 1999.
5. Carranza FA: *Glickman's clinical periodontology,* Philadelphia, 1979, WB Saunders.
6. Chan DC: Current methods and criteria for caries diagnosis in North America, *J Dent Educ* 57(6):422-7, 1993.
7. Chasen AI: Controversies in occlusion, *Dent Clin N Am* 34:1, 1990.
8. Colston BW et al: Imaging of hard- and soft-tissue structure in the oral cavity by optical coherence tomography, *Appl Optics* 37(16):3582-85, 1998.

Continued

9. Colston BW et al: Non-invasive diagnosis of early caries with polarization sensitive optical tomography (PS-OCT). In Featherstone JDB, Rechmann P, Fried D, editors: *Proceedings of Lasers in Dentistry V,* Vol. 3593, San Jose, Calif, January 24-25, 1999, The International Society for Optical Engineering.

10. Eakle WS et al: Mechanical retention versus bonding of amalgam and gallium alloy restorations, *J Prosthet Dent* 72(4):351-4, 1994.

11. Ekstrand KR et al: Relationship between external and histologic features of progressive stages of caries in the occlusal fossa, *Caries Res* 29(4):243-50, 1995.

12. Ekstrand KR, Ricketts DN, Kidd EA: Reproducibility and accuracy of three methods for assessment of demineralization depth of the occlusal surface: an in vitro examination, *Caries Res* 31(3):224-31, 1997.

13. Fusayama T, Terashima S: Differentiation of two layers of carious dentin by staining, *Bulletin of Tokyo Medical and Dental University* 19(1):83-92, 1972.

14. Galil KA, Gwinnett AJ: Three-dimensional replicas of pits and fissures in human teeth: scanning electron microscopy study, *Arch Oral Biol* 20:493-5, 1975.

15. Goldman HC, Cohen DW: *Periodontal therapy,* St Louis, 1980, Mosby.

16. Hall AF et al: Dye-enhanced laser fluorescence method. In Stookey GK, editor: *Early detection of dental caries: proceedings of the 1st Annual Indiana Conference,* Indianapolis, 1996, Indiana University.

17. Kidd EA: Diagnosis of secondary caries. In Stookey GK, editor: *Early detection of dental caries: proceedings of the 1st Annual Indiana Conference,* Indianapolis, 1996, Indiana University.

18. Kidd EA: The diagnosis and management of the 'early' carious lesion in permanent teeth, *Dent Update* 11(2):69-70, 72-4, 76-8 (passim), 1984.

19. Kidd EA, Joyston-Bechal S, Beighton D: Marginal ditching and staining as a predictor of secondary caries around amalgam restorations: a clinical and microbiological study, *J Dent Res* 74(5):1206-11, 1995.

20. Kidd EA, Joyston-Bechal S, Beighton D: The use of a caries detector dye during cavity preparation: a microbiological assessment, *Br Dent J* 174(7):245-8, 1993.

21. Kidd EA et al: The use of a caries detector dye in cavity preparation, *Br Dent J* 167(4):132-4, 1989.

22. Kidd EA, O'Hara JW: The caries status of occlusal amalgam restorations with marginal defects, *J Dent Res* 69(6):1275-7, 1990.

23. Kidd EA, Toffenetti F, Mjör IA: Secondary caries, *Int Dent J* 42(3):127-38, 1992.

24. Kleier DJ, Hicks MJ, Flaitz CM: A comparison of Ultraspeed and Ektaspeed dental x-ray film: in vitro study of the radiographic and histologic appearance of interproximal lesions, *Quintessence International* 18(9):623-31, 1987.

25. Kleter GA: Discoloration of dental carious lesions [review], *Arch Oral Biol* 43:629-32, 1998.

26. Levinkind M: Electrochemical impedance strategies for early caries detection. In Stookey GK, Beiswanger B, editors: *Indiana Conference 1996: early detection of dental caries,* Indianapolis, 1996, Indiana University.

27. Loesche WJ, Svanberg ML, Pape HR: Intraoral transmission of *Streptococcus mutans* by a dental explorer, *J Dent Res* 58(8):765-70, 1979.

28. Lussi A: Validity of diagnostic and treatment decisions of fissure caries, *Caries Res* 25(4):296-303, 1991.

29. Mjör IA: Frequency of secondary caries at various anatomical locations, *Oper Dent* 10(3):88-92, 1985.

30. Mount GJ, Hume WR: A new cavity classification, *Aust Dent J* 43(3):153-9, 1998.

31. Mount GJ, Hume WR: *Preservation and restoration of tooth structure,* St Louis, 1998, Mosby.

32. Ramfjord SP, Ash MM: *Occlusion,* Philadelphia, 1983, WB Saunders.

33. Ricketts DN, Kidd EA, Beighton D: Operative and microbiological validation of visual, radiographic and electronic diagnosis of occlusal caries in non-cavitated teeth judged to be in need of operative care, *Br Dent J* 179(6):214-20, 1995.

34. Ricketts DN et al: Histological validation of electrical resistance measurements in the diagnosis of occlusal caries, *Caries Res* 30(2):148-55, 1996.

35. Ricketts DN et al: Clinical and radiographic diagnosis of occlusal caries: a study in vitro, *J Oral Rehab* 22(1):15-20, 1995.

36. Ricketts D et al: Hidden caries: what is it? does it exist? does it matter?, *Int Dent J* 47(5):259-65, 1997.

37. Ricketts DN, Kidd EA, Wilson RF: The electronic diagnosis of caries in pits and fissures: site-specific stable conductance readings or cumulative resistance readings, *Caries Res* 31(2):119-24, 1997.

38. ten Bosch JJ: General aspects of optical methods in dentistry, *Adv Dent Res* 1(1):5-7, 1987.

39. ten Bosch JJ, Angmar-Mansson B: A review of quantitative methods for studies of mineral content of intra-oral incipient caries lesions, *J Dent Res* 70(1):2-14, 1991.

40. ten Cate JM, van Amerongen JP: Caries diagnosis, conventional methods. In Stookey GK, editor: *Early detection of dental caries: proceedings of the 1st Annual Indiana Conference,* Indianapolis, 1996, Indiana University.

41. Thurow RC: *Atlas of orthodontic principles,* St Louis, 1977, Mosby.

42. van Dorp CS, Exterkate RA, ten Cate JM: The effect of dental probing on subsequent enamel demineralization, *ASDC J Dent Child* 55(5):343-7, 1988.

43. Wenzel A, Larsen MJ, Fejerskov O: Detection of occlusal caries without cavitation by visual inspection, film radiographs, xeroradiographs, and digitized radiographs, *Caries Res* 25(5):365-71, 1991.

44. Yassin OM: In vitro studies of the effect of a dental explorer on the formation of an artificial carious lesion, *ASDC J Dent Child* 62(2):111-7, 1995.

45. Zander HA, Polson AM: Present status of occlusion and occlusal therapy in periodontics, *J Periodontol* 43:540-4, 1977.

CHAPTER 17

Radiographic Evaluation *and* Utilization

Judith Qualtieri, Deedee L. McClain

Chapter Outline

Selection of Radiographs
Case Study: Radiographic Evaluation: Essential
   to Patient Care
Radiographic Evaluation
   Errors in technique
   Errors in exposure and processing
   Patient protection
Patient Assessment
   Structural findings
   Pathological findings
   Periodontal findings

Treatment Planning
Patient Education
New Radiographic Techniques

Key Terms

Charged-coupled device (CCD)
Condensing osteitis
Diagnostic quality
Elongation

Film contrast
Film density
Foreshortening
Furcation involvement

Horizontal bone loss
Interproximal caries
Overlapping
Periapical lesions

Selection criteria
  (radiographic)
Vertical bitewings
Vertical bone loss

Learning Outcomes

1. Select the appropriate radiographic series for a given patient.
2. Identify factors that may contribute to poor radiographic quality.
3. Analyze radiographs to determine possible pathologic processes and disease states.
4. Develop a dental hygiene care plan and contribute information to the dentist for the formulation of a restorative treatment plan.

5. Discuss the use of radiographs in the provision of patient education, treatment, and evaluation of treatment.
6. Discuss the use of digital radiography in dental hygiene patient care.

Case Study — Radiographic Evaluation: Essential to Patient Care

Jorel Courtland, a 32-year-old Caucasian man, presents to the dental office for an initial examination.

Health History

Mr. Courtland's health history states that he is currently being treated with a calcium channel blocker for high blood pressure and that the condition has been well maintained for the past 6 years. Vital signs at the visit are all within normal limits. Mr. Courtland reports that he smokes approximately 10 cigarettes per day and has for the past 2 years.

Dental History

Mr. Courtland's dental history indicates that he is experiencing sore gums, some sensitivity in the maxillary left quadrant, and occasional bleeding during brushing. He says that he brushes once per day, rinses with mouthwash occasionally, and uses floss when he notices that material is lodged between his teeth. His last reported dental visit was 7 years ago.

Clinical Examination Data

The periodontal evaluation reveals generalized bleeding on probing with localized 4- to 6-mm of attachment loss in the posterior region. Mr. Courtland has generalized marginal gingivitis. His plaque score is 90%, and his existing restorations appear to be in good condition; however, several areas of marginal discrepancy are noted. Sensitivity in the maxillary right posterior region is noted upon exploration.

Dental radiographs are essential in the assessment, education, treatment planning, therapy, and evaluation of the patient. The dental hygienist uses radiographs in conjunction with the comprehensive health and dental history, clinical examination data, and patient symptoms to appropriately interpret the patient's condition and develop a plan for dental hygiene treatment and home self-care instruction. The radiographs used to interpret current conditions must be high in quality. *Diagnostic quality* is evident in a film that presents enough information to accurately diagnose an existing pathologic process. This type of quality can be affected by errors in technique, exposure, and processing. According to one source:[7]

> *Accurate radiographic assessment depends on films with good diagnostic quality and the ability of the hygienist to recognize the appearance of normal periodontal tissues as well as the periodontium in a diseased state.*

Box 17-1 outlines steps for consideration in the treatment of each patient.

This chapter introduces a case study and describes the steps listed in Box 17-1 as they relate to the case findings.

SELECTION OF RADIOGRAPHS

Selecting the appropriate radiographic series for the patient helps ensure an accurate diagnosis while keeping radiation exposure to the patient at a minimum level. Dental practices often rely on a generalized radiographic protocol that is the same for each patient. Screening films are not recommended for use on new patients because studies have shown that the chance that they will disclose occult disease in the asymptomatic individual is extremely small.[19] Dental practices should rely on guidelines published by professional organizations to determine the radiographic series after the patient's health and dental history and clinical examination data are examined. The guidelines shown in Table 17-1 were developed by an expert panel of representatives from the Academy of General Dentistry; American Academies of Dental Radiography, Periodontology, Oral Medicine, Pediatric Dentistry; and the American Dental Association. This *selection criteria (radiographic)* is a set of guidelines based on an examination of scientific literature (and is not a requirement by law or a regulation).[5]

Case Application

The clinical examination data on Mr. Courtland seem to indicate the presence of early periodontal disease, poor oral hygiene, several restorations, and carious lesions. Based on the clinical data, the guidelines in Table 17-1 and Boxes 17-2 and 17-3, a full-mouth intraoral radiographic examination would be appropriate for this patient. The clinical documentation also reveals the presence of localized periodontal pockets; therefore *vertical bitewings* should be exposed in the posterior areas. Vertical bitewings provide extended vertical coverage of the interalveolar bone and roots, which help assess the extent of the patient's periodontal condition.[10] The full-mouth radiographic examination of Mr. Courtland is shown in Fig. 17-1.

RADIOGRAPHIC EVALUATION

Radiographic quality must be assessed to ensure an appropriate interpretation and diagnosis. Factors that can diminish film quality include errors in technique, use of inappropriate exposure settings, and errors in film processing. Poor radiographic quality can lead to misinterpretation of findings and affect the quality of patient care provided. In addition, poor-quality radiographic images leading to an inaccurate diagnosis also can have legal implications for the practice.

17-A
17-B

TABLE 17-1

Guidelines for prescribing dental radiographs

	CHILD		ADOLESCENT	ADULT	
Patient category	**Primary dentition (before eruption of first permanent tooth)**	**Transitional dentition (after eruption of first permanent tooth)**	**Permanent dentition (before eruption of third molars)**	**Dentulous**	**Edentulous**
New patient* All new patients to assess dental diseases and growth and development	Posterior bitewing examination if proximal surfaces of primary teeth cannot be visualized or probed	Individualized radiographic examination consisting of periapical/occlusal views and posterior bitewings *or* panoramic examination and posterior bitewings	Individualized radiographic examination consisting of posterior bitewings and selected periapicals. A full mouth intraoral radiographic examination is appropriate when the patient presents with clinical evidence of generalized dental disease or a history of extensive dental treatment.		Full mouth intraoral radiographic examination *or* panoramic examination
Recall Patient* Clinical caries or high-risk factors for caries†	Posterior bitewing examination at 6-month intervals *or* until no carious lesions are evident	Posterior bitewing examination at 6-month intervals *or* until no carious lesions are evident	Posterior bitewing examination at 6- to 12-month intervals *or* until no carious lesions are evident	Posterior bitewing examination at 12- to 18-month intervals	Not applicable
No clinical caries and no high-risk factors for caries†	Posterior bitewing examination at 12- to 24-month intervals if proximal surfaces of primary teeth cannot be visualized or probed	Posterior bitewing examination at 12- to 24-month intervals	Posterior bitewing examination at 18- to 36-month intervals	Posterior bitewing examination at 24- to 36-month intervals	Not applicable
Periodontal disease or a history of periodontal treatment	Individualized radiographic examination consisting of selected periapical and/or bitewing radiographs for areas where periodontal disease (other than nonspecific gingivitis) can be demonstrated clinically	Individualized radiographic examination consisting of selected periapical and/or bitewing radiographs (other than nonspecific gingivitis) can be demonstrated clinically	Individualized radiographic examination consisting of selected periapical and/or bitewing radiographs for areas where periodontal disease (other than nonspecific gingivitis) can be demonstrated clinically		Not applicable
Growth and development assessment	Usually not indicated	Individualized radiographic examination consisting of a periapical/occlusal *or* panoramic examination	Periapical *or* panoramic examination to assess developing third molars	Usually not indicated	Usually not indicated

Modified from *Guidelines for prescribing dental radiographs.* Pub. No. N-80A. Rochester, NY, 1988, Eastman Kodak.

*See Box 17-2.

†See Box 17-3.

BOX 17-2

Clinical Situations for which Radiographs May Be Indicated

Positive Historical Findings
Previous periodontal or endodontic therapy
History of pain or trauma
Familial history of dental anomalies
Postoperative evaluation of healing
Presence of implants

Positive Clinical Signs and Symptoms
Clinical evidence of periodontal disease
Large or deep restorations
Deep carious lesions
Malposed or clinically impacted teeth
Swelling
Evidence of facial trauma
Mobility of teeth
Fistula or sinus tract infection

Clinically suspected sinus pathology
Growth abnormalities
Oral involvement in known or suspected systemic disease
Positive neurologic findings in the head and neck
Evidence of foreign objects
Pain and or dysfunction of the temporomandibular joint
Facial asymmetry
Abutment teeth for fixed or removable partial prosthesis
Unexplained bleeding
Unexplained sensitivity of teeth
Unusual eruption, spacing or migration of teeth
Unusual tooth morphology, calcification or color
Missing teeth with unknown reason

Modified from *Guidelines for prescribing dental radiographs.* Pub. No. N-80A. Rochester, NY, 1988, Eastman Kodak.

BOX 17-3

Potential Findings in Patients at High Risk for Dental Caries

High level of caries experience
History of recurrent caries
Existing restoration of poor quality
Poor oral hygiene
Inadequate fluoride exposure
Prolonged nursing (bottle or breast)
Diet with high sucrose frequency

Poor familial dental health
Developmental enamel defects
Developmental disability
Xerostomia
Genetic abnormality of teeth
Many multisurface restorations
Chemo radiation therapy

Modified from *Guidelines for prescribing dental radiographs.* Pub. No. N-80A. Rochester, NY, 1988, Eastman Kodak.

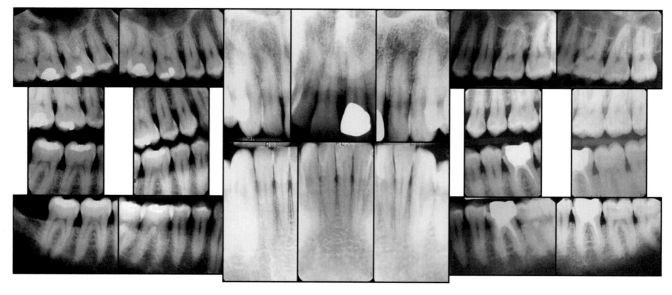

FIG. 17-1 Full-mouth radiographic series.

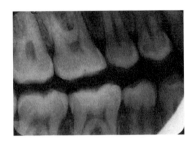

FIG. 17-2 Cone cut.

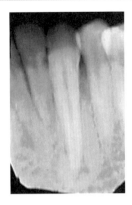

FIG. 17-3 Elongation.

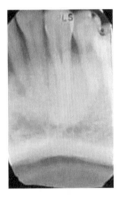

FIG. 17-4 Foreshortening.

ERRORS IN TECHNIQUE

Films placed too far anteriorly or posteriorly in the mouth can result in an inability to capture the mesial and distal structures. Films also can be placed too high or low in the mouth or at an improper angle, resulting in an inability to capture the occlusal-most or apical-most portion of the tooth on the radiograph. Errors in placement can result in incomplete radiographic coverage of the entire dentition and the loss of valuable diagnostic information.

 Case Application

Fig. 17-1 demonstrates film placement errors in the maxillary right molar film and the mandibular left molar film, one of the most common errors made in intraoral radiography.[16]

Other common technique errors that diminish diagnostic quality include improper vertical angulation of the cone and failure to cover the entire film packet with the x-ray beam. Failure to cover the entire film packet with the tray beam results in clear areas on the film called *cone cuts,* or *cone clips* (Fig. 17-2). ***Elongation*** is an error caused by the use of insufficient vertical angulation, which results in a stretched or elongated image and the visual absence of apical structures (Fig. 17-3). Another error, ***foreshortening,*** is caused by excessive vertical angulation and can result in a dwarfed image or an image visually lacking incisal or occlusal structures (Fig. 17-4).

Incorrect horizontal angulation of the cone is the cause of overlapping and can interfere with the detection of ***interproximal caries.*** The central ray of the x-ray beam must be directed between the interdental spaces for contacts to appear open. An open contact appears as a dark vertical line between the teeth, allowing a visual inspection of the interproximal enamel surfaces of the teeth (see Fig. 17-1, maxillary left molar).

 Case Application

A horizontal angulation error also is evident in the maxillary right and left lateral incisor and canine radiographs in Fig. 17-1. In the maxillary left molar radiograph the contacts between the teeth are ***overlapped.***

ERRORS IN EXPOSURE AND PROCESSING

Most x-ray machines today have variable exposure settings that can be selected for different areas within the mouth.

Settings also vary for patient age and the presence or absence of teeth. Failure to use the appropriate exposure time results in a film with poor film density, which describes the overall darkness of the film. A short exposure time setting can result in a film that is too light, whereas a long exposure time setting can result in a film that is too dark. Film quality also can be affected by changes in ***film contrast,*** which refers to the difference between the dark and light areas on the film (Fig. 17-5). Changing the kilovoltage peak (kVp) setting on the control panel alters film contrast.

 Case Application

The ***film density*** of the left molar bitewing in Fig. 17-1 appears low. This error was the result of the use of an improper exposure time setting on the control panel.

Poor density and contrast quality also can be the result of errors in film processing. Overdevelopment of a film or development at higher-than-normal temperatures can increase film density. Underdevelopment of a film or the use of exhausted solutions can decrease film density. Light leaks into the darkroom can cause "film fog," which negatively affects both the film density and the film contrast (Fig. 17-6). Poor radiographic contrast and density make distinguishing among the various structures on the film difficult and reduce the likelihood of an accurate diagnosis.

PATIENT PROTECTION

Poor film quality results not only in the loss of diagnostic information, as has been discussed, but also in an increase

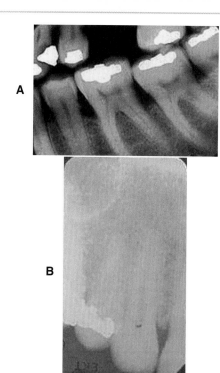

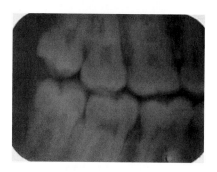

FIG. 17-5 A, Good film contrast. **B,** Poor film contrast.

FIG. 17-6 Film fog.

in patient exposure to radiation. The literature suggests that protection of patients during an intraoral radiographic procedure is best achieved with appropriate radiographic selection criteria for patients, methods of dose limitation, and development of quality assurance programs.[8] The use of guidelines for the selection of radiographs as a means of patient protection from excess radiation has been discussed (see Table 17-1). Dose limitation for the operator and the patient can be achieved by the evaluation of equipment function, as well as the use of E-speed film, rectangular collimation, a lead apron and a thyroid collar, improved processing quality, and annual training.[1,13] One underused method of dose limitation currently available is the use of E-speed or Ektaspeed film. Despite the reduction in radiation levels by approximately 50%, many clinicians still prefer D-speed or Ultraspeed film because of its image clarity.[14,18] Complaints of a grainy image appearance with E-speed film have hindered its overall acceptance in dentistry.

Quality assurance programs pull together all aspects involved in operator and patient protection, along with

methods used to produce diagnostic films. According to one research team:[9]

> *Quality assurance is defined as the planning and carrying out of procedures to assure high quality radiographs with maximum diagnostic information (yield) while minimizing the exposure to dental patients and personnel.*

Selection criteria, methods to reduce patient and operator exposure, infection-control procedures, proper equipment registration, maintenance, and labeling are all vital components of a quality assurance program in the dental office.

PATIENT ASSESSMENT

Radiographs provide information not visible in the clinical examination, information that is required to complete the patient's restorative and periodontal record. The dental hygienist interprets the radiographs by describing the conditions present on each film. The dentist then considers this information, along with the clinical documentation and patient symptoms, to diagnose the existing conditions and restorative needs. The dental hygienist's ability to differentiate between normal anatomical landmarks and diseased conditions is important in the provision of optimal care.

STRUCTURAL FINDINGS

Teeth should be thoroughly examined both clinically and radiographically to detect abnormalities in structure, including impacted, missing, and supernumerary teeth.

 Case Application
In Fig. 17-1 Mr. Courtland is missing tooth #32. These findings are included on his dental chart.

PATHOLOGICAL FINDINGS

Radiographs also are examined for signs of pathological processes, including carious lesions of the teeth, *periapical lesions,* and changes in the density of the alveolar bone. Carious lesions can be detected radiographically on various surfaces on the tooth. Interproximal enamel caries appears as a radiolucent notch in the enamel on the proximal surface of the tooth. Radiolucent notches located below the CEJ are referred to as *root caries.* Recurrent caries appears as a radiolucency around or under an existing restoration. Pit and fissure caries are generally not visible radiographically until they reach the dentin. When that much tooth structure is destroyed, the area appears as a radiolucency extending along the dentinoenamel junction (DEJ).

Case Application
The faulty restoration, a lack of routine dental care, and poor oral hygiene noted in Mr. Courtland are all considered contributing factors to the development of the carious lesions present. Carious lesions can be seen radiographically in the following teeth in Fig. 17-1: #4, #12, #14, and #19.

Periapical lesions can begin as a widening of the periodontal ligament space in the apical area and extend to a large rounded radiolucency around the apex of the root. A

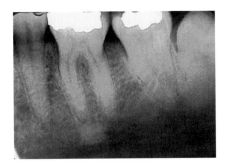

FIG. 17-7 Condensing osteitis.

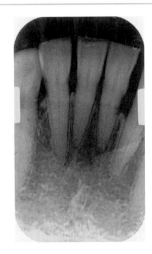

FIG. 17-8 Horizontal bone loss. (From White SC, Pharoah MJ: *Oral radiology: principles and interpretation,* ed 4, St Louis, 2000, Mosby.)

periapical lesion is commonly the result of a bacterial invasion of the pulp tissues and is referred to as an *abscess.* The mental foramen, a normal anatomical landmark found in the mandibular premolar area, has the same rounded radiolucent appearance as an abscess. A sound knowledge of anatomical landmarks commonly found in the oral cavity helps the dental hygienist prevent interpretation errors.

Alveolar bone can increase in density in response to a chronic periapical infection. This condition is called *condensing osteitis* and appears as an increase in the radiopacity of the bone around or below the radiolucent lesion (Fig. 17-7). Increases in bone density not associated with an infection are generally normal, but changes should be noted at supportive care appointments.

PERIODONTAL FINDINGS

Interpretation of radiographs involves an examination of the current periodontal condition and identification of factors that may contribute to the disease process.[2] The crest of the alveolar bone normally appears 1 to 1½ mm below the cementoenamel junction (CEJ).[11] Patterns of bone loss may take on horizontal or vertical appearances. *Horizontal bone loss* is evident when the degree of bone loss between adjacent teeth is similar (Fig. 17-8) and is seen often throughout the mouth (generalized).[5] A *vertical bone loss* defect, however, appears as a localized triangular radiolucency (Fig. 17-9). Bone loss also may extend into the space between the roots of the molar teeth, which is referred to as *furcation involvement* (Fig. 17-10).

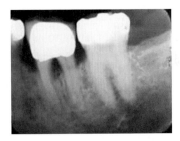

FIG. 17-9 Vertical bone loss.

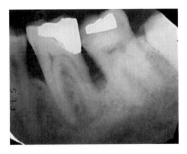

FIG. 17-10 Furcation involvement.

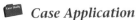 *Case Application*

In Mr. Courtland's radiographic series in Fig. 17-1 a pattern of generalized horizontal bone loss appears as an indistinct fuzziness of the crestal lamina dura. The crestal lamina dura is the most coronal portion of the alveolar bone that lies between the teeth.[5]

The bone loss evident in Fig. 17-1 indicates a history of periodontal disease. The active state of disease is determined by the clinical examination. During this examination, radiographs can be used to help determine the patient's periodontal classification according to the guidelines developed by the American Academy of Periodontology (AAP; see Chapter 15). Based on the clinical and radiographic data and the

guidelines located in Chapter 15, Mr. Courtland can be classified as having *generalized chronic periodontitis.*

Examination of the periodontium also includes detection of predisposing or contributing factors that can contribute to periodontal destruction. Faulty restorations, calculus, and malpositioned teeth can play a role in the progression of periodontal disease.

Case Application

Mr. Courtland's radiographic series in Fig. 17-1 exhibits an abundance of supragingival and subgingival calculus deposits seen as radiopaque areas interproximally along the root surfaces. A defective restoration can be noted on tooth #19, which can act as a haven for bacterial plaque and debris. This faulty restoration also may make flossing difficult, resulting in an accumulation of subgingival plaque in this area. Identification of such conditions is useful as the treatment plan is developed.

TREATMENT PLANNING

Developing a treatment plan for the patient involves close communication between the dental hygienist and the dentist. The treatment plan is developed for dental hygiene care and for restorative needs. This section focuses on the dental hygiene care plan.

Case Application

Mr. Courtland's clinical and radiographic evaluation revealed the presence of generalized bleeding, horizontal bone loss, calculus deposits, and interproximal caries. His health and dental history revealed treatment for high blood pressure with a calcium channel blocker and a smoking habit. Based on this information, quadrant scaling with local anesthesia is indicated. The health and dental history, clinical examination data, and radiographs help determine not only the treatment plan but also the proper preventive aids and techniques for Mr. Courtland. Oral self-care instruction in this case should include brushing with the modified Stillman's technique, use of a fluoridated dentifrice, daily flossing, and limited nutritional counseling. Because smoking has been shown to significantly increase both general bone loss and vertical bone defects in adult patients, a smoking-cessation program should be recommended for Mr. Courtland.[17]

PATIENT EDUCATION

Radiographs are useful as a visual aid to describe to the patient the extent and severity of that individual's current condition. After discussing the periodontal disease process and the effect that smoking has on the alveolar process, the dental hygienist should show the patient where the normal level of bone should be in relation to its current level. The radiographs can be used to describe reasons for the necessity of treatment, such as scaling and root debridement, by noting calculus deposits located below the gingival surface. Relating clinical data such as pocket depth and bleeding to the radiographic appearance of calculus and bone loss helps the patient gain a better understanding of the overall disease process and the reason the current treatment plan has been recommended. Radiographs also can be used to help the patient understand which areas may need added attention in oral self-care procedures. In addition, the dental hygienist can use radiographs to help the patient visualize areas of decay and faulty restorations, as well as calculus deposits and bone loss, allowing the patient to make an informed decision regarding the need for restorative, preventive, and periodontal treatment.

Case Application

Treatment
Quadrant or sextant scaling with localized anesthesia is the recommended periodontal treatment for Mr. Courtland. His radiographs were examined before scaling began to identify the location of calculus deposits and bony defects that require more extensive scaling, such as the maxillary and mandibular molar areas in Fig. 17-1. The radiographs helped the hygienist select the appropriate instruments for the procedure and were accessible during the appointment for confirmation of these conditions and to help differentiate

among calculus deposits, overhanging amalgam restorations, and carious lesions.

Evaluation
At the completion of all phases of the care plan, Mr. Courtland was placed on a 4-month supportive care plan. Vertical bitewings will be taken at appropriate evaluation intervals. The bitewing is recommended over the periapical film because it shows a more accurate view of the bone level.[6,15]

The guidelines listed in Table 17-1 indicate that selected periapicals and bitewing films should be taken on a recall basis for Mr. Courtland, who exhibited high risk factors for dental caries and a history of periodontal disease. These selected radiographs should show any remaining calculus deposits, new deposits, and new carious lesions. Examination of the radiographs, in conjunction with clinical data, will help determine whether the treatment was successful. If the periodontal condition appears stable, then Mr. Courtland will remain in the maintenance phase of treatment. If the condition has not improved or actually has deteriorated, a referral to a specialist may be indicated.

NEW RADIOGRAPHIC TECHNIQUES

A new technology used increasingly in dental offices is digital radiography. Radiographs exposed with the use of digital radiography are comparable to traditional radiographs in image quality and clarity. However, digital imaging greatly reduces the amount of radiation the patient receives.

The most commonly used system, direct digital imaging, uses a detector called a *charged-coupled device (CCD)* (Fig 17-11). The CCD receptor is placed intraorally in the same position that traditional films would be placed for a paralleling technique.[12] A standard x-ray machine is used with a low-exposure time setting. Instead of appearing on film, the images appear on a computer screen and can be printed or stored electronically.

Advantages of this technology include the ability to produce an image that can instantly be viewed by the patient and the dental team. Digital radiography provides the options to change contrast or color and to measure or amplify a specific area of the image.[1] Digital subtraction is used frequently as a diagnostic aid in endodontic and periodontal treatment. The digital processing method changes the light areas to dark and the dark to light, options that can help the dental team educate the patient and help the patient understand and accept necessary

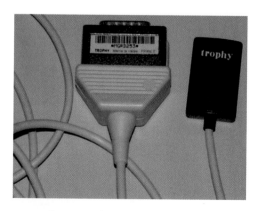

FIG. 17-11 Close-up of charged-coupled device sensor.

treatment. Another advantage of digital radiography is the reduction in radiation to the patient. Use of this technology reduces the amount of radiation received through traditional radiographic techniques by as much as 50% to 80%.[4] Other advantages include decreased costs associated with the purchase of dental film, film processing chemicals, processing equipment, and processing equipment maintenance. Digital imaging also allows the dental team to conduct remote consultations with other dental specialists because digital images can be transferred electronically to any location.

The primary disadvantage of digital radiography is the initial cost of equipment and set-up. The "average" figure for set-up and equipment is approximately $10,000 to $15,000 per treatment room.[3] Although this cost may seem prohibitive, it is offset by the cost savings in the purchase of film and processing chemicals, film storage, darkroom space, and labor. Another disadvantage of a digital system is that of a lack of infection control because the digital sensor cannot be heat sterilized; however, the use of barrier techniques prevent cross-contamination of the sensors. Patient discomfort during placement of the digital sensor also may be an issue. The sensors tend to be thicker than standard film and may feel bulky to the patient; impingement on the soft tissue and gagging are problems that may be encountered during the procedure. Concerns regarding the viability of digital radiographs used in litigation have become an area of debate. Because the image produced by a digital radiography unit can be easily manipulated, its use in legal proceedings has been questioned. To overcome this obstacle, major manufacturers have produced software within the system to indicate when an image has been altered.[3,4]

As major advancements continue in the area of dental radiography, technologies such as digital radiography will become an integral part of all future dental practices.

RITICAL THINKING ACTIVITIES

1. Select several series of radiographs from clinic patients and identify in writing the technique errors and pathologic process(es) in each set.
2. Using the radiographs selected in the first critical thinking activity, locate periodontal abnormalities and deposits and determine the AAP case type of each patient.
3. Determine a course of care a dental hygienist might take, given the conditions observed on each series of radiographs (those used in the previous two activities).
4. Given a case history and clinical findings, determine the type and number of films to be exposed according to the guidelines for radiographic exposure presented in Table 17-1.
5. Retrieve four radiographic surveys from patient files. Review the radiographs for the following:

   Density   Calculus
   Placement error   Bone loss
   Contrast

6. Using the radiographs selected in the previous activity (#5), what conclusions can you draw regarding the patient's history just by looking at the x-rays?
7. With a group of three or four colleagues, determine the patient protection in place in your school's clinic setting.
8. When a patient refuses to have dental x-ray films exposed, what is the policy your clinic follows? Role-play with a classmate and regarding ways you could address a patient's overradiation concerns.
9. Compare the radiographic criteria used by your school's clinic with those presented in this chapter.

REVIEW QUESTIONS

Questions 8 and 9 refer to the case study presented at the beginning of the chapter.

1. Which of the following are considered factors that affect the diagnostic quality of intraoral films?
   a. Exposure errors
   b. Technique errors
   c. Film selection errors
   d. All of the above
2. Your 1 PM patient is a 30-year-old female who exhibits good oral hygiene, has one occlusal restoration, and has no current carious lesions. According to the selec-

tion criteria guidelines in Table 17-1, which of the following would be an appropriate film series interval?
   a. A full mouth survey every year
   b. A posterior bitewing survey every 6 months
   c. A posterior bitewing survey every 12 to 18 months
   d. A posterior bitewing survey every 2 to 3 years

Continued

REVIEW QUESTIONS—cont'd

3. Your 2 PM patient received four quadrants of periodontal debridement 1 year ago and presents for a 3-month preventive care interval. Which of the following radiographic surveys would be appropriate for this appointment?
   a. A full mouth survey
   b. A posterior horizontal bitewing survey
   c. A posterior vertical bitewing survey
   d. A panoramic survey

4. Film contrast is due to which of the following items?
   a. The difference between the dark and light areas on the film and the overall darkness of the film
   b. The overall darkness of the film and the kVp peak setting
   c. The kVp peak setting and the exposure time setting
   d. The difference between the dark and light areas on the film and the kVp peak setting

5. Improper horizontal alignment of the cone results in which of the following?
   a. Elongation
   b. Foreshortening
   c. Overlapping
   d. Cone cutting

6. Which of the following results in a dwarfed image of the teeth and is caused by excessive vertical angulation of the cone?
   a. Overlapping
   b. Foreshortening
   c. Elongation
   d. Cone cutting

7. An overhanging amalgam restoration on the distal of tooth #19 may be a contributing factor to which of the following conditions?
   a. Vertical bone loss
   b. A periapical abscess
   c. Horizontal bone loss
   d. Condensing osteitis

8. A smoking-cessation program was recommended for Mr. Courtland, whose radiographs can be seen in Fig. 17-1, to help prevent or reduce which of the following oral conditions?
   a. Interproximal carious lesions
   b. Horizontal bone loss
   c. Gingival enlargement
   d. None of the above. The recommendation was made to improve general health only.

9. In Mr. Courtland's maxillary right premolar film in Fig. 17-1, the thin radiopaque line appearing above the roots of the molar and premolar teeth is which of the following?
   a. Zygomatic process of the maxilla
   b. Internal oblique ridge
   c. Posterior floor of the nasal cavity
   d. Floor of the maxillary sinus

10. Direct digital imaging systems use a detector called which of the following?
    a. Charged-coupled device
    b. Magnetic-coupled device
    c. Storage phosphor
    d. Both *a* and *c*

SUGGESTED AGENCIES AND WEB SITES

Because of the ever-changing nature of the Internet, some of the web sites listed here may have changed since publication. Please refer to Mosby's Evolve web site for the most current information.

Eastman Kodak Company: http://www.kodak.com

Kodak Radiography Series ("Successful intraoral radiography; Exposure and processing for dental radiography; Radiation safety in dental radiography"): http://www.kodak.com

Martindale's Health Science Guide 2001: The "Virtual" Dental Center: http://www-sci.lib.uci.edu

National Center for Dental Hygiene Research: http://jeffline.tju.edu

Procter & Gamble, Global Dental Resources: http://www.dentalcare.com

Pathology Services, Inc., 640 Memorial Drive, Cambridge, MA 02139: http://www.pathsrv.com

Teledentistry Network Newsletter, University of North Carolina at Chapel Hill, School of Dentistry: http://www.dent.unc.edu

ADDITIONAL READINGS AND RESOURCES

Bryan, JN: *Flash cards for radiology,* Anaheim, Calif, 1999, Bryan Edward [Bryan Edward Publications, 1284 East Katella, Anaheim, CA 92805].

Darby ML: *Mosby's comprehensive review of dental hygiene,* ed 4, St Louis, 1998, Mosby.

Nelson DM: *Review of dental hygiene,* Philadelphia, 2000, WB Saunders.

Qualtieri J: *Identifying anatomical landmarks on periapical radiographs; Mounting dental radiographs; Interpretation of dental radiographs* [radiographic series]. Charlotte, NC, 1998, Educational Software Systems [Education Software Systems, 6960 Forest Manor Drive, Denver, NC 28037].

Thomson-Lakey E: *Exercises in oral radiography techniques: a laboratory manual,* Upper Saddle River, NJ, 2000, Prentice Hall.

REFERENCES

1. Button TM, Moore WC, Goren AD: Causes of excessive bitewing exposure: results of a survey regarding radiographic equipment in New York, *Oral Surg Oral Med Oral Path Oral Radiol Endod* 87(4):513-7, 1999.

2. Bragger I: Radiographic diagnosis of periodontal disease progression, *Curr Opin Periodontol* 3:59-67, 1996.

3. Frommer H: *Radiology for dental auxiliaries,* St Louis, 2001, Mosby.

4. Haring JI, Jansen L: *Dental radiography: principles and techniques,* Philadelphia, 2000, WB Saunders.

5. Haring JI, Lind LJ: *Radiographic interpretation for the dental hygienist,* Philadelphia, 1993, WB Saunders.

6. Hausmann E et al: Effect of x-ray beam vertical angulation on radiographic alveolar crest level measurement, *J Periodontal Res* 24(1):8-19, 1989.

7. Herzog A, Paarmann C: Enhancing accurate assessment of periodontal disease by improving radiographic interpretation, *Probe* 31(4):130-5, 1997.

8. Horner K: Radiation protection in dental radiology [review article], *Br J Radiol* 67(803):1041-9, 1994.

9. Johnson ON, McNally MA, Essay CE: *Essentials of dental radiography for dental assistants and hygienists,* ed 6, Stamford, Conn, 1999, Appleton & Lange.

10. Langland OE, Langlais RP: *Principles of dental imaging,* Baltimore, 1997, Williams & Wilkins.

11. Mauriello SM, Overman VP, Platin E: *Radiographic imaging for the dental team,* Philadelphia, 1995, JB Lippincott.

12. Miles DA et al: *Radiographic imaging for dental auxiliaries,* Philadelphia, 1999, WB Saunders.

13. Nakfoor CA, Boork SL: Compliance of Michigan dentists with radiographic safety recommendations, *Oral Surg Oral Med Oral Pathol Oral Radiol Endod* 73(4):510-3, 1992.

14. Nesbit S et al: Comparing E- and D-speed film: the effects of various storage conditions on fogging, *J Am Dent Assoc* 126 (2):205-10, 1995.

15. Overman VP: Use of radiographs as an assessment tool with periodontal patients, *Access* 12:22, 1998.

16. Patel JR, Greer DF: Evaluating student progress through error reduction in intraoral radiographic technique, *Oral Surg Oral Med Oral Pathol Oral Radiol Endod* 62(4):471-4, 1986.

17. Persson RE, Hollender LG, Persson GR: Assessment of alveolar bone levels from intraoral radiographs in subjects between ages 15 and 94 years seeking dental care, *J Clin Periodontol* 25(8):647-54, 1998.

18. Platin E, Janhom A, Tyndall D: A quantitative analysis of dental radiography quality assurance practices among North Carolina dentists, *Oral Surg Oral Med Oral Pathol Oral Radiol Endod* 86(1):115-20, 1998.

19. Stephens RG et al: A critical view of the rationale for routine, initial and periodic radiographic surveys, *J Can Dent Assoc* 58(10):825-8,831-2,835-7, 1992.

CHAPTER 18

Nutritional Assessment

Cynthia A. Stegeman

Chapter Outline

Case Study: Effects of Nutrition on Oral Health
Nutrition in Dental Hygiene Practice
Effects of Nutrition on the Oral Cavity
    Hard and soft tissue formation
    Dental caries
    Periodontal disease
    Saliva
Effects of Oral Complications on Nutrition
Diet and Dietary Habits Contributing to Dental
  Caries
    Fermentable carbohydrates
    Physical form of fermentable carbohydrates
    Frequency of fermentable carbohydrates

Nutritional Assessment
    Health, dental, and social history
    Anthropometric evaluation
    Laboratory evaluation
    Dietary intake evaluation
    Treatment plan
    Evaluation

Key Terms

Ameloblast
Anticariogenic
Cariogenic
Demineralization

Disaccharides
Enamel hypoplasia
Monosaccharides
Nonacidogenic

Nonnutritive sweeteners
Nutritive sweeteners
Odontoblast

Polypharmacy
Polysaccharides
Remineralization

 ## Learning Outcomes

1. Discuss dental anomalies associated with nutrient imbalances.
2. Outline conditions in the oral cavity that create a reduction of food intake.
3. Describe conditions under which fermentable carbohydrates are cariogenic.
4. Assess the dental patient to determine whether nutritional care is needed and the type and amount of nutritional intervention required.

5. Develop strategies to provide the highest-quality health care that will lead to correction of the diet-related dental situation.
6. Evaluate the effectiveness of nutritional intervention in a dental patient.
7. Perform a dietary evaluation.

Effects of Nutrition on Oral Health

John Chen, a 14-year-old boy, has been seen for routine supportive care appointments since age 4. His health history is unremarkable. Throughout the years, his dental history has included several discussions on the importance of adequate plaque removal due to poor oral hygiene. His periodontal health has been acceptable, and he has not exhibited dental caries.

At the most recent supportive care appointment, the dental hygienist records 6 new areas of decay that were not noted 6 months previous, as well as several incipient carious lesions. On further investigation, John states that he does not floss but tries to remember to brush daily. His oral hygiene is fair.

John began high school this year. He thinks it is "so cool" to be able to drink sodas during class and notes that soda machines are present in almost every hall. He also carries a roll of mints to keep his breath fresh. On further questioning, the hygienist determines that John consumes 8 to 10 mints during the day.

Table 18-1 outlines information obtained from his 24-hour food recall.

TABLE 18-1
John's 24-hour food recall

Meal	Food and quantity	Location
Breakfast	5 Glazed doughnuts 16-oz. Chocolate milk	Car
Snack	20-oz. Soda	Classroom
Lunch	2 Cheeseburgers Large French fries with ketchup 20-oz. Soda	School cafeteria
Snack	20-oz. Soda 2 Small bags potato chips Mints (throughout day)	Classroom Car
Dinner	Medium cheese pizza 3 Breadsticks 16-oz. Lemonade	Local restaurant
Snack	3 to 4 Scoops chocolate-chip ice cream	Bedroom

NOTE: Did not brush or floss this day.

NUTRITION IN DENTAL HYGIENE PRACTICE

Nutrition has a tremendous impact in both oral and overall general health. Dental hygienists must recognize the relationship among dental health, prevention and wellness, and nutrition.

The oral cavity presents many characteristic abnormalities of nutritional discrepancies (deficiencies and ex-

cesses) during growth, development, and maintenance of oral tissues. Often, signs and symptoms of nutritional challenges first are observed in the oral cavity and used as a foundation to determine a diagnosis or medical cause. This chapter discusses the assessment process involved in the identification of nutrition-related disorders necessary to treat and refer patients to the appropriate health professionals.

The dental profession is in a unique patient-care situation. A patient may not visit his or her physician for routine physicals but may maintain intervals of regular supportive care. Dental hygienists are often the first to recognize medical abnormalities for which their patients should seek further medical treatment, making the dental hygienist an integral part of the healthcare team. Addressing that point specifically are the goals of any dental hygienist: to enhance health promotion and disease prevention and to provide comprehensive patient care.

Examples of oral conditions related to nutrition include soft tissue lesions, dental caries, salivary gland dysfunction, or ***polypharmacy.*** Disease states or conditions such as eating disorders, diabetes, human immunodeficiency virus/acquired immunodeficiency syndrome (HIV/AIDS), and the effects of cancer treatment are additional diet-related dental concerns. Dental hygienists are important information sources on general health for patients, including accurate and current nutrition information and information to dispel myths or fads. General nutrition counseling is a meaningful component of the comprehensive dental services offered to the patient.

EFFECTS OF NUTRITION ON THE ORAL CAVITY

Nutritional challenges change from decade to decade. Nutritional deficiencies can occur in a variety of circumstances—in medically compromised individuals during periods of rapid growth, in the elderly, in inner-city or rural areas of the United States, and in developing countries. Often today's nutrition-related complications are the result of overconsumption of food or supplements.

The oral cavity reflects many indiscretions related to an individual's nutrient intake. Table 18-2 presents a list of oral complications and links to nutrition. Growth, development, maintenance, and repair of oral tissues also are compromised because of improper nutritional balance. Periodontal tissues are metabolically active throughout life, and nutrients are regularly needed for such tissue maintenance. In many instances, clinical signs and symptoms of deficiencies or excesses are not noted until the problem is in an advanced state. An observant and knowledgeable dental hygienist can recognize subtle changes in an oral examination related to nutrition and work toward a solution before such changes become uncontrolled and/or cause irreparable damage.

In general, B vitamins (Box 18-1) are necessary daily, and a deficiency affects primarily the tongue and oral mucosa. Cheilosis, gingival hypertrophy, and stomatitis are other common occurrences from a vitamin-B deficiency. Deficiencies seldom occur in isolation but instead in combination with other vitamins within the B complex. Deficiencies can be a result of a low dietary intake; inadequate absorption or use; or increased body requirements, excretion, or destruction. Smoking, the consumption of

TABLE 18-2

Nutrition-related complications of the oral cavity

Nutrient	Deficiency symptoms
Thiamin (B$_1$)	Increased sensitivity and burning sensation of oral mucosa, burning tongue, loss of taste and appetite
Riboflavin (B$_2$)	Angular cheilosis, blue-to-purple mucosa, inflamed mucosa, glossitis, magenta tongue, enlarged fungiform papilla, atrophy and inflammation of filiform papilla, burning tongue
Niacin (B$_3$)	Glossitis, ulcerations of tongue, atrophy of papilla, cheilosis, thin epithelium, burning of oral mucosa, stomatitis, erythemic marginal and attached gingiva, loss of appetite
Pyridoxine (B$_6$)	Cheilosis, glossitis, atrophy and burning of tongue, stomatitis
Cobalamin (B$_{12}$)	Stomatitis, hemorrhaging, pale-to-yellow mucosa, glossitis, atrophy and burning of tongue, altered taste, loss of appetite
Folic acid	Glossitis with enlargement of fungiform papilla, ulcerations along edge of tongue, gingivitis, erosion and ulcerations on buccal mucosa, pale mucosa
Biotin	Glossitis, patchy atrophy of papilla, gray mucosa
Vitamin C	Odontoblast atrophy, porotic dentin formation, gingival inflammation with easy bleeding, deep-red–to–purple gingiva, ulceration and necrosis, delayed wound healing, muscle/joint pain, defects in collagen formation, petechia
Vitamin A	Ameloblast atrophy, faulty bone and tooth formation, accelerated periodontal destruction, hypoplasia, xerostomia, cleft lip, keratinization of epithelium, drying and hardening of salivary glands, impaired taste *Toxicity symptoms:* Hypertrophy of bone, cracking and bleeding lips, thinning of epithelium, erythemic gingiva, cheilosis
Vitamin D, calcium, and phosphorus	Failure of bones to heal, mild calcification to enamel hypoplasia, loss of alveolar/mandibular bone, delayed eruption, increased caries rate, loss of lamina dura around roots of tooth
Phosphorus	*Toxicity symptoms:* Poor tooth formation and bone demineralization
Vitamin K	Gingival hemorrhaging
Iron	Painful oral cavity; stomatitis; thinned buccal mucosa with ulcerations; pale-to-gray mucosa, lips, and tongue; angular cheilosis; burning tongue; reddening at lips and margins of tongue; atrophy of filiform papilla
Zinc	Thickening of epithelium, thickening of tongue with underlying muscle atrophy, impaired taste, atrophy of filiform papilla
Protein	Smooth, edematous tongue; angular cheilosis; fissures on lower lip; smaller teeth; delayed eruption; delayed wound healing; dental caries
Selenium	*Toxicity symptoms:* Dental caries
Fluoride	Dental caries *Toxicity symptoms:* Enamel fluorosis
Magnesium	Retardation in dentin formation, enamel hypoplasia, atrophy of ameloblasts and odontoblasts, enamel hyperplasia

Modified from Mahan LK, Escott-Stump S: *Food, nutrition, and diet therapy,* ed 10, Philadelphia, 2000, WB Saunders; Tonger-Decker R, Sirvis DA: Physical assessment of the oral cavity, *Support Line* 5:1-6, 1996; Davis I, Stegeman C: *The dental hygienist's guide to nutritional care,* Philadelphia, 1998, WB Saunders.

BOX 18-1

Water- and Fat-Soluble Vitamins

Water-Soluble Vitamins

B complex
    Thiamin (B$_1$)
    Riboflavin (B$_2$)
    Niacin (B$_3$)
    Pyridoxine (B$_6$)
    Cobalamin (B$_{12}$)
    Biotin
    Pantothenic acid
    Folic acid (folate, folacin)
Vitamin C (ascorbic acid)

Fat-Soluble Vitamins

Vitamin A
Vitamin D
Vitamin E
Vitamin K

large quantities of alcohol or caffeine, certain medications, and reactions to stress can increase the need for vitamins. A thorough evaluation of the patient's medical, dental, and social history can help identify an individual's risk factors for nutritional imbalance (Box 18-2), which will require close assessment by the dental hygienist.

HARD AND SOFT TISSUE FORMATION

The role of nutrition and diet begin with tooth bud formation, approximately 6 weeks in utero. Most structures of the craniofacial area are developed during the first trimester of pregnancy.[16] Even just one incidence of mild to moderate malnutrition during the first 12 months of life is associated with an increased risk for caries in deciduous and permanent teeth.[1] The systemic properties of nutrition continue until calcification is complete. Thus the development of enamel, dentin, cementum, and pulp are connected to dietary intake.

Vitamins A, D, and C and fluoride are among those nutrients considered important to preeruptive tooth growth and development. *Enamel hypoplasia,* delayed tooth

BOX 18-2

Groups at Nutritional Risk

Elderly
Dentate status
Medical problems
Polypharmacy
Psychosocial issues
Xerostomia
Osteoporosis
Low income
Individuals undergoing periods of rapid growth
Pregnant and lactating women
Infants and children
Individuals receiving inadequate calories or protein
Eating disorders
Long-term dieting
Medically compromised individuals
HIV infection
Cancer
Diabetes
Certain medications or polypharmacy
Alcoholics

BOX 18-3

Foods that Protect against Dental Caries

Cheese
Milk
Nuts
Products made with xylitol
Meat, fish, poultry, and eggs
Fat
　Butter
　Cream
　Cream cheese
　Margarine
　Oils
　Sour cream

eruption, tooth spacing, improper formation or atrophy of *ameloblast,* and *odontoblasts* that affect enamel, dentin, and pulp development, as well as resistance to decay, are common results of improper nutrition during craniofacial development.

Collagen is present throughout the periodontium as the principal connective tissue fiber in the gingiva, the periodontal ligament, and the major organic component of alveolar bone. Collagen requires protein; vitamin C; iron; zinc; and copper for growth, development, and maintenance. Defective collagen negatively affects the mineralization of enamel, creating structural defects of the teeth.

Mineralization occurs after collagen formation. This process involves the deposition of inorganic materials into an inorganic matrix and requires the nutritional elements of protein, carbohydrates, fat, calcium, phosphorus, magnesium, sodium, and potassium. Therefore the integrity of the entire tooth structure relies on adequate nutrition.

DENTAL CARIES

Although posteruptive nutrition has less of a systemic impact on tooth formation, nutrients do continue to support tooth maintenance. Systemic and topical fluoride help prevent dental caries in all age groups. Throughout the lifespan, fluoride is implicated in reducing the growth of *cariogenic* bacteria, inhibiting *demineralization,* and enhancing the *remineralization* of enamel.[6] Fat, protein, phosphorus, calcium, and sugar alcohols have local *anti-cariogenic* properties. These nutrients do not cause dental caries and may actually help prevent caries because they do not lower plaque pH. Box 18-3 provides examples of such protective foods.

Consumption of sugar and other fermentable carbohydrates is a significant factor in the progression of dental decay—not only because of acid formation but also be-

cause of the production of plaque. An increase in the consumption of soft drinks in the United States, particularly among teenagers, is responsible for a rise in the caries rate for this population group, as well as an increased risk of malnutrition. According to the National Soft Drink Association, carbonated soft drinks account for approximately one of every four beverages consumed by Americans.[14]

Case Application

As presented in the case study, John is a representative of the most avid consumer group for carbonated soft drinks (boys and men, ages 12 to 29).[8,24] From a health standpoint, John may be at risk for malnutrition. Sodas contain little to no nutrient value yet are high in calories (excepting diet drinks). The caffeine in some soft drinks actually interferes with the absorption of nutrients consumed in foods. Consuming a large number of sodas daily correlates with low consumption of milk (which provides calcium, protein, and riboflavin) and other vitamins and minerals that otherwise would be obtained from consumption of alternative, nutrient-rich foods.[9] In addition, carbonated beverages (diet or regular) reduce salivary pH, resulting in demineralization of enamel.[20] John's incidence of caries may be related to the constant "bathing" of the tooth surface in cariogenic carbohydrates.

PERIODONTAL DISEASE

Although inadequate nutrition alone does not cause a periodontal problem, it can be a factor influencing the severity of disease and wound healing.[5,18] Systemically, optimal nutrition is associated with the host defense mechanism, whereby the body can react more rapidly to healing and prevent or minimize infections. When a surgical procedure is required, an adequate nutrient reserve is essential for the individual to withstand the stresses incurred by the procedure. Nutrient needs actually can double in such situations due to blood loss, increased catabolism, tissue repair, and host defense mechanisms.

Another factor influencing the relationship between nutrition and periodontal disease is food texture. Soft, sticky, retentive foods cling to teeth and provide an environment conducive to plaque formation. Often such foods are carbohydrate-rich foods, such as bread or raisins. Such fermentable carbohydrates provide a substrate for bacterial growth. Therefore the role of the dental hygienist is to educate the patient on nutrient-rich food choices that do not promote plaque formation, as well as proper oral self-care techniques.

SALIVA

The development and secretory function of salivary glands are affected by nutrients, particularly vitamin A and protein. However, nutrient intake does not significantly affect saliva composition, volume, or antibacterial properties unless the patient is malnourished. The action of chewing and the taste of sour stimulate saliva flow, which is beneficial for control of the caries rate.

EFFECTS OF ORAL COMPLICATIONS ON NUTRITION

Inadequate nutritional intake or use can result from any inhibitive oral condition that causes pain or a reduced ability to chew or swallow food. Often individuals modify food selection and quantity to accommodate compromising oral conditions. Therefore maintaining optimal oral health is essential in the promotion and maintenance of overall health.

Poor eating habits, inadequate nutrient intake, sense of taste, and gastrointestinal disorders are associated with reduced masticatory ability.[3] The number of teeth, existence of a prosthesis, and/or function of the prosthesis often dictate food choices, particularly in the texture of food and quantity consumed. Individuals with such concerns often choose softer foods, which are frequently high in carbohydrates and low in nutrient value, simply for ease and safety. These foods adhere to teeth, encouraging plaque growth and creating an unhealthy oral environment.

When the taste buds responsible for sour and bitter sensations, located on the palate, are covered by a full upper denture, a decrease in taste sensations occurs. As the number of sensations for food (taste, texture, and temperature) decreases, the level of interest in eating declines, resulting in an increase risk of malnutrition.

In addition, xerostomia creates an unpleasant and often difficult eating situation to the extent that it becomes difficult for an individual to enjoy food. Functions of saliva include lubricating and moistening food to ease swallowing. A reduced salivary flow makes chewing and swallowing difficult. Without the protective buffering components of saliva, the individual with diminished saliva flow is at risk for increased incidence of caries and periodontal disease, just as the individual with a dry mucosa has difficulty removing oral debris. Xerostomia is most common in the elderly and is a side effect of numerous prescriptions and over-the-counter (OTC) medications.[4] Box 18-4 provides possible causes for xerostomia that the dental hygienist can use to further evaluate the patient.

A painful, sore tongue; oral lesions; inflamed gingiva; tooth sensitivity; and dental caries are examples of complications that result in a reduced ability and diminished desire to eat.[22] Box 18-5 identifies oral issues related to dietary intake. Poor oral health may be an important contributing factor of involuntary weight loss and compromised nutrient intake.[23]

BOX 18-4

Risk Factors for Xerostomia

Medications
Cancer treatment
Systemic conditions (Sjögren's syndrome, diabetes)
Stress and depression
Significant vitamin deficiency
Liquid diets (due to lack of mastication)
Dehydration

Modified from Davis J, Stegeman C: *The dental hygienists' guide to nutritional care,* Philadelphia, 1998, WB Saunders.

BOX 18-5

Common Oral Health Problems Associated with Food Intake

Glossitis
Xerostomia
Inability to chew or swallow
Inadequately occluding teeth
Temporomandibular joint (TMJ) difficulties
Infection or inflammation
Lesions or ulcerations
Pain or soreness
Bleeding on chewing or brushing
Caries
Tooth mobility
Dentinal sensitivity
Fractured teeth
Root tips
Prosthesis-related problems
Inadequate fit or lack of retention of prosthesis
Denture sores
Alveolar ridge resorption

Modified from Steinberg L: The impact of oral health on diet, *Nutrition and the MD* [newsletter], 23:1, 1997.

DIET AND DIETARY HABITS CONTRIBUTING TO DENTAL CARIES

The dental hygienist is the expert in the prevention and treatment of dental disorders. They become the primary educators in many dental issues that involve diet and diet behaviors and are alert to circumstances that may require collaboration with other members of the healthcare team.

Nutrition and dietary practices are the main ingredients for the development of dental caries. The presence of cariogenic bacteria in the dental plaque, the amount and quality of saliva, fluoride status, oral hygiene regime, and genetics are other etiological factors associated with the development of caries. When isolated, none of these factors significantly affects oral health. Only when all the factors interact can dental caries develop.

FERMENTABLE CARBOHYDRATES

Candy, cookies, soda, ice cream, and other food products containing sucrose can cause enamel demineralization;

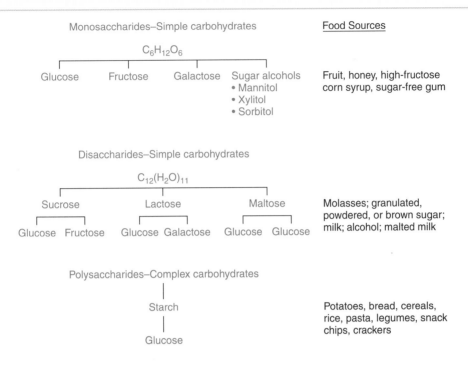

Monosaccharides–Simple carbohydrates

Food Sources

$C_6H_{12}O_6$

Glucose   Fructose   Galactose   Sugar alcohols
• Mannitol
• Xylitol
• Sorbitol

Fruit, honey, high-fructose corn syrup, sugar-free gum

Disaccharides–Simple carbohydrates

$C_{12}(H_2O)_{11}$

Sucrose   Lactose   Maltose

Glucose Fructose   Glucose Galactose   Glucose Glucose

Molasses; granulated, powdered, or brown sugar; milk; alcohol; malted milk

Polysaccharides–Complex carbohydrates

Starch

Glucose

Potatoes, bread, cereals, rice, pasta, legumes, snack chips, crackers

• Food sources metabolized by oral bacteria to produce acids.

FIG. 18-1 Fermentable carbohydrates. (Modified from Kandelman D: Sugar, alternative sweeteners, and meal frequency in relation to caries prevention, *Br J Nutr* 77(suppl)121-8, 1997 and American Dietetic Association: Use of nutritive and non-nutritive sweeteners [position statement], *J Am Diet Assoc* 98:580-7, 1998.)

this is a well-established fact. In addition, several other factors or behaviors relating to food intake must be addressed.

Nutritive Sweeteners

Creation of an Acidic Environment

All **nutritive sweeteners** and any sugar that contains calories have the potential to drop plaque pH to an acidic range, causing dissolution of enamel. Therefore **monosaccharides, disaccharides,** and **polysaccharides** are all considered fermentable carbohydrates. With the exception of sugar alcohols, each carbohydrate provides 4 calories per gram. A fermentable carbohydrate is any carbohydrate that has the potential to reduce plaque pH from neutral (approximately 7.0) to a critical level (5.5 or lower). Once pH is lowered, it remains at an acidic level for 20 to 40 minutes until the buffering capabilities of saliva return the pH to the neutral level. Dental researchers have defined a high-sugar food as one that contains 15% sugar by weight.[11]

Monosaccharides

Monosaccharides are single-unit carbohydrates (Fig. 18-1). Fructose, for example, is the primary carbohydrate in fruit. Unless eaten in excessive quantities, fruit is not cariogenic, with the exceptions of bananas and dried fruit. Because most fruits are fibrous, more chewing is required, increasing saliva flow and decreasing the chance for caries development. In addition, the high water content of most fruit can dilute its fructose. The exception to this statement, however, is illustrated in the individual with early childhood caries who sips fruit juice at will from a baby bottle,

a practice that permits the fluid to pool around the teeth for hours, producing an acidic environment and increasing the risk of decay.

Sugar Alcohols

Sugar alcohols (sorbitol, mannitol, xylitol) are nutritive sweeteners that typically do not promote decay. Each provides a small level of calories (1½ to 2½ calories per gram). Sugar alcohols are most commonly found in sugar-free candy and chewing gum. The use of sugar-free gum, especially one containing xylitol, has actually been recognized as **nonacidogenic,** that is, such gums do not raise the plaque pH to an acidic range.[10,12] The action of chewing, which stimulates saliva flow, in combination with the sugar alcohol promotes a healthier environment in the oral cavity.

However, because they contain calories, sugar alcohols can be cariogenic in some circumstances. One example of such an instance is the individual who experiences xerostomia and uses hard candy, sweetened with sugar alcohols, to relieve the dryness. The small amount of fermentable carbohydrate in the absence of the protective components of saliva can create an acidic environment. When recommending a product containing a sugar alcohol, the dental hygienist should inform the patient that such products may produce gastrointestinal distress and can have a laxative affect with as few as five to six pieces.

Disaccharides

Disaccharides are a combination of two carbohydrate units. Larger molecules of carbohydrates need to be hydrolyzed or broken down into the monosaccharide glucose before they can be digested and absorbed. Lactose, or milk sugar, is the least cariogenic of all disaccharides. The protective qualities of the protein, phosphates, and calcium lend milk its low cariogenic potential. As with juice, however, when milk is permitted to sit on teeth for hours, a cariogenic environment is created.

Polysaccharides

Polysaccharides are actually many monosaccharides, combined. A starch contains only glucose units. A starch molecule is large and cannot penetrate plaque. As salivary enzymes begin to hydrolyze starch to glucose, saliva can neutralize the acids easily. A cooked starch, such as instant oatmeal, is more readily hydrolyzed than a raw starch and lowers plaque pH, but at a slower rate than sucrose.[13] The combination of a starch and sucrose, such as jelly on toast, creates an even greater cariogenic potential than toast alone.

 Case Application

John had eaten glazed donuts for breakfast, another example of a combination of sucrose and starch, which contributes to his increased caries rate.

To label certain foods as cariogenic in all situations can be challenging because the multifactorial caries model acknowledges that an increase or decrease in any one factor can alter the cariogenic potential significantly. No food is cariogenic in all instances.

Nonnutritive Sweeteners

High intensity, **nonnutritive sweeteners** (saccharin, aspartame) do not provide energy and do not promote dental caries.[19] Saccharin can cross the placenta and has a slow clearance rate from fetal tissue. Although little research exists and its actual effects are unknown, use during pregnancy is not recommended.[17]

PHYSICAL FORM OF FERMENTABLE CARBOHYDRATES

The demineralization potential of any fermentable carbohydrate is most related to the length of tooth exposure, the sticky and retentive nature of the carbohydrate, and the point at which it is consumed, not just the amount of fermentable carbohydrate present in food or in a meal. Therefore some foods are considered destructive to enamel due to their sucrose content (e.g., soft drinks) but may not be as cariogenic as a food lower in sugar (e.g., potato chips).

The physical form (solid or solution) of the fermentable carbohydrate affects its cariogenicity. Typically, a fermentable carbohydrate in solution form, such as a fruit drink, is less cariogenic than a solid because it is readily cleared from the oral cavity. A drop in pH can occur within 2 to 4 minutes and last up to 20 minutes for liquids until the buffers in saliva return the pH in plaque to a neutral level. A softening of enamel can occur in as little as an hour.[20] A drink containing sucrose—such as soda, coffee or tea with sugar, sports drink—is even more damaging than fruit juice or milk.

Soft, sticky, or chewy fermentable carbohydrates are retained longer on the tooth surface and are therefore more cariogenic. The oral cavity can have a lowered pH for as long as 40 minutes with a retentive food, such as bread, raisins, or bananas.

 Case Application

A solid food with a liquid fermentable carbohydrate can be as cariogenic as a solid alone. Vanilla ice cream, for example, is cleared readily from the oral cavity (within 20 minutes). However, the chips in chocolate-chip ice cream, as consumed by John, can adhere to the tooth surface, creating an even greater cariogenic potential. In addition, the soda with the snack chips that John had as an afternoon snack is more cariogenic than the soda alone.

FREQUENCY OF FERMENTABLE CARBOHYDRATES

The point at which the fermentable carbohydrate is actually consumed is a second factor to consider in caries potential. A fermentable carbohydrate consumed as a snack alone, with no other protective food, is more harmful than the same food consumed with a meal.

 Case Application

The soda that John drank as a morning snack has a greater cariogenic potential than the same amount of soda he drank during his lunch. The protein, lipids, calcium, and phosphorus in the cheeseburger he ate for lunch provided a buffer to help neutralize plaque pH. If the soda, however, was consumed at the very end of the meal, then John would have gained little to no benefit from the protective foods.

The moment at which the fermentable carbohydrate is eaten during the meal affects the cariogenic potential significantly.[2] When a fermentable carbohydrate is ingested over a period of time, the number of minutes of acid exposure increases.[21]

 Case Application

If John drank his soda in the morning all at once, then he would have had only 20 minutes of acid exposure. If, however, he took the drink to class and sipped it all morning, the acid exposure would easily add up to many hours, leading to enamel demineralization. To determine the best intervention strategy for John's increased caries rate, an observant dental hygienist would question him further regarding his diet and eating behaviors. One example would be as follows:

Do you typically drink soda during your classes?

Consulting John's food record in Table 18-1, are there any other areas of concern related to the frequency of John's intake of fermentable carbohydrates?

Finally, fermentable carbohydrates consumed at bedtime are more cariogenic than those consumed at another time during the day. Salivary flow is reduced during sleep, resulting in less saliva to protect the teeth.

The goal of the dental hygienist should not be to eliminate all fermentable carbohydrates in any patient's dietary intake. A recommendation to reduce sugar or other fermentable carbohydrates is not effective and actually may lead that individual to select foods higher in protein or fat. Making the patient aware of the cariogenic potential of his or her existing diet, helping to modify the dietary intake, suggesting healthy snack alternatives, and recommending appropriate times to consume fermentable carbohydrates are considerations for patient education. Tailoring the information to the patient and changing the existing diet as little as possible results in a greater compliance rate, and thus a greater success rate. Above all, proper oral hygiene techniques need must be emphasized.

NUTRITIONAL ASSESSMENT

B-A
B-B

All dental patients can benefit from nutrition counseling. The goal of this section is to recognize those individuals at greatest risk for diet-related dental issues. To identify these patients and provide the highest quality and most appropriate care, the dental team must complete a thorough assessment. Analyzing the information provided ensures appropriate direction and helps prevent misinterpretation of the diet and dental situations. Fig. 18-2 provides a summary of this process. A nutritional assessment involves four basic components: a clinical evaluation, an anthropometric evaluation, laboratory evaluations, and a dietary intake evaluation.

HEALTH, DENTAL, AND SOCIAL HISTORY

A thorough health, dental, and social history notes risk factors suggestive of nutritional problems. A health history identifies those individuals with conditions that can lead to malnutrition, such as polypharmacy. Extraoral and intraoral examinations can detect such problematic physical signs and symptoms as malnutrition, dentate status, poor fit of dentures, and difficulty with chewing and swallowing. To gain further insight into dietary habits, the dental hygienist should ask open-ended questions to clarify or understand the patient's lifestyle. For example, the dental hygienist may have asked John from the case study how often he eats at home versus out and who prepares those meals.

ANTHROPOMETRIC EVALUATION

An anthropometric evaluation measures the physical characteristics of the body, such as height and weight. Most concerning is the patient who has unintentionally lost or gained 10% or greater of his or her body weight in a 6-month period. Other measures are either impractical or irrelevant to dentistry.

LABORATORY EVALUATION

Findings from standard saliva tests, plaque-control indices, and caries risk-assessment activities are examples of laboratory evaluations that can target those individuals at risk for diet-related dental problems. Biochemical tests, such as a complete blood count (CBC), although beneficial, are unrealistic in dental settings.

DIETARY INTAKE EVALUATION

The final element of the nutrition assessment process is to record a patient's food intake. Obtaining a food diary for 3 to 7 days allows a dental hygienist and the patient to evaluate individual food habits, consumption of fermentable carbohydrates, food preferences, and nutrient adequacy.

Case Application

Gathering data by patient interview and asking the patient to list the foods eaten the previous day is called a *24-hour recall*. John's case provides an example of this type of nutrition assessment (see Table 18-1).

Collecting data this way is easy, requires little time, and allows for an analysis of the foods. The greatest disadvantage is that a 24-hour recall only represents 1 day of food consumption and may not represent a person's true food intake pattern. A 3-day or 7-day food record, on the other hand, covers more days and is more representative of that individual's diet. The patient completes a food record through the stated period and returns it to the dental hygienist. Completing a 3-to-7-day food record allows patients to take responsibility for their personal health care by taking an active role. Dietary indiscretions are easier to observe when more days are recorded.

Analysis of Dietary Intake Data

Nutrient intakes from the diet history can be compared to a dietary standard, such as the United States Department of Agriculture (USDA) Food Guide Pyramid[7] and the Dietary Guidelines for Americans (Box 18-6).[15] The principles underlying these educational tools are appropriate for healthy Americans older than 2 years. Table 18-3 provides a comparison of the food intake of John from the case study to the Food Guide Pyramid. The results identify nutrition elements in which John is doing well and areas he needs to modify. When fermentable carbohydrate intake

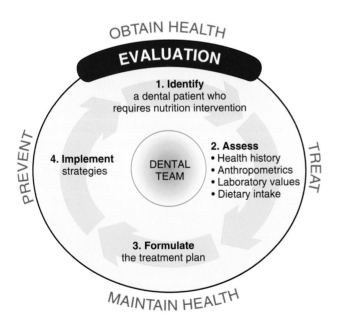

FIG. 18-2 Each of the components of the inner ring are to be conducted by the dental team to promote and encourage the components on the outer ring. Both rings revolve around the dental team. Evaluation is ongoing and is performed at each step.

BOX 18-6

Dietary Guidelines for Americans

Aim for Fitness
Aim for a healthy weight.
Be physically active each day.
Build a Healthy Base
Let the Pyramid guide food choices.
Choose a variety of grains daily, especially whole grains.
Chose a variety of fruits and vegetables daily.
Keep food safe to eat.
Choose Sensibly
Choose a diet low in saturated fat and cholesterol and moderate in total fat.
Choose beverages and foods to moderate intake of sugars.
Choose and prepare foods with less salt.
If consuming alcoholic beverages, do so in moderation.

Data from U.S. Department of Agriculture and Department of Health and Human Services: Nutrition and your health: dietary guidelines for Americans, ed 5, *Home and Garden Bulletin,* No. 232, Washington, DC, 2000, Superintendent of Documents.

increases the caries risk, as in the case study, the dental hygienist or the patient should circle or highlight these items on the food record.

TREATMENT PLAN

Once all the assessment information has been gathered, the dental team and patient can determine a realistic treatment plan that best suits the patient's needs. The counseling message therefore is tailored to the patient, and only information relevant to that individual needs to be discussed. This approach not only eliminates the standardized diet instruction but also increases patient compliance. Therefore each diet instruction is different.

Concise documentation is essential and provides a means of communication among members of the dental team. Documentation may include the patient's goal(s), expected compliance, and summary of the diet-related dental issue(s).

EVALUATION

At dental hygiene supportive care or other appointments, the dental team can monitor the patient's progress. The dental hygienist is there to support the positive changes

---

TABLE 18-3

Comparison of 24-hour recall to the Food Guide Pyramid

Food and quantity	Food group
5 *Glazed doughnuts*	5 Bread, fat
16-oz. *Chocolate milk*	2 Milk, sweet
3 20-oz. *Sodas*	Sweet
2 *Cheeseburgers*	4 Bread, 2 meat, 2 milk
Large *French fries*	2 Bread, fat
Ketchup	Sweet
2 Small bags *potato chips*	2 Bread, fat
Mints	Sweet
Medium cheese *pizza*	8 Bread, 3 milk, fat
3 *Breadsticks*	3 Bread, fat (if buttered)
Lemonade	Sweet
3 to 4 Scoops *ice cream*	3 to 4 milk, fat

Food group	Recommended	Actual	Comparison
Bread, cereal, rice, and pasta	6 to 11 Servings	24	Over
Fruit	2 to 4	0	Under
Vegetable	3 to 5	0	Under
Milk, yogurt, and cheese	4	10-11	Over
Meat, poultry, fish, dry beans, eggs, and nuts	2 to 3	2	OK
Fats, oils	Sparingly		Over
Sweets	Sparingly		Over

A comparison of John's 24-hour recall to the Food Guide Pyramid was used to estimate his nutrient adequacy and eating patterns. The fermentable carbohydrates are typically highlighted or circled. (They appear in *italics* within the table.) Note that all the foods John consumed this day are fermentable carbohydrates.

made, review material as needed, and revise or add goals. As with all phases of patient care, the evaluation process is ongoing.

Clearly, every dental patient can benefit from nutrition counseling. The members of each dental environment must determine a philosophy as to which patients are appropriate candidates for more intense education. Medically compromised patients require a referral to a dietitian or the primary care practitioner for nutrition intervention. The dental hygienist's role is that of an oral health expert who is part of a healthcare team. The dental hygienist can report findings related to positive or negative changes observed in the oral cavity and serve as an educational resource to others on the healthcare team.

RITICAL THINKING ACTIVITIES

1. Write down everything you consume for 3 consecutive days, including 1 weekend day. Compare your intake to the Food Guide Pyramid. In which groups are you within range? Which groups do you need to modify? List at least two realistic changes that you can make to improve your dietary intake.

2. Compare your lifestyle and eating to the USDA's dietary guidelines. Which guidelines do you follow? Which guidelines can you improve?

CRITICAL THINKING ACTIVITIES—cont'd

3. Interview a partner to establish that individual's intake from the previous day. Which questions did you need to ask to clarify the person's food intake? Circle the fermentable carbohydrates in red, and determine which aspects of each meal or snack are cariogenic.
4. Poll the class members at a local high school to establish the average number of sodas they consume each day. Provide education to the class concerning the nutritional issues related to increased soda intake. Brainstorm appropriate substitutions or alternative behaviors. To reinforce the topic, place an extracted tooth in soda for a week before the presentation and share the results with the class.

REVIEW QUESTIONS

1. Which of the following provides the most reliable data collection regarding nutritional intake?
   a. 24-Hour recall
   b. 3-to-7-Day diet survey
   c. Evaluation of food textures over 1 week
   d. Evaluation of times of carbohydrate consumption
2. Which of the following groups of foods are considered protective to the oral cavity against caries development?
   a. Cheese, milk, foods with saccharin
   b. Nuts, fats, foods with xylitol
   c. Milk, fruit juice, raisins
   d. Meat, fish, poultry, and peanut butter
3. Positive responses to which of the following items on a health history could indicate xerostomia?
   a. Depression
   b. Liquid diet
   c. Diabetes
   d. Medications
   e. All the above
4. Which of the following groups of individuals is/are at nutritional risk?
   a. Infants
   b. Elderly with osteoporosis
   c. Alcoholics
   d. Pregnant women
   e. All the above
   f. All except *a*
5. Posteruptively, which of the following is the most significant dietary influence on the development of dental caries?
   a. Fermentable carbohydrate content of the diet
   b. Overall vitamin content of the diet
   c. Mineral content of the diet
   d. Protein content of the diet
6. In which of the following ways can inadequate nutritional intake contribute to periodontal disease?
   a. Delays in wound healing
   b. Interference with collagen maintenance and repair
   c. Increases in bleeding on probing
   d. All the above
   e. Only *a* and *b*
7. Once consumed, a fermentable carbohydrate eaten alone can produce a drop in salivary pH in approximately which of the following amounts of time?
   a. 2 to 4 Minutes
   b. 20 to 30 Minutes
   c. 1 Hour
8. Once plaque pH has been affected by the resulting acid production of oral bacteria, how long will the lowered (acidic) pH remain before being buffered by the saliva?
   a. 2 to 4 Minutes
   b. 20 to 30 Minutes
   c. 1 Hour
9. Which of the following statement(s) concerning nutrition is/are true?
   a. Each dental hygienist should develop a list of cariogenic foods as a patient handout.
   b. Nonnutritive sweeteners produce dental caries.
   c. Nutrient intake has a significant impact on salivary composition.
   d. Sugar alcohols are never cariogenic.
   e. All the above
   f. None of the above
10. Which of the following numbers identifies a plaque pH capable of promoting demineralization?
    a. 2.0
    b. 5.5
    c. 7.0
    d. 10.0
    e. 12.5

SUGGESTED AGENCIES AND WEB SITES

Because of the ever-changing nature of the Internet, some of the web sites listed here may have changed since publication. Please refer to Mosby's Evolve web site for the most current information.

American Dietetic Association: http://www.eatright.org

American Journal of Clinical Nutrition: http://www.faseb.org

Consumer information from the Dental Hygienist Association: http://www.adha.org

Department of Health and Human Services *(Healthy People 2010):* http://web.health.gov

Ethnic food pyramids: http://www.oldwayspt.com

Institute of Medicine: *Dietary reference intakes for calcium, phosphorus, magnesium, vitamin D, and fluoride,* Washington, DC, 1997, National Academy Press: http://www.nap.edu

National Dairy Council: http://www.dairyinfo.com

Tufts University Nutrition Navigator: http://www.navigator.tufts.edu

United States Department of Agriculture ("Dietary guidelines for Americans"): http://www.usda.gov

United States Department of Agriculture ("Food pyramid" [United States and other countries]): http://www.nal.usda.gov

United States Department of Health and Human Services, consumer information: http://www.healthfinder.gov

Vegetarian Resource Group: http://www.vrg.org

ADDITIONAL READINGS AND RESOURCES

de la Torre M, Mobley C: Dental-nutrition case study, *Access* 13(6):50-3, 1999.

Morrison G, Hark L: *Medical nutrition and disease,* ed 2, Cambridge, Mass, 1999, Blackwell Science.

Russell R, Rasmussen H, Lichtenstein A: Modified Food Guide Pyramid for people over 70 years of age, *J Nutr* 129:751-3, 1999.

REFERENCES

1. Alvarez J: Nutrition, tooth development, and dental caries, *Am J Clin Nutr* 61(suppl):410-6, 1995.
2. Boyd L, Dwyer J: Guidelines for nutrition screening, assessment and intervention in the dental office, *J Dent Hyg* 72:31-43, 1998.
3. Brodeur J et al: Nutrient intake and gastrointestinal disorders related to masticatory performance in the edentulous elderly, *J Prosthet Dent* 70:468-73, 1993.
4. Davis J, Stegeman C: *The dental hygienists' guide to nutritional care,* Philadelphia, 1998, WB Saunders.
5. Enwonwu C: Interface of malnutrition and periodontal disease, *Am J Clin Nutr* 61(suppl):430-6, 1995.
6. Featherstone J: Prevention and reversal of dental caries: role of low level fluoride, *Community Dent Oral Epidemiol* 27:31-40, 1999.
7. U.S. Department of Agriculture, Human Nutrition Information Service: Food Guide Pyramid: a guide to daily food choices, *Home and Garden Bulletin* No. 232, Washington, DC, 1992, The Department.
8. Guthrie J, Morton J: Food sources of added sweeteners in the diets of Americans, *J Am Diet Assoc* 100:43-51, 2000.
9. Harnack L, Stang J, Story M: Soft drink consumption among U.S. children and adolescents: nutritional consequences, *J Am Diet Assoc* 99:436-41, 1999.
10. Jensen M: Diet and dental caries, *Dent Clin North Am* 43:615-33, 1999.
11. Kandelman D: Sugar, alternative sweeteners, and meal frequency in relation to caries prevention, *Brit J Nutr* 77(suppl 1):121-8, 1997.
12. Makinen K et al: Chewing gum and caries rate: a 40-month cohort study, *J Dent Res* 74:1904-13, 1995.
13. Mormann J, Muhlemann H: Oral starch degradation and its influence on acid production in human dental plaque, *Caries Res* 15:166-75, 1981.
14. National Soft Drink Association: *About soft drinks* [Internet], Washington, DC, 2001, The Association [http://www.nsda.org].
15. U.S. Department of Agriculture and Department of Health and Human Services: Nutrition and your health: dietary guidelines for Americans, ed 4, *Home and Garden Bulletin* No. 252, Washington, DC, 1995, Superintendent of Documents.
16. Pinkham J: *Pediatric dentistry: infancy through adolescence,* ed 3, Philadelphia, 1999, WB Saunders.
17. Pitkin R et al: Placental transmission and fetal distribution of saccharin, *Am J Obstet Gynecol* 111:280-6, 1971.
18. American Dietetic Association: Oral health and nutrition [position statement], *J Am Diet Assoc* 96:184-9, 1996.
19. American Dietetic Association: Use of nutritive and nonnutritive sweeteners [position statement], *J Am Diet Assoc* 98:580-7, 1998.
20. Steffen J: The effects of soft drinks on etched and sealed enamel, *Angle Orthod* 66:449-56, 1996.
21. Stegeman C, Carroll D, Schierling J: The battle of the fermentable carbohydrates, *Access* 12:38-40, 1998.
22. Steinberg L: The impact of oral health on diet, *Nutrition and the MD* [newsletter] 23:1, 1997.
23. Sullivan D et al: Oral health problems and involuntary weight loss in a population of frail elderly, *J Am Geriatr Soc* 41:725-31, 1993.
24. U.S. Department of Agriculture: *Nationwide food consumption survey, 1977-78; continuing survey of food intakes by individual, 1987-88, 1994-96,* Washington, DC, 1998, The Department [http://www.usda.gov].

CHAPTER 19

Intraoral Photographic Imaging

Lorie Holt

Chapter Outline

Theory
Case Study: Intraoral Images Enhance Treatment
  Acceptance
Types of Intraoral Photographic Imaging Systems
    Components of the 35-mm camera system
    Intraoral video imaging systems
    Components of intraoral video imaging systems
    Digital cameras
Selection Process for an Intraoral Photographic
  Imaging System
    Ease of use
    Image clarity and color
    Focus

Esthetics
Size and feel
Aseptic oral components
Expansion and upgrade capabilities
Equipment durability
Service
Price
Photographic Accessories
    Cheek, lip, and tongue retractors
    Intraoral mirrors
Photographic Exposures
Future Trends

Key Terms

Analog
F-stop (aperture setting)
Focal length
International Organization for Standardization (ISO)
Shutter release

Learning Outcomes

1. Recognize and understand the reasons for the use of intraoral photographic imaging in dentistry.
2. Become familiar with the types of intraoral photographic imaging equipment and accessories required for the documentation of intraoral anatomy.
3. Apply the necessary theory for exposure of intraoral photographic images.
4. Document intraoral anatomy with the appropriate intraoral photographic imaging.
5. Use intraoral photographic imaging to gather assessment information and develop an appropriate care plan.

*T*he latest technology in dentistry gives patients an inside look at their teeth and a better image and understanding of the condition of their oral health. For years clinicians have used intraoral photography in the dental setting for the main purpose of case documentation. With the development of new and improved equipment, intraoral photographic imaging (IPI) has taken on a new dimension in dentistry. IPI is changing the way clinicians practice. Patients today are more educated about and interested in dentistry than they were 10 to 20 years ago. They are also more interested in taking an active roll in their health care, including oral care.

The way in which dental hygienists communicate with their patients is often a crucial factor in treatment acceptance. Helping patients fully understand their current oral health needs is vital to patient acceptance of a comprehensive care plan, and IPI is one of the most useful, modern adjuncts to dental care available today. IPI can help dental professionals in their diagnosis, help patients visualize their oral health problems, help illustrate options during the treatment conference, and provide valuable documentation for dental insurance claims.[7,8] In this image-conscious society, the power of the visual aid as a tool of persuasion and education cannot be understated.

THEORY

19-A
19-B
Most of the traditional uses for IPI capitalize on one of the most fundamental benefits of intraoral photographic technology—magnification. Virtually all commercially available IPI systems have the ability to provide up to 40× magnification.[11] IPI enhances the practice of dentistry in the following ways:

- *It gives patients a sense of ownership of their mouth.* By taking a tour of the mouth, patients can explore the state of their own dental health, as illustrated in the case study.
- *It helps locate signs and symptoms of oral disease with greater speed and detail.* The visual presentation supports a higher level of self-awareness for the patient.
- *It facilitates patient education, which is one of the most important and fastest growing uses of IPI.* The use of IPI allows patients to take an active role in the care of their oral health.
- *IPI often facilitates enhanced patient acceptance of treatment recommendations.* It helps identify and visualize worn-out, leaking, or defective restorations; decay; aesthetic problems; periodontal disease; plaque and calculus; and other pathologic processes. The case described at the beginning of this chapter demonstrates that "seeing is believing."
- *IPI is an excellent aid that shows the condition of the patient's mouth before and after dental therapy.* It reinforces the need for consistent scheduling of professional care and adds value to the care provided.
- *IPI permits more accurate diagnoses with its improved magnification and increase in image detail.*
- *It aids in the development of appropriate intervention strategies because actual images of a patient's intraoral condition can be viewed.*
- *Videotapes of intraoral structures can be sent to specialists for professional peer evaluation.* This step helps with accurate treatment planning.

 Intraoral Images Enhance Treatment Acceptance

Sigorney Winston, a 45-year-old bank teller, comes into your clinical setting for the first time. As part of the patient interview, you learn that the patient has been told that she has periodontal disease but has not pursued treatment because she was not experiencing any pain. As part of the initial comprehensive examination, you take Ms. Winston on a video tour of her mouth. During this video tour, you recognize areas of the periodontium that exhibit disease. For the first time Ms. Winston can see the results of her disease process and is shocked. As you explain your observations and their meaning to the health of her teeth and gums, she becomes convinced that it is time to seek treatment. Ms. Winston agrees to the needed treatment and is motivated to comply with the necessary oral self-care to restore optimal health.

- *IPI makes the saving and storage of important patient documents easier.* This advantage facilitates paperless record keeping.
- *It aids dental insurance reports.* IPI objectively records intraoral conditions that may need further documentation to legitimize a claim or that may be difficult to describe in written notation.
- *Dental practices that use IPI are often viewed as being on the leading edge of dentistry and technology.* This advantage goes a long way toward building a practice and increasing patient satisfaction.*

TYPES OF INTRAORAL PHOTOGRAPHIC IMAGING SYSTEMS

A number of different camera systems are available today that can be used in dental practice. Camera systems range from the traditional 35-mm intraoral camera to the latest in computer-generated, video imaging, and digital imaging systems.

The 35-mm intraoral camera has been the gold standard in dentistry for many years (Fig. 19-1). Initially, 35-mm intraoral cameras were cumbersome and sometimes difficult to use; however, the newer 35-mm cameras are designed to provide an all-in-one system for highly detailed intraoral photographic images. All functions of the camera, from film advancement to film rewind and **shutter release,** are performed electronically, allowing the user to take excellent intraoral images without changing camera settings.

COMPONENTS OF THE 35-MM CAMERA SYSTEM

Lens

Every great photograph starts with the camera's lens. Because the lens transmits the image to the film, it is the single most important part of a camera. The 105-mm

---

*References 1, 3, 6, 9, 10, 12.

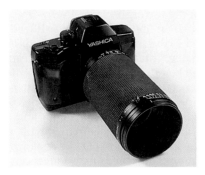

FIG. 19-1 A 35-mm camera. (Courtesy Kyocera Optics, Inc., Somerset, N.J.)

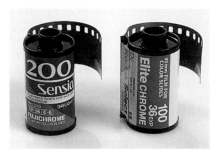

FIG. 19-2 ISO 100 or 200 film.

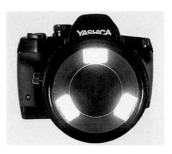

FIG. 19-3 Ringlight flash. (Courtesy Kyocera Optics, Inc., Somerset, N.J.)

macro lens is the best *focal length* lens for close-up clinical photography. The longer focal length permits a better working distance from the subject, thereby making intraoral posterior photography easier for the clinician and more comfortable for the patient. This lens length allows an appropriate distance between the camera and the sterile environment. Most importantly, the lens yields distortion-free facial photography.

Shutter Release

The shutter speed is the period of time the shutter remains open; thus the speed determines the amount of light that strikes the film. The higher the shutter speed, the more efficiently it "stops" the action of the subject. The typical shutter release speed for IPI is 1/800 to 1/10,000. The shutter needs to be open long enough so that the entire piece of film is uncovered at the same time. The newer-generation 35-mm cameras have the shutter speed automated so that adjustment is not needed during the taking of intraoral photographs.

F-Stop (Aperture Setting)

The *F-stop,* or *aperture setting,* is important because it determines the depth of field, or the areas of the image in which all objects are in focus. The smaller the aperture opening is, the greater the depth of field. The largest F-stop number indicates the smallest aperture opening. The F-stops usually range from F-4 (a wide opening) to F-32 (a small opening). Again, with the automated 35-mm cameras, this feature is preset to facilitate IPI.

Film

Photographic film is given an *International Organization for Standardization (ISO)* number, which refers to its light sensitivity. This term describes the amount of time the film needs to be exposed to light to create a high-quality image and is also called the *film speed.* Exposure is based on time and intensity. A fast film with a high ISO number, such as 1000, indicates that the film is extremely sensitive to light. These types of film are not necessary to take intraoral photographs. The typical film speed for IPI is 100 or 200 ISO (Fig. 19-2).

When intraoral photographic images are taken that are to be processed as slides versus color prints, Ektachrome-

or Kodachrome-type film is necessary. Film with the suffix *chrome* indicates that it is a slide film. Ektachrome slide film is easily processed; however, the processing of Kodachrome film is involved, and few laboratories actually process it.

Flash

Appropriate lighting can make all the difference in the quality of intraoral photographs. The direction and power of the light in IPI play a crucial role in determining the contrast of the intraoral image to the background. Light sources can vary in IPI from a single-point source flash on the top of the camera, to a ringlight surrounding the lens of the camera, or a combination of the two. The ringlight is a shadowless light that is called a *true clinical light* because it illuminates the entire area (Fig. 19-3). The ringlight reveals the total subject without any shadows and is best used for posterior intraoral pictures, intraoral mirror pictures, and pathologic photography. A point-source light flash, located on the end of the lens, is a shadow-casting light, and it can be rotated 360 degrees (Fig. 19-4). Pointlight creates a shadow on the subject that reveals topography, shape, and contour. It is best used for shape and profile pictures; orthodontic anterior views; or wherever shape, contour, and depth of the subject are of greatest importance.

INTRAORAL VIDEO IMAGING SYSTEMS

Intraoral video imaging systems have been used in dentistry since the early 1990s. These systems usually consist of a microcamera, typically in the shape of a wand, that can be held like a hand instrument and can be positioned in the mouth to take images of the oral cavity. The images can be viewed on a monitor, stored on a computer disk, or printed on a hard copy. Until recently, all intraoral video imaging systems were based on ***analog*** technology, allowing images to either be displayed on a monitor or printed. Analog imaging systems produce a continuous video signal that can be controlled with mechanical buttons, switches, and/or dials and viewed on any television monitor (Fig. 19-5). These first-generation analog systems can be used to either display full-motion or still (frozen) images on a video monitor. The images can be displayed in either a single-frame (Fig. 19-6) or four-plex format (Fig. 19-7). To permanently store an analog image, either a print must be made or the image must be stored on a videotape or a video floppy disk. Saving the images electronically involves conversion of the image to a digital format through the use of specialized software. Images then can be reviewed on floppy disks with a still video recorder. Images must be labeled, stored, and tracked. The inconvenience of analog storage in this particular camera should be considered before purchase for use in the dental office.

Second-generation intraoral imaging systems have typically been identified as digital or computerized systems but are actually a hybrid between analog and digital technology. The video camera itself remains the same and is essentially an analog system, but the analog output is fed into a computer that contains a video capture board. These systems provide benefits in the storage, organization, and refining of clinical images but require a computer to acquire the images.[4] The use of the digital/analog intraoral video imaging system requires the clinician to attain a minimal level of competence with the patient record software before learning how to use its camera. Once this level of expertise is attained, the clinician can concentrate on using the camera and not on operating the software. Thus the current digital/analog video imaging systems contain two components—the patient record software and the camera. Unlike the analog video imaging systems, the digital/analog systems are designed to store high-quality images, making the storage of images convenient. The computer can automatically "label" the image

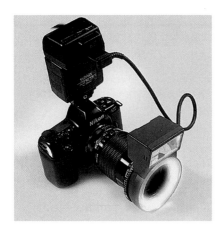

FIG. 19-4 Pointlight flash on the end of lens (shadow-casting lens). (Courtesy Dine Corporation, Palm Beach Gardens, Fla.)

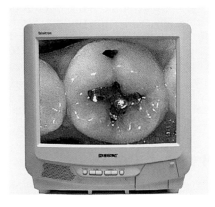

FIG. 19-6 Single-frame intraoral video image.

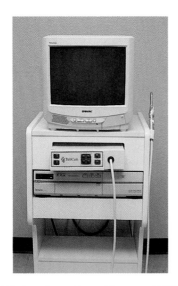

FIG. 19-5 Full-view Accu-Cam. (Courtesy TeliCam, Westlake Village, Calif.)

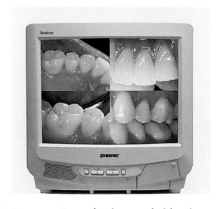

FIG. 19-7 Four-plex intraoral video image.

and permanently store it on a computer, thus simplifying the storage of intraoral images that document diseases and/or treatments and helping to create a paperless documenting system.

COMPONENTS OF INTRAORAL VIDEO IMAGING SYSTEMS

Camera

The microcamera itself is contained within a slender handpiece in the shape of a wand. One or more handpieces may come with the video imaging system. Some handpieces are designed with interchangeable adapter heads that allow different views to be captured. The different handpiece adapters provide various angles of view. The most common is the 0-degree handpiece, which is useful for both extraoral and intraoral images[5] (Fig. 19-8).

Lighting

System-supplemental light sources are located within the handpiece of the imaging system. The in-handpiece light is typically lightweight and thermally cool.

Automatic Iris

The light that enters the intraoral video imaging camera is automatically regulated. Because intraoral lighting conditions vary, cameras that automatically adjust are better and easier than those requiring the dentist to constantly adjust the iris setting.

Focusing Mechanism and Depth of Field

The distance from the lens at which all objects appear to be in focus is called the *depth of field*. The camera's optics, lenses, and iris opening determine the depth of field. Most intraoral video imaging systems require the clinician to focus the camera. Focusing is typically achieved through adjustment of a focal-length control ring on the wand handpiece (see Fig. 19-8). Focal depth values are usually preadjusted at the factory for maximal clarity of intraoral images.

Monitor

The monitor should be of adequate size to allow for easy viewing. The monitor size is often dictated by the availability of storage space.

Printer

For analog intraoral camera systems, the printer serves as the central storage area. It determines whether a system shows or prints a single image or multiple side-by-side images. The capture and manipulation of an image (freezing and printing) requires control of the printer. A foot pedal or voice-activated control are used for this purpose. Although the voice-activated controls are easier to use, voice recognition can pose problems in some models. The digital/analog camera systems require only that the image be saved to the computer system. Printing a hard copy of the image can be done at the clinician's discretion.

DIGITAL CAMERAS

Image capture in the consumer industry has led to yet another option for the expansion and development of IPI technology in dentistry—the use of a self-contained, portable digital camera (Fig. 19-9). Although many of the self-contained digital cameras used today for dental purposes lack high-quality facial and intraoral imaging, the technology is advancing rapidly. These digital cameras are not attached to a computer and are therefore highly portable. They use 1 to 4 megabytes (MB) of internal memory or a removable personal computer (PC) card for image storage.[4] Although convenient to use, wireless cameras are somewhat subject to electronic interference from other dental equipment and fluorescent lights, often making them unreliable in the dental office.

With the growing popularity of digital video cameras and readily available economical "digitizing" tools and storage media, the move toward a totally digital networking system is gaining momentum. The major benefits of digital cameras are their potential for easy and simple storage and retrieval. Although digital technology is expensive, vast improvements in digital camera technologies and lower prices are expected in the future.

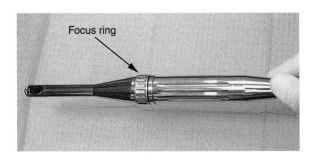

FIG. 19-8 Video wand and focus ring.

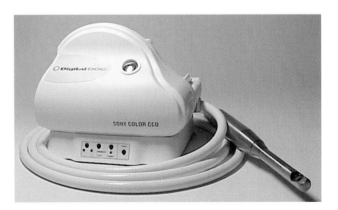

FIG. 19-9 Digital Doc wireless camera. (Courtesy Digital Doc, Inc., El Dorado Hills, Calif.)

Case Application

A digital video camera was used to show Ms. Winston the areas of concern in her mouth. This "real time" look was very revealing to Ms. Winston.

SELECTION PROCESS FOR AN INTRAORAL PHOTOGRAPHIC IMAGING SYSTEM

Although numerous intraoral video imaging systems with multiple functions seem to do everything, these cameras can often be complicated and difficult to use. Selecting an appropriate intraoral video imaging system for your needs is essential. The qualities discussed in the following sections are important is the decision-making process.[2]

EASE OF USE

A camera that is difficult to operate often gathers dust in the corner of the treatment room. User-friendliness is critical to realize the full range of benefits of IPI-device ownership. In-office training for all staff members often is necessary to ensure effective use of the equipment.

IMAGE CLARITY AND COLOR

Quality is key in the search for small fracture lines and areas of decay. Sharp images and color trueness are qualities to look for in an IPI device.

FOCUS

The camera lens should have a 1-mm-to-infinity focal range with good depth of field. In addition, the focal distance should be flexible enough to accommodate all the different views.

ESTHETICS

The patient's focus is often on the system itself. An IPI system that has clean lines, is easy to maintain, and is aesthetically pleasing gives the patient a sense of confidence about the equipment.

SIZE AND FEEL

The handpiece should be weighted and balanced so that it is comfortable to hold. Items such as external mirrors, extraneous gadgets, or anything else that could make the device awkward to use should be minimized.

ASEPTIC ORAL COMPONENTS

Appropriate infection control precautions should be taken. Typically, either autoclavable metal casings or, more commonly, disposable plastic sheaths are used.

EXPANSION AND UPGRADE CAPABILITIES

A system will have a longer life in the practice when it is fully integrated into the office software and is readily updated as the practice's needs expand.

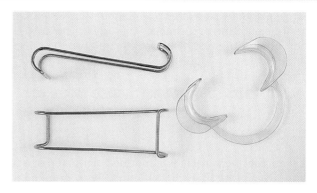

FIG. 19-10 Plastic and metal cheek retractors.

EQUIPMENT DURABILITY

Handpieces, cables, and other components made of solid, high-quality materials that are durable enough to withstand constant use add to the system's longevity.

SERVICE

Local service and support from manufacturers is essential to protect the practice's investment.

PRICE

Identifying a price range makes the choice of an IPI system easier. Because a wide range of prices exist for IPI equipment—with the traditional 35-mm system as the least expensive and the newer digital imaging systems as the most expensive—a practice can find a system that meets its budget and needs.

Identifying and prioritizing the various functions of the cameras considered are necessary. No single camera system fulfills all functions. Each camera has unique features, and different clinicians prefer different cameras for different reasons.

PHOTOGRAPHIC ACCESSORIES

CHEEK, LIP, AND TONGUE RETRACTORS

To improve visibility and establish a clear field of view for IPI, the use of various intraoral devices is often necessary to retract the cheeks, lips, and tongue. Cheek and lip retractors are available in a variety of shapes and sizes to accommodate most mouths. They are available in either clear plastic or metal and in either single-ended or double-ended styles (Fig. 19-10). All photographic accessories should be sterilized before intraoral use. Fig. 19-11 demonstrates various techniques used to retract the lips, cheeks, and tongue.

INTRAORAL MIRRORS

Intraoral mirrors often are necessary to capture an image of an area that is difficult to access (i.e., palatal aspect of the maxillary molars). Most intraoral mirrors used for this

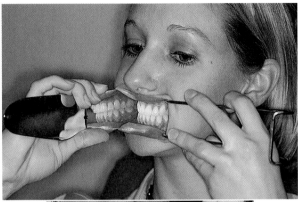

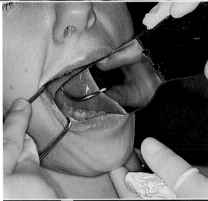

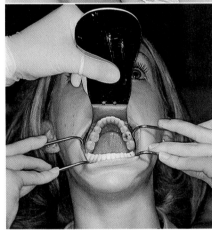

FIG. 19-11 Cheek and lip retractors in use.

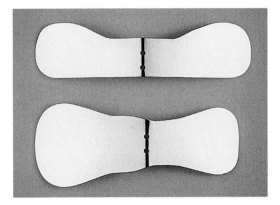

FIG. 19-12 Intraoral mirrors.

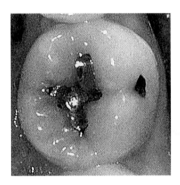

FIG. 19-13 Single-tooth intraoral image, as would be used when the clinician is focused on only one tooth.

needs. If the focus is on a single tooth, then only one intraoral photographic image may be necessary (Fig. 19-13). However, if a comprehensive set of intraoral images is necessary, then a series of approximately 12 images may be needed (Fig. 19-14).

FUTURE TRENDS

Dental practices have become increasingly sophisticated in their use of computer technology. As this sophistication increases, yet another generation of digital intraoral cameras will be developed. No longer will a camera be stored on a cart with a printer and storage device. Instead, the camera handpiece likely will be located alongside the air and suction hoses. Camera monitors will be located so that the practitioner and patient can simultaneously view the image. The camera will be connected via a computer network to the computer system, and, depending on the command given by the practitioner, images will be stored in the patient's records, printed at a central printer, attached to the bill submitted for third-party payment or retrieved for viewing. All these capabilities will be in every treatment room.

Questions have been posed concerning the possible use of notebook computers for IPI technology. Prototype laptop IPI devices have been developed that combine a camera with a computer the size of the older, portable computers. The laptop IPI system has the capability for

purpose are metal and have a highly polished reflective surface. Intraoral mirrors come in a variety of shapes to facilitate IPI in a wide variety of mouths (Fig. 19-12). These mirrors also must be sterilized before intraoral use. Fig. 19-11 demonstrates techniques used to take IPI with an intraoral mirror. If the mirror fogs, the clinician should spray compressed air directly onto the mirror and ask the patient to breath through the nose as much as possible. Intraoral mirrors are seldom needed when an intraoral video imaging system is used.

PHOTOGRAPHIC EXPOSURES

The number of different intraoral images required for clinical purposes can vary greatly based on the clinician's

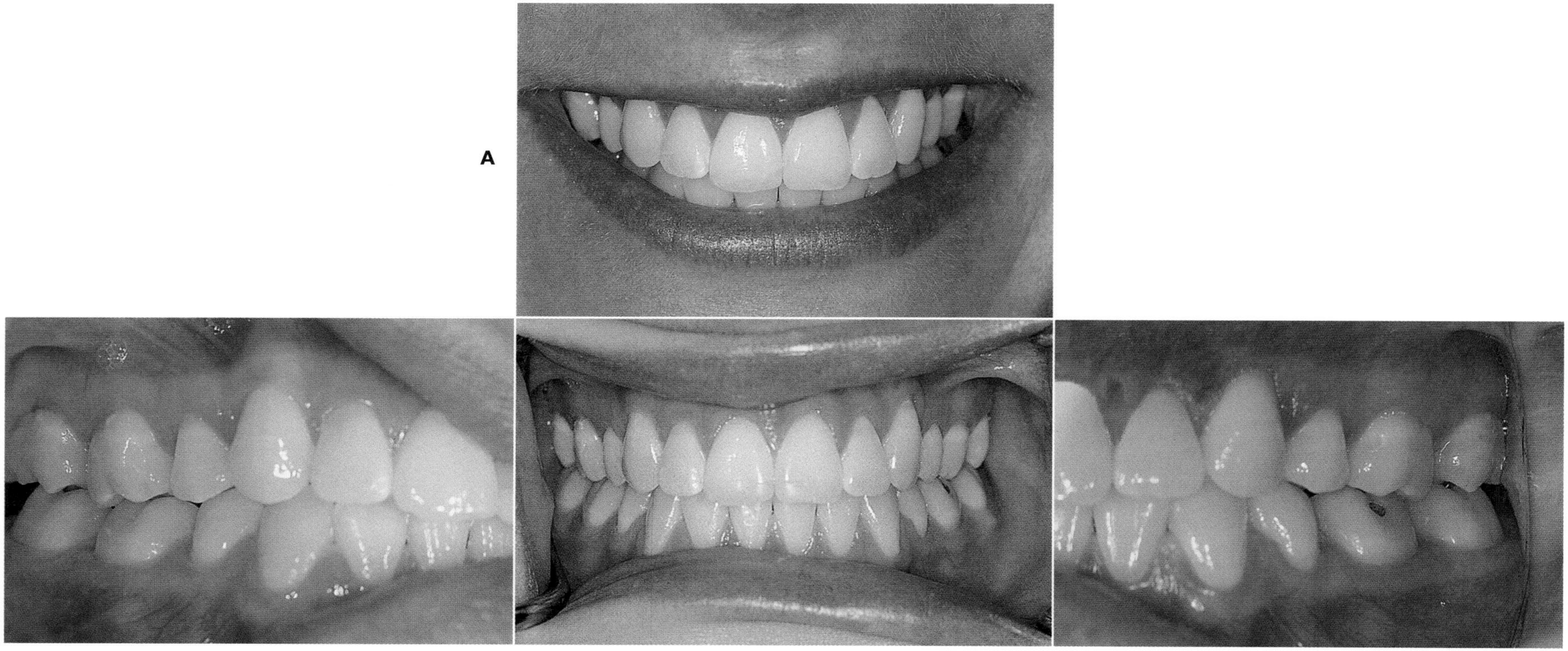

A

B, C

D

FIG. 19-14 Examples of a comprehensive set of intraoral images (set of 12 images): **A-D,** Facial views. **A,** Close-up of smile. **B,** Maxillary and mandibular right posterior facials. **C,** Maxillary and mandibular anterior facials. **D,** Maxillary and mandibular left posterior facials.

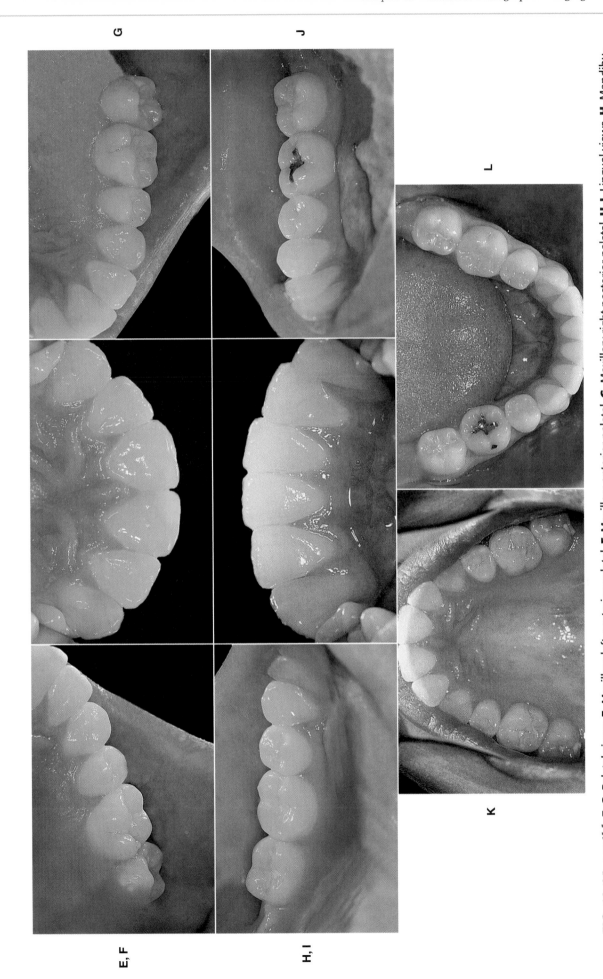

FIG. 19-14, cont'd **E-G,** Palatal views. **E,** Maxillary left posterior palatal. **F,** Maxillary anterior palatal. **G,** Maxillary right posterior palatal. **H-J,** Lingual views. **H,** Mandibular left posterior lingual. **I,** Mandibular anterior lingual. **J,** Mandibular right posterior lingual. **K-L,** Occlusal views. **K,** Maxillary occlusal. **L,** Mandibular occlusal.

real-time video display and can be attached to the delivery arm while the computer screen can be flipped down and out of sight when not in use.[4]

New advancements, refinements, innovations, and methodologies of IPI are setting the stage for a better and more practical product at a more affordable price. New and advanced systems continue to flood the market, and with each new product come different mechanisms of action and methods of application. Reading the manufacturer's directions will be critical to understanding how best to use these IPI systems in the dental practice.

 CRITICAL THINKING ACTIVITIES

1. Expose a roll each of Ektachrome and Kodachrome film. Compare the color of the oral tissues.
2. Work in groups of three with a 35-mm camera. One student acts as the patient; one operates the camera; and one places the intraoral mirrors. Each student should take at least three intraoral photographs; two should be mirror images. Practice placing cheek retractors and mirrors for each intraoral photograph.
3. Review intraoral photographs for technique errors and photograph composition.
4. Practice the placement of the intraoral video camera wand to achieve images of all areas of the mouth.

 REVIEW QUESTIONS

1. Which of the following is the most ideal lens for intraoral photography?
   a. 105-mm Macro lens
   b. Macro lens with bellows
   c. 55-mm Portrait lens
   d. All the above
2. Which of the following is the typical film speed used in 35-mm intraoral photography?
   a. 1000 ISO
   b. 100 ISO
   c. 200 ISO
   d. 400 ISO
   e. Both b and c
3. The pointlight is best used to capture which of the following images?
   a. Posterior images
   b. Mirrored images
   c. Orthodontic anterior images
   d. Any pathologic image
4. Which of the following is the major disadvantage in first-generation intraoral video imaging?
   a. Image clarity
   b. Image color
   c. Wand size
   d. Analog image storage
5. Adjusting the focus on an intraoral video imaging system is accomplished through which of the following actions?
   a. The wand's focal length must be adjusted.
   b. The focus must be synchronized with the light source.
   c. Focusing is not necessary, because it is done automatically.
   d. The adjustment depends on the model.
6. Selection of an IPI system appropriate for use would include a consideration of all of the following elements *except* which one?
   a. Cost
   b. Clarity of image
   c. Technical support
   d. Ease of use
   e. All the above

 SUGGESTED AGENCIES AND WEB SITES

Because of the ever-changing nature of the Internet, some of the web sites listed here may have changed since publication. Please refer to Mosby's Evolve web site for the most current information.

Dentsply: http://www.dentsply.com
Digital Doc, Inc.: http://www.digi-doc.com/
Lester A. Dine, Inc./Niamtu Imaging Systems: http://www.niamtu.com
The University of Iowa College of Dentistry, in collaboration with the Virtual Hospital ("A systematic evaluation of intraoral cameras"): http://www.vh.org
Yashica Corporation: http://www.yashica.com

ADDITIONAL READINGS AND RESOURCES

Dafoe B: Intraoral photography. In Woodall IR: *Comprehensive dental hygiene care,* ed 4, St Louis, 1993, Mosby.

REFERENCES

1. Baker CM: Introducing dentistry to the 21st century via the intraoral camera, *Dent Today* 15(10):94-95, 1996.
2. Blaisdell L: One practice's intraoral camera success story, *Dent Econ* 85(1):48-54, 1995.
3. Dresen B: A picture is worth more than a thousand words, *Access* 8(3):53-58, 1994.
4. Farr C: Intraoral cameras: dentistry's pursuit of wow, *Dent Today* 16(4):100-105, 1997.
5. Freedman G: Intraoral cameras: a tool for every operatory, *Dent Today* 16(4):106-109, 1997.
6. Johnson L: A systematic evaluation of intraoral cameras, *J Calif Dent Assoc* 22(11):34-47, 1994.
7. Levin R: Increasing treatment acceptance with the intraoral camera, *Dent Econ* 84(11):84, 1994.
8. Reis-Schmidt T: Intraoral video cameras show increased visibility and usefulness in U.S. general practices: survey report, *Dent Prod Report* 31(9):19-29, 1997.
9. Sagara J, Seltzer S: Motivate and educate patients utilizing your intraoral camera, *Pract Hyg* 7(4):52-53, 1998.
10. Tekavec C: Using your intraoral camera, *Dent Econ* 88(3):84-85, 1998.
11. Weisman G: Dental practitioners experimenting, broadening applications of intraoral video cameras, *Dent Prod Report* 32(4):154-161, 1998.
12. Woodall IR: *Comprehensive dental hygiene care,* ed 4, St Louis, 1993, Mosby.

CHAPTER 20

Supplementary Aids

George M. Taybos, Nelson L. Rhodus

Chapter Outline

Case Study: Role of Supplementary Aids in
    Diagnosis
Review of Examination Techniques
    Visual inspection
    Palpation
    Percussion
    Probing
    Auscultation
    Aspiration
    Diascopy
    Evaluation of function
Supplementary Aids
    Study casts

Tooth Sensitivity
    Dental caries
    Cracked tooth syndrome
    Pulpal disease
    Periodontal disease
Oral Mucosa
    Vital staining
    Biopsy
    Radiographic examination
Systemic Diagnostic Aids
    Anemia
    Bleeding problems
    Diabetes mellitus

Key Terms

Biopsy
Cracked tooth syndrome
Electric pulp tester
Endodontic lesion

Ethyl chloride
Gutta-percha
Insulin-dependent diabetes
    mellitus (IDDM)

Non–insulin-dependent
    diabetes mellitus (NIDDM)
Pulpitis
Vital staining

 ## Learning Outcomes

1. Determine the appropriate supplementary diagnostic aids needed based on a patient's subjective description of the condition and a clinical examination.
2. Correlate a patient's medical history to the intraoral findings and blood chemistry presented in this chapter.

3. Sequence the use of diagnostic aids based on a patient's condition.
4. Appreciate the role of the dental professional in promoting total body health.

The basic examination techniques are standard regardless of whether the dental professional examines the extraoral structures or the intraoral structures. The fine points of these examination techniques are discussed in greater detail in the chapters on Physical and Extraoral Examinations (Chapter 11), Intraoral Examination (Chapter 13), Periodontal Examination (Chapter 15), Hard Tissue Examination (Chapter 16), and Radiographic Evaluation and Utilization (Chapter 17). This chapter briefly reviews these techniques and creates a strong base from which to discuss supplementary diagnostic aids and techniques.

REVIEW OF EXAMINATION TECHNIQUES

VISUAL INSPECTION

Visual inspection is the thorough observation of the patient, beginning at the initial patient encounter and continuing through the interview and physical examination. The visual examination detects changes in the skin or mucous membranes or changes in the morphology of the musculature and skeleton. Intraorally, the visual examination detects the presence of plaque, caries, fractured teeth, fractured restoration, gingival inflammation, sinus tract drainage, and/or recession; however, of greater importance, the intraoral examination also detects any early squamous cell carcinoma.[1]

PALPATION

Palpation may be performed with two digits of the same hand (bidigital palpation) or through the manipulation of structures between the digits from both hands (bimanual palpation).[1] The dental hygienist feels and presses the structures to ascertain the following qualities:

- *Surface texture:* smooth, rough, or pebbly
- *Surface dimensions:* depth, shape, and contour
- *Consistency:* firm, fluctuant, or compressible
- *Temperature:* hot, warm, or cold
- *Functional events:* vascular lesion (e.g., bruit, thrill) and tooth mobility

PERCUSSION

Percussion is the striking or tapping of tissues with an instrument or fingers. The dental hygienist assesses the resulting sounds and observes the patient's response to the percussion. Extraorally, the sinuses are evaluated by percussion; intraorally, this technique assesses for periapical or periodontal pathology.[1]

PROBING

Probing is the use of an instrument during the performance of an examination. For the dental hygienist, the periodontal probe is an indispensable instrument. The probe is used to measure the depth of the periodontal sulcus. The dental explorer is used to detect carious lesions in the pit and fissure surfaces of the teeth, "open" margins around crowns, and, to some extent, interproximal carious lesions. The dental explorer and periodontal probe also confirm the presence of calculus. If a draining sinus is present in the oral cavity, a ***gutta-percha*** point can be

Case Study

Role of Supplementary Aids in Diagnosis

Mr. Banji Messina is 48 years old and overweight. His medical history reveals non–insulin-dependent diabetes mellitus (NIDDM) since age 42 that is treated with the oral hypoglycemic agents glipizide (Glucotrol) 15 mg bid and metformin HCl (Glucophage) 850 mg bid. During the clinical examination the following are noted: missing teeth #19, #20, and #30; attachment loss greater than 5 mm on the maxillary first molars; and extensive carious lesions on teeth #2, #14, and #18. With further examination a white, 1- × 1.5-cm lesion with a red ulcerative component is identified in the right anterior floor of the mouth.

placed into the tract, and a radiograph made, pinpointing the source of the draining infection.[1]

AUSCULTATION

During auscultation sounds in the body are listened to with the ear or a stethoscope. The use of the stethoscope to monitor blood pressure is obvious. The flat diaphragm of the stethoscope is used to detect high-pitched sounds. Low-pitched sounds are detected with the bell portion. Crepitus in the temporomandibular joint (TMJ) and bruits in tissues overlying vascular lesions are high-pitched sounds detected with the stethoscope's diaphragm.[1]

ASPIRATION

Aspiration is the removal of fluid from a body cavity. The area aspirated may be a soft-tissue lesion or a lesion central in bone. A purulent aspirate indicates an inflammatory or infectious process; yellow, straw-colored fluid is consistent with a cyst; a predominance of blood indicates a vascular lesion such as hemangioma; little or no aspirate may indicate a traumatic bone cyst or air embolism.[1]

DIASCOPY

Diascopy is the examination technique in which a glass slide is used to compress tissue. This is used to determine whether a lesion is vascular in origin. The glass slide is pressed evenly over the lesion. If the lesion is vascular, it blanches on diascopy and returns to its original color when the pressure is released.[1]

EVALUATION OF FUNCTION

Because the oral cavity is the site of numerous activities, the dental hygienist must be aware of these activities and assess their function during the oral examination. A decrease or compromised function of these activities may be the chief oral complaint for the patient: dry mouth caused by decreased salivary production, altered taste, pain in the temporomandibular joint, and difficulty in chewing as a result of missing teeth.[1]

SUPPLEMENTARY AIDS

20-A A variety of diagnostic aids are available in dentistry that
20-B goes beyond what traditional intraoral examination and
radiographs provide. To properly evaluate a patient's current oral health status or to provide documentation of a
specific disease, several of the following supplementary assessments can be used:

> Biopsy procedures
> Disclosing dyes
> Microbiological assays
> Pulp-testing devices
> Salivary tests
> Selective pressure applicators
> Study models
> TMJ images

 Case Application

As you read and study the supplementary aids presented in
this chapter, identify which items could be used to care for
Mr. Messina.

STUDY CASTS

Study casts, or models, are the most commonly used diagnostic aid. These reproductions of the teeth and gingival
and adjacent structures are also used as visual aids for treatment planning and patient education. The study casts not
only provide a permanent record of the patient's present
condition but also allow views of the dentition that are not
possible intraorally, such as the lingual, distal, and palatal
aspects (Fig. 20-1). Study casts provide observations of variations and departures from normal and a baseline from
which to assess changes during subsequent visits. Specialty
practices routinely use study casts to monitor phases of
treatment (e.g., orthodontic movement), presurgical evaluation (e.g., implant placement), and prosthesis design.

Most clinical practices use alginate, an irreversible hydrocolloid impression material, to obtain the negative impression for study casts. This negative impression is then
filled with a plaster or stone material that, when hard-
ened, provides the positive likeness of the patient's teeth.

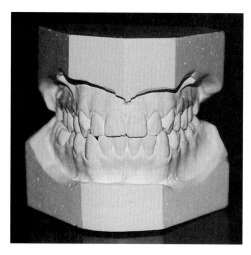

FIG. 20-1 A set of study casts used for diagnostic
purposes.

 Case Application

Study casts could be used to help chart Mr. Messina's missing teeth, gingival recession (if present as part of the attachment loss), and possibly the large carious lesions.

TOOTH SENSITIVITY

A patient with a sensitive tooth should be questioned as to
the stimuli involved, frequency of occurrence, and duration and type of pain. A sensitive tooth can indicate carious
lesions, *endodontic lesions, cracked tooth syndrome,* periodontal lesions, or sensitivity related to dentinal exposure.

DENTAL CARIES

Recognition of dental caries is accomplished by visual,
tactile, and radiographic means (Fig. 20-2). An intraoral
hard tissue examination accompanied by radiographs is
the best tool to diagnose caries. Thorough plaque control still remains the best method of prevention. Various
dental caries risk assessment methods and activity tests
are available, but these are primarily used as educational
and motivational tools to help patients realize the effects of an effective oral care regimen. These assessment
methods may include those presented in the following
sections.

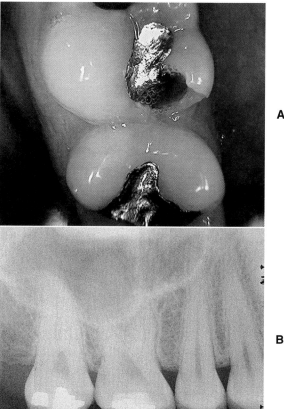

FIG. 20-2 Diagnosis of carious lesions with visual **(A)** and
radiographic **(B)** imaging.

Case Application

Note in Mr. Messina's case which methods would be used to detect his carious lesions.

Disclosing Agents

Disclosing agents are available as a liquid to be swabbed onto the dentition or as a tablet or wafer that may be chewed, swished, and then rinsed. Used either in the clinician's office before a prophylaxis or at home by the patient as a self-evaluation tool, a disclosing agent can help the patient visualize the location of plaque deposits.

Snyder Colorimetric Test

The Snyder colorimetric test requires the patient to chew a piece of paraffin. The resulting saliva is expectorated into a sterile bottle. The paraffin sample is then processed, allowed to solidify, and incubated. The sample is examined daily for three days, and color changes are recorded. Color changes from green to yellow indicate the amount of pH change, indicative of caries activity. Variations of the Snyder colorimetric test use either a wire loop or swab to collect saliva.

Salivary Reductase Test

In the salivary reductase test a saliva sample is mixed with a dye, and the color change is noted. The caries conduciveness is rated as nonconducive, slightly conducive, moderately conducive, highly conducive, extremely conducive, or caries.

Methyl Red-Plaque-Sugar Test

A sample of the patient's plaque is placed on a ceramic tile, covered with two to three drops of methyl red indicator, and then sprinkled with sugar in the methyl red-plaque-sugar test. Color changes from red to yellow indicate the degree of acid production.

Streptococcus mutans Count

A tongue depressor is used to collect saliva, which is deposited on an agar plate and incubated for the *S. mutans* count. The colony units are counted. A plaque sample may also be used. A comparison is then made by matching of the results to a predetermined scale of colony numbers and caries activity.

Salivary Flow

Similar to the collection methods used in the Snyder colorimetric test, unstimulated saliva is first collected and then measured during a specific time period. The test is repeated, measuring stimulated salivary flow. Results are compared, and a flow rate is determined.

Transillumination

Transillumination is an aid used to detect anterior interproximal carious lesions. A strong, direct light is focused on the labial surfaces of the anterior teeth, and a dental mirror is placed on the lingual or palatal surfaces. Defects in the enamel can be seen with this technique.

Laser Detection Device

Often, caries on the occlusal surfaces are hidden beneath the intact enamel surface. The KaVo DIAGNOdent (KaVo America, Lake Zurich, Ill.) is a new laser light system with a defined wavelength that helps detect demineralized tooth structure (Fig. 20-3). This device allows detection of a lesion without radiographic exposure.

Fluoride Level Detection Kits

Fluoride level detection kits measure the level of fluoride in the water supply and can be purchased or obtained through the particular state's health department. In addition, these kits may be available through the local dental office.

CRACKED TOOTH SYNDROME

To identify a cracked tooth, selective pressure is applied to the suspected cusp. To isolate the suspected cusp, rubber wheels, tongue blades, or orange woodsticks may be used. The patient's biting pressure reproduces the pain experienced while eating. Transillumination also may aid in the diagnosis of a cracked tooth. Light reflected from more than one direction indicates the presence of a fracture. If the fracture is deep, a disclosing dye penetrates into the fracture and visually reveals its presence.

PULPAL DISEASE

The status of the pulp is determined through the use of the *electric pulp tester* or by the application of heat or cold to the tooth in question (Fig. 20-4). When the electric pulp tester is used, the tooth must be dry to prevent the electrical impulses from being transmitted through the saliva to the gingival tissue. Most electric pulp testers require that the circuit be closed, which is achieved when the patient places a hand on the pulp tester wand. The electric pulp tester does not interfere with the activity of pacemakers.[3] Initial testing of a tooth assumed to be normal is recommended, allowing

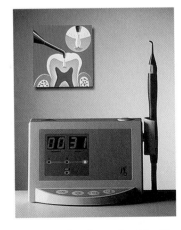

FIG. 20-3 The DIAGNOdent is used to identify subsurface carious lesions. (Courtesy KaVo American Corp., Lake Zurich, Ill.)

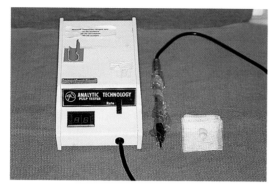

FIG. 20-4 The electric pulp tester is used to identify the tooth's vitality. (Courtesy Dr. Robert S. Gatewood, Jackson, Miss.)

the patient to anticipate the procedure to come. When the teeth are tested, the clinician should increase the stimulus until the patient reports a slight pain and instruct the patient to release contact with the wand when experiencing pain. Heat is applied to the tooth with a warm piece of gutta-percha, and cold is applied with either a piece of ice or a cotton-tipped applicator sprayed with *ethyl chloride.* In a healthy pulp the pain sensation disappears within five seconds after the stimulus is removed; a *pulpitis* results in persistent pain long after the stimulus is removed; a nonvital pulp does not respond to the temperature stimuli. The accurate assessment of the status of the pulp is difficult. Good communication and understanding between the patient and the examiner is required, and the results must be carefully interpreted.

PERIODONTAL DISEASE

Periodontal disease, similar to carious lesions, is most commonly detected through visual and radiographic examination. The American Academy of Periodontology (AAP) has recommended that all patients be screened for periodontal disease. The recommended method, Periodontal Screening and Recording (PSR) system, is designed to provide a quick and cost-effective means of periodontal assessment for every patient. A periodontal probe is used around all gingival crevices, and a scoring system of 0 to 4 is used to record the assessment. The highest score is recorded for each sextant; the test does not provide a tooth-by-tooth assessment for subsequent comparison but instead provides a tool to determine when a patient needs a full periodontal examination.

Case Application
Given Mr. Messina's periodontal description, what do you think his PSR score would have indicated?

Microbial monitoring of periodontal pockets can detect specific bacteria, which helps the dental hygienist select appropriate therapeutic interventions. Microbial testing methods currently available include the following:

Microscopic Techniques

Phase-contrast or darkfield microscopic examination of a plaque sample is an effective tool in plaque control assessment and patient motivation. It does not provide in-

formation related to treatment options but can help monitor the effects of treatment.

Culture Techniques

A plaque sample is collected, placed onto a transport medium, and sent to a laboratory for culturing. The culture is tested for its susceptibility to assorted antibiotics.

Immunological Assays

Enzyme-linked immunosorbent assay (ELISA) can detect specific antibodies that bind to selected bacterial antigens. The primary antibody is detected through colorimetric reaction. This technique is currently used in dental research and is not available commercially.

DNA Probe Assays

Samples are collected on a sterile paper point and sent to a laboratory where the strands of deoxyribonucleic acid (DNA) are split into single-stranded DNA. A single strand is marked or labeled with a radioactive isotope and serves as the probe. This strand is reintroduced and incubated with the other single-stranded DNA from the sample. If binding of the DNA probe occurs, it is detected through the marker, and the organism is identified.

Enzyme-Based Assays

Benzol-arginine naphthylamide (BANA) detects an enzyme produced primarily by *Porphyromonas gingivalis, Treponema denticola,* and *Bacteriodes forsythus.* The reaction of the plaque sample to the colorimetric substrate is proportional to the concentration of these bacterial species found in the plaque sample.

Evaluation techniques, including clinical and technological methods for the assessment of the periodontium's condition, are presented in Chapter 15.

ORAL MUCOSA

The diagnosis of oral lesions requires review of the patient's comprehensive health history, including lesion and social histories (i.e., use of tobacco and alcohol, sexually transmitted diseases, and human immunodeficiency virus [HIV]). Visual examination and palpation of the lesion provide important diagnostic information.

VITAL STAINING

Vital staining of the lesion is performed with toluidine blue, a dye that stains the nuclear and intracellular material of neoplastic cells but not normal cells. Penetration of the dye through many layers of haphazardly arranged neoplastic cells also results in staining of a neoplasia. Using this dye may reveal oral neoplasms not detected by visual examination. The diagnostic value of vital staining lies in its immediate reinforcement to your clinical suspicion. Vital staining also serves as a locator for neoplastic cells in a diffuse area of erythroplakia. This identifies the "best" area to biopsy. A strong clinical suspicion mandates a biopsy regardless of the results of the vital staining. Box 20-1 describes the vital staining technique.

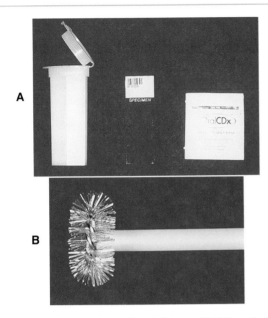

FIG. 20-5 The Oral CDx brush biopsy kit **(A)** and close-up of the brush contained in the kit used to obtain a tissue sample **(B)**.

Technique for Vital Staining

1. Rinse the mouth twice with water for 20 seconds.
2. Rinse the mouth vigorously with 1% acetic acid for 20 seconds.
3. Gently dry the areas with gauze.
4. Apply the 1% toluidine blue vital stain to the lesion.
5. Rinse with the acetic acid solution for 1 minute to remove the excess stain.
6. Rinse with water.

BIOPSY

A *biopsy* is a surgical procedure that removes tissue for the purpose of microscopic examination. The biopsy specimen must contain a representative sample of the lesion. Vital staining may help identify the area of the lesion with neoplastic activity. The biopsy may be either incisional where only a portion of the lesion is removed or excisional where the entire lesion is removed.

The oral brush biopsy technique was developed to assist healthcare providers in the identification of the early stages of oral cancer. This procedure is performed with the use of the Oral CDx kit (Oral Scan Laboratories, Inc., Suffern, N.Y.; Fig. 20-5). Box 20-2 outlines the necessary steps of the oral brush biopsy technique. The laboratory classifies the specimens into one of four categories: (1) *negative,* or no epithelial abnormality; (2) *atypical,* or abnormal epithelial changes of uncertain diagnostic significance; (3) *positive,* or definitive cellular evidence of epithelial dysplasia or carcinoma; or (4) *inadequate,* or incomplete transepithelial biopsy specimen. The sensitivity rate, defined as a measure of the likelihood that a patient with dysplasia or carcinoma will have an abnormal Oral CDx result, is 100%. The specificity rates, defined as a measure of the

BOX 20-2

Technique for Oral Brush Biopsy

1. Place the sterile brush against the surface of the lesion.
2. With firm pressure, rotate the brush five to ten times. The tissue should appear pink or demonstrate pinpoint bleeding.
3. Transfer the sample of cells to the glass slide.
4. Flood the sample with the fixative agent.
5. Place the dried slide in the plastic container and mail to the appropriate laboratory for computerized image analysis.

likelihood that a patient with a lesion determined to be benign by histology will not have an abnormal Oral CDx result, are 100% for positive results and 92.9% for atypical Oral CDx results. The Oral CDx brush biopsy is not a substitute for a histological examination; it identifies oral lesions that require the histological examination.[4]

 Case Application

Would a brush biopsy be appropriate for Mr. Messina? Why or why not?

RADIOGRAPHIC EXAMINATION

If a patient describes swelling in the maxilla or mandible, a portion of a lesion may be present on the bitewing or periapical radiograph. A radiographic survey that reveals the entire dimensions of the lesion is needed. The panoramic, lateral jaw, and/or occlusal radiograph individually or in combination reveal the total dimensions of a bony lesion in the maxilla or mandible (Figs. 20-6, 20-7, and 20-8). The dental hygienist should approach the radiographic interpretation of the bony lesion through the isolation of the disease process in general terms such as the following:

Radiolucency/radiopacity
Monostotic/polyostotic
Dimensional changes in the surrounding bone
Peripheral outline of the lesion
Trabecular pattern of the bone
Position and shape of associated tooth roots

SYSTEMIC DIAGNOSTIC AIDS

The physical examination of the dental patient was reviewed in Chapter 11. That chapter briefly discussed the extraoral and intraoral occurrences of numerous medical and dental diseases or conditions. During the treatment of a patient, an underlying medical problem may be suspected or the patient may identify a medical problem, which prompts the need to obtain more specific medical information for patient management. This discussion is limited to the specific medical problems presented in the following sections.

ANEMIA

Physical findings of a patient reveal a decreased amount of vasculature on the conjunctiva and alveolar mucosa.

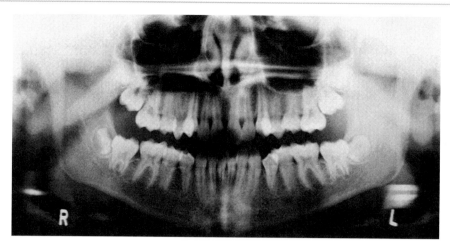

FIG. 20-6 A panoramic film. (From Haring JI, Jansen L: *Dental radiography principles and techniques,* ed 2, Philadelphia, 2000, WB Saunders.)

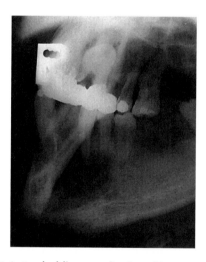

FIG. 20-7 Lateral oblique projection. (From Frommer HH: *Radiology for dental auxiliaries,* ed 7, St Louis, 2001, Mosby.)

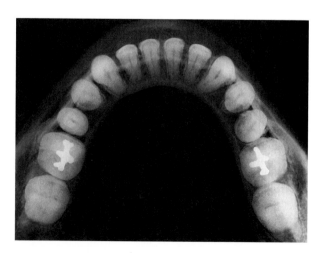

FIG. 20-8 Mandibular occlusal projection. (From White SC, Pharaoh MJ: *Oral radiology principles and interpretation,* ed 4, St Louis, 2000, Mosby.)

BOX 20-3

Laboratory Tests Used to Detect Anemia

Hypochromic Microcytic Anemia
Normal RBC count
Cause of iron deficiency: decreased MCV
Chronic blood loss: decreased MCHC, decreased hematocrit
Normochromic Normocytic Anemia
Decreased RBC count
Cause of acute blood loss: normal MCV
Hemodialysis: normal MCHC
Hemolysis: decreased hematocrit, decreased/increased reticulocyte count
Macrocytic (Megaloblastic) Anemia
Normal RBC count
Cause of folate deficiency: increased MCV
B_{12} deficiency: normal MCHC
Chronic alcoholism: decreased reticulocyte count

RBC, Red blood cell; *MCV,* mean corpuscular volume; *MCHC,* mean corpuscular hemoglobin concentration.

The patient also mentions feelings of fatigue. The dental professional suspects that this patient may be anemic. This patient should be referred to a physician. The laboratory tests used to determine the presence of anemia are shown in Box 20-3.

BLEEDING PROBLEMS

If the patient states that he or she bruises easily, takes a long time to stop bleeding, has liver disease, or takes an anticoagulant agent (i.e., warfarin sodium [Coumadin]),the dental professional should recognize that this patient may have a bleeding problem. Hemostasis has four phases: vascular, platelet, coagulation, and fibrinolysis. Tests assess each phase. The laboratory tests that evaluate the patient's ability to stop bleeding (hemostasis) are listed in Box 20-4.

BOX 20-4

Laboratory Tests for Hemostasis

Vascular Phase

In this phase the endothelial cells that line the blood vessels restrict the blood cell elements to the vessel. If there is a defect in the vessel wall integrity, blood cell elements may pass between the endothelial cells into the connective tissue. To evaluate the vessel integrity, place a blood pressure cuff in the normal position and inflate to 90 to 100 mm Hg. Leave the cuff at that pressure for 5 minutes. Then count the number of petechiae that occur within a circular area of 2.5-cm diameter (approximately 1 inch). This is called the *tourniquet test,* and a normal value is less than 10 petechiae.

Platelet Phase

If the vessel is damaged, platelets adhere to the exposed subendothelial tissues, continue to aggregate, and ultimately form a mechanical plug. Platelets can fail to form the plug if there is either a decrease in number or a decrease in activity. It is reported that aspirin and nonsteroidal antiinflammatory drugs (NSAIDs) alter the activity of the platelets; however, patients who take aspirin daily for cardiovascular benefit do not have bleeding times outside the normal range. The bleeding time is determined by either the Duke's or Ivy's method. In the Duke's method, a lancet cuts the earlobe; in the Ivy's method, a lancet cuts the forearm. The cut is blotted every 30 seconds until bleeding stops.

Platelet count: normal 100,000 to 400,000 platelets per mm^3
Bleeding time: less than 5 minutes

Coagulation Phase

This phase can be initiated by either the extrinsic or intrinsic pathways. The extrinsic pathway is the first to be activated, and it is initiated by the action of the tissue thromboplastin in combination with calcium (factor IV) and factor VII. The intrinsic pathway is initiated by contact between the Hageman's factor (factor XII) and the negatively charged endothelial surface. Several clotting factors require vitamin K for their production in the liver. Coumadin and other warfarin derivatives are similar in structure to the vitamin K–producing chemical factors but are nonfunctional in clotting activities. The International Normalized Ratio (INR) tests the extrinsic pathway and the partial thromboplastin time (PTT) tests the intrinsic pathway. The INR is used to measure the effects of Coumadin.*
INR: 1.2 to 1.4
PTT: 35 to 50 seconds

Fibrinolysis Phase

The fibrinolytic system is required to prevent the coagulation activity in areas far removed from the site in injury and also to dissolve the clot after it has served its hemostatic purpose. This process involves plasminogen that is converted to plasmin. The plasmin splits large and small pieces from the fibrin clot and stops the activity of the coagulation factors.*

*Data from Little JW et al: *Dental management of the medically compromised patient,* ed 6, St Louis, (in press), Mosby.

BOX 20-5

Signs and Symptoms of Insulin-Dependent Diabetes Mellitus

Polydipsia	Loss of strength
Polyphagia	Loss of weight
Polyuria	

BOX 20-6

Signs and Symptoms of Non–Insulin-Dependent Diabetes Mellitus

Blurred vision	Paresthesias
More than 40 years of age	Postural hypotension
Overweight	Urination at night

DIABETES MELLITUS

Diabetes mellitus (DM) is a microvasculature disease with a metabolic component, elevated glucose, and vascular components. The hyperglycemia is related to an absolute lack of insulin, such as that found in patients with *insulin-dependent diabetes mellitus (IDDM),* or the body's inability to use insulin, such as that found in patients with *non–insulin-dependent diabetes mellitus (NIDDM).* An understanding of DM is important in dentistry because dental professionals are in a position to detect new cases and are also responsible the treatment of patients who have the disease. The signs and symptoms suggestive of IDDM can be found in Box 20-5.[2] Usual symptoms or profiles for those with NIDDM are shown in Box 20-6, and laboratory tests that help diagnose DM are provided in Box 20-7.

In-office monitoring for the evaluation of suspected patients with diabetes or the evaluation of known patients

BOX 20-7

Laboratory Tests for the Diagnosis of Diabetes Mellitus

Fasting blood glucose: normal range 60 to 100 mg/dl
2-Hour postprandial: abnormal greater than 200 mg/dl
Glycosylated hemoglobin: normal range 3% to 6%

with diabetes can be accomplished with blood glucose meter systems. One such device is the Glucometer Elite (Bayer Corp, Ekhardt, Ind.; Fig. 20-9). The patient's skin is punctured with a lancet device, and a drop of blood is placed on the test strip. The test result is displayed within 30 seconds. Box 20-8 outlines the criteria for diabetes.

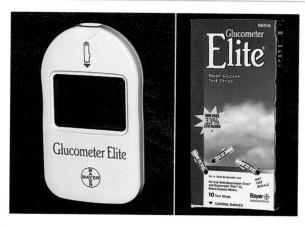

FIG. 20-9 The glucometer is used to test the concentration of sugar in the blood. The Elite is one type of glucometer available for this purpose.

BOX 20-8

Criteria for Diabetes

Normal
Fasting* less than 110 mg/dl
2-Hour postprandial
Random Plasma Glucose less than 140 mg/dl
Impaired
Fasting greater than 110 and less than 126 mg/dl
2-Hour postprandial
Random Plasma Glucose greater than 140 and less than 200 mg/dl
Diabetes
Fasting greater than 126 mg/dl
2-Hour postprandial
Random Plasma Glucose greater than 200 mg/dl

Fasting refers to no food intake for 8 hours before the blood sample is taken.

CRITICAL THINKING ACTIVITIES

1. With a peer, role-play, explaining the different supplementary aids that can be used in the examination of a patient with pain caused by the following:
   a. Carious lesion
   b. Cracked tooth
   c. Pulpitis
2. Given a certain set of patient conditions, medical history, and clinical findings, discuss within a small group the sequence of diagnostic aids that could be used to diagnose the patient's problem. Provide rationales for your decisions.
3. A patient who is noncompliant with plaque removal seeks treatment from you. Clinical examination indicates decalcification along the gingival margin of several teeth; overall plaque status is high. Generate in writing or role-play with a peer the presentation you would make to this patient to positively affect his or her oral self-care practices. Include the diagnostic aids you would select and provide rationales for your selections.
4. In groups of three, make a list of reasons for the use of supplementary aids in dentistry. Trade your list with another group's, and compare and contrast the two rationales.

REVIEW QUESTIONS

1. Which of the following supplementary aids can be used in the detection of dental caries?
   a. Visual examination
   b. Probing with an explorer
   c. Bitewing radiographs
   d. Transillumination
   e. All the above
2. To determine whether a lesion is vascular in origin, a glass slide can be used to compress the tissue to observe vascularity. Which of the following examination techniques does this statement describe?
   a. Aspiration
   b. Probing
   c. Diascopy
   d. Palpation
   e. Percussion
3. Which of the following supplementary aids *cannot* be used to evaluate the status of the dental pulp?
   a. Electric pulp tester
   b. Auscultation
   c. Heat
   d. Cold
   e. Radiograph
4. All of the following diagnostic aids assist in the detection of oral cancer *except* which one?
   a. Visual examination
   b. Bitewing radiograph
   c. Biopsy
   d. Vital staining
   e. Oral brush biopsy

REVIEW QUESTIONS—cont'd

5. All the following supplementary aids can be used to detect a periapical/pulpal infection *except* which one?
   a. Tooth mobility
   b. Periapical radiographs
   c. Transillumination
   d. Electric pulp tester
   e. Sinus tract drainage

6. Which of the following findings suggests that the patient might be anemic?
   a. Decreased red blood cell (RBC) count
   b. Decreased mean corpuscular volume (MCV)
   c. Decreased vasculature on oral mucosa
   d. Decreased hematocrit
   e. All the above

7. A patient with a platelet count of 100,000 to 400,000 per mm^3, a bleeding time of 4 minutes, and a tourniquet test of seven petecchiae would be considered to have which of the following?
   a. Anemic
   b. Diabetic (NIDDM)
   c. A hemophiliac
   d. Normal

8. Which of the following items does *not* pertain to the patient's ability to stop bleeding (hemostasis)?
   a. Vascular phase
   b. Iron deficiency
   c. Platelet phase
   d. Coagulation phase
   e. Fibrinolysis

9. Which of the following conditions does *not* pertain to diabetes mellitus?
   a. Elevated serum glucose
   b. Insulin
   c. More than 40 years old and overweight
   d. Increased thirst (polydipsia) and increased urination (polyuria)
   e. Folate and B$_{12}$ deficiency

10. The patient has the following clinical signs and symptoms:
    - Large amalgam restoration on tooth #13
    - Fleeting, sharp pain of short duration while chewing
    - Sensitivity to cold and heat

    Which of the following is the most definitive diagnostic aid for this patient?
    a. Radiograph
    b. Electric pulp tester
    c. Selective pressure with a rubber wheel
    d. *Streptococcus mutans* count

SUGGESTED AGENCIES AND WEB SITES

Because of the ever-changing nature of the Internet, some of the web sites listed here may have changed since publication. Please refer to Mosby's Evolve web site for the most current information.

American Academy of Oral Medicine ("Publications" [monographs]): http://www.aaom.com

KaVo America Corporation: http://www.kavousa.com

Naval Postgraduate Dental School, Comprehensive Dentistry ("Diagnosing and restoring the cracked tooth"): http://nnd40.med

Professional Results, Inc. ("Cracked teeth: why do we get them; how do we treat them?"): http://www.toothslooth.com

Professional Results, Inc. ("Products"): http://www.toothslooth.com

RxList: The Internet Drug Index: http://www.rxlist.com

ADDITIONAL READINGS AND RESOURCES

Bates B: *A guide to physical examination and history taking,* ed 6, Philadelphia, 1995, JB Lippincott.

Coleman G, Nelson J: *Principles of oral diagnosis,* St Louis, 1992, Mosby.

Mecklenburg RE et al: *How to help your patients stop using tobacco,* National Cancer Institute: NIH Pub No 98-3191, Bethesda, Md, 1993, National Institutes of Health.

REFERENCES

1. Bricker SL, Langlais RP, Miller CS: *Oral diagnosis, oral medicine and treatment planning,* ed 2, Philadelphia, 1994, Lea & Febiger.
2. Little JW et al: *Dental management of the medically compromised patient,* ed 6, St Louis, (in press), Mosby.
3. Miller CS, Leonelli FM, Latham E: Selective interference with pacemaker activity by electrical dental devices, *Oral Surg* 85(1):33-6, 1998.
4. Sciubba JJ: Improving detection of precancerous and cancerous oral lesions, *JADA* 130:1445-1457, 1999.

PART IV

Chapter 21
Devices for Oral Self-Care

Chapter 22
Fluoride and the Reversal of Dental Caries

Chapter 23
Dentifrices

Chapter 24
Chemotherapeutics

Chapter 25
Dentinal Sensitivity

Chapter 26
Sealants

Chapter 27
Prevention and Emergency Management of Dental Trauma

Chapter 28
Care of Appliances and Dental Prostheses

Competency Statements

The learner is expected to possess knowledge, skills, judgments, values, and attitudes to develop the listed competencies.

Core Competencies
- Apply a professional code of ethics in all endeavors.
- Adhere to state and federal laws, recommendations, and regulations in the provision of dental hygiene care.
- Provide dental hygiene care to promote patient health and wellness using critical thinking and problem solving in the provision of evidence-based practice.
- Use evidence-based decision making to evaluate and incorporate emerging treatment modalities.
- Assume responsibility for dental hygiene actions and care based on accepted scientific theories and research as well as the accepted standard of care.
- Promote the profession through service activities and affiliations with professional organizations.
- Provide quality assurance mechanisms for health services.
- Communicate effectively with individuals and groups from diverse populations both verbally and in writing.
- Provide accurate, consistent, and complete documentation for assessment, diagnosis, planning, implementation, and evaluation of dental hygiene services.
- Provide care to all patients using an individualized approach that is humane, empathetic, and caring.

Health Promotion and Disease Prevention
- Promote the values of oral and general health and wellness to the public and organizations within and outside the profession.
- Respect the goals, values, beliefs, and preferences of the patient while promoting optimal oral and general health.

Courtesy American Dental Education Association, Washington, DC.

Disease-Prevention Therapy: Professional *and* Self-Care

- Refer patients who may have a physiologic, psychological, and/or social problem for comprehensive patient evaluation.
- Identify individual and population risk factors and develop strategies that promote health related quality of life.
- Evaluate factors that can be used to promote patient adherence to disease prevention and/or health maintenance strategies.
- Evaluate and utilize methods to ensure the health and safety of the patient and the dental hygienist in the delivery of dental hygiene.

Community Involvement

- Assess the oral health needs of the community and the quality and availability of resources and services.
- Provide screening, referral, and educational services that allow clients to access the resources of the healthcare system.
- Provide community oral health services in a variety of settings.
- Facilitate client access to oral health services by influencing individuals and/or organizations for the provision of oral health care.
- Evaluate reimbursement mechanisms and their impact on the patient's/client's access to oral healthcare.
- Evaluate the outcomes of community-based programs and plan for future activities.

Patient Care

- Select, obtain, and interpret diagnostic information recognizing its advantages and limitations.
- Recognize predisposing and etiologic risk factors that require intervention to prevent disease.
- Obtain, review, and update a complete medical, family, social, and dental history.
- Recognize health conditions and medications that affect overall patient care.
- Identify patients at risk for a medical emergency and manage the patients' care in a manner that prevents an emergency.
- Perform a comprehensive examination using clinical, radiographic, periodontal, dental charting, and other data collection procedures to assess the patient's needs.
- Determine a dental hygiene diagnosis.
- Identify patient needs and significant findings that impact the delivery of dental hygiene services.
- Obtain consultations as indicated.
- Prioritize the care plan based on the health status and the actual and potential problems of the individual to facilitate optimal oral health.
- Establish a planned sequence of care (education, clinical, and evaluation) based on the dental hygiene diagnosis, identified oral conditions, potential problems, etiologic and risk factors, and available treatment modalities.
- Establish a collaborative relationship with the patient in the planned care to include etiology, prognosis, and treatment alternatives.
- Make referrals to other healthcare professionals.
- Obtain the patient's informed consent based on a thorough case presentation.
- Perform dental hygiene interventions to eliminate and/or control local etiologic factors to prevent and control caries, periodontal disease, and other oral conditions.
- Control pain and anxiety during treatment through the use of accepted clinical and behavioral techniques.
- Determine the outcomes of dental hygiene interventions using indices, instruments, examination techniques, and patient self-report.
- Evaluate the patient's satisfaction with the oral healthcare received and the oral healthcare status achieved.
- Provide subsequent treatment or referrals based on evaluation findings.
- Develop and maintain a health maintenance program.

Professional Growth and Development

- Access professional and social networks and resources to assist entrepreneurial initiatives.

CHAPTER 21

Devices *for* Oral Self-Care

Victoria C. Vick, Joan I. Gluch

Chapter Outline

Oral Self-Care Recommendations
    The challenge
    Patient expectations
    Evidence-based decision making
Case Study: Specific Oral Self-Care
    Recommendations
Anatomical Considerations and Physical
    Challenges to Oral Self-Care
        Anatomical considerations
        Physical challenges

Oral Self-Care Devices
    Disclosing solution
    The toothbrush
    Toothbrush replacement and care
    Tongue brushing
    Interdental cleaning

Key Terms

Anatomical considerations
Dental floss
Dental tape
Disclosing solution
End-rounded bristles
End-tufted toothbrush
Evidence-based decision
  making

Floss holder
Floss threader
Gingival architecture
Handle design
Head design
Interdental brush
International Organization for
  Standardization (ISO)

Interproximal embrasure
  classification
Multitufted
Patient compliance
Plaque control
Powered toothbrush
Textured floss

Tooth-brushing methods
  Bass
  Rolling stroke
  Modified Stillman's
  Charters'
  Fones'
  Horizontal/scrub

 ## Learning Outcomes

1. Describe and explain the appropriate use of oral health indicators for the following categories of oral self-care devices: toothbrushes and interdental cleaners.
2. Provide a rationale for oral self-care product selection based on evidence-based decision making, patient need, and anatomical considerations.
3. Explain the role of self-evaluation in plaque control.
4. Monitor and recommend modifications for patient use of oral self-care products based on therapeutic intervention planning and subjective indicators of health.

ORAL SELF-CARE RECOMMENDATIONS

THE CHALLENGE

Plaque control is the single most important factor in obtaining and sustaining optimal oral health. Daily cleaning with a toothbrush and other interdental aids is the most dependable way to achieve and maintain this status. Your role and professional responsibility as a dental hygienist is to provide oral health education and skill development to each patient as part of each and every appointment—without exception. That instruction should be tailored to lifestyles and abilities of children, adults, and the elderly so that they are able to adopt an oral self-care regimen that best suits their needs.

PATIENT EXPECTATIONS

Patients look to the dental healthcare professional for knowledge. Patients gain confidence when they are provided with professional recommendations and counseling. The positive impact that oral care product recommendation and oral self-care instruction have in patients' overall long-term oral health is significant. *What the dental health-care professional says and does makes a difference to a patient's life-long oral health.*

Far too often the importance of the role dental health-care professionals play in the recommendation of oral care products and techniques is overlooked. Dental patients appreciate the same kind of brand- and formula-specific recommendation regarding dental products so they can eliminate that same confusion when they walk down the pharmacy or grocery aisle faced with the hundreds of product choices.

EVIDENCE-BASED DECISION MAKING

The number of oral care products available for patients to choose from and for professionals to recommend is rapidly growing. Dental hygienists must acknowledge the core of information that needs to be reviewed in order to stay current regarding oral care products. It is a professional responsibility to maintain access to and stay current with the literature and scientific knowledge regarding any newly introduced product.

In the scientific community decisions based upon review of the literature are referred to as "evidence-based" decisions. All dental hygiene treatment decisions and oral self-care recommendations should be formulated from an evidence-based perspective. This requires access to professional journals and frequent searches on med-line (the National Library of Medicines database of medical abstracts) and will also require evaluation of the applicable and credible literature to determine if the studies are well designed, executed, and appropriate (see p. 409 for evaluation criteria). Some studies conducted by manufacturers are quite legitimate; in other cases they merely demonstrate what the manufacturers want them to, and are not based in fact. This type of fact-finding also requires trips to the pharmacy to stay current with patients and what they purchase. In other words, it requires a resolute and ongoing effort from the dental professional to know and to understand the dental products marketplace.

This chapter covers oral care products and self-care methods that patients expect and deserve to receive at each appointment as well as the use of oral anatomical features in determining which oral care products best meet their needs. (See also Chapter 22: Fluoride and the Reversal of Dental Caries, Chapter 23: Dentifrices, Chapter 24: Chemotherapeutics, Chapter 25: Dentinal Sensitivity, and Chapter 39: Cosmetic Whitening for additional oral care recommendations.)

ANATOMICAL CONSIDERATIONS AND PHYSICAL CHALLENGES TO ORAL SELF-CARE

ANATOMICAL CONSIDERATIONS

Plaque control includes the consistent removal of dental plaque from teeth and gingival surfaces. Although research does not consistently show significant differences in gingival scores and bleeding indices when using one manual brush versus another, the oral architecture does

merit examination as a foundation of oral self-care recommendations.

Ease of use and confidence in an oral care product's effectiveness are factors that can make a substantial difference in patient compliance. Understanding the topography and oral architecture of the oral cavity for each patient treated is the first step in recommending oral self-care products and procedures that are easy to use and effective.

Just as an individual presents with unique histories and experiences, each person's oral physiology presents challenges and distinct cues in selecting products and procedures to help achieve optimal oral self-care. When looking at the oral cavity architecture as a guide, the dental healthcare professional has several specific elements to evaluate that can help make the appropriate recommendations: Lips, alveolar architecture and tooth position, tori, tongue mobility, gingival architecture, and interproximal embrasures.

Lips

The width and elasticity of the opening to the oral cavity can affect the size and shape of the toothbrush head and type of interproximal cleaning procedures recommended. For example, if the lips are very tight and nonelastic, which makes the opening to the oral cavity small, it would be inadvisable to recommend a toothbrush with a large, square head and an interproximal cleansing method that requires a patient to see at least some posterior proximal surfaces.

To facilitate oral self-care procedures, the lip elasticity and oral opening should allow a patient to see at least the mesial of the first molars; to place a toothbrush in the vestibular areas, both anterior and posterior; and to manipulate an interproximal cleaning device/product to the distal of the distal-most tooth present. Based on this type of parameter, appropriate oral self-care devices can be recommended.

Alveolar Architecture and Tooth Position

The next step in selecting an appropriate oral self-care device is to evaluate the following factors: size and shape of the teeth, the overall alveolar architecture of the attached and unattached gingiva, and the teeth as a unit.

A review of the vertical dimension of the teeth and alveolar process as a unit from the facial perspective should also be completed. Questions to ask oneself during this evaluation include the following:

Do the teeth appear to be constricted at the neck or gingival one third of the tooth to the extent that a plaque-retentive area is formed?

Are teeth malpositioned thus creating plaque traps?

Will a typical brush stroke, if not appropriately placed, miss the critical area of plaque retention?

What size brush head will be the easiest for this patient to manipulate?

Teeth with no adjacent neighboring tooth, resulting in an unusual interdental space and interdental papilla configuration, require special brushing instructions and interdental cleaning recommendations. Teeth with no opposing tooth, crowded teeth, and teeth with large diastemas pose challenges to oral care recommendations as well.

The brushing plane of a toothbrush, or the surface used to actually perform the cleaning, varies from a fairly flat

Case Study: Specific Oral Self-Care Recommendations

Mrs. Ann Cronin, also a patient on the CD-ROM, is a 70-year-old retired seamstress. She is a new patient who has recently moved and is living in a multi-generational environment with her daughter and family. She is concerned that her small monthly pension will not cover her dental needs. She is arthritic, for which she takes Celebrex 100 mg twice a day, and is menopausal, for which she takes Premarin 1.25 mg once a day. On her prevention survey, she reports that she has sensitive teeth, a dry mouth, and a partial denture that doesn't fit. Her current oral hygiene measures include brushing once daily with a medium toothbrush, rinsing with a mouthrinse, and using whatever dentifrice her daughter buys

for the grandchildren—which she reports as fluoridated. Her dental status reveals missing teeth; multiple restorations including crowns, amalgams, and composites; rotated teeth; a 47% plaque index; and periodontal involvement of several teeth. She feels that prevention is important but that she is more likely than the "average person" to have oral problems. She does not see how she could change a habit at this time and does not believe she has control over the conditions in her mouth. Please access the patient schedule on the CD-ROM accompanying this textbook for the intraoral images, radiographs, periodontal and dental chartings of Mrs. Ann Cronin.

---

plane, a gently curved one, or one that is completely uneven. Although there is little evidence that any brushing plane is superior to another, the ADA's Council on Scientific Affairs points out that a brush must conform to an individual's needs.[20]

The position of the facial, lingual, and palatal surfaces in relationship to the alveolar mucosa should be considered when selecting the most appropriate toothbrush and tooth-brushing method. Teeth that are tilted toward the palatal surface of the maxilla or the lingual surface of the mandible require close scrutiny when selecting a brush, selecting a brushing method, and in brush placement. When tilted in this fashion, the palatal areas at the gingival one third of the tooth surface are more plaque retentive than teeth that are more vertically aligned.

Tori

Large mandibular tori may require anterior positioning of a very small toothbrush head, such as a child's brush, to clean mandibular lingual surfaces. Maxillary tuberosities on the facial aspects of the alveolus likewise should be evaluated in toothbrush and brushing method selection.

Tongue Mobility

The mobility of the tongue is important to functions of speech, mastication, and self-evaluation of plaque removal. A patient's inability to place his or her tongue at the distal-most surface of the distal-most tooth in either arch significantly alters the ability to determine successful plaque removal and will require suggestions for alternative methods of oral self-care evaluation.

Gingival Architecture and Interproximal Embrasures

Gingival recession, clefting, and rolled gingival margins are not only the result of inappropriate plaque removal techniques but create plaque-retentive areas difficult to reach without special and very specific instructions. Each area needs to be carefully evaluated and solutions discussed with the patient.

The anatomical factors affecting the selection of interdental cleaning aids include:
* Size and shape of the embrasure
* Tooth position and alignment
* Contour and consistency of gingival tissues

The shape of the interdental space can vary from tooth to tooth and can range from no recession and a tight, healthy papilla to no papilla present at all. Selecting the best interproximal cleaning aid will be based on efficiency in removing plaque from the interproximal space and the consistency of the gingival tissues.

The following embrasure classifications can be used in selecting oral self-care products:

Class I–presents with no gingival recession with the interdental papilla filling the space.

Class II–presents with moderate papillary recession.

Class III–presents with a complete loss of the interdental papilla.

 Case Application

The intraoral examination of Mrs. Cronin reveals several significant findings that will have an impact on oral self-care device recommendations. Her crusted commissures, xerostomia, and sensitive teeth in concert with the anatomical observations should lead to numerous questions for the dental hygienist. What questions would you have concerning her oral architecture as you think about oral self-care recommendations?

The hygienist working with Mrs. Cronin had the following observations: Will her lips be elastic enough to allow the hygienist to easily reach the distal of the maxillary second molars with a cleaning device? How much room is there between the cheeks and the gingival one third of the tooth? How can Mrs. Cronin be guided to more effectively clean the gingival margins? What questions would you have regarding tooth positions, recession, clefting, rolled margins, and interproximal embrasure spaces?

PHYSICAL CHALLENGES

Following a careful evaluation of the oral architecture for the acceptance and selection of an oral cleaning device, the hygienist should assess the patient's dexterity and eyesight. Conditions such as arthritis can make oral self-care difficult and painful. Diminished eyesight in an aging patient can cause a previously low plaque score to increase. Difficulty accessing a bathroom sink and/or standing may require modifications of methods for oral self-care.

Device Modifications

Modifications can be made to the handles of most oral care devices to allow a more secure grip. Suggestions for this type of modification include the use of a foam wrap, a soft rubber ball, a Velcro strap, and soft tubing. A toothbrush handle can be angled by placing it under hot running water and can provide an additional modification. The handles on most powered toothbrushes are larger and can therefore provide a more secure grip.

 Case Application

Mrs. Cronin, a retired seamstress, has arthritis evident in both hands, predominantly in her fingers. The oral self-care devices selected will probably have to be modified to accommodate this physical challenge. The degree of difficulty she will experience will have to be assessed.

ORAL SELF-CARE DEVICES

DISCLOSING SOLUTION

Disclosing agents are used by both the dental professional and the patient to determine the exact location of plaque. Patients should be encouraged to check their oral self-care with a disclosing agent on a regular basis. The recommendation of a small disposable mouth mirror along with a disclosing agent for patient self-assessment is an excellent way to encourage thorough plaque removal. Tissue assessment should be complete before disclosing; otherwise the tissues will also be stained from the solution, resulting in a misdiagnosis.

Composition and Lips

Disclosing agents are used to make plaque biofilm visible and are usually comprised of an erythrosine dye. They are manufactured as solutions, tablets, or on a swab. Some agents stain plaque biofilm pink or red, and others are two-toned and show mature plaque in purple or violet and immature plaque in red or pink.

Disclosing agents can be used to educate patients about the etiology of disease, to provide motivation for self-cleaning, and for evaluation of oral self-care. Patients cannot see plaque and are often unaware that red and bleeding gingiva are a result of the bacteria present within the plaque biofilm. Educating the patient about the presence of disease or plaque and the removal or disturbance of the bacteria is essential.

THE TOOTHBRUSH

The toothbrush remains the most effective and widely used dental plaque removal device. Approximately 80% to 90% of people in industrialized countries brush their teeth at least once a day.[13,27] A global patent search be-

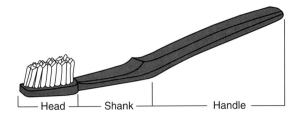

FIG. 21-1. Standard parts of a toothbrush.

tween 1963 and 1998 reveals about 3000 toothbrush patents—a seemingly endless variation in design. In the United States, more than 50 million toothbrushes are sold each year.[30]

Efficacy

It is still a matter for debate as to whether one toothbrush is better than another—or whether it can be proven to be so, and while some studies demonstrated a difference between patients, it is often the methods used that create the variance in plaque scores.[6,7,29]

This conflict of opinion highlights the dental professional's ongoing challenge to remain informed about current oral care products and to thoroughly review the related literature for scientific depth, reliability, and sound methodology. At the end of the day the dental professional has to make the judgment call as to the credibility of product claims and whether current and new developments should be incorporated into patient care and recommendations.

Attributes and Design

All toothbrushes, regardless of brand name, have the same standard design features: head, shank, and handle (Fig. 21-1). The ideal toothbrush should be easy to use and clean, effective and safe for cleaning all tooth surfaces and gingiva, able to reach all areas of the oral cavity, the right size and shape for the specific patient's oral architecture and dexterity, and durable. The ADA's Council on Dental Therapeutics has released guidelines for toothbrushes. Toothbrush manufacturers must adhere to good manufacturing practices and must use standard nylon bristles with a specific International Organization for Standardization (ISO) rating.[20] The ISO rating standard is important for bristle softness, which varies within an acceptable range to ensure safety of the teeth and gingival tissues during brushing.

Head and Handle Design

The most important requirements for the toothbrush head are size, and a shape that is free of any feature that might cause injury to the soft tissue. Shapes range from rectangular to oval and diamond shaped. A small head, no larger than 1 inch by ½ inch facilitates access to all areas of the oral cavity. The toothbrush handle needs to be ergonomically designed so that it is comfortable and easy for the patient to hold and manipulate throughout the mouth. For the most part, toothbrushes used to have a straight handle, but many are now designed with an angle and a rubberized grip, which make brushing easier. In studies evaluating levels of plaque removal based on variations in toothbrush handle design, long, contoured handles have performed better than short, non-contoured, straight handles.[21]

Bristles and Brushing Plane

Bristles are the topic of much concern in dentistry today. The original sharp-ended tip configurations have been replaced by end-rounded tip configurations, which is less abrasive to soft tissue. The degree of end-rounding of toothbrush bristles and firmness varies among brands.[8]

The rationale for recommending soft, end-rounded bristles is that they are more flexible than hard bristles and they are able to reach and clean more effectively interproximally and subgingivally.[3] Hard-bristled brushes and improper brushing methods have often been associated with gingival recession and cervical notching.[3,24] The degree of softness is rated and classified by the ISO (International Standards Organization) using the Stiffness Index. A soft brush is rated at an ISO index of 3, a medium at an ISO index of 5, and a hard-bristle brush at an ISO index of 7.[20] The length of the filament, the diameter of the filament, the size of the hole into which the tufts are inserted, the number of tufts per area, and the number of filament per tuft are all factors that determine stiffness.[19] Thinner filaments are softer and more resilient.

Toothbrush bristles are grouped in tufts that are arranged in rows. A heavily multitufted brush contains more bristles and has better cleaning potential than a brush with fewer bristles. Multitufted bristles are also less traumatic to the gingival tissues.[23] Bristle and tuft configurations have also undergone significant changes in recent times. The model suggested by Dr. Charles Bass in 1948 (three rows of bristles, six tufts to the row, evenly spaced, 80 bristles to the tuft, each with a diameter of 0.007, straight trimmed, finished to 13/32-inch length) would be difficult to locate in today's oral care market.[3] Bristles are now available in concave, convex, multilevel/rippled, and multi-angle configurations and may also include an outside row of rubber fingers designed to massage the gingival area during brushing.

Powered Toothbrushes

Powered toothbrushes, including sonic brushes, provide alternatives to manual brushes and are becoming increasingly popular. Recent papers by Moritis and Heanue support the powered toothbrush's superior efficacy in plaque removal and gingivitis reduction when compared to a manual toothbrush. Powered toothbrushes have been shown to be safe and effective, resulting in improved plaque and stain removal when compared to manual toothbrushes used for the same time period.[15,33] A recent study with the sonic brush has demonstrated effectiveness in reducing both plaque and bleeding scores as compared to a manual brush in the maintenance of dental implants.[36]

Because of its faster mode of brushing, 2 minutes of powered brushing is equal to approximately 5 to 6 minutes of manual brushing. The bristle motion of powered toothbrushes varies. The bristle action may be reciprocating (back-and-forth motion), accurate (filaments move up and down in an arc motion), orbital (circular motion), vibratory (sonic designs), elliptical (a combination of reciprocating and accurate motion), and dual motion (two or more of the previous actions). Powered brushes may have options such as multiple speeds, replaceable brush heads, timers, and rechargeable or replaceable batteries.

Indications for the Use of a Powered Toothbrush

Patients who find manual brushing difficult may especially benefit from powered toothbrushes, but their effectiveness still depends on brush and bristle placement, patient compliance, and proper use.[33] Evidence suggests that powered toothbrushes may provide increased benefits over manual toothbrushes in patients with limited mobility and special needs.[2,5,16,33] A wide variety of powered toothbrushes are available to consumers today[2,5,11,15,33] (Table 21-1).

Oral healthcare providers should request that patients bring in their powered toothbrushes for instruction concerning the most effective product use.[14,26,35] Due to the various actions of the powered brushes, it is helpful to become familiar with the suggested action of the brand recommended by your practice. Professional instruction is extremely important for a positive patient reaction to the use of powered toothbrushes.[29] Videotapes or instruction booklets do not take the place of professional, one-on-one instruction. Demonstrating the use of the powered brush on your patient followed by the patient

TABLE 21-1
Examples of powered toothbrushes

Product and company	Description
Oral B Braun 3-D Plaque Remover Oral B Laboratories Iowa City, Iowa	Oscillating, small circular brush head. Some units include dual oscillating and back-and-forth motion.
Butler GUM Pulse Plaque Remover John O. Butler Co. A Sunstar Company Chicago, Ill.	Brush tufts move up and down. Uses disposable AA batteries rather than rechargeable battery.
Colgate Actibrush Colgate-Palmolive Co. New York, N.Y.	Small, round soft bristle head with oscillating movement
Crest Spin Brush Procter & Gamble Cincinnati, Ohio	The brush head is a combination of stationary bristles on the posterior two-thirds and small, round oscillating bristles on the anterior one third of the head. Disposable AA batteries are used to operate the brush.
Interplak Powered Brush Bausch & Lomb Tucker, Ga.	Individual brush tufts rotate and counter-rotate. Choice of either large or small brush head.
Rotadent Prodentec Batesville, Ark.	Small rotating brush. Choice of flat or pointed brush head.
SynchroSonic Waterpik Technologies Fort Collins, Colo.	Brush head vibrates with sound.
Sonicare Philips Oral Healthcare Snoqualmie, Wash.	Brush head vibrates with sound.

repeating this action in his/her mouth can be a useful tool in acceptance and effectiveness of the powered toothbrush.

Toothbrushing Techniques

It is important to (1) instill in individuals the importance and goals of tooth brushing, (2) teach a brushing method or combination of methods that will meet the needs of that specific patient, and (3) assess thorough and effective tooth brushing as part of a total oral hygiene preventive program.[37] The dental hygienist should recognize the need to evaluate specific design attributes of the oral care device being recommended (Box 21-1) and patient factors (Box 21-2). Each patient will need specific technique instructions.

Brushing Sequence

If patients report areas that are particularly difficult for them to reach, the dental hygienist might suggest that they start with those areas first.

A specific brushing sequence should be recommended to patients so that they develop a brushing pattern. Patients should be instructed to begin on the distofacial surface of the distal-most tooth in the maxillary arch on their domi-

---

BOX 21-1

Brush Attributes to Consider in Making Oral Self-Care Recommendations

Does the brush have tufted bristles that will increase interproximal cleaning?
Are the bristles end-rounded?
Does the angulation of the brush head aid in accessing difficult-to-reach areas?
Is the size of the brush head appropriate for the size and age of the patient?
Does it have soft bristles to reduce the potential for tissue abrasion caused by over-aggressive brushing?
Does the design of the brush handle make it easier to use?

BOX 21-2

Patient Factors to Consider in Making Oral Self-Care Recommendations

Does the patient have any physical challenges that might require modifications to oral self-care devices or regimens?
Is the brush the right size for the patient's mouth?
What anatomical considerations need to be accommodated?
Is the current brushing style safe and effective?
Is the current brushing frequency sufficient?
Does the patient's age affect brush selection?
How motivated is the patient to comply with brushing instructions or what needs to be done to change level of motivation?
Are the patient's expectations for plaque removal consistent with those of the dental professional?

---

nant side and to continue around the arch including the occlusal and incisal surfaces until they have reached the distal-most surface of the distal-most molar on the opposite side. They should then repeat the same sequence on the palatal surfaces. This process is then repeated on the mandibular arch.

Occlusal Surfaces

The occlusal surfaces may be cleaned by a short, back-and-forth motion, which forces the bristles to reach (as much as possible) pits and fissures, followed by a sweeping motion to remove debris. A long sweeping stroke is not suggested because it does not allow the bristle tips to penetrate sufficiently into pits and fissures.

Anterior, Lingual, and Palatal Surfaces

A vertically positioned brush allows the best access to the anterior lingual and palatal areas. The heel of the brush should then be placed at the gingival margin, brought forward, and repeated several times.

Frequency

A common patient question is, "How frequently should and for how long should I brush?" The most commonly accepted recommendation among dental professionals is brushing twice a day.[10,16,21] Research has documented that thorough plaque removal every 48 hours is the longest interval that will control gingivitis.[10] The ADA recommends that patients brush "regularly" and that oral hygiene routines be customized for patients based on their thoroughness of plaque removal and history of adherence to recommended protocols.[1]

Duration

The length of brushing time for individual patients should be determined by the length of time it takes to thoroughly remove plaque. For some patients, brush placement and tooth-brushing procedures are fairly easy. For others, malposed teeth and other anatomical and physical challenges may require a longer brushing session. Rather than proscribing a time, it is best to observe a patient during a tooth-brushing procedure and assess the results. Research has demonstrated that unsupervised brushing by patients results in brushing times of 1 minute or less, even though they report their brushing times to be between 2 and 3 minutes.[13,17,37] Some dental hygienists recommend that patients use an egg timer to time their brushing duration or to brush for the length of one song on the radio. Brushing time can also be customized based on the patient's oral health status and history of adherence to oral hygiene programs.[37] Other factors, such as the tendency to accumulate plaque, psychomotor skills, and clearance of foods and bacteria with saliva all affect the amount of time needed by individuals to thoroughly brush their teeth.

Case Application

Mrs. Cronin's hygienist initially selected an ultrasoft, small, oval-headed toothbrush with multitufted, end-rounded bristles in a flat plane configuration. Using a large hand mirror, she showed Mrs. Cronin the areas of plaque retention in her mouth and how the ultrasoft brush and the Modified Stillman's brushing method easily removed the disclosed plaque. When Mrs. Cronin was asked to demonstrate the

TABLE 21-2
Tooth-brushing methods

Method	Description	Considerations	Initial brush placement
Bass	• Bristles placed directly into sulcus at 45-degree angle to the tooth. • Gentle short strokes in sulcus. • Followed by "rolling stroke" method since Bass method cleans only sulcus.	• Good plaque removal from gingival margin and sulcus. • Limited cleaning on remainder of tooth surface. • Easy to learn.	
Rolling stroke	• Bristles are placed against attached gingiva at a 45-degree angle to the tooth. • Brush is rolled slowly by flexing wrist to drag bristles against tooth with gentle, firm motion. • Brush is rolled at least five times for each area.	• Used for removing plaque at gingival margin and clinical crown. • Limited plaque removal at the gingival margin.	
Modified Stillman's	• Bristles are placed onto the attached gingival at a 45-degree angle to the tooth. • Bristles pressed (enough to cause slight gingival blanching) and vibrated to promote circulation. • A rolling stroke is added to cleanse the tooth. • The action is repeated sequentially throughout the mouth. • In the anterior lingual area place the heel or toe of the brush on the gingival, rotating and sweeping toward incisal edges.	• Good gingival stimulation. • Good (clinical crown) coronal and interproximal cleaning. • Limited sulcular cleaning. • Dexterity required	
Charters'	• Side of brush is placed against tooth with bristles facing occlusally. • Brush is slid to a 45-degree angle at the gingival margin. • Bristles are then pressed into the margin and proximal areas and vibrated for at least 10 strokes for each area of the mouth. • A "rolling stroke' is recommended before use of this technique to cleanse the coronal surface.	• Good interproximal cleaning. • Limited sulcular cleaning. • Useful around orthodontic bands, fixed prostheses.	
Fones'	• With teeth closed, brush is placed against the cheek with bristles directed to the posterior teeth. • Circular motions are used in a quick sweeping motion. • Anterior teeth are placed end-to-end and cleansed in the same manner. • In-and-out strokes are used to cleanse the palatal and lingual areas.	• Easy to learn first technique for children. • Possibly detrimental for vigorous adult brusher.	
Horizontal/ Scrub	• Bristles are placed at a 90-degree angle to the tooth, and brush is moved back and forth or in a large circular motion.	• Removes plaque successfully from facial and lingual surfaces (unless a hard brush is used). • If a hard brush is used there is the potential for damage to the tooth structure and to the soft tissues. • Inability to access interproximal areas.	

technique, she did so quite slowly and with apparent difficulty. After five or six brushing repetitions, Mrs. Cronin dropped the toothbrush. Following a flushed apology, she stated, "I guess these old hands just don't want to work today." Looking at Table 21-2, can you determine which consideration the hygienist overlooked in selecting this brushing recommendation? What method would you have recommended? Would a powered toothbrush have been a better recommendation?

Methods

Although patients have a wide variety of acceptable toothbrushes to choose from in the marketplace, they can only remove plaque thoroughly when the toothbrush is used routinely and effectively in a manner that does not harm the oral tissues. Table 21-2 summarizes the following six brushing methods that are most commonly taught to patients: Bass method, rolling stroke method, modified Stillman's method, Charters' method, Fones' method, and horizontal/scrub method.[4,12,32,37]

The dental hygienist should assess a patient's oral health status and observe the tooth-brushing technique before recommending a particular method. If a patient has healthy gingiva and few plaque deposits, arbitrarily recommending a change is counterproductive. This patient should merely be coached to continue a safe, effective pattern of brushing.[14]

When teaching patients new oral hygiene protocols, dental hygienists should provide information and skills training in combination with motivational messages to ensure an appropriate level of understanding.[9] Patients should be given written materials to reinforce concepts presented in the oral health lesson.[17] Sample patient education pamphlets are available from a variety of dental organizations and product manufacturers. Dental hygienists should note in the chart the exact instructions given to the patient so that they can be reviewed at the next visit. Not all patients will remember the exact instructions that they were given.

TOOTHBRUSH REPLACEMENT AND CARE

If a toothbrush is to remain effective, it must be replaced periodically. The wear exhibited by toothbrushes is determined more by the brushing method and force than how often the brush is used. Wear can be exhibited in many ways—bristles can become splayed, bent, or even broken. Although the average manual toothbrush lasts approximately 3 months, this time span can vary widely because of differences in brushing habits. Other reasons to replace a toothbrush include illness, continuous exposure to water or other foreign substances, and damage to the handle.[23,34,37]

After each use, the toothbrush should be cleaned by placing it under a stream of warm water, which forces any debris or remaining dentifrice from between the bristles. The brush handle should then be tapped against the sink top to remove any remaining water. Brushes should be kept with the head upright in the open air to enhance drying and minimize the development of bacterial growth. Brushes should not be kept in contact with other toothbrushes because this proximity is a rich source of bacterial cross-contamination.

TONGUE CLEANING

Patients often complain of mouth odor without realizing that it may be caused by bacterial accumulation on their tongue. Papillae on the tongue provide a perfect place to harbor bacteria and debris that can lead to the development of bad odor. Unless they are instructed to do so, patients often do not know that they should clean their tongue, much in the same way as they clean their teeth. Tongue brushing can be accomplished by placing the side of the toothbrush near the middle of the tongue. The brush is then swept forward and this step repeated several times. A dentifrice may be used to improve cleansing if it does not prove unpleasant to the patient. Plastic tongue scrapers are also available, and patients with elongated papilla and deep grooves may find this type of device beneficial. Place the scraper on the posterior portion of the tongue and pull forward to "scrape" the coating off of the tongue. The tongue scraper is rinsed and the process repeated until the tongue is cleansed. As with a toothbrush, the tongue scraper should be rinsed after the final use and allowed to air dry.

INTERDENTAL CLEANING

Self-care of the structures within the oral cavity requires more than cleaning the tooth surfaces with a toothbrush. Although some toothbrush bristles may reach proximal surfaces, not all surfaces, including the contact and subgingival areas, are cleansed with tooth brushing alone. Recommendations for self-care interdental cleaning aids should be based on the architecture of the oral anatomy at the proximal embrasure space and the dexterity of the patient. Interdental cleaning aids vary in size, shape, use, and cost.

Dental Floss

Self-cleaning of the proximal tooth surfaces for Class I embrasures can usually be accomplished with dental floss (Box 21-3). Dental floss is a thin-diameter thread that slides easily into tight contacts and is available as a waxed or unwaxed product. Unwaxed floss can occasionally fray when inserted or removed from tight contacts or when overlapping of teeth is present. Waxed floss and polytetrafluoroethylene (PTFE) coated dental floss can be inserted between contacts more easily than an unwaxed flossing product. The thin diameter of dental floss allows easy subgingival insertion to cleanse the proximal surface.

Floss and Tape

Dental floss is manufactured in single-use units (Fig. 21-2) and on spools of several yards. Dental flossing is usually done manually held by the fingers of both hands; however, it is also manufactured as a single-use unit attached to a holder, or the floss can be placed onto a floss holder (Fig. 21-3). Dental tape, a flattened and wider form of dental floss, is recommended for cleaning Class I to Class II embrasures.

Textured

Super floss, tufted, or textured floss are products available for cleaning proximal surfaces and subgingival areas and offer additional features to the traditional floss vari-

BOX 21-3

Traditional Use of Floss

Flossing Technique

- When using both hands, a sufficient supply of floss (approximately 16 inches) is removed from the spool
- Wrap one end of the floss loosely on the middle finger of one hand enough to secure the floss (4-5 inches).
- Wrap the remainder of the floss on the middle finger of the other hand (loosely so as not to cut off the circulation) leaving 2 to 3 inches between the fingers.
- The middle fingers act in a scroll-like fashion holding the floss, wrapping and unwrapping to provide a clean area on the floss for each proximal area. *Using the same piece of floss from one proximal area to the next can introduce bacteria from one area to another.*
- Using the first finger and thumb, grasp the floss that has been left between the two middle fingers. The first finger and the thumb provide stability by keeping the floss tight for insertion between the teeth.
- Insert the floss between the teeth with a gentle back-and-forth (sawing) motion until the floss has moved apical to the contact.
- Slide the floss gently apically under the gingival tissue without cutting the gingival tissues, and encircle the proximal surface onto the line angles.
- Move the floss coronal to the contact and then apically along the proximal surface at least two times to remove soft deposits.

- Remove the floss from the proximal area, wind the used portion of the floss on the middle finger, unwind on the finger with the most floss, and then move to the next proximal area.
- If the floss gets caught in the contact, do not force the floss coronally; release one end of the floss, pull the other end facially, and slide the floss out of the proximal area. If there is floss remaining in the contact, try to reinsert the floss or have waxed floss or PTFE-coated floss to assist in removal of the floss threads.
- Discard floss when finished flossing.

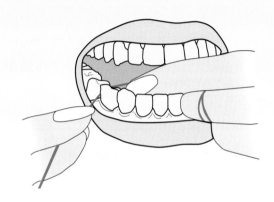

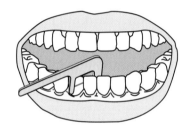

FIG. 21-2. Single-use floss unit.

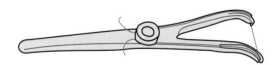

FIG. 21-3. Rethreading of floss is necessary with some floss handles.

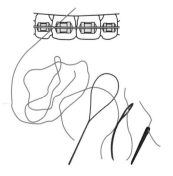

FIG. 21-4. Floss threaders and precut floss units.

eties (Fig. 21-4). Dental floss is available in flavors, fluoride coatings, and whitening components. Several floss manufacturers have added a spongy or textured surface to floss to assist in proximal cleaning for Class II and III embrasures. Although some of these product features may be appropriate for use in a Class I embrasure, the use will depend on a patient's oral anatomy. Super floss is designed to remove plaque from orthodontic appliances; fixed bridges; and Class I, II, and III embrasures. It is dispensed in a single strand with three components: a threader end, textured floss in the middle, and regular dental floss on the opposite end. Recommending super floss when only Class I embrasures are present is not efficient because there is a limited amount of the dental floss portion on the super floss strand. However, when a patient has multiple needs, such as bridgework, this aid can be sufficient.

Flossing Technique

In order to clean the proximal surfaces and line angles that may not be sufficiently cleaned with a toothbrush, floss or tape has to be placed into this area regardless of the technique used. The insertion and motion of the manual technique and the use of a flossing aid are identical. A step-by-step technique for flossing can be seen in Box 21-3.

Floss Holder

A floss holder can assist individuals whose dexterity or oral architecture cannot accommodate manual flossing with finger-held floss (see Fig. 21-3). Floss is wound around a central button, guided between two "fingers," then secured around the button. The taught floss in the holder can thus be substituted for the use of fingers. New floss can be pulled into place for the next proximal surface with the floss holder. The single unit floss variety, however, does not permit the use of a clean area of floss for each proximal surface.

Floss Threader

Certain conditions, such as orthodontics and fixed bridges, require the use of a floss threader (see Fig. 21-4). In both cases, the insertion of floss through the proximal contact area is not possible. A floss threader is strong and flexible enough to be easily threaded underneath the contact area. The threader looks like a sewing needle; floss is inserted into the eye of the threader, and the opposite end is then inserted underneath the contact. The dental floss is then used to cleanse each proximal surface. In fixed bridges, the floss will be passed underneath the pontic; for removal of soft deposits, the floss will be passed on the underside of the pontic.

Encouraging an orthodontic patient to use a floss threader to remove plaque around arch wires is as challenging as it is rewarding. Although flossing in these cases may take longer than normal, it is essential because these dental appliances harbor bacterial plaque that can be responsible for gingivitis and dental caries if left undisturbed.

Interdental Brushes

Interdental brushes are appropriate for Class II and III embrasures, furcations, and tooth surfaces adjacent to missing teeth and posterior to the distal-most molar where space is limited. The interdental brush handle is designed with contra-angled ends that provide a place for insertion of a disposable brush. These brushes come in two shapes (cylindrical and cone-shaped) and are available in varying diameters (Fig. 21-5). The recommendation of the most appropriate size and shape of interdental brush will depend on a careful examination of the oral architecture and tooth anatomy.

End-Tufted Brushes

An end-tufted brush holds tufts of bristles affixed to the end of a handle and is best used to clean proximal surfaces of teeth where an adjacent tooth is missing or in the posterior, distal-most surface in the mouth.

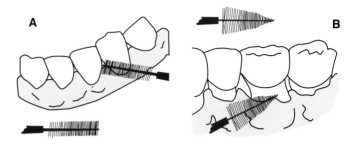

FIG. 21-5. Cylindrical **(A)** and tapered **(B)** interproximal brushes.

Use of Interdental and End-Tufted Brushes

To clean the proximal surfaces of a class II or III embrasure, an interdental or end-tufted brush is placed underneath the contact into the interproximal space and moved back and forth across the proximal surface. The brush should be rinsed when the procedure is finished and allowed to air dry. Floss may also be inserted into the area to ensure subgingival plaque removal.

Other Proximal Cleaning Aids

The following aids can also be used for proximal cleaning. Selection is based on oral architecture, dental anatomy, patient skill, or the lack of availability of other new products manufactured for oral care.

- Knitting yarn, pipe cleaners, and gauze strips are used for Class II and III embrasures and open spaces.
- Perio aids—A round, wooden toothpick is inserted into the end of the handle, broken off flush with the handle, and the point end is used to clean around the gingival margin and into the proximal surfaces of Class II and II embrasures as well as around into furcations.
- Stimudents are used to clean proximal surfaces of Class II and III embrasures and around furcations.
- Toothpicks are used to remove food debris from between teeth. Repeated incorrect use will result in blunted interdental papilla.

 Case Application

An evaluation of the proximal plaque retention and the embrasure configuration coupled with Mrs. Cronin's dexterity problems leave the hygienist with several concerns. What would your concerns be?

 RITICAL THINKING ACTIVITIES

1. Interview and/or survey 10 individuals regarding their oral self-care activities. Record and summarize the findings and discuss the expected and unexpected results.
   a. Evaluate the design of each toothbrush (head and handle shape, bristle configuration and type, and wear). How many need replacing?
   b. Determine the number of times each individual brushes per day and the average length of time each spends on brushing.
   c. Determine how and when each individual uses interdental cleaning products.
   d. Inquire about the method each individual uses for self-assessment of plaque removal.
   e. Record the instructions received from the oral healthcare provider. Determine which dental professional gave the instructions.
2. Evaluate five patient charts for the type of dental cleaning recommendations given. Summarize the results and discuss the expected and unexpected results.

REVIEW QUESTIONS

Questions 1 through 6 refer to the case study presented at the beginning of the chapter. Questions 7 to 14 refer to another patient, Mrs. Katrina Darcy, and her family.

1. Mrs. Cronin cannot take her powered toothbrush on vacation. Which of the following toothbrushes would you recommend she purchase?
   a. Large handle, multitufted small head
   b. Regular handle, flat-bristle medium head
   c. Child-size toothbrush
   d. Large handle, multitufted large head

2. Respond to Mrs. Cronin's question: "My sister loves to use waxed dental floss, but she heard that unwaxed floss is better. What do you think?"
   a. "Both work well. She should use the floss that is easiest for her."
   b. "Unwaxed is better because it is easier to use."
   c. "Unwaxed is better because it is thinner."
   d. "Waxed floss leaves a wax residue, so don't use it."

3. Mrs. Cronin has asked, "How frequently should I replace the head on my powered toothbrush?" How do you respond?
   a. "Every 3 months."
   b. "When the brush begins to show wear."
   c. "After you have been ill, especially after a cold."
   d. All of the above.

4. Mrs. Cronin's 12-year-old granddaughter has normal gingival tissue and tight contacts and several rotated teeth. Which of the following interdental aids is the best recommendation for her?
   a. Unwaxed floss
   b. Waxed floss
   c. Proximal brush
   d. Triangular wood stick

5. Mrs. Cronin's son-in-law just purchased a natural bristle toothbrush. Which of the following bristle types would you recommend as a replacement?
   a. Soft, natural bristle
   b. Medium, natural bristle
   c. Soft, nylon bristle
   d. Medium, nylon bristle

6. After Mrs. Cronin brushes, she uses a disclosing solution to check her plaque control. She reports that she notices a thin band of plaque remaining at the gingival margin. Which of the following recommendations should be made?
   a. Use an interproximal brush.
   b. Use waxed floss.
   c. Brush for a longer period of time.
   d. Angle the head of the toothbrush so the initial placement is against the gingiva at the gingival one third of the tooth.

7. Which of the following brushing methods is best recommended for Mrs. Cronin's 6-year-old grandson?
   a. Scrub brush method
   b. Fones' method
   c. Modified Bass method
   d. Rolling stroke method

8. Mrs. Cronin's son-in-law, Peter, has returned for a supportive care visit. He has a history of periodontal surgery and presents with healthy gingiva, large interproximal spaces, and slight plaque deposits. He says he enjoys using a wooden toothpick to clean between his teeth. How should you proceed?
   a. Coach Peter on the effective use of a toothpick.
   b. Substitute a proximal brush for the toothpick.
   c. Demonstrate the benefit of dental tape for the wide embrasure spaces.
   d. Review his tooth-brushing technique.

 ## SUGGESTED AGENCIES AND WEB SITES

Because of the ever-changing nature of the Internet, some of the web sites listed here may have changed since publication. Please refer to Mosby's Evolve web site for the most current information.

American Dental Association: http://www.ada.org
American Dental Hygienists' Association: http://www.adha.org
American Academy of Periodontology: http://www.perio.org
American Society of Dentistry for Children: http://www.asdc.org
Colgate Oral Pharmaceuticals, (800) 2-COLGATE: http://www.colgate.com
John O. Butler Company, (800) JBUTLER: http://www.jbutler.com
Johnson & Johnson, (800) 257-9508: http://www.jnj.com

National Institute of Dental and Craniofacial Research (NIDCR): http://www.nidcr.nih.gov
Oral B, (800) 446-7252: http://www.oralb.com
Procter and Gamble Company, (800) 997-8337: http://www.dentalcare.com
Warner Lambert (division of Pfizer), (800) 973-2000: http://www.warner-lambert.com

ADDITIONAL READINGS AND RESOURCES

Cohen LK, Gift HC, editors: *Disease prevention and oral health promotion,* Copenhagen, 1995, Munksgaard.

DeBiase CB: *Dental health education,* Philadelphia, 1991, Lea & Febiger.

Harris NO, Garcia-Godoy F: Primary preventive dentistry, ed 5, Stamford, Conn, 1999, Appleton & Lange.

Schou L, Blinkhorn AS, editors: *Oral health promotion,* Oxford, 1993, Oxford University Press.

REFERENCES

1. American Dental Association Seal-of-Acceptance Program: The ADA Seal of Acceptance Program [Internet], Chicago, 1999, American Dental Association http://www.ada.org

2. Bader HI: Review of currently available battery-operated toothbrushes, *Compend Cont Educ Dent* 13:1162, December 1992.

3. Bass CC: The optimum characteristics of toothbrushes for personal oral hygiene, *Dent Items Int* 70: 697-718, 1948.

4. Bass CC: An effective method of personal oral hygiene, II, *J Louisiana State Med Soc* 108:100-112, 1954.

5. Boyd RI: Clinical and laboratory evaluation of powered electric toothbrushes: review of the literature, *J Clin Dent* 8 (3 Spec No): 67-71,1997.

6. Claydon N et al: Comparative professional plaque removal study using 8 branded toothbrushes, *J Clin Periodontol* 29:310-316, 2002.

7. Claydon N, Addy M: Comparative single-use plaque removal by toothbrushes of different designs, *J Clin Periodontol* 23: 1112, 1996.

8. Checchi L, Minguzzi S, Franchi M, Forteleoni G: Toothbrush filaments end-rounding:stereomicroscope analysis, *J Clin Periodontol* 28:360-364, 2001.

9. Choo A, Delac, Messer LB: Oral hygiene measures and promotion: review and considerations, *Aust Dent Jr* 46:166-173, 2001.

10. Corbet EF, Davies WR: The role of supragingival plaque in the control of progressive periodontal disease: a review, *J Clin Periodontol* 20:307-313, 1993.

11. Emling RC, Yankell SL: The application of sonic technology to oral hygiene: the third generation of powered toothbrushes, *J Clin Dent* 8:1-3, 1997.

12. Fones AC: Home care of the mouth. In Fones AC, editor: *Mouth hygiene,* ed 4, Philadelphia, 1934, Lea & Febiger.

13. Fransden A: Mechanical oral hygiene practices. State-of-the-science review. In Loe H and Kleinman DV, editors: *Dental plaque control measures and oral hygiene practices. Proceedings for a state of the science workshop,* Oxford, 1986, IRL Press Ltd, pp. 93-116.

14. Glutch-Scranton J: *Collaboration and empowerment in educational activities during dental hygiene care,* Ann Arbor, Mich, 1992, University Microfilms.

15. Grossman E et al: A comparative study of extrinsic stain removal with two electric toothbrushes and a manual brush, *Am J Dent* 9:25-29,1996.

16. Hancock EB: Prevention. In Genco RJ, Newman MG, editors: *Annals of periodontology;* Chicago, 1996, American Academy of Periodontology.

17. Heaseman PA, Jacobs DJ, Chapple IL: An evaluation of the effectiveness and patient compliance with plaque control methods and prevention of periodontal disease, *Clin Prev Dent* 11:24-28, 1989.

18. Heanue M, Deacaon SA: Manual versus powered toothbrushing for oral health, *Cochrane Database Syst Rev* (1):CD002281, 2003.

19. Hine M: Toothbrush, *Int Dent J* 6:15, 1956.

20. International Organization for Standardization Dentistry–stiffness of the tufted area of toothbrushes, Reference ISO 8627: 1987 (4-page guideline document).

21. Jepson S: The role of manual toothbrushes in effective plaque control. In Lang NP, Attstrom R, Loe H, editors: *Proceedings of European workshop on mechanical plaque removal,* Chicago, 1998, Quintessence Books.

22. Moritis K, Delaurenti M: Comparison of the Sonicare Elite and a manual toothbrush in the evaluation of plaque reduction, *Am J Dent* (15 Spec No): 23B-25B, 2002.

23. Nelson D: *Review of dental hygiene,* Philadelphia, 2000, Saunders.

24. Nemcovsky CE, Artzi Z: Erosion-abrasion lesions revisited, *Compend Cont Educ Dent* 17: 516-523, 1996.

25. O'Neil HW: Opinion study comparing attitudes about dental health, *J Am Dent Assoc* 109:910-915, 1984.

26. Renton-Harper P, Addy M, Newcombe RG: Plaque removal with the uninstructed use of electric toothbrushes: comparison with a manual brush and toothpaste slurry, *J Clin Periodontol* 28:325-330, 2001.

27. Ring ME: *Dentistry—An Illustrated History,* New York, 1985, Abradale Press, Harry N. Abrams, Inc. Publishers, pp. 34-141.

28. Ring ME: The "electric" toothbrush of one hundred years ago, *Periodont Clin Invest* 21(1):23,1999

29. Saxer U: Impact of improved toothbrushes on dental diseases. II. *Quint Int* 28(9):573-593, 1997.

30. Sembera HW: Evolution and analysis of the toothbrush, www.org/mechanicaladvantage/March2001/toothbrush.html

31. Smith C: Toothbrush technology-even the pharaohs brushed their teeth, J Dent Tech 17(4):26-27, 2000.

32. Stillman PR: A philosophy of the treatment of periodontal disease, *Dent Digest* 38:315-319, 1932.

33. Van der Weijden GA et al: The role of electric toothbrushes: advantages and limitations. In Lang NP, Attstrom R, Loe H, editors: *Proceedings of European workshop on mechanical plaque removal,* Chicago, 1998, Quintessence Books.

34. Warren PR et al: A clinical investigation into the effect of toothbrush wear on efficacy, *J Clin Dent* 13:119-124, 2002.

35. Westfelt E: Rationale of mechanical plaque control, *J Clin Periodontol* 23:263-267,1996.

36. Wolf L, Kim A: Effectiveness of a sonic toothbrush in maintenance of dental implants, *J Clin Periodontol* 25:821-828, 1998.

37. Yankell SL, Saxer UP: Toothbrushes and toothbrushing methods. In Harris NO, Garcia-Godoy F, editors: *Primary preventive dentistry,* ed 6, Stamford Conn, 2004, Appleton & Lange.

CHAPTER 22

Fluoride *and the* Reversal *of* Dental Caries

Douglas A. Young, John D.B. Featherstone

Chapter Outline

Caries and Oral Hygiene
Case Study: Remineralization of the Early Carious
   Lesion
The Caries Process
   Demineralization
   Remineralization
   Composition of tooth mineral
Flouride
   Topical versus systemic uptake
   Role in saliva
   Mechanisms of action
Management of Dental Caries
   Team approach and the dental hygienist
   Caries management by risk assessment
   Caries risk assessment

Salivary analysis
Patient involvement
Management of a carious lesion
Reevaluation period
Clinical Implications: Fluoride-Delivery Systems
Professional Applications
   Patient education
   Traditional paint-on technique
   Fluoride varnish
   Fluoride trays
   Patient monitoring
Fluoride Toxicity
Self-Applied Topical Fluoride Products
Fluoride Supplements in Caries Prevention

Key Terms

Acidogenic bacteria
Body of the lesion
Buffering
Carbonated apatite
Caries management by risk
   assessment (CAMBRA)

Caries risk assessment
   (CRA)
Cavitation
Cavity
Demineralization
Dental caries

Diffusion channels
Fluorapatite
Fluoride
Fluorosis
Hydroxyapatite

Lactobacilli (LB)
Mutans streptococci (MS)
Parts per million (ppm)
Remineralization
White spot lesion

Learning Outcomes

1. Use caries risk assessment data to develop caries prevention and disease intervention strategies for patients.
2. Recommend the appropriate fluoride products for the patient's use.
3. Select appropriate therapeutic strategies for implementation in the dental office.

4. Establish an appropriate interval for evaluation of the suggested strategies.
5. Work with other oral healthcare providers in the management of dental caries.

Chapter 16 emphasizes the detection of *dental caries* as part of the hard tissue evaluation. This chapter focuses on the molecular mechanisms of dental caries and the management of this infectious disease, including preventive and conservative treatment protocols and chemical treatment of early lesions. The chemical aspects of *demineralization* and *remineralization* and the role of *fluoride* are discussed to solidify the scientific basis for caries management by risk assessment. Fluoride products and their proper use also are reviewed.

CARIES AND ORAL HYGIENE

Studies in the 1950s implied that oral hygiene programs reduced the incidence of dental caries, which explains the traditional approach of "drilling and filling" with improvements in oral hygiene. Later clinical studies that compared fluoride-containing dentifrice to placebo dentifrice reported caries reductions of approximately 30%, clearly showing that the addition of fluoride was important for beneficial anticaries effects related to tooth brushing.[80]

Dental caries remains a major problem in many developing countries. Although declining in most Western countries over the past two decades, caries continues to be the principal reason for dental treatment and tooth loss.[47,87] Interestingly, 80% of caries in U.S. children is found in 25% of the population.[47] Dental caries also remains a major problem in U.S. adults, with 94% reporting caries in one survey.[87] The reasons for the reported reductions in tooth decay during the last 20 years have not been determined precisely, but evidence indicates that the use of fluoride products is the major reason.[44,46] Such products include fluoride toothpaste, fluoride mouthrinses, and topical fluorides in the dental office. In addition to fluoride products, many public water supplies are fluoridated, resulting in a reported 40% to 70% reduction in dental caries.[13,66,68,69]

THE CARIES PROCESS

The basic process of dental decay is simple in concept. A biofilm called *pellicle,* derived from saliva, is strongly bound to the tooth surface. This coating has many beneficial effects, including protecting the surface from direct acid exposure and thus inhibiting demineralization. The pellicle, however, is in turn covered by the bacteria that form the dental plaque.[59,61] If the bacterial plaque contains significant numbers of the bacterial groups *mutans streptococci (MS)* or *lactobacilli (LB),* the by-products of their metabolism will be organic acids, such as formic, lactic, acetic, and propionic acids. MS includes several species, classified into serotypes, especially *Streptococcus mutans* and *S. sobrinus,* that occur in humans. These acid-producing bacteria are called *acidogenic bacteria.* That is, they produce acids when they metabolize fermentable carbohydrates.[59,61,68] Any fermentable carbohydrate, such as glucose, sucrose, fructose, or cooked starch, can be metabolized by these bacteria to produce acid as a by-product of their metabolism,[41] dispelling the myth that only "sweets" containing sucrose cause dental caries.

DEMINERALIZATION

The organic acids produced by pathogenic bacteria can dissolve the calcium phosphate mineral of the tooth

 Remineralization of the Early Carious Lesion

Frances Svensen, a 25-year-old sixth-grade teacher, reports to your dental office for a supportive care appointment. She and her husband have recently relocated to the area because of her husband's job transfer. She has brought her previous set of bitewing radiographs, which was taken 3 years before the current appoinment, at which a current set is ordered. Review her radiographs for signs of hard tissue disease (Fig. 22-1, *A*).

In comparing the radiograph taken 3 years ago with that taken at the current appointment (Fig. 22-1, *B*), what do you notice about the following teeth?

Tooth	*3 Years Ago*	*Now*
#11 Distal	Incipient lesion	Incipient lesion unchanged
#12 Mesial	Incipient lesion	Lesion progressed through dentinoenamel junction (DEJ)
#13 Distal	Incipient lesion	Lesion remineralized
#14 Mesial	Carious lesion	Lesion restored
#15 Mesial	No lesion noted	Carious lesion evident
#18 Occlusal	Recurrent caries	Caries restored
#21 Distoocclusal	Caries evident	Caries restored

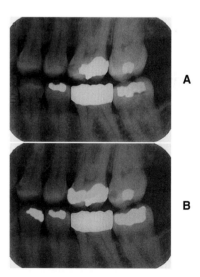

FIG. 22-1 Frances Svensen's previous **(A)** and current **(B)** radiographs.

enamel or dentin through the process of *demineralization.*[23,31,35] When taken into the mouth, fermentable carbohydrate is metabolized by the bacteria, creating acid as a by-product. The acid then diffuses from the *plaque fluid* (the water-based fluid among the bacteria in dental plaque) through the pellicle covering the tooth and into the tooth itself. Surprisingly to many, the enamel is porous to small molecules and ions, such as calcium, phosphate, fluoride, and the organic acids. Movement of these small molecules and ions into the tooth is driven by passive diffusion from an area of high concentration to an area of low concentration. Thus the diffusion of molecules follows a simple concentration gradient and continues until the concentration reaches equilibrium. The organic acids readily diffuse, following the concentration gradient into the enamel (or dentin if exposed), and dissociate to produce hydrogen ions as they travel.[22,35] The dissociated hydrogen ions then dissolve the mineral, freeing calcium and phosphate into solution, which can then diffuse from the tooth through a similar concentration gradient.

If demineralization is not halted or reversed, the caries lesion progresses and can eventually lead to a *cavity* or *cavitation.* The spaces between the enamel crystals that allow these small molecules to diffuse are called *diffusion channels* (see the section on composition of tooth mineral later in this chapter). This process of demineralization continues until equilibrium again is reached.

REMINERALIZATION

If the acid is neutralized and the concentration of calcium and phosphate ions becomes higher outside the tooth than inside, the calcium and phosphate ions reverse direction and diffuse back into the tooth, again through a concentration gradient. This replacement of mineral back into the tooth is called *remineralization.*[23,82,83] The saliva plays numerous roles, including neutralizing the acid, or *buffering,* and providing the minerals (calcium and phosphate ions) that can replace those dissolved from the tooth during a demineralization challenge.

The earliest clinically detectable sign of dental caries is the *white spot lesion* of enamel. This lesion consists of a demineralized region called the *body of the lesion* just below what appears to be an intact surface layer.[78] This subsurface area may have lost up to 50% of its mineral and can be distinguished in the laboratory by specialized histological techniques such as microradiography or polarized light microscopy. Clinically the lesion appears white because the loss of mineral changes the refractive index compared with that of the surrounding translucent enamel. The ability to recognize a white spot lesion clinically is a valuable asset for the clinician. A shiny white spot is usually a sign of arrested or remineralized lesions, and a dull appearance may indicate that the lesion is still actively demineralizing (see Chapter 16).

Why does the surface layer remain intact, or does it? In the early stages of caries the surface crystals are partially dissolved by the plaque acids, and during subsequent repair they are partially remineralized as subsurface demineralization progresses. This process makes the surface appear "intact," and the mineral is less soluble than it was originally. This remineralized surface accounts for the apparently intact surface layer seen by microradiography or polarized light microscopy in an early enamel lesion. This surface generally "feels" sound to gentle probing by the dental explorer.

COMPOSITION OF TOOTH MINERAL

Enamel is the hardest substance of the human body. The enamel and dentin of a tooth comprise millions of tiny

TABLE 22-1

Approximate composition of enamel and dentin

	ENAMEL		DENTIN	
Tissue component	% by Weight	% by Volume	% by Weight	% by Volume
Mineral: carbonated hydroxyapatite	96	85	70	47
Protein/lipid	1	3	20	33
Water	3	12	10	20

mineral crystals embedded in a protein-lipid matrix. The individual crystals of enamel are only about 40 nm in diameter, about $\frac{1}{1000}$ of the thickness of a human hair. These small crystals lie approximately perpendicular to the tooth surface and are clustered into enamel rods about 4 to 5 μm in diameter.[37] The tiny spaces or pores between the individual crystals and the larger spaces between the enamel rods are filled with protein, lipid, and water, which make up small passageways called *diffusion channels.* The diffusion channels between enamel rods form larger passageways than the channels between the individual crystals. The rod channels are large enough to allow the passage of small molecules and ions, such as hydrogen, calcium, phosphate, fluoride, and the organic acids produced by MS and LB, but are too narrow to allow entry of bacteria. Mature enamel is about 85% by volume mineral and 15% lipid, protein, and water; thus 15% is the volume available for diffusion (Table 22-1). The percent by volume is relevant to the diffusion processes that are the basis of dental caries progression. As the enamel is demineralized during caries progression, the mineral removed makes the carious enamel even more porous.[78] Dentin and cementum are roughly 47% by volume mineral and 53% lipid, protein, and water, illustrating their more porous nature.

For years the dental profession has referred to the tooth mineral as *hydroxyapatite,* even though pure hydroxyapatite does not exist in real teeth. Rather than "pure," the mineral of enamel, dentin, and bone may be viewed as "contaminated" by carbonate and other minerals, making the substance much more soluble in acid. Thus tooth mineral can be described best as a highly substituted *carbonated apatite.*[54,55] Although related to hydroxyapatite $[Ca_{10}(PO_4)_6(OH)_2]$, carbonated hydroxyapatite differs from pure hydroxyapatite in two ways. First, carbonated apatite is calcium deficient, with some calcium replaced by sodium, magnesium, zinc, and other substitutes. Second, some of the phosphate ions in the crystal lattice are replaced by carbonate, which can be as much as 3% to 6% by weight.* All these substitutions occur during tooth development, when the mineral is first laid down. The carbonate-rich areas represent major defects in the crystal structure. The three-dimensional size and shape of the carbonate ion differs from the phosphate ion, causing major crystal imperfections that are more susceptible to acid attack during demineralization.[29,32] The calcium substitutions (e.g., sodium, magnesium, zinc) also cause similar

---

*References 12, 15, 16, 30, 34, 54, 55.

defects in the crystal lattice, although to a lesser extent than the carbonate defects. The combined effect of tooth mineral being calcium deficient and carbonate rich is that the carbonated hydroxyapatite is much more soluble in acid than pure hydroxyapatite.

Just as the previously discussed substitutions make the crystal less perfect and more soluble, the fluoride ion (F^-) can substitute for the hydroxyl ion (OH^-) of hydroxyapatite and make the crystal more perfect and less soluble. This improved crystal is called **fluorapatite** [$Ca_{10}(PO_4)_6F_2$], which is very resistant to dissolution by acid. The solubility differential can be ranked as follows:
1. *Dental mineral, or carbonated hydroxyapatite:* most soluble in acid
2. *Hydroxyapatite:* less soluble in acid
3. *Fluorapatite:* least soluble in acid

The composition of crystal surfaces in remineralized enamel is a blend of hydroxyapatite and fluorapatite, and the remineralized crystals are therefore much less soluble than the original mineral.[83]

In summary, dental mineral is readily dissolved by acid unless it can be protected in some way, as with fluoride. The overwhelming reason for caries reduction in the United States is the use of topical fluoride.

FLUORIDE

TOPICAL VERSUS SYSTEMIC UPTAKE

Another misconception in dentistry is that the major caries-inhibiting effect of fluoride is caused by its systemic uptake and incorporation into the enamel during tooth development before eruption. This misconception led to water fluoridation and the use of oral fluoride supplements prescribed for children without access to fluoridated water. As the mechanism of dental caries was elucidated in the 1970s and 1980s, the importance of fluoride in caries prevention became apparent. However, the effects were found to be *topical* via the surface of the tooth, not systemic.* *Topical uptake* means the fluoride diffuses into the surface of the enamel of an erupted tooth rather than being incorporated preeruptively during development (systemic incorporation). Surprisingly, this fact is still not widely known, and the standard of care still recommends "dietary fluoride supplements" for children in nonfluoridated communities. Why then is fluoride still added to the drinking water? The simple answer is that fluoride in the drinking water works primarily by "topical" mechanisms and continues to be an effective public health measure for adults and children. From a public health standpoint, fluoridation of public water supplies is a good way to deliver fluoride to lower socioeconomic populations that may not otherwise have access to topical fluoride products, such as fluoridated dentifrice and mouthrinse.

Fluoridated water and prescription supplements incorporate insufficient amounts of fluoride systemically into the dental mineral to play a significant role in caries prevention.[40,83] Systemic delivery incorporates only about 1000 to 2000 **parts per million (ppm)** of fluoride in the outer enamel surface and 20 to 100 ppm of fluoride below the surface, depending on the fluoride ingestion during tooth de-

---

BOX 22-1

Groups of Salivary Components

1. Proteins that form pellicle and protect the tooth surface (proline-rich proteins, statherins, histatins, cystatins)
2. Proteins that maintain the calcium and phosphate in solution in a supersaturated state (proline-rich proteins, statherins)
3. Proteins with antifungal and antibacterial properties (histatins, lysozyme, lactoferrin, lactoperoxidase)
4. Immunoglobulins (IgG, IgA)
5. Lipids that form part of the pellicle
6. Minerals, including calcium, phosphate, fluoride, and bicarbonate, that keep the teeth intact and buffer acids produced in the plaque
7. Proteins with other functions, such as inhibition of proteases (cystatins), lubrication (mucins), and neutralization of acids (peptides)

---

velopment.[74] Other experiments showed that systemic uptake of fluoride during tooth development resulted in no measurable benefit against acid-induced dissolution.[23,36,67,83] In contrast to systemic delivery, topical sources of fluoride can deliver as much as 30,000 ppm to the surfaces of the individual crystals of enamel, which significantly reduces mineral solubility in acid.[23] Thus the effect of systemically ingested fluoride on caries is negligible compared with topical uptake. Prescription supplements are still the standard of care for children in nonfluoridated communities, but considering the risks of **fluorosis** (disturbance of enamel formation by fluoride during tooth development), use of systemic fluoride supplements soon may be questioned. Currently, if prescribed, fluoride supplements should be used as a topical delivery system, with patients sucking or chewing tablets or lozenges before ingestion.

ROLE IN SALIVA

Saliva may represent the single most important group of components in the maintenance of oral health because it contains many protective proteins and minerals and keeps them available in solution (Box 22-1). Laboratory studies have shown that a very low level of fluoride in the saliva (0.04 ppm) is sufficient to produce beneficial anticaries effects through remineralization.[23,26,33] As the fluoride concentration increases above 0.04 ppm, the amount of remineralization also increases, with an optimum level at 0.08 ppm or greater. Clinically this data indicate that small increases in the background level of fluoride in saliva and plaque fluid may provide important caries protection for erupted teeth of both children and adults.

When topical fluoride products are used in the mouth—whether a dentifrice (toothpaste), a fluoride mouthrinse, or prescribed agent—the increased fluoride levels in the saliva diminish over time as the fluoride is cleared from the mouth. Beneficial levels of fluoride between 0.03 and 0.1 ppm can be sustained for as long as 2 to 6 hours, depending on the product and the individual.[11] For example, researchers have shown that a 0.05% sodium fluoride (NaF) mouthrinse (225 ppm fluoride) used for

1 minute not only provided increased salivary levels of fluoride for 2 to 4 hours but also remained in plaque for much longer.[90] Other researchers also demonstrated that daily use of both a fluoride-containing dentifrice and a 0.05% NaF topical rinse could prevent formation of white spot lesions completely (early demineralization) around orthodontic brackets *in vivo* (on human patients).[71] Thus simple use of a fluoride mouthrinse for 1 minute twice a day can extend the preventive effects of fluoride day and night. In fact, people with xerostomia (lack of saliva), who are at great risk for caries, can retain elevated levels of fluoride for longer because of their low salivary flow (slow clearance effect).[8] The beneficial effects of a 0.05% NaF mouthrinse on xerostomic patients have been demonstrated clearly.[63]

Reviewing the success of topical fluoride in both access to the public and in reduction of the incidence of caries is interesting. Before fluoride in toothpaste was commonplace, the salivary fluoride concentrations reported in early studies were about 0.005 to 0.01 ppm fluoride. As fluoride use became more common in the late 1980s, clinical studies involving 7- to 12-year-old children in the United States reported mean baseline fluoride concentrations in saliva of 0.02 to 0.04 ppm in both fluoridated and nonfluoridated drinking water areas.[56,57] Clearly these higher salivary fluoride levels were achieved from topical fluoride sources other than the public water supplies; thus the salivary fluoride concentration (from all sources) rather than drinking water concentration is predictive of caries status.[56] In the 1990s similar studies on 7- to 12-year-old children reported slightly higher mean salivary levels of about 0.05 ppm fluoride, but again, this mean was the same for both fluoridated and nonfluoridated communities.[76,77] Not surprisingly, these studies also showed that children with high individual salivary fluoride (0.075 ppm or greater) were more frequently caries-free.

MECHANISMS OF ACTION

Topical fluoride prevents and inhibits caries progression in three ways: (1) inhibition of demineralization; (2) enhancement of remineralization, including the deposition of a more caries-resistant surface (fluorapatite) on the remineralized individual crystals; and (3) inhibition of bacterial activity.* These fluoride mechanisms rely on the fluoride being available in solution at the surface of the tooth.

Inhibition of Demineralization

When present in solution among the carbonated apatite (enamel mineral) crystals inside the tooth, fluoride inhibits demineralization by strongly *adsorbing* to the surfaces of these crystals, acting as a barrier against acid dissolution of surface sites. Thus when cariogenic bacteria generate acid, the fluoride present in the plaque fluid (even at low levels) travels with the acid into the subsurface of the tooth, adsorbs to the crystal surface, and protects it from being dissolved.[23,83]

---

*References 4, 23, 38, 42, 82, 83.

Enhancement of Remineralization

Fluoride enhances, or "speeds up," remineralization by adsorbing to the crystal surfaces and attracting calcium ions, which attract phosphate ions, leading to rapid crystal growth. The acid created by the plaque bacteria is neutralized slowly by the buffering components (bicarbonate, phosphate, and peptides) in healthy saliva as it flows over the plaque, causing the pH to increase toward neutral (Fig. 22-2). This buffering action eventually halts the subsurface dissolution of the mineral.

Along with the buffering components, the saliva is supersaturated with calcium and phosphate, acting as a reservoir until the chemistry (pH and concentration) is conducive for these essential minerals to diffuse back into the tooth and *remineralize,* or regrow a new crystal surface on the already partially demineralized surface of the crystal remnants inside the carious lesion. The partially dissolved crystals act as nucleators for new crystal formation, and fluoride adsorption to the crystal's surface greatly accelerates the entire process.

Incorporation of fluoride as phosphate instead of carbonate during remineralization creates a more perfect crystal, with a highly acid-resistant surface similar to the mineral called *fluorapatite.* During remineralization the newly forming crystal surface preferentially takes up fluoride and phosphate from the surrounding solution and excludes carbonate.[83] Therefore this veneer has a composition between hydroxyapatite and fluorapatite, as described previously. Fluorapatite contains about 30,000 ppm fluoride through topical fluoride uptake, creating a new surface that is fluorapatite-like in its properties and less soluble in acid than the more highly soluble carbon-

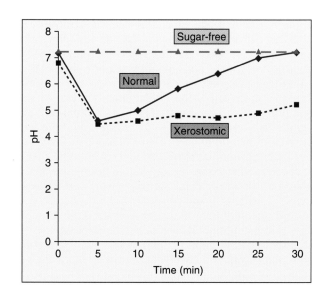

FIG. 22-2 Typical pH curve in dental plaque *(normal)* after ingestion of fermentable carbohydrate, characterized by a fall in pH due to generation of plaque acids and a return to neutral due to buffering by salivary components. Typical pH–time curves for a xerostomic subject and a normal subject with a sugar-free test are shown for comparison. (Modified from Featherstone JDB: Prevention and reversal of dental caries: role of low level fluoride, *Community Dent Oral Epidemiol* 27(1):31-40, 1999.)

ated apatite of the original crystal surface.[23] Fig. 22-3 outlines the demineralization–remineralization process.

Inhibition of Bactericidal Activity

After it enters the cell, fluoride is toxic to plaque bacteria because it both acidifies the cytoplasm and interferes with key enzyme pathways. Fluoride, in its ionized form (F^-), cannot cross the bacterial cell wall and membrane. Fluoride can travel rapidly through the cell wall and into the cariogenic bacteria only in the form of undissociated hydrofluoric acid (HF).[42,84,86] The cariogenic bacteria produce acids during metabolism of fermentable carbohydrates, causing a fall in the pH (see Fig. 22-2). A portion of the fluoride (F^-) present in the plaque fluid then combines with hydrogen ions (H^+) to form HF, which then can diffuse rapidly into the cell, effectively drawing more HF from the outside, and so on (Fig. 22-4). Once inside the cell, the HF dissociates again, acidifying the cell and releasing fluoride ions, which interfere with enzyme activity

(e.g., enolase, ATPase) in the bacterium. F^- and H^+ become trapped in the cell, and the process is cumulative, eventually becoming toxic to the bacterium.

In summary, fluoride from topical sources is taken up by the bacteria when they produce acid, thereby inhibiting essential enzyme activity. This process is the third topical mechanism of action of fluoride against the progression of dental caries.

MANAGEMENT OF DENTAL CARIES

Dental caries was once a life-threatening disease and even 22-A today remains a major problem in many developing countries. Although declining in the United States over the past two decades, dental caries continues to be the major reason for dental treatment and the primary cause of tooth loss.[47,87] Thus from a public health standpoint, identification and targeting of appropriate treatment to those individuals at greatest risk makes sense. Treatment of dental caries in the United States is beginning to change from the conventional "surgical" approach proposed by Black in the early 1900s to more contemporary methods. Research has elucidated clearly the mechanism of dental caries,* and the literature has suggested that dentists change the way they manage this infectious disease.[1,2,52] Newer methods include (1) treatment based on caries risk assessments, (2) treatment of caries as a curable and preventable infectious disease, and (3) nonsurgical, chemical approaches to early lesions, using new diagnostic methods.† Although their adoption has been slow in the United States, these new methods have been used in European countries with great promise. Lack of acceptance in the United States may be a result of inadequate compensation for preventive procedures by insurance companies and patients. However, "cosmetic" procedures initially had the same problem, which was helped by the increasing consumer demand and education of third-party payers. A similar approach in addition to more clinical trials scientifically proving the benefits may help in the adoption of new caries-management techniques.

TEAM APPROACH AND THE DENTAL HYGIENIST

The dental profession is advancing beyond the days when dentists are merely "drilling and filling," assistants are simply passing instruments, and hygienists are exclusively cleaning teeth. The traditional view held that the hygienist was only vital to the periodontal management of patients and played little or no role in caries management. The modern dental office, however, emphasizes expanded duties for staff members, with the dental hygienist focusing on patient satisfaction, providing service, and promoting oral health. Modern caries management requires all dental team members, including the patient, to be actively involved in prevention and early intervention. Although surgical restorative repair always will be needed in many cases, at least in the near future, the goal is to minimize this role through elimination of the source of the disease through patient education and chemical therapies.

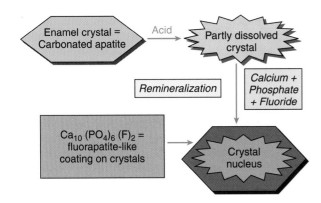

FIG. 22-3 Demineralization and remineralization processes that lead to remineralized crystals with surfaces rich in fluoride and low in solubility. (Modified from Featherstone JDB: Prevention and reversal of dental caries: role of low level fluoride, *Community Dent Oral Epidemiol* 27(1):31-40, 1999.)

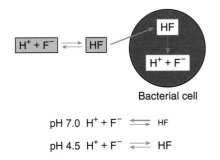

FIG. 22-4 Fluoride enters a bacterial cell in the form of hydrofluoric acid (HF) at lower pH values, dissociates, and thereby provides H^+ and F^- ions inside the cell. At pH 7.0, almost no HF is present. (Modified from Featherstone JDB: Prevention and reversal of dental caries: role of low level fluoride, *Community Dent Oral Epidemiol* 27(1):31-40, 1999.)

*References 4, 23, 26, 37, 39, 82, 83.
†References 2, 5, 25, 45, 53, 70, 72, 81.

Before a diagnosis can be made, dental personnel must provide information and gather data through patient education, oral hygiene instruction, dietary counseling, salivary testing, caries risk assessment, dental charting, and the bringing of suspect lesions to the dentist's attention. Once the dentist has made the diagnosis and outlined the treatment plan, other staff members can perform much of the implementation. For example, dental hygienists can place sealant, perform fluoride therapies, and provide chlorhexidine instruction in many states; clinicians should check local regulations for their state. In addition, the dental hygienist is uniquely positioned to implement remineralization strategies and plays a major role in preventing damage to these early lesions through unnecessary root planing, coronal polishing, or improper hand instrumentation. The dental hygienist and dental assistant must participate in the team approach to modern caries management.

CARIES MANAGEMENT BY RISK ASSESSMENT

The etiology of caries is multifactorial and involves plaque microorganisms, fermentable dietary carbohydrates (including frequency of ingestion), saliva, and the tooth surface itself.[64] The specific plaque hypothesis[58] states that only a limited number of organisms in plaque can cause disease. The primary organisms involved in human caries are MS and LB.[59] These organisms should be targeted, as with any bacterial infection in the human body. Filling teeth does not eliminate infection, and oral hygiene alone has not been proven to eliminate caries.[88] The medical model of dental care involves treatment of the disease, not the symptoms.[1,2] Treatment should be directed at reduction or elimination of MS and LB, not just tooth restoration. Management of caries requires a multifaceted approach.

Dental caries is an infectious disease transmissible from mother to child[14] and even iatrogenically transferred from one carious site to a previously uninfected site.[17,60] Therefore the clinician must use more "sterile" techniques during examination and restorative procedures.

The traditional surgical method used to treat dental caries often included only the restoration of carious teeth, the teaching of oral hygiene, and perhaps advice to avoid eating sweets. In the last decade, researchers and clinicians have demonstrated that these traditional methods alone do not guarantee oral health. Restorative dentistry and oral hygiene have not proven adequate to eliminate dental caries. Newer management techniques treat caries based on a risk assessment of the patient. This type of caries management has several names in the literature, suggesting the need for common nomenclature. In this text the term *caries management by risk assessment (CAMBRA)* is used because it accurately describes the process in which clinicians deal with caries as an infectious disease first by gathering information about the patient's caries risk status (risk assessment) and then by planning intervention or treatment (caries management) based on that risk. Whereas traditional methods treat the consequences of infection (the carious lesions), CAMBRA treats those at risk by the dentist first identifying these individuals and then treating the infection (the pathogenic bacteria). Dentists no longer need to wait until teeth are

damaged to begin caries treatment. CAMBRA is a major step toward prevention and elimination of dental caries disease.

CARIES RISK ASSESSMENT

Caries risk assessment (CRA) begins with an understanding of the chemical nature of the demineralization–remineralization process and the way in which it is affected by fluoride, saliva, pellicle, diet, and the bacterial environment.[37] Xerostomia, a high-sucrose diet, frequent snacking, a lack of fluoride, and the presence of pathogenic organisms can affect the patient's caries risk status. In each individual the unique balance between these pathological and protective components determines risk and ultimately disease (Fig. 22-5). Under average conditions, with an individual whose protective components are not compromised, this delicate balance is tipped either way several times a day. The goal of CAMBRA is to assess the risk of each patient and devise a management plan that tips the balance between protective and pathological components toward health.

The demineralization–remineralization process is a simple, reversible chemical reaction that can be manipulated (through its pathological and protective components) to benefit patient health.[26] To perform CRA, the dentist qualitatively weighs the pathological and protective factors of the patient. The dentist uses all the information available, including the medical history, when interviewing and examining the patient. See Appendix C for an example of a caries risk assessment form. Pathological factors include the amount of pathogenic (cariogenic) bacteria and adequacy of salivary flow, both of which can be determined by saliva testing (see following section). The dietary interview helps the clinician to assess the amount and frequency of fermentable carbohydrate intake. Also, lack of saliva (xerostomia) is a major pathological factor that may be caused by damaged salivary glands secondary to radiation therapy or certain medications (e.g., antidepressants).[43] On the other side of the caries balance,

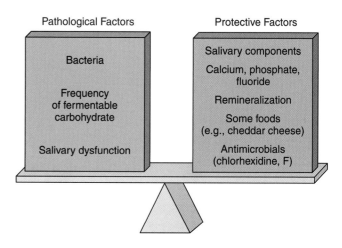

FIG. 22-5 Balance between protective and pathological factors in caries. (Modified from Featherstone JDB: Prevention and reversal of dental caries: role of low level fluoride, *Community Dent Oral Epidemiol* 27(1):31-40, 1999.)

adequate amounts of saliva (e.g., calcium, phosphate, fluoride), use of fluoride products, use of antimicrobial agents, and good dietary habits constitute the major protective components. Caries is an ever-changing balance between pathological and protective factors.

The next step in CRA is a thorough patient interview in the context of the medical and dental histories, including dietary habits, frequency of eating, complaints of xerostomia, oral hygiene, and fluoride use. Although many forms and formulas have been proposed to document the CRA quantitatively, most are time-consuming and intimidating and can deter clinicians from performing the CRA. Again, except for the quantitative saliva test, each patient's CRA may better be thought of qualitatively as a scale that balances protective factors on one side and pathogenic factors on the other to determine whether the balance is favoring health or disease (see Fig. 22-5).

SALIVARY ANALYSIS

For the salivary analysis the clinician measures the stimulated salivary flow rate and bacterial loading for both MS and LB. Stimulated saliva provides samples from the whole mouth and reflects the cariogenic bacteria in the plaque on the teeth. Some commercially available kits also include a pH test to evaluate the buffering capacity of the saliva. Although the ability of salivary buffers to neutralize acid in the mouth is an important protective function of saliva, caution should be used in the interpretation of this test because the overriding influence is sufficient salivary flow to buffer and provide calcium, phosphate, and protective proteins. In other words, the patient could have a normal pH test but simply not enough saliva. To diagnose xerostomia, the clinician collects saliva in a small measuring cup from the patient who chews on paraffin for 5 minutes, then divides the quantity selected by 5 to obtain stimulated salivary flow rate (in milliliters) per minute. A rate of 1 ml/minute or greater is normal; a rate less than 0.5 ml/minute indicates salivary dysfunction and risk of caries progression.

Bacterial testing is needed to determine whether cariogenic pathogens are present both before and after caries treatment and at what level these bacteria are present in the mouth. Although pathogenic organisms are present with an active carious lesion and it may seem that pretreatment bacterial testing is unnecessary, a baseline measurement is always better for comparison at the posttreatment recall visit. Furthermore, placement of a restoration after removal of the active lesion does not reduce the bacterial loading in the rest of the mouth.[88] Testing is beneficial even in patients without other signs of caries risk but where the lesion is supicious because these individuals may have early enamel lesions that are identifiable only by a positive result for pathogens in a bacterial test for MS and LB. In this case, chlorhexidine treatment may be instituted before any visible signs of demineralization. Bacterial testing for both MS and LB can be easily performed with one test with commercially available kits. The Ivoclar Vivacare system (Ivoclar North America, Amherst, N.Y., and Vivadent Co., Liechtenstein, Germany) uses selective media to provide counts of MS and LB and requires a 2-day incubation period to obtain the results. More rapid chairside methods that use monoclonal antibodies to surface antigens on the cariogenic bacteria are currently in development and will become available in the next few years.[75] Both groups of organisms should be tested because it is possible to have a low count of one organism and a very high count of the other and still have a high bacterial challenge. By definition, infection and caries can be diagnosed based on a high bacterial count of MS or LB and qualitative risk assessment alone. This approach indicates chemical and preventive treatment of early lesions that might otherwise be missed.

PATIENT INVOLVEMENT

Once the patient is diagnosed with an active infection of caries, CAMBRA begins with extensive patient education. Proper risk assessment permits early diagnosis without visible evidence of a carious lesion. The patient's understanding of the disease process is pivotal because successful treatment depends on patient involvement in treatment recommendations and preventive strategies. Without patient involvement, efforts to minimize pathological factors and to maximize protective factors would be difficult because patients are ultimately responsible for dietary, fluoride, and chlorhexidine compliance.[3] Patients can begin active involvement by complying with dietary recommendations and topical fluoride use. Topical fluoride is an important step in the management of patients at risk for caries, as described previously. Topical fluoride can come from multiple sources, such as fluoridated water, fluoridated toothpaste, fluoridated home rinses and gels, professional office gels, and varnishes. Recommendations on which fluoride product to use are based on an estimate of patient compliance; in other words, the product the patient is more likely to use is the best product for that patient. Very low concentrations (0.04 ppm or greater) of fluoride in saliva are all that is required for the beneficial effects during remineralization.[24,37,38]

MANAGEMENT OF A CARIOUS LESION

If CRA and salivary testing reveal that the patient is at high risk for caries, CAMBRA requires clinicians to decide whether to treat lesions chemically or surgically.[2] Chemical treatment modalities consist of topical fluoride and chlorhexidine. The location and extent of a lesion, whether it is cavitated, and whether it is active or inactive all help the dentist determine whether a lesion should be restored or remineralized. The absence of cavitation is significant because an intact enamel surface prevents bacteria from penetrating the tooth; the smaller enamel diffusion channels do not allow bacteria to enter. Thus noncavitated lesions can be remineralized. If the surface is substantially cavitated or presents a cosmetic problem, the tooth should undergo restorative treatment.

Location is important because the three sites on a tooth (pits and fissures, proximal, and cervical) are each unique and should not be treated the same. For example, most pits and fissures cannot be cleaned and are associated with poor caries-detection techniques and no reliable way to monitor remineralization procedures; therefore relying on remineralization therapy on the occlusal surface currently is problematic. In contrast, remineralization on early, proximal, smooth-surface enamel lesions offers better results because these lesions do not have deep occlusal anatomy and can be monitored more easily with bitewing radiographs. Finally, cervical carious lesions often involve the root surface, are difficult to restore compared with enamel lesions, and respond well to fluoride and preventive treatments.

Chemical Treatment with Topical Fluoride

A high-risk patient should be actively involved immediately in his or her treatment and intervention strategies (decisions) and remineralizing techniques initiated. The patient is educated about the disease process and CRA. Diagramming a personalized scale for the patient (see Fig. 22-5) showing the balance between pathological and protective factors may prove helpful. This tool is quite powerful in the review of dietary habits, oral hygiene, and pathogenesis, as well as in remineralization strategies. The patient is instructed in the use of a topical fluoride product personally selected based on compliance. In most cases the use of daily home fluoride products, such as an over-the-counter (OTC) 0.05% NaF rinse, is preferable. The daily fluoride application for remineralization is discontinued only if the patient is to receive a 2-week chlorhexidine treatment, so as not to confuse the patient with two different rinse therapies. The strongly cationic (positively charged) chlorhexidine rinse should not be combined with the strongly anionic (negatively charged) fluoride rinse, especially in the same bottle, because of some negating effect based on charge. Fluoride rinses should not be used in children under age 6 years to reduce the risk of excess fluoride ingestion by young children.

Management of the Occlusal Surface

Because of the large amount of surrounding sound tooth tissue, conventional radiography cannot detect lesions in occlusal surfaces until they are well advanced. Because pit and fissure lesions are now the most common type and currently cannot be monitored for remineralization, the first step in restorative procedures should be surgical caries control (temporary or permanent), with conservative preparations when possible, along with use of pit and fissure sealants to eliminate potential niches for pathogenic bacteria to thrive. The clinician may inspect any areas of possible caries (e.g., deeply stained pits or fissures) using the DIAGNOdent (KaVo America Corp., Lake Zurich, Ill.) caries detector. This fluorescence device detects and measures bacterial by-products in subsurface lesions, providing a number to indicate whether to "open up" the area. If this device is not available and the clinician suspects a hidden lesion, a caries biopsy is appropriate, a process that entails removal of the smallest amount of enamel with a ¼-round bur (or perhaps a laser or air abrasion) to determine the presence or absence of hidden caries. If caries is found, only the caries is removed. Then the clinician selects an appropriate restorative material and the proper preparation, often a conservative preventive resin restoration or flowable composite.

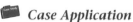 *Case Application*

Of the new caries-detection devices, which would you recommend for use on Mrs. Svensen?

This approach is the opposite of conventional methods, in which the material is chosen first and the tooth prepared with the G.V. Black "extension for prevention" philosophy (to include all pits and fissures in the outline form to a depth of at least 1.5 mm) even before the presence or extent of caries is determined. If the caries biopsy identifies no active infection, a sealant is placed with a filled, flowable composite resin. The benefits of dental sealants have been well described in the dental literature* but remain underused in clinical dentistry. If the patient is at high risk for dental caries and aggressive preventive treatment is indicated, sealants can be used to seal all pits and fissures and marginal discrepancies in adults as well as children.

Management of the Proximal Surface

As stated previously, early enamel lesions without cavitations are the best candidates for successful remineralization techniques. The task is much easier if the lesions are on a smooth enamel surface that is easily visible, such as a white or brown spot lesion on the facial or lingual enamel surfaces. However, many smooth-surface lesions occur in the proximal area directly below the proximal contact and are not visible with direct visual inspection. Until better detection methods are available, dentists must rely on bitewing radiographs and good clinical judgment. One recommended "rule of thumb" is to use remineralization therapies on radiographic E1 (enamel) lesions, and only those "touching" or penetrating the dentinoenamel junction (DEJ) should be restored. More accurate quantitative methods in the near future should improve these crude guidelines. One adjunct to the radiograph that is available now is the use of digital imaging fiber-optic transillumination (DIFOTI) (see Chapter 16). Although very sensitive at picking up early surface changes, studies have not demonstrated that DIFOTI can assess lesion depth.

Once surgical repair is chosen, the priority shifts to confirmation of the extent of both cavitation and active caries progression into dentin through a caries biopsy. One method for a proximal lesion is to start from an area close to the marginal ridge, such as a mesial or distal pit, then use a small dental bur, laser, or micro–air abrasion to tunnel internally to the DEJ area of the lesion. Often this process reveals only affected dentin (stained but hard dentin) and no sign of cavitation. In this case the dentist can simply back-fill with an occlusal composite. If caries is found, only the caries is removed; a restorative material is selected; and the cavity preparation is chosen for the selected material. Preferably a conservative approach can be implemented, such as a "slot prep" or "tunnel prep." A *slot preparation* is simply the proximal box of a traditional Class II Black preparation (without the dovetail and isthmus) and is as retentive as the traditional Black preparation.[18] In a *tunnel preparation* the caries biopsy continues from the DEJ through the proximal enamel, following the cavitation from the inside to the outside. Although these contemporary restorative materials and conservative preparations, sometimes called *micro dentistry,* are aesthetic and minimize loss of tooth structure, they are not yet accepted as the standard of care.

---

*References 3, 9, 10, 20, 51, 73, 85.

Management of the Cervical Region

If pit and fissure lesions are the most difficult lesions to detect and smooth-surface lesions the most easily remineralized, cervical lesions can be characterized as the most difficult to restore. All these differences result from the lesion's location. Although remineralization on a root surface is possible, this approach carries more inherent risk because of the high porosity of the root surface compared with enamel, proximity if the root to the pulp, vulnerability of exposed collagen in the tooth root to collagenase,[49] and low mineral content of cementum and dentin. In addition, the porous structure of dentin or cementum makes placement of restorations difficult and leakage of the restoration probable. For these reasons, treatment of cervical lesions requires special consideration.

As the number of elderly patients increases, more root caries will occur. Root caries is caused by the same bacteria that cause caries in enamel—MS and LB.[21,89] Ideally, cementum was designed to be covered by attached gingiva, and therefore an exposed root surface is at risk for caries.[48] Preventive strategies are essential in root caries because infections usually are severe and teeth difficult to restore. Lesions may not be readily visible or may be advanced by the time they are visible. As mentioned previously, bacterial enzymes such as collagenase can dissolve the collagen matrix of the root surface after partial loss of mineral by bacterially generated organic acids in the early stages of root caries. Despite the drawbacks, the demineralization–remineralization process in roots is similar to that of enamel, and fluoride still has beneficial effects on roots. However, the most effective concentration and frequency of fluoride use for root caries remain undetermined. Fluoride dentifrice is very effective in the prevention of root caries, as are OTC fluoride rinses (0.05% NaF) and higher-concentration fluoride gels.

Clinically, active caries on the root should be distinguished from inactive or arrested caries. If no active caries is evident, the lesion may be a result of abfraction or abrasion (see Chapters 15 and 16). In the absence of active caries, removal of tooth structure should be minimized, often restricted to simple "roughening up" of the surface, especially if bonding techniques are being used with composite resins, glass ionomers, or compomers. Clearly, classic Black retention preparations should be rethought in light of current bonding studies and the porous nature of cementum and dentin, which makes leakage probable. Deep preparations in areas already close to the pulp and with a high chance of leakage are problematic. In the United States, controversy surrounds which material is best for the cervical area, although composite resin is popular now because of its superior aesthetic results. However, composite shrinkage during the curing phase and subsequent gap formation have challenged the integrity of the cervical margin in these restorations.[50] Thus an aesthetic result is negated if the cervical margin leaks. Glass ionomers are very popular in other countries[65] and may be the material of choice because of enhanced fluoride release and lack of shrinkage.[7]

Because no ideal restorative material has yet been found for the cervical area, dentists may better serve patients by educating them and offering a second treatment option involving the use of glass ionomer as a fluoride delivery device that does not leak, rather than the traditional "permanent" aesthetic restoration.[6,7] Dentists should rethink the ways these cervical restorations are marketed to the patients.

Chemical Treatment with Chlorhexidine

Chlorhexidine is used in caries treatment in two ways. First, it is a "cavity cleanser" to reduce the chance of bacteria remaining in the cavity preparation. No evidence indicates that this practice is clinically beneficial, but it does seem logical because bacteria have been observed in dentinal tubules by microscopy. Second, chlorhexidine is used to reduce the number of bacteria in caries patients with high bacterial challenge. As soon as gross caries and cavitations are eliminated by caries-control procedures, the patient is given a prescription for 0.12% chlorhexidine gluconate oral rinse with instructions to rinse ½ oz for 1 minute twice a day for 14 days. The goal is to reduce the number of remaining pathogens, especially MS, to a safe level for that patient.[52] Once this goal is accomplished, the chlorhexidine rinse is discontinued, as in any other antibacterial treatment of infection. The chlorhexidine treatment usually is followed by daily topical fluoride, such as mouthrinse (0.05% NaF) and a dentifrice.

REEVALUATION PERIOD

Treatment with chlorhexidine does not guarantee that the patient will remain disease-free; that individual should be evaluated for risk indefinitely, just as in the prevention of periodontal disease. CRA with saliva testing is usually done in 3 months to evaluate for reinfection. Unlike the traditional approach, in which the next caries intervention would not be until another carious lesion is detected, the CAMBRA approach relies on immediate early intervention if pathogens are detected at recall. This procedure permits chemical reversal of demineralization that is not yet visible, resulting in a surface that is caries-resistant, as described previously. The patient is either placed on another 3-month caries recall if that individual is considered low-risk on CRA or given additional chlorhexidine and preventive treatments if bacterial test results are high.[1,3] Using CRA and salivary testing results to determine the next caries reevaluation period is an improvement over the use of unrelated periodontal maintenance schedules.

CLINICAL IMPLICATIONS: FLUORIDE-DELIVERY SYSTEMS

Fluoride is one of several protective factors and part of an overall plan to manage and prevent caries occurrence and progression.[27] Small adjustments can tip the caries balance one way or the other (see Fig. 22-5), leading to caries arrestment, reversal, or progression. The delivery of fluoride to the surfaces of the teeth on a frequent (at least daily) basis is essential. The topical effects of fluoride are overriding, whereas the systemic incorporation of fluoride in the tooth mineral has no major benefit.[26,27,40] Dentists must use this information to deal with caries more effectively in both adults and children. Fluoride in drinking water reduces dental caries but does not eradicate it. Fluoride in the drinking water provides fluoride at levels in the mouth that can inhibit demineralization and enhance remineralization, tipping the caries balance toward protection provided the challenge is not too great. However, concentration of fluoride in dental enamel and dentin provided systemically by fluoridation of drinking water or by natural fluoride water levels alone is insufficient to provide complete protection against caries. The mechanism of action of fluoride in the drinking water therefore is an effective topical delivery system.

Fluoride-containing products such as dentifrice, mouthrinse, and topically applied gels provide caries-preventive benefits through the topical mechanisms described previously. The effects involve the mechanisms of inhibition of demineralization, enhancement of remineralization, and action on the bacteria. With high bacterial challenge and xerostomia or salivary dysfunction, even high levels of fluoride therapy may be insufficient to balance the effect of the pathological factors and caries progression. Each individual has some level of challenge beyond which fluoride is insufficient to swing the balance. Fluoride products used frequently can maintain salivary fluoride levels in excess of 0.04 ppm, thereby providing marked caries protection. The major problem with the home-use products is the need for daily patient compliance.

Case Application

Mrs. Svensen's prevention survey indicates that she has been exposed to a number of sources of fluoride. She was raised and lived in a community with fluoridated water until 12 months ago, when she moved to a rural area. Currently her primary source of water is from a well, and her usual beverage of choice during the day is bottled water. She is using dentifrice with fluoride and brushes once a day. Mrs. Svensen does not use an oral rinse.

What recommendations would you suggest for Mrs. Svensen based on the previous information, as well as her clinical and radiographic findings?

PROFESSIONAL APPLICATIONS

PATIENT EDUCATION

The benefits of topical fluoride include prevention of demineralization, remineralization of early decay, decrease in enamel solubility, and maximization of enamel resistance to decay. Professionally applied fluoride is effective in the reduction of coronal caries by 30%. Fluoride treatments, however, are not limited to use on children. Many adults with high caries rates or root exposure also can benefit from professional and self-care topical fluoride applications.

Fluoride solutions for professional application, available as gels, rinses, or foams, include 1.2% NaF, 8% stannous fluoride, and 1.23% acidulated phosphate fluoride (APF). APF gel or solution is used most often and has a concentration of 1.23% sodium fluoride plus 0.1 M orthophosphoric acid. The gel form also contains a thixotropic agent, which maintains the gelatinous state, becoming fluidlike under stress. This property allows the material to adhere to the teeth while flowing into inter-

dental areas. Although the use of APF and stannous fluoride is safe on all tooth surfaces because of their acidic pH levels, a neutral NaF gel or solution should be used on patients with porcelain or composite restorations to prevent surface etching of these materials. Stannous fluoride is available in solution and gel form; the gel is recommended as an at-home, brush-on therapy, and the solution is available in combination with APF as a professional rinse. In addition, acidic fluoride (APF and stannous) can cause severe erosion of tooth structure if used routinely at home in devices that restrict salivary clearance, such as custom trays or nightguards, and should not be used.

The gel and foam fluoride formulas are applied to the teeth through use of a tray or can be painted on with cotton-tipped applicators.

TRADITIONAL PAINT-ON TECHNIQUE

The paint-on technique to apply fluoride formulas requires isolation of the treatment area(s) with cotton rolls. With the patient in an upright position, one half of the mouth is isolated with cotton rolls, which are placed in holders for the mandibular arch and by hand for the maxillary arch. The teeth are dried with compressed air, and the fluoride gel or solution is painted onto the teeth with a cotton-tipped applicator. A saliva ejector should be positioned near the cotton roll holder. A timer is set for 4 minutes, and the surfaces remain wet for this period. After 4 minutes the clinician removes the saliva ejector and cotton rolls, then wipes off the superficial gel or solution, allowing the patient to expectorate. The opposite side of the mouth then is isolated and fluoride applied. After the fluoride paint-on procedure is complete, the patient is instructed not to rinse, eat, drink, or brush the teeth for at least 30 minutes.

FLUORIDE VARNISH

Recently, fluoride varnish products have been approved by the Food and Drug Administration (FDA). They are applied as discussed in the previous section but are not wiped off the teeth after application. Once painted on dry teeth, the varnish gels and is removed after 4 hours by tooth brushing and expectoration.

FLUORIDE TRAYS

A variety of fluoride tray designs are available for professional application. Most are constructed of disposable foam with a spongelike lining or molded interior. Trays are single-arch design or hinged for dual-arch applications, and sizes include child, small, medium, and large. The dentition is evaluated to ensure proper tray selection. The tray should cover the most distal tooth and provide enough depth and width for gel contact against the tooth surface.

Amount of Fluoride

A maximum 2 ml of fluoride per tray is recommended for an application. Most commercial fluorides are supplied in dispensing bottles. Use of a graduated medicine cup to dispense and place 2 ml of fluoride into the application tray can help the clinician determine the appropriate amount for future applications.

Insertion of Tray

After the tray is selected and loaded with fluoride gel, the patient should be prepared for the application, seated in an upright position. Using compressed air, the teeth should be dried thoroughly. The clinician then should insert the tray (or trays), using light pressure to ensure gel contact with the teeth. The saliva ejector should be placed between the trays. Allowing the patient to close down gently against the saliva ejector helps maintain the adaptation of the gel to the tooth surfaces. A timer then is set for 4 minutes. On completion, the clinician should remove the trays and use the saliva ejector and gauze to remove excess fluoride, instructing the patient to expectorate thoroughly. Although a 4-minute application is recommended for optimal benefits, some manufacturers recommend 1-minute applications. Research is insufficient to support the claim that a 1-minute application is as effective as a 4-minute application. Again, the patient should be instructed not to rinse, eat, drink, or brush for 30 minutes after the fluoride application.

PATIENT MONITORING

As with any dental procedure, the patient should be monitored closely while the fluoride application is in progress. The tray or paint-on application may elicit a gag response. Leaning forward during the application allows the patient to feel that the gel is not flowing down the throat. Other gag-control techniques include deep nasal breathing and toe wiggling. The clinician also must ensure that the patient does not swallow the fluoride during or on completion of the application, possibly by allowing the patient to hold or move the saliva ejector during application.

If a stannous fluoride solution is used, gingival sloughing may occur, particularly if the gingival tissues were inflamed before application.

FLUORIDE TOXICITY

Fluoride is safe when used as directed but can prove to be damaging in chronic overexposure or in acute excess dosages. Chronic overexposure to fluoride in children under age 6 years through excessive ingestion of fluoride dentifrice or OTC fluoride rinses can lead to fluorosis. *Fluorosis* is enamel hypomineralization and appears as a white stain that later may become discolored and brown. Excessive fluoride ingestion during tooth development can produce a pitted or mottled enamel surface.

Abuse of high-concentration gels or solutions and accidental ingestion of a concentrated fluoride preparation can lead to an acute toxic reaction. Acute fluoride poisoning is rare. The amount of fluoride likely to cause death is the certainly lethal dose (CLD). The safely tolerated dose (STD) is the amount that can be consumed without producing symptoms of serious acute toxicity; STD is one-fourth the CLD (Box 22-2 and Table 22-2).

BOX 22-2

Lethal and Safe Doses of Fluoride for Adults (70 kg)

Certainly Lethal Dose (CLD)
5 to 10 g of sodium fluoride
or
32 to 64 mg fluoride/kg
Safely Tolerated Dose (STD)*
1.25 to 2.5 g of sodium fluoride
or
8 to 16 mg fluoride/kg

*One quarter of CLD.

TABLE 22-2

Lethal and safe doses of fluoride for children and adolescents (18 years)

Age (year)	Weight (lb)	CLD (mg)	STD (mg)
2	22	320	80
4	29	422	106
6	37	538	135
8	45	655	164
10	53	771	193
12	64	931	233
14	83	1206	301
16	92	1338	334
18	95	1382	346

From Heifetz SB, Horowitz HS: The amounts of fluoride in current fluoride therapies: safety considerations for children, *ASDC J Dent Child* 51(4):257, 1984.
CLD, Certainly lethal dose; *STD*, safely tolerated dose.

SELF-APPLIED TOPICAL FLUORIDE PRODUCTS

Self-applied topical fluoride products are available for patients with increased rates of caries, rampant enamel or root caries, xerostomia, exposure to radiation therapy, root-surface sensitivity, or orthodontic bands or bonded appliances. Topical fluoride is available by prescription or OTC for lower concentrations.

Self-applied fluoride methods include the use of a custom tray, rinsing, or tooth brushing; the method should be selected based on the patient's ability to follow the prescribed method of application. A mouth tray requires dexterity to place and remove, adherence to the correct amount of gel to be dispensed, correct timing, and expectoration. Fluoride mouthrinses are easy to dispense and use but are contraindicated in children under 6 years of age. Fluoride brush-on gels are used after normal toothbrushing and flossing. The gel is applied with a toothbrush and brushed on for 1 minute. The APF and stannous formulas should not be used on porcelain or composite restorations or allowed to remain in contact with teeth for extended periods of time when salivary clearance is impeded (with custom trays and nightguards).

FLUORIDE SUPPLEMENTS IN CARIES PREVENTION

The so-called fluoride supplements (tablets, lozenges, and drops) initially were used as a dietary supplement to make up for inadequate fluoride ingestion and thus protect against caries by incorporation into the tooth. For the reasons described previously, however, this is not the case. To be effective against caries, fluoride supplements should be thought of as a means to supplement the topical mechanisms of fluoride action and not the (minimal) systemic action of fluoride. To illustrate this concept, several researchers gave fluoride tablets to children in Scotland either to swallow or hold in the mouth (sucking or chewing).[62,79] The groups who dissolved the fluoride in the mouth and thereby "applied" fluoride topically had dramatic caries reductions (approximately 80%) compared with those who swallowed the tablets. Prescribed fluoride supplements should have instructions that the product be chewed or sucked to provide a caries-protective benefit.

When fluoride tablets are swallowed, fluoride returned via the plasma to the saliva may be sufficient to provide a "topical" benefit. Research shows that after ingestion of a fluoride tablet, fluoride is elevated in the plasma only transiently.[19] Levels in saliva resulting from once-a-day fluoride tablet ingestion are not likely to have much, if any, topical benefit on their own, although they add to topical fluoride from other sources. This point further illustrates the need to use fluoride supplements directly as a fluoride topical delivery mechanism if they are to be effective.

> The anticaries effects of fluoride are primarily topical for children and for adults. The mechanisms of action of fluoride are (1) inhibition of demineralization at the crystal surfaces, (2) enhancement of remineralization at the crystal surfaces, and (3) inhibition of bacterial activity. The systemic effects of fluoride are minimal.

RITICAL THINKING ACTIVITIES

1. Perform a fluoride history on five patients, one of whom is at least 65 years old. Identify the sources of fluoride and review the caries history in the patient's record. Compare the patient's exposure to fluoride with the history of caries.
2. Perform the following experiment when you have not consumed food, drink, or gum for 1 hour:
   a. Using a pH narrow-range indicator test strip (pH of 4 to 7), remove a small amount of plaque from your teeth with a toothpick and use it to moisten the strip. Check the pH and graph your reading.
   b. Eat your favorite sugar-containing candy.
   c. Moisten another pH test strip with your plaque.
   d. Continue this procedure every 10 minutes for 1 hour or until the pH returns to baseline, approximately 7.0.
   e. Repeat the exercise, but this time after eating the candy and checking pH, rinse with water and recheck the pH.
3. Take an egg at room temperature and paint half of it with topical fluoride. Allow the fluoride to dry. Immerse the egg in vinegar overnight (24 hours). Check results on the egg, and draw conclusions about the effect of fluoride.

REVIEW QUESTIONS

1. All the following statements about enamel are true *except* which one?
   a. Enamel is the most mineralized structure in human body.
   b. Enamel contains carbonated apatite crystals arranged in rods.
   c. Enamel is porous.
   d. Replacement of phosphate ion by carbonate ion increases enamel's strength.
2. When fluorapatite is formed from hydroxyapatite, the fluoride ion substitutes for which of the following ions?
   a. Hydroxide ion
   b. Phosphate ion
   c. Calcium ion
   d. Magnesium ion
   e. None of the above

3. Fluoride is antibacterial and an anticaries agent. However, ingesting more fluoride than prescribed can cause serious health problems.
   a. Both statements are true.
   b. Both statements are false.
   c. The first statement is true; the second is false.
   d. The second statement is true; the first is false.
4. Salivary analysis for caries risk assessment consists of measurement of the stimulated salivary flow rate and bacterial loading for both MS and LB. Placement of a restoration in an active lesion does not reduce the bacterial loading in the remainder of the mouth.
   a. Both statements are true.
   b. Both statements are false.
   c. The first statement is true; the second is false.
   d. The first statement is false; the second is true.

REVIEW QUESTIONS—cont'd

5. Which of the following is *not* a mechanism of fluoride action?
   a. Inhibits plaque bacteria
   b. Reduces stains from enamel
   c. Inhibits demineralization
   d. Enhances remineralization and creates fluorapatite-like surface

6. Demineralization is initiated after a rise in pH. Demineralization and remineralization may occur several times a day on the surfaces of teeth.
   a. The first statement is true; the second is false.
   b. The first statement is false; the second is true.
   c. Both statements are true.
   d. Both statements are false.

7. Enamel is protected initially from the acid of pathogenic bacteria by which of the following components?
   a. Plaque
   b. Pellicle
   c. Interprismatic layer
   d. None of the above

8. Which of the following choices best describes the process of demineralization?
   a. Acid-induced dissolution of enamel
   b. Diffusion of ions along their concentration gradients
   c. Active transport of ions into gingival crevicular fluid
   d. Both *a* and *b*
   e. Both *a* and *c*

9. Which of the following factors is the most important in remineralization?
   a. Fluoride
   b. Carbonate
   c. Saliva
   d. Oral hygiene

10. All the following statements about dental caries are true *except* which one?
    a. The etiology of caries is multifactorial.
    b. Dental caries is a site-specific disease affecting different teeth and different surfaces of teeth.
    c. Dental caries cannot be iatrogenically transferred from one carious site to a previously uninfected site.
    d. The DMF index is the single standard method for assessing dental caries in a population.
    e. Dental caries is an infectious disease that is transmissible from mother to child.

11. In a classic experiment, Keyes and Jordan noted that one strain of hamsters naturally exhibited caries, whereas a second strain of hamsters did not. The difference in disease susceptibility occurred when the strains were housed separately but fed the same diet. However, when the investigators housed the strains together in the same cages, both strains exhibited caries. What is the most likely explanation for these observations?
    a. Housing the animals together stressed the animals and decreased saliva secretion.
    b. Caries pathogens were transmitted from one strain to another.
    c. The change in caries susceptibility is caused by alterations in grooming behaviors.
    d. Fluoride exposures were decreased in housing the animal strains together.
    e. Eating behaviors changed in the second strain.

 # SUGGESTED AGENCIES AND WEB SITES

Because of the ever-changing nature of the Internet, some of the web sites listed here may have changed since publication. Please refer to Mosby's Evolve web site for the most current information.

Academy of General Dentistry ("Consumer information; Fluoride"): http://www.agd.org

American Dental Association ("Fluoride and fluoridation"): http://www.ada.org

American Dietetic Association ("The impact of fluoride on health"): http://www.eatright.org

Department of Health, Dental Health Division (fact sheet: fluoride used for dental caries prevention): http://www.anamai.moph.go.th/factsheet

Family Gentle Dental Care ("Fluoride"): http://www.dentalgentlecare.com

Fluorides: questions and answers: http://www.jcomisi.com

Harris County (Texas) Public and Environmental Services ("Fundamental facts on optimal use of fluorides for prevention of tooth decay"): http://www.hd.co.harris.tx.us

International Society for Fluoride Research ("Fluoride"): http://www.fluoride-journal.com

IVillage.com ("Enamel: de- and remineralization"): http://www.parentsplace.com

P&G Dental Resource Net: Consumer Information ("The role of fluoride and calcium in the demineralization/remineralization process"): http://www.dentalcare.com

Journal of Clinical Dentistry ("Remineralization by fluoride enhanced with calcium and phosphate ingredients"): http://www.jclindent.com

University of Chicago School of Dentistry ("Enhancing remineralization"): http://www.uic.edu

Web site of Kurt A. Butzin, DDS ("Fluoride and tooth decay"): http://www.butzin.com

Web site of Joel B. Schilling, DDS ("Ideal daily fluoride dosages"): http://www.jbschilling.com

ADDITIONAL READINGS AND RESOURCES

Fejerskov O, Ekstrand JAN, Burt B, editors: *Fluoride in dentistry,* ed 2, Copenhagen, 1996, Munksgaard.

Schneiderman A, Elbaum M, Shultz T, Keem S, Greenebaum M, Driller J: Assessment of dental caries with Digital Imaging Fiber-Optic Trans Illumination (DIFOTI): *In vitro* study. Caries Res 1997; 31:103-110.

REFERENCES

1. Anderson MH, Bales DJ, Omnell K-A: Modern management of dental caries: the cutting edge is not the dental bur, *J Am Dent Assoc* 124:37-44, 1993.
2. Anusavice KJ: Treatment regimens in preventive and restorative dentistry, *J Am Dent Assoc* 126(6):727-43, 1995.
3. Anusavice KJ: Chlorhexidine, fluoride varnish, and xylitol chewing gum: underutilized preventive therapies? *Gen Dent* 46(1):34-8, 40, 1998.
4. Arends J, ten Bosch JJ: In vivo de- and remineralization of dental enamel. In Leach SA, editor: *Factors relating to demineralization and remineralization of the teeth,* Oxford, 1995, IRL Press.
5. Benn DK et al: Standardizing data collection and decision making with an expert system, *J Dent Educ* 61:885-94, 1997.
6. Billings RJ: Restoration of carious lesions of the root, *Gerodontology* 5(1):43-9, 1986.
7. Billings RJ, Brown LR, Kaster AG: Contemporary treatment strategies for root surface dental caries, *Gerodontics* 1(1):20-7, 1985.
8. Billings RJ, Meyerowitz C, Featherstone JDB: Retention of topical fluoride in the mouths of xerostomic subjects, *Caries Res* 33:306-10, 1988.
9. Bohannan HM: Caries distribution and the case for sealants, *J Public Health Dent* 43:200-4, 1983.
10. Bohannan HM, Disney JA, Graves RC: Indications for sealant use in a community-based preventive dentistry program, *J Dent Educ* 48(2 suppl):45-55, 1984.
11. Bruun C, Givskov H, Thylstrup A: Whole saliva fluoride after toothbrushing with NaF and MFP dentifrices with different F concentrations, *Caries Res* 18:282-8, 1984.
12. Budz JA, LoRe M, Nancollas GH: Hydroxyapatite and carbonated-apatite as models for the dissolution behavior of human dental enamel, *Adv Dent Res* 1:314-21, 1987.
13. Burt BA, Fejerskov O: Water fluoridation. In Fejerskov O, Ekstrand J, Burt BA, editors: *Fluoride in dentistry,* ed 2, Copenhagen, 1996, Munksgaard.
14. Caufield PW, Cutter GR, Dasanayake AP: Initial acquisition of mutans streptococci by infants: evidence for a discrete window of infectivity, *J Dent Res* 72(1):37-45, 1993.
15. Curzon MEJ, Cutress TW, editors: *Trace elements and dental disease,* Littleton, NY, 1983, Wright-PSG.
16. Curzon MEJ, Featherstone JDB: Chemical composition of enamel. In Lazzari EP, editor: *Handbook of experimental aspects of oral biochemistry,* Boca Raton, Fla, 1983, CRC Press.
17. D'Hondt DG, Pape H, Loesche WJ: Reduction of contamination on the dental explorer, *J Am Dent Assoc* 104:329-30, 1982.
18. Eakle WS, Staninec M, Yip RL, Chavez MA: Mechanical retention versus bonding of amalgam and gallium alloy restorations, *J Prosthet Dent* 72(4):351-4, 1994.
19. Ekstrand J: Fluoride metabolism. In Fejerskov O, Ekstrand J, Burt BA, editors: *Fluoride in dentistry,* Copenhagen, 1996, Munksgaard.
20. Ekstrand KR et al: Detection, diagnosing, monitoring and logical treatment of occlusal caries in relation to lesion activity and severity: an in vivo examination with histological validation, *Caries Res* 32(4):247-54, 1998.
21. Ellen RP, Banting DW, Fillery ED: *Streptococcus mutans* and *Lactobacillus* detection in the assessment of dental root surface caries risk, *J Dent Res* 64(10):1245-9, 1985.
22. Featherstone JDB: Diffusion phenomena and enamel caries development. Paper presented at the Cariology Today International Congress, Zurich, 1983, 1984.
23. Featherstone JDB: An updated understanding of the mechanism of dental decay and its prevention, *Nutr Q* 14:5-11, 1990.
24. Featherstone JDB: Fluoride, remineralization and root caries, *Am J Dent* 7:271-4, 1994.
25. Featherstone JDB: Clinical implications of early caries detection: new strategies for caries prevention. Paper presented at the 1st Annual Indiana Conference: Early Detection of Dental Caries, 1996.
26. Featherstone JDB: Prevention and reversal of dental caries: role of low level fluoride, *Community Dent Oral Epidemiol* 27(1):31-40, 1999.
27. Featherstone JDB: The science and practice of caries prevention, *J Am Dent Assoc* 131(7):887-99, 2000.
28. Featherstone JDB, Glena R, Shariati M, Shields CP: Dependence of in vitro demineralization and remineralization of dental enamel on fluoride concentration, *J Dent Res* 69:620-5, 1990.
29. Featherstone JDB, Goodman P, MacLean JD: Electron microscope study of defect zones in dental enamel, *J Ultrastruc Res* 67:117-23, 1979.
30. Featherstone JDB, Mayer I, Driessens FCM: Synthetic apatites containing Na, Mg, and CO_3 and their comparison with tooth enamel mineral, *Calcif Tiss Int* 35:169-71, 1983.
31. Featherstone JDB, Mellberg JR: Relative rates of progress of artificial carious lesions in bovine, ovine and human enamel, *Caries Res* 15:109-14, 1981.
32. Featherstone JDB, Nelson DGA, McLean JD: An electron microscope study of modifications to defect regions in dental enamel and synthetic apatites, *Caries Res* 15:278-88, 1981.
33. Featherstone JDB, O'Reilly MM, Shariati M, Brugler S: Enhancement of remineralization *in vitro* and *in vivo.* In Leach SA, editor: *Factors relating to demineralization and remineralization of the teeth,* Oxford, 1986, IRL Press.
34. Featherstone JDB, Pearson S, LeGeros RZ: An IR method for quantification of carbonate in carbonated-apatites, *Caries Res* 18:63-6, 1984.
35. Featherstone JDB, Rodgers BE: The effect of acetic, lactic and other organic acids on the formation of artificial carious lesions, *Caries Res* 15:377-85, 1981.
36. Featherstone JDB, Shields CP, Khademazad B, Oldershaw MD: Acid reactivity of carbonated-apatites with strontium and fluoride substitutions, *J Dent Res* 62:1049-53, 1983.
37. Featherstone JDB, Silverstone LM: The caries process: morphological and chemical events. In Nikiforuk G, editor: *Understanding dental caries,* Basel, 1985, Karger.
38. Featherstone JDB, Ten Cate JM: Physicochemical aspects of fluoride-enamel interactions. In Ekstrand J, Fejerskov O, Silverstone LM, editors: *Fluoride in dentistry,* Copenhagen, 1988, Munksgaard.

39. Featherstone JDB, Zero DT: Laboratory and human studies to elucidate the mechanism of action of fluoride-containing dentifrices. In Embery G, Rolla R, editors: *Clinical and biological aspects of dentifrices*, Oxford, 1992, Oxford University Press.

40. Fejerskov O, Thylstrup A, Larsen MJ: Rational use of fluorides in caries prevention, *Acta Odontol Scand* 39:241-9, 1981.

41. Geddes DAM: Acids produced by human dental plaque metabolism in situ, *Caries Res* 9:98-109, 1975.

42. Hamilton IR, Bowden GHW: Fluoride effects on oral bacteria. In Fejerskov O, Ekstrand J, Burt BA, editors: *Fluoride in dentistry*, Copenhagen, 1996, Munksgaard.

43. Handelman SL, Baric JM, Saunders RH, Espeland MA: Hyposalivatory drug use, whole stimulated salivary flow, and mouth dryness in older, long-term care residents, *Spec Care Dent* 9:12-8, 1989.

44. Hargreaves JA, Thomson GW, Wagg BJ: Changes in caries prevalence in Isle of Lewis children between 1971 and 1981, *Caries Res* 17:554-9, 1983.

45. Hume WR: Need for change in dental caries diagnosis. Paper presented at the 1st Annual Indiana Conference: Early Detection of Dental Caries, 1996.

46. Jenkins GN: Recent changes in dental caries. *Br Med J* 291:1297-8, 1985.

47. Kaste LM, Selwitz RH, Oldakowski RJ: Coronal caries in the primary and permanent dentition of children and adolescents 1-17 years of age: United States, 1988-1991, *J Dent Res* 75:631-41, 1996.

48. Katz RV: Assessing root caries in populations: the evolution of the root caries index, *J Public Health Dent* 40(1):7-16, 1980.

49. Kawasaki K, Featherstone JDB: Effects of collagenase on root demineralization, *J Dent Res* 76:588-95, 1997.

50. Kemp-Scholte CM, Davidson CL: Marginal sealing of curing contraction gaps in Class V composite resin restorations, *J Dent Res* 67:841-5, 1988.

51. Kidd EA, Joyston-Bechal S: Update on fissure sealants, *Dent Update* 21(8):323-6, 1994.

52. Krasse B: Biological factors as indicators of future caries, *Int Dent J* 38:219-25, 1988.

53. Lagerlof F, Oliveby A: Clinical implications: new strategies for caries treatment. Paper presented at the 1st Annual Indiana Conference: Early Detection of Dental Caries, 1996.

54. LeGeros RZ: Calcium phosphates. Oral biology and medicine, *Monogr Oral Sci* 15:1-201, 1991.

55. LeGeros RZ, Trautz OR, LeGeros JP, Klein E: Carbonate substitution in the apatite structure, *Bull Soc Chim Fr* (Special issue):1712-8, 1968.

56. Leverett DH et al: Caries risk assessment by a cross-sectional discrimination model, *J Dent Res* 72:529-37, 1993.

57. Leverett DH et al: Caries risk assessment in a longitudinal discrimination study, *J Dent Res* 72:538-43, 1993.

58. Loesche WJ: Chemotherapy of dental plaque infections, *Oral Sci Rev* 9(9):65-107, 1976.

59. Loesche WJ: Role of *Streptococcus mutans* in human dental decay, *FEMS Microbiol Rev* 50:353-80, 1986.

60. Loesche WJ: Antimicrobials in dentistry: with knowledge comes responsibility, *J Dent Res* 75:1432-1433, 1996.

61. Loesche WJ, Hockett RN, Syed SA: The predominant cultivable flora of tooth surface plaque removed from institutionalized subjects, *Arch Oral Biol* 17:1311-25, 1973.

62. McCall D, Stephen KW, McNee SG: Fluoride tablets and salivary fluoride levels, *Caries Res* 15:98-102, 1981.

63. Meyerowitz C et al: Use of an intra-oral model to evaluate 0.05% sodium fluoride mouthrinse in radiation-induced hyposalivation, *J Dent Res* 70:894-8, 1991.

64. Moss ME, Zero DT: An overview of caries risk assessment, and its potential utility, *J Dent Educ* 59(10):932-40, 1995.

65. Mount GJ, Hume WR: *Preservation and restoration of tooth structure*, St Louis, 1998, Mosby.

66. Murray JJ, Rugg-Gunn AJ, Jenkins GN: *Fluorides in caries prevention*, ed 3, London, 1992, Wright.

67. Nelson DGA, Featherstone JDB, Duncan JF, Cutress TW: Effect of carbonate and fluoride on the dissolution behaviour of synthetic apatites, *Caries Res* 17:200-11, 1983.

68. Newbrun E: *Cariology*, ed 3, Chicago, 1989, Quintessence.

69. Newbrun E: Effectiveness of water fluoridation, *J Public Health Dent* 49:279-89, 1989.

70. Nyvad B, Fejerskov O: Assessing the stage of caries lesion activity on the basis of clinical and microbiological examination, *Community Dent Oral Epidemiol* 25:69-75, 1997.

71. O'Reilly MM, Featherstone JDB: De- and remineralization around orthodontic appliances: an in vivo study, *Am J Orthod* 92:33-40, 1987.

72. Pitts NB: Patient caries status in the context of practical, evidence-based management of the initial caries lesion, *J Dent Educ* 61:895-905, 1997.

73. Ricketts D, Kidd E, Weerheijm K, de Soet H: Hidden caries: what is it? Does it exist? Does it matter? *Int Dent J* 47(5):259-65, 1997.

74. Robinson C, Kirkham J, Weatherell JA: Fluoride in teeth and bone. In Fejerskov O, Ekstrand J, Burt BA, editors: *Fluoride in dentistry*, ed 2, Copenhagen, 1996, Munksgaard.

75. Shi W, Jewett A, Hume WR: Rapid and quantitative detection of *S. mutans* with species specific monoclonal antibodies, *Hybridoma* 17:365-71, 1998.

76. Shields CP, Moss ME, Billings RJ, Featherstone JDB: A longitudinal chemical analysis of saliva, *J Dent Res* 76(Special issue, IADR meeting), 1997.

77. Shields CP et al: Chemical analysis of saliva: a longitudinal study, *J Dent Res* 74:15, 1995.

78. Silverstone LM: The structure of carious enamel, including the early lesion, *Oral Sci Rev* 3:100-60, 1973.

79. Stephen KW, Campbell D: Caries reduction and cost benefit after 3 years of sucking fluoride tablets daily at school: a double blind trial, *Br Dent J* 144:202-6, 1978.

80. Stookey GK: Are all fluoride dentifrices the same? In Wei SHY, editor: *Clinical uses of fluorides*, Philadelphia, 1985, Lea & Febiger.

81. Suddick RP, Dodds MW Jr: Caries activity estimates and implications: insights into risk versus activity, *J Dent Educ* 61:876-84, 1997.

82. ten Cate JM, Duijsters PPE: Influence of fluoride in solution on tooth demineralization. II. Microradiographic data, *Caries Res* 17:513-9, 1983.

83. ten Cate JM, Featherstone JDB: Mechanistic aspects of the interactions between fluoride and dental enamel, *CRC Crit Rev Oral Biol* 2:283-96, 1991.

84. Van Louveren C: The antimicrobial action of fluoride and its role in caries inhibition, *J Dent Res* 69:676-81, 1990.

85. Weintraub JA et al: A retrospective analysis of the cost-effectiveness of dental sealants in a children's health center, *Soc Sci Med* 36:1483-93, 1993.

86. Whitford GM, Schuster GS, Pashley HD, Venkateswarlu P: Fluoride uptake by *Streptococcus mutans* 6715, *Infect Immun* 18(3):680-7, 1977.

87. Winn DM et al: Coronal and root caries in the dentition of adults in the United States, 1988-1991, *J Dent Res* 75:642-51, 1996.

88. Wright JT et al: Effect of conventional dental restorative treatment on bacteria in saliva, *Community Dent Oral Epidemiol* 20:138-43, 1992.

89. Zambon JJ, Kasprzak SA: The microbiology and histopathology of human root caries, *Am J Dent* 8(6):323-8, 1995.

90. Zero DT et al: Fluoride concentrations in plaque, whole saliva and ductal saliva after applications of home-use fluoride agents, *J Dent Res* 71:1768-75, 1992.

CHAPTER 23

Dentifrices

Margaret Hill, Regan L. Moore

Chapter Outline

Composition of Dentifrice
Adverse Effects
Safety and Efficacy
Case Study: Selecting the Correct Dentifrice
Evaluating Clinical Studies
    Study design
    Duration
    Study population
    Efficacy claims
    Examiner reliability

Dentifrice Formulations
    Anticaries
    Sensitivity control
    Calculus control
    Whitening benefit
    Antigingivitis
    Other agents

Key Terms

Chemotherapeutic
Chlorhexidine

Dentifrice
Sanguinarine

Sodium fluoride
Stannous fluoride

Triclosan

Learning Outcomes

1. Discuss compatibility of ingredients in a dentifrice and what makes each critical to the formulation.
2. Describe several adverse effects associated with use of a dentifrice.
3. Explain the process necessary for a new product to receive U.S. Food and Drug Administration (FDA) approval for marketing.
4. Discuss the process necessary for a product to receive the American Dental Association's (ADA) Seal of Acceptance.
5. Differentiate between the roles of FDA and ADA in product marketing.
6. Describe the different types of studies used to evaluate chemotherapeutic agents in dentifrice.
7. List the chemotherapeutic agents used in dentifrice for treatment of caries, sensitivity, gingivitis, calculus, and stain.
8. Recommend appropriate dentifrices for patients based on individual needs.
9. Become familiar with the types of dentifrice products available in your market.

Daily use of a *dentifrice,* usually a paste or gel, is one of the most beneficial recommendations that dental professionals can make to their patients in preventing and controlling dental diseases. Use of fluoride dentifrice, beginning in the late 1950s, is widely acknowledged as a major reason for the decrease in dental caries in many parts of the world.[27] Over the years, dental professionals have helped patients realize the benefits of oral hygiene, specifically by recommending a toothbrush and toothpaste for mechanical plaque re-moval. Together with toothbrushes, dentifrices are the most widely recommended and used oral hygiene products, and they offer increased oral health benefits beyond simple mechanical plaque removal.[13] In more recent years, various *chemotherapeutic* agents, such as fluoride, pyrophosphate, and triclosan, have been added to dentifrice formulations to enhance the benefits of the dentifrice delivery system.

When patients shop for toothpaste, they are faced with an overwhelming array of products with various claims.

Distinguishing products with proven therapeutic effects from those with only cosmetic benefits is difficult for patients and the dental care team. As part of individualizing prevention strategies, the dental professional must be prepared to help patients make informed choices about oral care purchases to maximize product benefits.

COMPOSITION OF DENTIFRICE

3-A *Dentifrice* is an inclusive term used to describe a powder, paste, or gel used with a toothbrush to aid in the removal of plaque, materia alba, and stain from teeth and soft tissues. The earliest commercial products were simple powder mixtures; modern dentifrices are generally toothpastes or gels that are complex formulations of many ingredients[68] (Table 23-1 and Fig. 23-1). Compatibility of the components in dentifrices is critical to ensure that the chemotherapeutic agents are stable during storage and are biologically active when used in the mouth.[14] Some early attempts to add chemotherapeutic agents to dentifrice were unsuccessful, largely because of reactions between ingredients.[66] As new agents are incorporated into dentifrices, such issues help explain the need for the extensive evaluations required by the U.S. Food and Drug Administration (FDA) before products can be released on the market.[64]

ADVERSE EFFECTS

Dental literature reports *allergic reactions* to many common ingredients in dentifrice formulations, most often contact-type reactions. The most common allergens are certain types of flavorings, detergents, and preservatives. Problems have been reported in 1.5% to 2.0% of users; immediate sensitivity reactions such as bronchospasm and asthma are rare.[58] Although fluoride has been implicated in allergy,[61] acnelike eruptions,[59] and ulcerative stomatitis,[19] it has been used safely for nearly 50 years. Reports

detail oral mucosal desquamative effects and increased gingival blood flow associated with the use of the detergent ingredient sodium lauryl sulfate (SLS).[30] Recurrent apthous ulcers may be related to SLS and cocoamidopropyl betaine detergents,[31] and perioral contact urticaria has been associated with sodium benzoate.[48]

Another concern is increased risk of *fluorosis* in children, which may be partly caused by ingestion of fluoride dentifrices during tooth development.[63] Improper use of fluoride supplements also can be a major contributing factor in fluorosis. The most critical time to avoid excess fluoride is during development of the anterior permanent teeth, which occurs up to age 3 years.[51] The American Dental Association (ADA) and the American Academy of Pediatric Dentistry have recommended that children less than age 3 should only use a "pea-sized" smear of fluoride dentifrice for brushing. Intentional ingestion of fluoride dentifrice should also be discouraged in children.

SAFETY AND EFFICACY

The FDA is responsible for protecting the public from unsafe products. All over-the-counter (OTC) and prescription drugs require research that demonstrates proof of product safety. The FDA recognizes two categories of approval for products.[64] *Cosmetic approval* requires only proof of safety and does not allow claims of therapeutic value. *Therapeutic approval* requires extensive testing that shows efficacy before products can be marketed. For a product with a new active ingredient and therapeutic claims, the manufacturer must undergo a formal new drug application (NDA) process with the FDA. The stages of the FDA approval process begin with *preclinical* research and development to prove safety related to allergenicity and carcinogenicity. After product safety is established, investigatory new drug approval is required before *clinical* research and development can be performed. Three phases of testing

---

 Case Study   **Selecting the Correct Dentifrice**

As a hygienist in a busy small town practice, you are the main resource for dental product information for your patients. One of the most common questions is "What is the best toothpaste?" Your stock answer is "It depends," and then you try to assess the needs of the patient and make an appropriate recommendation. With current patients, however, the answer is more complex.

Cynthia Courtland has been a patient in the practice for several years, along with her husband, Cal; daughter, Amber; and son, Brandon. Mrs. Courtland is 45 years old, and you enjoy her routine supportive care visits. She has some localized areas of mild gingivitis, mostly due to infrequent flossing. Today, she has some concerns that she wants to discuss with you.

At his last appointment, you needed to give Mr. Courtland extensive oral self-care reinstruction. He is 52 years old and has a history of periodontitis that has been successfully con-

trolled for about 10 years. He has some exposed root surfaces that are vulnerable to root caries and occasionally complains of cold sensitivity. Amber's dental care team is concerned for her oral health. She just had her orthodontic appliances removed because she has not been compliant with oral self-care or diet. Generalized enamel demineralization is present, as well as several carious lesions that need to be restored. Brandon, age 5, had no caries or plaque at his last visit, and he has his first loose tooth.

Mrs. Courtland wants to help her family maintain an optimal level of dental health, but she is confused by all the options when she shops for dental care products. She asks, "Which toothpaste should we use?" You pause as you consider the individual needs of the family members, and you realize that this situation may require more than a simple, single-product recommendation for the whole family.

TABLE 23-1

Basic dentifrice ingredients

Component	Purpose	Percent	Examples	Comments
Abrasives	Varying particle sizes create an abrasive system that cleans and polishes	20 to 40	Calcium carbonate, calcium pyrophosphate, aluminum oxide, silicone oxides, bicarbonate, chalk	Must be compatible with other ingredients; must not damage teeth or soft tissues
Detergents	Help loosen debris; foaming action; act as surfactant moisture	1 to 2	Sodium lauryl sulfate (SLS), sodium lauryl sarcosinate	Some patients may have mucosal reaction to SLS
Water		20 to 40		
Humectants	Maintain moisture and consistency	20 to 40	Sorbitol, glycerine, propylene glycol, mannitol	Some humectants also add a sweet taste; require preservative to prevent bacterial and mold growth
Binders (thickeners)	Prevent separation of ingredients	2	Alginate, gums, synthetic celluloses	Higher percentage in gel formulations
Preservatives	Prevent mold and bacterial growth	<1	Alcohols, sodium benzoate, dichlorinated phenols	Contact allergens in some patients
Sweetening agents	Imparts pleasant flavor	2	Saccharine, sorbitol, mannitol, xylitol, glycerine	Some also act as humectants
Flavoring agents	Give immediate pleasant taste sensation that lingers as an aftertaste	2	Essential oils (peppermint, spearmint, wintergreen, cinnamon), menthol	Contact allergens in some patients
Coloring agents	Give attractive and desirable appearance	2	Vegetable dyes	Must not stain teeth or soft tissues

Data from Wilkins EM: *Clinical practice of the dental hygienist,* ed 8, Philadelphia, 1999, Lippincott Williams & Wilkins.

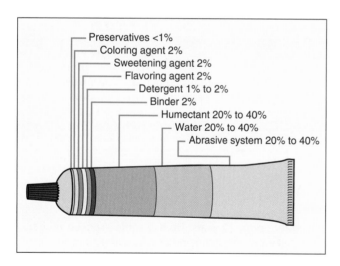

— Preservatives <1%
— Coloring agent 2%
— Sweetening agent 2%
— Flavoring agent 2%
— Detergent 1% to 2%
— Binder 2%
— Humectant 20% to 40%
— Water 20% to 40%
— Abrasive system 20% to 40%

FIG. 23-1 Dentifrice ingredients.

are performed: (1) pilot studies to determine safe doses for humans, (2) larger human studies to prove efficacy and define the effective dosage range, and (3) large, long-term, double-blind controlled clinical trials. The manufacturer then submits all this data to the FDA as part of the NDA and eventually receives approval from the FDA to market the product. The approval requires a period of postmarketing surveillance once the product is made available to the general public.[28]

The FDA also has established the monograph process to allow manufacturers to market dentifrices that meet specified compositional and technical requirements without going through the expensive and time-consuming NDA process. For example, one anticaries monograph permits dentifrices with either sodium fluoride, stannous fluoride, or sodium monofluorophosphate to be marketed as long as the fluoride level is 1000 to 1100 ppm. The manufacturer also must generate data showing acceptable fluoride stability. Other ingredients (e.g., pyrophosphate) can be added to a fluoride dentifrice without the need for an NDA, as long as the ingredient is present for a cosmetic benefit and has an established safety pedigree for oral use. In addition, a desensitization monograph exists that allows the use of 5% potassium nitrate in conjunction with fluoride in a dentifrice.

The manufacturer can apply for the ADA Seal of Acceptance. This program is administered by the ADA's Council on Scientific Affairs (CSA) and is designed to help dental professionals advise patients and the public worldwide. The ADA Seal of Acceptance is a voluntary process and often requires an exhaustive review of the product, depending on the amount of preexisting information on products of similar formulation. The manufacturer must reapply for the seal every 3 years, and the review committee can withdraw acceptance at any time. The seal applies to products used in the practice of dentistry and those sold commercially to the public. When used on labeling, the seal is meaningful only for those specific therapies for which acceptance has been issued. Both dental professionals and patients can be assured that products receiving the seal have been shown to be safe and effective when used as directed, based on the rigorous standards that the ADA has developed and continues to revise since the Council on Dental Therapeutics (predecessor to the Council on Scientific Affairs) was formed in 1930.[54]

EVALUATING CLINICAL STUDIES

Dental professionals and patients rely on the FDA to regulate availability of products based on safety and effectiveness and on the ADA for additional scrutiny of products. In addition to these extensive product evaluations, dental professionals also must be able to evaluate clinical studies performed on products. Data from well-designed clinical trials are invaluable as the dental professional attempts to select appropriate products to meet each patient's unique needs. Studies involving chemotherapeutic agents for the control and prevention of oral diseases require appropriate analysis using specific criteria to assess credibility and to prevent unfounded conclusions.

STUDY DESIGN

Accepted study designs use randomized, controlled clinical trials to evaluate chemotherapeutic agents in dentifrices, usually through efficacy studies or superiority studies. *Efficacy studies* compare a product to a placebo. *Superiority studies* compare products to one another, one of which has an accepted therapeutic value (positive control). The study design is usually either *parallel,* with groups of patients assigned to one treatment for the duration of the study, or *crossover,* when treatment groups are reversed midway through the study. Crossover studies require a period for the groups to return to baseline levels before starting the other treatment and are difficult to interpret because of a possible carryover effect from one treatment to the other.[21] Patients are assigned to treatment groups in a randomized fashion, and the groups are stratified to balance groups for factors such as age and disease severity.[33] The end points of the study should address the variable of interest.[26]

Observed changes in plaque accumulation can occur hourly and gingival changes within days, but periodontal attachment level changes take months to years to be observed clinically. Chemotherapeutic dentifrice studies usually evaluate plaque and gingival changes but not attachment level changes. Some studies monitor the oral microflora to assess changes; others assess supragingival calculus accumulation. Evaluation of all the potential changes in the mouth resulting from use of the chemotherapeutic agent is demanding and challenges researchers to select the appropriate indices.

Safety issues must also be addressed in the study design, with emphasis on standardized monitoring and reporting. Side effects in human studies can be difficult to assess; some effects are seen immediately, whereas others may take months or years to develop. Side effects are usually reported as adverse events, both serious and nonserious, and must be considered relative to the benefit of the agent.[49]

DURATION

Duration of the study depends on the agent being studied and the intended use. Well-designed studies of plaque and gingival changes usually last at least 3 months; the ADA guidelines for the Seal of Acceptance program require studies that last 6 months.[54]

STUDY POPULATION

The population chosen for the study is also a critical point of the study design. To demonstrate effectiveness of the chemotherapeutic agent, the study population must represent the consumer population. That is, patients must have the same level of the disease as the intended users of the product.[49]

EFFICACY CLAIMS

Conclusions about the effects of a chemotherapeutic agent are of significant value for the population studied, but extension of these effects to a general population is not always possible or appropriate.[32] Efficacy or superiority claims can be extrapolated theoretically to the larger group only when the population studied in a clinical trial of an agent in a dentifrice formulation is similar to the population who will use the drug. Variations in populations studied are present in long-term controlled clinical trials for formulations containing chemotherapeutic agents. These variations make comparisons between studies difficult, and claims of efficacy may be difficult to apply to populations other than the specific study population.

EXAMINER RELIABILITY

Few controlled clinical trials on chemotherapeutic agents in dentifrices reported in the literature contain statistical information or confirmation of examiner calibration. Calibration of examiners in the use of the indices is important to ensure consistency and validity of results.[22] Some studies use only one examiner for all clinical evaluations during the study, but intraexaminer reliability should be reported to allow for appropriate statistical analysis. In studies that use multiple examiners, interexaminer reliability is also needed.[53] Without confirmation of examiner calibration, it is difficult to interpret the overall reliability of the studies.

Blinding, or protecting the examiner from knowledge of information concerning the specific groups in the study, is also critical to protect the validity of the results. Ideally, neither the patient nor the examiner or clinician knows the treatment identity (double-blind design). In single-blind study designs, only the examiner is unaware of the treatment identity.

Evaluating all factors that may influence the outcome of a study is difficult. Ensuring that the results truly reflect the activity of the chemotherapeutic agent alone is challenging, especially in complex disease entities such as caries or gingivitis, which can be influenced by many factors. Studies analyzing chemotherapeutic agents in dentifrice formulations based on well-designed clinical trials are useful for the dental practitioner. Each study should be carefully evaluated, however, according to the inherent problems with applying information based on a specific population to an individual patient.

DENTIFRICE FORMULATIONS

With the wide availability of effective chemotherapeutic agents in dentifrice products, all patients can benefit from

23-B

appropriate use. Although these products will enhance mechanical hygiene, they clearly are not a substitute for constant vigilance in oral self-care efforts. Patients with special needs—such as contact allergies, high caries rates, sensitivity, calculus, stain, or periodontitis—require the best efforts of the dental hygienist to advise them in the use of specialized products.

ANTICARIES

As early as 1942, fluoride added to drinking water was found to reduce the incidence of dental caries. Early attempts to add fluoride to dentifrices were not successful, mostly because of the tendency of abrasives used at that time to inactivate the fluoride.[45] Continued testing found that *stannous fluoride,* when used with a compatible abrasive system, inhibited the formation of carious lesions. The ADA recognized the value of stannous fluoride dentifrice as an anticaries agent by granting the Seal of Acceptance to Crest in 1960. Problems with shelf life and staining for products containing stannous fluoride led to further research on additional fluoride formulations. As a result, products containing sodium monofluorophosphate and *sodium fluoride* were recognized as equally effective or slightly more effective anticaries agents. Dentifrices containing these types of fluoride are desirable because of stability and compatibility with many abrasive systems.[50]

Topical fluoride acts as an effective caries-preventive agent in several ways. Fluoride acts in conjunction with the calcium and phosphate in saliva to remineralize the earliest stages of caries, the hypomineralized or *white spot* enamel. Fluoride also exhibits some *substantivity,* or the ability to be held in reservoirs within the oral cavity, where it is released over time, creating continuous exposure of hypomineralized enamel to fluoride. Several areas of the mouth can be considered fluoride reservoirs, including oral mucosa, plaque, and enamel. Rinsing with water after brushing is not recommended; the greater the concentration of fluoride left in the mouth to form a reservoir, the less the chance of decay.[46] Frequent exposure to fluoride dentifrice is the most effective preventive method for caries in both children and adults.

The fluoride concentration of most dentifrices in U.S. OTC products is 1000 to 1100 parts per million (ppm). High-potency dentifrices also are available by prescription that contain fluoride at up to 5000 ppm. Caries prevention is directly proportional to fluoride concentration, and compliance improves with use of a paste rather than a fluoride gel because patients only have to use one product.[17] For populations at risk for severe caries, a high-potency fluoride dentifrice is an appropriate choice.

SENSITIVITY CONTROL

Dentin sensitivity is characterized by a localized, sharp, and instant pain, usually elicited when cold or other stimuli contact the cervical area of a tooth. Other oral conditions can mimic sensitivity, but the examiner can rely on the patient to point to the area. A short puff of air from the air/water syringe usually confirms the exact location, which is associated with an area of exposed root surface.

The accepted theory of pain transmission in dentin sensitivity involves delivery of stimuli through hydrodynamic movement of fluid in the dentinal tubule, activating pulpal tissues and inducing the sensation of pain.[43] Any procedures involving root surfaces can cause dentin sensitivity. Patients may complain of dentin sensitivity after periodontal debridement or restorative procedures. Others experience sensitivity after consumption of acidic foods or a period of poor oral hygiene. The concern that some ingredient in tartar-control dentifrice formulations may promote dentin sensitivity[2] has not been substantiated by clinical studies.

Because dentin sensitivity is associated with exposed dentinal tubules at the root surface, a course of treatment sometimes is directed at blocking or obfuscating the opening to the tubules. If untreated, dentin sensitivity may subside. Otherwise, treatment usually begins with specific plaque control instructions on use of a sensitivity-control dentifrice formulation. The most common active ingredient in commercial sensitivity-control dentifrices is potassium nitrate. Other salts of potassium have also demonstrated effectiveness.[43] Sensitivity-control dentifrices take time to be effective, so a common technique is to combine an in-office application of a dentin-blocking agent with use of a sensitivity-control dentifrice at home. If these methods do not produce relief after 4 to 6 weeks, more aggressive means include in-office applications of bonding agents, placement of permanent restorations, and gingival grafting for root coverage.

CALCULUS CONTROL

Dental professionals expend much time and effort in the removal of supragingival calculus deposits. Patients often see supragingival calculus as an aesthetic problem, and dental professionals are concerned about the role of supragingival calculus in the development of gingivitis. The rough surface of calculus can retain bacterial plaque close to the gingival tissues, and calculus is often located in areas that are difficult for patients to clean thoroughly.[4] Supragingival calculus can easily become discolored, and many extrinsic stains on teeth are actually stained calculus deposits.

For patients who form supragingival calculus, daily application of an anticalculus dentifrice to inhibit calculus deposition can be beneficial. Several active ingredients added to dentifrice formulations have anticalculus capabilities. The most effective ingredient appears to be sodium hexametaphosphate, which may inhibit calcification in the conversion of amorphous calcium phosphate to hydroxyapatite. The next most effective ingredient is pyrophosphate (3.3%-5%), usually comes in one of three forms: tetrasodium, disodium dihydrogen, or tetrapotassium pyrophosphate.[56] In addition, 1% to 2% *Gantrez,* a copolymer of methoxyethylene and maleic acid, provides some very modest anticalculus properties. Additionally, 2.0% zinc chloride and 0.5% zinc citrate are used alone or combined with other anticalculus chemicals.[70]

In evaluating anticalculus claims, the dental hygienist must realize that the major impact of these agents is only on supragingival calculus, and subgingival calculus is unaffected. Also, both pyrophosphates and zinc salts contribute some minor abrasiveness. Use of anticalculus dentifrices may be indicated in patients with supragingival calculus, which may result in a reduced need for calculus removal during dental treatment.[67]

WHITENING BENEFIT

Tooth discoloration is a patient concern that is addressed by various methods, both in-office treatments and at-home bleaching techniques. Intrinsic stains, such as fluorosis or tetracycline staining, can be treated using in-office vital bleaching techniques, with bleaching containing hydrogen peroxide or carbamide peroxide. The patient also can use bleaching trays for a few hours daily at home.[29] Newer products, such as whitening strips, allow the patient convenient, comfortable options to whiten teeth. Extrinsic stains can be removed by scaling and polishing in the office, but controlling the staining at home has always been difficult for patients. Many dentifrices use "whitening" in labeling, but until recently, no consistent guidelines existed for claims of whitening dentifrices. CSA criteria for whitening dentifrices call for demonstration of change in tooth color of two or more shades on a value-ordered shade guide over 6 months. The ADA Seal of Acceptance has been awarded to few OTC tooth-whitening dentifrices. The first accepted product has a mild abrasive that removes extrinsic stains by a gentle polishing action and also contains a tartar-control ingredient.[3]

ANTIGINGIVITIS

Most patients receiving treatment in a dental care setting have some level of gingival inflammation. Gingivitis is prevalent in the general population at a high rate, with as few as 15% of individuals free of signs of periodontal diseases.[10] Development of periodontitis usually is preceded by gingivitis, but not all sites with gingivitis progress to periodontitis. Currently, no way exists to predict the likelihood of developing attachment loss, and no evidence shows that control of gingivitis with topical agents decreases the progression of periodontitis or affects eventual tooth loss. Treatment of all gingivitis generally is recommended to prevent periodontitis. Dentifrices with chemotherapeutic agents that are successful in controlling or eliminating gingivitis, when combined with mechanical therapy, can improve oral health.

Stannous Fluoride

Stannous fluoride was the first chemotherapeutic agent added to a dentifrice formulation, but the usefulness of stannous fluoride was limited because of difficulties in formulation and short shelf life. Early stannous fluoride products also have had the potential for stain and taste side effects. Stannous fluoride has not only anticaries effects but also antiplaque and antigingivitis effects, probably due to effects of the tin ion.[11] A more stable form of stannous fluoride dentifrice with bioavailability comparable to nonaqueous gel and mouthrinse formulations has shown significant reductions in gingivitis scores and gingival bleeding but no decrease in plaque scores.[7] A stannous fluoride dentifrice could be a good choice for patients who need help with gingivitis and caries control.

Sodium Bicarbonate and Hydrogen Peroxide

In the 1970s, many patients pursued a new, widely publicized treatment for periodontitis as an alternative to periodontal surgery. The controversial *Keyes' technique* used a paste of baking soda, hydrogen peroxide, and salt as a dentifrice, combined with irrigation with a saturated salt solution. Scaling and root planing were also performed; microbiological monitoring with phase-contrast microscopy was used; and tetracycline was prescribed if indicated.[35] Compared with conventional oral hygiene techniques, the Keyes' technique demonstrated no statistically significant difference in clinical effectiveness. The extensive claims of this technique as an alternative to conventional periodontal therapy were unsubstantiated by controlled clinical trials, and patients may have been at risk for inadequate or ineffective treatment of their periodontal diseases.[25]

Sodium bicarbonate, or baking soda, is an abrasive and may also produce a mild antibacterial effect. In a dentifrice, bicarbonate is incorporated into both toothpastes and gels, sometimes in combination with hydrogen peroxide. Patient acceptance of baking soda products may be related to an increasing interest in natural products or in taste and texture. Hydrogen peroxide has been used for years, mostly in short-term treatment of acute gingival conditions and in bleaching products. The safety of long-term hydrogen peroxide use has been debated, especially regarding effects on healing and potential co-carcinogenicity.[65] However, it is generally accepted that the use of hydrogen peroxide in oral care products presents no long-term safety concerns. One marketed dentifrice containing peroxide, baking soda, and fluoride has not shown additional benefits over a dentifrice containing only peroxide.[8]

Chlorhexidine

Chlorhexidine is widely acknowledged as an extremely effective antiplaque and antigingivitis agent.[39] It has been studied mostly in mouthrinse formulations and is safe and effective[6], but staining, calculus formation, and taste alteration are problems with long-term use.[41] Early attempts to develop an effective dentifrice formulation containing chlorhexidine were not highly successful because chlorhexidine tends to react with the other components and is easily inactivated.[38] Recent efforts to produce a more stable dentifrice formulation containing chlorhexidine have been more successful, but none is currently available commercially in the United States. Studies on chlorhexidine dentifrice formulations have shown significant differences in plaque and gingivitis scores and in bleeding sites compared with controls. Staining, increased calculus formation, and taste alterations occurred less frequently with the chlorhexidine dentifrice than with the mouthrinse.[60,69] The use of chlorhexidine in a dentifrice that is appropriately formulated to provide bioavailability may offer an alternative delivery system that decreases the undesirable side effects of an otherwise highly effective chemotherapeutic agent for plaque control and treatment of gingivitis.

Triclosan

Triclosan is a bisphenol with broad-spectrum antimicrobial activity and no major side effects. First used in soaps and antiperspirants, it is considered safe for use in oral healthcare products.[18] In dentifrice formulations, triclosan has been combined with several other active ingredients, including sodium fluoride for caries control, a copolymer of vinylmethylether–maleic acid (PVM-MA) to increase substantivity, and pyrophosphates to add anticalculus properties.[44] The addition of the PVM-MA copolymer acts as a retention aid for triclosan in the mouth, increasing the potential duration of the antimicrobial effects of the triclosan on plaque bacteria. The PVM-MA copolymer also has been shown to have some anticalculus properties[23] but is not as effective as formulations containing zinc citrate or pyrophosphates.[20] The results of multiple long-term studies typically show significant reductions in plaque, gingivitis, and calculus in patients using triclosan and PVM-MA copolymer dentifrice compared with controls.* Some published articles do not support triclosan as an effective therapeutic agent.[20] A dentifrice formulation containing triclosan, PVM-MA copolymer, and sodium fluoride has been ADA-approved as a decay-preventive dentifrice that also helps to prevent and reduce gingivitis, plaque, and calculus.[1]

OTHER AGENTS

Over the years an amazing variety of ingredients has been added to dentifrice formulations to attempt to treat various dental conditions. Products that consumers perceive as "natural" or "alternative medicine" therapies are of particular interest. One of the most studied natural ingredients is *sanguinarine*, an alkaloid plant extract. It is currently used in both dentifrice and mouthwash formulations. Several studies have had conflicting reports of efficacy. Six-month studies using the dentifrice and mouthwash in combination show reduction in plaque and gingivitis. The formulations that contain zinc may show improved results.[37] Other agents evaluated in short-term studies include enzyme systems such as amyloglucosidase–glucose oxidase,[47] lactoperoxidase,[36] triclosan combined with silicon oil,[57] and cetylpyridinium chloride in a foam formulation.[5] It is difficult to draw any conclusions about the efficacy of these products from these studies. Further research is needed to explore alternative therapies in controlled clinical trials to prove their potential efficacy.

---

*References 9, 12, 15, 16, 24, 26, 32, 34, 40, 42, 52, 55, 62.

 Case Application

All four members of the Courtland family have different needs that may not be met by one dentifrice product. Your familiarity with the family enables you to decide how receptive each of them will be to compliance issues. Also, you will be estimating their ideal frequency of recall based on each of their patterns of disease history and their ability to stay motivated to practice optimal oral self-care.

Mrs. Courtland appears to maintain her oral health well from recall to recall except for localized areas of gingivitis. If you believe she is performing optimal oral self-care but is having problems managing specific areas, she might benefit from an antigingivitis toothpaste. Options would include a product that uses triclosan or stabilized stannous fluoride as the active ingredient. Mr. Courtland has a history of periodontal disease and sensitive root surfaces. Because root caries is also a concern, a desensitizing dentifrice that contains fluoride would address both the root caries and the sensitivity issues.

Amber and Brandon may present the most challenging problems. Amber's needs are multifactorial; your counseling services will involve maximum efforts at improving oral self-care motivation as well as dietary intervention to reduce the effects of fermentable carbohydrates. You should also be alert to the possibility of an eating disorder such as bulimia, which is common in this age group and can lead to decalcification of enamel surfaces. Before orthodontics can be reconsidered, Amber should be receiving in-office fluoride treatments as well as daily concentrated-fluoride applications at home in the form of a high-potency fluoride dentifrice. The dentist must prescribe this and probably needs to do some restorative work in the meantime.

Although some of Amber's problems are still reversible or at least reparable, she and Brandon both have future preventive needs. Both will benefit from oral hygiene counseling services. Brandon needs to establish the lifelong habit of regular daily plaque removal using a simple, pleasant-tasting, agreeably textured fluoride dentifrice. Amber's high-fluoride dentifrice is not appropriate for Brandon. Eventually, when Amber has improved her compliance with oral self-care and diet and her caries problem is controlled, she might benefit from a whitening dentifrice that contains fluoride, which would meet all her other needs and at the same time appeal to her need for increased self-esteem.

RITICAL THINKING ACTIVITIES

Survey 20 "consumers" (i.e., nondental professionals) to gain the following insight:

1. Does the consumer recall the last oral care product purchased? If yes, what was it?
   a. Dentifrice
   b. Toothbrush
   c. Floss
   d. Other _____

2. Regarding the last purchase of a dentifrice, does the consumer recall a specific brand name purchased? If yes, what was it? _____

3. Does the consumer recall the type of store where the purchase was made? If yes, what was it?
   a. Grocery
   b. Pharmacy
   c. "Superstore" (e.g., K-Mart, Sam's Club, Wal-Mart)

RITICAL THINKING ACTIVITIES—cont'd

4. What was the main reason for purchasing that particular brand?
   a. Professional recommendation
   b. Price
   c. Personal preference
   d. Advice of friend
5. Do they consider themselves to be "loyal" to a specific brand of dentifrice (that is, they repeatedly purchase the same dentifrice)?
   a. Yes
   b. No
6. If the oral care provider recommended a specific self-care product to purchase, how likely would the consumer be to comply (1 being least likely, 5 being most likely)?
   a. 1
   b. 2
   c. 3
   d. 4
   e. 5
7. Go to the local supermarket where you do your grocery marketing. If *your* oral care provider sent you to this store and told you to purchase the following products, how many choices would you have (*a* to *d*), and what selections would you make (*e* to *f*)?
   a. Tartar-control dentifrice _____
   b. Antigingivitis dentifrice _____
   c. Desensitizing dentifrice _____
   d. Whitening dentifrice _____
   e. Tartar-control selection: _____
   f. Antigingivitis selection: _____
   g. Desensitizing selection: _____
   h. Whitening selection: _____

 REVIEW QUESTIONS

1. Currently the ADA Seal of Acceptance is *not* given to any product as effective against which of the following?
   a. Gingivitis
   b. Periodontitis
   c. Caries
   d. Dentin sensitivity
2. A commercial dentifrice can be found in all the following forms *except* which one?
   a. Paste
   b. Gel
   c. Rinse
   d. Powder
3. People reporting allergic reactions to components of dentifrices are generally reacting to which one of the following groups?
   a. Abrasives
   b. Humectants
   c. Flavorings
   d. Coloring agents
4. The ADA Seal of Acceptance is currently administered by which one of the following groups?
   a. Council on Dental Research
   b. Council on Scientific Research
   c. Council on Scientific Affairs
   d. Committee of Studies Applications
5. The FDA regulates marketing of dentifrices by demanding evidence of all the following except which one?
   a. No carcinogenicity
   b. No allergenicity
   c. High customer approval ratings
   d. Proof of effectiveness
6. Large dentifrice trials that compare one active ingredient against another in coded containers are referred to as which one of the following groups?
   a. Efficacy studies
   b. Superiority studies
   c. Placebo-based studies
   d. Pilot studies
7. Stannous fluoride is an effective chemotherapeutic for all the following conditions except which one?
   a. Caries
   b. Dentin sensitivity
   c. Diminished salivary flow
   d. Gingivitis
8. The anticalculus ingredient that appears to be most effective in dentifrice preparations is which of the following?
   a. Zinc citrate
   b. Enzymes
   c. Pyrophosphate
   d. Gantrez copolymer
9. Salts used in dentin sensitivity preparations include all the following *except* which one?
   a. Potassium nitrate
   b. Sodium chloride
   c. Sodium monofluorophosphate
   d. Sodium bicarbonate
10. Nonperoxide-type tooth whiteners act by which one of the following mechanisms?
   a. Mild abrasives and polishers along with a tartar-control ingredient
   b. Mildly acidic base material
   c. Enamel-penetrating chemicals
   d. Increased amounts of detergents

SUGGESTED AGENCIES AND WEB SITES

Because of the ever-changing nature of the Internet, some of the web sites listed here may have changed since publication. Please refer to Mosby's Evolve web site for the most current information.

Academy of General Dentistry ("Consumer information," "Toothpaste"): http://www.agd.org

American Academy of Periodontology: http://www.perio.org

American Dental Association: http://www.ada.org

The American Dental Hygienists' Association (ADHA online): http://www.adha.org

Chid Online: The Combined Health Information Database: http://chid.nih.gov

Clinical Research Associates: Clinician's Guide to Dental Products and Techniques: http://www.cranews.com

Colgate-Palmolive: http://www.colgate-palmolive.com

Dental Hygienist News ("Orthodontic patients: implications for dental hygiene therapy"): http://www.dentalhygienistnews.com

Journal of Clinical Dentistry ("The effect of a triclosan/copolymer/ fluoride dentifrice on plaque formation and gingivitis: a six-month clinical study"): http://www.jclindent.com

[The] Journal of Contemporary Dental Practice: http://www.thejcdp.com

P&G Dental Resource Net: Poster Presentations ("Dentifrice effects on plaque regrowth: digital plaque image analysis"): http://www.dentalcare.com

P&G Dental Resource Net: Poster Presentations ("Dentifrice enhancement of plaque removal by manual toothbrushing"): http://www.dentalcare.com

PPG Industries, Inc: Silicas ("Dentifrice abrasive silicas"): http://www.ppg.com

PPG Industries, Inc: Silicas ("Dentifrice thickening silicas"): http://www.ppg.com

Procter & Gamble Global Dental Resources: http://www.dentalcare.com

 ADDITIONAL READINGS AND RESOURCES

Addy M, Moran J, editors: Toothpaste, mouthrinse and other topical remedies in periodontics, *Periodontology 2000* 15, 1997.

American Dental Association Seal Directory: ADA Council on Scientific Affairs, Chicago, 312-440-2500.

Harris NO, Christen AG, editors: *Primary preventive dentistry,* ed 4, Stamford, Conn, 1995, Appleton & Lange.

 REFERENCES

1. Luz C: First whitening dentifrice gets Seal, *ADA News* 30(20):14, 1999.
2. FDA okays gingivitis-fighting toothpaste for U.S. market, *ADA News* 28(15):3, 1997.
3. Hypersensitivity reports requested, *ADA News* 27(16):1, 1996.
4. Addy M, Koltai R: Control of supragingival calculus—scaling and polishing and anticalculus toothpastes: an opinion, *J Clin Periodontol* 21:342-6, 1994.
5. Addy M, Moran J: The effect of a cetylpyridinum chloride (CPC) detergent foam compared to a conventional toothpaste on plaque and gingivitis, *J Clin Periodontol* 16:87-91, 1989.
6. Baker K: Mouthrinses in the prevention and treatment of periodontal disease, *Curr Opin Periodontol* 89-96, 1993.
7. Beiswanger BB et al: The clinical effect of dentifrices containing stabilized stannous fluoride on plaque formation and gingivitis: a six-month study with ad libitum brushing, *J Clin Dent* 6(Special issue):46-53, 1995.
8. Beiswanger BB et al: The comparative efficacy of stabilized stannous fluoride dentifrice, peroxide/baking soda dentifrice, and essential oil mouthrinse for the prevention of gingivitis, *J Clin Dent* 8:46-53, 1997.
9. Bolden TE et al: The clinical effect of a dentifrice containing triclosan and a copolymer in a sodium fluoride/silica base on plaque formation and gingivitis: a six-month clinical study, *J Clin Dent* 3:125-31, 1992.
10. Brown LJ, Oliver RC, Loe H: Periodontal diseases in the U.S. in 1981: prevalence, severity, extent, and role in tooth mortality, *J Periodontol* 60:363-70, 1989.
11. Ciancio SG: Agents for the management of plaque and gingivitis, *J Dent Res* 71(7):1450-4, 1992.
12. Cubells AB et al: The effect of a triclosan/copolymer/fluoride dentifrice on plaque formation and gingivitis: a six-month clinical study, *J Clin Dent* 2:63-9, 1991.
13. Cummins D: Vehicles: how to deliver the goods, *Periodontology 2000* 15:84-5, 1997.
14. Cummins D, Creeth JE: Delivery of antiplaque agents from dentifrices, gels, and mouthwashes, *J Dent Res* 71(7):1439-49, 1992.
15. Deasy MJ et al: Effect of a dentifrice containing triclosan and a copolymer on plaque formation and gingivitis, *Clin Prev Dent* 13(6):12-19, 1991.
16. Denepitiya JL et al: Effect upon plaque formation and gingivitis of a triclosan/copolymer/fluoride dentifrice: a 6-month clinical study, *Am J Dent* 5:307-11, 1992.
17. DePaola PF: The benefits of high-potency fluoride dentifrices, *Compend Cont Educ Dent* 18(2):44-50, 1997.
18. DeSalva SJ, Kong BM, Lin YJ: Triclosan: a safety profile, *Am J Dent* 2:185-96, 1989.
19. Douglas TE: Fluoride dentifrice and stomatitis, *Northwest Med* 56:1037-9, 1957.
20. Fairbrother KJ et al: The comparative clinical efficacy of pyrophosphate/triclosan, copolymer/triclosan, and zinc citrate/triclosan dentifrices for the reduction of supragingival calculus formation, *J Clin Dent* 8:62-6, 1997.
21. Fleiss JL: General design issues in efficacy, equivalency, and superiority trials, *J Periodontal Res* 27(Special issue):306-13, 1992.

22. Fleiss JL et al: A study of inter- and intra-examiner reliability of pocket depth and attachment level, *J Periodontal Res;* 26: 122-8, 1991.

23. Gaffar A, Esposito A, Afflitto J: In vitro and in vivo anticalculus effects of a triclosan/copolymer system, *Am J Dent* 3:S37, 1990.

24. Garcia-Godoy F et al: Effect of a triclosan/copolymer/fluoride dentifrice on plaque formation and gingivitis: a 7-month clinical study, *Am J Dent* 3:S15-S26, 1990.

25. Greenwell H, Bissada NF: A dispassionate scientific analysis of Keyes' technique, *Int J Perio Rest Dent* 3:65-75, 1985.

26. Hancock B: Prevention, *Ann Periodontol* 1:223-55, 1996.

27. Hargreaves JA, Thompson GW, Wagg BJ: Changes in caries prevalence of Isle of Lewis children between 1971 and 1981, *Caries Res* 17:554-9, 1983.

28. Harris NO, Christen AG: *Primary preventive dentistry,* ed 4, Stamford, Conn, 1995, Appleton & Lange.

29. Haywood VB et al: Effectiveness, side effects and long-term status of Nightguard vital bleaching, *J Am Dent Assoc* 125: 1219-26, 1994.

30. Herlofson BB, Barkvoll P: The effect of two toothpaste detergents on the frequency of recurrent aphthous ulcers, *Acta Odontol Scand* 54:150-3, 1996.

31. Herlofson BB, Brodin P, Aars H: Increased human gingival blood flow induced by sodium lauryl sulfate, *J Clin Periodontol* 23:1004-7, 1996.

32. Hujoel PP: Logical and analytical issues in dental/oral product comparison research, *J Periodontal Res* 27(Special issue): 362-3, 1992.

33. Hyman FN, Welch ME, Cheever JR: Regulatory issues for evaluation of therapies to prevent or arrest disease progression, *Ann Periodontol* 2:166-75, 1997.

34. Kanchanakamol J et al: Reduction of plaque formation and gingivitis by a dentifrice containing triclosan and copolymer, *J Periodontol* 66:109-12, 1995.

35. Keyes P, Wright W, Howard S: The use of phase contrast microscopy and chemotherapy in the diagnosis and treatment of periodontal lesions: an initial report, *Quint Int* 9:51-6, 1978.

36. Kirstila B, Lenander-Lumikari M, Tenovuo J: Effects of a lactoperoxidase–system-containing toothpaste on dental plaque and whole saliva in vivo, *Acta Odontol Scand* 52:346-53, 1994.

37. Kopczyk R et al: Clinical and microbiological effects of a sanguinaria-containing mouthrinse and dentifrice with and without fluoride during 6 months of use, *J Periodontol* 62:617-22, 1991.

38. Kornman KS: The role of supragingival plaque in the prevention and treatment of periodontal diseases: a review of current concepts, *J Periodontal Res* (Suppl):5-22, 1986.

39. Lang NP, Brecx MC: Chlorhexidine digluconate: an agent for chemical plaque control and prevention of gingival inflammation, *J Periodontal Res* (Suppl):74-89, 1986.

40. Lindhe J et al: The effect of a triclosan-containing dentifrice on established plaque and gingivitis, *J Clin Periodontol* 20:327-34, 1993.

41. Mandel ID: Chemical agents for control of plaque and gingivitis, Committee on Research, Science and Therapy, American Academy of Periodontology, Chicago, 1994.

42. Mankodi SM et al: Clinical effect of a triclosan-containing dentifrice on plaque and gingivitis: a six-month study, *Clin Prev Dent* 14(6):4-10, 1992.

43. Markowitz K: Tooth sensitivity: mechanisms and management, *Compend Cont Educ Dent* 14(8):1032-45, 1997.

44. Marsh PD: Dentifrices containing new agents for the control of plaque and gingivitis: microbiological aspects, *J Clin Periodontol* 18:462-7, 1991.

45. Mellburg JR: Fluoride dentifrices: current status and prospects, *Int Dent J* 41:9-16, 1991.

46. Mellburg JR: The mechanism of fluoride protection, *Compend Cont Educ Dent* 18(2):37-43, 1997.

47. Moran J, Addy M, Newcombe R: Comparison of the effect of toothpastes containing enzymes or antimicrobial compounds with a conventional fluoride toothpaste on the development of plaque and gingivitis, *J Clin Periodontol* 16:295-9, 1989.

48. Munoz FJ et al: Perioral contact urticaria from sodium benzoate in a toothpaste, *Contact Dermatitis* 35:51, 1996.

49. Newman MG: Design and implementation of clinical trials of antimicrobial drugs and devices used in periodontal disease treatment, *Ann Periodontol* 2:180-98, 1997.

50. O'Mullane DM: Introduction and rationale for the use of fluoride for caries prevention, *Int Dent J* 44:257-61, 1994.

51. Osuju OO et al: Risk factors for dental fluorosis in a fluoridated community, *J Dent Res* 67:1488-92, 1988.

52. Palomo F et al: The effect of three commercially available dentifrices containing triclosan on supragingival plaque formation and gingivitis: a six-month clinical study, *Int Dent J* 44:75-81, 1994.

53. Polson AM: The research team, calibration, and quality assurance in clinical trials in periodontics, *Ann Periodontol* 2:75-82, 1997.

54. Products of excellence: ADA Seal Program, *J Am Dent Assoc* (Suppl):1-2, 1997.

55. Renvert S, Birkhed D: Comparison between 3 triclosan dentifrices on plaque, gingivitis, and salivary microflora, *J Clin Periodontol* 22:63-70, 1995.

56. Ripa LW et al: Clinical study of the anticaries efficacy of three fluoride dentifrices containing anticalculus ingredients: three-year (final) results, *J Clin Dent* 2:29-33, 1990.

57. Rolla G, Gaare D, Ellingsen JE: Experiments with a toothpaste containing polydimethylsiloxan/triclosan, *Scand J Dent Res* 101:130-2, 1993.

58. Sainio E, Kanerva L: Contact allergens in toothpastes and a review of their hypersensitivity, *Contact Dermatitis* 33:100-5, 1995.

59. Sanders MA: Fluoride toothpastes: a cause of acne-like eruptions, *Arch Dermatol* 111:793, 1975.

60. Sanz M et al: The effect of a dentifrice containing chlorhexidine and zinc on plaque, gingivitis, calculus and tooth staining, *J Clin Periodontol* 21:431-7, 1994.

61. Shea JJ, Gillispie SM, Waldbott GL: Allergy to fluoride, *Ann Allergy* 25:388-91, 1967.

62. Svatun B et al: The effects of three silica dentifrices containing triclosan on supragingival plaque and calculus formation and on gingivitis, *Int Dent J* 43:441-52, 1993.

63. Szpunar SM, Burt BA: Trends in the prevalence of dental fluorosis in the United States: a review, *J Public Health Dent* 47:71-9, 1987.

64. Trummel CL: Regulation of oral chemotherapeutic in the United States, *J Dent Res* 73(3):704-8, 1994.

65. Weitzman SA et al: Chronic treatment with hydrogen peroxide: is it safe? *J Periodontol* 55(9):510-11, 1984.

66. White DJ: A "return" to stannous fluoride dentifrices, *J Clin Dent* 6(Special issue):29-36, 1995.

67. White DJ et al: Qualicalc assessment of the clinical scaling benefits provided by pyrophosphate dentifrices with and without triclosan, *J Clin Dent* 7:46-9, 1996.

68. Wilkins EM: *Clinical practice of the dental hygienist,* ed 6, Philadelphia, 1989, Lea & Febiger.

69. Yates R et al: A 6-month home usage trial of a 1% chlorhexidine toothpaste. I. Effects on plaque, gingivitis, calculus and tooth staining, *J Clin Periodontol* 20:130-8, 1993.

70. Yiu CK, Wei SH: Clinical efficacy of dentifrices in the control of calculus, plaque, and gingivitis, *Quint Int* 24:181-8, 1993.

CHAPTER 24

Chemotherapeutics

Katharine R. Stilley

Chapter Outline

Case Study: Selecting a Chemotherapeutic Agent
  Based on Patient Need
Delivery Systems
  Rinsing
  Irrigation
Antimicrobials: General Considerations and
  Specific Agents
    Qualities of the ideal antimicrobial agent
    Selection
    Patient considerations
    Concentration, effect, and resistance
Agents
  Water
  Chlorhexidine
  Essential oils
  Tetracycline and its analogs
  Sanguinarine
  Stannous fluoride

Nonsteroidal antiinflammatory agents
Triclosan
Oxygen
Povidone–iodine
Quaternary ammonium compounds
Baking soda
Prebrushing rinse
Controlled Drug-Delivery Systems
  Advantages
  Cautions
  Actisite
  PerioChip
  Atrigel
  Arestin
Systemic Delivery
Quality Assurance
Evaluation of Success

Key Terms

Antimicrobial
Cannula
Cationic
Chemotherapeutic
Controlled-delivery device

Delivery system
Essential oil
Irrigation
Lumen
Marginal irrigation

Pulsating
Rinsing
Side-ported
Site-specific
Subgingival irrigation

Substantivity
Supragingival irrigation
Sustained release
Systemic
Topical

 ## Learning Outcomes

1. Discriminate among various chemotherapeutic agents
   and delivery systems to select the optimum intervention
   for individual patients.
2. Determine the appropriate time in the treatment
   sequence to recommend supplemental control of
   periodontal diseases through antimicrobial therapy.

3. Demonstrate irrigation and the procedures for the
   various controlled drug-delivery modalities.
4. Evaluate the effectiveness of chemotherapeutic
   intervention.
5. Understand the need to stay informed regarding
   developments and changes in the standards for
   nonsurgical periodontal therapy.

*T*he first, most basic, historical and indispensable method in the treatment of periodontal diseases is thorough mechanical plaque control, including both daily personal plaque control and periodic professional supportive periodontal care. Careful, daily disruption of plaque, especially interproximally and at the gingival margins, is an essential oral health habit for health maintenance; however, it is a tedious and uninteresting task for the average individual. As a result, most people do not clean their mouths as thoroughly as they should. In fact, dental hygienists are probably one of the few groups excited about plaque control. However, even with good daily, personal plaque control and regular professional debridement, some periodontally involved patients are unable to attain and maintain periodontal stability.

When mechanical disruption of the plaque is insufficient to control gingival inflammation, the use of chemotherapeutics should be considered. Chemotherapeutics and pharmacotherapeutics are broad terms encompassing agents that may affect microorganisms and hard and soft tissues in the oral cavity. *Chemotherapeutic* agents are used to eliminate, reduce, or alter the effect of microorganisms in the oral cavity, preferably the pathogenic microorganisms, or to effect a change in the host response. The term *antimicrobial* is narrower and refers to agents that kill microbes or affect the growth and multiplication of microorganisms.[5]

Chemotherapeutic agents have been demonstrated to lessen gingivitis, plaque, and gingival bleeding when used daily. Evidence is still not sufficient to state to what degree chemotherapeutics in clinical practice affect the deeper periodontal tissues such as bone height and attachment level. Differences in periodontal pockets after the use of *irrigation* or chemotherapeutics have been reported, typically by attachment gain and change in the pocket microflora. Currently, however, the use of pharmacotherapeutics is still considered *adjunct* therapy, not a substitute for thorough, frequent professional debridement and daily personal plaque control.

A new arena for the use of chemotherapeutics in dentistry is to cause a change in the host response to periodontal infections, rather than to affect the microbial status. This is accomplished with the use of a subantimicrobial concentration of certain chemotherapeutic agents (e.g., tetracycline derivatives). This concept is discussed more fully in the section on *systemic* delivery.

When oral health clinicians speak of the benefits of chemotherapeutics, they are most often referring to the effect on the periodontal status of the mouth. Yet chemotherapeutics are useful for more than the prevention and control of periodontal diseases. For example, fluoride, chlorhexidine, and essential oils are used in the control of dental caries and cariogenic microbes. However, this chapter focuses on the use of chemotherapeutics in periodontal diseases—the *delivery systems* and the agents.

DELIVERY SYSTEMS

The delivery of therapeutic chemical agents to the site of infection is accomplished either systemically or locally and may be used during the presurgical, surgical, or supportive phases of periodontal care. The means by which the agent is applied or made available to the oral site is termed the

 Case Study

Selecting a Chemotherapeutic Agent Based on Patient Need

Ms. Chlöe Tevus, a 29-year-old, apparently healthy Caucasian female was diagnosed with generalized chronic periodontitis. She denies any medical problems, takes no medication, and does not smoke. As a teenager she had active orthodontics and retains 24 teeth. The first premolars and the third molars were sound and were previously extracted for orthodontic reasons. She has occlusal amalgams on her molars, occlusal wear, and interproximal restorations between some of the posterior teeth.

Her private law practice specializes in contract law. She is the sole caregiver for her elderly parent.

Ms. Tevus completed periodontal therapy 18 months ago and has been seen every 3 months alternately by the hygienists at her periodontist and general dentist's offices. She demonstrates capable technique with the toothbrush and the interdental brush. Her bleeding-on-probing percentage has varied between 23% and 32% at the 3-month intervals, generalized to interproximal sites. She has also developed a probe depth of 7 mm on the palatal of #10. O'Leary's Plaque Control Record has resulted in average scores of 15% to 20%, particularly on the facial and palatal of the maxillary molars.

delivery system and includes the drug carrier or vehicle, the route, and the target. Systemic or enteric delivery allows agents to course through the body until reaching the diseased or intended site. Ingestion and intramuscular injection are common means of systemic delivery.

Topical drug-delivery systems deliver chemotherapeutic agents to the surface of mucosa or gingiva—for example with rinsing—or several millimeters below the gingival margin during supragingival irrigation. Site-specific delivery is accomplished with vehicles such as impregnated fibers, discs, and gels. *Site-specific* includes *sustained release* and controlled delivery of a chemotherapeutic agent to a specified area of the mouth. Sustained release refers to systems and agents that are most active (provide drug delivery) for less than 24 hours, whereas controlled delivery means the agent is active longer than 1 day.[5] Controlled delivery is indicated for periodontal pockets deeper than 5 mm, and treatment is usually over a period of 7 to 10 days. In addition to rinsing, irrigation, and controlled delivery, vehicles such as lozenges, chewing gum, and sprays also have been employed to deliver chemotherapeutic agents.

RINSING

Rinsing is the action of swishing liquid forcefully around the mouth and between the teeth through the muscle action of the checks, lips, and tongue to dislodge particles and debris and to disperse agents. Antimicrobial agents reach mucosal and gingival surfaces effectively through a good rinsing pattern. However, rinsing is ineffective against the subgingival flora, because the chemotherapeutic agent is not

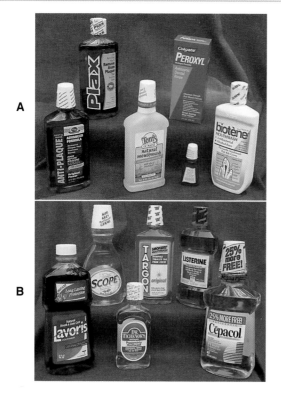

FIG. 24-1 Mouthrinses. **A,** Two prerinses *(left)* and several non–alcohol-containing mouthrinses *(right).* **B,** Familiar brands of mouthrinses containing alcohol ranging from 8% to 27%. (Courtesy Dr. W.B. Stilley II, Brandon, Miss.)

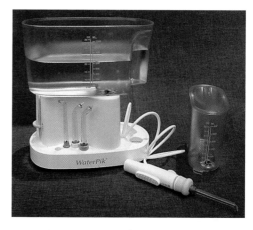

FIG. 24-2 Irrigator. Unit is shown with supragingival and marginal irrigation tips and two reservoirs. The larger reservoir is on top of the unit and is designed for water. The smaller reservoir is designed for chemotherapeutic agents (for example, chlorhexidine) and is tinted to reduce light degradation (Courtesy Waterpik Technologies, Fort Collins, Colo.)

TABLE 24-1

Oral irrigators with ADA Seal of Acceptance

Manufacturer	Model
Gillette Oral Care (Boston, Mass.)	Braun Oral-B Oral Care Center
	Braun Oral-B Oral Irrigator
Hydro-Pik (Miami, Fla.)	Hydro Pik
Waterpik Technologies (Fort Collins, Colo.)	Water Pik Family Dental System (WP-70W)
	Water Pik Personal Dental System (WP-60W)
	Waterpik Plus Plaque Control System (WP-90W)
	Water Pik Professional Dental System (WP-72W)
	Water Pik Travel Dental System (WP-350W)

From American Dental Association: *The ADA Seal of Acceptance, consumer products: by category* [Internet], Chicago, 1995-2001, The Association [http://www.ada.org].

directed into the gingival margin. Additionally, some patients are able to rinse well, whereas other patients do not have adequate muscle action to move liquids around their mouth effectively.

Mouthrinses frequently contain alcohol as a common ingredient. Alcohol is used to dissolve the flavoring agents used to mask the taste of the active ingredient or to dissolve the active ingredient and stabilize the product. Patients who have reduced salivary flow or xerostomia, alcohol-dependency problems, or tissues that are sensitive to alcohol should use an alcohol-free mouthrinse (Fig. 24-1).

IRRIGATION

Irrigation is the application of liquid under pressure via the use of an appliance. Powered irrigators emit a *pulsating* steam of water, whereas water-pressure driven appliances hook onto a faucet and deliver a steady stream of water (Table 24-1). A pulsating stream has been shown to be superior to a steady stream of water.[9] Irrigators permit delivery of liquid agents into the interproximal areas and submarginally into sulci and pockets (Fig. 24-2). With all oral irrigation, the tip is kept in motion, not held in one spot, to avoid trauma to cells or tissue. Pulsed irrigation has been available to patients since the early 1960s and has been proven safe.[15]

Tip design determines access in the periodontal area; thus irrigation is divided into three categories of irrigation according to the design of the tip: supragingival, marginal (at the gingival margin), and subgingival (Fig. 24-3).

Supragingival irrigation is accomplished by using a plastic tip with a wide *lumen,* or opening. The stream of irrigant is directed at right angles to the tooth just above the gingival margin with 9% to 54% of the liquid deflected into the sulcus (Fig. 24-4). Supragingival irrigation has been shown to have a beneficial effect on gingivitis and reduces bleeding when used with periodontal maintenance patients.[35] However, considerable research is still necessary to learn just how and to what degree the adjunctive use of *subgingival irrigation* actually affects the periodontal clinical indicators.

Marginal irrigation utilizes a flexible rubber tip with a lumen at the end (end-ported) or on the sides *(side-ported)* of the tip. The rubber tips are available in a short conical shape or *cannula* shape. The soft tip is placed below the gingival margin and directed at a 45-degree angle

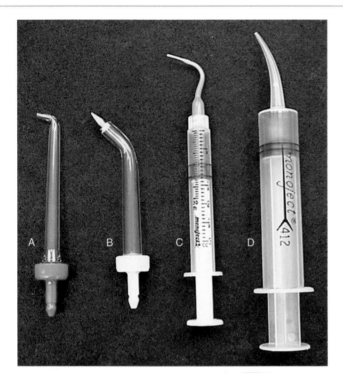

FIG. 24-3 Irrigation tip styles. Supragingival *(A)* and marginal *(B)* tips are designed to attach to a powered irrigator. The two tips on the right are attached to simple syringes. Tip *C* is a marginal irrigator tip. Tip *D* has the most difficult fit because the tip becomes progressively wider. (Courtesy Dr. W.B. Stilley, II, Brandon, Miss.)

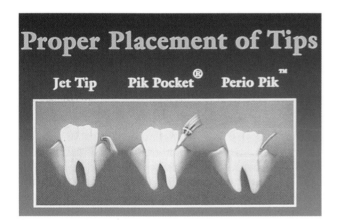

FIG. 24-4 Proper placement of tips. (Courtesy Waterpik Technologies, Fort Collins, Colo.)

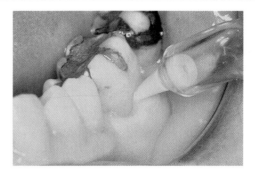

FIG. 24-5 Marginal tip in place. (Courtesy Waterpik Technologies, Fort Collins, Colo.)

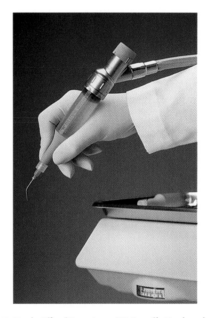

FIG. 24-6 PerioPik. (Courtesy Waterpik Technologies, Fort Collins, Colo.)

apically (Fig. 24-5). The patient should be instructed to use the lowest pressure power setting to avoid possibly tearing inflamed junctional epithelium and diseased pocket lining.

With the exception of patients for whom antibiotic or prophylactic premedication is indicated, supragingival and marginal irrigation is safe and effective for patients to use daily. Manipulation of oral tissues, including tooth brushing, has been shown to produce a transient rise in bacteria in the blood stream. However, it is beneficial to irrigate subgingivally before ultrasonic scaling when a patient has been covered by antibiotic premedication.[19] Guidelines have not been established for daily irrigation for patients who require antibiotic premedication; therefore irrigation is presently recommended only during antibiotic coverage.[31]

Subgingival irrigation is indicated for deep periodontal pockets and is performed by inserting a rigid metal cannula into the pocket and then releasing the irrigant. This is performed by an oral health professional either before scaling, simultaneously with scaling, or directly after scaling (Fig. 24-6). Occasionally, a patient may demonstrate sufficient psychomotor skills to use a rigid cannula for isolated areas requiring daily subgingival irrigation. Research has measured minimal benefit in professional irrigation; maximum therapeutic benefit is obtained with daily irrigation.[34]

Irrigation should be considered when bleeding has not been eliminated through regular (typically every 3 months) professional debridement and when personal care is being performed to the patient's best ability. Patient instruction, professional monitoring, and evaluation of the results are essential when irrigation is recommended to the patient.

ANTIMICROBIALS: GENERAL CONSIDERATIONS AND SPECIFIC AGENTS

QUALITIES OF THE IDEAL ANTIMICROBIAL AGENT

An ideal antimicrobial agent should possess certain qualities. The agent should be effective against specific microbes, inhibit the overgrowth of other organisms, and should not cause an increase in bacterial resistance. The antimicrobial must be nontoxic to oral tissues and acceptable to the patient—for example, in taste, ease of use, and cost. A valuable quality for an antimicrobial is *substantivity,* or the persistence of antimicrobial activity[18], the ability of an agent to remain in an area or site and resist becoming diluted or washed away by gingival crevicular fluid or salivary action. Substantivity is accomplished by adherence to the soft tissues in the oral cavity, which allows the agent to continue its antimicrobial action over a period of hours. Substantivity is assessed by measuring of the changes in duration and numbers of bacteria.[18] Chlorhexidine[7] and tetracycline have excellent substantivity. The usefulness of antimicrobials must be evaluated by site, concentration, and time (Box 24-1).[24] In other words, the agent must be in a form capable of being delivered to the site in an effective concentration and work for a sufficient length of time.

SELECTION

Ideally, the clinician should determine the specific type of periodontal pathogens present and then select the optimal antimicrobial. In actual practice, testing of periodontal pathogens has not been readily utilized by clinicians before the initiation of antimicrobial therapy. One reason is that the antimicrobial recommendations are not yet specific enough for most oral periodontal pathogens. Another is that specific bacteria are implicated for only a few of the various types of periodontal infections, although periodontal research efforts continue to search for putative microbes. Although the in-office tests take only minutes of the clinician's time, the cost to the patient for these tests is significant. However, the ability to identify and target oral pathogens would permit clinicians to choose an antimicrobial with more narrow selectivity. Antimicrobial selectivity enhances microbial effectiveness and reduces antimicrobial resistance, thus improving patient care outcomes.

PATIENT CONSIDERATIONS

The use of an antimicrobial involves several patient considerations:

1. Determine whether any patient sensitivity exists
2. Determine whether the entire dentition should receive antimicrobial therapy or only isolated areas
3. Inform the patient of the following aspects regarding the recommended antimicrobial:
   a. Name of the agent
   b. Method of use
   c. Anticipated benefits
   d. Possible side effects
3. Establish a date for follow-up evaluation of the antimicrobial therapy
4. Evaluate the results of chemotherapeutic use

CONCENTRATION, EFFECT, AND RESISTANCE

Chemotherapeutic agents should be used in the lowest concentration that achieves a benefit. Concentrations that are too low may be ineffective and increase the chance of microbial resistance, whereas excessive concentrations or length of use may have untoward tissue effects and be more costly. Local delivery allows high concentrations with less side effects yet has a seemingly effective kill.

AGENTS

WATER

Researchers caution about the overuse of antibiotics; therefore the introduction of a stream of intermittent (pulsed) water first is the least invasive procedure. Although irrigation does not actually remove plaque, pulsed irrigation with ordinary water has been shown to alter plaque quality and to reduce bleeding and gingival inflammation.[12,13,21] A powered, intermittent stream of water does not remove plaque but evidently reduces the quantity and alters the quality of plaque, rendering it less pathogenic by dilution or removal of the bacterial toxins.[35] The pulsating effect of water on bacteria in animal models has ruptured bacterial cell walls and production of bacterial ghosts, which are intact cell walls with no content, and imploded bacterial cell walls.[9] Research has demonstrated that a 14-day regimen of water irrigation produced therapeutic benefits in the gingiva and was accompanied by a reduction in the inflammatory cytokines in the gingival crevicular fluid.[7] In some cases, daily pulsed irrigation with water is the extra help a patient needs to achieve healthy gingiva.

Caution regarding use of antimicrobials is more often in reference to systemic use, yet the potential for bacterial mutation and adaptation is also present when microorganisms are affected by local administration of antimicrobials.[38] The overgrowth of *Candida* organisms has not been a problem with the more common local antimicrobials. Recommending first the daily use of water in a pulsed irrigator is reasonable. If bleeding has not stopped

---

BOX 24-1

Desirable Characteristics of Oral Chemotherapeutic Agents

Low toxicity
High potency
Good permeability
Intrinsic efficacy
Substantivity

From Goodson JM: Pharmacokinetic principles controlling efficacy of oral therapy, *J Dent Res* 68(Special issue):1625-32, 1989.

and other clinical parameters have not adequately improved, irrigation with an antimicrobial agent should be considered.

CHLORHEXIDINE

Chlorhexidine digluconate (CHX) has been used in mouthrinses and dentifrices over the counter in Canada and Europe for a number of years. In the United States it was first obtainable for oral use as a 0.12% prescription mouthrinse, Peridex (Zila Professional Pharmaceuticals, Antioch, Ill.) and PerioGard (Colgate Oral Pharmaceuticals, Canton, Mass.). Peridex was awarded the ADA Seal of Acceptance in 1988 for the reduction of supragingival plaque and gingivitis. Chlorhexidine gluconate is a *cationic* bisbiguanide and the most widely studied of the oral antimicrobials. Its mechanism of action is the rupture of the bacterial cell membrane and precipitation of the cytoplasmic contents. CHX can reduce the adherence properties of *Porphyromonas gingivalis,* a known periopathogen.[27] CHX binds well to oral tissues and continues to be released in its active form for up to 5 hours.[10] *In vitro* is evidence that 0.12% chlorhexidine is cytotoxic to fibroblasts.[39] Specific protective factors may protect the fibroblasts in the oral tissues. Because its substantivity is superior to that of other known products, CHX is the recommended positive control in oral chemotherapeutic studies.[30]

Although disadvantages exist for CHX use, not every patient manifests all the undesirable side effects. As a rinse, reported side effects of CHX are listed in Box 24-2. The stain and calculus accumulation can be removed professionally; the other side effects disappear when use of the product is discontinued. Stain from a CHX rinse can also be lessened by rinsing concomitantly with an oxidizing agent.[28] The side effects are lessened when CHX is used in an irrigant rather than as a rinse.

Patients should be instructed to rinse with 15 mL for 30 seconds twice a day.[2] For professional irrigation, 0.12% chlorhexidine is generally recommended, with 0.06% for at-home, daily irrigation.[21]

CHX interacts with and is inactivated by sodium lauryl sulfate and other positively charged detergents in dentifrices. Therefore patients should wait a minimum of 30 minutes between using a dentifrice and rinsing with CHX.[7] Also, rinsing with water immediately after rinsing with CHX is to be avoided because a bitter taste results.

Another use of chemotherapeutics has been advanced in the concept of whole mouth disinfection: debridement and antimicrobial therapy of the entire mouth within a 24-hour period.[40] Unlike the familiar quadrant scaling over a series of appointments at 1- or 2-week intervals, this 24-hour approach is designed to reduce the possibility of cross-infection and reinfection in areas that were treated.

To date, chlorhexidine is the only antimicrobial that has been used for full mouth disinfection. Scaling and root planing were accomplished within a 24-hour period and the mouth was disinfected using CHX in professional subgingival irrigation 1%, brushing of tongue 1% CHX gel, and rinsing 0.2% for 2 minutes daily for 2 weeks. A significant improvement was observed microbiologically and clinically after 2 months. Beneficial bacteria were found in periodontal pockets, with significantly fewer spirochetes and motile rods, and probing depths in deep pockets were reduced.[40] Further studies found beneficial clinical outcomes 8 months after a 1-day full-mouth scaling and root planing and disinfection[32] and a reduction in the microbial load.[41] The side effect of most interest was the temporary and slight increase in temperature experienced by some patients a day or two after the therapy. Investigation of the benefits of full-mouth disinfection should receive more attention and research in the future.

ESSENTIAL OILS

Formulations of phenol-related essential oils include thymol and eucalyptol with menthol and methylsalicylate. *Essential oil* rinses have a neutral electrical charge. The mechanism of action of the phenolics is to disrupt the bacterial cell wall and inhibit bacterial enzyme production. The most familiar essential oil mouthrinse is Listerine (Warner-Lambert Company, Morris Plains, N.J.), which was awarded the ADA Seal of Acceptance in 1988 for the control of plaque and gingivitis.

Recommended use is to rinse with 20 ml full strength for 30 seconds.[42] Studies have reported plaque reductions from 20% to 34% and gingivitis reductions from 28% to 34% with twice daily use after tooth brushing.[1] After more than a century of use of essential oils, no evidence exists of the emergence of opportunistic pathogens or resistant strains with the regular use of these rinses. Some individuals experience an initial burning sensation and an unpleasant taste with essential oil mouthrinses. Listerine antiseptic has a 26.9% alcohol content, whereas Listermint has a 21.6% alcohol content.

Concerns over the carcinogenic potential of preparations with a high alcohol content have been expressed. Studies reporting such carcinogenic potential have been fraught with problems—for example, inclusion of pharyngeal cancer, controlling for other use of alcohol, and frequency and length of rinsing.[12] After comment from the National Cancer Institute, the American Dental Association has stated that insufficient evidence exists to link oral cancer and mouthrinses containing alcohol in humans. The few studies available are not consistent in the findings on the relationship between smoking and the use of alcohol-containing mouthrinses.[12]

TETRACYCLINE AND ITS ANALOGS

The benefits of tetracycline (TCN) and its analogs, chemically modified tetracycline molecules (CMTs), are remarkable. Tetracyclines can be used either as bacteriostatic agents to inhibit protein synthesis in the bacterial cells or, at subantimicrobial (lower) concentration, to modulate

---

BOX 24-2

Disadvantages of Chlorhexidine Digluconate (CHX)

Extrinsic brown staining of teeth and tongue
Temporary alteration in taste perception
Increase in supragingival calculus accumulation
Some mucosal desquamation

the host response.[50] Two useful properties of tetracycline are its ability to concentrate in gingival crevicular fluid and its long-established safety record in low systemic doses. The CMTs inhibit the destructive activity of mammalian collagenases and possess a powerful ability to inhibit osteoclastic activity, thus reducing bone loss.[51] Tetracycline should not be administered to pregnant women or young children whose teeth are still calcifying because tetracycline's affinity for mineralizing tissue causes intrinsic staining in teeth.

As an irrigant, tetracycline (250-mg capsule in distilled water 53° C) was reported to achieve clinical healing similar to scaling and root planing with an average attachment gain of 1.3 mm when the irrigant was delivered for 5 minutes per site.[11,48] If the entire mouth is periodontally involved, the use of tetracycline as an antimicrobial irrigant is not practical because of the long application time. However, as an alternative to fiber placement in an isolated site, the authors suggested this time and concentration of TCN irrigant. Uses of tetracycline and its analogs systemically and in controlled delivery are discussed later in the chapter.

SANGUINARINE

Sanguinarine is an alkaloid extract obtained from the bloodroot plant *Sanguinaria canadensis* and is the active ingredient in both a rinse and a dentifrice for the treatment of gingivitis. No benefits were obtained when only one of the products was used, but a decrease in plaque and gingivitis has been shown when both the dentifrice and mouthrinse were used together regularly. The mechanism of action is not well understood. The only reported side effect has been a mild burning sensation when initially used.[12]

STANNOUS FLUORIDE

Studies have shown an adverse bacterial effect[46] and a reduction in plaque and gingivitis for a short period. The antigingivitis action of stannous fluoride is believed to be primarily through the stannous (tin) ion. However, a pilot study involving 70 sites in 10 patients found positive results using a 2.0% neutral gel as part of a supportive periodontal therapy program.[14]

The primary disadvantage is the extrinsic black stain produced when stannous fluoride is used as a mouthrinse. The stain is removable with an oral prophylaxis. In 1999 an untoward reaction of tissue necrosis after deep scaling and root planing and subgingival irrigation of 2% stannous fluoride solution was reported.[47] Until further safety and efficacy studies are conducted, the researchers present two arguments against the use of fluorides in professional irrigation: (1) the epithelial surfaces are not intact after scaling and (2) professional irrigation after quadrant scaling has shown no superior benefit.

NONSTEROIDAL ANTIINFLAMMATORY AGENTS

Indomethacin was the first nonsteroidal antiinflammatory agent (NSAID) used in periodontal animal research that showed a reduction in the amount of gingival inflammation and a decrease in alveolar bone resorption. Further animal studies also have investigated flurbiprofen, ibuprofen, naproxen, and prioxicam.[44] By their action in the arachidonic acid pathway, NSAIDs block the production of prostaglandins, which are proinflammatory mediators, and thereby slow the rate of progression of periodontal diseases. Even though NSAIDs lack substantivity when delivered locally and have side effects when delivered systemically, they still possess a potential role in the mediation of periodontal disease. Their disadvantages are primarily in gastrointestinal disturbances and bleeding, with some effects on the liver and kidneys. More research is necessary to determine the effectiveness of NSAIDs locally in conjunction with antimicrobial agents.

TRICLOSAN

This broad-spectrum antibiotic is a bisphenol and a nonionic germicide with low toxicity. It possesses a strong positive charge and therefore does not bind well to oral sites. The dentifrice Total (Colgate Oral Pharmaceuticals, Inc., Canton, Mass.) contains triclosan and Gantrez, a copolymer of polyvinylmethyl and maleic acid (PVM–MA). It is the first dentifrice sold in the USA to receive the ADA's Seal of Acceptance for the reduction of plaque and gingivitis. In the United States, triclosan for oral benefit is currently available only in a dentifrice.

OXYGEN

Oxygenating agents such as urea peroxide, hydrogen peroxide, gaseous oxygen, and redox agents release oxygen for the resulting deleterious effect on anaerobic pathogens.[45] For periodontal problems, oxygenation is not retained sufficiently long in the pockets and produces untoward side effects. Oxygenating agents alter normal healing, have produced soft tissue lesions, and have been cocarcinogenic in an animal model.[12] The general belief is that overuse of oxygenating rinses, hydrogen peroxide in particular, causes the overgrowth of opportunistic organisms such as Candida species. In most studies, results of the use of oxygenating agents are similar to those of the placebo. However, use of the redox agent methylene blue in a slow-release (controlled-delivery) device showed improvement in clinical and microbial pocket parameters beyond debridement alone.[37]

Rather than releasing oxygen, some oral antimicrobial agents such as Listerine, doxycycline, tetracycline HCL, and sanguinarine have an antioxidant effect in the tissue, thus decreasing gingival inflammation.[20] This is not the same concept as that of oxygenation. Periopathogenic microbes produce oxygen-free radicals (O⁻) that are toxic to the gingival tissues. An antioxidant chemically reacts with these oxygen free radicals, thus reducing the inflammatory tissue response.

POVIDONE–IODINE

Clinicians have generally avoided iodine preparations for their known caustic effect on tissue, staining, and the possibility of a sensitivity reaction to iodine. However, a low concentration of povidone–iodine is effective as a mouthrinse (in combination with hydrogen peroxide), a subgingival irrigant, and as a preprocedural rinse.[26]

QUATERNARY AMMONIUM COMPOUNDS

The most common quaternary ammonium compound is cetylpyridinium chloride 0.05%. This cationic compound binds to oral tissues but less strongly than CHX. Its mechanism of action is to rupture cell walls and alter cytoplasmic contents. Reported side effects are some staining, increased calculus formation, and an occasional burning sensation and epithelial desquamation.[12] Cepacol (Merrell Dow Pharmaceuticals, Inc., Kansas City, Mo.) and Scope (Procter & Gamble, Cincinnati, Ohio) are familiar brands.

BAKING SODA

Keyes repopularized baking soda as an oral product in the 1970s when he used it as part of his recommended regimen of oral care. Research has so far not indicated any improvement in gingival/periodontal health through the use of baking soda with what is called the Keyes' Technique.[3] However, baking soda is a common household product and popular with consumers and is now an ingredient in several dentifrices for its tooth whitening effect.

PREBRUSHING RINSE *No benefit*

Plax (Pfizer, New York, NY) is a detergent–sodium benzoate mixture sold as a prebrushing rinse. Although a reduction in plaque has been shown in short-term studies, no long-term studies have been conducted. Generally, no benefit accrues because results from using the prebrushing rinse appear to be similar to placebo use.[33]

Local antimicrobials are an evidence-based option in periodontal care. Research efforts continue in the arena of antimicrobials in patient care, with the result that formulary changes, newer antimicrobials, new uses of familiar antimicrobials, and recommendations about how chemotherapeutics should be utilized are changing and growing. Thus the dental hygienist must continue learning in the dynamic area of chemotherapeutics.

CONTROLLED DRUG-DELIVERY SYSTEMS

Before considering site-specific therapy, clinicians should evaluate the efficacy of initial therapy. The effect of mechanical interventions should be given time to produce a positive change in the health of the periodontium. These interventions include the proven effectiveness of professional debridement and improved daily personal oral hygiene care. If this change is not sufficient to stabilize the periodontal conditions and the condition is not generalized, then a *controlled-delivery device* should be considered for localized problem sites. Currently, Actisite, Perio-Chip, Atridox, and Arestin are the three controlled-delivery systems available in the United States.

ADVANTAGES

A controlled-delivery system has several advantages. First, the patient does not have to remember to "take the medicine" because the dose and timing are part of the delivery system. Second, dosage concentration can be much greater, permitting a greater microbial kill rate and less

opportunity for microbial resistance to develop. Third, side effects are often reduced because the agent is delivered to a particular site and not distributed throughout the mouth. Finally, the systemic effect on the body is also lessened because the agent is delivered locally rather than systemically.

CAUTIONS

Controlled delivery is not recommended for the entire *Not* mouth because, by definition, it targets specific areas of the mouth. Also, controlled-release delivery is not recommended for pockets 5 mm or less. Because clinical trials have not included children under 18, pregnant women, and medically compromised individuals, controlled-delivery therapy is not recommended for these cohorts. Finally, individuals may respond differently to controlled-delivery systems, ranging from a worsened condition (infrequent) to gradual improvement. No single therapy is guaranteed, and all therapy should be monitored.

ACTISITE

The first controlled-delivery system available in the United States was a nonresorbable fiber impregnated with 12.7 mg tetracycline hydrochloride. Actisite (Johnson & Johnson, Greenwich, Conn.) is a 23-cm (9-inch) monofilament of ethylene acetate copolymer, 0.5 mm in diameter. Research has shown continuous release of the bacteriostatic agent into the periodontal pocket resulted in a mean gingival fluid concentration of 1590 µg/mL. Tetracycline is released for 10 days in the pocket, at which time the fiber should be removed by an oral healthcare professional. Reported side effects during clinical trials included discomfort during placement (10%) and local erythema at removal (11%).[36]

PERIOCHIP

In 1998 the first subgingival sustained-release delivery system containing chlorhexidine became available to U.S. practitioners. PerioChip (Astra USA, Inc., Westborough, Mass.) is literally a small, pale orange chip, 4 mm × 5 mm × 350 µm, weighing 7.4 mg. The prescription chip contains 2.5 mg of chlorhexidine gluconate, a broad-spectrum antimicrobial, in a biodegradable matrix of hydrolyzed gelatin cross-linked with glutaraldehyde, glycerin, and water. Gingival crevicular fluid concentration appears to be biphasic and varies among patients, peaking at 4 hours (more than 1000 µg/mL) after insertion of the chip into the pocket, and then again at 72 hours (more than 480 µg/mL). Release of CHX lasts from 7 to 10 days. In patients with 5- to 8-mm pockets, depth reductions of 2 mm or more over scaling and root planing alone were reported in a 9-month period.[29]

Insertion of the chip with forceps is simple, quick, and comfortable. Bacterial resistance to chlorhexidine in studies up to 2 years has not been observed.[10] Also the customary side effects of chlorhexidine are not evident, most likely because chlorhexidine is released below the gingival margin.[6]

ATRIGEL

The delivery system Atrigel (Atrix Laboratories, Inc., Ft. Collins, Colo.) contains Atridox (Block Drug Corporation,

Jersey City, N.J.), a 10.0% concentration of doxycycline hyclate for controlled delivery subgingivally in the treatment of chronic adult periodontitis. Marketed in the United States since 1998, Atridox is available by prescription and carries the ADA Seal of Acceptance. The polylactic acid gel and drug are mixed at chairside and delivered to the bottom of the pocket via a small cannula. The gel then solidifies, releasing doxycycline for a period of seven days. Clinical trials have resulted in an increase in clinical attachment averaging 0.8 mm and a reduction of probe depths averaging 1.3 mm in a 9-month study.[22] Headache, common cold, and some toothache and gingival discomfort were the most common side effects. Interestingly, the difference in improvement between two groups, smokers and nonsmokers, was not evident when Atridox was used.[43]

ARESTIN

Minocycline HCl is available in a controlled-delivery system with the brand name of Arestin (OraPharma, Inc., Warminster, Pa.). This TCN derivative is incorporated in a bioresorbable polymer in the form of a powder of bioadhesive microspheres and marketed in 1-mg unit-dose cartridges with accompanying delivery syringes. In clinical trials conducted by OraPharma in 2001, retreatment occurred at 3 and 6 months; at 9 months the greatest pocket depth reductions occurred with scaling and root planing (SCRP) and Arestin, rather than SCRP alone or SCRP with a vehicle. Patients are cautioned not to eat hard or sticky foods for 1 week after placement of the microspheres.

SYSTEMIC DELIVERY

With the systemic delivery of antimicrobials, the drug affects the entire body rather than just the local area of interest (Box 24-3). The advantage of a systemic antibiotic, assuming patient compliance in taking the oral medication, is that the drug reaches bacteria in deep periodontal pockets, gingival tissue, and other oral sites and leaves no reservoir or niche of microbes. The disadvantages of systemic delivery are the adverse side effects, such as gastrointestinal imbalance, nausea, diarrhea, and rash; the risk of producing antimicrobially resistant microbes; and

---

BOX 24-3

Potential Concerns with Systemic Antimicrobials

Interference with the body's normal microbial flora
Side effects
Drug pharmacokinetics (absorption, distribution, metabolism, and excretion)
Drug pharmacodynamics (how the drug affects the body)
Potential for development of microbial resistance
Drug interactions
Concerns with special populations (pregnant women, children, elderly, ethnicity, gender, general health status)
Likelihood of increasing drug sensitivity
Adherence/compliance to daily medication regimen

---

patients not taking the pills as prescribed.[50] Another concern is that systemic antibiotics to treat periodontal infections are not sufficiently narrow. Ideally, the putative organism should be identified so that the appropriate antibiotic can be selected. Because the causative organism(s) and the destructive processes in periodontal diseases are not yet fully understood, it is difficult to select an antibiotic with a sufficiently narrow spectrum.

Mechanical debridement should be completed and its effects judged before the selection of a systemic antimicrobial is considered. Systemic antibiotics may be prescribed as a single drug, used in combination with another drug, or used sequentially. They are either bacteriocidal or bacteriostatic.[50] The most familiar systemic agents in the treatment of periodontal diseases are tetracycline, metronidazole, clindamycin, ciprofloxacin, and the penicillins.

The general recommendation is that systemic antimicrobials are inappropriate in the treatment of chronic adult periodontitis but may be used in the treatment of acute problems or refractory conditions. However, tetracycline specifically affects *Actinobacillus actinomycetemcomitans* (Aa) and is recommended for use in the treatment of localized juvenile periodontitis (LJP).

In 1999 results with azithromycin administered systemically appeared positive. After a regimen of 500 mg per day for 3 days, significantly higher concentrations of the drug were found in oral pathological tissue than in healthy gingiva. High concentrations were evident in healthy gingiva, saliva, and diseased periodontal tissue for up to 6½ days after administration of the last dose.[8]

Systemically, metronidazole is effective against obligate anaerobic organisms, spirochetes, and bacteroides and reduces the amount of gingival crevicular fluid. Because periodontal infections often include a mixed microflora, metronidazole is usually prescribed with another antibiotic.[25]

With the appearance of microbes resistant to antibiotics, concern has been expressed regarding what some consider excessive prescribing and the public's inappropriate demand and use of antibiotics. Serendipitously, a newer approach to systemic drug use in the treatment of periodontal disease is to effect a change in the host response to the infection. Theorists have shown that some low doses of antibiotics alter the host response to the effects of a bacterial infection without affecting the bacteria themselves, thus possibly reducing or avoiding the development of antimicrobial resistance.

Research conducted on diabetic rats first identified the anticollagenase property of tetracycline (TCN) in the gingival crevicular fluid (GCF).[23] The TCN derivatives doxycycline and minocycline have greater anticollagenase effects than TCN. Based on this research, Periostat (CollaGenex Pharmaceuticals, Inc., Newton, Penn.) became available in 1998 as the first oral product to effect change at the subantimicrobial level. The low drug level of doxycycline hyclate in Periostat is insufficient to treat an infection or to affect pathogens. Its subantimicrobial action is designed instead to suppress enzymes, specifically to reduce the increased collagenase found in gingival crevicular fluid.

The recommended dose of Periostat is one 20-mg capsule taken twice daily, 1 hour before mealtime. In this subantimicrobial concentration, Periostat has been shown to reduce pocket depth and promote attachment level gain beyond scaling and root planing alone in patients with chronic adult periodontitis.[16] The customary precautions with the use of systemic tetracycline resulting from its affinity for mineralizing dentition and patient sensitivity should be followed when Periostat is being considered.

QUALITY ASSURANCE

Evaluation of the effect of the antimicrobial is essential. It begins with the Food and Drug Administration (FDA) and the manufacturers, then may voluntarily move to the ADA Council on Scientific Affairs' Seal of Acceptance program, and is ultimately the purview of the clinician and the patient. (Refer to Chapter 20 for further discussion on the roles of the FDA and the ADA seal program.) Until 2000 only consumer products that claimed a therapeutic benefit were eligible for approval through the ADA Seal program.

EVALUATION OF SUCCESS

Evaluation of the efficacy and the effects of irrigation and use of chemotherapeutics is ultimately the responsibility of the clinician. Patients should be placed on a chemotherapeutic agent for a finite period of time and then return to the office for an evaluation. Several clinical signs currently considered indicative of periodontal health include (1) absence of signs of inflammation—erythema, edema, exudate, and bleeding; (2) maintenance of a functional periodontal attachment over time; and (3) immobile dental implants[4] (Box 24-4). If these effects are not demonstrated when the use of irrigation and antimicrobials has been added to the patient's regimen, the clinician should consider a number of possibilities, including the following:

- Was the agent used?
- Was the agent used as directed?
- Did pus, blood, calculus, or debris inactivate or block the action of the antimicrobial?
- Would a different chemotherapeutic agent be more effective?

If these questions do not provide some insight, the clinician must reinvestigate the oral circumstances and probe further into the patient's general health and well-being. Adverse personal circumstances such as increases in patient stress, a change in health status not reported by the patient, or an undiagnosed medical condition may contribute to the regression of the oral status. Although people are keeping their teeth longer—even seriously involved periodontal teeth—not every case always results in complete absence of bleeding and absence of attachment loss. Remembering the goal of regrowing or restoring alveolar bone, currently the most significant parameter of success, is a gain in clinical attachment.

 Case Application

What areas of concern do you have for Ms. Tevus' oral health? What treatment options could you offer her? Use a decision-tree diagram to illustrate your choices. (A decision tree is a pathway or diagram of lines indicating, at each problem point, the available choices or paths.) Some considerations to guide your thoughts may include the following:

- Is the level of plaque control Ms. Tevus is attaining adequate?
- Explain to Ms. Tevus (role-play) the type of therapy you would recommend.
- Which chemotherapeutic agent would you recommend for the treatment of tooth #10?

If irrigation does not stabilize the attachment loss and bleeding on tooth #10 after she has been irrigating for 3 months, what options would you suggest for that tooth? What are the advantages and disadvantages in not discussing a controlled-delivery approach to tooth #10 during the initial broaching of irrigation?

BOX 24-4

Measurable Outcomes in Periodontal Therapy

Probing depths
Clinical attachment levels
Visual signs of inflammation
Bleeding on probing
Alveolar bone height and density
Changes in subgingival microflora
Flow and composition of gingival crevicular fluid

From: Consensus reports from the 1996 World Workshop in Periodontics, *J Am Dent Assoc* 129(Suppl):1S-64, 1998.

RITICAL THINKING ACTIVITIES

1. Watch instructional videotapes on the manipulation of various chemotherapeutic delivery systems. Using a typodont, practice the insertion and removal (if nonresorbable) techniques with fibers (for example, dental floss), gels, irrigation, chips, and powders.
2. Select the appropriate irrigation tip and use an oral irrigator in your own mouth.
3. Obtain the drug insert sheet on different oral antimicrobial agents. These are frequently available on the Internet. Compare the recommendations for use, the advantages and disadvantages, and reported precautions.
4. Develop a brochure for the patient to take home on each of the controlled-delivery systems. Such information may be obtained directly from the manufacturer, the company's web site, or the package insert.
5. With the aid of a microbiologist, culture saliva or plaque. Investigate the effects of various antimicrobials. (Saliva is easier to culture than plaque.)

Continued

CRITICAL THINKING ACTIVITIES—cont'd

6. Track the efficacy of each intervention used in #5.
7. Select a patient with periodontal probe depths of less than 4 mm. Take preirrigation and postirrigation samples to examine under the microscope. Keep preirrigation and postirrigation bleeding indices over a period of time. Do the same for each controlled-delivery system used.
8. Role-play with a student partner the roles of Ms. Tevus (from the case study presented at the begin-

ning of this chapter) and the dental hygienist. Explain the role a chemotherapeutic agent could play in Ms. Tevus' oral health.
9. Use the AAP web sites to access position papers pertaining to pharmacotherapeutics in periodontal diseases.
10. Select one irrigation tip or one chemotherapeutic agent to research in-depth and report to your class.

REVIEW QUESTIONS

The following review questions refer to the case study presented at the beginning of the chapter.

1. For the profile that does not indicate an increase in generalized bleeding, which of the following approaches would you select for Ms. Tevus at this appointment?
   a. Appoint her for care every 2 months instead of at 3-month intervals
   b. Take a sample to culture for suspected periodontopathogens
   c. Place her on a pulsed-water irrigator
   d. Refer her to the periodontist
2. Which of the following types of infection do you suspect that Ms. Tevus has?
   a. Necrotizing ulcerative gingivitis (NUG)
   b. Plaque-associated periodontitis
   c. Linear gingival erythema
   d. Hormonal gingivitis
3. Which of the following conditions seems to be Ms. Tevus' most obvious problem?
   a. Inadequate plaque control
   b. Noncompliance
   c. An immunocompromised system
   d. Stress
4. Of the following categories of irrigation, which one would you teach Ms. Tevus?
   a. Supragingival
   b. Marginal
   c. Subgingival
5. At this appointment, which of the following irrigants would you recommend for Ms. Tevus?
   a. CHX
   b. TCN

   c. Essential oils
   d. Water
6. If water irrigation reduces but does not control Ms. Tevus' bleeding, which of the following options would be your next choice?
   a. Irrigate with CHX
   b. Irrigate with stannous fluoride
   c. Use the chlorhexidine chip
   d. Use TCN impregnated fibers
7. Which of the following treatment options would you consider for tooth #10?
   1. Debride
   2. Wait to see what changes irrigation might produce
   3. Use site-specific therapy such as Arestin, Atridox, or the PerioChip
   4. Refer to a periodontist
   a. All the above
   b. 3
   c. 2, 3, and 4
   d. 4
8. Assume that Ms. Tevus required debridement due to residual calculus on #10. After debridement, a subgingival irrigant is use. Which of the following agents would the hygienist least likely select?
   a. TCN
   b. CHX
   c. Stannous fluoride
   d. Water

 SUGGESTED AGENCIES AND WEB SITES

Because of the ever-changing nature of the Internet, some of the web sites listed here may have changed since publication. Please refer to Mosby's Evolve web site for the most current information.

American Academy of Periodontology (position papers of AAP): http://www.perio.org

Blue Cross and Blue Shield of Massachusetts (chlorhexidine mouthrinses, information for patients): http://www.ahealthyme.com

CollaGenex Pharmaceuticals, Inc. (information about Periostat): http://www.collagenex.com

Dental Products.net (extensive list of manufacturers, with searching capabilities for product information): http://www.dentalproducts.net

SUGGESTED AGENCIES AND WEB SITES—cont'd

GlaxoSmithKline (information about Atridox): http://www.block drug.com.

OraPharma Inc. ("Arestin"): http://www.arestin.com.

Pfizer/Warner-Lambert Consumer Group—Listerine (for information about Listerine and other Pfizer/Warner-Lambert products): http://www.listerine.com.

 ADDITIONAL READINGS AND RESOURCES

Greenstein G, Rethman M: The role of tetracycline—impregnated fibers in retreatment, *Perio 2000* 12:33-9, 1996.

Jones CG: Chlorhexidine: is it the gold standard? *Perio 2000* 15:55-62, 1997.

Killoy WJ, Polso AM: Controlled local delivery of antimicrobials in the treatment of periodontitis, *Dent Clin N Amer* 42(2):263-83, 1998.

Rams TE, Slots J: Local delivery of antimicrobial agents in the periodontal pocket, *Perio 2000* 10:139-59, 1996.

 REFERENCES

1. American Dental Association, Council on Dental Therapeutics: Council on dental therapeutics accepts Listerine, *J Am Dent Assoc* 117:515-6, 1988.
2. American Dental Association, Council on Dental Therapeutics: Council on dental therapeutics accepts Peridex, *J Am Dent Assoc* 117:516-7, 1988.
3. American Academy of Periodontology: Current understanding of the role of microscopic monitoring, baking soda and hydrogen peroxide in the treatment of periodontal disease, *J Periodontol* 69:951-4, 1998.
4. American Academy of Periodontology: Guidelines for periodontal therapy, *J Periodontol* 69:405-8, 1998.
5. American Academy of Periodontology: The role of controlled drug delivery for periodontitis, *J Periodontol* 71:125-40, 2000.
6. *Astra monograph and full prescribing information* [brochure], Wilmington, Del, 1998, AstraZenica Pharmaceuticals.
7. Barkvoll P, Rølla G, Svendsen AK: Chlorhexidine interactions with sodium lauryl sulfate in vivo, *J Dent Res* (Special issue):1722-3, 1989.
8. Blandizzi C et al: Periodontal tissue disposition of azithromycin in patients affected by chronic inflammatory periodontal diseases, *J Periodontol* 70:960-6, 1999.
9. Brady JR, Gray WA, Bhaskar SN: Electron microscopic study of the effect of water jet lavage device on dental plaque, *J Dent Res* 52:1310-5, 1973.
10. Briner WW, Kayrouz GA, Chanak MX: Comparative antimicrobial effectiveness of a substantive (0.12% chlorhexidine) and a nonsubstantive (phenolic) mouthrinse in vivo and in vitro, *Compend Contin Educ Dent* 15:1158-68, 1994.
11. Christersson LA, Morderyd OM, Puchalsky CS: Topical application of tetracycline-HCL in human periodontitis, *J Clin Periodontol* 20:88-95, 1993.
12. Ciancio SG: Chemical agents: plaque control, calculus reduction and treatment of dentinal hypersensitivity, *Perio 2000* 8:75-86, 1995.
13. Ciancio SG et al: Effect of a chemotherapeutic agent delivered by an oral irrigating device on plaque, gingivitis, and subgingival microflora, *J Periodontol* 60:310-5, 1989.
14. Cleveland S, McLey L, Jones J: Irrigation of nonresponding periodontal pockets with neutral fluoride gel: a pilot study, *Prac Hyg* 6(2):21-5, 1997.
15. Cobb CM, Rogers RI, Killoy WJ: Ultrastructural examination of human periodontal pockets following the use of an oral irrigation device *in vivo*, *J Periodontol* 59:155-9, 1988.

16. Package insert, Newtown, Pa, CollaGenex Pharmaceuticals.
17. Cutler CW et al: Clinical benefits of oral irrigation for periodontitis are related to reduction of pro-inflammatory cytokine levels and plaque, *J Clin Periodontol* 27:134-43, 2000.
18. Elworthy A et al: The substantivity of a number of oral hygiene products determined by the duration of effects on salivary bacteria, *J Periodontol* 76:572-6, 1996.
19. Fine DH, Korik I, Furgang D, et al: Assessing pre-procedural subgingival irrigation and rinsing with an antiseptic mouthrinse to reduce bacteremia, *J Am Dent Assoc* 127:641-6, 1996.
20. Firatli E et al: Antioxidative activities of some chemotherapeutics. A possible mechanism in reducing gingival inflammation, *J Clin Periodontol* 21:680-3, 1994.
21. Flemmig TF et al: Supragingival irrigation with 0.06% chlorhexidine in naturally occurring gingivitis. I. 6 month clinical observations, *J Periodontol* 61:112-7, 1990.
22. Garrett S et al: Two multi-center studies evaluating locally delivered doxycycline hyclate, placebo control, oral hygiene, and scaling and root planing in the treatment of periodontitis, *J Periodontol* 70:490-503, 1999.
23. Golub LM et al: Tetracyclines inhibit tissue collagenase activity. A new mechanism in the treatment of periodontal disease, *J Perio Res* 19(6):651-5, 1984.
24. Goodson JM: Pharmacokinetic principles controlling efficacy of oral therapy, *J Dent Res* 68(Special issue):1625-32, 1989.
25. Greenstein G: The role of metronidazole in the treatment of periodontal diseases, *J Periodontol* 64:1-15, 1993.
26. Greenstein G: Povidone-iodine's effects and role in the management of periodontal diseases: a review, *J Periodontol* 70:1397-1405, 1999.
27. Grenier D: Effect of chlorhexidine on the adherence properties of *Porphyromonas gingivalis*, *J Clin Periodontol* 23:140-2, 1996.
28. Gründemann LJMM et al: Stain, plaque and gingivitis reduction by combining chlorhexidine and peroxyborate, *J Clin Periodontol* 27:9-15, 2000.
29. Jeffcoat MK et al: Adjunctive use of a subgingival controlled-release chlorhexidine chip reduces probing depth and improves attachment level compared with scaling and root planing alone, *J Periodontol* 69:989-97, 1998.
30. Lang NP, Brecx MC: Chlorhexidine digluconate, an agent for chemical plaque control and prevention of gingival inflammation, *J Periodontal Res* 21:74-89, 1986.

Continued

31. Lockhart PB: The risk for endocarditis in dental practice, *Perio 2000* 23:127-135, 2000.

32. Mongardini C et al: One stage full- versus partial-mouth disinfection in the treatment of chronic adult or generalized early-onset periodontitis, I. Long-term clinical observations, *J Periodontol* 70:632-45, 1999.

33. Moran J, Addy M: The effects of a cetylpyridinium chloride prebrushing rinse as an adjunct to oral hygiene and gingival health, *J Periodontol* 62:562-4, 1991.

34. Newman HN: Periodontal pocket irrigation as adjunctive treatment, *Curr Opin Periodontol* 4:41-50, 1997.

35. Newman MG et al: Effectiveness of adjunctive irrigation in early periodontitis: multi-center evaluation, *J Periodontol* 65:224-9, 1994.

36. Newman M, Kornman K, Doherty F: A 6-month multi-center evaluation of adjunctive tetracycline fiber therapy used in conjunction with scaling and root planing in maintenance patients: clinical results, *J Periodontol* 65:685-91, 1994.

37. Ower PC et al: The effects on chronic periodontitis of a subgingivally-placed redox agent in a slow release device, *J Clin Periodontol* 22:494-500, 1995.

38. Pallasch TJ: Antimicrobials and periodontal disease: *quo vadis?, Intl J Perio Rest Dentistry* 18(3):212-3, 1998.

39. Pucher JJ, Daniel JC: The effects of chlorhexidine digluconate on human fibroblasts in vitro, *J Periodontol* 62:526-32, 1993.

40. Quirynen M et al: Full- versus partial-mouth disinfection in the treatment of periodontal infections: short-term clinical and microbiological observations, *J Dent Res* 74:1459-67, 1995.

41. Quirynen M et al: One stage full- versus partial-mouth disinfection in the treatment of chronic adult or generalized early-onset periodontitis. II. Long-term impact on microbial load, *J Periodontol* 70:646-56, 1999.

42. Ross NM et al: Effect of rinsing time on antiplaque-antigingivitis efficacy of Listerine, *J Clin Periodontol* 20:279-81, 1993.

43. Ryder M et al: Effects of smoking on local delivery of controlled-release doxycycline as compared to scaling and root planning, *J Clin Periodontol* 26:683-91, 1999.

44. Salvi GE, Williams RC, Offenbacher S: Nonsteroidal anti-inflammatory drugs as adjuncts in the management of periodontal diseases and peri-implantitis, *Curr Opinion Periodontol* 4:51-8, 1997.

45. Schlagenhauf U et al: Repeated subgingival oxygen irrigations in untreated periodontal patients, *J Clin Periodontol* 21:48-50, 1994.

46. Schmid E, Kornman KS, Tinanoff N: Changes of subgingival total colony-forming units and black pigmented bacteroides after a single irrigation of periodontal pockets with 1.64% SnF$_2$, *J Periodontol* 56:330-3, 1985.

47. Sjöström S, Kalfas S: Tissue necrosis after subgingival irrigation with fluoride solution, *J Clin Periodontol* 26:257-60, 1999.

48. Stabholz A et al: Clinical and antimicrobial effects of a single episode of subgingival irrigation with tetracycline HCL or chlorhexidine in deep periodontal pockets, *J Clin Periodontol* 25:794-800, 1998.

49. Stelzel M, Florès-de-Jacoby L: Topical metronidazole application compared with subgingival scaling, *J Clin Peridontol* 23: 24-9, 1996.

50. Van Winkelhoff AJ, Rams TE, Slots J: Systemic antibiotic therapy in periodontics, *Perio 2000* 10:45-78, 1996.

51. Vernillo AT et al: The nonantimicrobial properties of tetracycline for the treatment of periodontal disease, *Curr Opinion Periodontol* 2:111-8, 1994.

CHAPTER 25

Dentinal Sensitivity

Shannon Mitchell

Chapter Outline

Etiology
Case Study: Treatment of Dentinal Sensitivity to
    Cold Stimuli
Stimuli that Elicit Pain Response
    Hydrodynamic theory
    Types of pain stimuli
Natural Defense Mechanisms

Treatment of Sensitivity
    Criteria for sensitivity agents
    Factors influencing studies of dentinal
      sensitivity agents
    Personal oral hygiene
    Commercially available products
    Professional products

Key Terms

Burnishing
Dentinal sensitivity
Desensitizing

Hydrodynamic theory
Odontoblast
Pain stimulus

Potassium nitrate
Smear layer
Sodium citrate

Strontium chloride
Tubules

Learning Outcomes

1. Understand the hydrodynamic theory of pain conduction.
2. Describe the three general categories of stimuli that elicit pain response and give examples of each.
3. Discuss the role of plaque in the prognosis of dentinal sensitivity treatment.
4. Describe desensitizing agents and products available for home care use.

5. Select office procedures for the treatment of sensitivity based on patient needs and evaluate their response to agents.
6. Evaluate a patient's plaque removal and dietary habits to make recommendations for the reduction of dentinal sensitivity.
7. Evaluate literature on desensitizing agents.

*I*t has been reported that approximately 40 million adults in the United States have *dentinal sensitivity* (20% to 30% of adults) at some time in their lives, and more than 10 million have chronic dentinal sensitivity.[39] Dentinal sensitivity is most common among patients aged 20 to 40 years, peaking during the third decade.[26,32] The condition has been reported to occur slightly more often in females than males; however, this finding has not been statistically significant.[6,8,36]

ETIOLOGY

Dentinal sensitivity is an adverse reaction or pain resulting from a thermal, chemical, or mechanical stimulus in one or more teeth.[5,19] Microscopic examination of clinically sensitive surfaces has shown that some areas of dentin are exposed by gingival recession, abrasion, erosion, periodontal therapy, defective restorations, or caries (Fig. 25-1). The *tubules* in these areas are also shown microscopically to be wider and more numerous than in nonsensitive areas.[1,2,62] Dentinal sensitivity is found almost exclusively on the facial surfaces of teeth at the cervical margins.[32] The relative frequency of sensitivity of different teeth has been reported as follows: premolars (38%), incisors (26%), canines (24%), and molars (12%).[47] The etiology of dentinal sensitivity is multifactorial. Stimuli that may elicit a pain response have been categorized as tactile, thermal, chemical, or osmotic.[9] Dental procedures

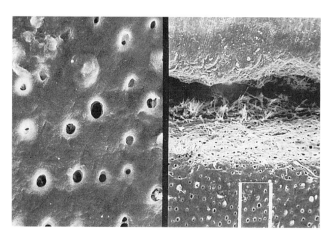

FIG. 25-1 Sensitive dentin under high magnification. Note the open tubules. (From Addy M: Etiology of clinical implications of dentine hypersensitivity, *Dent Clin North Am* 34[3]:510, 1990.)

 Case Study

Treatment of Dentinal Sensitivity to Cold Stimuli

You have just seated your 10 AM appointment, a 6-month supportive care patient, Suki Yamagashi, a 28-year-old Asian female who appears to be in good physical health. Her health history reveals she is single, an attorney at one of the town's law firms, and she has no contraindications to dental treatment. Upon your clinical examination all extraoral conditions are within normal limits. All intraoral findings are also within normal limits, except for two areas of localized 3-mm recession on the facial surfaces of teeth #6 and #12. When you gently probe these areas, Ms. Yamagashi is in noticeable pain and asks you to stop. On questioning about these areas, she tells you that they have been sensitive to cold for several years; however, in the past few months she has noticed that she feels pain in these areas even if something is slightly cold. Ms. Yamagashi has stopped eating ice cream and does not even try to have ice in her drinks.

can contribute to or initiate the onset or progression of sensitivity.

 ## STIMULI THAT ELICIT PAIN RESPONSE

25-A ### *HYDRODYNAMIC THEORY*

Historically, several theories have tried to explain the mechanism of transmission of pain from the dentin to the pulp. As early as the mid-nineteenth century, the work of Dr. Neill of Philadelphia was reviewed and published by Blandy (1850-1851). Dr. Neill originally postulated the following:[12]

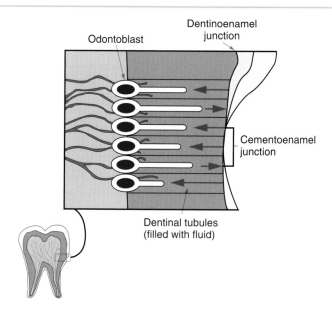

FIG. 25-2 Hydrodynamic theory of dentinal sensation, as described by Brannström.

> *... dentin consists of hollow tubules, filled with fluid secreted by the pulp, and pressure applied without, by compressing the enamel and the fluid of the tubules, affected the nervous pulp within, by subjecting the latter to a species of hydrostatic pressure, the amount of which can be measured. Whatever reduces the thickness of the enamel or uncovers any portion of the dentin, increases the painful impression caused by external pressure.*

Approximately 100 years later, Kramer proposed the "hydrodynamic" theory. This theory was later expanded by Alfred Gysi; however, it was not until the late 1950s with the work of Martin Brannström that the theory was accepted by the dental profession. Dr. Brannström conducted a series of experiments asking the following questions:
- How could an area of tooth that has no obvious signs of decay sometimes be so sensitive to the slightest stimulus?
- Why would exposure to a mere blast of air elicit pain?
- Why would exposure to sugar or salty foods cause pain when many chemical agents known to stimulate nerve fibers do not produce a response when applied to exposed dentin?

The **hydrodynamic theory** is based on the observation that fluid within the dentinal tubules can flow in either an outward or an inward direction depending on the pressure variations in the surrounding tissues (Fig. 25-2). The rapid movement of fluid in the open dentinal tubules may subsequently deform the **odontoblast** or its process and therefore elicit the transmission of a pain-causing stimulus.[16] This theory of hydrodynamics helps explain the reason why so many different stimuli can elicit the same pain response.

TYPES OF PAIN STIMULI

Mechanical

The clearest example of the hydrodynamic theory and a mechanical stimulus is exhibited in the dehydration of dentin (i.e., by air blast). The air causes dehydration, which causes the dentinal fluid to move in an outward direction by capillary action. This would, in turn, pull the odontoblastic process farther into the tubule, stimulating sensory pulpal nerves.[16] A direct mechanical stimulation may occur during dental instrumentation (e.g., during exploratory procedures or scaling). Mechanical trauma may result from brushing, especially when toothbrushes with firm bristles are combined with an overzealous brushing technique. Incorrect brushing may cause gingival recession and root surface abrasion, which may account for the high incidence of dentinal sensitivity on facial surfaces, particularly in teeth at the corners of the arch, a region susceptible to toothbrush trauma.[47]

 Case Application

Ms. Yamagashi reports symptoms similar to those described previously. Therefore the dental hygienist should evaluate her tooth-brushing technique.

Patients who chronically clench and grind their teeth often complain of tooth sensitivity. Enamel loss through occlusal wear caused by bruxing can expose dentinal tubules and cause pain.[52]

Thermal

The second type of stimulus that elicits dentinal sensitivity is thermal. Pain accompanying exposure to cold air or beverages is the most frequently reported patient complaint. Responses may occur when hot and cold foods or liquids are consumed or when cold air reaches the exposed dentinal areas. For example, heat applied to the dentin results in an expansion of the fluid, putting pressure on the odontoblast, which again stimulates a pain response.[16] In the case presented at the beginning of this chapter, the patient complains when she eats something cold; therefore the hygienist can explain to her that the *pain stimulus* is thermal in nature.

Chemical or Osmotic

Chemical stimuli also may cause pain, especially with sweet, sour, or highly acidic foods. Tubular fluid movements also may explain pain produced when sugar or salted solutions are placed in contact with exposed dentin. Fluids of a low osmolarity (i.e., the dentinal tubule fluid) have a tendency to flow toward solutions of a higher osmolarity (i.e., salty or sugar solutions).[11] This outward flow of fluid elicits a pain response. Some highly acidic foods (e.g., lemons) may chemically dissolve the enamel, exposing underlying dentin. Sensitivity also has been reported in cases of bulimic individuals because of the repeated exposure of the enamel to highly acidic gastric juices.[45] Chemically induced pain also has been attributed to production of lactic acid by bacteria present in plaque. Conversely, others have found less tooth sensitivity to be associated with the presence of plaque. Addy and colleagues[6] reported greater sensitivity in an area of the mouth with the least plaque. In this study, the subjects who were right-handed had less plaque but greater sensitivity on the left side than the right side. This negative association may be due to the patient's vigorous brushing at the cervical margin, which resulted in less plaque but greater abrasion of

the exposed dentin. Evaluation of the patient's diet would be appropriate by performing a diet analysis as described in Chapter 18.

Periodontal Procedures

Certain periodontal procedures result in a pain response from mechanical and thermal stimuli. Periodontal therapy may create or increase the exposure of root surfaces, and it is recommended that concepts of dentinal sensitivity be explained to the patient when such procedures as supragingival and subgingival debridement have been planned. The root surface is covered with cementum, which is softer than calculus and often is removed by hand or ultrasonic instruments, exposing the dentinal surface. Anatomically, those teeth in which the cementum and enamel may not meet at the CEJ (5% to 10%) may be predisposed to developing dentinal sensitivity in the presence of gingival recession.[8]

Although root instrumentation has been reported to increase root sensitivity,[6,25] one study reported that root instrumentation produced partially occluded dentinal tubules and a *smear layer* comprising microcrystals of cementum and dentin. Therefore this partial occlusion may decrease the conduction of a painful stimulus through the dentinal tubule.[2] More often, however, a painful stimulus results from the exposure of root surfaces after periodontal surgery than from root debridement.[55]

What makes one type of dentinal exposure respond to painful stimuli more than the other? The difference is analogous to the difference between an acute and chronic wound. That is to say that dentin, once it has been exposed and traumatized, over time develops a reparative dentin, and the tooth becomes less susceptible to the debriding stimulus. However, after periodontal surgery, which results in apically positioned gingival tissues in conjunction with root debridement, dentin is newly exposed and the root becomes acutely sensitive to stimuli until reparative dentin can form.

One study investigated the difference in root sensitivity between the air powder polisher and the rubber cup polisher. The dentinal tubules remained open with the air powder polish, whereas the rubber cup polish left a smear layer that partially occluded the tubules. Therefore an increase in sensitivity was reported among the group receiving the air powder polish.[23]

Restorative Procedures

Some restorative procedures also may elicit sensitivity. Dental caries or crown preparations have resulted in dental sensitivity. This sensitivity may result if temporary filling materials are in contact with the dentin for too long after a cavity preparation has been performed. This postoperative sensitivity may be avoided if a varnish and base material are placed beneath restorations and crown preparations.[15] The varnish helps seal the dental tubules, and the base provides additional insulation from the restorative material.

NATURAL DEFENSE MECHANISMS

The pulp has several natural defenses to protect itself from irritating stimuli. One of these, reparative dentin, was discussed in the previous section. The tooth also may produce secondary dentin in response to calcification in the pulp chamber from stimuli.[42] Dental sclerosis, if not caused by caries or attrition, may be associated with the aging process affecting the cervical region of the tooth late in life. This process is evidenced by mineralization in the peritubular dentin that may partially or completely block the patent tubule and prevent the passage of painful impulses.[4] Yoshiyama and colleagues[62] reported the presence of rhomboidal-shaped crystals in dentinal tubules from naturally desensitized dentin. The majority of treatments for dentinal sensitivity attempt in some way to block fluid flow in the tubules. The following section describes some of the common agents and the difficulty of assessing their effects.

TREATMENT OF SENSITIVITY

25-B   Although many products are available for use either by the patient or in a professional office, no one accepted modality gives maximum or consistent benefit.* Identification of the cause of a patient's pain response is important. The differential diagnosis to determine dentinal sensitivity requires the generation of a list of reasons the patient may perceive pain. The dental professional must rule out various sources as the cause of pain to arrive at dentinal sensitivity as the diagnosis. Box 25-1 lists conditions that may cause dentinal sensitivity.

CRITERIA FOR SENSITIVITY AGENTS

Many agents have been tested for treating sensitive teeth. Grossman[36] developed the essential criteria used to select agents to be tested (Box 25-2). These criteria apply to both professional and over-the-counter (OTC) products. Decision making for managing dentinal sensitivity should follow a hierarchy of treatment methods, which are based on using the most conservative treatments first and saving the most aggressive treatment options until after others have been given time to be effective and are professionally evaluated (Fig. 25-3).

---

*References 17, 18, 24, 33, 50, 58, 59.

FACTORS INFLUENCING STUDIES OF DENTINAL SENSITIVITY AGENTS

Clinical studies to determine the effectiveness of agents or products for desensitization have been difficult to conduct because of the following factors:
• Use of subjective evaluations
• Lack of proper controls
• Lack of objective measurements
• Strong placebo effect in control groups

Historically, many evaluations have been based on subjective reactions. In these studies, the person's reaction to the products being tested has been based on impressions of whether improvement was poor, fair, good, or excellent. In addition, several studies have been based on the patient's evaluation under unsupervised use and without a placebo or control product (i.e., a product containing no known effective agent).

A major problem with testing *desensitizing* agents or products can be the high degree of reduction in sensitivity that occurs in groups treated with control products. This may be associated with improved cleaning by patients who are seen routinely by the dental professional or the result of a general decline over a period of time (often observed with sensitivity problems). Some researchers are attempting to improve the designs of dentinal sensitivity studies by adding wash-in periods of 4 to 6 weeks when all patients use a control substance such as toothpaste, then retesting the patients for sensitive teeth that meet the inclusion study criteria before starting the active phase of the study.[3]

PERSONAL ORAL HYGIENE

Personal oral hygiene should be emphasized as a primary factor in the treatment of sensitivity. Adequate plaque control procedures should be well developed by the patient before professional treatments are started[17,33,34,50,58] and for long-term success.[58] In addition to proper brushing, interdental cleaning with floss and other aids to remove plaque should be initiated. Hygienists should discuss diet with the patient and, if necessary, elimination of acidic or sour foods, as well as those that are fermentable carbohydrates, which can produce acids in plaque (Fig. 25-4).[6,21] Brushing with a soft or ultrasoft toothbrush and use of a minimum abrasive dentifrice, or one formulated to reduce sensitivity is recommended.

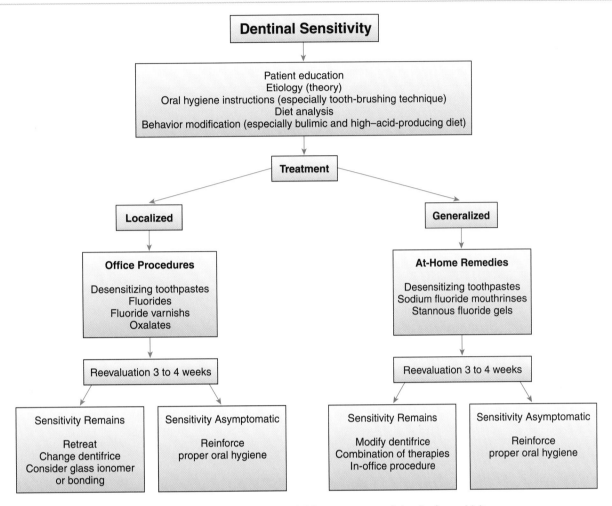

Dentinal Sensitivity

Patient education
Etiology (theory)
Oral hygiene instructions (especially tooth-brushing technique)
Diet analysis
Behavior modification (especially bulimic and high–acid-producing diet)

Treatment

Localized

Generalized

Office Procedures

Desensitizing toothpastes
Fluorides
Fluoride varnishs
Oxalates

At-Home Remedies

Desensitizing toothpastes
Sodium fluoride mouthrinses
Stannous fluoride gels

Reevaluation 3 to 4 weeks

Reevaluation 3 to 4 weeks

Sensitivity Remains

Retreat
Change dentifrice
Consider glass ionomer
or bonding

Sensitivity Asymptomatic

Reinforce
proper oral hygiene

Sensitivity Remains

Modify dentifrice
Combination of therapies
In-office procedure

Sensitivity Asymptomatic

Reinforce
proper oral hygiene

FIG. 25-3 Decision-making model for treatment of dentinal sensitivity.

No toothbrush bristle standard exists to guide manufacturers; one manufacturer's soft bristles may be firmer than another manufacturer's medium bristles.[60] Toothpaste abrasiveness is difficult to monitor clinically, and the dental professional should recommend an appropriate dentifrice for each patient (see Chapter 23). Regardless of desensitization methods used, reports exist of tooth sensitivity being reduced with improved personal oral hygiene procedures.[31,37]

COMMERCIALLY AVAILABLE PRODUCTS

Desensitizing toothpastes are widely promoted to both the dental profession and the public. Crest Sensitivity Protection (Procter & Gamble Co., Cincinnati, Ohio), Colgate Sensitive Maximum Strength (Colgate-Palmolive Co., New York, N.Y.), Promise Sensitive Teeth Toothpaste, Sensodyne F Toothpaste for Sensitive Teeth, and Mint Sensodyne (Block Drug Co., Inc., Jersey City, N.J.), all contain 5% *potassium nitrate* as the active ingredient and have been found to be an effective agent in some clinical studies. The exact mechanism of action of potassium nitrate is not known. Some postulate that it, like most other ingredients, reduces dentin permeability by partially occluding the tubule. Others believe it has a desensitizing action on the fine nerve fibers at the dentinal-pulpal junction.

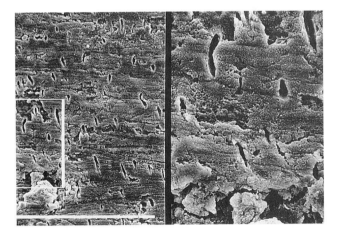

FIG. 25-4 Organic acids open tubules in minutes from dietary acid. (From Addy M: Etiology of clinical implications of dentine hypersensitivity, *Dent Clin North Am* 34[3]:510, 1990.)

Aconite and aconitine, albargine, aluminum salts, ammoniacal silver nitrate, Anderson's remineralizing powder, anesthetic agents (general), anodyne cement, arsenic and arsenious acid, asbestos, atropia

Benzyl alcohol, Buckley's desensitizing paste

Calcium hydroxide, calcium lactate, calcium orthophosphate complex, calcium sucrose phosphate, Campho-Phenique, carbolic acid, carbolized potash, cataphoresis apparatus, caustic agents, cavity varnish, chloral hydrate, chloro-carboline, chloroform, chromic acid, chromium sesquichloride, cocaine phenate, collodion, composite resins, corticosteroids, creosote, cyanoacrylates

Dr. Dowsley's dental obtundent

Electrical osmosis, erythrophicin, ether, ethyl chloride, eucain, eucalyptus, eugenol

Fluoride iontophoresis, formalin, Fowler's solution

Gold, Gottlieb's solution

Hartmann's desensitizer (alcohol, thymol, sulfuric ether), HEMA, hemicrania, hot water, hydrochlorate of cocaine

Iodine, kreosotum, lactophosphate of lime

Magnesium hydroxide, menthol, methyl chloride, morphine, Myer's obtundent

Nervocidine, novocaine, oleate of cocaine, orthoform, oxide of lime

Paraform, phenol, phosphoric acid, potassium carbonate–sodium carbonate, potassium nitrate, potassium oxalate, potassocaine, prednisolone

Quinine sulfate, Robinson's remedy

Siloxane ethers, silver iodine, silver nitrate, small dentine obtundent, sodium dioxide, sodium fluoride, sodium monofluorophosphate, sodium silicofluoride, stannous fluoride, stenocarpin, strontium chloride, strontium sequestrant salts, style obtunding device, sulfuric acid, syrup of the phosphates

Tar water, The Herbst obtunder, The Rahinator, thymol, trichloroacetic acid

Unslaked lime, Van Wyck obtundent, vapocain, varnishes and cements, veratra

Weaver obtundent, Wilcox obtunder, zinc chloride, zinc oxychloride

FIG. 25-5 Agents reported in the literature to reduce dentinal sensitivity. (Modified from Rosenthall MW: Historic review of the management of tooth hypersensitivity, *Dent Clin North Am* 34:403, 1990.)

Thermodent (Lee Pharmaceuticals, South El Monte, Calif.) contains 10% *strontium chloride* as the active ingredient, and some clinical studies support its effectiveness.[46] These products require patient cooperation for daily application and are effective over time, not giving immediate relief of discomfort. A suggestion for more rapid relief in patients with severe generalized dentinal sensitivity is to use a custom soft mouthguard as a carrier for the desensitizing medicament and as protection from stimuli.[7,18,30]

Another product, Protect (John O. Butler Co., Chicago, Ill.), contains dibasic *sodium citrate* in a pluronic gel. Its action is thought to be derived from the polyglycoid's precipitation of dentinal or salivary proteins. Studies have not shown significant improvement in desensitization.[20]

PROFESSIONAL PRODUCTS

More than 100 different agents used to reduce dentinal sensitivity have been reported in literature (Fig. 25-5). Many of these agents were detrimental to the pulp or discolored the tooth surface. Most modern products used today by dental professionals have not changed significantly, nor have the method(s) of application changed profoundly since they were comprehensively reviewed by Everett, Hall, and Phatak in 1966,[24] and as described in many textbooks and review articles since[17,33,50] (Box 25-3). The American Dental Association (ADA) has granted its Seal of Acceptance to the following desensitizing dentifrices:

- Crest Sensitivity Protection
- Colgate Sensitive Maximum Strength
- Sensodyne Maximum Strength Tartar Control and Whitening

Treatment of sensitive teeth should be targeted at reducing the size of the tubules to limit fluid movement. One of the following strategies may be used[40]:

1. Forming a smear layer by burnishing the exposed root surface
2. Applying topical agents that produce insoluble precipitates in the tubules
3. Occluding the tubule opening with plastic resin
4. Sealing the tubules with bonding agents

Initial preparation of the teeth must be done before any desensitizing agent is professionally applied. Teeth must be free of all hard and soft deposits. In addition, 3% hydrogen peroxide may be applied to the teeth with a cotton pellet for further cleansing. The clinician should rinse the teeth with warm water, dry, and isolate before treatment. Care should be taken to use air lightly or to dry the sensitive areas with cotton rolls.

Most desensitizing agents are applied with a *burnishing* action. One study reported the action of burnishing with an orangewood stick alone to be as effective as burnishing with sodium fluoride.[49] Still another found the action of burnishing with water to reduce dentinal sensitivity.[22] The reduction in sensitivity can be attributed to partial occlusion of the dentinal tubules by a smear layer that results from burnishing. Although a smear layer can exist, it may be dissolved in an acidic environment or worn away from abrasion or attrition. The ingredients and application claims of desensitizing agents are outlined in Table 25-1.*

*References 10, 13, 14, 18, 25, 27, 29, 35, 38, 41, 43, 44, 48, 49, 53, 54, 57, 61, 63.

BOX 25-3

Professional Products Used to Treat Dentinal Sensitivity

Products or Agents that Partially Occlude Dentinal Tubules
Burnishing
Calcium hydroxide
Dibasic calcium phosphate
Iontophoresis
Fluoride compounds
  Sodium fluoride
  Sodium silicofluoride
  Stannous fluoride
Formalin
Potassium oxalate
Silver nitrate
Strontium chloride
Zinc chloride–potassium ferrocyanide
Surface-Sealing Agents
Bonding agents
Cements
Resins
Varnishes

Modified from Trowbridge HO, Silver DR: A review of current approaches to in-office management of tooth hypersensitivity, *Dent Clin North Am* 34:561, 1990.

Certain claims exist that formalin reduces sensitivity when in a concentration of 40% and applied to a sensitive area, using a cotton pellet and burnishing with a porte polisher or toothpick. (See Chapter 32 for a description of the use of the porte polisher.) A 10% formalin solution was reported to be ineffective in decreasing hydraulic conductance.[35] (*Hydraulic conductance* refers to the ability of a substance or stimuli to produce fluid movement in the tubules.) This agent should not come into contact with the mucosa because a reaction (precipitation of protein) with the tissues will occur, resulting in soft tissue irritation.

A solution of basic or ammoniated silver nitrate is alleged to decrease dentinal sensitivity. This solution is applied directly to the sensitive area and then is precipitated with a reducing agent such as eugenol. The solution acts to partially occlude the tubules and therefore decrease hydraulic conductance. This particular preparation may be irritating to soft dental tissue and cause tooth discoloration.

Calcium hydroxide is another agent that decreases dentin permeability. This product produces a precipitate inside the dentinal tubule.[43] The effectiveness of this precipitate is negatively influenced by an acidic environment. Acids dissolve the calcium hydroxide crystals within the tubules.

Another product found to be effective in decreasing sensitivity is dibasic calcium phosphate. It is burnished into the dentinal surface, depositing minerals into the tubules. Dibasic calcium phosphate therefore reduces the opening and subsequently the effects of painful stimuli.

Solutions of 40% zinc chloride and 20% potassium ferrocyanide are used in a two-step process. The solution of

TABLE 25-1

Professional treatment of dentinal sensitivity

Agent	Claim
Glutaraldehye and hydroxyethyl methacylate	One-step chairside procedure
	Very expensive
	Effective
	Very irritating to gingival tissues
Formalin	40% Applied with cotton pellet + burnishing
	10% Ineffective
	Irritating to soft gingival tissues
Silver nitrate	Applied directly + eugenol as reducing agent
	Irritating to gingival tissues
	Possible tooth discoloration
Calcium hydroxide	Applied mixed with sterile water + burnishing
	Fair effectiveness
	Acids dissolve calcium hydroxide crystals in tubules
Resin adhesives	Procedure technique-sensitive
	Fair to good effectiveness
	Seals dentin well
Sodium fluoride	Teeth free of deposits
	Localized or generalized sensitivity
	Paint technique
	Patient may dislike initial yellow film.
Stannous fluoride	Paint and burnish technique
	Prescription home-applied gel (patient compliance required)
	Taste must be considered
Oxalates	Teeth free of deposits
	No burnishing required
	Fair, short-term relief
Iontophoresis	Negative fluoride ion enhanced by electrical current
	May promote secondary dentin formation
	May be coupled with fluoride therapy for improved results
	Patient may experience brief pain during procedure.
Lasers	Nd:YAG and CO_2 showing encouraging results
	Expensive equipment
	Long-term studies needed to determine pulpal effects
Composite bonding	Permanent restorative procedure
	Procedure technique-sensitive
	Expensive
	Nd:YAG, Neodymium: yttrium aluminum garnet; CO_2, carbon dioxide.

zinc chloride is applied with a moist cotton pellet or porte polisher and rubbed vigorously into the tooth surface. Excess solution is removed from the gingival margin. While the teeth are still moist, the second solution of potassium ferrocyanide is applied. This solution is rubbed vigorously until an orange, curdy precipitate forms. After 1 minute (during which time the reaction should occur), the excess is removed from the gingival margin. Scanning electron microscopy revealed a crystalline deposit on the dentinal surface; however, most of the crystals appeared to be too large to enter the tubule. Therefore the reduction in sensitivity with the use of this product may be attributed to the burnishing action.

Professional products consisting of fluoride gels, varnishes, and solutions for caries treatment are used to treat sensitivity.[28,61] The teeth should be free of deposits before fluoride treatment. With generalized sensitivity or many areas of gingival recession, tray or painting procedures are used. If specific teeth are sensitive, fluoride may be burnished into the area with a porte polisher. Also available are fluoride products with claimed desensitization properties. The first contains equal amounts of sodium fluoride, kaolin, and glycerin. This product is rubbed into the dried isolated sensitive area with a porte polisher for 1 to 5 minutes. The mechanism of action is attributed to the deposition of insoluble salts. Two products are available that contain sodium silicofluoride. The first of these is a saturated solution containing 0.7% in cold water or 0.9% in hot water. This preparation is rubbed into sensitive areas for 5 minutes. A calcium gel forms, which is stated to be an improved insulating barrier.

Sodium silicofluoride also is contained with calcium hydroxide in a two-step procedure. Initially, the sodium silicofluoride is applied and allowed to react for 1 to 2 minutes. Then the area is painted with 5% calcium hydroxide and allowed to stand for 1 minute. This combination treatment is claimed to reduce the tubule opening.

Stannous fluoride, in various percentages and forms (solution or gel), has been found to provide relief from dentinal sensitivity. Solutions of 10% and 0.717% when burnished into the sensitive area have reduced sensitivity.[13,53] A prescription home-applied gel of 0.4% stannous fluoride has been reported to produce satisfactory results when used for at least 4 weeks and has "accepted" status by the ADA as a desensitizing agent. Stannous fluoride works by occluding the dentinal tubules with tin and fluoride.[14,51,54]

Oxalate solutions have shown a reduction in sensitivity and can be applied without the need for burnishing, which is often painful to the patient. Researchers reported a 96% decrease in dentin permeability with the use of a 3% solution of oxalic acid.[49] The dentinal tubules were occluded and the surface covered with an acid-resistant layer of calcium oxalate crystals. This could provide a less painful method of achieving desensitization.

Iontophoresis is another method of treating dental sensitivity. The purpose of this procedure is to enhance movement of ions by electric currents. With this system, a negative ion such as fluoride would be pushed away from the toothbrush surface and encouraged to penetrate dental enamel.[29] Iontophoresis may result in the formation of secondary dentin, resulting in a decrease in sensitivity. Several clinical studies have been reported on the use of iontophoresis alone or coupled with the use of fluoride material or a strontium chloride preparation. In general, iontophoresis alone has been claimed to be effective against sensitivity; when this procedure has been coupled with an active agent, an enhanced benefit has been reported.[48]

Several professional iontophoresis units are available, and two are discussed here. The first is the Chayes-Siemon apparatus, which contains a 9-volt battery and an ammeter that must register 20, or about 0.4 milliampere, to ensure ion transfer. The patient holds the grip, or positive pole, of the equipment. The dental professional then applies the negatively charged end of the equipment, a sable brush dipped into a 1% sodium fluoride solution, in contact with the sensitive area for 1 minute. Because of a fairly high current, the patient may experience slight pain on initial contact.

The second apparatus is the barrel-shaped Lemonstron apparatus with a sable brush at one end. The clinician moistens the brush with a 2% sodium fluoride solution and applied this to the sensitive tooth area.[41] The circuit is completed by the clinician touching the patient. The brush is allowed to contact the sensitive area for one minute. Because this unit operates with two penlight batteries and no ammeter is used, the clinician is unsure of the quantity of the current being dispensed.

Surface-sealing agents such as varnishes, resins, and cyanoacrylate are useful in treating sensitivity when other agents are ineffective. Great success has been found using fluoride varnishes and unfilled resins to cover the outside of the patent tubules.[19,28] More recently, acid etching and bonding have been employed to reduce areas of cervical sensitivity.[27] Another clinician recommends the use of glass ionomer cements followed by bonding as an alternative for dentinal sensitivity.[18,44] A promising product called *cyanoacrylate* has been shown in clinical studies to have an immediate and long-lasting effect on sensitive dentin. Data indicates that it is 33% more effective than sodium fluoride.[10,38]

GLUMA (Bayer-Dental, D-509 Leverkusen, West Germany) is a bonding agent system of a 5% glutaraldehyde primer and 35% HEMA (hydroxyethyl methacrylate). Carefully applied to the sensitive tooth surfaces with a cotton-tip applicator, with care taken to prevent contact with gingival tissues, GLUMA has been found to be effective when other methods of treatment fail to provide relief.[54,56]

Corticosteroid products also are available for dentinal sensitivity. These products are used primarily for sensitivity resulting from cavity preparations but also are used for dentinal sensitivity. Usually the agent is administered by being rubbed into the sensitive site. The mode of action is considered to be that of decreasing pulpal inflammation. This action implies that sensitivity is linked to pulpal inflammation. More research is needed to investigate the existence of this relationship.

Research in the use of lasers to reduce dentinal sensitivity is underway. One study reported no significant difference in the reduction of sensitivity with the use of lasers as compared with conventional methods.[57] Studies have reported success with the use of lasers in desensitization.[63] Both Nd:YAG and CO_2 lasers have been studied and the results are encouraging, but the equipment is expensive, and the long-term pulpal effects have not been investigated relative to desensitizing treatments.[63]

 Case Application

Review Ms. Yamagashi's case and, using the decision tree in Fig. 25-3, determine which path you would take to determine both the reason for her sensitivity and the appropriate home and in-office therapies.

CRITICAL THINKING ACTIVITIES

1. Determine whether members of the class have areas of gingival recession or tooth sensitivity.
   a. Test both areas with the following: ice, a blast of air, cold water, hot water, and a sharp probe.
   b. What is the most severe reaction in terms of speed of reaction and pain?
   c. Do areas of recession and sensitivity differ? Why?
   d. What parameters do you think would be best for testing a new antisensitive agent?
2. Review two publications on desensitizing products, before and after 1990. Comment on the occurrence of placebo effect and on the measurements used.

REVIEW QUESTIONS

1. Which of the following areas of the tooth are considered most sensitive from various stimuli?
   a. Occlusal, incisal
   b. Cervical, proximal
   c. Lingual, cervical
   d. Facial, cervical
2. Dentinal sensitivity is caused by all of the following professional procedures *except* which one?
   a. Periodontal instrumentation
   b. Periodontal surgery
   c. Cosmetic polishing
   d. Periodontal probing
3. Dentinal sensitivity is a multifactorial condition. Stimuli of a thermal, tactile, chemical, or osmotic nature can result in pain.
   a. The first statement is true; the second is false.
   b. The first statement is false; the second is true.

   c. Both statements are true.
   d. Both statements are false.
4. Desensitizing agents primarily work by which of the following ways?
   a. Occluding the dentinal tubules
   b. Changing the surface ions
   c. Interfering with neurological responses
   d. Inhibiting the osmotic pressure between membranes
5. Regardless of the type of treatment, improved oral hygiene can reduce dentinal sensitivity. In fact, the placebo effect often occurs in treating sensitivity.
   a. The first statement is true; the second is false.
   b. The first statement is false; the second is true.
   c. Both statements are true.
   d. Both statements are false.

SUGGESTED AGENCIES AND WEB SITES

Because of the ever-changing nature of the Internet, some of the web sites listed here may have changed since publication. Please refer to Mosby's Evolve web site for the most current information.

National Center for Dental Hygiene Research:
    http://jeffline.tju.edu/DHNet
Procter & Gamble Global Dental Resources:
    http://www.dentalcare.com

Block Drug Company, Inc.: http://www.blockdrug.com
Colgate-Palmolive: http://www.colgate.com

 ## ADDITIONAL READINGS AND RESOURCES

Council on Dental Therapeutics: Acceptance of Promise with fluoride and Sensodyne toothpastes for sensitive teeth, *J Am Dent Assoc* 113:673, 1986.

Kim S: Hypersensitive teeth. Part II: treatment, *J Prosthet Dent* 56(3):307, 1986.

Parr OD, Brokaw WC: Economical iontophoresis for dentistry, *Quint Int* 20(11):841-5, 1989.

Perno M, Murray-Ryder ML: Lasers: no longer the wave of the future (Part 1), *Access* 15(9):30-7.

Snyder RA, Beck FM, Horton JE: The efficacy of a 0.4% SnF_2 solution on root surface hypersensitivity, IADR/AADR Abstracts 237, 1985.

Thrash W, Dorman HI, Smith FD: A method to measure pain associated with hypersensitive dentin, *J Periodontol* 54:160, 1983.

Wilder-Smith P: The soft laser: therapeutic tool or popular placebo? *Oral Surg* 66(6):654, 1988.

 ## REFERENCES

1. Absi EG, Adams D, Addy M: The patency of dentinal tubules in hypersensitive and non-sensitive dentine, *J Dent Res* 65(4): 497, 1986.

2. Absi EG, Addy M, Adams D: Dentine hypersensitivity: a study of the patency of dentinal tubules in sensitive and non-sensitive cervical dentine, *J Clin Periodontol* 14(5):280, 1987.

3. Absi EG, Addy M, Adams D: The dentine hypersensitivity: the development and evaluation of a replica technique to study sensitive and nonsensitive cervical dentine, *J Clin Periodontol* 16(3):190-5, 1989.

4. ADA Council on Dental Therapeutics: *Accepted products categorical listing*, Chicago, 1992 (Jan 27), American Dental Association.

5. Addy M: Etiology and clinical implications of dentine hypersensitivity, *Dent Clin North Am* 34(3):503, 1990.

6. Addy M, Absi EG, Adams D: Dentine hypersensitivity: the effects in vitro of acids and dietary substances on root-planed and burred dentine, *J Clin Periodontol* 14(5):274, 1987.

7. Addy M, Mostafa P: Dentine hypersensitivity. II. Effects produced by the uptake in vitro of toothpastes onto dentine, *J Oral Rehab* 16:35-48, 1989.

8. Addy M, Mostafa P, Newcombe RG: Dentine hypersensitivity: the distribution of recession, sensitivity and plaque, *J Dent* 15(6):242, 1987.

9. Addy M, Mostafa P, Newcombe RG: Effect on plaque of five toothpastes used in the treatment of dentin hypersensitivity, *Clin Prevent Dent* 12(4):28, 1990.

10. Bahram J: Cyanoacrylate—a new treatment for hypersensitive dentin and cementum, *J Am Dent Assoc* 114:216, 1987.

11. Berman L: Dentinal sensation and hypersensitivity, *J Periodontol* 56(4):216, 1984.

12. Blandy AA: On the sensibility of teeth. *Am J Dent Sci* 1:22, 1850-1851.

13. Blank LW, Charbeneau GT: Urgent treatment in operative dentistry, *Dent Clin North Am* 30:489, 1986.

14. Blong MA et al: Effects of a gel containing 0.4 percent stannous fluoride on dentinal hypersensitivity, *Dent Hyg* 59:489, 1985.

15. Brannstrom M: The hydrodynamic theory of dentinal pain: sensation in the preparations, caries, and the dentinal crack syndrome, *J Endodont* 12(10):453, 1986.

16. Brannstrom M, Astrom A: A study of the mechanism of pain elicited from the dentine, *J Dent Res* 43:619, 1964.

17. Chasens AI: The management of tooth pain and sensitivity. In Chasens AI, Kaslick RS, editors: *Mechanisms of pain and sensitivity in the teeth and supporting tissues,* Rutherford, NJ, 1974, Fairleigh Dickinson University.

18. Christensen GJ: Desensitization of cervical tooth structure, *J Am Dent Assoc* 129(6):765-6, 1998.

19. Clark DC: The effectiveness of a fluoride varnish and a desensitizing toothpaste in treating dentinal hypersensitivity, *J Periodont Res* 20:212, 1985.

20. Clark DC, Al-Joburi W, Chan ECS: The efficacy of a new dentifrice in treating dentin sensitivity: effects of sodium citrate and sodium fluoride as active ingredients, *J Periodont Res* 22(2):89, 1987.

21. Clark DC et al: The influence of frequent ingestion of acids in the diet on treatment for dentin sensitivity, *Can Dent Assoc J* 56(12):1101-3, 1990.

22. Cooley RL, Sandoval VA: Effectiveness of potassium oxalate treatment on dentin hypersensitivity, *Gen Dent* 37(4):316, 1989.

23. Dederich DN, Gulevich T, Reid A: The effect of rubber cup vs an air-powder abrasive system on root surfaces, *Canadian Dent Hyg/Probe* 23(3):135, 1989.

24. Everett FG, Hall WB, Phatak NM: Treatment of hypersensitive dentin, *J Oral Ther Pharmacol* 2:300, 1966.

25. Fischer C et al: Clinical evaluation of pulp and dentine sensitivity after supragingival and subgingival scaling, *Endod Dent Traumatol* 7:259, 1991.

26. Flynn J, Galloway R, Orchardson R: The incidence of hypersensitive teeth in the West of Scotland, *J Dent* 13:230, 1985.

27. Fusayama T: Etiology and treatment of sensitive teeth, *Quint Int* 19(12):921, 1988.

28. Gaffer A: Treating hypersensitivity with fluoride varnishes, *Compend Contin Educ Dent* 19(11): 1088-97,1998.

29. Gangarosa LP et al: Double-blind evaluation of duration of dentin sensitivity reduction by fluoride iontophoresis, *Gen Dent* 37(4):316, 1989.

30. Gangarosa LP: Current strategies for dentist-applied treatment in management of hypersensitive dentine, *Arch Oral Biol* 39(suppl):101-6, 1994.

31. Gedalia I et al: The effect of fluoride and strontium application on dentin: in vivo and in vitro studies, *J Periodontol* 49: 269, 1978.

32. Graf H., Galasse R: Morbidity, prevalence, and intraoral distribution of the hypersensitive teeth, *J Dent Res* 56(Special issue A):162, 1977 (abstract 479).

33. Grant DA, Stern IB, Everett FG: *Periodontics: in the tradition of Orban and Gottlieb,* ed 5, St Louis, 1979, Mosby.

34. Green BL, Green ML, McFall WT Jr: Calcium hydroxide and potassium nitrate as desensitizing agents for hypersensitive root surfaces, *J Periodontol* 48:667, 1977.

35. Greenhill JD, Pashley D: The effects of desensitizing agents on the hydraulic conductance of dentin in vitro, *J Dent Res* 60:686, 1981.

36. Grossman LI: A systematic method for the treatment of hypersensitive dentin, *J Am Dent Assoc* 22:592, 1935.

37. Hiatt WH, Johansen E: Root preparation, I: obturation of dentinal tubules in treatment of root hypersensitivity, *J Periodontol* 43:373, 1972.

38. Javid B, Barkhordar RA, Bhinda SV: Cyanoacrylate—a new treatment for hypersensitive dentin and cementum, *J Am Dent Assoc* 114:486, 1987.

39. Kanapka JA: A new agent, *Compend Contin Educ Dent* 3:S118, 1982.

40. Kanapka JA: Over-the-counter dentrifices in the treatment of tooth hypersensitivity, *Dent Clin North Am* 34(3):545, 1990.

41. Kern DA et al: Effectiveness of sodium fluoride on tooth hypersensitivity with and without iontophoresis, *J Periodontol* 60(7):386, 1989.

42. Krauser JT: Hypersensitive teeth. Part I. Etiology, *J Prosthet Dent* 2:153, 1986.

43. Levin MP, Yearwood LL, Carpenter WN: The desensitizing effect of calcium hydroxide and magnesium hydroxide on hypersensitive dentin, *Oral Surg* 35:741, 1973.

44. Markowitz K: Tooth sensitivity—mechanisms and management, *Compend Cont Educ Dent* 14(8):1032-45,1997.

45. Miles DA: Dental management and reported cases of bulimic erosion, *Can Dent Assoc J* 51(10):757, 1985.

46. Minkoff S, Axelrod S: Efficacy of strontium chloride in dental hypersensitivity, *J Periodontol* 58(7):470, 1987.

47. Ong G, Strahan D: Effect of a desensitizing dentifrice on dentinal hypersensitivity, *Endod Dent Traumatol* 5:213-8, 1989.

48. Orchardson R, Collins WJN: Clinical features of hypersensitive teeth, *Br Dent J* 162:253, 1987.

49. Pashley DH, Leibach JG, Horner JA: The effects of burnishing NaF/kaolin/glycerin paste on dentin permeability, *J Periodontol* 58(1):19, 1987.

50. Pashley DH: Mechanisms of dentin sensitivity, *Dent Clin North Am* 34(3):449, 1990.

51. Peden JW: Dental hypersensitivity, *J West Soc Periodontol* 25: 75, 1977.

52. Silverman G et al: Assessing the efficacy of three dentifrices in the treatment of dental hypersensitivity, *J Am Dent Assoc* 127(1):191-201,1996.

53. Smith BA, Ash MM Jr: Evaluation of a desensitizing dentifrice, *J Am Dent Assoc* 68:639, 1964 (a).

54. Tachibana Y: Dentin hypersensitivity following grinding of vital teeth, *Shikai Tenbo* Aug(Special no):153, 1985.

55. Thrash WJ: Long-term effects of a gel containing 0.4 percent stannous fluoride on dentinal hypersensitivity as compared to placebo and no treatment control. Unpublished manuscript, 1992.

56. Trowbridge HO, Silver DR: A review of current approaches to in-office management of tooth hypersensitivity, *Dent Clin N Am* 34(3):561-81, 1990.

57. Wallace JA et al: Pulpal and root sensitivity rated to periodontal therapy, *Oral Surg Oral Med Oral Pathol* 69(6):743, 1990.

58. Wycoff SJ: Current treatment for dentinal hypersensitivity: in-office treatment, *Compend Contin Educ Dent* 3(suppl):S113, 1982.

59. Yankell SL: At home treatment, *Compend Contin Educ Dent* 3(suppl):S115, 1982.

60. Yankell SL, Emling RC: Understanding dental products: what you should know and what your patient should know, *Contin Dent Educ* 1:(7), 1978.

61. Yates R, West N, Addy M, Marlow I: The effects of a potassium citrate, cetylpyridinium chloride, sodium fluoride mouth rinse on dentine hypersensitivity, plaque and gingivitis. A placebo-controlled study, *J Clin Periodontol* 25(10): 813-20,1998.

62. Yoshiyama M et al: Scanning electron microscopic characterization of sensitive vs insensitive human radicular dentin, *J Dent Res* 68(11):1498, 1989.

63. Zhang C et al: Effects of CO_2 laser in the treatment of cervical dentinal hypersensitivity, *J Endod* 24(9):595-97, 1998.

CHAPTER 26

❧
Sealants

Colleen R. Schmidt

Chapter Outline

Case Study: Pediatric Considerations for Sealant
    Application
Action and Effectiveness of Sealants
    Indications for placement
    Contraindications to placement
Sealant Composition and Types

Armamentarium and Application
    Application technique
Retention, Wear, and Replacement
Potential Estrogenicity
Future Applications

Key Terms

Acid etching
BIS-GMA
Bonding
Curing

Estrogenicity
Filled resin sealants
Monomers

Pits and fissures
Polymers
Polymerization

Retention
Viscosity
Wear

Learning Outcomes

1. Discuss the indications for the use of pit and fissure sealants.
2. Describe the appropriate technique for application of sealant.
3. Identify teeth for sealant placement based on selection criteria.
4. Discuss the clinical characteristics of dental sealant materials, including types, properties, retentive characteristics, and potential estrogenicity.

5. Describe how sealants can prevent recurrent decay from developing adjacent to margins of dental restorations by sealing the open margins of both amalgam and composite restorations.
6. Outline the role of the dental hygienist in the prevention of new carious lesions and recurrent dental decay.
7. Recognize that sealants are a primary preventive means of reducing the need for future restorative treatment.
8. Cite three reasons for dental practitioners' underuse of sealants.
9. Develop a community-based sealant program.

*R*esearch has shown that use of resin sealants to treat dental *pits and fissures* is a successful primary preventive procedure.* Dental hygienists must be familiar with the scientific evidence regarding dental sealants to use them properly and to recommend sealants for patients as preventive dental procedures. Dental pit and fissure sealants have three primary preventive effects: (1) they provide a mechanical barrier in the pit

and fissure of the tooth; (2) they eliminate the environment conducive to *Streptococcus mutans;* and (3) they make the occlusal pit and fissure easier to clean by tooth brushing and mastication.[8,59,64]

The decline in the rate of dental caries assessed in the general population can be directly related to the availability and efficacy of fluoride. Fluoride efficacy occurs primarily on smooth tooth surfaces, leaving occlusal pits and fissure at higher risk for dental disease. Numerous epidemiological studies have evaluated the role of dental sealant in the declining rate of dental decay.[57,58,68-70]

---

*References 1, 2, 15, 41, 58, 69, 70.

Dental sealants provide a barrier between the enamel pits and fissures (areas inaccessible to toothbrush bristles) and fermentable carbohydrates and *S. mutans*. With appropriate and conscientious placement and maintenance, sealants have been highly effective in preventing new pit and fissure decay since their introduction in the late 1960s.* Sealants effectively eliminate sites of bacterial proliferation by blocking the exposed areas of the occlusal surface. Research indicates clinicians could approach 100% caries prevention in pits and fissures with repeated sealant application.†

As part of a comprehensive preventive dental program, sealants significantly reduce the incidence of new pit and fissure decay as well as the need for future restorative treatment. Other preventive measures (e.g., oral hygiene instructions, dietary analysis and modification) are still required for beneficial patient outcomes, and other treatment modalities are still necessary for teeth and tooth surfaces not protected by dental sealants. Also, patients want additional preventive measures in dental care. These factors should increase the current placement rate of dental pit and fissure sealants. In addition, specific population groups are in particular need for preventive measures (e.g., immigrant populations, institutionalized individuals, disabled persons, low-income families). Dental sealants provide a simple and effective means to reduce the incidence of occlusal caries and increase the prevalence of healthy habits, which ultimately leads to improved quality of life.[79]

ACTION AND EFFECTIVENESS OF SEALANTS

Fluorides, both systemic and topical, increase enamel resistance to dental decay. However, pit and fissures do not benefit from this effect as do smooth enamel surfaces. Dental pit and fissure sealants provide a physical barrier from the oral environment and change the occlusal anat-

omy. This barrier prevents oral bacteria and their nutrients from creating an environment conducive to the initiation of carious lesions. Due to the occlusal anatomy of posterior teeth and resultant topographical concavities, acidogenic microorganisms accumulate, with the potential to demineralize enamel (Fig. 26-1). The application of a liquid resin to these caries-susceptible zones fills the areas not cleansed by tooth brushing. Clinical research studies provide sufficient evidence of sealant efficacy when the pits and fissures of posterior teeth remain completely sealed.* In fact, caries protection approaches 100% with use of pit and fissure resin sealants.[78]

In order for resin sealants to be mechanically retained within the pit and fissure, the enamel surface requires pretreatment with a phosphoric acid etchant. Michael Buonocore developed the system of *acid etching* in the 1950s (Fig. 26-2). Focusing on the *bonding* of materials to enamel, Buonocore discovered that the enamel surface could be sufficiently roughened by the application of a

---

*References 25, 42, 55, 69, 70, 78.

---

*References 21, 23, 24, 61, 62, 75.
†References 6, 20, 28, 69, 70, 78.

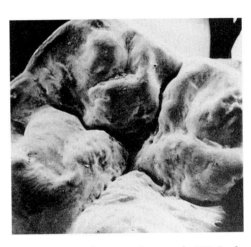

FIG. 26-1 Scanning electron micrograph (SEM) of occlusal pits and fissures.

Pediatric Considerations for Sealant Application

Meghan Kopel, 6 years old, presents to the office for routine cleaning and examination. The clinical evaluation reveals that all four first molars are partially erupted. Brown stain is evident in the mandibular molar fissures, but no explorer resistance or enamel opacity is evident in any of the four permanent molars. The radiographic examination reveals no incipient interproximal decay and sound tooth surfaces. The patient has not had restorative treatment in any of her primary teeth. Her snacking habits consist of moderate amounts of sweets, including chocolate, licorice, and bubble gum. Her oral hygiene habits include brushing in the morning before school and at night, "when my mom reminds me." Meghan is rambunctious and interested in everything around her.

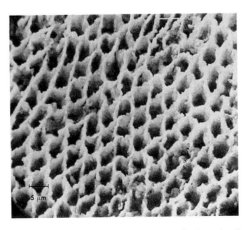

FIG. 26-2 Scanning electron micrograph (SEM) of etched enamel surface after 60-second acid conditioning.

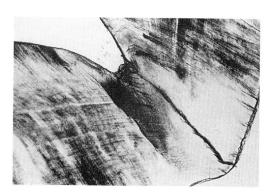

FIG. 26-3 Scanning electron micrograph (SEM) of wide V-shaped fissure.

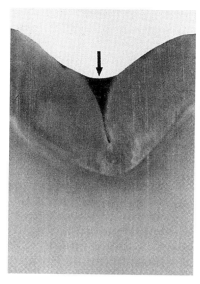

FIG. 26-4 Scanning electron micrograph (SEM) of penetration of resin sealant into occlusal fissure.

phosphoric acid solution, which enhanced the ***retention*** of the applied dental material.[23] When the enamel surface is prepared in this manner, a low-viscosity resin sealant material can flow more easily into the pit and fissures of the tooth because the enamel pores have been enlarged or opened by the acidic conditioning agent.

It is imperative that the resin sealant has contact with or has bonded within the pit and fissures of the tooth during placement. *Mechanical bonding* results when the material becomes physically entrapped within the widened enamel pores. The application of a phosphoric acid solution removes inorganic materials and creates micropores, which increase the surface area of the enamel and form a strong bond between the resin and the enamel. Provided the area conditioned with the acid is subsequently covered with the resin sealant, the tooth surface will remineralize. Once the tooth is reexposed to the minerals naturally found in saliva, the tooth surface structure is replenished.

Two factors must be taken into consideration regarding sealant placement. First, if the resin cannot contact the base of the fissure, no bonding occurs to that specific area. Second, because of the inability to access the base of the fissure completely during the cleansing procedure, caries may develop under the sealant in the depths of the occlusal fissure (Figs. 26-3 and 26-4). Many clinical investigations have shown that resin pit and fissure sealants can be safely placed over early carious lesions.[27,30,42,44-47] Occlusal fissures vary greatly in their anatomy; both wide and narrow fissures can be assessed. The ***viscosity*** of the resin sealant and the width of the enamel fissure affect the ability for the resin to penetrate to the depth of the fissure itself.

Routine clinical evaluations are necessary to determine whether resealing of teeth is necessary in cases of sealant loss due to poor retention. This issue reflects the sensitive nature of the application technique. Any form or amount of moisture contamination can influence the overall effectiveness and resultant use of a sealant intraorally,

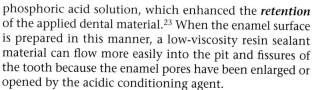

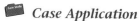

BOX 26-1
Factors in Sealant Placement
Tooth anatomy
Location
Contours, depth, and irregularity of pits and fissures
Age of tooth
Tooth's proximity to other restorations
Future caries risk
Eruption patterns

which diminishes its overall benefit to the patient. Rubber dam isolation is the most thorough means of isolating tooth surfaces to be sealed. Sealant placements with cotton roll isolation and adequate evacuation have also been successful.

Case Application

The reader should refer to the case of 6-year-old Meghan while reading this section and consider how to apply this content to her situation.

INDICATIONS FOR PLACEMENT

Three major factors must be considered before placement of dental sealants (Box 26-1). First, the clinician must assess the anatomy of the tooth (Fig. 26-5); deep occlusal fissures, fossa, cingula, and pits are ideal surfaces on which to place sealant materials. Second, with regard to tooth selection, the clinician must evaluate the location, the contours of the pits and fissures, the depth and irregularity of the pits and fissures, the age of the tooth, and its proximity to another restoration. Each patient's conditions should be evaluated for risk of future caries. In determining a patient's caries risk, the dental hygienist must include an analysis of the patient's dietary patterns and cur-

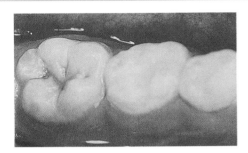

FIG. 26-5 Fully erupted permanent first molar. (From Ryan JP: The clinical benefits of dental sealants, *J Pract Hyg,* 6:13-7, 1997.)

<table>
<tr><td>

BOX 26-2

Classification of Sealants

Filled
Unfilled
Fluoride-releasing
Autopolymerized
Photopolymerized (light polymerized)

</td></tr>
</table>

rent and past fluoride exposure. These risk factors may predispose an identified tooth for future caries or for sealant placement challenges. If a restoration exists on an adjacent tooth, the tooth assessed for sealant placement may already be at even greater caries risk and may not benefit from the sealant. Third, in evaluating a mixed dentition, the clinician should be aware of the progression of dental eruption and note the position of teeth for ease of access during sealant placement.

A review of the previous factors shows that three conditions are optimal choices for the placement of pit and fissure sealants: (1) newly erupted posterior teeth, (2) lingual surfaces of anterior teeth with fissures, and (3) occlusal surfaces of teeth in older persons with reduced salivary flow. Restorative margins, both amalgam and composite, require reassessment at each supportive care appointment. Because these areas are susceptible sites for recurrent caries, sealing of these restorations' margins may improve marginal integrity.*

Patient population groups that benefit from the placement of dental sealants because of their intraoral status include (1) children with newly erupted teeth with pits and fissures; (2) children whose lifestyle, developmental, or behavioral patterns or lack of fluoride exposure make them susceptible to caries; (3) older individuals with reduced salivary flow; and (4) other persons who desire sealant application and for whom sealant therapy is technically feasible.† The clinician must also determine the depth of the pit and fissures and patients' future caries risk, dietary patterns, current and past exposure to fluoride, and ability to cooperate during the proposed treatment.

CONTRAINDICATIONS TO PLACEMENT

Contraindications to sealant placement include patients with behavioral characteristics, clinically evident dental caries, proximal decay, insufficiently erupted teeth, and primary teeth with short life expectancy. The patient's cooperation during the sealant placement procedure also must be considered because proper placement and maintenance of sealants require a well-isolated, dry field. With radiographic evidence of interproximal caries or in cases

of self-cleaning pits and fissures, sealant placement provides no additional patient benefit. Dental professionals and the public should not view dental pit and fissure sealants as a substitute for other caries-control measures. Pit and fissure sealants are an additional component to the patient's overall preventive oral self-care habits.

SEALANT COMPOSITION AND TYPES

Dental sealants are composed of polyurethane, cyanoacrylates, resin (filled or unfilled), and ***BIS-GMA,*** or bisphenol A–glycidyl methacrylate.[18,53,59,72] Sealant materials may also contain glass ionomer, resin-modified glass ionomer, fluoride, and color.* Most commercial sealants are BIS-GMA, in which ***polymerization*** is accelerated by light or another chemical compound.[13,14] Through the process of polymerization, ***monomers*** found in sealant resin become cross-linked ***polymers,*** adding strength to material. Most sealant materials contain up to 50% inorganic filler to improve the material's durability[13,14] (Box 26-2).

When handling resin sealant materials, clinicians must follow specific guidelines. The resin materials must not be exposed to air or light to prevent evaporation and maintain the proper fluidity of the material and its ability to penetrate into the enamel pores. For optimal pit and fissure sealant placement it is important to use fresh materials and a well-maintained armamentarium.

A variety of delivery systems is available to clinicians. With a chemically cured system the clinician physically mixes the base and catalyst, then applies the mixture to the tooth surface. The resin cures, or hardens, as a result of the chemical reaction between the base and the catalyst. The *photopolymerized system* requires exposure to ultraviolet light to cure the material. Currently, a one-step delivery system is available in which a light-protected syringe tip has been preloaded with resin material, ready for direct application to the prepared tooth surface, followed by ultraviolet light activation.

ARMAMENTARIUM AND APPLICATION

In preparation for placing a sealant on a tooth, a clinician must have the proper materials for the procedure (Box 26-3 and Figs. 26-6 to 26-8). The most important aspect of sealant placement procedures is appropriate and adequate isolation equipment and techniques. Adequate preparation before the patient appointment ensures efficiency and effectiveness during the procedure. Although many

26-A
26-B

---

*References 4, 16, 17, 32, 42, 44-47, 56.
†References 4, 10, 11, 15, 21, 62, 66, 71, 81.

*References 6, 7, 19, 26, 31, 33, 34, 38-40, 48, 52, 60, 68, 80.

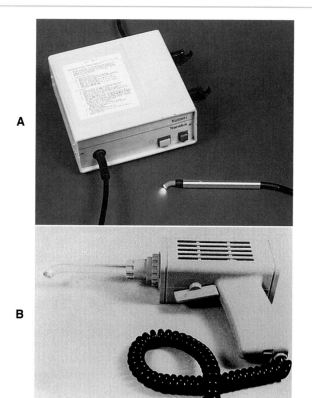

FIG. 26-6 A, Visible white light wand. **B,** Visible white light.

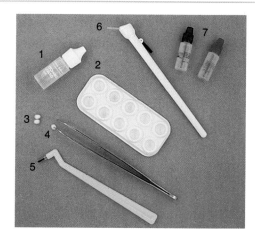

FIG. 26-7 Armamentarium for sealant application: acid etchant *(1)*, dappen dish *(2)*, cotton pellets *(3)*, cotton pliers *(4)*, brush *(5)*, sealant applicator *(6)*, and sealant materials *(7; base and catalyst)*.

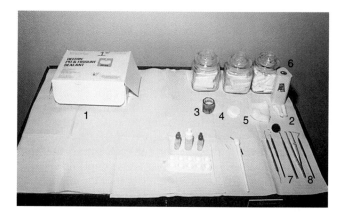

FIG. 26-8 Armamentarium for sealant application and evaluation: pit and fissure sealant kit *(1)*, cotton rolls *(2)*, pumice *(3)*, dry angles *(4)*, cotton gauze *(5)*, floss *(6)*, mirror *(7)*, explorer *(8)*.

BOX 26-3

Armamentarium for Sealant Application

Acid etchant
Air/water syringe tip
Articulating paper
Brush applicator
Cotton pliers
Cotton rolls
Explorer (shepherd's hook)
Gauze
High-volume suction
Light (ultraviolet)
Light shield
Liquid resin
Protective eyewear for operator and assistant
Rubber dam, including armamentarium (optional)

BOX 26-4

Application Technique for Dental Sealant

1. Tooth surfaces cleansed
2. Tooth isolated
3. Surfaces dried and etched
4. Acid washed away and surfaces dried
5. Sealant applied according to manufacturer's instructions
6. Sealant properly cured for polymerization
7. Sealant examined for appropriate placement
8. Patient evaluated for finishing and sealant bonding
9. Topical fluoride application

---

different sealant materials are available through various manufacturers, the steps involved in sealant application are similar (Box 26-4).

APPLICATION TECHNIQUE

1. *Cleanse the tooth surfaces* of hard and soft debris with a prophylactic brush on a slow-speed handpiece or with an air polisher. When the tooth is cleansed with an air polisher, the mechanical interlocking of the resin to the enamel surface improves, with increased retention

of the sealant material.[9] Cleansing agents containing oil or fluoride inhibit sealant retention and therefore should be avoided in the tooth preparation process.[18] The cleansing agent should be rinsed from the tooth surface with water and high-speed evacuation.

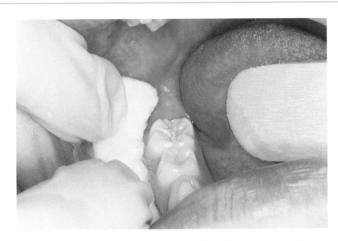

FIG. 26-9 Isolate cleansed tooth with cotton roll and tongue depressor.

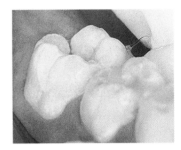

FIG. 26-11 Rinse and dry etched surfaces. (From Ryan JP: The clinical benefits of dental sealants, *J Pract Hyg*, 6:13-7, 1997.)

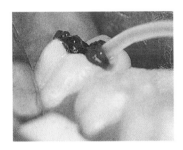

FIG. 26-10 Apply acid etchant to enamel surface. (From Ryan JP: The clinical benefits of dental sealants, *J Pract Hyg*, 6:13-7, 1997.)

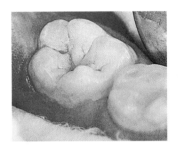

FIG. 26-12 Thoroughly dry surface until frosty white. (From Ryan JP: The clinical benefits of dental sealants, *J Pract Hyg*, 6:13-7, 1997.)

2. *Properly isolate the tooth* to prevent any moisture contamination. The clinician may use a triangular cotton isolation over the parotid papilla, known as *Driangles* (Dental Health Products, Youngstown, N.Y.), cotton rolls held with a metal clamp, or cotton roll holders and suction. Isolation may require placement of a rubber dam for application to multiple teeth in a quadrant (Fig. 26-9).

3. *Apply the phosphoric acid (30% to 50%) enamel conditioner,* covering all areas of the enamel surface to be sealed (Fig. 26-10). Apply the etchant 1 full minute with a brush-tipped applicator or a cotton pellet, then thoroughly rinse with water using high-speed evacuation (Fig. 26-11). It is important to avoid contact between the acid and oral mucosal tissues because it may cause tissue discomfort and sloughing. The conditioning process may need to be repeated if an area of the tooth becomes contaminated with water or saliva on drying. In this case, repeat the conditioning process for 10 seconds, and completely dry the reconditioned surface(s).

4. *Evaluate the tooth surfaces* for a frosty, white appearance of the areas to be sealed. This appearance ensures that the enamel fissures have been opened and made available to the sealant material (Fig. 26-12). Again, take precautions to avoid salivary contamination of the conditioned surface.

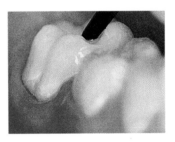

FIG. 26-13 Apply sealant to conditioned surface. (From Ryan JP: The clinical benefits of dental sealants, *J Pract Hyg*, 6:13-7, 1997.)

5. *Apply the sealant material* according to the manufacturer's directions (Fig. 26-13). Concentrate the sealant material in the central pit and fissure, and trace the resin material with an explorer to encourage flow into the prepared fissures. Even coverage on the maxillary

> Overmanipulation of the resin material can lead to entrapment of air bubbles, leading to decreased material retention and voids on the sealant surface.

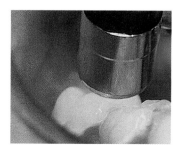

FIG. 26-14 Polymerize with visible white light for the manufacturer's recommended exposure time. (From Ryan JP: The clinical benefits of dental sealants, *J Pract Hyg*, 6:13-7, 1997.)

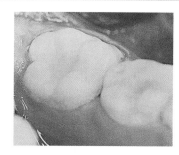

FIG. 26-15 Occlusal sealant in place. Rinse thoroughly, evaluate occlusion, and assess interproximal areas with floss. (From Ryan JP: The clinical benefits of dental sealants, *J Pract Hyg*, 6:13-7, 1997.)

molars is difficult because of patient positioning and the resultant mesial to distal flow of the material. Take care not to flow the material into the contact area.

6. *Ensure proper sealant curing.* Polymerization of the sealant occurs through either light or chemical **curing** (Fig. 26-14). If a light-cured material is being used, the visible light must be correctly placed over the material and exposed for the required time (refer to manufacturer's instructions). The placement and timing of the light source must be properly maintained for successful material curing. The effectiveness of the light source diminishes once materials begin to accumulate on the light wand (see Fig. 26-6). Both the patient and the clinician require protection from the intensity of the curing light. The sealant must not be disturbed until polymerization is complete. If a material requiring chemical polymerization is used, it is imperative to follow the manufacturer's directions for proper and complete manipulation of the materials. The sealant must remain undisturbed until the polymerization process is complete, whether this is a result of chemical or light polymerization. Once the sealant has been light or chemically cured, wipe the surface with a wet cotton roll to remove the oxygen-inhibited layer of unpolymerized resin; this also prevents an unpleasant taste.

7. *Examine the sealant* with an explorer for voids, undercuring, and proper extension into pits and fissures. With the explorer, attempt gentle removal of the sealant to determine whether an adequate bond exists between the sealant and the tooth.

8. *Evaluate the patient's occlusion* with articulating paper, and smooth out any high areas with a finishing bur or a fine stone. Often high areas are removed during masticatory action. Evaluate the interproximal space to ensure the resin has not closed it. Any unnecessary resin material may require removal with a scaler (Fig. 26-15).

9. *Administer a neutral sodium fluoride treatment* to ensure remineralization of the previously etched tooth surfaces before patient dismissal.

RETENTION, WEAR, AND REPLACEMENT

Adequate retention in conjunction with the application technique is the principal predictor of dental sealant suc-

cess. Retention rates 1 year after application are 85% or greater and after 5 years are at least 50%.[69,70] Short-term sealant loss is often a result of technical application error rather than inadequate mechanical bonding.[12,70,78] The inability to maintain a dry field is the most frequent cause of sealant failure; often sealants cannot be placed on the surfaces where they would be of most benefit. Also, poor isolation and improper acid etching contribute to short-term sealant loss.[12] The majority of sealant materials used today are composed of the monomer BIS-GMA, with titanium dioxide added to improve clinical identification and assessment.[70]

The two major factors affecting sealant durability are filler content and glass ionomer content. A number of studies have confirmed that unfilled resin sealant materials are as effective as *filled resin sealants*.[19,31,48] Two advantages of glass ionomer materials include (1) the ability to adhere chemically to the tooth surface and (2) the ability to release fluoride.[59] Theoretically, fluoride is incorporated into the surrounding tooth structure to prevent and arrest dental caries. Studies have shown the greatest fluoride release occurs 24 hours after application and steadily decreases with time.[59,60,67,73] Fluoride release from glass ionomer materials inhibits both dentinal and recurrent marginal caries,[26] although it may not be the primary factor in caries prevention within enamel pits and fissures.[7] Other investigators state the caries-preventive effect of glass ionomer sealant depends on both sealant retention and fluoride release.[34]

Again, retention is the prime determinant of dental sealant success.[58] The bond between the sealant and the enamel surface prevents significant marginal leakage.[58] Application of acid etchant before sealant placement enhances mechanical retention of sealants. Proper acid-etch bonding produces a mechanical bond strong enough to retain restorations, orthodontic brackets, bridges, and sealants.[53] This mechanical bond is unlikely to fail if the materials have been properly applied. Poor retention and excessive wear are frequently cited reasons for the current limited use of pit and fissure sealants.[54]

Fissure penetration is a result of both capillary action and the viscosity of the sealant material. If the site is well cleansed, etched, rinsed, and dried, the acrylic monomers such as BIS-GMA tend to wet, or spread, across the enamel surface. Sealant penetration only into the neck region (top opening) of the fissure has also shown clinically acceptable results; therefore complete fissure penetration is not critical.[13,14]

Evaluating the retention and effectiveness of sealants, researchers reported clinical success after one application.[70] Of all sealants placed, 27% were completely retained after 15 years and 35% partially retained. Of unsealed teeth surfaces, 82% became carious and 31% exhibited signs of decay. The author concluded that if sealants were reapplied when appropriate, 100% cavity protection could be realized.[78] Another researcher developed a similar conclusion provided teeth remain completely sealed. Typical sealant retention rates have been reported to be 60% at 2 years and 42% at 5 years.[57] After sealant placement the rate of dental decay can be reduced by 80% after 1 year and 70% after 2 years. The decreased rate is a result of progressive loss of material over time.[57] It has been proposed that if a sealant could endure 30 months of use, progressive change was unlikely while the sealant continued to provide sufficient fissure protection from bacterial invasion.[54]

Other investigators report that most sealant losses occur shortly after placement, with the greatest loss and wear during the first 6 months of application.[7,23,32,54] Controversy has ensued regarding the clinical relevance of the observed volume of sealant loss. If anatomically critical areas remain safely obturated, the amount of material loss may not be critical.[54]

The effectiveness of sealants improves when lost or partially lost sealants are repaired or replaced at subsequent visits. Therefore, with regularly scheduled maintenance appointments, clinicians should use explorers to examine the margins of sealants to determine whether the bond strength is still adequate or whether the sealant should be partially or completely replaced.

Wear is a natural process resulting from movement between surfaces, which creates a damaged layer and subsequent loss of material.[8,36] Information is limited on the wear resistance of sealant materials.[6,12,35,65] Air polishing used during regular prophylaxis has been shown to increase the amount of wear of resin sealants.[29] Air polishing can also create resin surface roughness, leading to future material breakdown. The amount of wear increases with the longer time and exposure to air abrasion.[29] If replacement of sealant materials becomes necessary because of inadequate bond strength or wear, any residual sealant material should be removed if possible, the tooth cleansed and re-etched, and a new resin placed and cured.

POTENTIAL ESTROGENICITY

Sealants and composites may contain unpolymerized or only partially polymerized monomers. Small amounts of unreacted monomer may remain within cured materials because light curing of plastic materials is inhibited by oxygen. Therefore the oxygen-inhibited layer often present on the sealant surface may contain unreacted monomers. Unreacted monomer may be able to diffuse out of the restoration into either dentin or saliva. The biological acceptability of these unpolymerized materials has been studied.[22,49-51] Evidence is insufficient to suggest that the low concentration of inactivated monomers found in resin sealants poses a direct risk to dental patients.[8] Also hypothetically, wear debris might be carried with food and saliva into the gastrointestinal tract. The amount of material is probably small, however, and the accompanying problem negligible.[51]

Pit and fissure sealants and traditional composite materials have been based on BIS-GMA or BIS-GMA–like monomers. These monomers are derived from glycidyl methacrylate reaction with bisphenol-A (BPA). BPA may be released from the resin matrix of sealants and composites.[50] Under laboratory research conditions, leachable components such as BPA from the unpolymerized monomers of resin sealant materials have mimicked the naturally occurring female hormone, estrogen.[49-51]

The safety of resin materials is a concern because of possible systemic absorption and carcinogenic properties *(estrogenicity).*[63] It is unclear what type of relationship exists between the elution of unpolymerized monomers from dental materials and their absorption into the bloodstream, resulting in physiological problems. With negligible clinical evidence on the estrogenicity of these materials, the current standards for sealant placement seem appropriate. The indications for the continued clinical application of these materials should be encouraged.

FUTURE APPLICATIONS

In addition to preventing caries in the pits and fissures of posterior teeth, sealants also protect the margins of dental restorations.[3,37,45,46] Marginal microleakage of dental composites is a potential concern because of material contraction during visible-light polymerization or debonding during tooth flexure or in situ occlusal loading. These gaps not only contribute to potential microleakage but also may result in marginal staining, recurrent decay, tooth sensitivity, and pulpal pathology.[76] Clinical researchers have investigated the potential use of unfilled resins in reducing marginal microleakage.[3,16,37,45,46] Researchers observed that sealed composite restorations were clinically superior to unsealed restorations in their ability to maintain marginal integrity.[16]

Preventive dental procedures before the manifestation or spread of disease can conserve tooth structure.[5,41,43,45,73] Studies on the use of sealant in alternative preventive and therapeutic applications have shown that restorations sealed with unfilled resin (1) have less microleakage, (2) arrest the progression of caries, (3) preserve existing restorations, (4) increase marginal integrity, and (5) preserve tooth structure.[3,37,45,46] Sealants are effective preventive materials when used simultaneously with amalgam and composite resin as surface sealants.[3,16,46,74] Clinical research has found that early carious lesions have been arrested up to 6 years after placement of sealants over composite resin and amalgam restorations.[16,17,45] Therefore pit and fissure sealants are effective in maintaining dental health and marginal integrity. Further, this type of treatment may substantially increase the longevity of the restoration, particularly if sealant reapplication occurs at 1-year intervals.

RITICAL THINKING ACTIVITIES

1. Practice sealant placement on dentiform or extracted teeth.
2. Organize or participate in a dental health fair. Develop pamphlets on dental pit and fissure sealants and caries prevention.
3. Place a sealant on a peer.
4. Develop a table clinic regarding the prevention of decay.
5. Organize and promote elementary school programs regarding sealant education.

 REVIEW QUESTIONS

Question 4 refers to the case study presented at the beginning of the chapter.

1. Proper acid-etch bonding produces which of the following bonds?
   a. Mechanical
   b. Chemical
   c. Both *a* and *b*
   d. None of the above
2. Which of the following best explains the underuse of sealants?
   a. Retention rate of sealants
   b. Fear of caries being buried under sealant
   c. Cost effectiveness of the procedure
   d. All the above
3. A 20-year-old female patient presents to your office for prophylaxis. She is primarily interested in having her teeth polished and requests that you use an air-powder polisher. She has sealants on all her molars and premolars. Which of the following statements is correct regarding air polishing of sealants?
   a. Does not harm pit and fissure sealants provided the power is on a low setting.
   b. Does not result in changes to the sealant surface.
   c. Is safe to use as a cleansing method before sealant placement.
   d. Is not contraindicated for use on resin sealants.
4. Approximately 3 months after Meghan's sealants were placed, none of the sealants were clinically evident. What is the most likely cause for the early loss of these materials?
   a. The etched enamel site was contaminated by oil or by water in the compressed air used for drying.

   b. Light wand was held too closely to the sealant surface.
   c. Sealant was overexposed to light polymerization.
   d. The acid etchant used was at a concentration of 40%.
5. At recall examinations, sealants may have a brown stain along some marginal areas. Which of the following is the cause of this finding?
   a. Inadequate enamel preparation at margin
   b. Contamination of site
   c. Overextension of sealant beyond etched preparation
   d. Occlusal forces producing stress at thin areas of sealant, exceeding bond strength
   e. All the above
6. One year after sealant placement, the dental hygienist's clinical examination reveals that the sealants on #3 and #14 are only partially intact. Both teeth are missing resin from the palatal groove. Which of the following statements is correct to replace the missing areas?
   a. Cleanse with fluoride, then etch, dry, and place the resin sealant.
   b. After scaling, cleanse the area, etch, dry, and apply the resin material.
   c. After scaling and polishing with paste containing fluoride, etch, dry, and place the resin sealant.
   d. Air-polish the entire tooth for 30 seconds, then place the resin sealant.

SUGGESTED AGENCIES AND WEB SITES http:

Because of the ever-changing nature of the Internet, some of the web sites listed here may have changed since publication. Please refer to Mosby's Evolve web site for the most current information.

American Academy of Pediatric Dentistry: http://www.aapd.org
American Dental Association: http://www.ada.org
Centers for Disease Control and Prevention: http://www.cdc.gov
Crest Dental Resource Net: http://www.dentalcare.com
National Institute of Dental and Craniofacial Research: http://www.nidr.nih.gov

National Library of Medicine [U.S.]: http://www.nlm.nih.gov
P&G Dental ResourceNet, Consumer Information ("Care of children's teeth: a guide from Crest"): http://www.dentalcare.com

ADDITIONAL READINGS AND RESOURCES

Arenholt-Bindslev D, Breinholt V, Preiss A, Schmalz G: Time-related bisphenol-A content and estrogenic activity in saliva samples collected in relation to placement of fissure sealants, *Clin Oral Invest* 3(3):120-5, 1999.

Chan DC et al: Evaluation of different methods for cleaning and preparing occlusal fissures, *Oper Dent* 24(6):331-6, 1999.

Croll TP: Simplified resin-based composite sealant, *ASDC J Dent Child* 67(3):182-5, 2000.

Croll TP, Sundfeld RH: Resin-based composite reinforced sealant, *ASDC J Dent Child* 66(4):233-7, 1999.

Deery C: The economic evaluation of pit and fissure sealants, *Int J Paediatr Dent* 9(4):235-41, 1999.

Deery C et al: General dental practitioners' diagnostic and treatment decisions related to fissure sealed surfaces, *J Dent* 28(5):313-8, 2000.

Dennison JB, Straffon LH, Smith RC: Effectiveness of sealant treatment over five years in an insured population, *J Am Dent Assoc* 131(5):597-605, 2000.

De Rego MA, de Araujo MA: Microleakage evaluation of pit and fissure sealants done with different procedures, materials, and laser after invasive technique, *J Clin Pediatr Dent* 24(1):63-8, 1999.

Fung EY et al: Pharmacokinetics of bisphenol-A released from a dental sealant, *J Am Dent Assoc* 131(1):51-8, 2000.

Ganss C, Klimek J, Gleim A: One year clinical evaluation of the retention and quality of two fluoride-releasing sealants, *Clin Oral Invest* 3(4):188-93, 1999.

Geiger SB, Gulayev S, Weiss EI: Improving fissure sealant quality: mechanical preparation and filling level, *J Dent* 28(6):407-12, 2000.

Hickham J: Single-operator sealant placement made easy, *J Am Dent Assoc* 131(8):1175-6, 2000.

Hicks MJ, Westerman GH, Flaitz CM, Powell GL: Surface topography and enamel-resin interface of pit and fissure sealants following visible light and argon laser polymerization: an in vitro study, *ASDC J Dent Child* 67(3):169-75, 2000.

Imai Y: Comments on "Estrogenicity of resin-based composites and sealants used in dentistry," *Environ Health Perspect* 107(6):A290-2, 1999.

Kozai K, Suzuki J, Okada M, Nagasaka N: In vitro study of antibacterial and antiadhesive activities of fluoride-containing light-cured fissure sealants and a glass ionomer liner/base against oral bacteria, *ASDC J Dent Child* 67(2):117-22, 2000.

Kumar JV, Siegal MD: A contemporary perspective on dental sealants, *J Calif Dent Assoc* 26(5):378-85, 1998.

Leinfelder KF: Will pit-and-fissure sealants be improved? *J Am Dent Assoc* 131(8):1185, 2000.

Murray J: Prevalence of dental caries: retrospect and prospect, *Dent Update* 25(9):374-8, 1998.

Rajic Z, Gvozdanovic Z, Rajic-Mestrovic S, Bagic I: Preventive sealing of dental fissures with Heliosil: a two-year follow-up, *Coll Antropol* 24(1):151-5, 2000.

Rethman J: Trends in preventive care: caries risk assessment and indications for sealants, *J Am Dent Assoc* 131(suppl):8S-12S, 2000.

Schafer TE, Lapp CA, Hanes CM, Lewis JB: What parents should know about estrogen-like compounds in dental materials, *Pediatr Dent* 22(1):75-6, 2000.

Schmalz G, Preiss A, Arenholt-Bindslev D: Bisphenol-A content of resin monomers and related degradation products, *Clin Oral Invest* 3(3):114-9, 1999.

Tarumi H et al: Estrogenicity of fissure sealants and adhesive resins determined by reporter gene assay, *J Dent Res* 79(11):1838-43, 2000.

Vrbic V: Retention of a fluoride-containing sealant on primary and permanent teeth 3 years after placement, *Quint Int* 30(12):825-8, 1999.

Werner CW, Pereira AC, Eklund SA: Cost-effectiveness study of a school-based sealant program, *ASDC J Dent Child* 67(2):93-7, 2000.

REFERENCES

1. ADA Council on Access, Prevention, and Interprofessional Relations: Intervention: pit and fissure sealants, *J Am Dent Assoc* 126:17-S, 1995.

2. ADA Council on Access, Prevention, and Interprofessional Relations, Council on Scientific Affairs: Dental sealants, *J Am Dent Assoc* 128(4):485-8, 1997.

3. Anderson KN, Anderson LE: *Mosby's pocket dictionary of medicine,* ed 3, St Louis, 1998, Mosby.

4. Anderson MH: Modern management of dental caries: the cutting edge is not the dental bur, *J Am Dent Assoc* 124(6):36-44, 1993.

5. Anusavice KJ: Treatment regimens in preventive and restorative dentistry, *J Am Dent Assoc* 126:727-43, 1995.

6. Aranda M, Garcia-Godoy F: Clinical evaluation of the retention and wear of a light-cured pit and fissure glass ionomer sealant, *J Clin Pediatr Dent* 19(4):273-7, 1995.

7. Arrow P, Riordan PJ: Retention and caries preventive effects of a GIC and a resin-based fissure sealant, *Community Dent Oral Epidemiol* 23:282-5, 1995.

8. Bayne SC, Thompson JY: Dental materials. In Roberson TM, Heymann HO, Swift EJ: *Sturdevant's art and science of operative dentistry,* ed 4, St Louis, 2001, Mosby.

9. Brockmann SL, Scott RL, Eick JD: A scanning electron microscopic study of the effect of air polishing on the enamel-sealant surface, *Quint Int* 21(3):201-6, 1990.

10. Brown LJ, Kaste LM, Selwitz RH, Furman LJ: Dental caries and sealant usage in U.S. children, 1988-1991: selected findings from the Third National Health and Nutrition Examination Survey, *J Am Dent Assoc* 127(3):335-43, 1996.

11. Brown LJ, Selwitz RH: The impact of recent changes in the epidemiology of dental caries on guidelines for the use of dental sealants, *J Public Health Dent* 55(5 spec):274-91, 1995.

12. Conry JP, Pintado MR, Douglas WH: Quantitative changes in fissure sealant six months after placement, *Pediatr Dent* 12(3):162-7, 1990.

13. Craig RG, Powers JM: *Dental materials: properties and manipulation,* ed 6, St Louis, 1996, Mosby.

14. Craig RG, Powers JM, Wataha JC: *Dental materials: properties and manipulation,* ed 7, St Louis, 2000, Mosby.

15. Dental sealants in the prevention of tooth decay, *NIH Consensus Statement,* 4(11):1-18, 1983.

16. Dickinson GL, Leinfelder KF, Mazer RB, Russell CM: Effect of surface-penetrating sealant on wear rate of posterior composite resins, *J Am Dent Assoc* 121:251-5, 1990.

Continued

17. Dickinson GL, Leinfelder KF: Assessing the long-term effect of a surface-penetrating sealant, *J Am Dent Assoc* 124:68-72, 1993.

18. Ferracane JL: *Materials in dentistry: principles and applications,* Philadelphia, 1995, Lippincott Williams & Wilkins.

19. Forss H, Saarni UM, Seppa L: Comparison of glass-ionomer and resin-based fissure sealants: a 2-year clinical trial, *Community Dent Oral Epidemiol* 22:21-4, 1994.

20. Futatsuki M et al: Early loss of pit and fissure sealant: a clinical and SEM study, *J Clin Pediatr Dent* 19(2):99-104, 1995.

21. Gilpin JL: Pit and fissure sealants: a review of the literature, *J Dent Hyg* 71(4):150-8, 1997.

22. Hamid A, Hume WR: A study of component release from resin pit and fissure sealants in vitro, *Dent Mater* 13:98-102, 1997.

23. Handleman SL, Shey Z: Michael Buonocore and the Eastman Dental Center: a historic perspective on sealants, *J Dent Res* 75(1):529-34, 1996.

24. Handelman SL, Washburn F, Wopperer P: Two-year report of sealant effect on bacteria in dental caries, *J Am Dent Assoc* 93(11):967-70, 1976.

25. Hicks MJ, Silverstone LM: Fissure sealants and dental enamel: a histological study of microleakage in vitro, *Caries Res* 16:353-60, 1982.

26. Houpt M, Fuks A, Eidelman E: The preventive resin (composite resin/sealant) restoration: nine-year results, *Quint Int* 25(3):155-9, 1994.

27. Houpt MI, Santucci E, Fabok J, Fuks AB: Compressive strength of fissure sealant applied over cavities, *Pediatr Dent* 6(3):125-7, 1984.

28. Houpt M, Shey Z: The effectiveness of a fissure sealant after six years, *Pediatr Dent* 5(2):104-6, 1983.

29. Huennekens SC, Daniel SJ, Bayne SC: Effects of air polishing on the abrasion of occlusal sealants, *Quint Int* 22(7):581-5, 1991.

30. Jeronimus DJ, Till MJ, Sveen OB: Reduced viability of microorganisms under dental sealants, *J Dent Child* 42(4):275-80, 1975.

31. Karlzen-Reuterving G, van Dijken JWV: A three-year follow-up of glass ionomer cement and resin fissure sealants, *J Dent Child,* 62:108-10: 1995.

32. Kawai K, Leinfelder KF: Effect of surface-penetrating sealant on composite wear, *Dent Mater* 9(3):108-13, 1993.

33. Kilpatrick NM, Murray JJ, McCabe JF: A clinical comparison of a light-cured glass ionomer sealant restoration with a composite sealant restoration, *J Dent* 24(6):399-405, 1996.

34. Komatsu H, Shimokobe J, Kawakami S, Yoshimura M: Caries-preventive effect of glass ionomer sealant reapplication: study presents three-year results, *J Am Dent Assoc* 125(5):543-9, 1994.

35. Lekka M, Papagiannoulis L, Eliades G: Porosity of pit and fissure sealants, *J Oral Rehabil* 18:213-20, 1991.

36. Mair LH: Wear in dentistry: current terminology, *J Dent* 20(3):140-4, 1992.

37. May KN Jr, Swift EJ Jr, Wilder AD Jr, Futrell SC: Effect of a surface sealant on microleakage of Class V restorations, *Am J Dent* 9:133-6, 1996.

38. McCarthy MF, Hondrum SO: Mechanical and bond strength properties of light-cured and chemically cured glass ionomer cements, *Am J Orthod Dentofac Orthop* 105:135-41, 1994.

39. McLean JW, Wilson AD: Fissure sealing and filling with an adhesive glass-ionomer cement, *Br Dent J* 136(4):269-76, 1974.

40. Mejare I, Mjor IA: Glass ionomer and resin-based fissure sealants: a clinical study, *Scand J Dent Res* 98:345-50, 1990.

41. Mertz-Fairhurst EJ: Current status of sealant retention and caries prevention, *J Dent Educ* 48(2 suppl):18-26, 1984.

42. Mertz-Fairhurst EJ, Schuster GS, Fairhurst CW: Arresting caries by sealants: results of a clinical study, *J Am Dent Assoc* 112:194-7, 1986.

43. Mertz-Fairhurst EJ et al: A comparative clinical study of two pit and fissure sealants: 7 year results in Augusta, GA, *J Am Dent Assoc* 109:252-5, 1984.

44. Mertz-Fairhurst EJ et al: Sealed restorations: 4-year results, *Am J Dent* 4:43-9, 1991.

45. Mertz-Fairhurst EJ et al: Cariostatic and ultraconservative sealed restorations: six-year results, *Quint Int* 23:827-38, 1992.

46. Mertz-Fairhurst EJ et al: Cariostatic and ultraconservative sealed restorations: nine-year results among children and adults, *J Dent Child,* 62:97-107, 1995.

47. Mertz-Fairhurst EJ et al: Ultraconservative and cariostatic sealed restorations: results at year 10, *J Am Dent Assoc* 129(1):55-66, 1998.

48. Moore BK, Winkler MM, Ewoldsen N: Laboratory testing of light-cured glass ionomers as pit-and-fissure sealants, *Gen Dent* 43:176-80, 1995.

49. Nathanson D et al: In vitro elution of leachable components from dental sealants, *J Am Dent Assoc* 128:1517-23, 1997.

50. Olea N et al: Estrogenicity of resin-based composites and sealants used in dentistry, *Environ Health Perspect* 104:298-305, 1996.

51. Olio F: Biodegradation of dental composites/glass-ionomer cements, *Adv Dent Res* 6:50-4, 1992.

52. Ovrebo RC, Raadal M: Microleakage in fissures sealed with resin or glass ionomer cement, *Scand J Dent Res* 98:66-9, 1990.

53. Phillips RW, Moore BK: *Elements of dental materials for dental hygienists and dental assistants,* ed 5, Philadelphia, 1994, WB Saunders.

54. Pintado MR, Conry JP, Douglas WH: Fissure sealant wear at 30 months: new evaluation criteria, *J Dent* 19:33-8, 1991.

55. Pope BD, Garcia-Godoy F, Summitt JB, Chan DDCN: Effectiveness of occlusal fissure cleansing methods and sealant micromorphology, *J Dent Child,* 63:175-80, 1996.

56. Reid JS, Saunders WP, Chen YY: The effect of bonding agent and fissure sealant on microleakage of composite resin restorations, *Quint Int* 22(4):295-8, 1991.

57. Ripa LW: Sealants revisited: an update of the effectiveness of pit-and-fissure sealants, *Caries Res* 27(suppl 1):77-82, 1993.

58. Ripa LW: The current status of pit-and-fissure sealants: a review, *J Can Dent Assoc* 51:367-80, 1985.

59. Roberson TM, Heymann HO, Swift EJ: *Sturdevant's art and science of operative dentistry,* ed 4, St Louis, 2001, Mosby.

60. Rock WP, Foulkes EE, Perry J, Smith AJ: A comparative study of fluoride-releasing composite resin and glass ionomer materials used as fissure sealants, *J Dent* 24(4):275-80, 1996.

61. Romcke RG, Lewis DW, Maze BD, Vickerson RA: Retention and maintenance of fissure sealants over 10 years, *J Can Dent Assoc* 56(3):235-7, 1990.

62. Rozier RG: The impact of recent changes in the epidemiology of dental caries on guidelines for the use of dental sealants, *J Public Health Dent* 55(5 spec):292-301, 1995.

63. Ruse ND: Xenoestrogenicity and dental materials, *J Can Dent Assoc* 63(11):833-6, 1997.

64. Ryan JP: The clinical benefits of dental sealants, *J Pract Hyg,* 6:13-7, 1997.

65. Scott L, Brockmann S, Houston G, Tira D: Retention of dental sealants following the use of air polishing and traditional cleaning, *Dent Hyg,* 62:402-6, 1988.

66. Selwitz RH, Winn DM, Kingman A, Zion GR: The prevalence of dental sealants in the U.S. population: findings from NHANES III, 1988-1991, *J Dent Res* 75:652-60, 1996.

67. Sidhu SK, Watson TF: Resin-modified glass ionomer materials: a status report, *Am J Dent* 8(1):59-67, 1995.

68. Simonsen RJ: Glass ionomer as fissure sealant: a critical review, *J Public Health Dent* 56(3 spec):146-9, 1996.

69. Simonsen RJ: Retention and effectiveness of dental sealant after 15 years, *J Am Dent Assoc* 122:34-42, 1991.

70. Simonsen RJ: Retention and effectiveness of a single application of white sealant after 10 years, *J Am Dent Assoc* 115(7):31-6, 1987.

71. Soderholm KM: The impact of recent changes in the epidemiology of dental caries on guidelines for the use of dental sealants: clinical perspectives, *J Public Health Dent* 55(5 [Special]):302-11, 1995.

72. Soderholm K, Mariotti AL: BIS-GMA–based resins in dentistry: are they safe? *J Am Dent Assoc* 130(2):201-9, 1999.

73. Souto M, Donly KJ: Caries inhibition of glass ionomers, *Am J Dent* 7(2):122-4, 1994.

74. Stadtler P: A 3-year clinical study of a hybrid composite resin as fissure sealant and as restorative material for Class I restorations, *Quint Int* 23:759-62, 1992.

75. Swift EJ Jr: The effect of sealants on dental caries: a review, *J Am Dent Assoc* 116(6):700-4, 1988.

76. Tjan AHL, Tan DE: Microleakage at gingival margins of Class V composite resin restorations rebonded with various low-viscosity resin systems, *Quint Int* 22(7): 65-73, 1991.

77. Waggoner WF, Siegal M: Pit-and-fissure sealant application: updating the technique, *J Am Dent Assoc* 127:351-61, 1996.

78. Weintraub JA: The effectiveness of pit-and-fissure sealants, *J Public Health Dent* 49(5):317-30, 1989.

79. Williams KB et al: Oral health–related quality of life: a model for dental hygiene, *J Dent Hyg* 72(2):19-26, 1998.

80. Winkler MM et al: Using a resin-modified glass ionomer as an occlusal sealant: a one-year clinical study, *J Am Dent Assoc* 127(10):1508-14, 1996.

81. Workshop on Guidelines for Sealant Use: Recommendations, *J Public Health Dent* 55(5 [Special]):263-73, 1995.

CHAPTER 27

Prevention *and* Emergency Management *of* Dental Trauma

Dennis N. Ranalli, Deborah Studen-Pavlovich

Chapter Outline

Case Study: Sports-Related Dental Trauma
Epidemiology
Developmental Etiology
Sports-Related Injury
   Risk assessment
   Predictive index
   Assessment of the trauma patient
   Dental evaluation of the trauma patient
Emergency Management of Dental Trauma
   Crown fracture
   Root fracture
   Luxation injury
   Avulsed teeth
   Mandibular fracture
   Soft tissue injury

Child Abuse and Neglect
   Historical perspective
   Definitions
   Demographic factors
   Evaluation of abuse
   Documentation and reporting
Prevention of Sports-Related Injury
   Mouthguards
Strategies for the Dental Hygienist
   Domestic violence
   Malpractice and abuse allegations
   Sports dentistry
   Community activities

Key Terms

Apexifiction
Apexogenesis
Avulsed tooth
Battered child syndrome

Child abuse
Crown elongation
Dental neglect
Incidence

Luxation
Mouthguards
Neglect

Orofacial trauma
Prevalence
Triage

Learning Outcomes

1. Discuss the epidemiology and etiology of dental trauma.
2. Perform appropriate physical and oral assessments of traumatized dental patients.
3. Describe appropriate protocols for emergency management or referral of patients with dental injuries.
4. Outline proper documentation for traumatized dental patients.

5. Understand strategies for the prevention of orofacial trauma, with particular emphasis on child abuse and sports-related dental injuries.
6. Identify risk prone behaviors and profiles for dental trauma.
7. Understand the child protection mandates and laws.

ental hygienists have been at the forefront in their efforts to promote the prevention of dental caries and periodontal diseases. Despite recent evidence that indicates almost one fourth of the U.S. population has experienced a traumatic dental episode to an anterior tooth, prevention of dental trauma has received little emphasis by the dental team. This chapter presents specific concepts to assist the dental hygienist in incorporating strategies for the prevention of dental trauma into a comprehensive program. The discussion focuses on the diagnosis and emergency management of dental injuries in children and adolescents. The emphasis is on the prevention, recognition, and reporting of *orofacial trauma* associated with child abuse and neglect, as well as the prediction, treatment, and prevention of sports-related dental injuries. Dental hygienists can help expand the scope of trauma prevention from the private practice setting into community activities to reach larger segments of the at-risk population.

EPIDEMIOLOGY

Traumatic dental injuries pose serious consequences, not only in terms of the pain, suffering, and financial burdens associated with emergency management and long-term treatment but also as a significant dental public health issue. One study of a large sample population reported that nearly one quarter (24.9%) of the U.S. population between 6 and 50 years of age had experienced dental trauma to one or more anterior teeth. The study confirmed that maxillary anterior teeth were more prone to injury than their mandibular counterparts. Also, males were more prone to dental injuries than females by a ratio of 1.5 to 1.0. No racial or ethnic factors were found to be significant when considering such injuries.[26]

Evaluation of this type of data from the scientific dental literature requires clarification of two terms that are often misused—incidence and prevalence. These terms are 27-A sometimes used interchangeably but have different meanings. *Incidence* refers to the number of new cases of trauma that occur during a specific time interval. *Prevalence* refers to the number of cases of trauma that exist at a given moment in time. Thus the information presented in the previous example represents trauma prevalence data.

DEVELOPMENTAL ETIOLOGY

The developmental etiology of traumatic dental injuries varies according to the patient's chronological age, level of activity, and state of maturity. For example, the most frequent and often devastating type of trauma to the primary dentition is the intrusive *luxation* of a primary anterior tooth (Fig. 27-1). Toddlers who are learning to walk are especially prone to intrusive luxations because primary anterior teeth are small and immature alveolar bone is relatively soft. Conversely, the most frequent type of dental injury to the permanent dentition is a crown fracture, because permanent anterior teeth are larger and mature alveolar bone is denser (Fig. 27-2). Dental injuries associated with child abuse are more likely in the primary dentition of young children, whereas sports-related trauma is more likely in the mixed or permanent dentitions of adolescents and young adults.

The developmental period between the primary and the permanent dentition phases is a time of significant change as a growing child progresses through the adolescent years toward adulthood. During these developmental periods the resorption and exfoliation of the primary teeth are accompanied by the timing and sequence of eruption of the permanent teeth until the adult dental occlusion has been established. The child first progresses from the primary dentition to the mixed dentition. The "ugly duckling" stage is the period from the eruption of the permanent lateral incisors to the eruption of the

Sports-Related Dental Trauma

Tonya Washington, a 16-year-old junior point guard, will be starting in her first high-school varsity basketball game. In her excitement about the upcoming competition, Tonya is focused and intense during the last practice before the start of the season. Tonya dribbles the ball down court and sees an opening for a shot. She stops and takes a jump shot from the top of the key. Tonya follows the shot to the basket and leaps for the rebound when the ball glances off the rim. As she comes down with the ball, the elbow of a taller teammate strikes Tonya in the mouth. Tonya is not wearing a mouthguard.

Tonya's right maxillary permanent central incisor is completely knocked out of the socket from the force of the trauma in a lingual to labial direction. The tooth flies out of Tonya's mouth and skids across the floor. Tonya drops down to her knees, hands clutching her mouth, as blood oozes from between her fingers and drips onto the floor. The coach rushes over to Tonya with ice wrapped in a towel and applies the compress over Tonya's mouth. Her teammates search for Tonya's *avulsed tooth* and find it under the team bench. The coach takes Tonya into the locker room and contacts Tonya's mother to inform her about the accident and to advise her to contact Tonya's dentist for an emergency appointment as soon as possible.

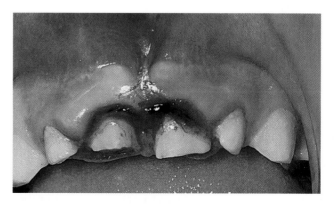

FIG. 27-1 Intrusive luxation of maxillary primary central incisors.

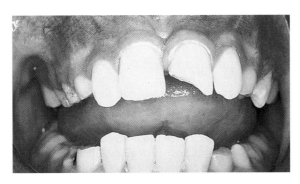

FIG. 27-2 Enamel-dentin fracture of maxillary left permanent central incisor.

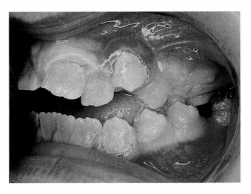

FIG. 27-4 Accident-prone dental profile in patient with marked gingival inflammation and dentinogenesis imperfecta.

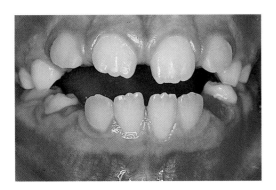

FIG. 27-3 "Ugly duckling" stage of mixed dentition.

permanent canines (Fig. 27-3). During this stage, unaesthetic space may develop between the maxillary permanent central incisors, and the crowns of the maxillary permanent lateral incisors may flare. When the maxillary permanent canines do erupt, anterior spacing generally closes, and tooth alignment becomes more aesthetic.

Other factors, such as genetics, tooth size, arch length, skeletal growth, and oral habits, also contribute to the ultimate occlusion in the adult permanent dentition. *Occlusion* can be classified broadly as Class I, II, or III based on the molar relationship of the maxillary permanent first molar to the mandibular permanent first molar. *Class I molar relationship* is characterized by the mesial cusp of the maxillary permanent first molar in occlusal alignment with the buccal groove of the mandibular permanent first molar. *Class II molar relationship* is characterized by the occlusion of the mesial cusp of the maxillary permanent first molar anterior to the buccal groove of the mandibular permanent first molar. This type of molar relationship may be accompanied by protrusion of the maxillary anterior teeth with lack of a protective lip seal. This situation is known as an *accident-prone dental profile* and places the patient at greater risk for dental injury (Fig. 27-4). Conversely, *Class III molar relationship* is characterized by the mesial cusp of the maxillary permanent first molar positioned posterior to the buccal groove of the mandibular permanent first molar. When a Class III molar relationship is accompanied by a protruding mandible, the mandibular arch is more vulnerable to dental trauma.

27-B

In summary, a variety of factors, including age, gender, occlusal development, vulnerability to abusive behavior, and level of activity (e.g., learning to walk, participating in sports), place an individual at risk for a traumatic dental injury.

SPORTS-RELATED INJURY

RISK ASSESSMENT

The dental hygienist is in a key position to identify patients who may be at risk for sustaining sports-related dental trauma. In addition to questions related to brushing, flossing, and dietary habits on the dental intake form, the dental hygienist should include the question, "Do you (Does your child) participate in sports?" A positive response allows a detailed discussion of the type of sport, level of participation, and appropriate recommendations for protective athletic equipment.[50]

PREDICTIVE INDEX

To better enable clinicians to determine the likelihood of a patient experiencing a sports-related dental injury, a predictive index has been developed.[22] The predictive index is based on a defined set of risk factors, as discussed previously. The index identifies risk factors in eight categories: (1) demographic information (e.g., age, gender, dental occlusion), (2) type and use of protective equipment, (3) velocity and intensity of the sport, (4) level of activity and exposure time, (5) level of coaching and type of sports organization, (6) player position in a contact or noncontact sport, (7) history of sports-related dental trauma, and (8) practice or game situation. An analysis of these factors can be used to identify an athlete who is at high risk for an orofacial injury and, more importantly, to recommend specific prevention strategies, such as a properly fitted athletic mouthguard.

ASSESSMENT OF THE TRAUMA PATIENT

Physical Assessment

Before initiation of dental treatment, it is essential to determine the physical status of the trauma victim. The dental injury may be relatively minor compared with a serious

27-

head injury. Thus the patient should undergo individual *triage* so that the most serious problems are prioritized for immediate attention. As a first priority the need for basic life support must be determined. Any life-threatening injury requires activation of the local emergency medical services system. Patients should be observed for signs of shock, and when required, airway management, breathing, and circulation (ABCs) must be maintained until help arrives.[8]

If a *concussion* is suspected, a rapid neurological assessment can be performed, including eye opening, verbal response, and motor responses. As with victims who have sustained other serious head injuries, patients with suspected concussions must be referred immediately to appropriate medical personnel.[19,27] Trauma patients with *seizure disorders* should be observed carefully before initiation of emergency dental treatment. The most recent dose of antiseizure medication should be determined. For trauma patients with *cardiac disease,* such as rheumatic and valvular conditions, antibiotics are required according to the American Heart Association guidelines for prevention of subacute bacterial (infective) endocarditis.[9] To avoid serious postoperative bleeding episodes or severe infections, patients with bleeding tendencies, those taking anticoagulant medication, and immunocompromised patients must be identified so that appropriate preoperative adjustments can be made.

Any drug allergies or current medications should be noted to prevent untoward reactions. Tetanus immunization status should be determined because many dental injuries involve intraoral blood and saliva. Appropriate referral to a physician for a tetanus booster within 48 hours of the accident should be made if the last dose of tetanus toxoid was administered more than 5 years ago. Antibiotic coverage and tetanus immunization status are important considerations in this chapter's sports dentistry case study.

Health History

A trauma victim who is new to the dental practice requires a complete health history, including vital statistics and vital signs. Current patients should already have a completed record and may require only an update of the health history and reassessment of blood pressure and pulse.

Before initiation of intraoral trauma evaluation procedures and treatment, *universal precautions* must be implemented to prevent the spread of infectious diseases through blood and body fluids.

DENTAL EVALUATION OF THE TRAUMA PATIENT

Accident History

Trauma is never convenient, so the dental office should be "trauma-ready" and receptive to patients with emergency dental needs.[2] The dental team members should keep in mind that a traumatic episode may be a child's first visit to the dental office. In addition, dental professionals also must recognize their legal and ethical responsibilities to patients of record.

The circumstances of the accident are noted, including how, when, and where the accident occurred. The time in-

terval between the accident and the initiation of treatment is especially important; the shorter the interval, the better the prognosis. Delays in treatment of traumatic dental injuries will adversely affect long-term outcome.

A previous history of dental trauma can help to distinguish between past and recent injuries. This differentiation is an important aspect in establishing an appropriate treatment plan. Repetitive patterned injuries also may raise the suspicion of child abuse or other forms of domestic violence.

Subjective symptoms reported by the patient can help the clinician establish a diagnosis. For example, dental sensitivity to touch, air, and cold might indicate a vital tooth with a dentin or pulp exposure. Conversely, sensitivity to percussion, mastication, and heat might indicate a tooth with periapical infection.

Intraoral Examination

The visual examination identifies the type and extent of the injury. *Transillumination* of the tooth can reveal cracks within an intact crown or pulpal hemorrhage into dental tubules. Caution should be exercised when considering palpation of a traumatized tooth. *Palpation* can assist the clinician to determine the degree of mobility of an intact tooth within the socket, the presence of a root fracture, or an alveolar bone segment fracture. *Percussion* of a recently traumatized tooth should be avoided because it adds little diagnostic information and may only exacerbate the existing trauma. *Vitality tests* for teeth are nondefinitive after recent trauma and should be postponed for several weeks to prevent further damage to the traumatized tooth.

Radiographic Examination

The type and extent of the radiographic examination depend on the age of the patient and the severity of the accident. Because of medicolegal and insurance reasons, it is advisable to expose double-pack film so that an original radiograph may be retained in the patient record.

The special concern with children's primary dentition is not only the condition of the traumatized primary anterior teeth but also the status of the underlying, developing permanent successors. Radiographic interpretation of trauma to primary teeth should include the presence of crown fractures, root fractures, or displacements, as well as the position and stage of root development of the underlying permanent incisors (Fig. 27-5).

In a young patient's permanent dentition the traumatized area should be evaluated radiographically for crown fractures, root fractures, displacements, and degree of root end closure, as well as alveolar bone fractures and the location of tooth fragments or foreign debris. Some patients should have a radiograph of the teeth in the opposing dental arch. Suspected maxillary or mandibular fractures may require panoramic or cephalometric radiographs. Patients also may be referred for computed tomography (CT) scans and magnetic resonance imaging (MRI) as needed.

Treatment Plan

Based on the health history and the clinical and radiographic examinations, the dentist is ready to establish a

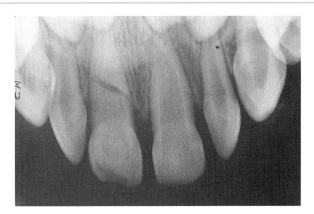

FIG. 27-5 Middle-one-third root fracture of maxillary right primary central incisor. Note the underlying, developing permanent teeth.

diagnosis and develop an appropriate treatment plan to maintain the traumatized tooth. Even minor dental trauma, however, may result in pulpal necrosis or tooth loss in the future. This information must be explained to the patient (or parent) and documented in the progress notes of the chart to indicate informed consent.

EMERGENCY MANAGEMENT OF DENTAL TRAUMA

For the purposes of this chapter, emergency management is described in terms of crown fractures, root fractures, luxation injuries, avulsed teeth, mandibular fractures, and soft tissue trauma.

CROWN FRACTURE

Enamel Only

Crown fractures that involve only the enamel usually are not painful and often are unnoticed by the patient. The fractured enamel may feel rough to the tongue. Enamel-only fractures are often discovered by the dental hygienist during a routine dental examination (Fig. 27-6). Minimal enamel fractures in both the primary and the permanent incisors may be aesthetically recontoured, followed by topical fluoride application.

Enamel and Dentin

Crown fractures involving the enamel and dentin are sensitive to air, touch, and cold. They have sharp edges and are unaesthetic (see Fig. 27-6). Emergency management of vital primary and permanent enamel-dentin fractures includes placement of a calcium hydroxide pulp-protecting medicament, followed by an acid-etched composite resin bandage or restoration.

Enamel, Dentin, and Pulp

Crown fractures that involve the enamel, dentin, and pulpal tissues of vital teeth represent a complex array of diagnostic and treatment possibilities[20] (see Fig. 27-6). In the

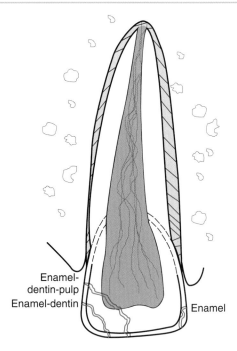

FIG. 27-6 Crown fractures: enamel only, enamel-dentin, enamel-dentin-pulp.

permanent dentition a vital pulp exposure of a tooth with a closed apex may be treated with a direct pulp cap and calcium hydroxide, followed by an acid-etched composite resin restoration. In a vital permanent tooth with an open apex, continued physiological root formation should be stimulated through *apexogenesis*, a calcium hydroxide pulpotomy technique. For a nonvital permanent tooth with a closed apex, conventional root canal therapy is indicated. A nonvital permanent tooth with an open apex requires *apexification*, a procedure to induce calcific root end closure.

Crown fractures involving the enamel, dentin, and pulp of primary anterior teeth are treated with a formocresol pulpotomy if the primary tooth is vital or with a pulpectomy sealed with resorbable paste if the primary tooth is nonvital. The final restoration may be either an acid-etched composite resin restoration or an aesthetic strip crown in more extensive fractures.

ROOT FRACTURE

Apical One-Third

If a root fracture occurs in the apical one third of a primary or permanent anterior tooth and there is no mobility, the tooth should be observed clinically and radiographically at recall appointments for signs of root healing (Fig. 27-7). Adverse sequelae, such as a widening of the periodontal ligament (PDL) space or periapical pathosis, must also be evaluated.

Middle One-Third

If the segments of a middle-one-third root fracture of a permanent tooth are displaced, the segments should be

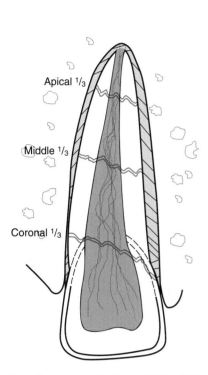

FIG. 27-7 Root fractures: apical one-third, middle one-third, coronal one-third.

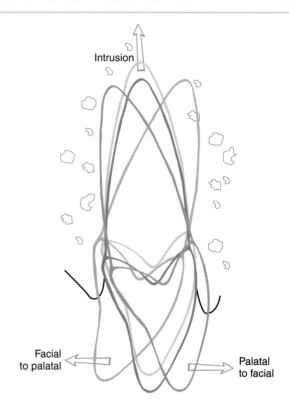

FIG. 27-8 Luxation injuries: intrusion, facial to palatal, palatal to facial.

repositioned and splinted for approximately 12 to 16 weeks (see Fig. 27-7). The patient's oral hygiene is critical while the acid-etched composite resin splint is in place. The dental hygienist should provide specific home care instructions for proper maintenance of the soft tissues surrounding the injured tooth as well as tissues in proximity to the splint. Chlorhexidine gluconate rinses may be beneficial for reducing the oral microflora.[17]

Coronal One-Third

Fractures of the root at the coronal one third are the most difficult to manage (see Fig. 27-7). Treatment may include root canal therapy, periodontal *crown elongation,* or orthodontic extrusion of the remaining root, usually followed by a post, core, and crown as a final restoration. Coronal-one-third root fractures often require extraction and prosthodontic replacement of the lost tooth.

Middle and coronal root fractures in primary teeth should be treated simply. If stable, the root segment should not be probed because probing may damage the underlying permanent tooth. The primary root fragment should eventually resorb.[37]

LUXATION INJURY

Primary and permanent teeth may be displaced in a lateral, intrusive, or extrusive direction (Fig. 27-8). The major concern with luxated primary teeth is possible damage to the underlying, developing permanent successor. Dis-

placed permanent teeth should be repositioned and splinted for approximately 2 weeks. Antibiotics may be prescribed, and meticulous oral hygiene procedures (as for middle-one-third root fractures) should be used for displaced, splinted permanent anterior teeth. The major concern with luxated permanent teeth is maintaining the viability of the PDL cells and preventing external root resorption.

AVULSED TEETH

Primary teeth that have been completely luxated out of the alveolar socket should not be reimplanted. Permanent teeth that have been avulsed should be reimplanted as soon as possible to maintain the viability of the PDL cells that remain on the cementum of the root (Fig. 27-9). The tooth should be splinted in place for approximately 2 weeks, antibiotics prescribed, and meticulous oral hygiene procedures followed. The longer the tooth remains outside the socket, the poorer the prognosis, due to subsequent external root resorption.

Case Application
What do you think might be the prognosis for Tonya?

The patient (or parent), school nurse, or coach should be instructed to reimplant the tooth as quickly as possible at the scene of the accident. Often, however, this can be an unrealistic expectation. As an alternative, the avulsed tooth should be placed in some type of solution for transport to the dental office or hospital emergency room. The

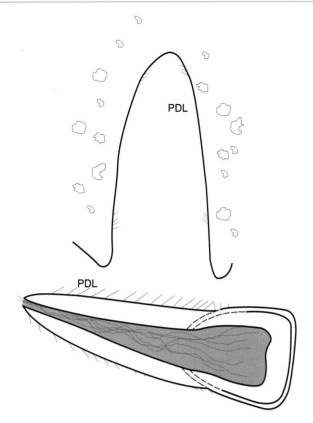

FIG. 27-9 Avulsed tooth. *PDL,* Periodontal ligament.

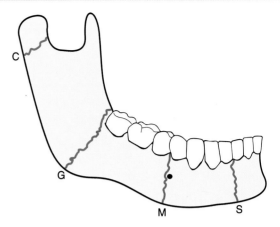

FIG. 27-10 Mandibular fractures. *C,* Condyle; *G,* gonial angle; *M,* mental foramen; *S,* symphysis.

tooth should not be transported in a dry gauze or paper towel. Liquids used for tooth transport, from most effective to least effective, include Hank's solution, milk, saline, saliva, and water.[4,29]

MANDIBULAR FRACTURE

Fracture to the mandible may occur at the condyle, gonial angle, mental foramen region, or mandibular symphysis (Fig. 27-10). If the fracture is displaced, the patient will be unable to occlude the teeth in a normal manner. Emergency management includes the removal of any intraoral debris to maintain the airway. The patient should be transported to a hospital emergency room (ER) for further evaluation and treatment.

SOFT TISSUE INJURY

Emergency management for soft tissue lacerations includes hemorrhage control, wound cleansing, suturing, and antibiotics as required. Tetanus immunization status should be reviewed.

CHILD ABUSE AND NEGLECT

 HISTORICAL PERSPECTIVE

27-D Child abuse and neglect are not new phenomena but recently have received heightened awareness because of educational programs for healthcare professionals and the general public. Severe punishment of children, infanti-

cide, and ritualistic killings have been reported in many cultures for thousands of years.

The Case of Mary Ellen

The first reported case of child abuse in the United States occurred in 1874 in New York City.[10] Mary Ellen, a 9-year-old girl, was being brutally beaten by her foster parents. At that time, no laws or organizations protected children from parents and guardians or provided removal of children from abusive homes. The social worker who rescued Mary Ellen was forced to have her declared an "animal" so that she could be protected under the auspices of the American Society for the Prevention of Cruelty to Animals (ASPCA). This early effort led to the beginning of the child protection movement in America and the founding of the first Society for the Prevention of Cruelty to Children in 1875 in New York City.

In the early 1900s, activist groups began to condemn many labor practices in factories, textile mills, and coal mines. Through their efforts the National Children's Bureau (NCB) was established in 1912 to provide information, resources, training, and legislation to child advocacy organizations. The creation of the NCB was the first time that the federal government officially recognized the need to protect children. Within several years the bureau succeeded in protecting children working in factories and coal mines by lobbying successfully for the passage of the Keating-Owen Act of 1916.[10]

Battered Child Syndrome

In 1961, Henry Kempe, a Colorado physician, used the term *battered child syndrome* to describe children with numerous unexplained injuries and to characterize child abuse as a diagnosable condition. The term became accepted by the courts as admissible evidence in child abuse cases and strengthened the court's ability to prosecute these cases successfully.[28]

Legislative Efforts

In 1962, states began to mandate child-abuse reporting, and by 1965 all 50 states had some laws for reporting child abuse. During the next decade, additional laws on the reporting of child abuse were developed. These laws defined those persons who would be required to report suspected cases of child abuse, designated as *mandated reporters*.[10] In 1974 the Child Abuse Prevention and Treatment Act (CAPTA) addressed many of the previous problems that interfered with protecting children. The act defined the terms *child abuse* and *neglect* for all states. Training programs for child welfare professionals were funded and financial incentives provided for states to implement child abuse and neglect awareness programs.

Currently, every state has laws that define child abuse and neglect, reporting mechanisms, and intervention protocols. The states' child protective services are responsible for investigating suspected child maltreatment and providing foster care for child safety.[21] Unfortunately, demand is much greater than the services that can be provided.

DEFINITIONS

Child abuse and neglect include various types of experiences that may be dangerous or life threatening to the child. The American Academy of Pediatric Dentistry[3] defines **child abuse** as physical or mental injury, sexual abuse, or negligent treatment of a child under age 18 by a person responsible for the child's welfare under circumstances that might indicate the child's health or welfare is harmed or threatened. *Neglect* refers to the condition in which any child under age 18 lacks adequate food, clothing, medical or dental care, supervision, or other essential care. **Dental neglect** is "willful failure of parent or guardian to seek and follow through with treatment necessary to ensure a level of oral health essential for adequate function and freedom from pain and infection."[3] These three definitions provide the dental team with parameters to identify the different types of child abuse and neglect that may be evident at the dental appointment.

DEMOGRAPHIC FACTORS

Children from all socioeconomic strata may be victims of child abuse or neglect, but the actual incidence remains unknown. Although professionals as mandated reporters are more aware of the problem, reluctance to report is still a concern. Approximately 50% to 65% of reported cases are neglect; 25% are physical abuse. Sexual abuse and emotional abuse constitute the majority of the remaining 10% to 25% of cases.[36] Often, children who are victims of one type of abuse may also be victims of other forms of abuse.

Although reported at all socioeconomic levels, child abuse and neglect are disproportionately higher among poor families, whether from poverty-related conditions or increased scrutiny by public agencies.[33] No significant correlation between race and the incidence, type, or severity of child abuse and neglect was identified in two national studies.[11] The greater proportion of abused children from minority families may be attributed to a higher rate of investigations in lower-income groups compared with more affluent families.

Children with disabilities are abused at twice the rate as children without disabilities.[49] Disabled children may be more vulnerable to abuse when parents become frustrated with the child's limitations. Also, the disabled child may be unable to express what has happened, so the details of the abuse remain unknown.

Demographic characteristics vary depending on the type of abuse or neglect. An estimated 3 million children were reported as abused or neglected in the United States in 1994, and 2000 children die annually from abuse.[34] The average age of the maltreated child is 7.4 years, although younger children are more susceptible to abuse because of parental reaction to behaviors associated with certain developmental stages, inability to escape from an angry parent, and defenselessness.[44]

Certain family situations also may contribute to child abuse and neglect, including substance abuse, stress, domestic violence, female-headed households, and families without support systems.[10] It is estimated that one third of persons who were physically abused or neglected as children will abuse or neglect their own children. Thus child abuse may be a learned behavior that becomes a cycle within a family. Although risk factors must be considered, every child is a potential victim.

EVALUATION OF ABUSE

Because about 65% of the cases of physical abuse are associated with craniofacial trauma (head, neck, and mouth), the dental team will likely treat patients who have been abused or currently are victims of abuse.[36] The dentist and dental hygienist must be receptive to a diagnosis of possible child abuse and neglect in order for it to be identified, reported, and substantiated properly. Identification may be aided by (1) a thorough medical history, (2) observation of the child's behavior with and without the parent or guardian, and (3) physical examination. Careful examination of appropriate body surfaces (e.g., head, neck, face, mouth) and documentation with appropriate radiographs and photographs are essential in all cases of suspected abuse.

Health History

The health history will help to determine whether the oral condition is the result of abuse or neglect, systemic disease, or accidental injury. Questions should include how and when the injury occurred. The dental team should indicate whether (1) the child has been similarly injured on several occasions in the past; (2) the child has a history of repeated hospitalizations, particularly at different sites; or (3) the parent or guardian has delayed seeking treatment. Details regarding any trauma should be complete and obtained from both the child and the parent or guardian. The dental team should be alert to discrepancies in the interview and history when the injury does not match the explanation. For example, an infant who is unable to walk is unlikely to have sustained a fractured femur from crawling.

Behavioral Observations

Specific behavioral changes may be attributed to child abuse and neglect. The child may react inappropriately to stimuli, such as invasion of personal space when the dental hygienist attempts to examine the child's dentition.

Also, the child may not make eye contact and may demonstrate fear of touch. The parent or guardian may be hostile, either blaming or claiming that the child is "different" or is a troublemaker. The child may state that the parent is responsible for an injury. Generally, if younger children accuse someone, it is usually the truth. In another type of reaction the child may not volunteer information for fear of repeated injury by the caregiver or separation from the family. Every child is unique, so the clinician must evaluate the child's behavior compared with that of children of similar maturity given a similar set of circumstances. When the dentist or the dental hygienist cannot find an adequate explanation for these types of behavior, child abuse and neglect should be suspected.

Physical Assessment

The physical status of the child tends to be a more objective measure than behavioral indicators of child abuse and neglect. Factors to consider include whether the child is dirty, is inappropriately dressed for the season, or has unexplained injuries. The child's general appearance may indicate the type of care provided by the parent or guardian. A child with a persistent skin disorder may not be receiving proper hygiene. Children who come to the dental office wearing a long-sleeved shirt in the summer may be concealing intentional trauma caused by an adult. Children dressed inadequately for cold weather may be victims of neglect at home. An assessment of overall appearance (posture, gait, clothing) should be performed routinely for every child entering the treatment room.

Injury Patterns

Because physical abuse generally leaves noticeable evidence, this form of child abuse is more easily recognized.[46] However, the dentist and the dental hygienist should not assume that all traumatic physical injuries are a result of abuse. Active children do experience normal bruising, and the dental team needs to be familiar with the usual sites of bumps and bruises. Typical sites for bruising are the bony protuberances, including the forehead, chin, elbows, hands, knees, and shins. Because of limited fat available to cushion them, these parts of the body may be more susceptible to injury. On the other hand, if a child exhibits bruising on the backs of the legs, abuse should be suspected; children generally injure themselves by running into objects, not backing into them. Likewise, an infant who is brought to the dental office with a black eye is most likely a victim of abuse.

Often in abuse, children are struck by objects that leave distinctive marks with recognizable injury patterns.[45] For example, a belt will leave a distinct mark where the strap or buckle struck the skin. Other objects used for discipline, such as hairbrushes, wooden spoons, coat hangers, electrical cords, and rulers, may also leave identifiable marks. The dental professional should examine the shape of the mark to see whether it resembles a known household object that may have been used to inflict the injury (Fig. 27-11).

While examining the shape of the mark, the dentist or dental hygienist should observe the color of the bruise to determine its age. Bruises in various stages of healing should alert the dental professional to possible abuse. Rate of healing depends on severity, location, depth, and amount of

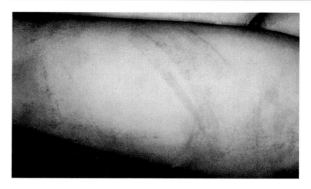

FIG. 27-11 Physical abuse of child. Note injury pattern resulting from a belt.

bleeding into the tissues.[45] Recording information in the progress notes on the color and age of bruises will help the clinician to document the suspicion of child abuse.

Inflicted Burns

Inflicted burns are another manifestation of physical abuse that may be observed during the general assessment of the child. Burns are involved in about 10% of physical abuse cases and are classified into three categories: immersion, pattern, and splash. *Immersion burns* are caused by placing a body part, typically the buttocks, feet, or hands, into a very hot liquid.[31] *Pattern burns,* such as cigarette or lighter burns, have an identifying pattern and are usually symmetrical and well defined. *Splash burns* occur when a hot liquid is poured over or thrown at a child. These burns tend to be more severe closer to the craniofacial complex and to become less severe toward the lower body because the liquid loses heat running down the skin.[31] Often, splash burns are accidental because curious children may pull hot liquids from a surface and onto themselves. The dental team should question the child on how the burn occurred to determine whether child abuse should be suspected.

The preceding descriptions of traumatic injuries and conditions are indicators that should alert the dental professional to suspect child abuse. The dental team then must decide whether the injury was accidental, self-inflicted, or an intentional assault by an adult.

Dental Evaluation of Perioral Structures

After completion of the general physical assessment, the dental professional should examine the perioral structures. Because most injuries from child abuse cases occur to the region of the head, neck, and mouth, the dental team is ideally suited to detect these cases. A thorough examination of the hard and soft tissues of the perioral structures may help to document and substantiate suspected cases of child abuse.

Soft Tissue Assessment

In child abuse the face is injured more often than any other part of the body.[13] Ready access to the face by the abuser and the psychological importance of the face and mouth for communication and nutrition are probable reasons. The cheeks are injured most often, followed by the eyes, ears, nose, and lips.[13] Bruises on the ears, especially bilaterally, are rarely accidental. The ears become injured from pinching or pulling, making them bruised or swollen.

The dental team can detect all these injuries if a thorough general assessment of the child is performed. Clinicians should inquire about any visible wounds, examine any exposed skin, and document the findings of possible traumatic assault in the progress notes of the chart. Identification of these injuries in the office may prevent further harm to the child at home.

Recognition of abusive injuries on the lips is usually easy to detect. Burns may originate from heated objects or cigarettes, and lacerations at the corners of the mouth may be caused by a rope or piece of cloth used as a gag. Injuries to the upper lip and maxillary frenum may result from blunt trauma from an instrument, a finger, or forced feeding. This type of traumatic injury is usually seen in young children 6 to 18 months old. A lacerated lingual frenum may be indicative of sexual abuse or forced feeding. These types of injuries should be diagnosed and documented during the soft tissue evaluation at the dental appointment.

Examination of the gingiva, tongue, and palate may reveal signs of physical and sexual abuse. Identification of sexual abuse in children may be difficult because it is rare and may occur without signs of physical abuse, and the dental team encounters oral sexual lesions infrequently.[18] Oral manifestations of sexual abuse include infections, venereal lesions, and traumatic injuries from oral sex (Fig. 27-12). Venereal lesions of gonorrhea, syphilis, herpes, candidiasis, and other viral infections are pathognomonic of sexual abuse in children.[18] The lesions may be sampled, cultured, and identified to substantiate the presence of a sexually transmitted disease. Palatal petechiae or bruising may also indicate sexual abuse by oral penetration. A diagnosis of sexual abuse must be considered when these lesions or injuries are observed at the dental appointment.

Hard Tissue Assessment
Radiographic examination may reveal healing and recurring facial fractures. When facial trauma indicates a possible fracture, the dental team should consider radiographic examination using several different views. Initial management requires attention to basic life support issues, such as airway maintenance, control of bleeding, and fluid management. A patient with a deviated mandible may have a condylar fracture, which may indicate trauma from child abuse. Nasal and symphyseal fractures may also result from child maltreatment. The dental team should remember that facial fractures are relatively uncommon in children and suggest abuse.[36]

The dentition may be a "permanent register" of child abuse and neglect. Even though abusive parents and guardians may avoid the same hospital or pediatrician's office for emergency care, they generally return to the same dental office. Thus the dental team must be aware of (1) unexplained missing teeth since the previous dental examination; (2) any signs of trauma around primary or permanent teeth; (3) avulsed, displaced, or mobile teeth; and (4) fractured teeth or roots.[5] Traumatic injuries in various stages of healing may indicate child abuse and neglect. Delay in seeking care for the trauma-

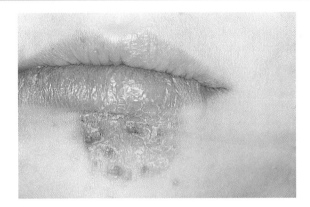

FIG. 27-12 A 4-year-old child with *Candida* infection resulting from sexual abuse.

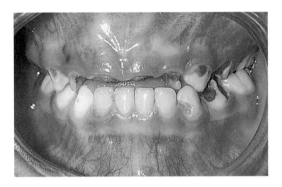

FIG. 27-13 A 3-year-old child with rampant caries associated with dental neglect.

tized child or a discrepant report of the trauma in addition to the dental injury should arouse suspicion of abuse.

Another aspect of the hard tissue assessment is the evaluation for dental neglect. Dental neglect can be identified by the presence of obvious dental disrepair along with the parents' or guardians' failure to provide adequate dental care. Indicators that may assist in the identification of dental neglect in children include (1) untreated, rampant caries that could be identified by a layperson; (2) untreated pain, infection, bleeding, or trauma affecting the orofacial region; and (3) history of a *lack of continuity of care* in the presence of previously identified dental pathology.[3] A complete and accurate dental history is essential in confirming suspicions of neglect. The common factor in dental neglect cases is the failure of the child's caregiver to obtain appropriate care for the child after identification of severe dental pathological conditions (Fig. 27-13).

The cruelty of physical abuse differs greatly from the debilitation associated with dental neglect. Many caregivers are unaware of the processes and effects of untreated dental disease. However, once the parents or guardians have been informed, the treatment goals explained, and the barriers to care removed, failure to follow through with the treatment plan is considered to be dental neglect. Because optimal oral health is a part of the overall physical health of a child, deliberate dental neglect must be reported because it can cause pain, infection, and possible disability.

When a child has trauma or dental neglect to the craniofacial complex, the dental team must consider child abuse and neglect. The goal of the evaluation is to document any trauma and then report any suspicion to the appropriate state child protective service agency.

DOCUMENTATION AND REPORTING

Collection of Evidence

One of the most important responsibilities of the dental team in cases of suspected child abuse or neglect is the systematic documentation and collection of physical evidence.[43] This phase is essential for proper identification, diagnosis, and eventual confirmation of abuse or neglect. An examination has little value unless the findings are recorded permanently and accurately in the dental chart for evaluation and comparison at a later date. This information constitutes legal documentation that may be subpoenaed as evidence in a court of law.

All information collected in the medical and dental histories and the physical assessment should be documented in a detailed and objective manner. Positive and negative findings should be recorded, but personal opinions and suppositions should be avoided. Another member of the dental team should be present as a legal witness during the physical assessment and documentation phases of suspected abuse or neglect.

Documentation

Injuries from suspected physical abuse may be documented through written observations, photographs, radiographs, and dental casts.[43] Written observations, including detailed descriptions of the injury, should be recorded in the progress notes using black or blue ink. The documentation should include a narrative that indicates the number, type, size, and location of the injury. Diagrams and drawings may be included in the description. Injuries observed on other body surfaces within accepted dental practice should be recorded, with all entries signed and dated by the examiner and recorder.

Photographs are valuable in the substantiation of child abuse and neglect. Ideally, color photographs should be taken with a 35-mm camera that has a dating option. Metric rulers, identification labels, and objects of known dimensions (e.g., coins) may be used to indicate the size of the injury (Fig. 27-14). Identification on the back of the photograph should include the name of the patient, date, and film type. Photographs of the patient and the injury should be taken at different angles.

Although the physical injury may not involve hard tissues such as the bones and dentition, a panoramic radiograph or a full-mouth series may be obtained to determine the presence of recent or previous hard tissue injuries to the craniofacial complex. Abnormal tooth development (e.g., dilacerated root, Turner's tooth) indicative of past trauma may be present. These dental anomalies may occur

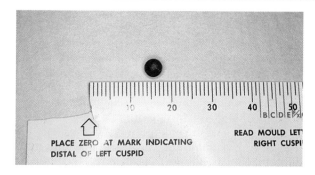

FIG. 27-14 Documentation of physical evidence (buckshot from buccal mucosa), with use of denture ruler as dimensional guide.

when primary roots are forced into the developing tooth buds from direct blows to the face. The same information as noted on the photographs should be placed on all properly mounted radiographs.

An impression of the injury can be taken using dental materials such as alginate or compound. The impression should be processed as soon as possible and labeled with the same information included on the photographs and radiographs. The impression and cast materials used should also be recorded. Dental casts may be helpful in the evaluation and identification of pattern injuries (e.g., bite marks) that involve tissue destruction.

In cases of suspected child abuse and neglect, parent/guardian informed consent is not required for documentation with photographs, radiographs, or dental casts.[43] The general consent obtained before the child's dental examination to perform diagnostic procedures is adequate because all this documentation is diagnostic in nature. Accuracy and presentation of this evidence are important to substantiate any suspicions of the dental team regarding abuse or neglect.

Professional Responsibilities

Reporting suspected child abuse and neglect to the proper authorities may protect the child from continued pain, suffering, or even death. Dentists are mandated and protected by law in all states to report suspected cases of child abuse and neglect. Presently, dental hygienists are mandated reporters in 40 of the 50 states (80%).[5] According to the American Dental Association's *Principles of Ethics and Code of Professional Conduct,* the dentist's role in identifying and reporting child abuse and neglect is (1) to observe and examine suspicious evidence that can be ascertained by the dental team in the office; (2) to record, per legal requirements, any evidence that may be helpful in the case review, including the physical evidence and comments from interviews; (3) to remain objective toward all parties; (4) to treat dental or orofacial injuries; (5) to establish/maintain a professional therapeutic relationship with the family; and (6) to become familiar with the signs of child abuse and neglect and to report suspected cases to the proper authorities consistent with state law.[48] The primary responsibility of the dental team is to identify and to report suspected cases of child abuse and neglect.

Reporting may result in a positive change in the home environment. By reporting suspicions to the proper agencies, the child may be protected from further abuse. In addition, reporting one child in a family may help to protect other children living in the home. In some cases an agency's investigation of child abuse or neglect may lead to the discovery of other problems within the home, which may enable the agency to provide the family with other appropriate and needed services.

Child abuse and neglect reporting laws may vary from state to state, but all contain specific guidelines for mandated reporters. Initially an oral report to the child protective agency is made, followed by a written report within 36 hours to 5 days depending on the state where the child resides.[10] State laws define what information the reports must contain, typically (1) the name, age, gender, address, and telephone number of the child; (2) the nature and extent of the suspected abuse or neglect; (3) the name, address, and telephone number of the parent/guardian; and (4) the mandated reporter's name, address, telephone number, profession, and relationship to the child. Non-mandated reporters may request anonymity. A description of the child's injuries, abuse, or neglect and any indication of prior maltreatment should also be reported.[5]

Once the report has been made, the child protective agency and the judicial system perform all subsequent investigations. This report will result in an investigation if any injury to a child occurs with one or more of the following conditions: (1) the explanation of the cause of the injury is inconsistent with the physical findings; (2) the injury is incompatible with the child's developmental age; (3) the injury seems to be older than the information given by the parent or guardian; and (4) the appearance of nutritional neglect is evident.[21]

Legal Considerations

When reporting a suspected case of child abuse or neglect, the dental team's ethical obligation is to be consistent with state law. Although all states require reports of suspected child maltreatment, the definitions of abuse vary by state, and not all states mandate the reporting of suspected child neglect. Additionally, laws have been enacted that penalize healthcare providers for failure to report suspected cases of child abuse and neglect. These penalties also vary by state.

Generally, mandated reporters are protected from legal liability if they make a report in accordance with state laws and in good faith.[14] *Good faith* implies that the report was made to protect the child and without malicious intent to do harm. With increased public awareness, continuing education courses for the dental team, and lectures on child abuse and neglect in dental and dental hygiene curricula, ignorance in the diagnosis, detection, and reporting of suspected child abuse and neglect is no longer an acceptable reason for not reporting.

Strict confidentiality of records must be maintained. Reports and any other information obtained in reference to a report are confidential and are available only to persons authorized by the juvenile courts.[14]

The most important step in reporting and documenting child abuse and neglect is *advance preparation*. The professional and ethical responsibility of the dental team is to prevent the continuation of pain and suffering of a child. The dental professional must be educated regarding the indicators of child abuse and neglect, understand the legal responsibilities in reporting suspected cases, and know whom to contact when abuse and neglect are suspected. The best action that the dental team can take for an abused or neglected child is to report suspected cases *immediately* to the appropriate agency.

This approach to child abuse prevention is intended to increase awareness among dental professionals regarding the clinical signs and appropriate reporting protocols to break the cycle of abuse. Likewise, prevention of sports-related dental trauma requires enhanced awareness of prevention strategies for patients who participate in competitive sports or vigorous recreational activities.

PREVENTION OF SPORTS-RELATED INJURY

Although sports-related traumatic dental injuries continue to occur, reason for optimism exists. Many of these injuries could be prevented with the use of protective athletic equipment. Studies demonstrate that in organized sports in which helmets, face masks, and **mouthguards** are required during practice and in competition, the number and severity of craniofacial and intraoral injuries are reduced significantly.[15,16,24,25,32]

MOUTHGUARDS

At present in most states, rules in five sports at the *amateur* level mandate the use of a mouthguard: boxing, football, ice hockey, men's lacrosse, and women's field hockey. The only sport at the *professional* level that requires a mouthguard is boxing.[40,41] In an effort to extend protection to a greater number of athletes, the American Dental Association (ADA) and the Academy for Sports Dentistry strongly recommend the use of a mouthguard in any sport or vigorous recreational activity that places an athlete at risk for contact or collision with a ball, bat (racquet), a teammate, or an opponent. Such "athletes" include the young soccer player, the high-school or college basketball player, and the "weekend warrior" who enjoys a rigorous game of racquetball.[7] This information is especially applicable to the female basketball player with the avulsed tooth in this chapter's case study.

Although mouthguards offer athletes protection from injury, many athletes choose not to wear them, even in sports that require mouthguards.[23] Some athletes complain that the mouthguard does not fit properly, that it makes them gag, or that it interferes with breathing and speech. All mouthguards are not of equal quality, and complaints are most often attributable to the poor quality of some mouthguards. Recommendations should be made for the use of a properly fitted mouthguard.[1]

Types

The American Society for Testing and Materials (ASTM) defines three types of mouthguards: Type I, or stock; Type II, or mouth-formed; and Type III, or custom-fabricated.[12]

Stock Mouthguards

Stock mouthguards may be purchased at many sporting goods stores. These over-the-counter mouthguards are the least expensive but offer the poorest fit. They must be held in place by clenching the teeth together. Type I mouthguards offer the least protection and interfere most with breathing and speech compared with Types II and III. They are not well tolerated by most athletes.[40,41]

Mouth-Formed Mouthguards

Most mouth-formed mouthguards may also be purchased over the counter. Often referred to as "boil-and-bite" mouthguards, they vary in price as well as quality. Often they are inadequately formed by the athlete self-fitting the softened material into the mouth. Retention of Type II mouthguards of better quality may be enhanced if the device is properly fitted by a dentist[1,40,41] (Fig. 27-15).

Custom-Fabricated Mouthguards

Custom-fabricated mouthguards are made over a stone dental cast of the maxillary arch for athletes with Class I or II malocclusion or over the cast of the mandibular arch for athletes with Class III malocclusion (Fig. 27-16). The two laboratory methods currently used to custom-fabricate a mouthguard are the *vacuum-forming technique* and the *heat-pressure-laminating technique*.[40,41] Because Type III mouthguards are made specifically for the indi-

vidual athlete using an impression, stone cast, and laboratory time and materials, they are the most expensive of the three types of mouthguards. Despite this expense, custom-fabricated mouthguards are superior for protection, comfort, and fit. They interfere least with breathing and speech and generally last longer than either stock or mouth-formed mouthguards.[40,41]

Inspection, Cleaning, and Storage

Mouthguards should be inspected throughout the course of the season to determine any distortions or bite-through problems, either of which will compromise the mouthguard's ability to protect the athlete. When these problems are detected, a new mouthguard is required for player safety.

Mouthguards should be cleaned and stored properly. They may be brushed with toothpaste or a toothbrush and rinsed with mouthwash or clear water. The water should be cold or lukewarm. Hot water or exposure to direct sunlight will cause the mouthguard to distort. The mouthguard should be stored in a plastic container when not in use.[12,40,41]

STRATEGIES FOR THE DENTAL HYGIENIST

A fundamental professional goal for dental hygienists is to preserve the health of the teeth and supporting structures as a significant component of the general health and well-being of the individual patient. Implicit in this goal is active rather than passive daily participation by the patient in preventive practices that will ensure optimal personal health. Further, this goal for the individual may be extended by dental hygienists to larger segments of the general population through dental public health initiatives and community service projects. This broad fundamental goal involves specific patient education objectives and appropriate clinical procedures used by dental hygienists to ensure the prevention of dental caries and periodontal diseases. Dental hygienists also play an important role in the prevention of traumatic dental injuries.

DOMESTIC VIOLENCE

Although this chapter focuses on issues related to child abuse and neglect, other forms of domestic violence may be encountered by the dental team in the clinical setting. These may include *spousal abuse, elder abuse,* or *date assault.* The dental team must be aware that any form of domestic violence may be seen in their practice. Similar to child abuse injuries, domestic violence injuries occur generally in the head and neck region. Therefore the dental team will likely observe these injuries.

Public awareness programs on all forms of domestic violence can be an effective way to publicize availability of services and to provide training programs for healthcare professionals. The key to prevention is education. The ADA and the American Dental Hygienists' Association have been active in their promotion of programs to educate dental professionals. In 1998 the ADA sponsored the Dentists C.A.R.E. (Child Abuse Recognition and Education) Conference in Chicago. One of the primary goals

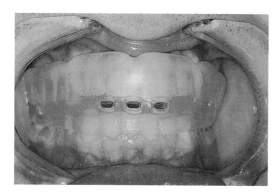

FIG. 27-15 Properly fitted Type II (mouth-formed, "boil-and-bite") mouthguard.

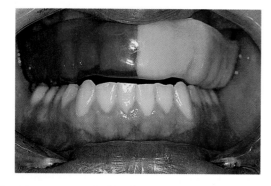

FIG. 27-16 Properly fitted Type III (custom-fabricated) mouthguard.

was to encourage dental professionals, through state and local societies, to form coalitions with public health professionals, child protective services personnel, and advocacy organizations to increase awareness of the incidence of child abuse and other forms of family violence.[6]

Another initiative, the Prevent Abuse and Neglect through Dental Awareness (PANDA) coalition, began in Missouri in 1992. Collaborations with dental professionals, public health agencies, dental insurers, and child protective agencies have made this program effective. Since the inception of this program, reporting rates by dentists have steadily increased.

In addition to the curricular guidelines in the ADA accreditation standards, mandatory continuing education courses in the recognition of child abuse and neglect should be recommended for relicensure of dentists and dental hygienists. Education may give professionals the confidence to make reports of suspected child abuse and neglect. Because studies have documented that a lack of knowledge about abuse and neglect resulted in the subsequent lack of reporting, educational efforts should be directed toward breaking the cycle of abuse by enhanced knowledge and active reporting.[13]

Another way to break this cycle of abuse is for the dental team to serve as an example. A concerned and compassionate atmosphere in the dental office may offer insight into suitable ways to manage children and adults. The dental professional should counsel patients on primary prevention practices and healthful nutrition habits. Primary prevention efforts should also be directed toward domestic violence.

As in all activities that involve children, some forms of child abuse may occur in youth sports.[35] Long practice hours without adequate rest or refueling, abusive language directed at poor performance, and pressure to win at all costs may be viewed as abusive situations to the child athlete.

The dental professional must demonstrate genuine concern for the patient's total health and show a willingness to help each patient to attain this goal. The dental team can make a difference against the escalating public health problem of domestic violence. Besides protecting children from abuse and neglect, the profession's attitude and actions may also save lives.

MALPRACTICE AND ABUSE ALLEGATIONS

Dentists traditionally have been protectors of children's health and well-being. Recently, however, this role has been challenged by an increased number of criminal and civil allegations against dentists during conventional patient care. Due to a lack of parental acceptance of certain behavioral management techniques, dentists are being sued for child abuse, assault, and battery. This litigious behavior appears to reflect two trends in society: an increase in malpractice claims against health professionals and an increase in charges of child abuse against persons who care for children.[47] Hand-over-mouth (HOM) techniques are arguable as assault and battery if used without parental or guardian consent. In addition, physical restraints such as the papoose board may instigate claims of false imprisonment if used without consent.

Prevention is the best defense against potential lawsuits. Communication is the key to prevention. Discussing treatment options and behavioral strategies with the parent or guardian before initiating more invasive care is recommended as an appropriate informed consent procedure and a risk management strategy.

SPORTS DENTISTRY

Trauma-Ready Office

Several private practice considerations related to sports dentistry are identified previously in this chapter. One particularly important consideration is to prepare the office and staff to be "trauma-ready" when a patient contacts the practice for an emergency appointment after a traumatic episode. Professional responsibility and expeditious scheduling of trauma patients are essential elements to successful patient management.

 Case Application

What steps could Tonya's dentist have taken to prepare for an emergency appointment such as hers?

Initial Interview

A second factor of particular importance for the prevention of sports-related dental trauma is to include on the dental history form a question related to participation in organized sports or recreational activities that might place the patient at risk for injury. On most dental history forms this type of information is not solicited, and patients often do not recognize the dentist's need to know unless clinicians ask the question.[39] A positive response allows the dental hygienist to initiate patient education strategies for the prevention of sports-related dental injuries.

Congenital Abnormalities and Orthodontic Considerations

Patients with a history of congenital abnormalities, such as the child with cleft lip or palate, the adolescent undergoing orthodontic treatment, or the adult who wears prosthetic dental appliances (e.g., implants), must be evaluated thoroughly by the dentist.[1,12] Once this intraoral examination has been completed, the dentist and dental hygienist are better prepared to make an appropriate recommendation for a specific type of mouthguard to meet the individual needs of the patient.

COMMUNITY ACTIVITIES

Dental hygienists have ample opportunities to use their expertise to enhance awareness of trauma prevention in the community by participating in educational activities and public service projects that promote player safety (Fig. 27-17). For example, the hygienist can advocate for the use of properly fitted mouthguards for athletes and volunteer for community programs to raise awareness of the benefits of mouthguard use.[1,30,42]

An excellent initial step for the dental hygienist, whether in a private practice, public health, or a school-based

A

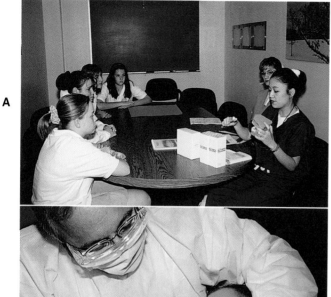

B

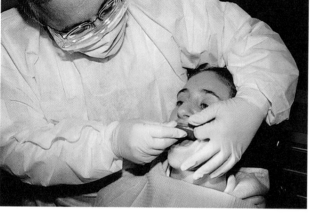

FIG. 27-17 A, Dental hygiene students presenting home-care instructions to high-school basketball players. **B,** Insertion of custom-fabricated mouthguard.

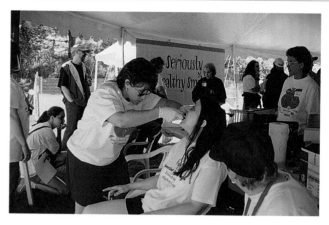

FIG. 27-18 Fitting of mouth-formed mouthguard in Special Olympics athlete, one of the activities in the Special Smiles program.

mental agencies. Scouting groups might welcome dental hygiene participation either by providing a forum for a presentation to the group or serving as a mentor for dental health–related projects for scouts to earn merit badges.[42]

Participating in the Special Olympics Special Smiles program provides an excellent opportunity for interested dental hygienists to use a variety of skills.[38] Special Olympic athletes may choose to participate in the Special Smiles program on-site at many of their events throughout the United States. Special Smiles includes a dental screening examination, referral for treatment as needed, oral hygiene instruction, and dietary counseling. In 1999 at selected sites, Special Smiles began to offer mouthguards to these special athletes in specified contact sports (Fig. 27-18). All participants in the Special Smiles Program receive a "goodies bag" containing a Special Olympics Special Smiles logo T-shirt and dental hygiene products such as toothpaste, toothbrush, and dental floss. Dental hygienists should use this opportunity to provide community services to an appreciative group of special athletes.

setting, is to enroll in continuing education courses in sports dentistry and trauma management. The hygienist might participate in the annual symposium sponsored by the Academy for Sports Dentistry. The well-informed dental hygienist will then be in a better position to begin to share this knowledge with others in the community, such as school nurses, athletic teams and coaches, or govern-

RITICAL THINKING ACTIVITIES

1. Fabricate a Type II "boil-and-bite" mouthguard. Evaluate the finished mouthguard for protective qualities.
2. Volunteer to participate in a local "mouthguard day." Observe the ages of those interested in information. In which sporting activities are they involved?
3. Participate in a local Special Olympics Special Smiles event.
4. Review course availability on domestic violence and child abuse. Prepare a handout for students and faculty to encourage them to attend a class.

5. Interview an abuse counselor. Determine his or her experiences with trauma to the head and neck region of abuse victims, differentiating between men, women, children, and the elderly.
6. Obtain a child abuse and neglect report from your appropriate local authority.
7. Review your state Dental Practice Act to determine your legal obligations in reporting suspected child abuse and neglect.

REVIEW QUESTIONS

Questions 2 through 5 refer to the case study presented at the beginning of the chapter.

1. Dental hygienists play a key role in primary care prevention in the dental office and through community service projects. Which of the following activities should be included in a total dental prevention program?
   a. Prevention of dental caries
   b. Prevention of periodontal diseases
   c. Prevention of traumatic dental injuries
   d. Prevention of child abuse and neglect
   e. All the above

2. When Tonya's mother contacts your trauma-ready dental office, which of the following sets of instructions should she be given to enhance the prognosis for Tonya's avulsed permanent incisor?
   a. Reinsert the avulsed tooth into the socket and bring Tonya to the dental office immediately.
   b. Place the tooth in milk and bring Tonya and her avulsed tooth to the dental office within the next 2 days.
   c. Control the bleeding, place the avulsed tooth in a dry paper towel and bring Tonya and her avulsed tooth to the dental office immediately.
   d. Control the bleeding and bring Tonya to the dental office within the next 2 days.

3. When Tonya arrives at the dental office, which of the following diagnostic procedures should *not* be performed in her case of an avulsed permanent incisor?
   a. Updated health history
   b. Clinical examination
   c. Percussion of avulsed tooth
   d. Periapical radiograph

4. After the dentist has repositioned and splinted the avulsed tooth in place, which of the following oral self-care instructions should the dental hygienist give to Tonya and her mother?
   a. Avoid brushing and flossing the traumatized tooth and soft tissue, but continue to brush and floss the remainder of the teeth.
   b. Vigorously brush and floss the traumatized tooth and soft tissue with a hard toothbrush, and use an interproximal dental stimulator.
   c. Avoid brushing and flossing for the 2 weeks the splint is in place.
   d. Gently brush and floss the traumatized tooth and soft tissue with a soft toothbrush, and use an intraoral rinse such as warm salt water or chlorhexidine. Maintain standard oral self-care for the remainder of the teeth.

5. Which of the following recommendation should be made to Tonya and her mother in terms of Tonya's future participation in athletic activities?
   a. Stop playing basketball.
   b. Play basketball less vigorously.
   c. Use a properly fitted mouthguard when playing basketball.
   d. Switch to a different sport, such as field hockey.

 ## SUGGESTED AGENCIES AND WEB SITES

Because of the ever-changing nature of the Internet, some of the web sites listed here may have changed since publication. Please refer to Mosby's Evolve web site for the most current information.

Academy for Sports Dentistry: http://www.acadsportsdent.org
American Academy of Pediatric Dentistry: http://www.aapd.org
National Clearinghouse on Child Abuse and Neglect Information: http://www.calib.com

National Oral Health Information Clearinghouse: http://www.nohic.nidcr.nih.gov
The American Society of Dentistry for Children: http://www.asdckids.org

 ## ADDITIONAL READINGS AND RESOURCES

American Humane Association (AHA), Children's Division, 63 Inverness Dr East, Englewood, CO 80112-5117. The AHA is a not-for-profit corporation and the oldest agency in the United States dedicated to the protection of children from abuse and neglect. Since the formation of the Children's Division in 1878, AHA has provided national leadership in the development of programs, policies, and services on behalf of abused and neglected children.

Jessee SA: Risk factors as determinants of dental neglect in children, *J Dent Child* 65(1), 1998.
Mouden LD: The dentist's role in detecting and reporting abuse, *Quint Int* 29(7), 1998.
Ranalli DN, editor: *Adv Sports Dent* 44(1), 2000 (entire issue).
Ranalli DN, editor: *Sports Dent* 35(4), 1991 (entire issue).

REFERENCES

1. Academy for Sports Dentistry: Position statement: a properly fitted mouthguard, Chicago, 1999, Board of Directors, The Academy.

2. Adair SM, Durr DP: Practical clinical applications of sports dentistry in private practice, *Dent Clin North Am* 35:757-70, 1991.

3. American Academy of Pediatric Dentistry: Reference manual, 1999-2000, *Pediatr Dent* 21:20, 25-7, 1999.

4. American Association of Endodontists: *Recommended guidelines for treatment of the avulsed permanent tooth,* Chicago, 1995, The Association.

5. American Dental Association: *The dentist's responsibility in identifying and reporting child abuse and neglect,* Chicago, 1995, The Association.

6. American Dental Association: *Proceedings of the Dentists C.A.R.E. Conference,* Chicago, 1998, The Association.

7. American Dental Association, Academy for Sports Dentistry: *Protect your smile with a mouthguard* (brochure), Chicago, 1999, The Association.

8. American Heart Association: Guidelines for cardiopulmonary resuscitation and emergency cardiac care, *JAMA* 268:2171-97, 1992.

9. American Heart Association: Guidelines for the prevention of bacterial endocarditis, *JAMA* 277:1794-1801, 1997.

10. American Humane Association: *Guidebook for the visual assessment of child abuse,* Englewood, Colo, 1996, The Association.

11. American Humane Association: *Trends in child abuse and neglect: a national perspective,* Englewood, Colo, 1984, The Association.

12. American Society for Testing and Materials: *Standard practice for care and use of mouthguards, designation F697-80,* Philadelphia, 1986, The Society.

13. Becker DB et al: Child abuse and dentistry: orofacial trauma and its recognition by dentists, *J Am Dent Assoc* 97:24-8, 1978.

14. Bross DC: Legal aspects of child abuse. In Sanger RE, Bross DC, editors: *Clinical management of child abuse and neglect,* Chicago, 1984, Quintessence.

15. Bureau of Dental Health Education: Mouth protectors for football players: the dentist's role, *J Am Dent Assoc* 64:419-21, 1962.

16. Bureau of Health Education and Audiovisual Services, Council on Dental Materials, Instruments and Equipment: Mouth protectors and sports team dentists, *J Am Dent Assoc* 109:84-7, 1984.

17. Camp JH: Management of sports-related root fractures, *Dent Clin North Am* 44:95-110, 2000.

18. Casamassimo PS: Oral facial lesions in sexual abuse. In Sanger RE, Bross DC, editors: *Clinical management of child abuse and neglect,* Chicago, 1984, Quintessence.

19. Croll TP et al: Rapid neurologic assessment and initial management for the patient with traumatic dental injuries, *J Am Dent Assoc* 100:530-4, 1980.

20. Diangelis AJ, Bakland LK: Traumatic dental injuries: current treatment concepts, *J Am Dent Assoc* 129:1401-14, 1998.

21. Dubowitz H, Newberger E: Sequelae of reporting child abuse, *Pediatr Dent* 8:88-92, 1986.

22. Fos PJ, Pinkham JR, Ranalli DN: Prediction of sports-related dental traumatic injuries, *Dent Clin North Am* 44:19-34, 2000.

23. Gardiner DM, Ranalli DN: Attitudinal factors influencing mouthguard utilization, *Dent Clin North Am* 44:53-65, 2000.

24. Garon MW, Merkle A, Wright JT: Mouth protectors and oral trauma: a study of adolescent football players, *J Am Dent Assoc* 112:663-5, 1986.

25. Godwin WC et al: The utilization of mouth protectors by freshman football players, *J Public Health Dent* 32:22-4, 1972.

26. Kaste LM et al: Prevalence of incisor trauma in persons 6-50 years of age: United States, 1988-1991, *J Dent Res* 75:696-705, 1996.

27. Kelley JP, Rosenberg JH: Diagnosis and management of concussions in sports, *Neurology* 48:575-80, 1997.

28. Kempe CH et al: The battered child syndrome, *JAMA* 181:17-24, 1962.

29. Krasner P, Rankow HJ: New philosophy for the treatment of avulsed teeth, *Oral Surg Oral Med Oral Pathol* 79:616-23, 1995.

30. Kumamoto DP, Winters JE: Private practice and community activities in sports dentistry, *Dent Clin North Am* 44:209-220, 2000.

31. Lenoski EE, Hunter KA: Specific patterns of inflicted burn injuries, *J Trauma* 17:842-6, 1977.

32. McNutt T et al: Oral trauma in adolescent athletes: a study of mouth protectors, *Pediatr Dent* 11: 209-13, 1989.

33. National Clearinghouse on Child Abuse and Neglect Information: *Executive summary: Study of national incidence and prevalence of child abuse and neglect,* Washington, DC, 1988, US Government Printing Office.

34. National Committee for Prevention of Child Abuse: *Think you know something about child abuse?* Chicago, 1996, The Committee.

35. National Institute for Youth Sports Administration: *Child abuse and youth sports: a comprehensive risk management program,* Palm Beach, Fla, 1996, The Institute.

36. Needleman HL: Orofacial trauma in child abuse: types, prevalence, management, and the dental profession's involvement, *Pediatr Dent* 8:71-80, 1986.

37. Nowak AJ, editor: *Pediatric dentistry handbook,* ed 2, Chicago, 1999, American Academy of Pediatric Dentistry.

38. Perlman S: Helping Special Olympic athletes sport good smiles: an effort to reach out to people with special needs, *Dent Clin North Am* 44:221-30, 2000.

39. Pollack BR: Legal considerations in sports dentistry, *Dent Clin North Am* 35:809-30, 1991.

40. Ranalli DN: Prevention of craniofacial injuries in football, *Dent Clin North Am* 35:627-46, 1991.

41. Ranalli DN: Prevention of sports-related traumatic dental injuries, *Dent Clin North Am* 44:35-52, 2000.

42. Ranalli DN: Sports dentistry in general practice, *Gen Dent* 48:158-64, 2000.

43. Sanger RG: Documentation and collection of physical evidence. In Sanger RE, Bross DC, editors: *Clinical management of child abuse and neglect,* Chicago, 1984, Quintessence.

44. Sanger RG: Oral facial injuries in physical abuse. In Sanger RE, Bross DC, editors: *Clinical management of child abuse and neglect,* Chicago, 1984, Quintessence.

45. Schmitt BD: Physical abuse: specifics of clinical diagnosis, *Pediatr Dent* 8:83-7, 1986.

46. Schmitt BD: Types of child abuse and neglect: an overview for dentists, *Pediatr Dent* 8:67-71, 1986.

47. Schumann NJ: Child abuse and the dental practitioner: discussion and case reports, *Quint Int* 18:619-22, 1987.

48. Sfikas PM: Reporting abuse and neglect, *J Am Dent Am* 130: 1797-9, 1999.

49. Waldman HB: Your next pediatric dental patient may have been physically or sexually abused, *J Dent Child* 60:325-9, 1993.

50. Winters JE: Sports dentistry: the profession's role in athletics, *J Am Dent Assoc* 127:810-1, 1996.

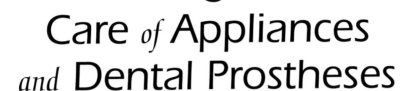

CHAPTER 28

Care *of* Appliances *and* Dental Prostheses

Kenneth Shay

Chapter Outline

Role of the Dental Hygienist
Case Study: Caring for the Prosthodontic Patient
Overview of Dental Appliances
    Fixed partial dentures
    Complete dentures
    Removable partial dentures
    Implant and implant-borne prostheses
    Orthodontic appliances
    Splints

Mouthguards, nightguards, fluoride carriers,
    and bleaching trays
Maxillofacial prostheses
Postsurgical stents and sleep apnea devices
Evaluating Oral Tissues Associated with Appliances
    Conditions associated with appliance wear
Care and Cleaning of Dental Appliances

Key Terms

Abutment
Circummandibular ligatures
Denture adhesive
Facial prosthesis
Fixed bridge

Full dentures
Gingiva/implant interface
Implant abutments
Implant-borne prostheses
Mouthguard

Nightguard
Obturator
Overdenture
Palatal lift
Partial denture

Pontic
Porcelain fused-to-metal bridge
Retainer
Surgical stent

Learning Outcomes

1. Correctly identify the following dental appliances: fixed partial denture, removable partial denture, complete removable denture, overdenture, splint, fluoride tray, bleaching tray, and maxillofacial prosthesis.
2. Evaluate a prosthesis for the type of deposits present and cleaning required.
3. Detail the instruments, products, and procedures that are used to clean removable dental prostheses.
4. Explain the need for daily self-care of implant abutments, and specify how and why particular care must be taken.

5. Correctly identify and explain the etiology of soft-tissue pathoses associated with improperly maintained dental prostheses.
6. Explain to a patient the reason and method for cleaning a dental appliance and the abutment teeth, regardless of whether it is fixed, removable, implant-borne, therapeutic, or prosthetic.
7. Observe fabrication of dental appliances and prostheses.

Intraoral appliances make up a varied, large, and important aspect of the practice of dentistry. Intraoral appliances may comprise the dental treatment itself, as with a denture or a *facial prosthesis.* They may also be the instrument by which care is effected, as with orthodontic appliances or bleaching trays. The appliance may play a key role in the prevention of disease, as with a fluoride carrier or a nightguard. Finally, appliances may be used as a temporary measure, as with a *surgical stent,* or a long-lived measure, as with a *fixed bridge.*

Care of dental appliances is as varied as the devices themselves. Some prostheses are cleaned intraorally (e.g., fixed bridges, *implant abutments*), whereas others must be cared for extraorally (e.g., dentures, orthodontic appliances). Some appliances require the regular application of a material to accomplish their tasks (e.g., fluoride carriers, bleaching trays), whereas other devices may benefit from the addition of a material but not all patients feel that is necessary (e.g., the use of *denture adhesive* for dentures and certain maxillofacial prostheses). The cleaning of dental prostheses can involve brushing, soaking, immersing in ultrasonic baths, using microwave radiation, or combining these procedures. A variety of mechanical and chemical products is available, generally as over-the-counter products, for the care of dental appliances. Thus patients need to be educated as to which methods and compounds are or are not suitable for their own needs.

Dental practices vary with respect to the role the dental hygienist is expected to play in the education of patients about the care of intraoral appliances (Fig. 28-1). Although the majority of a dental hygienist's training and professional practice is generally devoted to the removal of deposits from the teeth, patient education in oral health is an important and indispensable duty. The large number of patients with oral prosthetic appliances—dentures, bridges, splints, and orthodontic devices—must be taught and periodically reminded of the techniques for and importance of proper care of their appliances. In addition, the dental hygienist plays an essential role in the assessment of the integrity of such devices and the tissues they contact and in the referral of developing and extant problems before they worsen.

Some dental practices delegate all discussion of appliance care to the dental assistant, reserving the dental hygienist's time exclusively for intraoral care. Other dentists prefer to retain sole responsibility for the instruction of patients about the care and use of all dental devices. Most dental practices fall somewhere in the middle of these two and have policies or practices that clarify the roles team members are expected to play with respect to the instruction of patients on the care of dental appliances.

ROLE OF THE DENTAL HYGIENIST

The dental hygienist must (1) be fully familiar with the range of dental appliances encountered in practice, (2) know how to keep all of them clean, (3) be able to detect current or impending problems, and (4) be able to distinguish between those clinical situations in which he or she is able to handle the patient's needs and those in which a dentist should be consulted. As a key member of the dental team, the dental hygienist is the team member considered most focused on issues of prevention and patient education. For this reason, patients commonly direct many questions about self-care issues to the hygienist. Even if the dental practice's custom is to have the dentist provide information on the care of prostheses, it may not be practical for a hygienist to defer the answers to a patient's question. The dental hygienist also must be familiar with dental appliances because no one in the dental office—except the dentist—devotes as much attention to detailed scrutiny of the oral cavity as does the hygienist. As such, the hygienist needs to be comfortable in the recognition of intraoral conditions that represent heightened need for oral self-care and in those situations that require a dentist's attention.

OVERVIEW OF DENTAL APPLIANCES

FIXED PARTIAL DENTURES

Fixed partial dentures, also commonly called *bridges,* are multitooth devices that replace one or more missing teeth (Fig. 28-2). Natural teeth, termed *retainers* or *abutments,* are located on either side of the artificial tooth (termed the *pontic*) or teeth and support the pontic(s), which the patient is not able to remove. Clinicians should be alert to the following four common problems to which bridges are prone:

1. The connection between an abutment and a pontic may break, which results in excessive and adverse forces on the other abutment. A break between a pontic and an abutment is readily visualized as an irregular linear separation, usually in the area that mimics the interproximal region. The fracture usually permits independent, visible movement of the parts on either side of the break, and therefore it must be brought to a dentist's attention without delay. Although some bridges are designed in such a way as to permit inde-

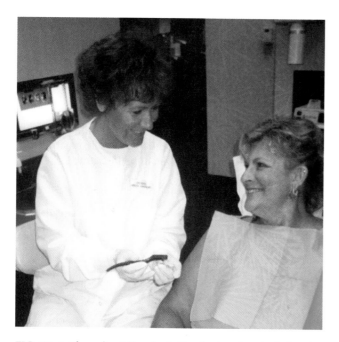

FIG. 28-1 The role of the dental hygienist often includes the education of patients about the care of intraoral appliances.

pendent movement of the pontic and one abutment, the connection in such a case is a *machined keyway* or *rest,* and the independent movements of the abutments are generally not visible.

2. Because bridges use natural teeth to withstand the forces on the pontic, the abutment teeth experience greater occlusal forces and are prone to trauma from occlusion. Mobility of a bridge abutment that is more exaggerated than mobility of teeth elsewhere in the mouth should be brought to a dentist's attention without delay.

3. Bridges are impediments to plaque control because they hinder the removal of plaque from the proximal surfaces of abutments and provide new surfaces on which plaque may collect, such as the side of the pontic facing the alveolar ridge tissue. In many cases this

---

Caring for the Prosthodontic Patient

You have just begun employment in a thriving prosthodontics group practice headed by three young, full-time dentists. You are the first hygienist to be employed by the practice because, until lately, most of the patients had general dentists who oversaw the cases and provided preventive services, as needed. But with the growth of the practice, the expanding number of patients with sophisticated oral reconstructions needing attentive preventive strategies have caused the partner dentists to realize that a dental hygienist dedicated to their patients would be an excellent patient service.

Your first patient illustrates the wisdom of their plan. Dr. Raj Basha, a 72-year-old retired professor of engineering at the nearby state university, has an edentulous maxilla that features a severely resorbed anterior ridge segment and a partially edentulous mandibular dentition. The maxillary arch is restored with a complete overdenture retained by a pair of implant-borne attachments that are connected with a gold bar that is in contact with the residual tissue. His mandibular dentition features a **porcelain fused-to-metal bridge** from cuspid to cuspid, full-coverage surveyed crowns with supragingival margins on all four premolars, and a removable **partial denture** that bilaterally replaces the molars. Dr. Basha is attuned to the "engineering" of his prostheses and takes good care of them, although he has noticed that the shiny silver metal of the lower partial is darkening and becoming dull.

Dr. Basha's mouth is rather dry, and the appearance of the periodontium around his remaining teeth is strongly suggestive of a history of resective periodontal surgery. The abundant exposed root surfaces are only moderately clean but appear free of caries. Despite the plaque, the gingiva appears healthy and features minimal bleeding on probing, and probe depths do not exceed 3 mm. Dr. Basha informs you that he uses a fluoride carrier each evening when he remembers to do so but admits that he dislikes the flavor of the topical fluoride he currently uses. He inquires as to whether you have a preferred type of fluoride gel and voices his hope that it might be a better-tasting product. Dr. Basha is familiar with floss, floss threaders, and interproximal brushes but prefers to use the latter in the mandible because of arthritic changes in his hands and right shoulder. The tissue around the splint bar in the anterior maxilla is inflamed, although the patient reports no discomfort in that area and seems confused when you inquire about his regimen for keeping the bar's tissue surface clean.

Dr. Basha is a rather obese man who is a mouth breather. He requests to have his prophylaxis completed with the chair only partly reclined because he has even greater difficulty breathing when flat on his back. Further questioning reveals that this same problem has plagued him and his wife at night and that episodes of labored or even interrupted nocturnal breathing recently led to one of the prosthodontists fabricating him a device to help manage his sleep apnea.

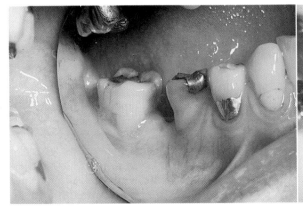
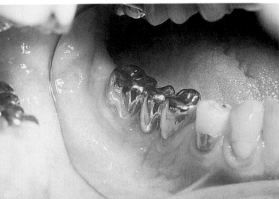

FIG. 28-2 A, A common prosthetic dental solution for a missing single tooth is the fixed bridge. **B,** A three-unit bridge made of cast gold has been cemented into place, which provides the patient with additional occlusal function—and also with some new hygiene challenges.

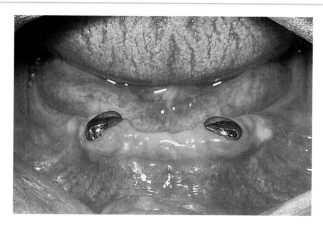

FIG. 28-3 Overdenture abutments may be unrestored, restored only at the endodontic access, or restored to a contour that is most favorable for the retention of the prosthesis.

side of the pontic has been designed for aesthetic reasons with concavities that make hygiene impossible; in other cases, the pontic is fully convex, but the patient does not keep its undersurface clean. In either of these situations the alveolar ridge tissue may be inflamed and can bleed spontaneously.

4. The pontic(s) of a fixed bridge undergo(es) a limited but still finite amount of bending under function. Porcelain is more inflexible than metal, so if deformation exceeds a certain level, the porcelain of a porcelain-to-metal fixed bridge may exhibit fracture, particularly in the pontic and embrasure areas.

COMPLETE DENTURES

Complete dentures replace all of the teeth of either the mandible, the maxilla, or both. Complete dentures (also called *full dentures*) may be seen by the hygienist if the patient is edentulous in only one arch (and therefore requires care of the natural teeth of the opposing arch). They may also be seen if some of the teeth have been endodontically treated and contoured flush or nearly flush with the alveolar ridge, with the denture (then termed an *overdenture*) resting over them. In this case the remaining teeth (the *overdenture abutments*) still require periodic scaling (Fig. 28-3).

An **overdenture** is fabricated much like a denture, but the resulting prosthesis is far more stable and retentive, which allows the patient to exert more bite force. An overdenture may be preferable to a removable partial denture when the abutments are mobile or badly broken down or when the abutments disrupt the plane of occlusion. Abutments are generally endodontically treated, but this is not necessary if the pulp is not exposed when the abutment is reduced occlusally. Abutments may be unrestored, restored only at the endodontic access, or restored to a contour that is most favorable for retaining the overdenture.

Case Application
Dr. Basha has an overdenture. As you continue to read, determine the steps you would take when caring for him.

Complete dentures are usually made of pink or clear acrylic resin, although some dentures may have metallic

inserts for strength and rigidity. The teeth of dentures may be made from a material that bonds with the pink denture base (acrylic or composite) or from porcelain, which necessitates some means for mechanically connecting the teeth to the denture. The tissue surface of some complete dentures may have a lining of a material more resilient than acrylic. These "soft liners" can be temporary (placed by a dentist as a "tissue conditioner" to reduce trauma to the soft tissues) or permanent (placed by a dentist or a dental laboratory). Equivalent products can be purchased over the counter by patients in pharmacies, but in most cases these cause oral trauma and irreparable damage to the denture itself.

As mentioned previously, some complete dentures are designed to sit over teeth that have been reduced (and sometimes crowned) to extend only slightly beyond the contour of the alveolar ridge. These overdentures may sit passively on the recontoured teeth or may actively engage some retentive device attached to the root face. In other cases complete dentures, usually only mandibular ones, may have most of the portion of the base that contacts the tissues made from chrome-cobalt alloy, which affords greater accuracy and better tissue reaction.

When caring for a patient with one or more removable complete dentures, the clinician needs to be alert to the following:

- Fractures in the acrylic base may readily reduce retention of the prosthesis, pinch the soft tissues, or cut the tongue. The flanges of dentures may have broken off if the appliance was dropped on a hard surface; the resulting sharp edges may traumatize adjacent tissues or the tongue. Fractures and dentures that are missing parts of their flanges need to be brought to the dentist's attention.
- Fractures in prosthetic teeth are common. Patients may be unaware of them, but they may be the source of vague complaints of poor chewing ability or impaired hygiene. Missing or damaged teeth need to be brought to the dentist's attention.
- Extreme wear of acrylic teeth, to the extent that mastication takes place against one or more areas of pink acrylic base material (which is much less resistant to wear), requires repair before perforation of the denture base occurs (Fig. 28-4). Perforation through the denture base may be responsible for claims of looseness (as the "seal" of an upper denture is lost) or soreness (as the source of the perforation now traumatizes the underlying tissue). Perforation generally necessitates remake or at least major modification of the prosthesis and definitely needs to be called to a dentist's attention.
- Stained prosthetic teeth are common if the denture was made with porcelain teeth. This is because there is no chemical bond—only an intimate fit prone to leakage—between porcelain teeth and the denture base, and thus stain accumulates along that interface (Fig. 28-5).
- Overdentures with retentive elements generally require that parts of those elements be replaced once or more each year. Overdentures that fail to engage their retainers or engage some retainers more strongly and others less tightly need to be called to a dentist's attention.
- Soft liners of dentures often peel away from the base, which leads to odor, stains, and irritation. Soft bases

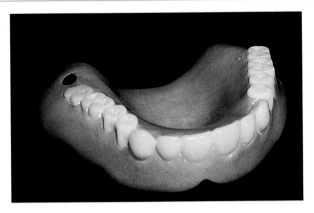

FIG. 28-4 If extreme wear is apparent in an area of the denture base, repair is required before perforation of the denture base and loss of retention occur.

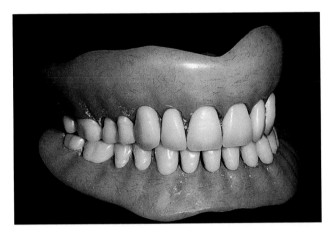

FIG. 28-5 Because porcelain denture teeth do not bond to the denture base, many years of use may result in unaesthetic staining that cannot be removed between the porcelain prosthetic teeth and the denture base.

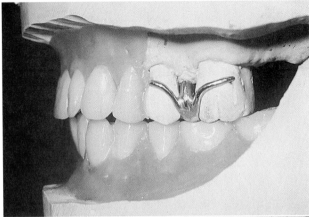

A

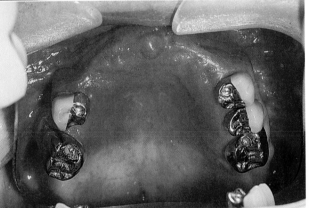

B

FIG. 28-6 A, Aesthetic results can be excellent, and the prosthesis allows natural teeth and soft tissues to distribute and share the added occlusal function. **B,** Removable partial dentures pose oral hygiene challenges by impeding the cleansing action of saliva and by placing large areas of soft and hard tissues in contact with materials that retain plaque and food debris.

may also be less resilient than when originally placed. Problems with soft liners should be brought to the dentist's attention.

REMOVABLE PARTIAL DENTURES

Removable partial dentures (RPDs), often termed *partials* or *removable bridges,* replace some, but not all, teeth in an arch. They generally attach to two or more remaining natural teeth with metallic clasps or wires or with soft plastic rings in the body of the denture that slip over the natural teeth. Partials are usually fabricated with a combination of metallic and acrylic elements. Some partials are wholly metal, with the prosthetic teeth made of porcelain, acrylic, or composite that is mechanically attached to the metal. Other partial dentures are wholly acrylic except for small wires that clip onto two or more natural teeth (termed *abutments* or *retainers,* as with fixed bridges). The simplest version of this form of partial denture is fabricated without any clasps and replaces one or a few anterior teeth. Called *flippers,* these devices stay in place with the engagement of small undercut areas on the palatal side of

maxillary teeth between lingual palatal gingival papillae and interproximal contact areas. The most common partial has a cast metal framework that is largely encased in pink acrylic to which the prosthetic teeth are attached. In this partial, highly polished metal pieces of the framework extend beyond the acrylic to attach the appliance to the abutment teeth (Fig. 28-6).

For a patient with removable partial dentures, the clinician needs to be alert to the following:

- Fractures within acrylic elements that pose a risk of laceration to the oral soft tissues
- Metal portions, particularly smaller ones, that have broken off and thus pose a laceration hazard to the soft tissues of the oral cavity and indicate that the prosthesis is exerting forces onto teeth and tissues that vary from those intended by the original design
- Fractured teeth, worn teeth, stained areas around teeth, and signs of wear through the base acrylic, as described for complete dentures in the preceding section

IMPLANT AND IMPLANT-BORNE PROSTHESES

Implants and **implant-borne prostheses** have become widely used in dentistry. Many of the care issues associated

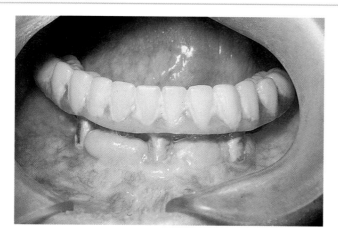

FIG. 28-7 Failure to remove plaque from implant abutments may result in a disease process termed *periimplantitis,* which is similar to periodontitis.

with this form of treatment are identical to ones already discussed. Specifically, if the case has been restored with fixed bridgework, the clinician needs to be alert for broken connectors, loss of porcelain, and the need for hygiene techniques to clean the surface of the prosthesis adjacent to alveolar ridge tissue. An additional consideration not present in tooth-borne fixed partial dentures is for the clinician to scrupulously assess the integrity of the screws that attach the fixed bridgework to the implants and to call to a dentist's attention any suspicious loosening or separation. If the case has been restored with a complete denture (specifically, an overdenture retained by attachments connected to the implants), most of the issues raised previously in connection with complete dentures apply (e.g., damage to the base, need to assess retention of retainers, wear or fracture or stain of prosthetic teeth).

The additional challenge that implants present to clinicians concerns the assessment and care of the ***gingiva/ implant interface.*** As with the gingiva/tooth interface, an epithelialized sulcus exists along the subgingival surface of the implant. But with implants, there is no junctional epithelium and no epithelial attachment. Failure on the part of the patient to fastidiously remove plaque from the supragingival and subgingival tissues around implants results in gingival inflammation (Fig. 28-7) that may, in some cases, develop into the implant equivalent of periodontitis, termed *periimplantitis.* Periimplantitis involves inflammatory cell infiltration of the bone, purulent exudate around the implant, loss of bony support, and, if not treated, eventual exfoliation of the implant. The clinician needs to devote the same level of meticulous assessment and removal of supragingival and subgingival deposits to implants as is expended on teeth. Instrumentation is slightly different, however. Special nonmetal scalers and curets are recommended for professional care of implants. Stainless steel instruments are contraindicated for instrumentation to eliminate the possibility of scratching or otherwise damaging the smooth, machined surface of the implants, which would lead to more rapid and tenacious plaque accumulation and greater hygiene difficulties.

ORTHODONTIC APPLIANCES

Orthodontic appliances may be fixed or removable and active or passive. The most common variety encountered outside of the orthodontic practice is the passive, removable variety, often called a *retainer* because its function is to retain the teeth in the position to which they were moved during the active phase of orthodontic therapy. Retainers are generally made from a tinted or colorless clear acrylic with one or more bent wire elements. Clinicians should examine retainers for sharp wires (usually an indication that an element has broken off as a result of metal fatigue) or cracks in the acrylic base. Either of these findings requires a dentist's attention.

SPLINTS

Splints are designed to take stresses off the temporomandibular joint by providing a more healthful interocclusal resting position for the mandible. Splints are generally made to lock onto the maxillary arch, covering the occlusal surfaces and incisal edges. They may be retained by extensions of the acrylic base that lock into interproximal areas, or with small ball clasps that extend beyond the acrylic. Splints are customarily made from clear acrylic and require periodic adjustment to continue to contact the mandibular teeth uniformly. As was specified for orthodontic appliances, a dentist needs to be informed when the hygienist finds sharp or broken wires and cracks or holes caused by excess wear in the acrylic base.

MOUTHGUARDS, NIGHTGUARDS, FLUORIDE CARRIERS, AND BLEACHING TRAYS

Mouthguards, nightguards, fluoride carriers, and bleaching trays are made for patients by dentists but are rarely seen again in the dental office. They are made by drawing a heated sheet of plastic over a plaster or stone model of a patient's arch through the use of a vacuum apparatus. When cooled, the plastic is then trimmed just short of the gingival margin (sometimes more, sometimes less) and removed from the model so that the trimmed areas can be smoothed. These devices are usually made from 0.050-inch flexible clear acrylic that deforms elastically to a degree that undercut areas may be engaged, providing retention. Mouthguards are generally made for patients who are at risk, usually in sports, for blows or shocks to the jaws and dentition. Nightguards are often recommended for bruxism. It is believed that the introduction of the additional occlusal material interrupts uncontrollable clenching and grinding or at least switches the trauma on irreplaceable tissues (teeth) to trauma on a material (the mouthguard) that is easier to replace. Patients with high rates of caries or with a risk for rampant caries should be considered candidates for fluoride carriers. Fluoride carriers and bleaching trays provide an intimate fit of appliance against teeth. In this way, when a small amount of remineralizing fluoride solution or an enamel-bleaching agent is placed into the tray before insertion, the desired chemical is brought into intimate contact with the teeth until the tray is removed (Fig. 28-8). After the carrier is

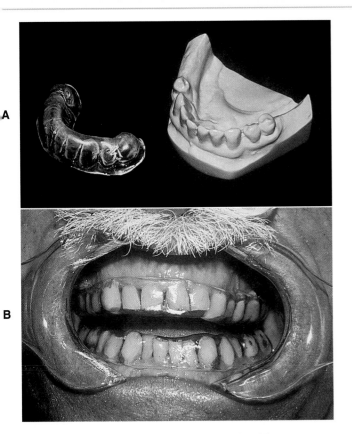

FIG. 28-8 A, A model of the patient's dentition serves as the template for a vacuum-formed appliance that covers all buccal, lingual, and occlusal surfaces along with the gingiva immediately adjacent to the teeth. **B,** At the recommended frequency (usually daily), the patient places a drop or less of fluoride gel into each tooth hollow in the carrier and then inserts the carrier for the recommended period.

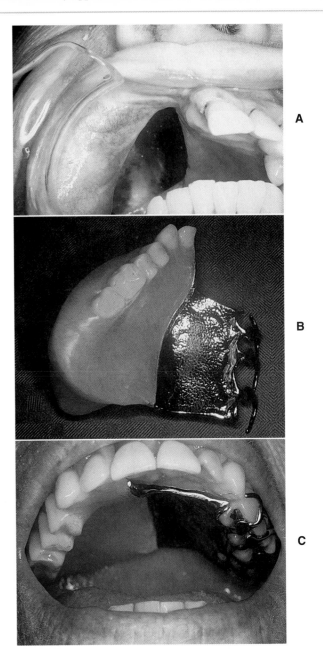

FIG. 28-9 A, Resection of a maxillary tumor has left a large defect that affects the palate and sinus and impedes speech, swallowing, and chewing. **B,** A unilateral removable partial denture has been combined with an obturator *(the acrylic portion on the lower left)* that replaces contours of the missing palatal and antral structures. **C,** This treatment allows the patient to function in a more normal manner.

removed, excess gel in the mouth is expectorated. The carrier should then be rinsed thoroughly (brushing with a denture brush is also acceptable) and stored in a safe place. The patient spits out the excess medicament (either fluoride gel or bleaching solution) and must not rinse, eat, or drink for at least 30 minutes.

MAXILLOFACIAL PROSTHESES

Maxillofacial prostheses encompass a wide variety of removable appliances that are used to replace missing anatomical structures (loss caused by trauma, surgical resection for malignancy, or congenital defect) other than teeth or, less commonly, to supplement insufficient neuromuscular control. Maxillofacial prostheses may be entirely intraoral, such as when a complete or partial denture has an attached *obturator* that replaces all or part of the palate or maxilla (Fig. 28-9) or has a posterior extension called a *palatal lift* that positions a flaccid soft palate superiorly and thereby aids speech and swallowing. The prosthesis may have both intraoral and extraoral components, such as when a maxillary prosthesis is connected to an extraoral piece that prosthetically replaces the nose, an eye, or another missing facial structures. Maxillofacial

prostheses may be exclusively extraoral, replacing an ear, a nose, part of an orbit, or a cheek.

It would be unusual for a patient with a maxillofacial prosthesis not to be under the care of a specialist, so the role the hygienist plays in the care of such prostheses is limited. Nevertheless, a hygienist should be alert to certain findings that are analogous to those of potential concern in the removable prostheses previously discussed (complete dentures, removable dentures). Thus perforations missing acrylic or metal elements, sharp edges of any material, peeling or flaking of a resilient material away from the more rigid base, and stains or cracks need to be brought to the dentist's immediate attention.

POSTSURGICAL STENTS AND SLEEP APNEA DEVICES

Two other varieties of prosthetic devices the hygienist encounters include postsurgical stents that protect graft sites or graft donor sites and sleep apnea devices that reposition the mandible anteriorly to ensure an open airway. Postsurgical stents may be removable, as when they cover a conservative graft site, such as the palatal donor site for a free gingival graft. They may be held in place with *circummandibular ligatures,* as is often the case following reconstructive oral surgery. Sleep apnea devices generally engage the coronal portions of both mandibular and maxillary teeth while flexibly directing the two jaws to relate in a slightly open, prognathic position.

Case Application
Dr. Basha had been given a sleep apnea device.

Postsurgical stents, whether removable or affixed by ligatures, are generally used for a few days or weeks and then discarded. The hygienist whose patient wears such a stent should be alert for sharp edges, mobile segments, and cracks. Sleep apnea devices are usually not brought to dental offices by patients unless the patient requires an adjustment. As with all acrylic devices, clinicians need to be alert for cracked or missing pieces and sharp edges in both the acrylic and metal components of the device.

EVALUATING ORAL TISSUES ASSOCIATED WITH APPLIANCES

Dental appliances should not cause discernible changes in the adjacent oral soft tissues when the devices have been fabricated properly and maintained appropriately, unless, as with an orthodontic appliance or a bleaching tray, such is the stated purpose. Oral tissues in contact with, or near dental appliances, often display signals that call for dental attention, patient education, or both. Dental appliances may directly affect oral tissues, such as when a sharp edge lacerates or an acrylic component exerts undue pressure. Effects may also be indirect, such as the greater plaque accumulation on abutment teeth of fixed or removable partial dentures (Fig. 28-10) or the reaction of gingival tissues to home-bleaching solutions. In the course of a thorough examination of the head and neck tissues, findings that may be attributable to dental appliances (e.g., erythema with or without edema, ulceration, hyperplastic tissue, microbial colonies, or desquamative lesions) will readily be identified. Yet the astute hygienist needs to be open as to the diagnosis of such findings until all data are collected: a poor-fitting denture that overlies a lesion may have caused the lesion or may be poor-fitting because the lesion has altered the intraoral anatomy. In either case, both the lesion and the suspicion regarding the appliance need to be called to the dentist's attention.

CONDITIONS ASSOCIATED WITH APPLIANCE WEAR

The most common condition associated with appliance wear is erythema, or redness of the tissues. Under close examination, erythematous tissue is seen to possess dilated vessels that account for its heightened color. Erythema may be associated with edema, caused by the passage of fluid out of the dilated blood vessels into the surrounding connective tissues, or edema may be absent. If erythema associated with an appliance is acute and localized, it is likely accompanied by the patient's complaint of discomfort and is probably a result of trauma from the appliance in the area of the redness. Less common possibilities include lesions that are coincidentally located in the area of the appliance or perhaps worsened by its presence, such as erosive lichen planus, early herpes simplex lesions, and bullous mucous membrane pemphigoid. Erythema, neither asymptomatic nor associated with pain, is probably chronic and caused by a candidal infection attributable to inadequate hygiene of the prosthesis. Other possible diagnoses, coincidentally in the area of the appliance, are squamous cell carcinoma or its predecessor, carcinoma *in situ.*

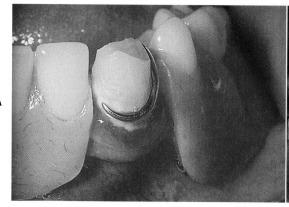
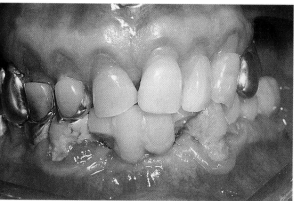

A

B

FIG. 28-10 A, The clasp arm of a removable partial denture readily retains plaque in the gingival third of abutment teeth. **B,** A damaged lower anterior bridge traps food debris and calculus.

Candida Infection

Many removable dental appliances, such as complete dentures, partial dentures, splints, and maxillofacial prostheses, are composed in large part of methyl methacrylate resin, a strong and stain-resistant material that is adjustable, polishable, and characterized to resemble oral mucosa. The curing process for methyl methacrylate resin results in a material that appears pockmarked upon microscopic examination. These surface irregularities and chemical properties of the material lead readily to its colonization by species of the common oral yeast candida, particularly *Candida albicans* and *Candida glabrata*. Adherent yeast organisms excrete metabolic byproducts that irritate the mucosa. If various factors permit the uncontrolled colonization of the denture surface with candida, the result is a condition of tissue erythema and edema called *candidiasis*, or more correctly—though less commonly used—*candidosis*. The most common form of candidosis specifically associated with the use of removable dentures is termed *acute atrophic candidiasis* and is characterized by striking erythema of the part of the tissue in contact with the prosthesis (Fig. 28-11). Two less common forms of candidosis are acute hyperplastic candidiasis and chronic hyperplastic candidiasis. Acute hyperplastic candidiasis, also termed *thrush,* is raised, loosely adherent, irregular white patches (composed of dead mucosal cells and colonies of the yeast organisms) that are disseminated across the surface of the tissue (Fig. 28-12). Chronic hyperplastic candidiasis, also termed *palatal hyperplasia,* occurs when the surface mucosa (usually of the palate, but the alveolar ridges may also be affected) is covered by a continuous mat of small, spherical projections of tissue that readily bleed under moderate pressure (Fig. 28-13).

In a healthy person, natural antifungal proteins in the saliva and the presence of other organisms stabilize the population of intraoral candida. However, the *Candida* organisms thrive under the following conditions:

- If an acrylic substrate is present, especially one that is worn continuously
- If saliva is reduced as a result of medications or disease
- If oxygen is sparse (a condition more easily attained between a prosthesis and the bearing mucosa)
- If a glucose source is plentiful (caused by poor oral hygiene or poorly controlled diabetes)
- If antibiotics have disturbed the natural balance of intraoral microorganisms
- If the host's immunological defenses are compromised (caused by chemotherapy, certain diseases, and certain medications)

The dental hygienist then needs to be observant for lesions of candida associated with dental appliance use not only to ensure optimal oral health but also because the presence of candidal lesions may indicate a more serious underlying health condition.[7]

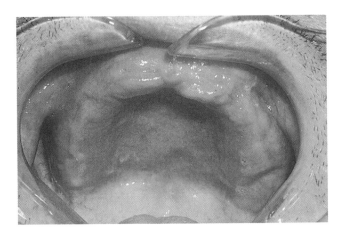

FIG. 28-11 Acute atrophic candidiasis, also called *denture stomatitis,* features edematous, red tissue (usually palatal) that is in direct contact with a denture.

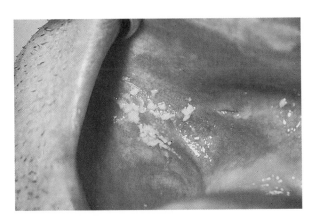

FIG. 28-12 Acute hyperplastic candidiasis (thrush) comprises raised white plaques that, when removed, reveal a raw, bleeding surface underneath.

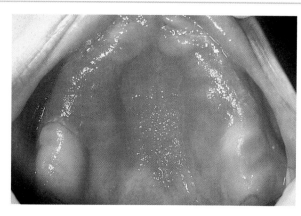

FIG. 28-13 This patient has chronic hyperplastic candidiasis (palatal hyperplasia), a condition in which small rounded projections of epithelialized tissue grow into the space between the palate and an ill-fitting maxillary denture.

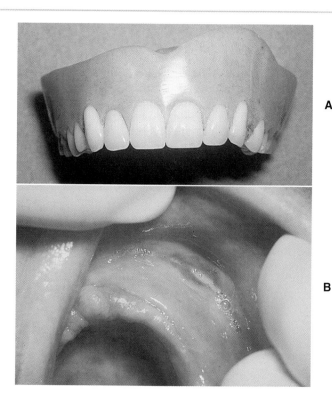

FIG. 28-14 If denture flanges are made too long **(A)** or become too long as the denture "settles" as a result of gradual loss of the supporting bone, a painful denture ulceration results **(B)**.

Erythema and Edema

Erythema and edema caused by bacterial plaque may be present beneath the pontic area of a fixed bridge, where their presence is essentially invisible unless floss is passed between the pontic and the underlying tissue (in which case slight bleeding occurs). Bacterially mediated erythema and edema at the gingival margin are also, of course, hallmark signs of gingivitis and are commonly seen on abutment teeth because the appliance disrupts the hygienic contour of the tooth surface itself. Similar changes are observed in the tissues surrounding implants if plaque deposits are not scrupulously removed.

Ulcerations and Lacerations

Ulcerations and lacerations are also conditions often associated with dental appliance use. Ulceration may occur as a result of repeated abrasion of soft tissue by a dental appliance or excess pressure against tissue, which results in a localized pressure necrosis. Laceration, or cutting of the tissue, results from a rough edge or other sharp element that causes a break in the mucosa. In all these cases, lesions are distinctly localized, with a reddish outline and a yellowish center that exposes the submucosal layer (Fig. 28-14). The tissue immediately adjacent to the lesion or laceration may be erythematous and slightly edematous, or it may be normal in color and contour. Some ulcerations and lacerations are painful, although others are not. When the causative agent of this sort of lesion is not addressed (because the lesions are asymptomatic or beneath the patient's threshold to seek help), the mucosa may heal but often does so accompanied by a proliferation of soft tissue, which is, itself, subsequently traumatized. Patients with removable dental appliances should always be carefully examined for signs of redundant tissue at the border areas where the appliance terminates against mucosal tissue.

Desquamation

Areas in which a thin mucosal layer has been sloughed away from the underlying tissue are described as *desqua-*

mative. Desquamative lesions in association with a dental appliance may be caused by direct trauma from the appliance before proper adjustment. Desquamative lesions associated with dental appliances are more likely caused by chemical burns (Fig. 28-15), such as a reaction to the surface of the appliance (e.g., when a denture has not been thoroughly rinsed after soaking in a disinfectant solution) or to its contents (e.g., home-bleaching solutions).

CARE AND CLEANING OF DENTAL APPLIANCES

Removable dental appliances should not be continuously worn in the mouth. Oral tissues—whether teeth, gingiva, or mucosa—need to have some extended period, each day, during which they are in unrestricted contact with salivary components. Saliva provides an environment of essential lubricating, antimicrobial, remineralizing, hydrating, oxygenating, and buffering properties that ensure optimal tissue health.

Regular cleaning of dental appliances is necessary to minimize unpleasant odors, sensations, and, in particular, unwanted tissue reactions. Fixed bridges and fixed bridgework over implants should be cleaned several times a day with a toothbrush, toothpaste, and one or more supplemental hygiene aids, such as a floss threader, interproximal brush, or superfloss (Fig. 28-16). The supplemental aids are necessary to clean the areas of the prostheses in contact with or facing the alveolar ridges. The hygienist

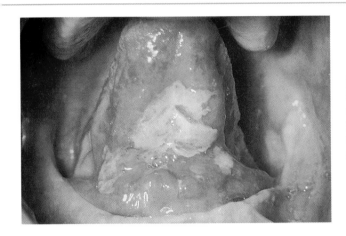

FIG. 28-15 This patient has a desquamative lesion on the ventral surface of the tongue. The patient failed to rinse the mandibular denture after it had been soaked in a bleach solution. The resulting chemical burn caused sloughing of the mucosa of the underside of the tongue. The lesion is painful but will resolve in 7 to 10 days without treatment.

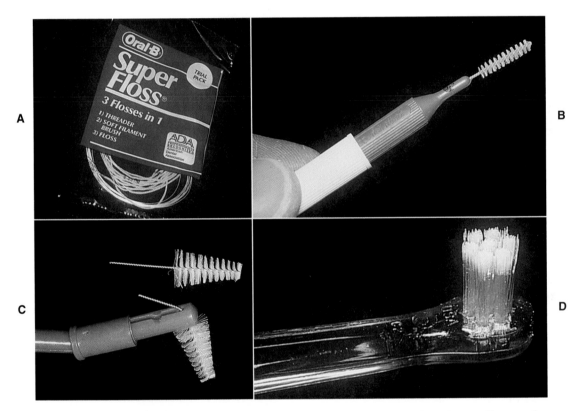

FIG. 28-16 Floss can be introduced under a bridge pontic with a floss threader or a floss product with a stiffer end **(A).** Interproximal brushes are also effective for cleaning between the pontic and the ridge tissue, whether held straight **(B)** or contraangled **(C).** End-tuft or uni-tuft brushes are also useful **(D).**

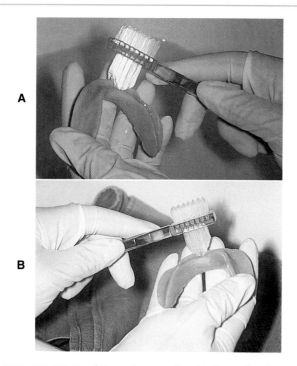

FIG. 28-17 Brushing a denture should always be done over water **(A)** or a towel **(B)** so that the denture is not damaged if it is dropped.

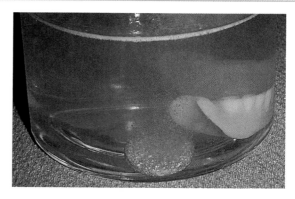

FIG. 28-18 Commercial soaking agents effectively clean dentures in 10 to 20 minutes.

needs to work closely with each patient to identify which hygiene aid or aids is or are most appropriate for a patient's dental needs, manual dexterity, and visual acuity and to train the patient in the correct technique.

Removable prostheses are cleaned outside the mouth. Patients should remove such appliances after every meal to rinse off adherent food and thereby minimize the substrate for development of bacterial plaque. Complete dentures, overdentures, and partial dentures should be gently but thoroughly scrubbed daily on all surfaces under running water, using a brush specifically designed for dentures. Patients should be instructed to always clean their oral prostheses over a sink in which several inches of water are present or in which a washcloth has been placed (Fig. 28-17) so that the appliance will not break if it is accidentally dropped while being cleaned. Toothpaste should not be used with the denture brush because the abrasive properties of normal dentifrice actually wear away acrylic over time. Patients who desire a "fresh" or "minty" flavor or sensation once they have cleaned their dental appliance should be directed to one or more commercial products, either foaming denture cleansing pastes or soaking agents, that feature such a flavor.

Brushing, even with a denture dentifrice, does not adequately remove organisms that tightly adhere to the appliance surface and are sheltered within the acrylic pores.[1] Placing an acrylic appliance in a small ultrasonic cleaning bath effectively removes all microorganisms in a few minutes.[5] Small cleansing units that cost less than $100 can be obtained for patient use, but they are not widely available and are used by only a small minority of patients. Soaking overnight in a cup of 10% home-bleaching solution, with or without a teaspoon of dishwasher detergent, is also effective in the eradication of microbes on removable appliances.[2] More than 75% of patients with com-

plete and removable dentures, however, use a commercial denture-soaking solution two or more times a week. In the United States, denture-cleaning products come as tablets that effervesce in water (Fig. 28-18) and release an effective bleach, chelation (for removal of calcium), and detergent solution, which effectively eradicates more than 99% of adherent microbes in less than 15 minutes.[8] When an appliance is left overnight in such a solution, virtual sterilization of the device occurs. Appliances with metal elements, such as partial dentures and orthodontic retainers, should not be left for more than 20 minutes in such solutions (or in home-bleaching solutions, for that matter) because the metallic parts darken and become dull as a result of the powerful oxidization effects of the bleach. A recent development in commercially available appliance-soaking solutions is the introduction of a product that both cleans the dental device and coats it with a thin, insoluble layer of silicone polymer. This silicone polymer inhibits subsequent candidal colonization of the surface but wears off during the course of a day. This "preventive" approach to hygiene of dental devices is novel and logical.

Several dental appliances either benefit from or actually require the use of materials that need periodic (usually daily or more frequent) reapplication or replenishment. Fluoride carriers are the best example; their proper use is dependent on the daily introduction of fluoride gel that is then held in proximity to the teeth by the appliance. The two most common formulations for topical fluoride gel are acidulated stannous fluoride (1100 ppm or 0.4%) and neutral sodium fluoride gel (5000 ppm or 1.1%). Much clinical and experimental data support the use of one or the other of these for a given clinical situation. The most compelling criterion concerns the acidity of the compounds—stannous fluoride gel is distinctly acidic (with a pH of approximately 4.5) and should not be left in contact with the teeth for more than 3 minutes daily. After fluoride trays have been in the mouth for the desired interval, they are to be removed, cleaned under running water with a denture brush, and stored in clean water.

An empiric regimen used is the introduction of a drop of fluoride gel into the areas of an overdenture that correspond to the retentive abutment (Fig. 28-19). Limited clinical data support this regimen, noting enhanced periodontal health and limited root caries in abutment teeth.[3]

As with fluoride trays, bleaching trays are specifically designed and used to place a therapeutic agent into contact with the dentition. Home-bleaching solutions are

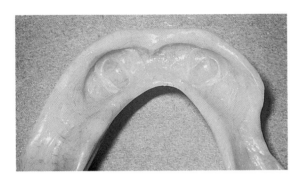

FIG. 28-19 The undersurface of an overdenture clearly shows where the abutment teeth sit. Daily application of a single drop of topical fluoride gel into each of these sites will suppress plaque growth and metabolism and therefore help to preserve abutment health and longevity.

used under a dentist's supervision, and thus the material, its amount, and all other patient instructions have been specified in advance. The dental hygienist's responsibility is to assess the surrounding soft tissues and, as necessary, counsel the patient on providing or enhancing the necessary daily hygiene of the appliance.

Certain removable dental appliances benefit from the use of products applied to keep the device in place. Some maxillofacial prosthetic devices, particularly those with extraoral components such as eyes, ears, noses, and cheekbones, may require or benefit from the use of solvent-dissoluble adhesives that ensure aesthetic, prolonged adaptation to the natural tissues. Increasingly such appliances rely on osseointegrated implants for retention but still may benefit from the ability of adhesive material to ensure a less apparent transition from prosthetic to genuine skin. The adhesive material and its solvent are generally available only by prescription.

Denture adhesive is an over-the-counter product that is used by approximately 25% of patients with complete dentures. Sparingly soluble in water or saliva, powder and cream denture adhesives work by flowing into spaces between the denture and the bearing tissues. This optimizes the "seal" that results from an intimate fit between the denture and the soft tissues. In addition, denture adhesive is sticky, thick, and effectively adheres to the tissues and the denture while also resisting disaggregation.[6] Use of denture adhesive improves the retention (resistance to displacement of the denture away from the bearing tissues) and stability (resistance to movement relative to the underlying bone, while being retained by the soft tissue) of all dentures, even well-fitting, new ones.[4] However, expense is involved in its use, and the product makes daily hygiene more complex because, by design, the material is not easily removed from either the denture or the oral tissues. Use of warm or hot water and a brush or washcloth assists in the removal of adhesive. Some dentists have strong feelings in opposition to patients' use of denture adhesive because of the provider's lack of familiarity with the high quality and efficacy of modern denture adhesives. For this reason, the dental hygienist needs to understand the practice's preference with respect to the use of denture adhesive before offering such a product to a patient.

 RITICAL THINKING ACTIVITIES

1. Visit a dental laboratory. Examine dentures as they are repaired and relined. What clues suggest whether the patient was effective at keeping the prosthesis clean? What methods do you suggest to clean the prosthesis before it is returned to the patient? What methods would you suggest to the patient to keep the prosthesis clean in the future?

2. At a dentist's office, examine the different designs of the pontics and the connectors of fixed partial dentures that have not yet been delivered to patients. Can you identify designs that would be easier than others for a patient to keep clean? For each case, what would be the device or material you would suggest to the patient to use at home to keep the new prosthesis clean?

3. Obtain some scrap orthodontic wire. Place it for a week in a glass cup with a solution of 9 oz of water and 1 oz of laundry bleach so that some of the wire is covered by liquid and some is not. How does the wire look at the end of the week?

4. Obtain a sample of denture cleanser (or buy a small package). Place a tablet of the material in a clear glass of water. What changes does the solution undergo during the next 20 minutes? How does this differ from what happens to a sample of a different denture cleanser?

5. Repeat the preceding experiment, but moisten a polished piece of dental acrylic with water. What does the wetted acrylic feel like to your fingers? Now drop the acrylic into one of the cleansing solutions for several minutes. Remove the acrylic with your fingers. What does it feel like now? How long do you need to rinse the acrylic in tap water before the solution's odor disappears? How long is it before the surface of the acrylic feels like it did before it was placed in the cleaning solution? How will this information help you educate patients?

6. Demonstrate the use of a tufted floss, such as superfloss, and a proxabrush to a patient who has just received a fixed bridge. When you next see that patient, compare the tendency for gingival bleeding around the prosthesis to the soft tissue behavior of another bridge patient who has not been instructed in the use of these products.

7. The next time you treat a patient who has a removable prosthesis, carefully examine both the tissue surface of the denture and the color and consistency of the mucosa on which it rested. What connection can you make between the appearances of the two?

REVIEW QUESTIONS

The following questions refer to the case study presented at the beginning of the chapter.

1. Which is the most likely reason that the metal framework of Dr. Basha's mandibular removal partial denture (RPD) is dark and dull?
   a. Dr. Basha fails to clean the RPD on a regular basis.
   b. One of the medications Dr. Basha uses probably causes the staining.
   c. The metal framework is an alloy of inferior quality.
   d. Dr. Basha soaks the partial denture too long in a commercial denture-cleansing solution.

2. Which of the following is the most likely reason that Dr. Basha dislikes the flavor of the fluoride solution?
   a. It is a neutral sodium fluoride preparation.
   b. It is a stannous fluoride preparation.
   c. It is an outdated solution.
   d. Dr. Basha may not clean the fluoride carrier between uses.

3. For which of the following arches has the fluoride carrier been prepared?
   a. The maxillary arch, to limit the effect of plaque on the implant abutments
   b. The mandibular arch, to prevent and remineralize incipient caries and to inhibit periodontal pathogens
   c. Either arch, because the increased concentration of fluoride in the oral cavity is effective throughout the mouth
   d. The maxillary arch, to limit the effect of the overdenture on the palatal tissues

4. The tissue underneath the implant splint bar is inflamed for which of the following reasons?
   a. Tissues beneath dentures are generally inflamed because of the pressure of the prosthesis.
   b. The presence of plaque between the splint bar and the mucosa is irritating to the soft tissue.

   c. Dr. Basha is likely allergic to nickel in the alloy of the splint bar.
   d. The tight fit of the overdenture causes blood to be brought to the surface of the mucosa whenever the appliance is removed.

5. Which of the following oral findings in a prosthodontic patient would you associate with Dr. Basha's dry mouth?
   a. The dentures are likely to be clean because so little saliva is present.
   b. The soft tissues beneath the dentures are likely to be inflamed because underhydrated acrylic is toxic.
   c. The soft tissues beneath the dentures are likely to be white and hyperkeratotic because underlubricated prostheses are more retentive.
   d. The soft tissues beneath the dentures are likely to display changes consistent with candidal infection because of the absence of saliva and its antimicrobial and lubricant properties.

6. Dr. Basha displays evidence of prior periodontal surgery. For which of the following reasons would you not insist on the use of dental floss on the lower teeth?
   a. He does an acceptable job with an interproximal cleaner.
   b. Dental floss may not be the best device for cleaning beneath a fixed bridge, depending on the contour of the undersurfaces of the contact area and pontics.
   c. Dr. Basha's medical condition dictates the use of a nonfloss alternative.
   d. All the above

 SUGGESTED AGENCIES AND WEB SITES

Because of the ever-changing nature of the Internet, some of the web sites listed here may have changed since publication. Please refer to Mosby's Evolve web site for the most current information.

Academy of Osseointegration (patient education materials on implants, partial dentures, dentures): http://www.osseo.org

American Academy of Implant Dentistry (frequently asked questions regarding dental implants): http://www.aaid-implant.org

Dental Hygiene Education: Margaret J. Fehrenbach and Associates (site by a dental hygienist and educator with brief, pragmatic patient information on dentures, partial dentures, bridges, implants, and orthodontic appliances): http://home1.gte.net

 ADDITIONAL READINGS AND RESOURCES

Banting D, Hill S: Microwave disinfection of dentures for the treatment of oral candidiasis, *Spec Care Dent* 21(1):4-8, 2001.

Shay K: Denture hygiene: review and update [Internet and journal], *J Contemp Dent Pract* 1(2):28, 2000 [http://www.thejcdp. com].

REFERENCES

1. Dills SS et al: Comparison of the antimicrobial capability of an abrasive paste and chemical-soak denture cleaners, *J Prosthet Dent* 60:467, 1988.
2. Ettinger RL, Bergman W, Wefel J: Effect of fluoride on over-denture abutments, *Am J Dent* 7(1):17, 1994.
3. Glass RT, Belobraydic KA: The dilemma of denture contamination, *Okla Dent Assoc J* 81(2):30, 1990.
4. Grasso JE, Rendell J, Gay T: Effect of denture adhesive on the retention and stability of maxillary dentures, *J Prosthet Dent* 72:399, 1994.
5. Gwinnett AJ, Caputo L: The effectiveness of ultrasonic denture cleaning: a scanning electron microscope study, *J Prosthet Dent* 50:20, 1983.
6. Shay K: Denture adhesives: choosing the right powders and pastes, *J Am Dent Assoc* 122:70, 1991.
7. Shay K, Renner RP, Truhlar MR: Oropharyngeal candidosis in the older patient, *J Am Geriatr Soc* 45:863, 1997.
8. Warner-Lambert Company: Discussion with product manager [oral communication], 1999.

PART V

Chapter 29
Oral Risk Assessment and Intervention Planning

Chapter 30
Individualizing Preventive and Therapeutic Strategies

Competency Statements

The learner is expected to possess knowledge, skills, judgments, values, and attitudes to develop the listed competencies.

Core Competencies
- Apply a professional code of ethics in all endeavors.
- Adhere to state and federal laws, recommendations, and regulations in the provision of dental hygiene care.
- Provide dental hygiene care to promote patient health and wellness using critical thinking and problem solving in the provision of evidence-based practice.
- Use evidence-based decision making to evaluate and incorporate emerging treatment modalities.
- Assume responsibility for dental hygiene actions and care based on accepted scientific theories and research as well as the accepted standard of care.
- Provide quality assurance mechanisms for health services.
- Communicate effectively with individuals and groups from diverse populations both verbally and in writing.
- Provide accurate, consistent, and complete documentation for assessment, diagnosis, planning, implementation, and evaluation of dental hygiene services.
- Provide care to all patients using an individualized approach that is humane, empathetic, and caring.

Health Promotion and Disease Prevention
- Promote the values of oral and general health and wellness to the public and organizations within and outside the profession.

Courtesy American Dental Education Association, Washington, DC.

Health Promotion
and Disease Prevention

- Respect the goals, values, beliefs, and preferences of the patient while promoting optimal oral and general health.
- Refer patients who may have a physiologic psychological, and/or social problem for comprehensive patient evaluation.
- Identify individual and population risk factors and develop strategies that promote health related quality of life.
- Evaluate factors that can be used to promote patient adherence to disease prevention and/or health maintenance strategies.
- Evaluate and utilize methods to ensure the health and safety of the patient and the dental hygienist in the delivery of dental hygiene care.

Community Involvement
- Evaluate reimbursement mechanisms and their impact on the patient's access to oral healthcare.

Patient Care
- Select, obtain, and interpret diagnostic information recognizing its advantages and limitations.
- Recognize predisposing and etiologic risk factors that require intervention to prevent disease.
- Obtain, review, and update a complete medical, family, social, and dental history.
- Recognize health conditions and medications that impact overall patient care.
- Identify patients at risk for a medical emergency and manage the patients care in a manner that prevents an emergency.
- Perform a comprehensive examination using clinical, radiographic, periodontal, dental charting, and other data collection procedures to assess the patient's needs.
- Determine a dental hygiene diagnosis.
- Identify patient needs and significant findings that impact the delivery of dental hygiene services.

- Obtain consultations as indicated.
- Prioritize the care plan based on the health status and the actual and potential problems of the individual to facilitate optimal oral health.
- Establish a planned sequence of care (education, clinical, and evaluation) based on the dental hygiene diagnosis; identified oral conditions; potential problems; etiologic and risk factors; and available treatment modalities.
- Establish a collaborative relationship with the patient in the planned care to include etiology, prognosis, and treatment alternatives.
- Make referrals to other healthcare professionals.
- Obtain the patient's informed consent based on a thorough case presentation.
- Perform dental hygiene interventions to eliminate and/or control local etiologic factors to prevent and control caries, periodontal disease, and other oral conditions.
- Control pain and anxiety during treatment through the use of accepted clinical and behavioral techniques.
- Determine the outcomes of dental hygiene interventions using indices, instruments, examination techniques, and patient self-report.
- Evaluate the patient's satisfaction with the oral healthcare received and the oral healthcare status achieved.
- Provide subsequent treatment or referrals based on evaluation findings.
- Develop and maintain a health maintenance program.

Professional Growth and Development
- Access professional and social networks and resources to assist entrepreneurial initiatives.

CHAPTER 29

Oral Risk Assessment
and Intervention Planning

Sherry A. Harfst, Victoria C. Vick

Chapter Outline

Case Study: Therapeutic Intervention with Risk
    Assessment
Patient-Specific Approach to Oral Care
    Oral risk assessment
ORA System
    ORA worksheet
ORA Application to Case Study
    Step 1: review
    Step 2: analyze
    Step 3: plan therapeutic intervention

Case Summary
    Step 1: review assessment data
    Step 2: analyze data for oral risk concerns
    Step 3: plan therapeutic intervention

Key Terms

Intervention	Risk	Risk factors
Prevention	Risk assessment	Therapeutic intervention strategy

Learning Outcomes

1. Determine a working definition for the following terms: intervention, oral risk assessment, prevention, risk, and risk assessment.
2. Compare and contrast a patient-specific approach to care with a standardized routine.
3. Give examples of patient-centered oral care.
4. Provide examples of therapeutic intervention and prevention strategies in dentistry and their overlap.

5. Describe the benefits of oral risk assessment.
6. State and explain the five steps in the ORA system.
7. Apply Steps 1, 2, and 3 of the ORA system to any clinic patient.
8. Develop a clinical goal, therapeutic intervention, and evaluation measure based on a given oral risk concern.

One of the more complex and ultimately rewarding functions the dental hygienist performs in patient care is in the diagnosis and planning of dental hygiene therapy. This function is complex because numerous physical and cognitive steps are involved that then must be carefully evaluated and weighed to arrive at an appropriate plan of therapy, education, and ongoing, supportive care.

Planning patient care is as rewarding as it is complex in that it affords dental hygienists the opportunity to touch a life and to impact the oral health—and potentially the systemic health—of those in our care. Dental hygienists may provide treatment, service, and care for individuals in a way they may have never before experienced. In the following case example, consider both the complexity and the opportunity to change a lifetime of dental pain.

PATIENT-SPECIFIC APPROACH TO ORAL CARE

29-A At first it might appear that a standard course of therapy can be applied to any patient exhibiting certain clinical criteria. To some extent, this is a true statement. For example, a patient with marginal gingivitis will be clinically treated to remove the bacterial plaque and associated toxins and provided with appropriate self-care techniques to prevent and lessen plaque accumulation to a level biologically acceptable so that health is promoted and maintained. As a "standard" of care, that treatment rationale is sound by today's criteria. However, every patient treated brings unique health histories (medical, dental, biological, psychological, sociological, and cultural), including prescription and over-the-counter medications, beliefs, behaviors, unique clinical and radiographic findings, and expectations—all of which must be factored in providing appropriate clinical and oral self-care therapy. Patient-centered care—the method of care driven by the person's specific needs—holds to the dictates of the surgeon general's *Report on Oral Health in America* (see Chapter 2), presents a holistic approach to care, and is the currently accepted method of patient care, planning, and delivery.[19]

ORAL RISK ASSESSMENT

Concept

One of the newest concepts in patient-centered care is oral **risk assessment**.[1,6,17,18,20] The basic premise of this concept states that each patient has a set of historical data—facts about genetic predisposition, previous oral and systemic disease experiences, medication regimens, fluoride history, habits, practices, behaviors, and beliefs. Each patient also has a specific set of current medical–dental data that reveal the patient's current oral status. Dental hygienists have the data necessary to complete an oral risk assessment when both the historical and current information is evaluated for a given patient. Once the data is evaluated, a clear picture of potential and clinical oral risk concerns begins to emerge. Not only can the oral conditions cur-

---

Please refer to the case study presented near the beginning of this chapter for background information concerning the patient discussed throughout the chapter.

Therapeutic Intervention with Risk Assessment

Robin Wallace, a 54-year-old woman who recently separated from her husband, arrives at your practice for a new patient examination. She has had inconsistent oral care during her lifetime and is currently experiencing pain caused by untreated dental caries. Ms. Wallace has no dental insurance at this time and, as evidenced by her clinical oral examination and radiographic survey, needs significant restorative dentistry. Periodontally, she exhibits generalized gingivitis characterized by marginal inflammation of the gingiva and bleeding on gentle probing. Horizontal bone loss is evident radiographically; loss of attachment is noted in the premolar region.

When asked about her normal oral self-care habits, she confides that her toothbrush was "lost" in her recent move when she and her husband separated and that she just has not cared much about her appearance. Ms. Wallace believes she has a promising job interview in a month, which she anticipates will offer dental insurance as a benefit. The job for which she is applying involves initial client contact for a major law firm in your community.

Think about the components involved in planning care for Ms. Wallace and the assessment steps that must occur before a plan is developed. How do you approach the pattern of dental neglect and lack of interest in self-care? What motivational factors can you isolate and use to help her gain optimal self-care? Where do you start? How do you individualize the treatment plan appropriate for this patient? This seemingly overwhelming function of dental hygiene diagnosis and patient care planning is manageable when broken down into a series of steps, particularly when the patient is involved as a participant.

---

rently in evidence for a given patient be determined, but a listing of *potential* oral risk concerns (conditions, manifestations) can also be provided. This listing is based on current and past health histories, including dental, for which therapeutic **intervention** strategies and personalized **prevention** strategies can be developed (Box 29-1).

Definition

Risk is defined as the probability that an event will occur, such as a loss or injury. ***Risk factors*** are those conditions or behaviors associated with risk occurrence.[3]

Applying the concept to health, the term *risk* can be further defined as the probability of a person experiencing a change in health status over time.[12] In risk assessment, knowledge of risk factors—known associates to specific diseases or conditions—is used to partially determine a course of therapy and to design self-care interventions, as appropriate to a given patient (Box 29-2).

Application to Medicine and Dentistry

Medicine has provided dentistry a model for the application of risk assessment. For decades, through the use of

---

BOX 29-1

Intervention and Prevention

An explanation of the terms *intervention* and *prevention* is warranted as the discussion on patient-care planning begins. Each term is clearly and distinctly defined; however, in dentistry these terms overlap, which makes their application less clear. For example, *to intervene* implies a step or a measure designed to halt or significantly alter the current course of an event. In the case of removing demineralized tooth structure and replacing it with a restorative material, the caries process has been arrested by the intervention of a restorative dental procedure. To give a periodontal example, debriding a 4-mm pocket should result in the elimination of gingival inflammation and in the arrest of bone loss and gingival attachment. Both are clear examples of intervention.

Likewise, *prevention* is defined as the method that stops or prevents an expected or anticipated outcome from occurring. Removal of plaque to biologically acceptable levels can prevent both dental caries and gingival or periodontal diseases. The application of topical fluoride can prevent demineralization and enhance remineralization. Again, this is a clear example of prevention.

However, understanding the way in which intervention and prevention can occur simultaneously, even from the therapeutic or self-care procedure, is required for the reader to grasp the entire picture. For example, when topical fluoride is applied to an incipient carious lesion, what happens?

The lesion remineralizes (intervention), and the caries process is arrested. At the same time, the tooth structure becomes less pervious to an acid challenge, preventing demineralization from occurring (see Chapter 22). Removal of plaque and associated toxins can be an intervention to a disease process, as in debridement, and a prevention of a disease process, as in daily oral self-care to prevent toxins from accumulating at the gingival margin (see Chapter 21).

This chapter uses these two terms in their simplest forms: intervention strategies are designed to stop the disease process, and prevention strategies are designed to ensure a disease process will not occur. However, it should be noted that many times intervention and prevention occur simultaneously.

BOX 29-2

Knowledge of Risk Factors

Benefits to be gained from risk assessment, as presented by Douglas, include four basic tenets. Knowledge of risk factors can facilitate the following:
1. Increase the chances of correctly predicting an oral disease instance (e.g., caries or periodontal disease)
2. Help identify individuals and groups who would benefit from targeted interventions
3. Stimulate increased clinician awareness and level of suspicion, which prompts increased acuteness in the assessment process
4. Provide a foundation for early disease recognition, which identifies candidates for new and emerging disease management technologies

From Douglas CW: Risk assessment in dentistry *J Dent Ed* 62(10): 756-761, 1998.

BOX 29-3

Five-Step Process in Oral Risk Assessment

1. *Review assessment data*: Step 1 reviews all patient data.
2. *Analyze data for oral risk concerns:* Step 2 analyzes patient data for potential oral concerns (oral risk).
3. *Plan:* Step 3 outlines goals of therapy for professional and patient self-care.
4. *Recommend*: Step 4 provides specific oral-care products and an oral self-care regimen.
5. *Evaluate/reevaluate*: Step 5 evaluates outcomes of clinical dental hygiene therapy and recommends alternatives as appropriate.

---

risk assessment, the medical community has targeted groups of individuals at risk for certain diseases (e.g., stroke, cancer, diabetes, heart disease), with intervention strategies specific to that disease.[4] This type of ***therapeutic intervention strategy*** is also appropriate for dentistry. Research has confirmed that certain subgroups are at an increased risk for certain oral disease populations. In planning appropriate dental hygiene care, clinicians need to be aware of these subgroups and realize that aggressive disease states are often defined by biological, psychological, and sociological components.[2,5,7,10]

Gathering, reviewing, and assessing patient data to perform a risk assessment can indeed be a time-consuming function for the oral healthcare provider, yet it is probably one of the most important functions integral to determining risk factors and potential oral conditions, designing appropriate supportive therapy, and planning patient self-care prevention strategies based on specific patient need. Use of a system-driven, clinical decision-making tool assists in the collection, assessment, and implementation of this process.

ORA SYSTEM

In dentistry, a clinical framework for risk assessment can be provided by the Oral Risk Assessment and Early Intervention System (ORA), an organizational tool that helps systematically review data, analyze risk, and provide appropriate oral-care recommendations. ORA helps to provide a more holistic approach to patient data collection and subsequent course of therapy, which can result in early disease intervention.[6,11,14]

ORA is a simple, clinical data-gathering and decision-making tool for chairside use. It incorporates a five-phase approach to the design of therapeutic intervention and prevention strategies, based on numerous health promotion stratagems and decision support systems.[6,8,11,14,15,16] The ORA system gathers data via a standard health history form and through the use of a specialized patient questionnaire termed the *Prevention Survey* (Fig. 29-1).

The five-step ORA process follows the traditional dental hygiene model of assessment, diagnosis, planning, implementation, and evaluation.[13] The difference is in the organizational tool—and a more formalized analysis of current and potential oral risk concerns (Box 29-3).

DENTAL HISTORY

Name _____   Date _____

1. **In the past two years, have you experienced any of the following symptoms?**
   (If yes, please check all that apply)
   ❏ Sensitive teeth ❏ Sore jaw ❏ Toothache ❏ Sore gums
   ❏ Bleeding gums ❏ Difficulty chewing ❏ Filling fell out ❏ Dry mouth
   ❏ Bad breath ❏ Burning sensation ❏ Abscess ❏ Swollen face
   ❏ Swelling inside mouth ❏ Tartar buildup ❏ Yellowing teeth ❏ Difficulty swallowing
   Comments _____

2. **When you look inside your mouth, do you know what to look for?**
	Yes	No
Tooth Decay	❏	❏
Oral Cancer	❏	❏
Gum Disease	❏	❏

3. **For the past two years, what is your best estimate of the number of times you have been to see a dental professional for each of the following:**
   _____ Checkups and cleanings
   _____ Other dental treatment such as fillings, gum treatment, crowns (caps), bridges, dentures
   _____ Dental emergencies

4. **Do you clench or grind your teeth in the daytime or at night?**
   ❏ Yes ❏ No
   If yes, do you wear a bite guard? _____ For how long? _____

5. **In the past two years, have you been concerned about the appearance of your teeth?**
   (If yes, please check all that apply)
   ❏ Yellowing/graying teeth ❏ Stains ❏ Crowded, crooked ❏ Spacing between teeth
   ❏ Other _____

6. **Check any of the following you regularly use at home:**
   ❏ Soft toothbrush ❏ Dental floss ❏ Floss threader ❏ Powered interdental cleaner
   ❏ Hard toothbrush ❏ Special brush ❏ Toothpick ❏ Powered brush
   ❏ Medium toothbrush ❏ Fluoride toothpaste ❏ Fluoride rinse or gel ❏ Other_____
   ❏ Oral irrigator ❏ Rubber tip ❏ Mouthrinse
   ❏ Denture adhesive ❏ Denture cleanser ❏ Whitening product

7. **Check the type of toothpaste you use:**
   ❏ Fluoride ❏ Tartar control ❏ Gum benefit ❏ Whitening
   ❏ Sensitivity protection ❏ Baking soda ❏ Peroxide ❏ Multiple benefit

8. **Estimate how long it takes you to clean your teeth and gums each time:**
   Please indicate your best and most reliable estimate.
   Brushing_____ Flossing_____
   (time)   (time)

9. **About how many times each day/week do you brush and floss?**
   I brush about _____ times per day OR _____ per week
   I floss about _____ times per day OR _____ per week

10. **Do you find it difficult to maintain an oral hygiene schedule due to your job/profession or other reasons?**
    ❏ No ❏ Yes

11. **Do any conditions make it difficult for you to adequately clean your teeth?**
    (If yes, please check all that apply)
    ❏ Hold a toothbrush ❏ Use dental floss ❏ Brush/floss for any length of time ❏ Don't see well

12. **Generally, how have you felt about your previous dental appointments?**
    ❏ Very anxious and afraid ❏ Don't care one way or the other
    ❏ Somewhat anxious and afraid ❏ Look forward to it

Prevention Survey

A

FLUORIDE HISTORY

1. ❏ Yes ❏ No Are you on a fluoridated public water system?
   If yes, for how long? _____

2. ❏ Yes ❏ No Do you use any type of water filter or bottled water for your main water source?
   If yes, what type of filter? _____
   If yes, what brand of water? _____
   For how long? _____

3. ❏ Yes ❏ No If you are on a fluoridated public water system, does your job/profession keep
   you away from home more than 4 days per week?
   If yes, do you use any fluoride supplements during that time?
   (For example: a fluoridated mouthrinse) ❏ Yes ❏ No

4. ❏ Yes ❏ No Do you drink bottled fruit juices? _____
   If yes, how many per day? _____

5. ❏ Yes ❏ No Do you currently use a fluoridated toothpaste?
   If yes, how often? _____
   If yes, for how many years? _____
   If yes, what brand? _____
   If no, why not? _____

6. ❏ Yes ❏ No Do you use an oral rinse containing fluoride?
   If yes, how often? _____
   If yes, what brand? _____

7. ❏ Yes ❏ No Do you use any additional sources of fluoride (such as mouthrinse, drops, tablets)?
   If yes, what sources? _____
   For how long? _____

For Child Patient

8. ❏ Yes ❏ No Are the children in your home in childcare, daycare or school where they **do not
   receive** fluoridated public water?
   If yes, how many days per week? _____

9. ❏ Yes ❏ No Do you or anyone in your home use a fluoridated supplement (drops or tablets?)
   If yes, what dosage? _____
   If yes, for how long? _____

B

FIG. 29-1 The ORA Prevention Survey is a specialized, four-part patient questionnaire used to gather data on dental history **(A)**, fluoride history **(B)**

Continued

BEHAVIORS

1. **Do you have an annual physical examination?**
   ❑ No   ❑ Yes

2. **When you are ill, do you?**
   ❑ See your physician?   ❑ Seek care in an emergency room?
   ❑ Wait to see if the condition goes away?

3. **When your physician recommends a change in health behavior, do you follow his/her advice?**
   ❑ No   ❑ Yes   ❑ Sometimes

4. **When your dental professional recommends a change in health behavior, do you follow his/her advice?**
   ❑ No   ❑ Yes   ❑ Sometimes

5. **When your dental professional recommends a specific oral care product or self-care regimen do you follow his/her advice?**
   ❑ No   ❑ Yes   ❑ Sometimes

6. **Do you have regular hobbies/interests outside of work?**
   ❑ No   ❑ Yes

7. **Do you strive to reach a balance between work and relaxation?**
   ❑ No   ❑ Yes

8. **Are your eating habits out of control?**
   ❑ No   ❑ Yes

9. **Do you feel your stress level has increased in the past 6 months?**
   ❑ No   ❑ Yes

10. **Do you use tobacco in any form? If yes, what form and frequency?**
    ❑ No   ❑ Yes   ❑ Sometimes Type _____ Frequency/Quantity _____
    For how long? _____

11. **Do you consume alcohol?**
    ❑ No   ❑ Yes   ❑ Sometimes Type _____ Frequency/Quantity _____

12. **Do you consume caffeine?**
    ❑ No   ❑ Yes   ❑ Sometimes Type _____ Frequency/Quantity _____

13. **Do you exercise daily?**
    ❑ No   ❑ Yes   ❑ Sometimes Type _____ Frequency/Quantity _____

14. **Do you participate in sports/recreation activities?**
    ❑ No   ❑ Yes   ❑ Sometimes Type _____ Frequency/Quantity _____

C

DIET SURVEY

Please indicate which sweets and cooked starches you eat between meals.

Food	Frequency	✓ if between meals
breath mints		
cough drops		
chewing gum		
dried fruits		
canned/bottled beverages		
sugared liquids		
chips		
crackers		
cookies		

D

BELIEFS

1. **In your opinion, compared to the average person, how likely do you think you are to have cavities or other problems with your teeth and/or gums?**
   ❑ Much more likely   ❑ About average   ❑ Much less than average
   ❑ More than average   ❑ Less than average

2. **How important is it for you to prevent cavities, gum problems or other diseases of the mouth?**
   ❑ Very important   ❑ Somewhat important   ❑ Not at all important

3. **Would you like your dental professional to make specific product recommendations to meet your oral care needs?**
   ❑ Yes   ❑ I am not sure   ❑ No

4. **There are times in our lives when it seems we have the energy and time to tackle new projects or to make changes.**
   At this time, I ❑ can   ❑ cannot imagine trying to change a habit.

5. **I believe that I have control over the condition of my mouth.**
   ❑ Firmly believe   ❑ Somewhat believe   ❑ Do not believe

FIG. 29-1, cont'd Health behaviors **(C)**, and diet recall and health beliefs **(D)**.

ORA WORKSHEET

The five columns on the ORA Worksheet (Fig. 29-2) provide a template for the clinician to record the following:

- Summary findings from the review of pertinent histories and current clinical findings
- Listings of current and potential oral symptoms and conditions based on oral risk
- Established goals of therapy (therapeutic intervention strategies) and patient self-care prevention goals, including appointment planning
- Specific oral-care recommendations
- Reevaluation

This chapter addresses Steps 1, 2, and 3 of the ORA system. Steps 4 and 5, which involve individualized prevention strategies, appointment planning and sequencing, and planning are discussed in Chapter 30.

Column I: Review

In Step 1 the clinician reviews and records a summary of all documented histories and clinical and radiographic findings (see Fig. 29-2, *Column A*).

Column II: Analyze

In Step 2 the patient information is assessed relative to both current and potential oral disease and conditions (see Fig. 29-2, *Column B*).

Column III: Plan Strategies for Therapeutic Intervention, Individualized Prevention, and Appointment Planning

Step 3 formalizes the process of the establishment of therapeutic intervention and prevention strategies essential to appointment planning and the reevaluation process (see Fig. 29-2, *Column C*).

Column IV: Recommend

In Step 4 the clinician actively recommends specific products and procedures to the patient for the implementation of prevention strategies (see Fig. 29-2, *Column D*).

Column V: Evaluate/Reevaluate

In Step 5 both clinical therapy and patient oral self-care must be evaluated or reevaluated after therapy and intervention recommendation. Oral-care habits can be evaluated for successful outcomes; new suggestions can be made as appropriate. Sometimes this reevaluation is done during the course of treatment, as in the case of multiple appointments, or it can occur at a subsequent supportive care appointment (see Fig. 29-2, *Column E*). Whatever the continuum of care, the reevaluation phase is critical to the delivery of competent oral care; the design of appropriate, individualized oral self-care prevention strategies; and the patient's involvement in the process of care. This step is addressed in Chapter 30.

The ORA Worksheet is a linear form that is used from the far left column to the far right column. The case study introduced earlier in this chapter now can be applied to the ORA system.

 Case Application

The patient, 54-year-old Ms. Wallace, has generalized, marginal gingivitis and dental caries. The data for this case were gathered through the use of the ORA Prevention Survey (see Fig. 29-1), which collects the patient's dental history, use of fluoride, health behaviors, and health beliefs. Because the ORA system uses a clinic's or practitioner's health history and clinical recording form, those portions of the patient's history and findings are reported in narrative. Ms. Wallace, who reported for a new patient examination, revealed the following information in her ORA survey.

Health History

- Her health history indicates she is being treated for cardiovascular disease, for which she takes diltiazem (Cardizem), a calcium channel blocker.
- Her blood pressure is 179/80 (right arm, sitting); her pulse is 82 BPM (strong and regular).

Prevention Survey

- Her self-reported prevention survey (Fig. 29-3) reveals the following:

DENTAL HISTORY

- Bleeding gingiva
- Calculus accumulation
- Toothache
- Unaware of signs of oral disease
- Irregular dental visits
- Indicates that her teeth appear yellow and that she would like them to be whiter
- Cannot find her toothbrush
- Does not use dental floss (unable to coordinate her fingers)
- Spends an inadequate amount of time in oral self-care
- Unsure of type of toothpaste used
- Seeks dental care only when in pain

FLUORIDE HISTORY

- Is not currently benefiting from fluoridated public water source
- Unsure whether her dentifrice contains fluoride; uses any sale brand (when she brushes)

HEALTH BEHAVIOR

- Seeks medical attention only on an emergency basis
- Occasionally follows medical and dental care providers' recommendations
- Feels stressed
- Does not use tobacco products
- Occasionally consumes alcohol
- Drinks six to eight caffeinated beverages a day
- Does not exercise

DIET SURVEY

- Consumes crackers between meals

HEALTH BELIEFS

- Feels she is more likely than others to have dental problems
- Believes prevention of oral problems is important

Text continued on p. 496

Oral Risk Assessment Worksheet

ORA Oral Risk Assessment Early Intervention System

Patient Name______________________________

Ⓐ Ⓑ

REVIEW

Health History	Medications & Dose Duration
❑ Cardiovascular (heart)	(prescription and OTC)
❑ Central nervous system (nerves)	
❑ Endocrine (endocrine glands)	
❑ Gastrointestinal (stomach, intestines)	
❑ Gentiourinary (sex organs, urinary tract)	
❑ Head, eyes, ears, nose, throat	
❑ Hematological (blood)	
❑ Integumentary (skin)	
❑ Musculoskeletal (muscles, bones, joints)	
❑ Psychological	
❑ Respiratory	
Vital Signs BP /	Pulse

PREVENTION SURVEY

Dental History				
❑ Sensitive teeth	❑ Sore jaw	❑ Toothache	❑ Sore gums	❑ Clenching
❑ Bleeding gums	❑ Difficulty chewing	❑ Filling fell out	❑ Dry mouth	❑ Grinding
❑ Bad breath	❑ Burning sensation		❑ Abscess	❑ Swollen face
❑ Swelling inside mouth	❑ Tartar buildup	❑ Yellowing teeth	❑ Difficulty swallowing	
❑ Adequate OH time	❑ Anxiety/Pain	❑ Oral self care difficulty		
Oral Health Products:				
Fluoride History				
❑ Fluoridated water	❑ Away from home >4 days/week		❑ Oral rinse w/fluoride	
❑ Water filter	❑ Bottled juice	Child:		
❑ Bottled water	❑ Fluoridated dentifrice	❑ In daycare w/out fluoride		❑ Supplements
Behaviors				
❑ Annual physical	❑ Balance work/relaxation	❑ Tobacco use		❑ Exercise
❑ Follows medical advice	❑ Eating habits controlled	❑ Alcohol use		
❑ Follows dental advice	❑ Increased stress	❑ Caffeine use		
Diet Survey	❑ Carbohydrate/Sucrose intake (excessive/moderate/minimal)			
Beliefs				
❑ Understands oral status	❑ Values prevention			
❑ Wants product recommendations	❑ Open to change	❑ Feels in control of oral condition		

Clinical and Radiographic Findings				
Intraoral/Extraoral Examination		❑ Within normal limits		❑ See chart
Caries	❑ Coronal	❑ Interproximal		❑ Root surface
Restorations/Prosthetics				
Restorations	❑ Amalgam	❑ Composite	❑ Crowns/inlays/onlays	❑ Bridges
Dentures	❑ Complete	❑ Partial		
Periodontium				
❑ Recession	❑ Plaque ❑ Bleeding on probing		❑ Loss of attached gingiva	❑ Pockets <3mm
❑ Mucogingival defects				
Occlusion/TMJ	❑ Traumatic occlusion		❑ Crepitus	
Bone Loss	❑ <25%	❑ 25-50%	❑ Horizontal	❑ Vertical

ANALYZE
Oral Risk Concerns

At risk for		Clinically Evident
	Hard Tissues	
❑	Abrasion/Attrition/Erosion	❑
❑	Bone Loss	❑
❑	Bruxism/Occlusal Trauma	❑
❑	Calculus	❑
❑	Caries: coronal/interproximal	❑
❑	Caries: root surface	❑
❑	Chipped broken teeth	❑
❑	Extrinsic staining	❑
❑	Fluorosis	❑
❑	Intrinsic staining	❑
❑	Malaligned teeth	❑
❑	Mobile teeth	❑
❑	Sensitive teeth	❑
❑	Trauma	❑
❑	Other	❑
	Soft Tissues	
❑	Abscess: carious	❑
❑	Abscess: periodontal	❑
❑	Atrophic ulcer	❑
❑	Apthous ulcer	❑
❑	Burning tongue/mouth	❑
❑	Candidiasis	❑
❑	Echymosis	❑
❑	Gingival recession	❑
❑	Gingival hyperplasia	❑
❑	Gingivitis	❑
❑	Herpetic lesions	❑
❑	Increased plaque	❑
❑	Leukoplakia	❑
❑	Lichen planus	❑
❑	Oral cancer	❑
❑	Periodontal disease	❑
❑	Petechiae	❑
❑	Salivation – increased	❑
❑	Salivation – decreased	❑
❑	Trauma	❑
❑	Xerostomia	❑
❑	Other__________	❑

Consult		Referral
❑	Consultation with physician	❑
❑	Consultation with dental specialist	❑

FIG. 29-2 Five columns of the ORA Worksheet, a form used to summarize, analyze, and plan patient treatment. *A,* Column I is used to summarize a review of patient data. *B,* Column II is used to analyze the assessment data reviewed in Column I for oral risk concerns.

Date_____

Ⓒ   Ⓓ   Ⓔ

PLAN			ORAL CARE RECOMMENDATIONS			EVALUATE
Clinical Goals	Therapeutic Intervention	Patient Goals	Prevention Strategy	**Toothbrush**	Product	Clinical Goals
				❑ Mechanical		
				❑ Child ❑ Youth ❑ Compact ❑ Full		
				❑ Soft ❑ Extra Soft		
				❑ Powered		
				Brushing frequency		
				Brushing duration		
				Interdental Cleaning Products		
				❑ Floss Type Frequency		
				❑ Oral Irrigator Frequency		
				❑ Interdental Brush Frequency		
				❑ Other		
				Dentifrice		
				❑ Fluoride ❑ Whitening		
				❑ Sensitivity ❑ Multiple Benefit		
				❑ Tartar Control ❑ Gingival Benefit		
				❑ Children's		
				Oral Rinse		
				❑ Fluoride		
				❑ Cosmetic		Patient Goals
				❑ Alcohol-free		
				❑ Tartar Control		
				❑ Chlorhexidine		
				❑ Essential Oil/Phenol Compound		
				Prosthodontic Care		
				❑ Adhesive ❑ Denture Brush		
				❑ Denture Bath/Cleanser		
				Self Evaluation		
				❑ Disclosing tablets or solutions		
				❑ Evaluate bleeding points		
				Other		

FIG. 29-2, cont'd *C,* Column III is used to plan therapeutic intervention. *D,* Column IV is used for specific product and procedure recommendations for patient oral self-care. *E,* Column V is used for therapeutic and patient-goal reevaluation.

D E N T A L   H I S T O R Y

Name _Robin Wallace_   Date _MM/DD/YY_

Prevention Survey (vertical side label, A)

1. **In the past two years, have you experienced any of the following symptoms?**
   (If yes, please check all that apply)
   - ☐ Sensitive teeth
   - ☑ Bleeding gums
   - ☐ Bad breath
   - ☐ Swelling inside mouth
   - ☐ Sore jaw
   - ☐ Difficulty chewing
   - ☐ Burning sensation
   - ☑ Tartar buildup
   - ☑ Toothache
   - ☐ Filling fell out
   - ☐ Abscess
   - ☐ Yellowing teeth
   - ☐ Sore gums
   - ☐ Dry mouth
   - ☐ Swollen face
   - ☐ Difficulty swallowing

   Comments _____

2. **When you look inside your mouth, do you know what to look for?**

	Yes	No
Tooth Decay	☐	☑
Oral Cancer	☐	☑
Gum Disease	☐	☑

3. **For the past two years, what is your best estimate of the number of times you have been to see a dental professional for each of the following:**
   - ____ Checkups and cleanings
   - ____ Other dental treatment such as fillings, gum treatment, crowns (caps), bridges, dentures
   - _3_ Dental emergencies

4. **Do you clench or grind your teeth in the daytime or at night?**
   ☐ Yes ☐ No
   If yes, do you wear a bite guard?_____ For how long?_____

5. **In the past two years, have you been concerned about the appearance of your teeth?**
   (If yes, please check all that apply)
   - ☑ Yellowing/graying teeth
   - ☐ Stains
   - ☐ Crowded, crooked
   - ☐ Spacing between teeth
   - ☐ Other

6. **Check any of the following you regularly use at home:**
   - ☐ Soft toothbrush
   - ☐ Hard toothbrush
   - ☐ Medium toothbrush
   - ☐ Oral irrigator
   - ☐ Denture adhesive
   - ☐ Dental floss
   - ☐ Special brush
   - ☐ Fluoride toothpaste
   - ☐ Rubber tip
   - ☐ Denture cleanser
   - ☐ Floss threader
   - ☐ Toothpick
   - ☐ Fluoride rinse or gel
   - ☐ Mouthrinse
   - ☐ Whitening product
   - ☐ Powered interdental cleaner
   - ☐ Powered brush
   - ☐ Other_____

   Lost my toothbrush

7. **Check the type of toothpaste you use:**
   - ☑ Fluoride
   - ☐ Sensitivity protection
   - ☐ Tartar control
   - ☐ Baking soda
   - ☐ Gum benefit
   - ☐ Peroxide
   - ☐ Whitening
   - ☐ Multiple benefit

8. **Estimate how long it takes you to clean your teeth and gums each time:**
   Please indicate your best and most reliable estimate.
   Brushing _15 seconds_ (time)   Flossing _0_ (time)

9. **About how many times each day/week do you brush and floss?**
   I brush about _1_ times per day OR _____ per week - _when I have a toothbrush_
   I floss about _0_ times per day OR _0_ per week

10. **Do you find it difficult to maintain an oral hygiene schedule due to your job/profession or other reasons?**
    ☐ No ☑ Yes _I don't have a toothbrush_

11. **Do any conditions make it difficult for you to adequately clean your teeth?**
    (If yes, please check all that apply) - _fingers don't work that way_
    - ☐ Hold a toothbrush
    - ☑ Use dental floss
    - ☐ Brush/floss for any length of time
    - ☐ Don't see well

12. **Generally, how have you felt about your previous dental appointments?**
    - ☐ Very anxious and afraid
    - ☐ Somewhat anxious and afraid
    - ☑ Don't care one way or the other
    - ☐ Look forward to it

    - _I go when I have a problem_

F L U O R I D E   H I S T O R Y

(B)

1. ☐ Yes ☑ No Are you on a fluoridated public water system?
   If yes, for how long? _____

2. ☐ Yes ☑ No Do you use any type of water filter or bottled water for your main water source?
   If yes, what type of filter? _____
   If yes, what brand of water? _____
   For how long? _____

3. ☐ Yes ☐ No If you are on a fluoridated public water system, does your job/profession keep you away from home more than 4 days per week?
   If yes, do you use any fluoride supplements during that time?
   (For example: a fluoridated mouthrinse) ☐ Yes ☑ No

4. ☐ Yes ☑ No Do you drink bottled fruit juices? _____
   If yes, how many per day? _____

5. ☐ Yes _?_ ☐ No Do you currently use a fluoridated toothpaste?
   If yes, how often? _not sure_
   If yes, for how many years? _____
   If yes, what brand? _____
   If no, why not? _____

6. ☐ Yes ☑ No Do you use an oral rinse containing fluoride?
   If yes, how often? _____
   If yes, what brand? _____

7. ☐ Yes ☑ No Do you use any additional sources of fluoride (such as mouthrinse, drops, tablets)?
   If yes, what sources? _____
   For how long? _____

For Child Patient

8. ☐ Yes ☐ No Are the children in your home in childcare, daycare or school where they **do not receive** fluoridated public water? _____
   If yes, how many days per week? _____

9. ☐ Yes ☐ No Do you or anyone in your home use a fluoridated supplement (drops or tablets)?
   If yes, what dosage? _____
   If yes, for how long? _____

FIG. 29-3 Prevention survey filled out by Robin Wallace, the case study patient, showing the dental history **(A)** and fluoride history **(B)** portions.

BEHAVIORS

1. Do you have an annual physical examination?
   ☒ No   ☐ Yes

2. When you are ill, do you?
   ☐ See your physician?   ☒ Seek care in an emergency room?
   ☐ Wait to see if the condition goes away?

3. When your physician recommends a change in health behavior, do you follow his/her advice?
   ☐ No   ☐ Yes   ☒ Sometimes

4. When your dental professional recommends a change in health behavior, do you follow his/her advice?
   ☐ No   ☐ Yes   ☒ Sometimes

5. When your dental professional recommends a specific oral care product or self-care regimen do you follow his/her advice?
   ☐ No   ☐ Yes   ☒ Sometimes

6. Do you have regular hobbies/interests outside of work?
   ☒ No   ☐ Yes

7. Do you strive to reach a balance between work and relaxation?
   ☒ No   ☐ Yes

8. Are your eating habits out of control?
   ☒ No   ☐ Yes

9. Do you feel your stress level has increased in the past 6 months?
   ☐ No   ☒ Yes

10. Do you use tobacco in any form? If yes, what form and frequency?
    ☒ No   ☐ Yes   ☐ Sometimes   Type _____ Frequency/Quantity _____
                                       For how long? _____

11. Do you consume alcohol?
    ☐ No   ☐ Yes   ☒ Sometimes   Type _*beer*_ Frequency/Quantity _*weekends only*_

12. Do you consume caffeine?
    ☐ No   ☒ Yes   ☐ Sometimes   Type _*coffee*_ Frequency/Quantity _*6-8 cups a day*_

13. Do you exercise daily?
    ☒ No   ☐ Yes   ☐ Sometimes   Type _____ Frequency/Quantity _____

14. Do you participate in sports/recreation activities?
    ☒ No   ☐ Yes   ☐ Sometimes   Type _____ Frequency/Quantity _____

C

DIET SURVEY

Please indicate which sweets and cooked starches you eat between meals.

Food	Frequency	✓ if between meals
breath mints		
cough drops		
chewing gum		
dried fruits		
canned/bottled beverages		
sugared liquids		
chips		
crackers *either peanut butter or plain*	*after breakfast, lunch, dinner, and snacks*	✓
cookies		

D

BELIEFS

1. In your opinion, compared to the average person, how likely do you think you are to have cavities or other problems with your teeth and/or gums?
   ☒ Much more likely   ☐ About average   ☐ Much less than average
   ☐ More than average   ☐ Less than average

2. How important is it for you to prevent cavities, gum problems or other diseases of the mouth?
   ☒ Very important   ☐ Somewhat important   ☐ Not at all important

3. Would you like your dental professional to make specific product recommendations to meet your oral care needs?
   ☒ Yes   ☐ I am not sure   ☐ No

4. There are times in our lives when it seems we have the energy and time to tackle new projects or to make changes.
   At this time, I ☒ can   ☐ cannot imagine trying to change a habit.

5. I believe that I have control over the condition of my mouth.
   ☐ Firmly believe   ☒ Somewhat believe   ☐ Do not believe

FIG. 29-3, cont'd Health behavior **(C)** and diet recall and health beliefs **(D)** portions of Robin Wallace's prevention survey.

- Likes to get recommendations from dental professionals
- Feels she can tackle a new project or make a change
- Somewhat believes she has control over her oral condition

Clinical and Radiographic Findings

- Extraoral and intraoral examination (Fig. 29-4) reveals several breaks in the integrity of the buccal mucosa at the line of occlusion (consistent with cheek biting).
- Root surface caries is noted in the mandibular premolar area (Fig. 29-5).
- Numerous restorations indicate previous carious experience; restorative materials present include amalgam, composite, and gold alloy (see Figs. 29-5 and 29-7).
- Periodontium exhibits recession, plaque, bleeding when probed, and loss of attached gingiva (Fig. 29-6).

- Horizontal bone loss is evidenced (Fig. 29-7).
- No pathological processes noted radiographically (see Fig. 29-7).

Although the case study concerning Ms. Wallace in this chapter may present a somewhat similar picture to many others, it presents a unique patient background and circumstances that provide clues necessary to the planning of appropriate therapeutic strategies. The design of both the clinical therapy and the patient intervention therapy is vastly different and unique to this patient's circumstances, an idea that becomes evident during the exploration of the basing of therapeutic strategies on the concepts of oral risk assessment.

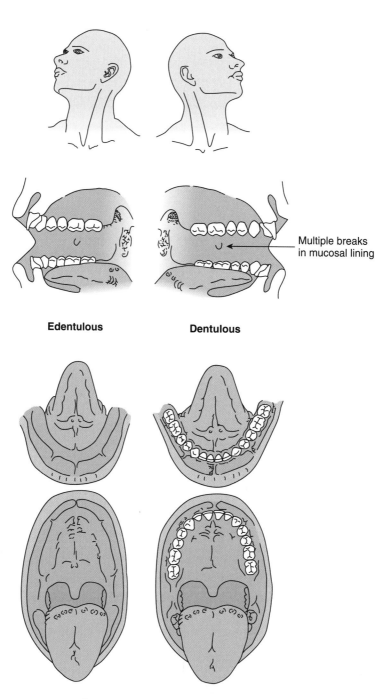

Edentulous   **Dentulous**

Multiple breaks in mucosal lining

FIG. 29-4 Intraoral–extraoral chart form.

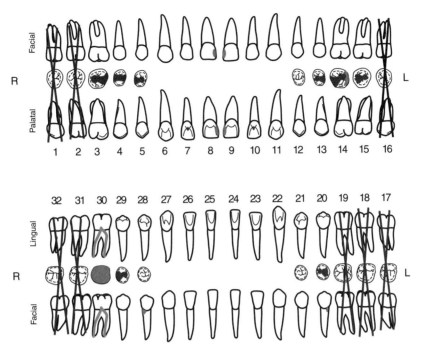

FIG. 29-5 Dental chart.

Patient Name: _Wallace, Robin_

Last First MI

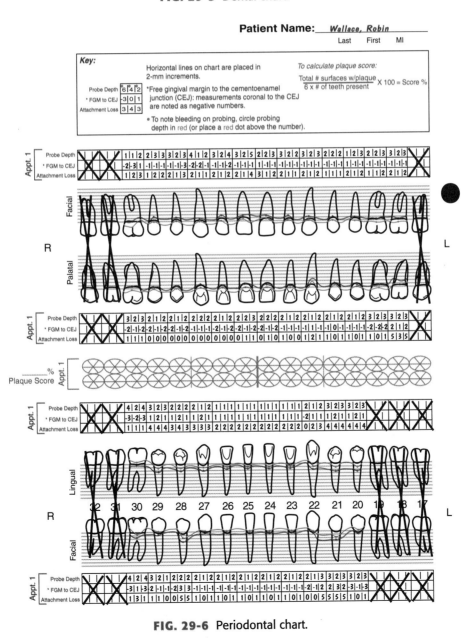

FIG. 29-6 Periodontal chart.

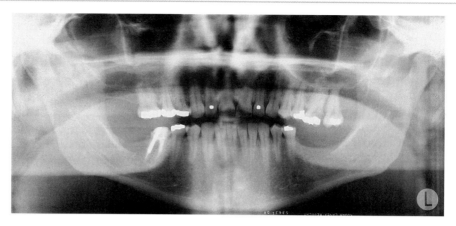

FIG. 29-7 Dental panoramic radiograph.

ORA APPLICATION TO CASE STUDY

STEP 1: REVIEW

Health History

Fig. 29-8
- Ms. Wallace's health history indicates she is being treated for cardiovascular disease, for which she takes diltiazem (Cardizem), a calcium channel blocker.

- Her blood pressure is 179/80 (right arm, sitting); her pulse is 82 BPM (strong and regular).

Health History	Medications & Dose	Duration
☑ Cardiovascular (heart)	(prescription and OTC)	
❏ Central nervous system (nerves)	*Cardizem*	
❏ Endocrine (endocrine glands)		
❏ Gastrointestinal (stomach, intestines)		
❏ Gentiourinary (sex organs, urinary tract)		
❏ Head, eyes, ears, nose, throat		
❏ Hematological (blood)		
❏ Integumentary (skin)		
❏ Musculoskeletal (muscles, bones, joints)		
❏ Psychological		
❏ Respiratory		
Vital Signs BP	*(RAS) 179/80* Pulse *82 bpm (S+R)*	

FIG. 29-8 Summary of information from health history applied to Column I of the ORA Worksheet.

Dental History

Fig. 29-9; see also Fig. 29-3, *A*
- Bleeding gingiva
- Calculus accumulation
- Toothache
- Unaware of signs of oral disease
- Irregular dental visits
- Indicates that her teeth appear yellow and that she would like them to be whiter

- Cannot find her toothbrush
- Does not use dental floss (unable to coordinate her fingers)
- Spends an inadequate amount of time in oral self-care
- Seeks dental care only when something hurts

Dental History				
❑ Sensitive teeth	❑ Sore jaw	☒ Toothache	❑ Sore gums	❑ Clenching
☒ Bleeding gums	❑ Difficulty chewing	❑ Filling fell out	❑ Dry mouth	❑ Grinding
❑ Bad breath	❑ Burning sensation		❑ Abscess	❑ Swollen face
❑ Swelling inside mouth	☒ Tartar buildup	☒ Yellowing teeth	❑ Difficulty swallowing	
❑ Adequate OH time *NO*	❑ Anxiety/Pain	☒ Oral self care diffuculty		
Oral Health Products: *No flossing, inconsistent brushing — can't find brush*				

FIG. 29-9 Dental history portion of the ORA Prevention Survey applied to Column I of the ORA Worksheet.

Fluoride History

Fig. 29-10; see also Fig. 29-3, *B*
- Is not currently benefiting from fluoridated public water source

- Unsure whether her dentifrice contains fluoride; uses any sale brand (when she brushes)

Fluoride History			
❑ Fluoridated water *NO*	❑ Away from home >4 days/week	❑ Oral rinse w/fluoride	
❑ Water filter *NO*	❑ Bottled juice *NO*	Child:	
❑ Bottled water *NO*	☒ Fluoridated dentifrice	❑ In daycare w/out fluoride	❑ Supplements

FIG. 29-10 Fluoride history portion of the ORA Prevention Survey applied to Column I of the ORA Worksheet.

Health Behavior

Fig. 29-11; see also Fig. 29-3, *C*
- Seeks medical attention when only appropriate
- Occasionally follows medical and dental care providers' recommendations
- Feels stressed

- Does not use tobacco products
- Occasionally consumes alcohol
- Drinks 6 to 8 caffeinated beverages a day
- Does not exercise

Behaviors			
❑ Annual physical *NO*	❑ Balance work/relaxation	❑ Tobacco use	❑ Exercise *NO*
❑ Follows medical advice *some*	❑ Eating habits controlled	☒ Alcohol use	
❑ Follows dental advice *some*	❑ Increased stress	☒ Caffeine use *6-8 cups a day*	

FIG. 29-11 Health behavior portion of the ORA Prevention Survey applied to Column I of the ORA Worksheet.

Diet Survey

Fig. 29-12; see also Fig. 29-3, *D*
- Consumes crackers between meals

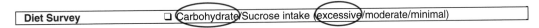

FIG. 29-12 Diet survey portion of the ORA Prevention Survey applied to Column I of the ORA Worksheet.

Health Beliefs

Fig. 29-13; see also Fig. 29-3, *D*
- Feels she is more likely than others to have dental problems
- Believes prevention of oral problems is important
- Likes to get recommendations from dental professionals
- Feels she can tackle a new project or make a change at this time
- Somewhat believes she has control over her oral condition

Beliefs		
❑ Understands oral status	☑ Values prevention	
☑ Wants product recommendations	❑ Open to change	☑ Feels in control of oral condition – *somewhat*

FIG. 29-13 Health beliefs portion of the ORA Prevention Survey applied to Column I of the ORA Worksheet.

Clinical and Radiographic Findings

Fig. 29-14; see also Figs. 29-4 through 29-7
- Extraoral and intraoral examination reveals several breaks in the integrity of the buccal mucosal at the line of occlusion (consistent with cheek biting).
- Root surface caries is noted in the mandibular premolar area.
- Numerous restorations indicate previous carious experience; restorative materials present include amalgam and composite.
- Periodontium exhibits recession, plaque, bleeding when probed, and loss of attached gingiva.
- Horizontal bone loss is evidenced.
- No pathological processes are noted radiographically.

Clinical and Radiographic Findings			
Intraoral/Extraoral Examination	❑ Within normal limits	*Cheek biting* ☑ See chart	
Caries	❑ Coronal	❑ Interproximal	☑ Root surface
Restorations/Prosthetics			
Restorations	☑ Amalgam	☑ Composite	☑ Crowns/inlays/onlays ❑ Bridges
Dentures	❑ Complete	❑ Partial	
Periodontium			
☑ Recession	☑ Plaque ☑ Bleeding on probing	☑ Loss of attached gingiva	❑ Pockets <3mm
❑ Mucogingival defects	*Bone loss – horizontal*		
Occlusion/TMJ	❑ Traumatic occlusion	❑ Crepitus	
Bone Loss	❑ <25%	❑ 25-50%	❑ Horizontal ❑ Vertical

FIG. 29-14 Clinical and radiographic findings portion of the ORA Prevention Survey applied to Column I of the ORA Worksheet.

STEP 2: ANALYZE

Based on the review of the patient findings recorded in Column I of the ORA Worksheet, some evidence-based assumptions of *potential* oral risk concerns can be made. The *first* analysis is for *potential,* not actual or clinically evident risk concerns. This process is now applied to Ms. Wallace.

Potential Risk Concerns

The health history findings for Ms. Wallace indicate she is taking a calcium channel blocker for cardiovascular disease. Based on pharmacological studies, several oral sequelae to that drug include xerostomia, lichenoid reactions, altered taste, gland pain, and gingival hyperplasia.[9] These oral risk concerns would be indicated on the left side of Column II of the ORA Worksheet (Fig. 29-15).

Based on the patient's dental history, gingivitis may be expected (she does not use dental floss). She reports bleeding gingiva and calculus accumulation, which indicate an oral risk concern for gingivitis, increased plaque, and periodontal disease. As potential oral risk concerns, these findings would be noted on the left side of Column II of the ORA Worksheet (see Fig. 29-15).

Reading her self-reported fluoride history, dental caries would be checked as a *potential* oral finding because she does not have access to a public fluoridated water source and she is unsure whether her toothpaste contains fluoride (when she brushes; see Fig. 29-15).

Ms. Wallace's diet survey indicates a source of refined carbohydrates consumed between meals, which potentially could contribute to both coronal and root surface caries (see Fig. 29-15).

Clinically Evident Concerns

Clinical and radiographic findings for this patient reveal the following:
- Loss of integrity of the oral mucosa (trauma)
- Root surface caries
- Gingivitis
- Periodontitis

FIG. 29-15 Potential oral risk concerns recorded in Column II of the ORA Worksheet.

FIG. 29-16 Completed oral risk concerns.

The clinical findings are recorded on the right side of Column II of the ORA Worksheet as *clinically evident* (Fig. 29-16). Based on this review and assessment, a sense is developed of the types of therapeutic intervention strategies that need to be planned and of the self-care measures that should be recommended based on specific patient need.

Now that a summarized picture of this patient's therapeutic needs has been developed, the therapeutic intervention can be mapped through definition of the goals of therapy.

STEP 3: PLAN THERAPEUTIC INTERVENTION

Strategies for therapeutic intervention follow the data review and assessment phase or risk assessment and begin with the establishment of goals of therapy (Box 29-4). Put in other terms, the first portion of this phase sets expected *clinical* outcomes.

When a patient's oral conditions are within normal limits of health, goals for clinical therapy will include maintenance of health and prevention of disease. This goal will be achieved when no change in oral health status occurs

---

BOX 29-4

Therapeutic Intervention

Identify patient needs.
Establish goals.
Plan executional tactics for those goals.
Define treatment sequence.
Reevaluate outcomes and modify goals as necessary.

---

within a stated evaluation period. Although this evaluation or reevaluation period should be established for every patient, it typically equates to a patient's next supportive care appointment at 3, 4, 6, or even 12 months. When active disease is present, goals become more complex and include broader categories such as the identification of disease etiology, elimination of the disease process, and establishment and maintenance of health.

Corresponding goals to address patient self-care health behavior and beliefs also need to be established (phase two of Step 3) and are addressed in the Chapter 30.

TABLE 29-1

Steps in therapeutic intervention planning

Oral risk concern	Clinical goal	Therapeutic intervention	Evaluation measure
Bone loss (*clinical finding*)	Arrest bone loss Prevent future bone loss	Periodontal therapy Patient goals (see Chapter 30)	No increase in attachment loss at supportive care intervals
Gingival recession (*clinical finding*)	Arrest gingival recession Prevent future recession	Patient goals (see Chapter 30) Periodontal therapy	No additional recession at supportive care intervals No increase in current recession
Gingival hyperplasia (*potential finding*)	Prevent future gingival hyperplasia (because problem is potential, *not* diagnostic)		
Gingivitis (*clinical finding*)	Arrest gingival inflammation	Periodontal debridement	No bleeding on probing at reevaluation interval Tissue color, contour, and consistency within normal limits
Increased plaque (*clinical finding*)	Reduce plaque quantity to biologically acceptable level	Patient goals (see Chapter 30)	No bleeding on probing at reevaluation interval Improved plaque index
Periodontal disease (*clinical finding*)	Arrest periodontal disease activity	Periodontal therapy	No bleeding on probing at reevaluation interval No increased probing depths at reevaluation interval No new evidence of radiographic bone loss at reevaluation interval
Coronal caries (*potential finding*)	Prevent future caries (because problem is potential, *not* diagnostic)	Patient goals (see Chapter 30)	No coronal caries at supportive care intervals
Root caries (*clinical finding*)	Arrest demineralization Promote remineralization	Plaque control Diet survey and discussion Fluoride application Oral self-care evaluation	No new caries at supportive care appointment Arrested/reversed caries process
Trauma (*clinical finding*)	Determine cause of trauma	Patient goals (see Chapter 30)	No evidence of trauma
Taste alteration (*potential finding*)	No treatment goal	Patient goals (see Chapter 30)	Patient interview
Xerostomia (*potential finding*)	No treatment goal	Patient goals (see Chapter 30)	Patient interview
Gland pain (*potential finding*)	No treatment goal	Patient goals (see Chapter 30)	Patient interview

Measurable Goals

Every phase of treatment has clinical goals that can be measured. Returning to the information in the case application, the reader should refer to the second column of the ORA Worksheet developed for Ms. Wallace. Note the following oral findings for which this patient is either *at risk* or for which she has exhibited *symptoms*: bone loss, coronal caries, root caries, gingival recession, gingival hyperplasia, gingivitis, increased plaque, periodontal disease, trauma, taste alteration, and gland pain. The clinical goal, therapeutic intervention, and evaluation goals for Ms. Wallace are charted in Table 29-1.

CASE SUMMARY

Designing therapeutic intervention is not an easy task, especially when therapy is based on individualized needs. With the use of an organized system, such as ORA, this complex task can be broken into a series of manageable steps.

STEP 1: REVIEW ASSESSMENT DATA

In applying this step to the patient, the ORA Worksheet has been completed for Ms. Wallace (Fig. 29-17). Her health history, prevention survey, and clinical and radio-

graphic findings were reviewed and then summarized in Column I of the ORA Worksheet (Fig. 29-17, *A*).

STEP 2: ANALYZE DATA FOR ORAL RISK CONCERNS

The data from Column I (see Fig. 29-17, *A*) was analyzed to make evidence-based assumptions about Ms. Wallace's *potential oral concerns* ("risk assessment," which was placed in Column II to the left of listing). Ms. Wallace's clinical and radiographic findings were reviewed to reveal her *current oral status*, which was also placed in Column II to the right of the listing (see Fig. 29-17, *B*).

STEP 3: PLAN THERAPEUTIC INTERVENTION

Based on the notations of oral risk, both potential and actual, the therapeutic intervention for the patient was planned (see Fig. 29-17, *C*, and Table 29-1).

This step completes the portion of patient care planning that involves primarily the clinician. It is now time to explore how the patient is involved in the management and prevention of oral conditions and disease, an aspect critical to gaining a successful outcome to therapy. To complete the ORA process, see Chapter 30 for Step 4: Recommend and Step 5: Evaluate/Reevaluate.

(A)

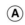

REVIEW

Health History	Medications & Dose	Duration
☒ Cardiovascular (heart)	(prescription and OTC)	
☐ Central nervous system (nerves)	*Cardizem*	
☐ Endocrine (endocrine glands)		
☐ Gastrointestinal (stomach, intestines)		
☐ Gentiourinary (sex organs, urinary tract)		
☐ Head, eyes, ears, nose, throat		
☐ Hematological (blood)		
☐ Integumentary (skin)		
☐ Musculoskeletal (muscles, bones, joints)		
☐ Psychological		
☐ Respiratory		

Vital Signs BP *(RAS) 179/80* Pulse *82 bpm (S+R)*

PREVENTION SURVEY

Dental History
- ☐ Sensitive teeth ☐ Sore jaw ☒ Toothache ☐ Sore gums ☐ Clenching
- ☒ Bleeding gums ☐ Difficulty chewing ☐ Filling fell out ☐ Dry mouth ☐ Grinding
- ☐ Bad breath ☐ Burning sensation ☐ Abscess ☐ Swollen face
- ☐ Swelling inside mouth ☒ Tartar buildup ☒ Yellowing teeth ☐ Difficulty swallowing
- ☐ Adequate OH time *NO* ☐ Anxiety/Pain ☒ Oral self care diffuculty

Oral Health Products: *No flossing, inconsistent brushing — can't find brush*

Fluoride History
- ☐ Fluoridated water *NO* ☐ Away from home >4 days/week ☐ Oral rinse w/fluoride *NO*
- ☐ Water filter *NO* ☐ Bottled juice *NO* Child:
- ☐ Bottled water ☒ Fluoridated dentifrice ☐ In daycare w/out fluoride ☐ Supplements

Behaviors
- ☐ Annual physical *NO* ☐ Balance work/relaxation ☐ Tobacco use ☐ Exercise *NO*
- ☐ Follows medical advice *some* ☐ Eating habits controlled ☒ Alcohol use
- ☐ Follows dental advice *some* ☐ Increased stress ☒ Caffeine use *6–8 cups a day*

Diet Survey ☒ (Carbohydrate)/Sucrose intake ((excessive)/moderate/minimal)

Beliefs
- ☐ Understands oral status ☒ Values prevention
- ☒ Wants product recommendations ☐ Open to change ☒ Feels in control of oral condition *somewhat*

Clinical and Radiographic Findings
- **Intraoral/Extraoral Examination** ☐ Within normal limits *Cheek biting* ☒ See chart
- **Caries** ☐ Coronal ☐ Interproximal ☒ Root surface

Restorations/Prosthetics
- Restorations ☒ Amalgam ☒ Composite ☒ Crowns/inlays/onlays ☐ Bridges
- Dentures ☐ Complete ☐ Partial

Periodontium
- ☒ Recession ☒ Plaque ☒ Bleeding on probing ☒ Loss of attached gingiva ☐ Pockets <3mm
- ☐ Mucogingival defects *Bone loss – horizontal*
- **Occlusion/TMJ** ☐ Traumatic occlusion ☐ Crepitus
- **Bone Loss** ☐ <25% ☐ 25-50% ☒ Horizontal ☐ Vertical

(B)

ANALYZE
Oral Risk Concerns

At risk for		Clinically Evident
	Hard Tissues	
☐	Abrasion/Attrition/Erosion	☐
☒	Bone Loss	☒
☐	Bruxism/Occlusal Trauma	☐
☐	Calculus	☐
☒	Caries: coronal/interproximal	☐
☒	Caries: root surface	☒
☐	Chipped broken teeth	☐
☐	Extrinsic staining	☐
☐	Fluorosis	☐
☐	Intrinsic staining	☐
☐	Malaligned teeth	☐
☐	Mobile teeth	☐
☐	Sensitive teeth	☐
☐	Trauma	☐
☐	Other	☐
	Soft Tissues	
☐	Abscess: carious	☐
☐	Abscess: periodontal	☐
☐	Atrophic ulcer	☐
☐	Apthous ulcer	☐
☐	Burning tongue/mouth	☐
☐	Candidiasis	☐
☐	Echymosis	☐
☐	Gingival recession	☒
☒	Gingival hyperplasia	☐
☒	Gingivitis	☒
☐	Herpetic lesions	☐
☒	Increased plaque	☒
☐	Leukoplakia	☐
☒	Lichen planus	☐
☐	Oral cancer	☐
☒	Periodontal disease	☒
☐	Petechiae	☐
☐	Salivation – increased	☐
☐	Salivation – decreased	☐
☐	Trauma	☒
☒	Xerostomia	☐
☒	Other *altered taste, gland pain*	☐

Consult	Referral
☐ Consultation with physician	☐
☐ Consultation with dental specialist	☐

FIG. 29-17 The completed ORA Worksheet showing Column I *(A)* and Column II *(B)*.

Continued

PLAN		
Clinical Goals	**Therapeutic Intervention**	**Patient Goals**
Bone Loss • Arrest bone loss. • Prevent future bone loss. Gingival Recession • Arrest gingival recession. • Prevent future recession. Gingival Hyperplasia • Prevention goal only Gingivitis • Arrest gingival inflammation. Increased Plaque • Reduce plaque quantity to a biologically acceptable level. Periodontal Disease • Arrest periodontal disease activity.	• Periodontal therapy • Debridement	• Acknowledge the signs of gingival disease. • Understand the role of plaque in gingival disease. • Understand the role of the host response in gingival inflammation. • Understand/demonstrate patient role in treatment and prevention of gingival disease. • Purchase and use recommended products for the treatment and control of gingival disease. • Understand personal role in compliance. • Appreciate the benefits of supportive care appointments.
Coronal Caries • Prevention goal only Root Caries • Arrest demineralization. • Promote remineralization. Trauma • Determine cause of trauma. Taste Alteration • No treatment goal Xerostomia • No treatment goal Gland Pain • No treatment goal	• Plaque control • Diet survey and discussion • Fluoride application • Oral self-care evaluation	• Understand the role of plaque, diet, and saliva in the caries process. • Acknowledge the difference between coronal and root surface caries. • Understand/demonstrate patient role in treatment and prevention of dental caries. • Purchase and use recommended products for the prevention of dental caries. • Understand personal role in compliance.

FIG. 29-17, cont'd The completed ORA Worksheet showing Column III *(C)*.

RITICAL THINKING ACTIVITIES

1. Together with a classmate, fill out an ORA Prevention Survey. In a role-playing format, perform Step 1 of the ORA system, using the ORA Worksheet. Were there any pertinent findings from this step that you previously overlooked? Did any biological, psychological, or sociological elements come to light that might impact the therapeutic and intervention strategies?

2. Make a list of all therapeutic intervention strategies that you perform as a dental hygienist. Determine whether each acts strictly as an intervention, prevention, or both.

3. Using the worksheet from Activity #1, perform Step 2 of the ORA system with a student partner. What types of oral concerns can you clinically document? Which are potential oral concerns?

4. Go online and review the surgeon general's report *Oral Health in America* (see the suggested agencies and web sites listed at the end of this chapter). In what ways does the ORA system support a more holistic approach to oral care?

5. If you are a first-year student, select a second-year student with whom to work. Ask to review the dental records of a patient that your partner is currently treating. After completing Steps 1 and 2 of the ORA system with the use of only the dental records provided, complete Step 3. Determine the clinical goal, therapeutic intervention, and evaluation method for each oral risk concern noted. Would this process have been more thorough with an ORA Prevention Survey?

REVIEW QUESTIONS

Questions 5 through 7 and Question 9 refer to the case study presented at the beginning of the chapter and discussed throughout.

1. A patient-specific approach to oral care includes which of the following approaches?
   a. Following a standard therapeutic intervention, individualizing the prevention aspects based principally on current patient knowledge
   b. Gaining an understanding of the unique patient needs from a clinical, biological, psychological, and sociological aspect before planning care
   c. Estimating patient expectations and building a care plan based on the patient's expressed needs so that compliance is increased
   d. All the above
   e. None of the above

2. Oral risk assessment is based on which of the following healthcare platforms?
   a. Health promotion
   b. Risk and risk assessment
   c. Intervention and prevention
   d. All the above

3. The benefits of a system-based, data-gathering tool for chairside use include all *except* which of the following?
   a. Provides a holistic approach to care
   b. Can provide for early disease intervention
   c. Provides oral risk concerns on which to build prevention strategies
   d. Predetermines insurance coding

4. To complete the assessment phase for a patient using the ORA system, which of the following information is *not* required?
   1. Health history
   2. Dental history
   3. Fluoride history
   4. Belief survey
   5. Clinical and radiographic findings
   a. 4 and 5
   b. All except 4
   c. 2, 3, and 4
   d. All elements listed are required.

5. For Ms. Wallace, the oral risk concern of gingival hyperplasia is based on which of the following assessment tools?
   a. Clinical findings
   b. Health history
   c. Patient concern of a specific symptom
   d. All the above

6. The evaluation of no bleeding on probing at a reevaluation appointment would be a measure of evaluation for which of the following oral risk concerns for Ms. Wallace?
   a. Bone loss
   b. Gingival recession
   c. Gland pain
   d. Gingival hyperplasia
   e. None of the above

7. The diet survey portion of the ORA Prevention Survey can provide clues in defining which oral risk concern for Ms. Wallace?
   a. Root caries
   b. Bone loss
   c. Trauma
   d. Gland pain

8. The terms *intervention* and *prevention* can be clearly defined; however, in dentistry, these terms often overlap.
   a. Both the statement and the clarification are true.
   b. The statement is correct; the clarification is incorrect.
   c. The statement is incorrect; the clarification is correct.
   d. Neither the statement nor the clarification is correct.

9. An example of a therapeutic intervention for Ms. Wallace would include which of the following?
   a. Fluoride treatment
   b. Debridement
   c. Diet discussion
   d. Discussion of the oral manifestations of her current medication
   e. All except d

10. Planning patient care is not considered a complex process because all patient care can be based on a standard, set routine.
    a. The statement is true; the rationale is false.
    b. Both the statement and the rationale are false.
    c. The statement is false; the rationale is true.
    d. Both the statement and the rationale are true.

SUGGESTED AGENCIES AND WEB SITES

Because of the ever-changing nature of the Internet, some of the web sites listed here may have changed since publication. Please refer to Mosby's Evolve web site for the most current information.

Centers for Disease Control and Prevention, National Center for Chronic Disease Prevention and Health Promotion ("Improving oral health: preventing unnecessary disease among all Americans"): http://www.cdc.gov

IPCS Harmonization: ("IPCS workshop on issues in cancer risk assessment"): http://www.ipcsharmonize.org

National Institutes of Health ("Oral Health in America: a report of the surgeon general"): http://www.nidr.nih.gov

University of Michigan School of Dentistry: http://www.dent.umich.edu

ADDITIONAL READINGS AND RESOURCES

Alanen P: Risks in risk definitions, *Community Dent Oral Epidemiol* 27:394-7, 1999.

Boyd LD, Dwyer JT: Guidelines for nutrition screening, assessment, and intervention in the dental office, *J Dent Hyg* 172(4): 31-43, 1998.

Burgess RC: Assessment of caries risk factors and preventive practices, *J Dent Educ* 59(10):962-71, 1995.

Galgut PN et al: The relationship between multidimensional health locus of control and the performance of subjects on a preventive periodontal programme, *J Clin Periodontol* 14(3):171-5, 1987.

Messer LB: Assessing caries risk in children, *Aust Dent J* 45(1):10-6, 2000.

Milgrom P et al: Oral hygiene instruction and health risk assessment in dental practice, *J Public Health Dent* 49(1):24-31, 1989.

Page RC, Beck JD: Risk assessment for periodontal diseases *Int Dent J* 47(2):61-87, 1997.

Papanou PN: Risk assessments in the diagnosis and treatment of periodontal diseases *J Dent Educ* 62(10):822-39, 1998.

Rayant GA, Sheiham A: An analysis of factors affecting compliance with tooth-cleaning recommendations, *J Clin Periodontol* 7(4):289-99, 1980.

Reich E, Lussi A, Newbrun E: Caries-risk assessment, *Int Dent J* 49(1):15-26, 1999.

Rotter JB: Generalized expectancies for internal versus external control of reinforcement, *Psychol Monogr* 80(1):1-28, 1966.

Schafer TE, Adair SM: Prevention of dental disease: the role of the pediatrician, *Pediatr Clin North Am* 47(5):1021-42, v-vi, 2000.

Tinanoff N: Dental caries risk assessment and prevention, *Dent Clin North Am* 39(4):709-19, 1995.

Wandera A, Bhakta S, Barker T: Caries prediction and indicators using a pediatric risk assessment teaching tool, *ASDC J Dent Child* 67(6):408-12, 375, 2000.

Wilson TG, Jr: Using risk assessment to customize periodontal treatment *J Calif Dent Assoc* 27(8):627-32, 634-9, 1999.

Yorty JS, Brown KB: Caries risk assessment/treatment programs in U.S. dental schools, *J Dent Educ* 63(10):745-7, 1999.

Zarvas AI, Edelstein BL, Vamvakidis A: Health care savings from microbiological caries risk screening of toddlers: a cost estimation model, *J Public Health Dent* 60(3):182-8, 2000.

REFERENCES

1. Beck JD: Risk revisited, *Community Dent Oral Epidemiol* 26(4):220-5, 1998.

2. Beck JD: Issues in assessment of diagnostic tests and risks for periodontal disease, *Perio 2000* 7:100-8, 1995.

3. Beck JD: Methods of assessing risk or periodontitis and developing multifactorial models, *J Periodontol* 65:468-78, 1994.

4. Beck JD, Kahout F, Hunt RJ: Identification of high caries risk adults: attitudes, social factors and diseases, *Int Dent J* 38(4):231-8, 1988.

5. Disney JA et al: The University of North Carolina Caries Risk Assessment Study: further developments in caries risk prediction, *Community Dent Oral Epidemiol* 20:64-75, 1992.

6. Douglas CW: Risk assessment in dentistry, *J Dent Ed* 62(10):756-61, 1998.

7. Edelstein BL: Case planning and risk management according to caries risk assessment, *Dent Clin North Am* 39(4):721-58, 1995.

8. Frank MS: Embodying medical expertise in decision support systems for health care management: techniques and benefits, *Top Health Inf Manage* 19(2):44-54, 1998.

9. Gage TW, Pickett FA: *Mosby's dental drug reference,* ed 6, St Louis, (in press), Mosby.

10. Hildebrandt GH: Caries risk assessment and prevention for adults *J Dent Educ* 59(10):972-80, 1993.

11. Karlsson D, Aspervall O, Forsum U: Concepts, contexts, and expert systems, *Stud Health Technol Inform* 68:713-5, 1999.

12. Kleinbaum D, Kupper L, Morgenstern H: *Epidemiologic research: principles and quantitative methods,* Belmont, Calif, 1982, Lifetime Learning Publications.

13. Dental hygiene process of care. In Mueller-Joseph L, Petersen M: *Dental hygiene process: diagnosis and care planning,* Albany, NY, 1995, Delmar.

14. Novak B: Intelligent systems in medical diagnosis, *Stud Health Technol Inform* 68: 700-2, 1999.

15. Saunders RP: What is health promotion? *Health Educ* 19(5):14-8, 1998.

16. Slavkin HC: Placing health promotion into the context of our lives, *J Am Dent Assoc* 129(1):91-5, 1998.

17. Stamm JW et al: Risk assessment for oral diseases, *Adv Dent Res* 5:4-17, 1991.

18. Stoddard JW: Caries risk assessment used as a determinant for caries management and prediction, *J Dent Educ* 59(10):957-61, 1995.

19. U.S. Department of Health and Human Services, National Institute of Dental and Craniofacial Research, National Institutes of Health: *Oral health in America: a report of the surgeon general,* U.S. Department of Health and Human Services, Rockville, Md, 2000.

20. Vick VC, Harfst SA: The Oral Risk Assessment and Early Intervention System: a clinician's tool for integrating the bio/psycho/social risk into oral disease interventions, *Compendium* 30(21 suppl):57-67, 2000.

CHAPTER 30

Individualizing Preventive *and* Therapeutic Strategies

Sherry A. Harfst, Victoria C. Vick

Chapter Outline

The Patient as a Clinical Partner
Case Study: Individualizing Prevention Strategies
Step 4: Recommend
    Oral risk concerns
    Patient goal
    Product recommendation

Prevention Strategy Implementation
    Treatment sequencing
Step 5: Reevaluation

Key Terms

Implementation
Prevention strategy
Therapeutic intervention

Learning Outcomes

1. State rationale for the engagement of the patient as a partner in the oral-care process.
2. Compare and contrast a therapeutic intervention and a prevention strategy.
3. Explain, by way of a patient example, four logical small steps in the process of recommending products and practices for oral self-care.
4. Differentiate between a goal and a strategy.
5. Cite several obstacles to seeking dental care.
6. Discuss components important to consider in planning oral care.
7. Defend the value of evaluation/reevaluation as a way of ensuring optimal oral health.
8. Map a patient's care plan in therapeutic intervention, prevention, and evaluation/reevaluation.
9. Apply Steps 4 and 5 of the ORA system to any patient.
10. Recognize the value of a systematized holistic approach to oral care.

THE PATIENT AS A CLINICAL PARTNER

The more a patient is involved in his or her dental hygiene therapy, and ultimately oral self-care, the greater the chances are for a successful outcome. Involving patients in their care implies that intervention strategies are individualized—again, a complex but ultimately rewarding process—which, to many clinicians, is the central core of dental hygiene care. To design successful clinical therapy and to realize a short-term goal of a successful initial clinical outcome is satisfying, but to witness the failure of therapy when the patient returns with the same—or even worse—level of disease causes frustration for dental hygienists and, ultimately, can lead to career burnout. Although individualizing prevention strategies and involving patients in their oral self-care cannot ensure 100% success, they do go a long way toward promoting optimal oral health for each patient, delivering on the promise and

Case Study

Individualizing Prevention Strategies

30-A

In the case application presented in Chapter 29, the following information from 54-year-old Robin Wallace's ORA Prevention Survey was noted under the section titled "Health Beliefs" (see Figs. 29-3, *E*, and 29-13):

Health Beliefs

- Feels she is more likely than others to have dental problems
- Believes prevention of oral problems is important
- Likes to get recommendations from dental professionals
- Feels she can tackle a new project or make a change at this time
- Somewhat believes she has control over her oral condition

Based on your knowledge of patient and human behavior, do you think that the outcome of prevention discussions with Ms. Wallace will be positive? What if Ms. Wallace did not believe prevention of oral problems was important? Would you address her needs differently? What if she did not feel she could make any changes in personal habits at this time? Would your course of action and or patient goals change?

---

the oath, and adding to the personal satisfaction of the healthcare provider.

The determination of *clinical treatment goals* and corresponding **therapeutic intervention** is more or less empirical—based on supporting evidence—and it addresses oral conditions present a time of therapy. The establishment of *patient goals* and course of action is based on dental science plus an understanding of each specific patient's needs, individual background, health beliefs, and health habits. It also addresses long-term patient intervention and prevention.

STEP 4: RECOMMEND

As Step 4 of the ORA (oral risk assessment) system is explored, it is important for dental hygienists to realize the crucial need to treat each individual patient based on his or her unique needs and circumstances.

Step 4: recommend, when broken into logical planning steps, does the following:

1. Reviews the oral risk concerns for the patient (Column II of the ORA Worksheet; see Fig. 29-16)
2. Determines the specific patient goal in managing the prevention of the risk concerns and designs the **prevention strategy** necessary to reach the goal, based on specific patient needs
3. Recommends specific products and procedures to help each patient reach the stated goals and records the recommendations on the Personalized Oral Care Recommendation form
4. Determines the measure of evaluation

This chapter is written in conjunction with Chapter 29, which the reader is advised to consult for prerequisite information.

ORAL RISK CONCERNS

By reviewing a patient's oral risk concerns, four main topic areas can be determined for which patient goals will be developed.

Periodontal Concerns

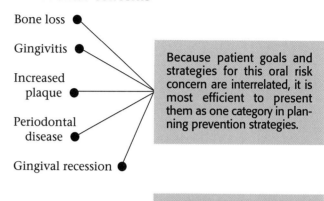

Bone loss
Gingivitis
Increased plaque
Periodontal disease
Gingival recession

Because patient goals and strategies for this oral risk concern are interrelated, it is most efficient to present them as one category in planning prevention strategies.

Dental Caries

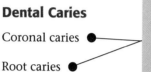

Coronal caries
Root caries

Because patient goals and strategies for this oral risk concern are interrelated, it is most efficient to present them as one category in planning prevention strategies.

Trauma

Medication-Induced Oral Risk Concerns

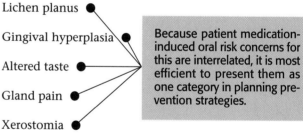

Lichen planus
Gingival hyperplasia
Altered taste
Gland pain
Xerostomia

Because patient medication-induced oral risk concerns for this are interrelated, it is most efficient to present them as one category in planning prevention strategies.

 Case Application
Based on Ms. Wallace's history and clinical findings, her oral risk concerns are examined in Table 30-1.

PATIENT GOAL

Addressing each area of oral risk concern involves understanding not only the clinical aspects of the therapeutic intervention strategy but also the biological, psychological, and sociological components as well.

 Case Application
It is clear from Ms. Wallace's prevention survey that she lacks a basic understanding of the following primary topics:
- The role of plaque in both gingival and hard tissue disease
- Her role in the prevention process
- The benefits of regular dental care
- Knowledge of products and practices used to promote the prevention of oral disease
- Awareness of a cheek-biting habit
- Potential side effects of prescription medications

TABLE 30-1
Application of Step 4 to Robin Wallace*

Oral risk concerns	Patient goal	Prevention strategy	Evaluation
Bone loss Gingivitis Increased plaque Periodontal disease Gingival recession	• Acknowledge signs of gingival disease • Understand role of plaque in gingival disease • Understand role of host response in gingival inflammation • Understand/demonstrate patient role in treatment and prevention of gingival disease • Purchase and use recommended products for treatment and control of gingival disease • Understand personal role in compliance • Appreciate benefits of supportive therapy appointments	• Discussion and discovery (with patient) of intraoral conditions contributing to gingival disease • Discussion of host response and immune defenses • Discussion with patient of oral self-care strategies for treatment and prevention of gingival disease • Recommendation of products for oral self-care for prevention of gingival disease • Demonstration of oral self-care techniques for treatment and prevention of gingival disease • Discussion and plan of supportive therapy appointments	*At appropriate supportive therapy appointment, patient should:* • Describe oral changes noticed in gingival inflammation, dental caries, and esthetics • Describe/demonstrate oral self-care regimen appropriate for disease prevention • Describe role plaque plays in process of oral disease • Present for appointment and book next one
Root caries Coronal caries	• Understand role of plaque, diet, and saliva in caries process • Acknowledge difference between coronal and root surface caries • Understand/demonstrate patient role in treatment and prevention of dental caries • Purchase and use recommended products for prevention of dental caries • Understand personal role in compliance • Appreciate benefits of supportive care appointments	• Discussion and discovery (with patient) of intraoral conditions that contribute to dental caries • Determination of habits that place patient at risk for dental caries • Discussion with patient of oral self-care strategies for treatment and prevention of dental caries • Recommendation of products for oral self-care for prevention of dental caries • Demonstration of oral self-care techniques for prevention of dental caries	*At appropriate supportive care appointment, patient should:* • Describe/document changes in diet and oral self-care that have contributed to reduction/prevention in dental caries
Trauma	• Understand result of trauma-inducing oral habits	• Discussion and plan of supportive care appointments • Discussion and discovery (with patient) of intraoral conditions that contribute to breaks in oral mucosa	*At appropriate supportive care appointment, patient should:* • Describe/demonstrate cessation of traumatic oral habit
Lichenoid lesions	• Understand result of trauma-inducing oral habits	• Discussion of possible oral effects of current medication	*At appropriate supportive care appointment, patient should:* • Evaluate occurrence/lack of occurrence of oral side effect
Taste alteration	• Raise patient awareness to oral side effects of current medication	• Discussion of possible oral effects of current medication	*At appropriate supportive care appointment, patient should:* • Evaluate occurrence/lack of occurrence of oral side effect
Gingival hyperplasia	• Raise patient awareness to oral side effects of current medication	• Discussion of possible oral effects of current medication	*At appropriate supportive care appointment, patient should:* • Evaluate occurrence/lack of occurrence of oral side effect
Xerostomia	• Raise patient awareness to side effects of current medication	• Discussion of possible oral effects of current medication	*At appropriate supportive care appointment, patient should:* • Evaluate occurrence/lack of occurrence of oral side effect
Gland pain	• Raise patient awareness to side effects of current medication	• Discussion of possible oral effects of current medication	*At appropriate supportive care appointment, patient should:* • Evaluate occurrence/lack of occurrence of oral side effect

*Refer to Chapter 29, this chapter's case study, and the case applications for more information.

Periodontal Concerns

Patient goals that address these oral risk concerns in the periodontal concerns category would include the following:

- Acknowledge the signs of gingival disease
- Understand the role of plaque in gingival disease
- Understand the role of the host response in gingival inflammation
- Understand and demonstrate the patient role in the treatment and prevention of gingival disease
- Purchase and use recommended products for the treatment and control of gingival disease
- Understand the personal role in compliance
- Appreciate the benefits of supportive therapy appointments

Prevention Strategy for Periodontal Concerns

The prevention strategy statements outline how the patient goals can be reached for each of the concern areas. For example, the prevention strategy that would be used to reach the patient goals for the category of periodontal concerns would include the following:

- Discussion and discovery (with patient) of intraoral conditions contributing to gingival disease
- Discussion of host response and immune defenses

- Discussion with patient of oral self-care strategies for the treatment and prevention of gingival disease
- Recommendation of products for oral self-care for the prevention of gingival disease
- Demonstration of oral self-care techniques for the treatment and prevention of gingival disease
- Discussion and planning of supportive therapy appointments

 Case Application

Review Table 30-1 to determine how such prevention strategies were applied to Ms. Wallace.

PRODUCT RECOMMENDATION

For a patient to fully comply with any given prevention strategy, he or she needs to know what tools (i.e., specific procedures and products) are recommend for use. Chapters 21, 23, 24, 25, and 28 outline personal self-care procedures and detailed product options. For Ms. Wallace, products and procedures are recommended in the following categories: toothbrush, interdental cleaning, dentifrice, oral rinse, and self-evaluation (Fig. 30-1).

To complete the product recommendation process, the patient can be provided with personalized, written instructions, as shown in Fig. 30-2.

ORAL CARE RECOMMENDATIONS

Prevention Strategy	Toothbrush	Product
• Discussion and discovery (with patient) of intraoral conditions	☐ Mechanical	
	☐ Child ☐ Youth ☐ Compact ☐ Full	
	☑ Soft ☐ Extra Soft	
	☑ Powered	*Spinbrush*
	Brushing frequency *2X daily*	
• Discussion of host response and immune defenses	Brushing duration *2 minutes*	
	Interdental Cleaning Products	
	☑ Floss Type *waxed* Frequency *1X day*	*OralB*
• Discussion with patient of oral self-care strategies	☑ Oral Irrigator *w/water* Frequency *1X day*	
	☐ Interdental Brush Frequency	
	☐ Other	
• Recommendation of products for oral self-care		
	Dentifrice	
	☐ Fluoride ☐ Whitening	*Crest*
• Demonstration of oral self-care techniques	☐ Sensitivity ☑ Multiple Benefit	*Multicare*
	☐ Tartar Control ☐ Gingival Benefit	*w/whitening*
	☐ Children's	
• Discuss and plan supportive care appointments.		
	Oral Rinse	
	☐ Fluoride	
• Discussion and discovery (with patient) of intraoral conditions	☐ Cosmetic	
	☐ Alcohol-free	
	☐ Tartar Control	
	☐ Chlorhexidine	
• Determine habits that place her at risk for dental caries.	☐ Essential Oil/Phenol Compound	
	Prosthodontic Care	
• Discussion with patient of oral self-care strategies	☐ Adhesive ☐ Denture Brush	
	☐ Denture Bath/Cleanser	
• Recommendation of products for oral self-care	**Self Evaluation**	
	☑ Disclosing tablets or solutions	
• Demonstration of oral self-care techniques	☑ Evaluate bleeding points	
	Other	
• Discuss and plan supportive care appointments.		
• Discuss possible oral effects of current medication.		

FIG. 30-1 Column V of the ORA Worksheet—Evaluate.

The process for personalizing prevention strategies is the same for each area of oral risk concern identified, as presented in Table 30-1.

PREVENTION STRATEGY IMPLEMENTATION

For *implementation,* important consideration needs to be made of how best to address patient goals. Discussing all patient goals at the first appointment can be overwhelming to the patient. Just as it is necessary to divide dental hygiene therapy between appointments, it is also important to address patient goals in small steps. Depending on patient success in mastering a goal, more goals can be added to subsequent appointments. When a patient has difficulty mastering concepts of oral self-care, goals can be revised. Again, depending on patient motivation, not all patients will take the recommended actions. Constant evaluation and revision of goals is necessary to provide optimal oral health care.

At this point in the planning stage, several elements can be taken into consideration that can significantly affect successful appointment planning: appointment flow, appointment times, and engagement of the patient in his or her oral care.

TREATMENT SEQUENCING

Determining appropriate clinical treatment planning involves the following:
- Identifying all necessary therapeutic interventions (see Chapter 29) and required armamentarium
- Understanding obstacles to care

Personalized Oral Care Recommendations

For *Robin Wallace*

Date *MM/DD/YY*

Services provided at today's visit:

☑ Oral hygiene instructions
☐ Prophylaxis (dental cleaning)
☐ Therapeutic debridement
☑ Fluoride treatment
☐ Sealant/Varnish
☐ Nutrition evaluation
☐ Other

Plaque was noted in the following areas

Along gum line · *Along gum line* · *Along gum line*

Your next scheduled visit with our dental hygienist should be in ___1___ months/(weeks)

Recommended oral care products

Toothbrush	Product
☐ Mechanical	
☐ Child ☐ Youth ☐ Compact ☐ Full	
☑ Soft ☐ Extra Soft	
☑ Powered	*Spinbrush*
Brushing frequency *2x day*	
Brushing duration *2 minutes*	
Interdental Cleaning Products	
☑ Floss Type *waxed* Frequency *1x day*	*Oral B*
☑ Oral Irrigator *w/ water* Frequency *1x day*	
☐ Interdental Brush Frequency	
☐ Other Frequency	
☐ Other	
Dentifrice	
☐ Fluoride ☐ Whitening	
☐ Sensitivity ☑ Multiple benefit *w/ whitening*	*Crest Multicare Whitening*
☐ Tartar control ☐ Gingival benefit	
☐ Children's	
Oral Rinse *none*	
☐ Fluoride	
☐ Cosmetic	
☐ Alcohol-free	
☐ Tartar Control	
☐ Chlorhexidine	
☐ Essential Oil/Phenol Compound	
Prosthodontic Care *none*	
☐ Adhesive ☐ Denture Brush	
☐ Denture Bath/Cleanser	
Self Evaluation	
☑ Disclosing tablets or solutions	*Use 1X a week*
☑ Evaluate bleeding points	*Check floss daily*
Other	

Crest

FIG. 30-2 Oral care recommendations for 54-year-old Robin Wallace, whose case is presented in the chapter's case study.

BOX 30-1

Obstacles to Obtaining Health Care

Ethnic and cultural beliefs	Confidence in treatment outcomes
Differences in terms used by professionals and nonprofessionals	Denial of illness
	Belief in personal invulnerability
Negative views of the medical setting	Differing opinions
Personal and group values	Risk of suggested procedure
Group memberships and attitudes	Transportation difficulties
Ineffective form and content of message delivery	Convenience
Illiteracy	Attitudes toward the body
Poverty	Fear and anxiety level
Lack of technical sophistication	Education level
Habit	Confusion regarding treatment options
Availability of services	Insincerity of educator or patient

From DeBiase CB: *Dental health education: theory and practice,* Philadelphia, 1961, Lea & Febiger.

- Planning appropriate appointment sequencing
- Gaining patient feedback in the reassessment process
- Reevaluating and retreating as appropriate

Identifying Armamentaria

Although this is not a crucial planning step, it is important to be certain that all necessary armamentaria are available for use. For example, being aware that only four air-polishing units are available for use among 16 clinicians can help prevent a potential problem in patient completion. If the patient appointment calls for special supplies, such as a sealant kit or a specific type of fluoride, it may be necessary to check supplies well in advance of the patient's arrival.

Understanding Obstacles to Care

Appointment planning is influenced by many variables—some patient-driven, some clinician-determined. Patients may face several obstacles to obtaining the health care they need, for valid reasons (Box 30-1). Being sensitive to these issues can help the clinician establish successful appointment habits.

Planning Appropriate Appointment Sequencing

Once appointment times have been established and possible obstacles have been examined and overcome, the dental hygienist must plan care for each patient visit. This process, once again, involves weighing variables to provide the necessary data upon which to plan appropriate treatment sequencing.

Gauging Patient Comfort or Pain

If a patient experiences oral pain and a diagnosis has been established in which dental hygiene therapy will help alleviate the discomfort, that section or area of the mouth might be treated first.

If, however, a patient does not experience oral discomfort, the therapy might be initiated in a specific, standardized sequence of either sextants (six oral divisions),

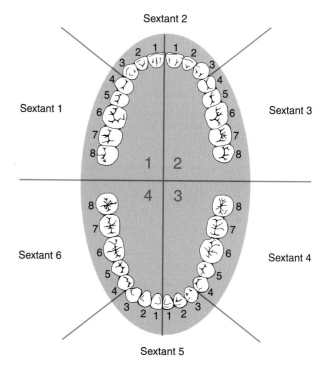

FIG. 30-3 Sextant divisions of the dentition. (Modified from Liebgott B: *The anatomical basis of dentistry,* ed 2, St Louis, 2001, Mosby.)

quadrants (four oral divisions), or half-mouth (maxillary and mandibular quadrants on one side). The selection of the sequencing depends on the disease classification, intraoral access, clinician proficiency, and patient factors (Figs. 30-3 through 30-5).

Using a Consistent Starting Point

By initiating dental hygiene therapy at a consistent location, record keeping and subsequent appointments can be more efficient. For example, for the right-handed clinician, begin on the upper right, at the posterior surface of

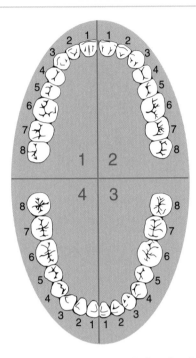

FIG. 30-4 Quadrant divisions of the dentition. (From Liebgott B: *The anatomical basis of dentistry,* ed 2, St Louis, 2001, Mosby.)

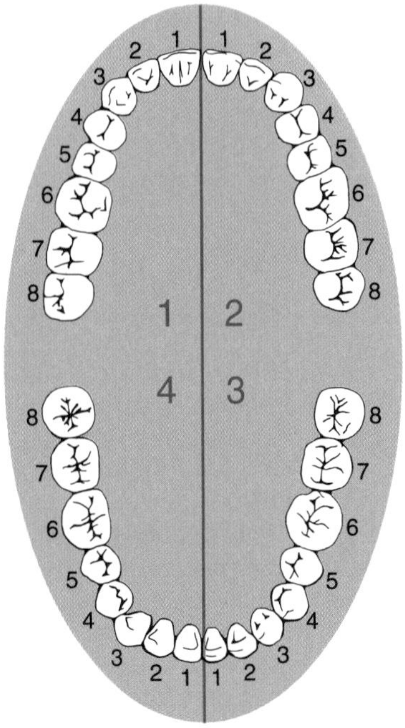

FIG. 30-5 Half-mouth division. (Modified from Liebgott B: *The anatomical basis of dentistry,* ed 2, St Louis, 2001, Mosby.)

the most posterior tooth (e.g., distobuccal of #1), or begin on the lower right, at the posterior surface of the most posterior tooth (e.g., distobuccal of #32). (Left-handed hygienists would begin on the opposite side). Clinical faculty may have additional suggestions and recommendations on this topic.

Determining the Degree of Difficulty

Occasionally, it can be determined from radiographic interpretation and clinical charting that the disease status in a specific area of the mouth is more advanced than others. By initiating dental hygiene therapy in the more advanced disease sites, the clinician can have more opportunity to reevaluate the success of therapy at sequential appointments.

Accommodating Patient Perceptions

A patient may direct where he or she wants the dental hygiene therapy started. Reasons a patient may provide these instructions could be aesthetic (e.g., unsightly stains or calculus on the anterior facials), or could be driven by discomfort. Although total patient-directed care is not encouraged, accommodating such requests may provide an opportunity for fuller patient participation in oral self-care.

Realizing the Goal of Therapy

Whatever appointment sequencing is established, it is important that the dental hygienist realize the goal of any dental hygiene therapy—to complete whatever therapy is initiated.

The goal of any dental hygiene appointment is to complete any areas initiated, for these two reasons:
1. Wound healing is improved. Once an area is biologically stressed from a bioburden and inflammatory standpoint, it is important to thoroughly remove all toxin and underlying gingival irritants so the tissue can respond quickly and efficiently.
2. Assessing outcomes of dental hygiene therapy is only accomplished when the therapy is complete. In that way, any area requiring retreatment is easily identified. Patient self-care can likewise be addressed, and goals can be changed as appropriate.

Planning the Time Allotment

Appointment times have been carefully established by most dental hygiene programs and will be modified as clinical competence is gained. Typically, longer appointment schedules are established at the beginning of the student experience. As clinical competence is gained, each successive clinic session will provide more challenges in that appointment times will be shorter, allowing more patients to be seen in a single clinic session. The goal of this chapter is to provide considerations for *planning the allotted time*—not in suggesting the length of time a specific procedure should take.

Listening to Patient Feedback

Patient-centered dental hygiene therapy delivers on the definition. Although patients do not *direct* the therapy, they clearly need to be active participants.

Setting expectations of treatment involves clinical judgment and establishment of the patient as a fully active participant in his or her oral self-care. Although it is a complex process, establishing and evaluating patient goals is not only rewarding and satisfying but also essential to provide and promote optimal oral health.

STEP 5: REEVALUATION

Evaluation/reevaluation of clinical outcomes (therapeutic intervention) and patient goals (prevention strategies) is the final step in dental hygiene care. Evaluation of the outcome is just as important as the first step and determines the type of supportive care each patent requires.

 Case Application

Ms. Wallace's, sextant #1 was debrided (see Fig. 29-6, on p. 497). At the end of 3 weeks, sextant #1 is evaluated for bleeding on probing and plaque accumulation. The recommendation for supportive care will differ based on the outcome (Fig. 30-6). For each of the following clinical outcomes, what supportive care recommendations would you make?
- Three sites that were initially charted as bleeding on probing were unchanged.
- Although no bleeding on probing is noted, a high plaque index is calculated, and the patient is unable to recall any signs of gingival inflammation.
- No bleeding on probing and no discernible plaque are noted.
- The patient is unable to demonstrate interdental cleaning, and three sites exhibit bleeding on probing.

Each of the examples in the previous case application requires a different form of supportive care. Taking the necessary time to evaluate outcomes is crucial to successful dental hygiene therapy, both in therapeutic intervention and prevention strategies.

Case Application

Initial treatment sequencing for Ms. Wallace now can be mapped. This appointment mapping uses the ORA Prevention Survey, clinical and radiographic findings, and the ORA Worksheet.

For this case, care has been divided into sextants, requiring seven total appointments: six for therapeutic intervention and prevention strategy implementation and a final one for reevaluation (Boxes 30-2 through 30-8).

Designing successful clinical therapy and appropriate personalized patient care requires the following careful steps:
- *Review* of all patient records
- *Analysis* of oral risk concerns
- *Planning* of therapeutic intervention and prevention strategies
- *Recommendations* of personalized oral self-care products and practices
- *Reevaluation* of all outcomes
The use of a system-based organization tool, such as the ORA system, can help dental students and clinicians reach a holistic, patient-centered approach to oral care, providing optimal oral health and clinician satisfaction.

EVALUATE
Clinical Goals

- Attachment loss does not increase as measured at supportive care intervals.
- No additional recession at supportive care intervals
- Current recession does not increase.
- No bleeding on probing at reevaluation interval
- Tissue color, contour, consistency within normal limits
- Improved plaque index
- No bleeding on probing at reevaluation interval
- No increased probing depths at reevaluation interval
- No new evidence of radiographic bone loss at reevaluation interval
- No coronal caries evident at supportive care intervals
- No new caries at supportive care appointment
- Arrested/reversed caries process
- No evidence of trauma
- Patient interview

Patient Goals

At the appropriate supportive care appointment, the patient will:

- Describe the oral changes the patient has noticed in the area of gingival inflammation, dental caries, and esthetics
- Describe/demonstrate an oral self-care regimen appropriate for disease prevention
- Describe the role plaque plays in the process of oral disease
- Have been present for the appointment and booked the next one
- Describe/document changes in diet and oral self-care that have contributed to a reduction/prevention in dental caries
- Describe/demonstrate a cessation of the traumatic oral habit
- Evaluate the occurrence/lack of occurrence of the oral side effect

FIG 30-6 Personalized instructions for 54-year-old Robin Wallace (whose case is presented in the chapter's case study) to take home.

BOX 30-2

Appointment #1

Dental Hygiene Therapy Therapeutic Intervention	Patient Discussion Prevention Strategy	Evaluation
• Review intraoral examination • Disclose patient • Engage patient in oral evaluation • Chart plaque index • Discuss patient education • Debride sextant #1 (assuming no variables need consideration in order of treatment of oral cavity) • Give postdebridement instructions	• Discussion and discovery (with patient) of intraoral conditions contributing to gingival disease • Discussion of host response and immune defenses • Discussion with patient of oral self-care strategies for treatment and prevention of gingival disease • Recommendation of products for oral self-care for prevention of gingival disease • Demonstration of oral self-care techniques for treatment and prevention of gingival disease • Asking/answering of any new questions as needed	Verbal feedback to gain additional goals, ensuring that communication is clear

BOX 30-3

Appointment #2

Dental Hygiene Therapy Therapeutic Intervention	Patient Discussion Prevention Strategy	Evaluation
• Review intraoral examination • Disclose patient • Engage patient in oral evaluation • Chart plaque index • Debride sextant #2 • Give postdebridement instructions	• Discussion and discovery (with patient) of intraoral conditions contributing to dental caries • Determination of habits that place patient at risk for dental caries • Determination of why patient feels more likely than others to have dental problems • Discussion with patient of oral self-care strategies for treatment and prevention of dental caries • Asking/answering of any new questions as needed	• Plaque index should be lower. • Patient should be able to articulate role of plaque in gingival disease. • Patient should be able to demonstrate compliance with recommendations.

BOX 30-4

Appointment #3

Dental Hygiene Therapy Therapeutic Intervention	Patient Discussion Prevention Strategy	Evaluation
• Review intraoral examination • Check BOP index on sextant #1 • Disclose patient • Engage patient in oral evaluation • Chart plaque index • Debride sextant #3 • Debride again any areas of BOP on sextant #1 • Give postdebridement instructions	• Determination of which oral changes patient may have noticed, such as: Improved gingival color, tone No bleeding on brushing No breath odor Teeth "feeling" better • Discussion of importance in following healthcare provider recommendations • Raising of patient awareness to side effects of current medication • Asking/answering of any new questions as needed	• Plaque index should be lower. • Patient should be able to articulate role of plaque in dental caries. • Patient should be able to discuss changes made to diet to reduce acid challenge to hard tooth structures. • Patient should be able to discuss why, in the past, she has experienced oral disease and how, in the future, she can control oral health. • Patient should be able to demonstrate compliance with recommendations.

BOP, Bleeding on probing.

BOX 30-5

Appointment #4

Dental Hygiene Therapy Therapeutic Intervention	Patient Discussion Prevention Strategy	Evaluation
• Review intraoral examination • Check BOP index on sextant #2 • Disclose patient • Engage patient in oral evaluation • Chart plaque index • Debride sextant #4 • Debride again any areas of BOP on sextant #2 • Give postdebridement instructions	• Progress of therapy • Compliance with recommendations • Asking/answering of any new questions as needed	• Patient should be able to self-evaluate for oral change and comply with recommendations. • Any BOP in sextant #2 needs careful notation and retreatment.

BOP, Bleeding on probing.

BOX 30-6

Appointment #5

Dental Hygiene Therapy Therapeutic Intervention	Patient Discussion Prevention Strategy	Evaluation
• Review intraoral examination • Check BOP index on sextant #3 • Disclose patient • Engage patient in oral evaluation • Chart plaque index • Debride sextant #5 • Debride again any areas of BOP on sextant #3 • Give postdebridement instructions	• Progress of therapy • Compliance with recommendations • Asking/answering of any new questions as needed	• Patient should be able to self-evaluate for oral change and comply with recommendations. • Any BOP in sextant #3 needs careful notation and retreatment.

BOP, Bleeding on probing.

BOX 30-7

Appointment #6

Dental Hygiene Therapy Therapeutic Intervention	Patient Discussion Prevention Strategy	Evaluation
• Review intraoral examination • Check BOP index on sextant #4 • Disclose patient • Engage patient in oral evaluation • Chart plaque index • Debride sextant #6 • Debride again any areas of BOP on sextant #4 • Give postdebridement instructions	• Progress of therapy • Compliance with recommendations • Asking/answering of any new questions as needed	• Patient should be able to self-evaluate for oral change and comply with recommendations. • Any BOP in sextant #4 needs careful notation and retreatment.

BOP, Bleeding on probing.

BOX 30-8

Appointment #7 (21 Days after Therapy)

Dental Hygiene Therapy Therapeutic Intervention	Patient Discussion Prevention Strategy	Evaluation
• Review intraoral examination • Check BOP index on all sextants • Disclose patient • Engage patient in oral evaluation • Chart plaque index • Debride any areas that BOP • Polish as appropriate • Apply topical fluoride • Establish supportive care interval	• Summary of all previous discussions, time for questions, and clarification of responses • Summary of dental hygiene therapy outcomes, with notation of progress on charts such as plaque index • Reinforcement of progress • Suggestions for improvement, where appropriate • Establishment of interval of supportive care	• Any BOP in any sextant needs careful notation and retreatment. • Changes in color, contour, consistency in gingiva should be noted. • Patient should be able to articulate own role in oral self-care for the prevention of gingivitis and caries. • Patient should be able to discuss signs and symptoms of oral disease. • Patient should be able to discuss recommended oral self-care regimens and products, specific to individual need. • Patient should acknowledge appropriate supportive care interval.

BOP, Bleeding on probing.

CRITICAL THINKING ACTIVITIES

1. Together with a classmate, complete an ORA Prevention Survey. In a role-playing format, perform Steps 1, 2, 3, and 4 of the ORA system using the ORA Worksheet. Were there any pertinent findings from this step that you previously overlooked? Did any biological, psychological, or sociological elements come to light that might planning prevention strategies?
2. Make as many prevention strategies as you can. Determine whether each acts strictly as a prevention strategy, therapeutic intervention or both.
3. Using the ORA Worksheet from Activity #1, perform Steps 4 and 5 of the ORA system on a student partner. What types of patient goals and prevention strategies can you document?

4. Select a student from the second-year class. Present different clinical outcomes and ask which supportive care steps he or she would recommend.
5. If you are a first-year student, select a second-year student with whom to work. Ask to review the dental records of a patient he or she is currently treating. After completing Steps 1, 2, and 3 of the ORA system with the use of only the dental records provided, complete Steps 4 and 5. Determine the clinical goal, therapeutic intervention, patient goal, prevention strategy, and evaluation method for each oral risk concern noted. Would this process have been more thorough with an ORA Prevention Survey?

REVIEW QUESTIONS

Questions 4-6, 8, and 10 refer to the case study presented at the beginning of the chapter.

1. Personalizing patient oral self-care instructions is characterized by which of the following?
   a. Important to engage the patient as a partner
   b. Part of patient-centered treatment philosophy
   c. Helpful to the hygienist in terms of job satisfaction.
   d. *a* and *b* only
   e. All the above
2. Which step in the ORA system recommends oral self-care products and practices?
   a. Step 1
   b. Step 3
   c. Step 4
   d. Step 2
   e. Step 5

3. Reevaluation of supportive care includes which of the following?
   a. Only the debrided portion of the treatment plan
   b. Patient compliance
   c. Caries rate
   d. Review of all aspects of the supportive care process, including both therapeutic intervention and prevention strategies
4. Oral risk concerns for Ms. Wallace include all of the following *except* which one?
   a. Increase in plaque
   b. Lichen planus
   c. Gingival hyperplasia
   d. Tooth mobility
   e. *a* and *c* only

Continued

REVIEW QUESTIONS—cont'd

5. Of the prevention strategies for Ms. Wallace, which of the following addresses the oral risk concern for gingival hyperplasia?
   a. Discussion of host defense mechanisms
   b. Discussion and plan of supportive care appointments
   c. Discussion of role of saliva in remineralization process
   d. Discussion of possible oral effects of her current medications
   e. None of the above

6. Which of the following obstacles to care should be considered in the planning of supportive care appointments for Ms. Wallace?
   a. Transportation
   b. Confusion about dental terminology
   c. Illiteracy
   d. Poor perception of dentistry
   e. None of the above

7. In determining the appropriate appointment sequencing, which of the following should be followed as a goal of therapy?
   a. Remove gross debris only at the first appointment so the patient tolerance will increase with time.
   b. Complete therapy that is initiated.
   c. Always begin on anterior teeth so the patient can see a difference.
   d. Follow the wishes of the patient.

8. Which reevaluation measure(s) are appropriate for Ms. Wallace in determining whether she has met the goal of understanding signs and symptoms of gingival disease?
   a. She can pick out a photo of diseased gingiva.
   b. She can point to any areas in her mouth that she feels are not responding to therapy.

   c. She can point out areas in her mouth that require polishing.
   d. She can cite the symptoms of gingival inflammation.
   e. *a, b,* and *d* only

9. The five steps in the ORA system include all *except* which of the following?
   a. Carefully reviewing all patient data
   b. Determining oral risk concerns
   c. Mapping each appointment
   d. Evaluating therapy
   e. Evaluating clinician satisfaction

10. Of the following factors for Ms. Wallace, which do you feel is the most important factor to address in helping provide her with a future of optimal oral health?
   1. Lack of oral self-care tools
   2. Not understanding the oral effects of prescription medication
   3. Not seeking regular dental care
   4. Lack of appreciation for her role in disease prevention
   5. Not spending adequate time in oral self-care
   a. 1 and 3
   b. 1, 4, 5
   c. 2 and 3
   d. All the above
   e. None of the above

SUGGESTED AGENCIES AND WEB SITES

Because of the ever-changing nature of the Internet, some of the web sites listed here may have changed since publication. Please refer to Mosby's Evolve web site for the most current information.

Centers for Disease Control and Prevention, *MMWR Weekly* 37(30):578-83, 1988 ("Perspectives in disease prevention and health promotion: progress toward achieving the national 1990 objectives for fluoridation and dental health"): http://www.cdc.gov
Dental Disease Prevention and Resources: http://www.holisticmed.com

National Institutes of Health, National Oral Health Information Clearinghouse ("Detection and prevention of periodontal disease in diabetes"): http://www.nohic.nidcr.nih.gov
The American Academy of Periodontology ("Tobacco use and periodontal disease"): http://www.perio.org

ADDITIONAL READINGS AND RESOURCES

Berg R, Garcia LT, Berky DB: Spectrum of care treatment planning: application of the model in older adults, *Gen Dent* 48(5):534-43, 2000.

Calley KH et al: A proposed client self-care commitment model, *J Dent Hyg* 74(1):24-35, 2000.

Chu R, Craig B: Understanding the determinants of preventive oral health behaviors, *Probe* 30(1):12-8, 1996 (review).

Edwab RR: When to modify treatment plans, *Dent Today* 17(11): 106-7, 1998.

Williams KB et al: Oral health-related quality of life: a model for dental hygiene, *J Dent Hyg* 72(2):19-26, 1998.

PART VI

Chapter 31
Powered Instrumentation in Periodontal Debridement

Chapter 32
Cosmetic and Therapeutic Polishing

Chapter 33
Periodontal Dressings and Suturing

Competency Statements

The learner is expected to possess knowledge, skills, judgments, values, and attitudes to develop the listed competencies.

Core Competencies

- Apply a professional code of ethics in all endeavors.
- Adhere to state and federal laws, recommendations, and regulations in the provision of dental hygiene care.
- Provide dental hygiene care to promote patient health and wellness using critical thinking and problem solving in the provision of evidence-based practice.
- Use evidence-based decision making to evaluate and incorporate emerging treatment modalities.
- Assume responsibility for dental hygiene actions and care based on accepted scientific theories and research as well as the accepted standard of care.
- Continuously perform self-assessment for life-long learning and professional growth.
- Provide quality assurance mechanisms for health services.
- Communicate effectively with individuals and groups from diverse populations both verbally and in writing.
- Provide accurate, consistent, and complete documentation for assessment, diagnosis, planning, implementation, and evaluation of dental hygiene services.
- Provide care to all clients using an individualized approach that is humane, empathetic, and caring.

Courtesy American Dental Education Association, Washington, DC.

Therapeutic Implementation

Health Promotion and Disease Prevention

- Promote the values of oral and general health and wellness to the public and organizations within and outside the profession.
- Respect the goals, values, beliefs, and preferences of the patient while promoting optimal oral and general health.
- Refer patients who may have a physiologic, psychological, and/or social problem for comprehensive patient evaluation.
- Identify individual and population risk factors and develop strategies that promote health related quality of life.
- Evaluate factors that can be used to promote patient adherence to disease prevention and/or health maintenance strategies.
- Evaluate and utilize methods to ensure the health and safety of the patient and the dental hygienist in the delivery of dental hygiene.

Patient Care

- Select, obtain, and interpret diagnostic information recognizing its advantages and limitations.
- Recognize predisposing and etiologic risk factors that require intervention to prevent disease.
- Obtain, review, and update a complete medical, family, social, and dental history.
- Recognize health conditions and medications that impact overall patient care.
- Identify patients at risk for a medical emergency and manage the patient care in a manner that prevents an emergency.
- Determine a dental hygiene diagnosis.
- Identify patient needs and significant findings that impact the delivery of dental hygiene services.
- Obtain consultations as indicated.
- Prioritize the care plan based on the health status and the actual and potential problems of the individual to facilitate optimal oral health.
- Establish a planned sequence of care (education, clinical, and evaluation) based on the dental hygiene diagnosis; identified oral conditions; potential problems; etiologic and risk factors; and available treatment modalities.
- Establish a collaborative relationship with the patient in the planned care to include etiology, prognosis, and treatment alternatives.
- Make referrals to other healthcare professionals.
- Obtain the patient's informed consent based on a thorough case presentation.
- Perform dental hygiene interventions to eliminate and/or control local etiologic factors to prevent and control caries, periodontal disease, and other oral conditions.
- Control pain and anxiety during treatment through the use of accepted clinical and behavioral techniques.
- Provide life support measures to manage medical and dental emergencies in the patient care environment.
- Determine the outcomes of dental hygiene interventions using indices, instruments, examination techniques, and patient self-report.
- Evaluate the patient's satisfaction with the oral healthcare received and the oral healthcare status achieved.
- Provide subsequent treatment or referrals based on evaluation findings.
- Develop and maintain a health maintenance program.

Professional Growth and Development

- Access professional and social networks and resources to assist entrepreneurial initiatives.

CHAPTER 31

Powered Instrumentation
in Periodontal Debridement

Susan J. Daniel, Bonnie Francis

Chapter Outline

Periodontal Debridement
   Goals of debridement
Case Study: Therapeutic Selections for the
   Periodontal Patient
Review of Pathogenesis and Wound Healing
   Wound healing
Powered Scaling Instruments
   Sonic scalers
   Ultrasonic scalers
Tip Selection and Application
   Universal tips
   Modified tips
Preparation of Powered Instruments
   Patient and operator preparation
   Therapeutic use of powered scalers

Fundamentals of Powered Instrumentation
   Patient and operator positioning
   Patient comfort
   Grasp
   Fulcrum
   Adaptation
   Insertion and activation
Evaluation of Debridement
   Posttherapy evaluation at 4 to 6 weeks
Coding for Periodontal Debridement

Key Terms

Air turbine
Antigens
Bioburden
Cavitational
Cycles per second (CPS)
Cytokines

Debonding
Hertz (Hz)
Host response
Interleukins
Lipopolysaccharides
Magnetostrictive

Mechanical
Microstreaming
Pathogenesis
Pericoronitis
Periodontal debridement

Piezoelectric
Power-driven
Prostaglandins
Sonic
Ultrasonic

Learning Outcomes

1. Select the appropriate instrument—manual or powered—
for periodontal debridement.
2. Discuss the process of pathogenesis and wound healing
in relationship to the need for periodontal debridement.
3. Select the appropriate tips for the debridement process,
based on patient need and access.

4. Set up a powered instrument for periodontal
debridement.
5. Determine the need for further therapeutic intervention
at the 4- to 6-week evaluation based on tissue response.
6. Understand the rate of wound healing of the oral tissues
and the role this plays in therapeutic intervention.

eriodontal debridement is the foundation of dental hygiene care. The goals of debridement are to arrest infection and return tissue to health by eliminating the deposits on the tooth and reducing the bioburden within the pocket. Providing therapeutic intervention that results in health of human tissue and maintenance of function is rewarding. Dental hygienists are gratified by seeing changes that occur because of the intervention and the compliant self-care regimen the patient has demonstrated under their guidance.

The hygienist determines the need for periodontal debridement and selects the appropriate manual or powered instruments to achieve the best clinical outcome and meet the goals established for each individual. Knowledge of powered instruments, tip selection, and fundamentals for use is critical to achieving the established goals. Evaluations of tissue response and bleeding are the most important factors in determining whether further intervention (professional or self) is required. Continuous and frequent monitoring of periodontally involved patients is necessary to prevent further tissue destruction; therefore placement on frequent intervals of supportive care may be necessary in providing optimal oral care.

The previous chapters provided a background of procedures and techniques used to thoroughly assess a patient's health, to develop therapeutic and preventive strategies, and to educate patients on appropriate preventive strategies. This chapter provides content on the procedures employed for therapeutic *periodontal debridement* delivered by the dental hygienist. Periodontal debridement refers to the physical removal of substance from the tooth surface with either hand or powered instruments. Design of hand and *ultrasonic* instruments was covered in Chapter 7, along with the technique for use of hand instruments. This chapter focuses on the use of powered instruments in periodontal debridement.

PERIODONTAL DEBRIDEMENT

Debridement is the process by which hard and soft deposits are removed from the supragingival and subgingival surfaces of the teeth, including the disruption of bacterial cell walls of nonadherent plaque.[35] Debridement ultimately reduces the *bioburden,* resulting in improvement and healing of the soft tissues.

Several methods reduce bioburden: brushing and interproximal cleaning, performing chemotherapeutics, using an exploratory, performing scaling and root-planing stroke, and polishing. The result of debridement is not necessarily a glassy and squeaky-smooth tooth surface, as was once the suggested result of root planing. Continued smoothing of the surface and excess removal of the root structure to obtain healthy soft tissue is not as dependent on deposit removal as it is on the individual patient's immune response. Those individuals who are immunocompromised may not respond to the same degree as someone who is in good health. Studies have concluded that it is the bacterial products within the nonadherent plaque that are most detrimental to the soft tissues. With removal of endotoxins and other noxious subgingival substances, tissue healing can occur.

The traditional approach to periodontal therapy through scaling and root planing was based on the theory that endotoxins (*lipopolysaccharides* released from gram-negative bacteria) were deeply embedded into cementum. Therefore it was thought to be critical to remove all diseased cementum.[4,7,20,33]

More recent research shows that complete cementum removal is not necessary to achieve a positive result with nonsurgical periodontal therapy. In fact, it can actually cause more harm than good. Without the use of powered instruments versus hand/*mechanical* root planing, endotoxin can be removed without removal of the cementum layer. Powered instruments create a *cavitational* action, which is produced as water hits the tip. This cavitation results in an acoustic *microstreaming* phenomena, whereby large hydrodynamic shear stress is produced close to oscillating objects. Within the sulcus or pocket the acoustic microstreaming phenomenon disturbs the integrity of the bacterial cell wall and removes lightly bound endotoxin. These actions have been proven effective in the reduction of bioburden and the production of a healing response.[18] From a biological standpoint, thorough plaque and calculus removal is the most desired outcome and rarely is complete removal achieved with any method.[5,6] However, soft tissue can be repaired and regenerated despite residual amounts of plaque and calculus, which makes the case for debridement over traditional scaling and root planing even more compelling.[2]

GOALS OF DEBRIDEMENT

Arresting infection, resulting in the healing of inflamed tissue, and preventing of further disease activity are the primary goals of debridement. This includes the prevention, arrest, and stabilization of periodontal disease by removing supragingival and subgingival bacterial plaque and its by-products. Although calculus removal is a secondary goal of the debridement process, the importance of its elimination cannot be overlooked because of its plaque-harboring qualities. Once the endotoxin is removed and inflammation subsides, greater patient comfort levels may be achieved and regeneration of the periodontium can begin.

Patient compliance, disease severity, and host immune response are among other major factors that may determine the success or failure of treatment. Additionally, the dental professional's expertise, proficiency, and use of various instrumentation devices also dictate the degree to which these goals can be attained.

If the overall goal of periodontal debridement is to produce healthy tissue, the processes of wound development and wound healing must be considered. The dental hygienist has several therapeutic options to assist in the process of wound healing—the primary one being to remove or reduce the bioburden from the tooth surface so that the *host response* or immune response can achieve the mission of producing healthy tissues.

This debridement process includes instrumentation of the supragingival and subgingival aspects of the tooth and reduction of viable bacteria within the periodontal pocket. Chemotherapeutic agents, both local and systemic, may be used in conjunction with instrumentation and have been noted to improve the outcome in patients with periodontitis as a manifestation of systemic disease.

To more fully appreciate the role of the host's immune response in periodontal therapy and the role of the dental

Therapeutic Selections for the Periodontal Patient

Mrs. Melba Ray is a 55-year-old Caucasian woman seeking supportive care for the first time in more than a year. She recently has moved to your area and indicates that she has had previous periodontal problems and that some areas of her mouth are sensitive. She also informs you that she has a tooth that is partially erupted palatal to an existing fixed bridge but that does not cause her any problems.

Mrs. Ray's health history reveals non–insulin-dependent diabetes mellitus (NIDDM) and mild hypertension. She takes 10 mg of glipizide daily for her diabetes and is not taking any medications for hypertension. Instead, she closely monitors her blood pressure, exercises, and modifies her diet to control both the hypertension and the diabetes.

The intraoral examination reveals a cheek bite on the right buccal mucosa, whereas the extraoral examination is within normal limits (WNL), or noncontributory.

Clinical and radiographic findings are presented in the images of the mouth in the periodontal charting. As you review these, use the process presented in Chapters 29 and 30 to identify risks and establish therapeutic and self-care strategies for patient care. This chapter will help you to apply a therapeutic strategy consistent with Mrs. Ray's needs.

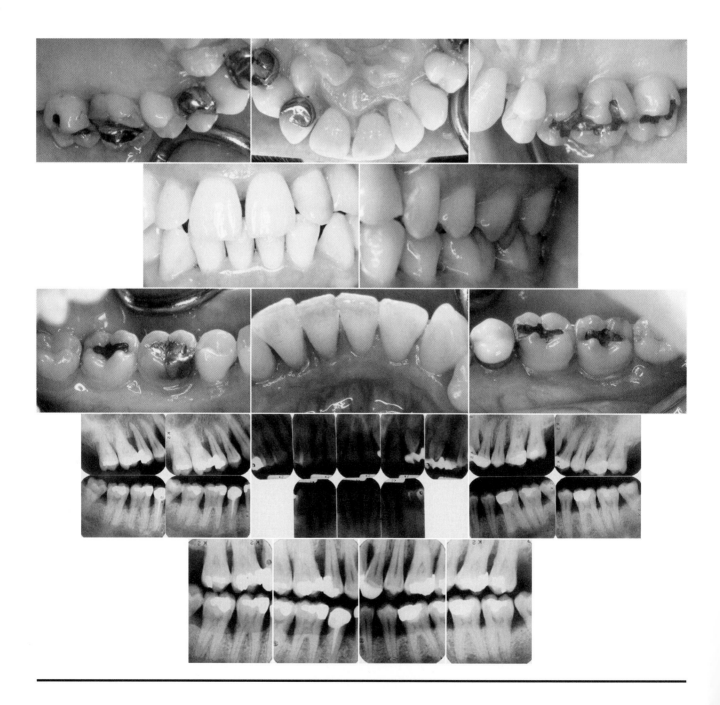

Case Study

Therapeutic Selections for the Periodontal Patient—cont'd

Periodontal Charting

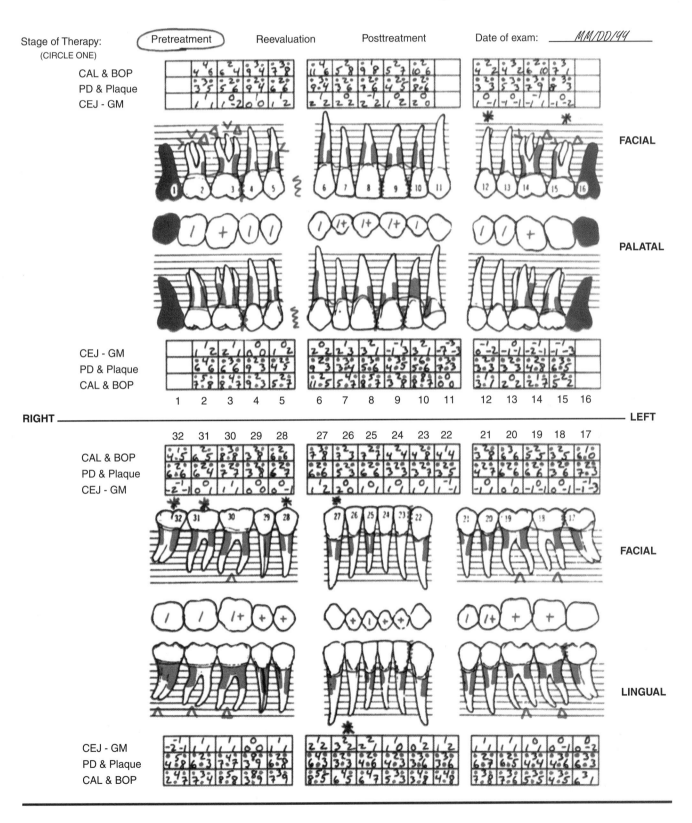

professional in therapy, an understanding of the process of wound development and wound healing is needed.

REVIEW OF PATHOGENESIS AND WOUND HEALING

As indicated in Chapter 15, the periodontal lesions known as gingivitis and periodontitis originate from the presence of bacterial plaque, which produces a bioburden on the host's immune system. Initially, plaque is deposited on the clinical crowns of teeth, primarily at the cementoenamel junction. When plaque remains undisturbed, it begins to migrate subgingivally. The two main forms of subgingival plaque are (1) adherent and (2) nonadherent. Both adherent subgingival plaque and the supragingival plaque comprise primarily gram-positive rods and cocci. These bacteria may include *Streptococcus mitis, Streptococcus sanguis, Actinomyces viscosus, Actinomyces naeslundii,* and *Eubacterium* species.

In contrast, the nonadherent or tissue-associated plaque is composed of both gram-positive and gram-negative species. These bacteria may include *Porphyromonas gingivalis, Prevotella intermedia,* and *Capnocytophaga ochracea.* Among the most common secretions of gram-negative bacteria is the potent endotoxin—lipopolysaccharide (LPS).[10]

Adherent plaque is dense, whereas the portion of plaque adjacent to the tissues (nonadherent) is more loosely organized and has been found to be much more virulent. When the nonadherent plaque becomes incorporated into the periodontal tissues, it may secrete a number of enzymes that can damage host tissues, invoking an immune response. These bacterial plaque produce **antigens** and lipopolysaccharides that trigger the body's immune response by releasing neutrophils, monocytes, and macrophages to attack the by-products of the bacterial plaque. If these defense cells cannot contain or reduce the bacterial bioburden they will trigger the release of inflammatory mediators such as **cytokines, interleukins,** and enzymes such as collagenase and proteinase (Fig. 31-1). **Prostaglandins** and interleukins are released to assist in the battle producing the inflammatory response seen clinically as erythema and edema accompanied by bleeding, increased temperature, and pain.[10] Table 31-1 shows the development of the periodontal lesion in stages (the Page and Schroeder model).

This cascade of events of the immune system causes tissue breakdown and destruction as they try to combat the bacterial bioburden located along the tooth surface and within the periodontal pocket. Destruction of the periodontal attachment involving the gingiva, junctional epithelium, and bone result when the bacterial bioburden is not reduced or removed.[10] Although plaque is not the only factor in the **pathogenesis** of periodontal disease, it is the primary etiology managed in debridement procedures. Other factors contributing to periodontal pathogenesis such as genetic factors[14] and systemic challenges[7,30] are covered in Chapter 15.

🔘 WOUND HEALING

31-A
31-B
Understanding of the process of wound healing helps the dental professional to visualize the activity occurring within the tissues and sets expectations during the evalu-

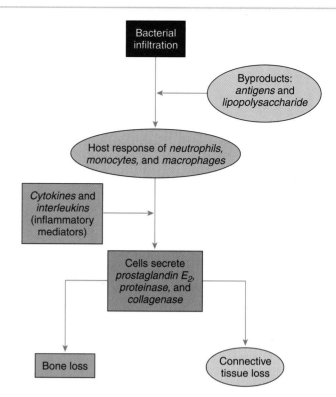

FIG. 31-1 The immune response to the presence of periodontal pathogens.

ation of a patient's tissues. Any debridement procedure essentially produces a wound, which goes through a natural healing phase. In *The Periodontic Syllabus,* Rapley[27] writes the following:

> *Healing is the phase of the inflammatory response that leads to a new physiological and anatomical relationship among the disrupted body elements.*

Histologically, periodontal wound healing is initiated after instrumentation when a small clot becomes interposed between the collagen fibers in the cementum and the collagen of the wound surface in the soft tissues. The healing wound surface consists of a base of moderately inflamed connective tissue covered with granulation tissue, a layered zone of neutrophils, and a clot. The epithelium begins to proliferate from the margins of the wound and migrates, cell by cell, at about 0.5 mm per day. During this time, fibroblasts in the granulation tissue begin to produce collagen. Granulation tissue penetrates the thin clot and permits the fibers extending from the cementum to unite with the new collagen formed by gingival fibroblasts. The epithelial attachment usually remains at its original position on the tooth, or it may migrate a few cells apically, producing a long junctional epithelial attachment.[27]

Thus periodontal debridement actually initiates soft tissue reattachment, regeneration, and remodeling. Awareness of the healing rate of the tissues involved in periodontal diseases is important in the monitoring of treatment outcomes. Epithelial tissue heals at a faster rate than connective tissue. Of the periodontal tissues bone takes the longest time to heal and regenerate. This knowledge is essential to the development of appropriate inter-

TABLE 31-1

Page and Schroeder model for development of the periodontal lesion

Lesion	Consecutive days of plaque exposure	Histological	Clinical
Initial	2 to 4 with plaque	PMNs, mononuclear cells subjacent to JE; decrease of some collagen fibers	Gingival fluid detectable in sulcus; vasculitis subjacent to JE
Early	4 to 7 with plaque	Dense lymphoid cell infiltrate in CT; reduction in collagen by 70% in areas of inflammation	More gingival fluid detectable and increase in vasculitis subjacent to JE; possible bleeding on probing
Established	2 to 3 weeks with plaque	Plasma cells predominant within CT, producing IgG	JE and sulcular epithelium; continuation of signs of proliferation, with thickening of epithelium; inflammation present; BOP
Advanced	Variable	Extensive destruction of collagen fibers; predominance of plasma cell; regeneration of transseptal fibers as lesion moves apically	Continued progression of gingivitis with attachment loss; crestal alveolar bone resorbing

PMN, Polymorphonucleositis; *JE,* junctional epithelium; *CT,* connective tissue; *IgG,* immunoglobulin G; *BOP,* bleeding on probing.

TABLE 31-2

Healing rates of periodontal tissues

Tissue type and location	Healing rate
Junctional epithelium	5 days
Sulcular epithelium	7 to 10 days
Gingival surface epithelium	10 to 14 days
Connective tissue	21 to 28 days
Bone	4 to 6 weeks

vention strategies and realistic expectations for clinical outcomes. Table 31-2 lists the tissues of the periodontium and associated healing rates. Healing of the underlying alveolar bone, particularly osseous infrabony defects that have occurred as a result of periodontal disease destruction, generally require surgical intervention and are not covered in this chapter.

Shifts in the composition of the subgingival microflora are found after periodontal debridement procedures. Organisms associated with periodontal health are more prominent with an increase in gram-positive rods and cocci species. Gram-negative organisms, spirochetes, and motile forms are consistently reduced but not always eliminated from the pocket. *Actinobacillus actinomycetemcomitans,* one of the most virulent and pathogenic oral microorganisms, is more resistant to mechanical debridement. Additional systemic antimicrobial therapy is often needed to completely manage the more aggressive diseases associated with this particular bacteria.*

Pocket depth reduction, decreased gingival inflammation, and less bleeding upon probing are measurable clinical indicators of healing. Pocket depth reduction results from tissue shrinkage and healing of the gingival structures, as evidenced by gingival recession and a gain

of clinical attachment. Recession may be assessed 1 week after debridement procedures. The amount of recession is generally related to the initial probing depths and the amount of inflammation in the tissues before treatment. In studies, deeper pocket depths exhibiting moderate to severe inflammation have exhibited greater healing and gain of clinical attachment, with the most gingival shrinkage occurring interproximally. Conversely, after instrumentation, a small amount of attachment loss has been noted in sites that are shallow with little or no inflammation.* Some loss of attachment does occur as a result of trauma inflicted during aggressive subgingival instrumentation. During the subsequent healing phase, however, this loss generally rebounds with attachment levels returning to the positions they held before instrumentation.[3]

Reducing the bioburden and creating an environment for tissue healing through therapeutic intervention is the dental hygienist's role in periodontal debridement. The selection of best method, technique, or procedure to reduce the bioburden is constantly under review, a thorough additional scientific inquiry generating knowledge and new questions. Continued advancements in dental technology and resulting therapies will add to the existing armamentarium in the provision of optimal periodontal health to all patients.

POWERED SCALING INSTRUMENTS

The two categories of powered instruments are sonic and ultrasonic. Periodontal debridement formerly was performed primarily by manual instrumentation. With today's advances in tip design offering longer shanks and smaller tips, powered scaling has become a more efficient option. The variations between the types of powered instruments and working tips available require attention to the specific mechanical and therapeutic characteristics of each (Table 31-3). The manufacturer's instructions for use

31-C

---

*References 11, 12, 15, 19, 21, 23, 28, 32, 34.

*References 11, 17, 22, 24, 25, 26.

TABLE 31-3

Comparison of characteristics of powered instruments

Type of instrument	Cycle per second/Hertz	Motion of tip
Sonic	2500 to 7000	Linear or elliptical
Magnetostrictive ultrasonic	8000 to 45,000	Elliptical
Piezoelectric ultrasonic	29,000 to 50,000	Linear

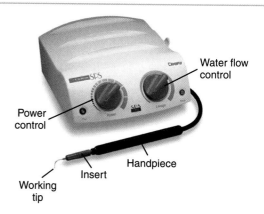

FIG. 31-3 Components of magnetostrictive unit. (Courtesy Dentsply, York, Pa.)

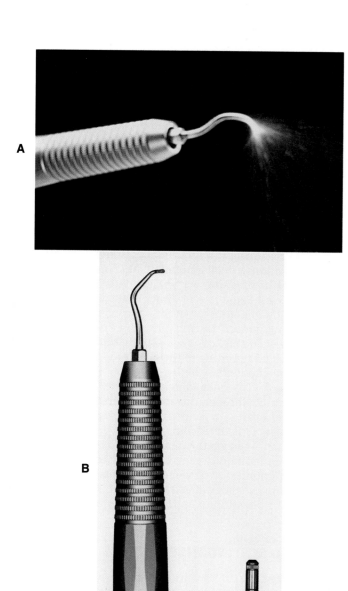

FIG. 31-2 A, Sonic instrument with fiber optics. **B,** Sonic tip connected to a fiber-optic coupler that connects to the dental unit air/water connection. (Courtesy KaVo America, Lake Zurich, Ill.)

and maintenance should always be consulted before use of any powered instrument.

SONIC SCALERS

Sonic scalers are **air turbine** units attached to a conventional high-speed handpiece connector on the dental unit. Some are equipped with fiber optics, as in the scaler pictured in Fig. 31-2. The sonic operates at a frequency of 3000 to 8000 *cycles per second (CPS)* and is cooled by the water from the dental unit. Sonics elicit a vibratory type of tip movement that is primarily linear or elliptical in direction. All surfaces of the tip are active.[1]

Sonic instruments have changeable tips. The tip design is based on the task to be performed and specific tooth anatomy. Most manufacturers' tips are designed to simulate curet and sickle scalers. Directions for use may vary slightly depending on the manufacturer. When cross-sectioned, some tips are round, whereas others may have angles, producing flat sides and requiring a slightly different tip to tooth adaptation.

ULTRASONIC SCALERS

An electrical current powers ultrasonic scaling instruments. The electricity is transformed within the unit, producing movement of the working tip. The two categories of ultrasonic scalers—*magnetostrictive* and *piezoelectric*—are based on the mechanism used for conversion of the electrical power to movement of the tip.

Magnetostrictive

The first and most prominent of ultrasonic instruments is the magnetostrictive (Fig. 31-3). With this mechanism of action, the working tip is part of an insert that fits into a handpiece located on the ultrasonic unit. The insert comprises either a "stack" of nickel alloy strips or a ferrous rod. One end inserts into the handpiece, and the other is a shaft where the working tip is connected (Fig. 31-4). Water flows around the stack to cool as the stack transfers a magnetic vibratory motion of 18,000 to 45,000 CPS or *Hertz (Hz)*. Magnetostrictive ultrasonic units are available in the older 25 kilohertz (kHz) or newer 30 kHz options. Magnetostrictive action produces an elliptical motion by the tip allowing for activation of all surfaces of the tip si-

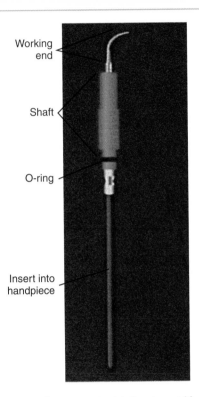

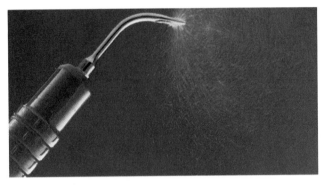

FIG. 31-5 Notice the halo appearance of the water as it contacts the instrument tip. (Courtesy Dentsply, York, Pa.)

FIG. 31-4 Parts of a magnetostrictive insert/tip. (Courtesy Dentsply, York, Pa.)

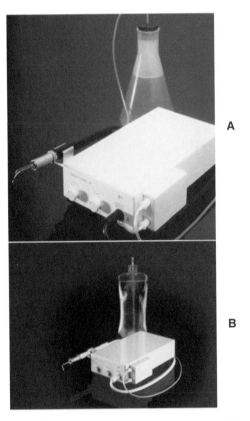

FIG. 31-6 The Odontoson piezoelectric powered instrument with water or chemotherapeutic agent **(A)** or sterile water **(B)**. (Courtesy Odonto-Wave, Fort Collins, Colo.)

multaneously. This provides the option to use the side, back, or front of the tip for adaptation to the root surface.[1]

In addition to a power switch on the unit, ultrasonics have frequency and water controls so that the power presented at the tip and water flow can be independently adjusted as needed. The power setting on the unit affects the length of stroke or amplitude of the vibrations. The higher power setting delivers a longer, more powerful stroke, and conversely, a lower power setting delivers a shorter, less powerful stroke. The frequency control on manually tuned units can be adjusted to fine tune the tip vibration or adjust the number of tip cycles per second. The water control adjusts the volume and temperature of the water flowing from the handpiece to cool the stack and insert tip. The water also lubricates the tip for easy insertion and acts as an irrigator that flushes debris from the treatment site. All of these factors come into play when instrumentation in initiated.

Before use and after connections, the unit waterline and reservoir must be flushed to remove/reduce waterborne bacteria and biofilm in the unit. Water should be run through the unit handpiece before tip insertion and water adjustment. To adjust water flow, the clinician should turn the handpiece parallel to the floor (over a sink), activate the unit, and observe the water flow from the tip. The water control knob is adjusted so that the handpiece emits contiguous drops. Once this has been achieved, the handpiece is held perpendicular to the floor and the unit is activated, which allows water to flow out of the handpiece to remove air bubbles from the line. Air bubbles in the line prevent the proper cooling of the metal stack and result in overheating of the tip during activation. While holding the handpiece in an upright position without activation of the unit, the clinician inserts

the selected tip by pushing downward with a slight twist until the O-ring is within the handpiece and the tip securely in place. Next, the appropriate power is selected. The unit is activated and the water spray observed. The spray should reflect off the working tip in a fine spray, forming a halo appearance (Fig. 31-5).

Piezoelectric

The second and most powerful ultrasonic is the piezoelectric (Fig. 31-6). The mechanism for conversion of electrical power to tip movement is by way of ceramic crystal vibrations. The vibratory motion of the crystals is transformed to the tip to produce a linear movement at 25,000 to 50,000 CPS. Unlike the magnetostrictive unit inserts, no magnetic field is present and little heat is generated.[9] The piezoelectric working tips screw onto the end of the handpiece and are available in an assortment of styles for the varying clinical applications. Because of the linear movement of the tip, the lateral surfaces are more active than the flat front or back of the tip. When adapted incorrectly, the different sound from the tip alerts the clinician to adjust the adaptation to allow the proper working end to be effective (Fig. 31-7).[1]

Water reservoirs, attached directly to each machine, can be interchanged with either water or various chemotherapeutic agents such as chlorhexidine, hydrogen peroxide, or phenolic compounds. It is important to read the manufacturer's instructions regarding use of chemotherapeutics for each machine. Cleaning the water reservoir and lines is still required before placement of the tip onto the handpiece. Power and water are adjusted after placement of the tip.

TIP SELECTION AND APPLICATION

Because of the wide variety of powered scaling instruments on the market, providing examples of all the tips available in the sonic and ultrasonic categories is an impossible task. Tip designs generally vary in length, shape, and diameter. Fig. 31-8 comparatively illustrates the sonic, magnetostrictive, and piezoelectric tips.

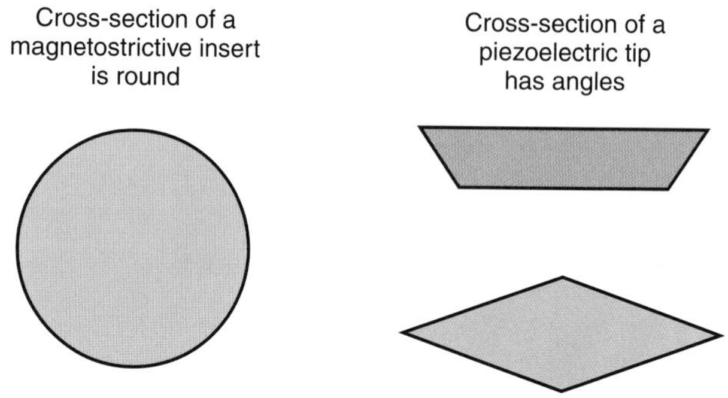

Cross-section of a
magnetostrictive insert
is round

Cross-section of a
piezoelectric tip
has angles

FIG. 31-7 Comparison of cross-sections of powered instrument working ends.

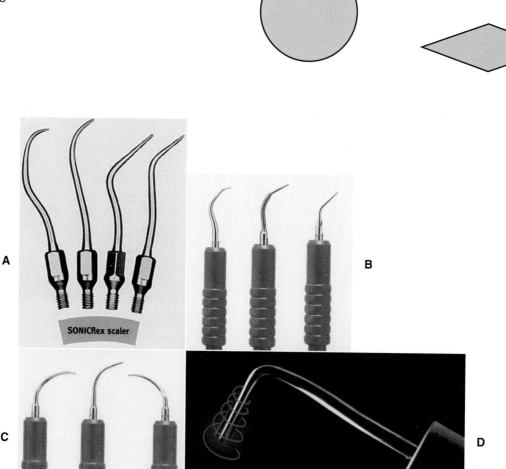

FIG. 31-8 Tips of sonic **(A)**, magnetostrictive **(B** and **C)**, and piezoelectric **(D)** for comparison. **(A,** Courtesy KaVo America, Lake Zurich, Ill.; **B** and **C,** Courtesy Dentsply, York, Pa.; **D,** Courtesy Odonto-Wave, Fort Collins, Colo.)

Dentsply (York, Pa.), maker of the Cavitron ultrasonic unit, developed inserts for the magnetostrictive instrument to meet various needs. These instruments were designed similarly to the manual instruments including shapes like the chisel, sickle, curet, probe, and a wide, flat instrument used for heavy stain removal. As various ultrasonic units became available, Hu-Friedy, an instrument manufacturing company, developed a product line with similar features as those of Dentsply. Initial inserts/tips featured an external water tube known as a *trombone* to provide water to the vibrating tip. With use and sterilization of the insert, the trombone can become bent and misaligned, sending the water spray away from the working tip. To facilitate deeper pocket placement and to avoid the problems with the trombone, manufacturers designed a lightweight resin handle with an internal water delivery source within the tip that can control the water source and provide increased ease of use. The resin handle allowed clinicians an increased tactile sensitivity and reduced hand fatigue. The most recent design improvement features a fixed external water delivery tube, allowing for a thinner tip design. Manufacturers have given these thinner tip designs various names, but the design dictates use.[16]

UNIVERSAL TIPS

The original standard diameter P-style, or #10 universal insert, is ideal for the removal of moderate to heavy supragingival deposits if the tissue permits tip entry into the pocket. This insert may be operated on a medium to high power setting, depending on the amount of power needed for the debridement procedure. Also included in this category is the #1000 triple bend and the #3 beaver tail. Both of these designs assist the clinician in removing heavier, hard-to-remove deposits and stain.

MODIFIED TIPS

Modifications were made to the original design resulting in a right and left insert and subsequently the 40% thinner and longer probelike (thin perio design) periodontal inserts. The new modified periodontal inserts feature a straight and right or left design and are longer and thinner than the standard designed tips. These inserts enhance access and adaptation in deeper periodontal pockets, particularly in posterior areas with complex anatomical features that may include concavities, convexities, and furcations. These modified perio designs feature a thinner tip (0.5 mm at the tip) and longer shank, which is ideal for debriding deep pocket areas. Fig. 31-9 shows a comparison of the standard and slimline tips. Adjusting the power is necessary when using these tips. Low to medium power is more than adequate for this thinner type of insert.

A furcation insert was also developed with a 0.8-mm ball end on the tip that reduces the likelihood of gouging the root surface. Furcation inserts are available in a straight, right, and left option, which allow access into the variety and complexity of furcation anatomical sites.

Inserts are offered in either the metal or resin handles. External or internal water source options are also available. Fig. 31-10 shows a series of tips from Dentsply of

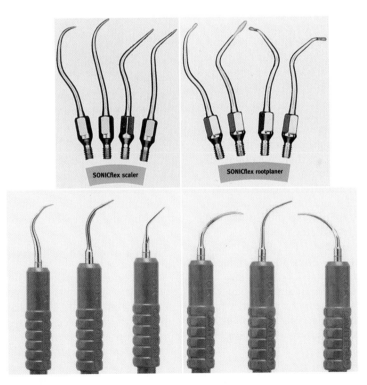

FIG. 31-9 The shape and size of the periodontal or slimline tips differ from the standard tip. Note these differences and their applications in periodontal debridement. (*Top,* Courtesy KaVo America, Lake Zurich, Ill.; *Bottom,* Courtesy Dentsply, York, Pa.)

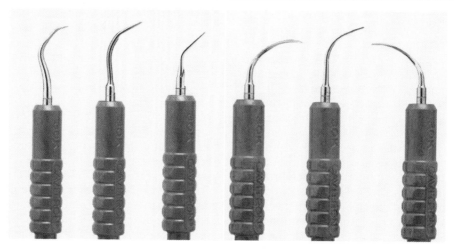

FIG. 31-10 The series of ultrasonic tips from one manufacturer provides a visual understanding of the application of tip selection criteria. (Courtesy Dentsply, York, Pa.)

various shapes and designs for powered instruments (see also Fig. 31-9, *C* and *D*).

PREPARATION OF POWERED INSTRUMENTS

PATIENT AND OPERATOR PREPARATION

Preparation of the operator and dental unit is the same as when one is providing any form of patient care. Universal precautions are followed, as outlined in Chapter 5. The additional PPE of a face shield is ideal during the use of ***power-driven*** instruments, and clinicians may also choose to wear a disposable head covering.

Preparation of the ultrasonic unit and patient is necessary when using powered instruments. Before use of the power instrument and possibly at the time of informed consent, the dental hygienist should explain the procedure to the patient, reason for use, action of the powered instrument, necessity of suction and drape, and any anticipated response.

Preparation of the unit with appropriate coverings to prevent contamination is also necessary. Chapter 5 discusses work practice controls and personal protective equipment (PPE) required for instruments that create aerosols. Providing protection and a drape for the patient or providing some form of barrier protection from the water spray is required. A cotton towel may be provided to the patient to be placed over the nose and upper face to prevent the area from being covered with spatter from the procedure and reduce the inhalation of aerosols. Fig. 31-11 illustrates patient, operator, and equipment readiness for use. Draping of the face and nose is optional; eyewear is essential.

Use of high-volume suction with an aerosol reduction device is recommended. Aerosol reduction devices have been shown to reduce aerosols when attached to various types of powered instruments, including ultrasonics.[13,29]

THERAPEUTIC USE OF POWERED SCALERS

31-E Before any therapeutic or preventive measure, a thorough health history must be obtained. Review of the assessment data, identification of oral and systemic risks, and a strate-

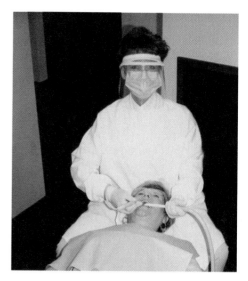

FIG. 31-11 The operator and patient are prepared for the debridement procedure with a powered instrument. Notice the infection-control measures in place and patient readiness.

gic plan must be developed (see Chapters 29 and 30). During this process the clinician identifies whether the patient has any medical or dental considerations that could prohibit use of powered instruments.

Health and Dental Considerations

Some concern surrounds the use of magnetostrictive ultrasonics on patients with pacemakers. In general, modern pacemakers are shielded against electromagnetic interference, but discussion with the patient's cardiologist prior to use is recommended. If use of the magnetostrictive ultrasonic is prohibited, a sonic or piezoelectric instrument may be used.

Other considerations for the use of powered instruments are patients with communicable diseases such as hepatitis, tuberculosis, or human immunodeficiency virus (HIV), primarily because of the amount of aerosols produced during the procedure and the immunocompromised status of these patients. Patients at an increased risk for infection because of medical conditions such as immunosuppression, diabetes, or organ transplants may exhibit complications from aerosols or contaminated dental-unit waterlines. Additional considerations include patients at risk for respiratory or breathing problems such as asthma, emphysema, cystic fibrosis, or pulmonary diseases. Because of the amount of aerosols and water produced during powered instrumentation, patients prone to gagging or dysphagia may not be good candidates.

Box 31-1 lists systemic conditions to consider in the decision of whether to use powered instruments. Universal precautions protect the clinician, and therefore the real concern when making the decision to use powered instruments is for the patient's health.[1]

Caution also should be exercised in the use of powered instruments with certain dental conditions (Box 31-2). Powered instrumentation is contraindicated on titanium implants unless a protective plastic sheath is used to cover the tip and to minimize the risk of damage. Certain restorative materials, including composite, porcelain, gold, and amalgam, can be damaged or scratched during instrumentation of the restored surface. The heat, water, and vibration associated with this technique also may aggravate sensitive areas such as exposed dentin or demineralization and is generally contraindicated in such areas to minimize sensitivity and further breakdown.[1]

Instrument Selection

As with all debridement procedures, powered instrumentation requires appropriate instrument selection. A variety of instruments is available for use with each of the powered units. Differences in tip curvature, shape, design, length, and diameter should be considered for each clinical application. Factors such as the state of health or disease of the periodontium, tooth and root anatomy, and types and location of deposits all impact powered instrument selection. The sturdier standard tips are designed for general deposit removal, whereas the modified periodontal tips with thinner and longer shanks are designed for periodontal pockets and finer debridement procedures. Diamond-coated tips are available and have been shown to be more efficient in removal of calculus in moderate to deep pockets than regular ultrasonic tips.[36] Furcation and curved tips are also favorable for site-specific debridement in the complex anatomy of multirooted teeth. Diamond-coated furcation instruments are also available for efficient removal of debris within the furcation.[31]

Case Application

Note the size, shape, and length of the tips in Fig. 31-10. Try to determine which tip is used in which area of the mouth and for which type of debridement. Now select the tip(s) you would choose for Mrs. Ray's debridement.

Adjusting Power and Water Volume

Depending on the unit used, power setting and water often need to be adjusted with each tip application. The sturdier tips can accommodate a higher power setting where the finer periodontally designed tips require less power. Medium- to high-power settings are recommended for heavy debris removal, and a low to medium setting is recommended for removing light debris and plaque. Water is essential at all times, regardless of power setting or tip used.

Indications for Use

Many clinical situations dictate the use of powered instruments for debridement, as follows[1]:
- Removal of deposits
  Moderate to heavy supragingival and subgingival calculus
  Moderate to heavy stain
- Reduction of bacterial bioburden in the following:
  Furcations and periodontal pockets
  Areas of infection, as in *pericoronitis*
- Removal of overhangs and excess cement
- *Debonding* procedures

FUNDAMENTALS OF POWERED INSTRUMENTATION

PATIENT AND OPERATOR POSITIONING

If no circumstances are modifying clinical procedures, the clinician can rely on the appropriate proprioceptive position for working in the selected area. Patient and clinician positioning are important in the achievement of the

TABLE 31-4

Fundamentals of powered instrumentation

Fundamental	Description
Patient/operator positioning	Proprioceptive positioning is used but with the back of the dental chair elevated slightly because of pooling of water and the need for direct visibility of certain areas.
Modified pen grasp	The powered instrument handpiece is grasped in a modified pen grasp at the junction of the handle and shank.
Fulcrum	A stable fulcrum is necessary with the powered instruments even though lateral pressure is not applied, as in manual instrumentation. Extraoral fulcrums are used more frequently in powered instrumentation.
Adaptation	The instrument anterior 2 to 3 mm of the tip is placed on the tooth surface at nearly a zero-degree angulation. A slight angulation of no greater than 15 degrees is sometimes used.
Insertion	The instrument tip is moved apically beneath the gingival tissue and to the extent of the pocket as the instrument is being activated for the working stroke.
Activation	Movement of the tip across the tooth surface is constant. Dividing the tooth surface into sections for thorough debridement is recommended. As the tip moves further into the pocket, another section of the tooth can be instrumented. After each section has been instrumented, joining the sections together in a longer stroke to prevent unevenness also is recommended.

correct instrumentation technique (Table 31-4). Given the water spray, use of the mouth mirror for indirect vision is minimal; however, the mirror may be used to reflect light to the area for better visibility. Slightly raising the back of the patient's chair also may be done to more easily manage water flow and provide better direct visibility.

PATIENT COMFORT

During powered debridement procedures, managing patient comfort is important. Power scaling can produce high-pitched sounds, increased tooth sensitivity, and excessive water that many patients may find uncomfortable. Communicating before starting the procedure is an important aspect of patient management. The clinician should explain to the patient what can be expected. Selecting the proper power setting and technique is also important. High power settings often cause excess heat and vibration, which can lead to patient discomfort. Effective evacuation control of the aerosols and water produced also increase patient comfort and acceptance of the procedure.

GRASP

Like manual instrumentation, powered instruments require use of a light, modified pen grasp (Fig. 31-12; see also Table 31-4). Light grasp increases tactile sensitivity, increases patient comfort, and reduces clinician fatigue.

Both sonic and ultrasonic handpieces are heavier than manual instruments. Additionally, weight from the cord causes drag and may require adjustments in cord placement. To reduce tension from the cord, many clinicians find it helpful to drape the cord around their necks, wrap it around their forearms, lay it across their laps, or grasp it between their fingers in the grasp (Fig. 31-13). Management of the cord is essential to support and correct adaptation of the instrument. Each clinician must find a personally preferred method.

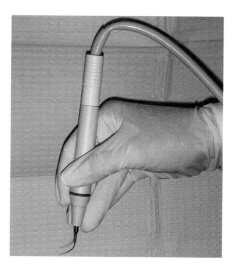

FIG. 31-12 The modified pen grasp of the powered handpiece.

FULCRUM

Establishing a fulcrum when using powered instruments is as important as when using manual instruments (see Table 31-4). Soft tissue external fulcrums are used more frequently in proprioceptive positioning and also during the use of powered instruments (Fig. 31-14; refer to Chapter 6 for positioning content). The bulk of the powered instrument handpiece and attached cord sometimes requires use of an extraoral fulcrum to maintain control of the instrument. An external fulcrum provides balance rather than strength. When using an external fulcrum, the clinician must carefully monitor the water.

ADAPTATION

Like manual instrumentation, adaptation of the anterior 2 to 3 mm of the tip is appropriate (Fig. 31-15; see also

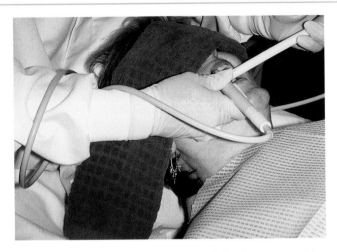

FIG. 31-13 Wrapping the cord around the forearm provides one way of controlling the weight and drag on the handpiece during application.

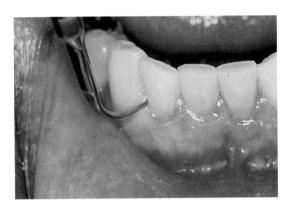

FIG. 31-15 The tip is adapted to the tooth at less than 15 degrees, close to 0.

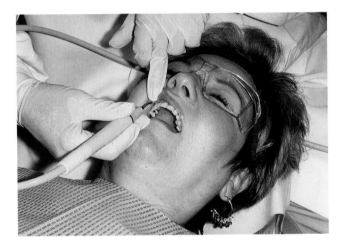

FIG. 31-14 Typical extraoral fulcrum used during powered instrumentation.

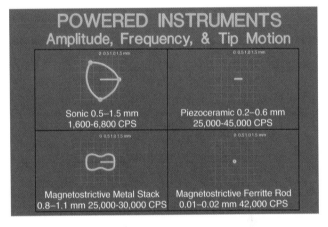

FIG. 31-16 Motion of different types of tips. (Courtesy Odonto-Wave, Fort Collins, Colo.)

Table 31-4). With some of the powered instruments, the tip is designed so that any portion of the tip can be used for debridement, not just the side tip. Other tips are designed so that the tip must be adapted in a certain manner to be effective in calculus removal. The manufacturer's instructions provide this information.

Powered instruments, like manual instruments, must be adapted properly. Keeping the tip parallel to the surface being treated keeps the tip adapted as close to 0 degrees as possible. Tip-to-tooth adaptation should not exceed 15 degrees. Improper adaptation of the tip (more than 15 degrees) causes gouging on the root surface and injury to the soft tissue surrounding the area.

INSERTION AND ACTIVATION

After the tip has been adapted to the tooth surface, the tip may be moved apically beneath the gingival tissue (see Table 31-4). The clinician activates the unit during this process and moves the tip across the tooth surface in a painting-like motion while also moving apically to the junctional epithelium. The tip is maintained in continuous motion; the clinician uses little or no lateral pressure while moving around the tooth to cover all surfaces (see Table 31-4). Lateral pressure against the tooth results in defects or gouged areas.[8] Fig. 31-16 depicts a comparison of the tip movement of various types of powered instruments.

Periodically, the clinician may stop activation of the unit, pause, and use an exploratory stroke to feel the tooth surface. If roughness or deposit is noted, immediate activation of the tip can occur, thus increasing time utilization. Tactile sensitivity develops with continued use of the powered instruments, as it does with the use of manual instruments. With an increased tactile sense, evaluation of the tooth surface can occur while the tip is activated. Finite evaluation of the tooth surface may be accomplished with an instrument designed for this purpose.

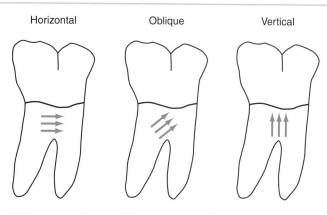

Horizontal   Oblique   Vertical

FIG. 31-17 Powered instrument strokes are vertical, horizontal, and oblique.

Strokes with powered instruments may be made in various directions: overlapping vertical, horizontal, and oblique (Fig. 31-17). Sometimes the use of strokes in each direction is required to complete the task in a given area. Even a probing action can be employed with certain tip designs to achieve the desired result. Regardless of the stroke direction used, constant movement of an adapted tip with minimal lateral pressure is required to prevent gouging of the tooth surface and injury to adjacent soft tissue.

If, during activation of the magnetostrictive instrument, the handpiece begins to feel warm, some adjustment is required. Increasing the water flow may reduce the heat; however, disadvantages are that this produces too much water for the clinician and patient and that the spray will no longer be directed onto the tip. Reducing the power setting may also decrease the generation of heat to the handpiece but may result in inefficient deposit removal. Minor adjustments to both water and power settings can sometimes solve the problem. Many times the reason for excess heat production is air bubbles in the waterline, preventing sufficient cooling of the stack. The best course of action is to remove the insert, bleed the waterline of air, and reinsert the tip.

EVALUATION OF DEBRIDEMENT

During the process of periodontal debridement, tactile evaluation is used. As previously mentioned, the nonactivated tip may be used during the procedure to evaluate the tooth surface. Feeling the tooth surface for deposit or roughness can be performed more definitively with an explorer or periodontal probe. All tissue tags should be removed and bleeding stopped before dismissal of the patient. At each appointment during the planned therapy, tissue response and self-care are evaluated. If an area still exhibits signs of bleeding and inflammation, the area may need further instrumentation and or closer self-care attention. A common side effect of healing tissue is exposed dentin, which produces dentinal sensitivity. When this situation occurs, refer to Chapter 25 for specific management techniques.

Clinical outcomes of therapy are best evaluated no sooner than 4 to 6 weeks after therapy. At this time, clin-

ical evaluation of soft tissue for signs of healing and reduction of disease are assessed.[20] Review of the general goals for periodontal debridement and patient-specific goals are needed to evaluate the success of the therapeutic procedure.

Asking patients for feedback about their oral conditions may be beneficial in the evaluation process. Often patients will feel differences in their tissue as healing occurs, as a response to professional therapy and self-care intervention measures. Patients also may identify trouble spots; areas not healing or still bleeding when providing self-care and areas that are difficult to clean. Discussing clinical outcomes of care and whether goals have been met can be encouraging and motivating to the patient. This action also can make the patient feel a part of the healthcare process.

POSTTHERAPY EVALUATION AT 4 TO 6 WEEKS

If tissue has not healed as expected at the end of the 4- to 6-week period, additional therapeutic intervention may be necessary.

 Case Application

In Mrs. Ray's 4- to 6-week evaluation, a new periodontal intervention (perioscope) was applied to detect the possible cause of the poor response on teeth #10 and #14.

Posttherapy evaluation revealed generalized healing of 2 to 3 mm with reduction of inflammation and bleeding on probing. Most areas had healed to a stage where oral self-care and routine supportive care could effectively maintain periodontal health, with the exception of teeth #10 and #14. Mrs. Ray had noticed less bleeding when brushing and seemed satisfied with the effort she was putting into her dental care.

Teeth #10 and #14 still exhibited probe depths of 7 to 8 mm with bleeding on probing and interproximal inflammation. The areas were evaluated under perioscopy with a new fiber-optic endoscopic instrument that fits onto specially designed periodontal explorers (Fig. 31-18). With 24- to 46-power magnification and fiberoptic illumination, this device allows clear visualization into deep subgingival pockets and in furcations. Remaining deposits in the buccal furcation, distobuccal line angle, and in this case, distal furcation of tooth #14 were visualized and subsequently thoroughly redebrided using manual and powered periodontal instruments. Tooth #10 had deposit remaining in the mesial palatal line angle, which was also visualized and removed.

After 2 weeks the site was evaluated for subsequent healing and desensitization of the treated areas. Healing was evident in all sites. Sensitive areas were treated with Ultradent UltraEz (Ultradent Products, Inc., South Jordan, Utah) for sensitivity, and Mrs. Ray was given Crest Sensitivity Protection dentifrice (Procter & Gamble, Cincinnati, Ohio) for self-care of the sensitivity.

Not all patients heal at the same rate. The healing response is also dependent on the immune system. Systemic conditions may decrease healing, and other intervention strategies may become necessary.

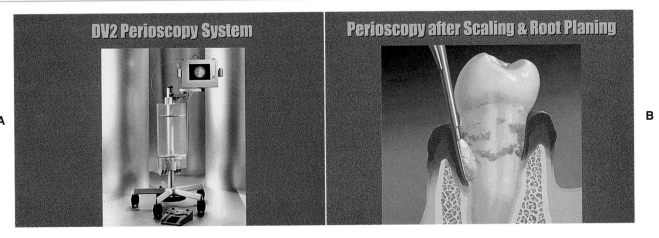

FIG. 31-18 The perioscope allows a view of the root surface and pocket wall to evaluate areas that are difficult to instrument. **A,** Full view of equipment. **B,** Section of tip within the pocket. (Courtesy DentalView, Inc., Irvine, Calif.)

TABLE 31-5	

Treatment codes for reimbursement purposes

Code	Description
1110	A dental prophylaxis performed on transitional or permanent dentition that includes scaling and polishing procedures to remove coronal plaque, calculus, and stains
4910	Periodontal supportive care (after active therapy) for patients who have been diagnosed with a type of periodontal disease and placed on a less-than-6-month supportive care interval (usually 3 months); including removal of bacterial flora from crevicular and pocket areas, scaling and polishing of the teeth, and review of patient's plaque control
4341	Periodontal debridement by sextants or quadrants and initial therapy for patients diagnosed with a type of periodontal disease; involving instrumentation of crown and root surfaces of the teeth to remove plaque and calculus; therapeutic in nature, not prophylactic
4355	Debridement to enable comprehensive periodontal evaluation and diagnosis; removal of subgingival and/or supragingival plaque and calculus; may be necessary more than once and may require multiple visits to complete

Modified from American Dental Association: *Current dental terminology version 2000: the code on dental procedures and nomenclature,* Chicago, 2000, The Association.

CODING FOR PERIODONTAL DEBRIDEMENT

Like medical diagnoses and treatment, dental diagnoses and treatments have specific codes that are provided to third-party reimbursement agencies for services rendered. Each treatment in periodontics must be preceded by a diagnostic code that explains the reason for the treatment rendered. The codes have specific descriptions so that the provider and third-party payer know what treatment has been provided. Fees for these services or treatments vary based on the type of treatment rendered. Therefore the dental hygienist must understand and use the appropriate treatment codes and fees for the type of treatment provided.

In health care, fees and codes for diagnoses and treatment are associated with specific descriptions, and usually the more complicated the treatment, the greater the fee for service. The dental hygienist provides different treatments for patients who have complicated periodontal conditions requiring a higher level of skill and intervention/prevention strategies than for those who have minimal to no gingivitis or periodontal diseases. Given the differences that exist among patients and the disease with which each may present for care, the dentist and dental hygienist must establish a reasonable fee structure given the type of disease and associated treatments the patient will receive. Once a fee has been established for a specific treatment code, adjusting that fee among patients with the same treatment for third party reimbursement is unethical and fraudulent.

Dental hygiene students should begin to understand the use of appropriate treatment codes. This provides an understanding of the differences in levels of care required among patients with varying types and degrees of disease. Table 31-5 lists and describes each periodontal debridement code for the adult patient. The dentist and/or office personnel establish fees for each of these periodontal debridement codes. Being a responsible dental professional includes contributing to patient care decisions and delivery and to the dental practice's management.

CRITICAL THINKING ACTIVITIES

1. Practice setting up and preparing an ultrasonic and sonic instrument for use.
2. Ask a classmate to relate specific clinical case scenarios. Determine the appropriate method of periodontal debridement and select the tip or tips to be used in the process.
3. Practice using a powered instrument on an extracted tooth or typodont and follow the fundamentals for instrumentation.
4. Assist a senior student or a practicing hygienist who is using a powered instrument and perform the following items:
   a. Help set up and prepare the unit and patient.
   b. Discuss with the operator the rationale for use of the powered instrument for periodontal debridement and specifics about the case.
   c. Help evacuate water and keep the patient dry. If an aerosol reduction device is available, place it on the high velocity evacuation tip and see if a visible reduction occurs in spray or spatter.
   d. Observe the tip(s) selected for use and determine the reason for selection.
   e. Observe the fundamentals of instrumentation and determine if the operator follows the fundamentals.
5. Role-play with a student partner to provide informed consent to periodontal therapy using powered instruments.

REVIEW QUESTIONS

1. Which of the following powered instruments uses an insert with a stack?
   a. Sonic
   b. Magnetostrictive
   c. Piezoelectric
   d. Manual instrument
2. All the following *except* which one can cause harm to the tooth?
   a. Lavage
   b. Lateral pressure
   c. Motionless tip
   d. No water
   e. Power setting too high
3. During preparation of the magnetostrictive ultrasonic for use, which of the following steps would be completed first?
   a. Insert the tip
   b. Bleed the waterline
   c. Adjust water flow
   d. Adjust power setting
4. Which of the following treatment codes is used for periodontal supportive care?
   a. 4341
   b. 4345

   c. 4910
   d. 1110
5. Which of the following powered instruments functions at the highest cycles per second?
   a. Magnetostrictive
   b. Sonic
   c. Piezoelectric
   d. Manual
6. Which of the following angles of tip adaptation best describes the angle required during activation of the powered instrument?
   a. 70 to 90 degrees
   b. 50 to 60 degrees
   c. 30 to 40 degrees
   d. 0 to 15 degrees
7. Which of the following best describes the term *microstreaming*?
   a. The process of microfilm breaking off a waterline
   b. Hydrodynamic sheer stress close to oscillating objects
   c. Small droplets occurring in a straight line from the tip
   d. Contiguous drops of water from the tip

 ## SUGGESTED AGENCIES AND WEB SITES

Because of the ever-changing nature of the Internet, some of the web sites listed here may have changed since publication. Please refer to Mosby's Evolve web site for the most current information.

Powered Instruments
Amadent (on web site of Satelec, Inc.): http://www.amadent.com
DentalView, Inc. (dental endoscope-perioscopy company): http://www.dentalview.com

Dentsply International (dental product company): http://www.dentsply.com *and* http://xray.essix.com [with entry of "cavitron AND ultrasonics" in the search box to find specifics on ultrasonic units available through Dentsply]

SUGGESTED AGENCIES AND WEB SITES—cont'd

Hu-Friedy Manufacturing Company, Inc. (dental instrument manufacturing company): http://www.hufriedy.com

KaVo America: http://www.kavousa.com

Pro-Dentec Pro-Select³ (ultrasonic scaler from Prodentec): http://www.prodentec.com)

Star Dental (Titan sonic scalers): http://www.dentalez.com

Continuing Education Courses in Periodontal Debridement

Dentsply Canada Limited ("Clinical education"): http://www.dentsply.ca

Dynamic Seminars ("Ultrasonics: the wave of the future") http://www.dynamicseminars.net

ErgoSonics (course descriptions): http://www.ergosonics.com

Odonto-Wave (Brain-*Wave* Education seminars on ultrasonic debridement): http://www.odontoson.com

University of Minnesota School of Dentistry Continuing Dental Education: ("Periodontal therapies I: a hands-on nonsurgical program"): http://www.dentalce.umn.edu

Periodontology

European Academy of Periodontology ("Periodontal disease entities"): http://www.od.mah.se

Periodontal Associates, Inc. ("Periodontics"): http://www.periodontal.com

The American Academy of Periodontology: http://www.perio.org

UCLA Periodontics Information Center: http://www.dent.ucla.edu

University of Pennsylvania and Temple University ("Histology of the periodontium"): http://www.temple.edu

W3 site of Periodontology and Oral Implantology ("Aesthetics"): http://www.paro.org

 ADDITIONAL READINGS AND RESOURCES

Checchi L et al: Plaque removal with variable instrumentation, *J Clin Periodontol* 24:715-7, 1997.

Clifford LR, Needleman IG, Chan YK: Comparison of periodontal pocket penetration by conventional and microultrasonic inserts, *J Clin Periodontol* 26:124-30, 1999.

Drisko CH: Root instrumentation—power-driven versus manual scalers—which one? *Dent Clin North Am* 42(2):229-44, 1998.

Drisko CH, Lewis LH: Ultrasonic instruments and antimicrobial agents in supportive periodontal treatment and retreatment of recurrent or refractory periodontitis, *J Periodontol* 12:90-115, 2000.

Hammerle CHF, Joss A, Lang NP: Short-term effects of initial periodontal therapy (hygiene phase), *J Clin Periodontol* 18:233-9, 1991.

Hughes TP, Caffesse RG: Gingival changes following scaling rooth planing and oral hygiene: a biometric evaluation, *J Periodontol* 49:245-52, 1978.

Jenkins WMM et al: Effect of subgingival scaling during supportive therapy, *J Clin Periodontol* 27:590-6, 1999.

Otero-Cagide FJ, Long BA: Comparative in vitro effectiveness of closed root debridement with fine instruments on specific areas of mandibular first molar furcations. I. Root trunk and furcation entrance, *J Periodontol* 68:1093-7, 1997.

Sandhu HS, Salloum IA, Stakiw JE: Scaling and root planing: hand versus power driven instruments, *J Can Dent Assoc* 64(4):269-75, 1998.

Schlageter L, Rateitshak-Pluss EM, Schwarz JP: Root surface smoothness or roughness following open debridement, *J Clin Periodontol* 23:460-4, 1996.

 REFERENCES

1. American Academy of Periodontology: Position paper: sonic and ultrasonic scalers in periodontics, *J Periodontol* 17:1792-801, 2000.

2. Badersten A, Nilveus R, Egelberg J: Effect of nonsurgical periodontal therapy. III. Single versus repeated instrumentation, *J Clin Periodontol* 11:114-24, 1994.

3. Claffey N, Egelberg J: Clinical characteristics of periodontal sites with probing attachment loss following initial periodontal treatment, *J Clin Periodontol* 21:670-9, 1994.

4. Cobb CM: Non-surgical pocket therapy: mechanical, *Ann Periodontol* 1:443-90, 1996.

5. Copulos TA et al: Comparative analysis between a modified ultrasonic tip and hand instruments on clinical parameters of periodontal disease, *J Periodontol* 64:694-700, 1993.

6. Dragoo MR: A clinical evaluation of hand and ultrasonic instruments on subgingival debridement, *Int J Periodont Rest Dent* 12:311-23, 1992.

7. Drisko CH: Trends in surgical and nonsurgical periodontal treatment, *J Am Dent Assoc* 131(6):31S-8S, 2000.

8. Flemming TF et al: Working parameters of a magnetostrictive ultrasonic scaler influencing root substance removal. In vitro, *J Periodontol* 69:547-53, 1998.

9. Flemming TF et al: The effect of working parameters on root substance removal using a piezoelectric ultrasonic scaler, *J Clin Periodontol* 25:158-63, 1998.

10. Greenstein G: Nonsurgical periodontal therapy in 2000: a literature review, *J Am Dent Assoc* 131:1580-92, 2000.

11. Greenstein G: Periodontal response to mechanical nonsurgical therapy: a review, *J Periodontol* 63:118-30, 1992.

12. Greenwell H, Bissada NF: Variations in subgingival microflora from healthy and intervention sites using probing depth and bacteriologic identification criteria, *J Periodontol* 55:391-7, 1984.

13. Harrel SK, Barnes JB, Rivera-Hidalgo F: Aerosol and splatter contamination from the operative site during ultrasonic scaling, *J Am Dent Assoc* 129(9):1241-9, 1998.

14. Hart TC, Korman KS: Genetic factors in the pathogenesis of periodontal disease, *Periodontal 2000* 14:202-15, 1997.

15. Hinrichs J et al: Effects of scaling and root planing on subgingival microbial proportons standardized in terms of the naturally occuring distrubution, *J Periodontol* 56:187-94, 1985.

16. *Instrument catalogue,* Chicago, 2001, Hu-Friedy, Inc.

Continued

17. Kaldahl WB et al: Evaluation of four modalities of periodontal therapy: mean probing depth, probing attachment levels and recession changes, *J Periodontol* 59:783-93, 1988.

18. Khambay BS, Walmsley AD: Acoustic microstreaming: detection and measurement around ultrasonic scalers, *J Periodontol* 70:626-31, 1999.

19. Kornman KS, Robertson PB: Clinical and microbiological evaluation of therapy for juvenile periodontitis, *J Periodontol* 56:433-46, 1985.

20. Low SB, Giancio SG: Reviewing nonsurgical periodontal therapy, *J Am Dent Assoc* 121:467-70, 1990.

21. Magnusson I et al: Recolonization of a subgingival microbiota following scaling in deep pockets, *J Clin Periodontol* 11:193-207, 1984.

22. Morrison EC, Ramfjord SP, Hill RW: Short-term effects of initial non-surgical periodontal treatment (hygiene phase), *J Clin Periodontol* 7:199-211, 1980.

23. Mousques T, Listgarten MA, Phillips RW: Effects of scaling and root planing on the composition of humans subgingival microbial flora, *J Periodontal Res* 15:144-51, 1980.

24. Pihlstrom BL, Oritz-Campos C, McHugh RB: A randomized four year study of periodontal therapy, *J Periodontol* 52:227-42, 1981.

25. Proye M, Caton J, Polson A: Initial healing of periodontal pockets after a single episode of root planing monitored by controlling probing force, *J Periodontol* 53:206-301, 1982.

26. Ramfjord S et al: Four modalities of periodontal treatment compared over 5 years, *J Clin Periodontol* 14:445-52, 1987.

27. Rapley J: Wound healing. In Fedi PF, Vernino AR, Gray JL, editors: *The periodontic syllabus*, ed 4, Philadelphia, 2000, Lippincott Williams & Wilkins.

28. Renvert S et al: Effect of root debridement on the elimination of *Actinobacillus actinomycetemcomitans* and *Bacteroides gingivalis* from periodontal pockets, *J Clin Periodontol* 17:345-50, 1990.

29. Rivera-Hidalgo F, Barnes JB, Harrel SK: Aerosol and splatter production by focused spray and standard ultrasonic inserts, *J Periodontol* 70:473-7, 1999.

30. Salvi GE et al: Influence of risk factors on the pathogenesis of periodontitis, *Periodontol 2000* 14:173-201, 1997.

31. Scott JB, Steed-Vellandis AM, Yukna RA: Improved efficacy of calculus removal in furcations using ultrasonic diamond-coated inserts, *Int J Periodont Rest Dent* 19:355-61, 1999.

32. Slots J, Rosling B: Suppressing the periodontopathic microflora in localized juvenile periodontitis by systemic tetracycline, *J Clin Periodontol* 10:465-86, 1983.

33. Smart GJ et al: The assessment of ultrasonic root surface debridement by determination of residual endotoxin levels. 1990, *J Clin Periodontol* 17:174-8.

34. van Winkelhoff AJ, van der Velden U, de Graff J: Microbial succession in recolonizing deep periodontal pockets after a single course of supra- and subgingival debridement, *J Clin Periodontol* 14:116-22, 1988.

35. Young NS, O'Heir TE, Woodall I: Periodontal debridement. In Woodall I, editor: *Comprehensive dental hygiene care*, ed 4, St Louis, 1993, Mosby.

36. Yukna RA et al: Clinical evaluation of the speed and effectiveness of subgingival calculus removal on single-rooted teeth with diamond-coated ultrasonic tips, *J Periodontol* 68:436-42, 1997.

CHAPTER 32

∾
Cosmetic *and* Therapeutic Polishing

Bonnie Francis, Susan J. Daniel

Chapter Outline

Assessment of Need
Case Study: Selecting the Appropriate Polishing
  Method
Theory
  Dental stains
  Stain evaluation

Professional treatment of extrinsic stains
Mechanical devices for polishing
Maintaining aesthetic restorations
Therapeutic polishing
Role of polishing in dental hygiene care

Key Terms

Abrasion
Abrasive
Esthetics
Air-powder polisher
Coronal polishing

Endogenous
Engine-driven polishing
Exogenous
Extrinsic
Grit

Hypoplasia
Intrinsic
Pounds per square inch (PSI)
Polishing
Polishing agent

Porte polisher
Pumice
Revolutions per minute (rpm)
Therapeutic polishing

Learning Outcomes

1. Explain to a colleague, patient, or an employer the relationship of polishing to the therapeutic and cosmetic goals for oral care.
2. Classify the various dental stains as either endogenous or exogenous and be able to determine whether the stain can be removed and, if so, which polishing procedure can remove the stain.
3. Select porte, engine, or air-powder polishing, and the appropriate polishing agent, based on the requirements of the patients' oral condition, their responses to care, and the equipment and time available.

4. Apply appropriate procedures for each of the polishing methods to remove stain without causing trauma to the oral structures and restorations or discomfort to the patient.
5. Summarize the research findings that suggest the limited therapeutic benefit for coronal polishing and the more relevant therapeutic value of root polishing.

A visit to the dental hygienist is often associated with the *polishing* procedure performed at the conclusion of the supportive care appointment. Polishing traditionally has been associated with the prophylaxis procedure in most dental practices, which patients know and expect. Patients prefer this procedure over debridement with instruments for many reasons. An important factor is that the patients respond positively to the smooth, clean feeling that polishing produces. It is

also less traumatic than scaling and less stressful and easier for a patient to understand and tolerate. Polishing often produces a benefit patients can see when they look in the mirror. Patients also know that polishing generally comes at the conclusion of the oral prophylaxis procedure. All of these factors play a role in the patient-operator interactions that take place daily in the dental office.

As with changing perspectives regarding scaling and root instrumentation, polishing principles have been reviewed and revised over time. Superficial polishing of the crown is now considered mainly cosmetic, with *minimal* therapeutic benefit. ***Therapeutic polishing,*** in contrast, refers to polishing of the root surfaces that are exposed during surgery to reduce endotoxin and the microflora on the cementum. Whether polishing for cosmetic or therapeutic benefit, an understanding of the polishing process and the resulting effects on the tooth surface and restorations is critical to dental hygiene professional development.

Polishing involves smoothing a surface to make it glossy or lustrous; *cleaning* is the act of removing of debris, impurities, or extraneous matter. Although the term *polishing* has been used to describe the professional removal of soft deposits and stain from tooth surfaces, in reality this includes both cleaning and polishing. Removal of deposits has usually been achieved by friction created with the use of an ***abrasive*** agent and some form of mechanical device. Plaque, stain, and acquired pellicle (which is the acellular bonding apparatus for plaque and stain) are all removed during polishing. Although polishing does remove plaque and therefore may inhibit the occurrence of gingivitis,[70] the same benefit can be accomplished with thorough plaque removal procedures at home. Therefore ***coronal polishing*** has questionable positive effects beyond creating a stain-free smile.[69]

Historically, teeth were polished to remove all soft deposits and stains before the application of topical fluorides, because clinicians believed that it would allow for greater fluoride uptake in the enamel. However, studies have repeatedly demonstrated that polishing does not improve the uptake of professionally applied fluoride, and therefore it is no longer a prerequisite to topical fluoride application.[59,65] At one time, polishing plaque off the patient's teeth and removing stains was considered the responsibility of the dental hygienist as opposed to a patient responsibility. As scientific knowledge has evolved, it has been demonstrated that professional polishing removes part of the fluoride-rich outer layer of enamel.[39,53] Even though remineralization of tooth structure does occur under normal oral conditions[72] and exposure to fluoride,[16,37] it is felt that continuous professional polishing over years of routine care may cause morphological changes in the teeth. Essentially, the tooth structure may be abraded by routine polishing, especially at the cervix of cementum and dentin.[17] It is therefore every dental hygienist's responsibility to understand the delicate balance between cosmetic and therapeutic polishing.

ASSESSMENT OF NEED

As part of a clinical assessment, an identification of the types and amount of soft deposits present on patients' teeth should be made to aid in establishing an effective treatment plan. Obviously, stain that cannot be removed by the patient is the primary factor that determines the need for cosmetic polishing. Once the type, amount, and distribution of stains have been assessed, the type of abrasive and mechanical device best suited for stain removal can be planned. With this information, a more appropriate treatment choice can be made to consider patients' expectations, effectiveness, and long-term effects of clinical decisions. This chapter assists the dental hygiene student in understanding stains, the professional treatment op-

Case Study   Selecting the Appropriate Polishing Method

Bill Smith, a 28-year-old healthy Caucasian man, reports that he is concerned with health, works out daily, and has a diet filled with fruits and vegetables. On his visit to the clinic, Mr. Smith's chief complaint is to get his teeth cleaned because he knows that his smoking habit is ruining his health and the way his teeth look, and he has noticed some staining. Mr. Smith reported he felt that getting his teeth cleaned would be a "good motivator to help me quit smoking."

The intraoral exam revealed stable periodontal status with generalized 2- to 3-mm pocketing and localized areas of slight recession. Gingival structures appear pink, firm, stippled, and healthy. Porcelain veneer restorations had been placed on the facial surfaces of teeth #6 through #11 to cover the tetracycline-stained anterior teeth. No other apparent tetracycline stain is noted. Moderate tobacco stain is present, primarily on the lingual and palatal surfaces. Mr. Smith reports that he has smoked one pack of cigarettes a day for the past 10 years but is aware of its impact on his health and is "ready to quit."

tions available to remove those stains, and the attentiveness necessary to maintain tooth structure and aesthetic restorations in the polishing process.

THEORY

DENTAL STAINS

Classification of Dental Stains and Tooth Discoloration

Tooth discoloration and dental stains are often associated with the ***exogenous, extrinsic*** staining effects from food, drink, tobacco, and drugs. Although this type of staining is common, staining or discoloration actually may be attributed to three main sources: (1) direct adherence to tooth surfaces by bonding to the acquired pellicle, (2) containment within calculus and soft deposits, and (3) staining integral to the actual tooth structure.

Tooth staining and discoloration are categorized as either ***endogenous*** or exogenous in nature.[56,68] Endogenous stains originate within the tooth from developmental and systemic disturbances, whereas exogenous stains originate outside the tooth from exposure to environmental agents. Exogenous staining can be subcategorized even further as extrinsic and ***intrinsic*** stains, based on their ability to be removed mechanically by either the individual or the dental professional. Extrinsic stains are those stains that are on the exterior of the tooth and can be removed. Intrinsic stains are of exogenous origin but become incorporated into the tooth structure and cannot be removed by mechanical means.

Because many patients are more concerned with ***esthetics*** than disease, the presence of these dental stains may be used to the patient's advantage as a motivating

32-A

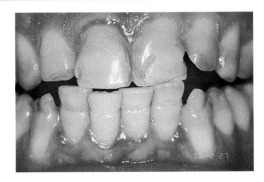

FIG. 32-1 Endogenous developmental stain: febrile illness. (Courtesy Dr. George Taybos, Jackson, Miss.)

TABLE 32-1
Endogenous stains: developmental

Type	Appearance	Etiology
Amelogenesis imperfecta	*Hypoplastic:* insufficient enamel ranging from pits and grooves to complete absence of enamel *Hypocalcification:* normal quantity of enamel but soft and friable; color variable, from white opaque to yellow to brown and darkening with age	Genetic disorder of enamel formation affecting both dentitions
Dentinogenesis imperfecta	Overall bluish translucence or opalescence; teeth variable in color from yellow-brown to gray; entire crown appearing stained because of underlying dentin malformation	Genetic disturbance in odontoblastic layer during dentin formation; may occur with osteogenesis imperfecta or as isolated trait
Dentin dysplasia	*Type I:* both dentitions normal color but have short roots or periapical inflammatory lesions *Type II:* opalescent primary dentition, normal permanent dentition	Genetic autosomal dominant trait affecting dentin
Congenital porphyria	Teeth appearing red to brown and fluorescing red with ultraviolet light; enamel, dentin, and cementum all affected	Genetic disorder of hemoglobin formation
Rh incompatibility	Primary teeth appearing green to brown	Maternal antibody destruction of fetal red blood cells
Liver disease Biliary atresia Neonatal hepatitis	Primary dentition affected; green discoloration; yellowish-brown color	Secondary to the deposition of bilirubin in developing enamel and dentin

factor to improve oral hygiene. A good example of is the case of Mr. Smith, who wants to get his teeth cleaned because of aesthetic concerns. Patients such as Mr. Smith may practice more thorough plaque removal and may be motivated to change some stain-promoting behaviors in an attempt to achieve a whiter and healthier appearance of the teeth. As coronal surfaces are polished to remove the stain, soft debris, and acquired pellicle, the fluoride-rich outer layer of the enamel is also affected and potentially removed. Because of this, clinicians should possess and understanding of the origins and manifestations of the various stains in determining whether stains can or cannot be removed by mechanical means.

Examples of stains that cannot be removed by mechanical means of scaling and polishing begin with endogenous developmental stains. These stains are the result of heredity, developmental disturbances, genetic factors, drugs, and trauma. Endogenous stains imbedded within the actual tooth structure often reflect the period of tooth development affected by the exposure. These stains manifest in newly erupted teeth and can be seen in both deciduous and permanent dentitions (Fig. 32-1). Examples of endogenous developmental stains are found in Tables 32-1 through 32-4.

Endogenous stains developmental in origin include stains from medications that the mother or child takes during tooth development (see Table 32-2). Such medications may cause staining that occurs as a result of the deposition of substances circulating systemically at that time. Tetracycline is one example of a medication that is known to cause developmental stains (Fig. 32-2). Exposure to tetracycline between the fifth month of fetal life and age 8 often results in discoloration and sometimes *hypoplasia* of permanent and deciduous teeth. Tetracycline discoloration results because the drugs have an affinity for calcifying tissue, which is active during tooth formation. Tetracyclines are incorporated chiefly into dentin but also may interfere with enamel formation. The tooth discolorations range from yellow through brown to gray and produce stains that are particularly visible on anterior teeth because of the thin enamel coating overlying the damaged tetracycline-stained dentin.[42]

TABLE 32-2

Endogenous stains: drug-induced

Etiology	Appearance	Tooth structure involved
Exposure to tetracycline between the fifth month of fetal life and age 8	Discolorations ranging from yellow through brown to gray; stains particularly visible on anterior teeth because of thin enamel coating overlying damaged tetracycline-stained dentin	Tetracycline's affinity for calcifying tissue incorporated chiefly into dentin but also may interfere with enamel formation; may affect permanent and deciduous teeth
Fluoride ingestion (dental fluorosis)	Mottled discoloration of enamel ranging from white flecks and chalky opaque areas of enamel to brown or black staining and pitted or overall corroded enamel appearance; more fluoride ingested at time of enamel formation, more severe staining and mottling	Can affect any permanent or primary teeth exposed to fluoride during development; affected teeth generally resistant to decay

---

TABLE 32-3

Endogenous stains: enamel hypoplasia

Etiology	Appearance	Tooth structure involved
Dental fluorosis: excessive repeated intake of fluoride during tooth development	See Table 32-2	See Table 32-2
Febrile illness (measles, chicken pox, scarlet fever) Vitamin deficiency (A, C, or D)	Pitting of enamel of teeth developing at time of illness or deficiency	Teeth that form during first year of life (permanent central incisors, laterals, cuspids, and first molars)
Local infections or trauma of primary teeth	Color of enamel possibly ranging from yellow to brown, or severe pitting and deformity; severity dependent on degree of infection or stage of underlying tooth development	Usually single tooth; permanent maxillary incisors and permanent mandibular premolars
Trauma during tooth maturation, endocrine, metabolic, or unknown causes	Enamel hypocalcification; localized chalky white flecks or spots in enamel, focally or linearly; normal amounts of enamel produced but hypomineralized; underlying enamel possibly soft and susceptible to caries	Possibly single tooth or all teeth being formed at time of disturbance

---

TABLE 32-4

Endogenous stains: environmental

Type	Appearance	Etiology
Incipient caries	White, chalky	Acid-producing bacteria
Active caries	Brown to black	Acid-producing bacteria
Secondary caries	White, gray to brownish-black around existing restorations	Marginal leakage of restorations and acid-producing bacteria
Pulpless teeth	Light yellow-brown, bluish-black, or black; possibly also tinted orange, pink, and green	Decomposed pulp tissue and hemoglobin penetrating dentin tubules
Pulpal necrosis	Yellowish-black	Trauma
Iatrogenic	Variable from gray-brown to pinkish hues	Usually result of restorative materials, exposure of dentin to bleeding, and other problems of unknown etiology

---

Endogenous staining exhibiting enamel hypoplasia can be found when factors such as local infections or trauma and congenital illness have altered tooth form or color. Enamel hypoplasia results from a disturbance of or damage to ameloblasts during enamel matrix formation and exhibits defective enamel of normal hardness (Fig. 32-3).

Examples are summarized in Table 32-3. Excessive repeated intake of fluoride during tooth development is a classic example of enamel hypoplasia that is often referred to as *dental fluorosis* (Fig. 32-4). This type of hypoplasia may cause tooth discoloration ranging from localized white flecks to irregular patterns of brown pitting of the

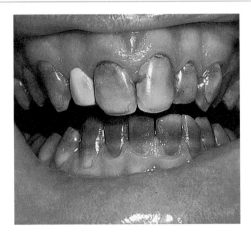

FIG. 32-2 Endogenous developmental stain: tetracycline. (Courtesy Dr. George Taybos, Jackson, Miss.)

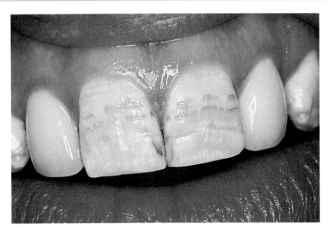

FIG. 32-4 Endogenous developmental stain: dental fluorosis. (Courtesy Dr. George Taybos, Jackson, Miss.)

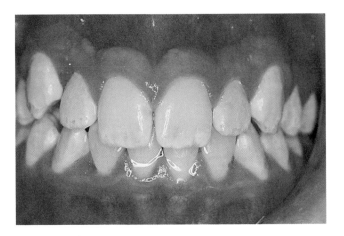

FIG. 32-3 Endogenous developmental stain: enamel hypoplasia. (Courtesy Dr. George Taybos, Jackson, Miss.)

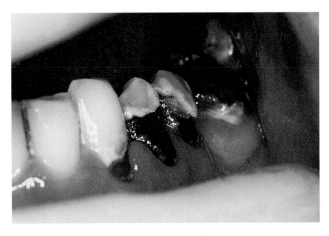

FIG. 32-5 Endogenous stain: cervical caries. (Courtesy Dr. George Taybos, Jackson, Miss.)

enamel, often referred to as *mottled enamel.* The more fluoride that is ingested at the time of enamel formation, the more severe the staining and mottling.

Another endogenous stain category includes stains that are environmentally induced. These stains are the result of pathological incursions into the tooth, such as dental caries or pulpal necrosis, metallic stains from dental restorations, or prolonged exposure to metals in the air or water (see Table 32-4). Stains associated with primary (initial lesions on unrestored tooth surfaces) and secondary (recurrent) caries transform over time with exposure to the harsh oral environment. Initial (incipient) carious lesions appear slightly whiter, chalky, and dull in comparison with unaffected enamel. With increased caries development, the decalcified areas become stained with food and bacterial debris, and the degree of discoloration is proportionate to the duration of active decay (Fig. 32-5). The second type of discoloration includes those stains adjacent to both intact and defective restorations. These stains may indicate the presence of secondary or recurrent caries and need to be closely monitored (Fig. 32-6). Stains resulting from the pigments of restorative material containing

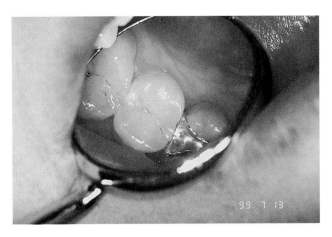

FIG. 32-6 Endogenous stain: secondary caries. (Courtesy Dr. George Taybos, Jackson, Miss.)

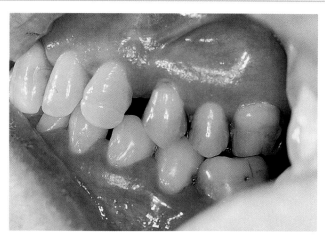

FIG. 32-7 Endogenous stain: amalgam restoration. (Courtesy Dr. George Taybos, Jackson, Miss.)

metal seeping into the dentinal tubules often reveal a gray shadow adjacent to the restoration (Fig. 32-7). Similar staining can occur as a result of leakage between the restoration and the tooth, which allows saliva and bacteria to penetrate and begin the process of recurrent caries. Recurring caries will appear as a gray or brown area adjacent to the margin of a defective restoration. Endodontically involved teeth often appear darker clinically (Figs. 32-8 and 32-9), whereas internal resorption often manifests as the classic "pink tooth" (Figs. 32-10 and 32-11). Careful inspection of the area with supportive radiographic diagnostic information is essential to determine the appropriate source of the staining.

All the endogenous stains previously discussed cannot be removed by simple polishing procedures. These stains are imbedded in the enamel and dentin matrix and require more complex restorative and cosmetic procedures to treat the affected areas. Methods for the cosmetic improvement of teeth affected by endogenous or intrinsic

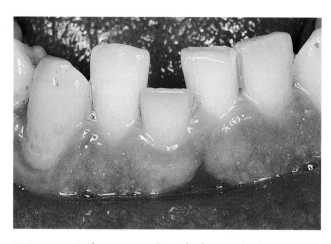

FIG. 32-8 Endogenous stain: pulpal necrosis. (Courtesy Dr. George Taybos, Jackson, Miss.)

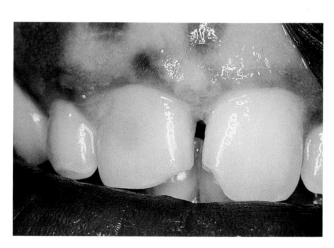

FIG. 32-10 Endogenous stain: internal resorption "pink tooth." (Courtesy Dr. George Taybos, Jackson, Miss.)

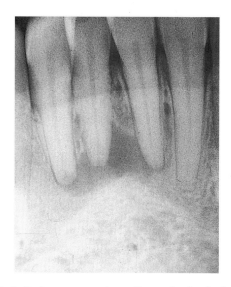

FIG. 32-9 Endogenous stain: radiograph of pulpal necrosis of Fig. 32-8. (Courtesy Dr. George Taybos, Jackson, Miss.)

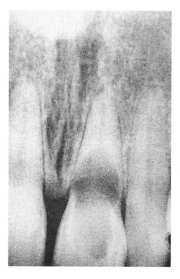

FIG. 32-11 Endogenous stain: radiograph of Fig 32-10. (Courtesy Dr. George Taybos, Jackson, Miss.)

stains include enamel microabrasion, vital and nonvital tooth bleaching, composite restorative materials bonded as overlays, laminate veneers, and combination treatments. Chapters 38 and 39 provide specific information on these procedures.

Stains that can be removed are most commonly categorized as *environmental exogenous* and *extrinsic* stains. These stains are associated with exposure to certain foods, tobacco, tea, coffee, and airborne particles and can be identified by color, distribution, and tenacity.[52] Individuals vary widely in the rate and amount of accumulated extrinsic stains. Certain factors are known to predispose a person to the accumulation of both dental deposits and stains; these include enamel roughness, organic salts in saliva, increased or decreased salivary flow, and poor oral hygiene. Most extrinsic stains may be removed by scaling and polishing procedures, discussed later in this chapter.

Some of the more common extrinsic stains are summarized in Tables 32-5 and 32-6. In the tables, stains are categorized by exposure elements and by color of appearance.

The most common extrinsic stains by an exposure element are tobacco and food stains. Tobacco stains range in appearance from tan to dark brown or black and cover approximately the cervical one third to one half of most affected teeth (Fig. 32-12). This type of staining occurs mostly on lingual and palatal surfaces and is commonly found in pits and fissures and other enamel irregularities. Tobacco staining has been found to be directly proportional to the number of cigarettes smoked per day.[46] Staining also may be found in individuals who smoke pipes or cigars and those who use smokeless tobacco (snuff or

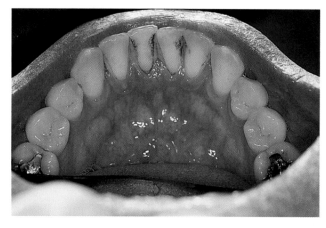

FIG. 32-12 Extrinsic stain: tobacco smoking. (Courtesy Dr. George Taybos, Jackson, Miss)

TABLE 32-5

Extrinsic stains: categorized by exposure

Category	Primary sites	Composition and appearance	Etiology
Tobacco	Cervical one third to one half of lingual surfaces: pits and fissures	Tars, pigments; light brown to dark-leathery, brownish-black	Smoking, chewing, dipping (tobacco)
Food	Cervical one third to one half of lingual surfaces: pits and fissures	Food pigments: brownish-pellicle type stain	Consumption of tea, coffee, cola drinks, red wine, berries, spices, betel leaves, nuts, and candy
Metallic	Cervical one third; primarily anterior teeth affected but possibly occurring on random surfaces	Associated with specific metals: copper or brass exhibiting bluish-green; iron and nickel showing greenish-brown	Environmental, food, water
Drug, therapeutic	Cervical one third: pits and fissures	Plaque bacteria, tin, reactions with food colors; usually brown in color	Extended antibiotic use, stannous fluoride, chlorhexidine

---

TABLE 32-6

Extrinsic stains: categorized by color

Category	Primary sites	Composition and appearance	Etiology
Black-line	Thin band along gingival margin on buccal or lingual surfaces; most common on posterior palatal	Ferric sulfide fine line following contour of gingival crest with no apparent thickness	Iron in saliva, gingival fluid, plaque or bacteria; affecting all ages; most common in female patients
Green	Cervical one third to one half of facial surfaces of maxillary anteriors	Inorganic elements, chromogenic bacteria; light- to dark-green; embedded in bacterial plaque	Poor oral hygiene, surface irregularities; most common in children
Gray-green	Cervical one third of labial surfaces	Oils, resin, and pigments; embedded in pellicle and bacterial plaque	Poor oral hygiene, marijuana smoking
Orange	Thin line; cervical one third of incisors	Chromogenic bacteria; usually orange or red stain on facial and lingual surfaces of anterior teeth	Poor oral hygiene; most common in children

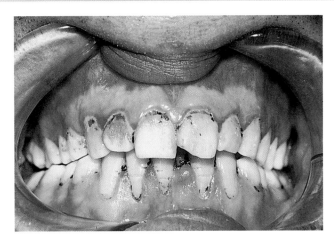

FIG. 32-13 Extrinsic stain: tobacco snuff. (Courtesy Dr. George Taybos, Jackson, Miss.)

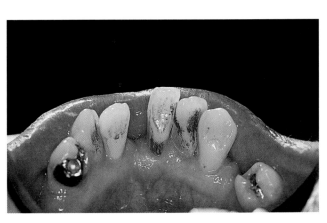

FIG. 32-16 Extrinsic stain: chlorhexidine. (Courtesy Dr. George Taybos, Jackson, Miss.)

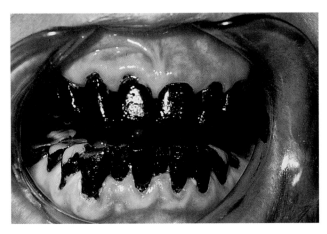

FIG. 32-14 Extrinsic stain: betel nut stain. (Courtesy Dr. George Taybos, Jackson, Miss.)

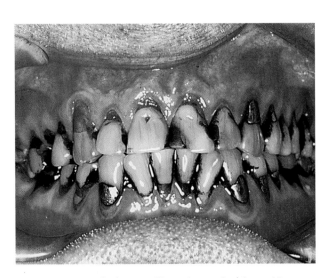

FIG. 32-15 Extrinsic metallic stain: topical iron. (Courtesy Dr. George Taybos, Jackson, Miss.)

chewing; Fig. 32-13). Tobacco stains may, over time, penetrate the enamel and become intrinsic.

Food staining is common in individuals who frequently drink coffee and tea. Other categories of food that may contribute to stain include cola drinks, red wine, berries such as raspberries and blueberries, spices, leaves and nuts of the betel plant, licorice and other candy-containing coloring agents. Stains resulting from ingestion of these foods range from tan to dark brown in color and occur over broad smooth tooth surfaces and in pits and fissures (Fig. 32-14).

Stains associated with metal exposure or drugs and therapeutic agents also have been identified. Metallic stains vary in color depending on the metal or the metallic salt that is ingested or inhaled. Green or blue-green colors result from copper or brass, whereas brown colors may result from an ingestion of materials or dust particles containing iron (Fig. 32-15). The majority of these stains have been attributed to industrial dust, but they may also be found in various foods and water.

Many drugs or therapeutic agents may cause tooth stains, only a few of which are described here. Surface discolorations and staining have occurred after extended topical or systemic antibiotic use or in studies of antibacterial agents with antiplaque activity.[42,57] These stains have been attributed to the direct effects of the agent on plaque bacteria. The most common and well-known antibacterial agent attributed to staining is chlorhexidine. A dark-brown stain beginning at the gingival margin can be noted shortly after beginning the daily use of a chlorhexidine regimen (Fig. 32-16). A brown to black pigmented stain in plaque-associated areas has also been reported in several clinical studies and is attributed to dentifrices containing stannous fluoride.[75] A summary of extrinsic exposure stains is shown in Table 32-5.

Stains categorized by color include black-line stain, green stain, gray-green stain, and orange stain, summarized in Table 32-6. Black-line stain usually occurs as a continuous thin band along the gingival margin and follows the crestal contour on lingual palatal and/or proximal sur-

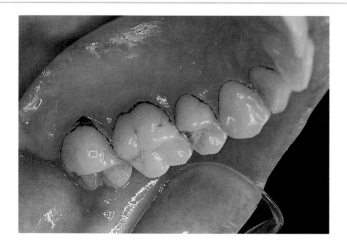

FIG. 32-17 Extrinsic stain: black line. (Courtesy Dr. George Taybos, Jackson, Miss.)

faces (Fig. 32-17). It occurs at all ages and is found more often in female patients. The primary cause of this deposit is iron compounds in saliva or gingival circular fluid that become embedded in the dental pellicle, plaque, and/or plaque bacteria. This stain is a ferric sulfide compound and is most often found in a relatively clean mouth.[52]

Green stain occurs primarily on cervical areas of the maxillary anterior teeth and is associated with the primary dental cuticle. It is usually crescent shape, close to the gingival margin, and colored light green to yellow-green to dark green. Green stains are usually a result of poor oral hygiene and are associated with chromogenic bacteria and gingival hemorrhage. The enamel beneath a green stain may become demineralized or carious as a result of cariogenic plaque accumulations. The roughened surface then encourages reaccumulation of plaque and recurrence of green stain. This stain is often difficult to remove with polishing agents. If the patient is not allergic to iodine, including a small amount of it in the *polishing agent* can aid in the removal of the green stain. Grey-green stain occurs around the gingival one third of teeth as a result of marijuana use. The stain is caused from oils, resin, and pigments found in marijuana. Orange stain is fairly rare. It occurs at the cervical third of incisor teeth and may be attributed to chromogenic bacteria.

STAIN EVALUATION

Clinically, stains are evaluated by severity and location. Light, moderate, or heavy stains may be generalized or localized in specific areas. Because these categories are simply observations and have no specific scientific guidelines, variations of conclusions between practitioners often result. Attempts have been made to develop scoring procedures to evaluate the extent of intrinsic and extrinsic staining for research purposes. One of the first attempts to evaluate stain clinically was the categorization of both the intensity and severity of the stain and the specific tooth area covered.[35] Other approaches attempted to quantify tooth stain by the use of plastic chips of various standardized colors[76] or grading stain on a stain/no-stain basis.[56] These measurements are commonly used in research to compare stain development or removal among treatment groups in clinical trials.

PROFESSIONAL TREATMENT OF EXTRINSIC STAINS

As part of the dental prophylaxis regimen, areas of stained **32-B** enamel and dentin are professionally polished with an abrasive agent following the appropriate debridement or scaling procedures. Polishing coronal surfaces includes the removal of stain and soft debris, acquired pellicle, and a small portion of fluoride-rich outer layer of enamel. This is an especially important factor to recall when polishing teeth in children because of the incomplete enamel mineralization of newly erupted teeth. During treatment planning, the dental hygienist must keep the following factors in mind:

- Selection of the least abrasive polishing agent possible that will thoroughly remove plaque and stain
- Use of proper techniques to reduce unnecessary iatrogenic *abrasion* on exposed enamel and dentinal surfaces during the procedure.

Varying factors of time, speed, and pressure (load) utilization also contribute to the clinical outcome. Therefore the clinician must have a thorough understanding of the basic principles and correct techniques that relate to selection of the abrasive agent, mechanical devices, and the specific procedures involved.

Abrasive Agents

Abrasive agents are incorporated into prophylaxis pastes for the purpose of cleaning and polishing. A dental abrasive changes the surface of the tooth by frictional grinding, rubbing, scraping, and abrading any surface irregularities. As this process proceeds from coarse abrasion (cleaning) to fine abrasion (polishing), the surface of the tooth passes through various stages—from irregular, to grooved, to finely abraded, with a concomitant increase in smoothness and light reflectance. The last stage is regarded as the polished surface.

Many prophylaxis pastes are available, each brand varying considerably in abrasiveness. The abrasives contained in these commercially available products are similar to those in dentifrice products.[14,47] The major difference is that the abrasive levels in professional products are much higher. Factors determining the abrasiveness and polishing potential of an agent include particle hardness, shape, size, and concentration. Abrasives vary markedly in inherent hardness and shape. Within the same polishing product, abrasive particle sizes are graded from fine to coarse. Harder, rough-shaped, large, particle-size compounds produce more abrasive action than particles that are soft, smooth-shaped, and small. Polishing products are also available that claim to change from a coarse polishing agent to a fine paste during use. The basic concept behind polishing is that as each of these factors (particle size, shape and hardness) decrease, surface abrasion is lessened and the surface becomes smooth or polished.

Polishing Agents

The two main abrasive polishing agents used in dental prophylaxis products or available as chemical compounds

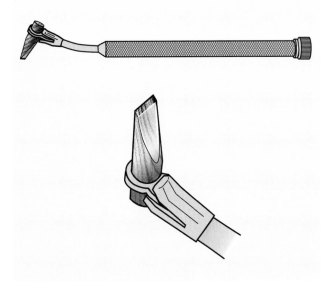

FIG. 32-18 Wooden point on porte polisher.

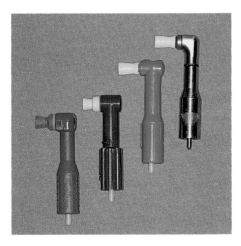

FIG. 32-19 Prophy angles: sterilizable *(right)* and disposable *(first through third from left).*

are *pumice* and calcium carbonate. Calcium carbonate may be purchased as chalk or whiting and is manufactured in several particle shapes and sizes and is less abrasive than pumice. Calcium carbonate produces minimal scratches and results in a smooth polished surface that reflects light. Pumice is also manufactured in a wide variety of particle sizes, and its use ranges from an abrasive stain-removal agent to fine polishing of acrylic dentures. Diamond and aluminum oxide polishing paste, rubber polishing cups, disks, or points are also available for polishing and maintaining aesthetic restorations.[38,40]

Most professional dental abrasive or polishing products have been categorized as fine, medium, or coarse, although no standardized definitions exist for these terms. One manufacturer's fine prophylaxis paste may be more abrasive than another manufacturer's medium paste. As a result, clinicians should use the least abrasive paste in the product line first. If it is determined that more abrasive is needed to remove a particular stain, the clinician should start the process with a medium or coarse paste, followed by the finer abrasive to finish the polishing. Additional factors must also be considered in the polishing procedure. These include the mechanical device used for polishing, indications and contraindications for use, and specific technique functions.

MECHANICAL DEVICES FOR POLISHING

Porte Polisher

The *porte polisher* is a simple, handheld device featuring a tapered orange-wood point. This instrument may be adapted to the various aspects of the teeth and rubs the abrasive agent against the tooth surface with a wedge-shaped, tapered, or pointed wooden point (Fig. 32-18). This technique requires considerable hand strength and control but the advantages of portability, ability to access obscured malpositioned tooth surfaces, generation of minimal fric-

tional heat, lack of engine noise, and minimal bacterial aerosol offer a valuable adjunctive instrument that should be the method of choice for selected patients. A more common device for polishing is the engine-driven polisher.

Engine-Driven Polishing

Engine-driven polishing is widely used in clinical practice because of its efficiency and efficacy. The power for engine-driven polishing may be derived from an electric motor or compressed air, which is the power source for most of today's dental units. A slow-speed handpiece is attached to the appropriate power source. The handpiece selected for use should be specifically designed for the system being used; it may screw, snap, lock, or clip onto the power source. Attached to the handpiece is the prophylaxis angle (prophy angle).

Prophy angles are designed with either straight or contraangled shanks. They can be either reusable after sterilization or disposable (Fig. 32-19). It has been shown that the disposable prophy angle works as effectively as the autoclavable angle, with the added benefit of eliminating any potential for cross-contamination between patients.[15] A rubber cup or brush is then attached to the prophy angle.

Prophy cups are designed with varying degrees of flexibility. The interior walls may have a ribbed-open, ribbed-webbed, or ribbed-turbine configuration. These ribs and webs permit retention of the prophy paste. Those cups without webs allow for greater flexibility of the rim. Brushes are designed with different shapes and degrees of flexibility. Most commonly, the cup or brush comes prepackaged and attached to the disposable prophy angle. If a sterilizable prophy angle is used, the cup or brush attaches by means of a mandrel that latches, screw, or snaps into place. Equipment and procedure preparation are summarized in Table 32-7.

Whatever mechanism or power source is used in any given clinical setting, the dental hygienist should become

TABLE 32-7

Engine-driven polishing: equipment and procedure preparation

Equipment piece	Use	Features
Handpiece	Low (or slow) speed: 6000 to 10,000 rpm; must supply adequate torque	Requires routine maintenance
Prophylaxis angle	Contraangle or right-angle attachment	Disposable or reusable and sterilizable
Attachments:		
Rubber cup		Rubber cup on all exposed tooth surfaces
Ribbed/webbed	*Ribbing:* facilitates holding of polishing agent	
Hard/soft	*Soft rubber cup:* more flexibility	
Latex-free		
Occlusal brush		Brush only on occlusal surfaces
Soft or hard	*Soft brush:* usually adequate for occlusal stain removal	
Abrasive agent	Least abrasive agent used to sufficiently remove stain	Fine grit or toothpaste agent should be used. If medium or coarse grit is needed for heavy stain removal, fine grit should follow its use.
Protective equipment	Safety glasses for patient	Protection from aerosol splatter to eyes
	Personal protective wear for operator	Protection from aerosols generated from procedure
Aerosol control	Saliva ejector and or high-speed suction	Excessive saliva produced during procedure
	Air/water syringe	Periodic rinsing of area completed

familiar with the operation and maintenance of the system and the knowledge to troubleshoot if the polishing instrument fails to properly function. The handpiece and the prophylaxis angle require proper care and maintenance. It is suggested to refer to specific manufacturer recommendations for such maintenance procedures.

Indications for Use

The engine-driven polisher is indicated for most clinical applications in which the operator has access to a slow-speed handpiece. Patient compliance and acceptance are high; it is often regarded the instrument of choice for patients and operators. Because of its association with "the drill," a thorough explanation of the procedure is warranted for apprehensive patients, first-time patients, and especially young children. A simple "show-and-tell" technique is generally sufficient to introduce the patient to the rotating action of the soft rubber cup and hear the mechanical action of the handpiece. The guidelines for engine-driven polishing include patient selection and preparation, unit and operator preparation, and actual clinical technique.

Patient Selection and Preparation

Patient medical history and treatment plan should always be reviewed for any possible contraindications to the procedure. Contraindications for this procedure include allergies to latex or fluoride. In such instances, the following are available: rubber-cup "latex-free" products, prophy pastes, and pumice slurry without fluoride. Safety glasses for the patient are recommended to ensure that pumice and/or aerosols do not contaminate the patient's eyes.

Offering the patient a tissue or wipe is appreciated, as is the option to manage the saliva ejector during the procedure. A thorough explanation of the procedure allows young children and those new to the engine-polishing method an idea of what to expect from the procedure. Children and some adults may be intimidated by the

sound of the handpiece, and a simple explanation or demonstration usually eases the apprehensions associated with the sound of "the drill."

Unit and Operator Preparation

Unit preparation includes obtaining the necessary equipment: handpiece and prophy angle with specific attachment (brush or cup) desired. The engine-polishing procedure requires adequate evacuation, as the polishing agent and the mechanical manipulation in the mouth stimulates salivary glands to secrete more saliva than normal. The air/water syringe must be available to rinse the area as each arch segment is completed. Finally, the selected polishing paste or abrasive (as indicated in treatment plan), dental floss, and disclosing solution complete the polishing armamentarium. Operator preparation emphasizes basic aerosol protection barriers such as a well-fitting mask, protective eye wear, and/or a face shield in addition to basic personal protective equipment discussed in Chapter 5.

Clinical Technique

All polishing procedures mandate proper patient-operator positioning. Using the modified pen grasp, the clinician rests the handpiece over the hand in the notch between the thumb and forefinger. This allows flexibility of motion of the handpiece and cord. The handpiece is manipulated outside the mouth first, by the application of light steady pressure on the rheostat to evaluate speed and proper function of the device. The clinician fills the rubber cup with polishing paste by slowly running the handpiece in the polishing agent or by dipping the rubber cup or brush into the abrasive-filled dappen dish or small prepackaged container. The stable fulcrum is established and the rheostat slowly activated so that the applicator rotates at a slow steady speed just before the cup or brush is placed against the tooth surface. The handpiece and angle must supply adequate torque to maintain the abrasive against the tooth for polishing. The rubber cup is refilled

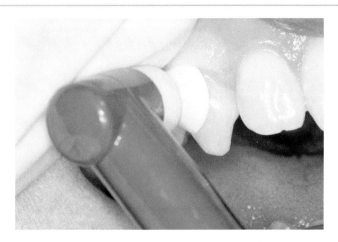

FIG. 32-20 Rubber cup: subgingival application.

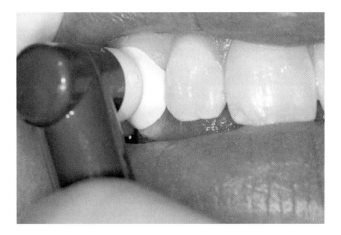

FIG. 32-21 Rubber cup: interproximal application.

with abrasive paste as necessary. The abrasive-filled container or dappen dish may be held in the nondominant hand for ready access. Also the abrasive may be applied directly to the teeth just ahead of the path of the rubber cup or brush.

Regardless of how the abrasive is placed on the tooth, adequate amounts must be used. Usually a full rubber cup of abrasive is sufficient for one or two teeth. A bare or saliva-laden cup void of polishing agent does not polish the teeth and generates heat.[58] The rubber cup is refilled as necessary, a stable fulcrum reestablished, the handpiece activated slowly, and the rubber cup placed on the tooth surface before polishing procedures continue.

A systematic approach increases efficiency and ensures all surfaces are adequately polished. Most surfaces can be polished in 2 to 3 seconds with the use of a light, steady speed in a patting motion, adapting the rubber cup smoothly to cover all exposed tooth surfaces. The lip of the cup can be flared and slipped slightly subgingival so that the most coronal aspects of the sulcus may be cleaned for therapeutic effects on the root surface (Fig. 32-20). The clinician should apply the rubber cup to proximal surfaces by sliding the lip of the cup as far proximally as possible and slightly under the contact point area (Fig. 32-21). Vertical,

oblique, or horizontal stroke direction is used as the rim of the cup is moved across the tooth surface. Adapting the lip of the cup into the occlusal grooves often suffices for stain removal from these difficult areas.

When the rubber cup does not remove occlusal stain adequately, the brush attachment should be considered. Brush attachments should be used *only* on occlusal surfaces and should not be used on any other tooth surfaces because they are highly abrasive, especially to soft tissues,[62] and difficult to control. Brushes are available with soft or firm bristles. The softer bristles are usually adequate for stain removal, and they hold an abrasive agent more readily. Clinical procedures are summarized in Tables 32-8 and 32-9.

Whether a cup or brush is being used, the attachment and abrasive should be used with moderate intermittent pressure.[64] Using intermittent pressure on the tooth allows the heat generated to dissipate between each stroke. Constant pressure of the rubber cup or brush on the tooth builds up frictional heat that may cause discomfort, pain, and possible pulpal damage. This is especially critical for anterior teeth, which provide minimal insulation for the pulp because of the lesser amount of dentin and enamel compared to that on posterior teeth. Clinicians may also observe the patient's facial expression carefully to detect signs of discomfort from heat. Patients apparently in pain should be asked if they sense heat. If so, the polishing procedure should be adjusted to reduce heat by the reduction of the duration of each application and/or pressure of the cup or brush on the tooth.

The speed of the cup is critical in both minimizing frictional heat and in ensuring effective polishing. Operating the cup at high speeds is both harmful and ineffective.[58] As it is rarely possible to determine the exact **revolutions per minute (rpm)** during operation, using the lowest possible speed that moves the cup or brush against the tooth without stalling is recommended. Sound also may provide a clue for determining whether the cup is rotating too rapidly. A high whine or whistle in the handpiece usually indicates excessive speed. To achieve the lowest possible speed, the rheostat may need to be activated to a high or medium speed and then backed down to a low speed before the tooth is touched with the attachment. Most dental units have a gauge that measures air pressure for each handpiece connector in **pounds per square inch (PSI).** Operating the handpiece at approximately 20 PSI seems to be sufficient for stain removal. Table 32-8 provides a summary of factors to consider in controlling the negative aspects of the polishing procedure.

At the completion of the polishing procedure, the patient's dentition should be rinsed thoroughly to remove all residual polishing agent. Proximal areas should then be flossed with either dental floss or dental tape. Inspection for remaining stain should be performed with good intraoral light, compressed air, mouth mirror, and a disclosing solution. Any remaining plaque or stain should be removed by either reinstrumenting the area or repolishing the surface. Finishing strips or dental tape rubbed with a small amount of prophy paste before flossing assists in the removal of residual interproximal stain. The type of deposit remaining determines which procedure is indicated. (See Table 32-12 later in the chapter for finishing and evaluating procedures.)

TABLE 32-8

Engine-driven polishing: procedures

Polishing considerations	Concerns	Recommended actions
Health history	Latex allergy	Use latex-free rubber cup.
	Fluoride allergy	Use nonfluoridated paste.
	Children	Do not use pumice slurry on primary teeth.
Treatment plan	Contraindication immediately after root planing procedure	
Grasp	Use of modified pen grasp	Rest handpiece and cord over outreached hand to ease manipulation.
Handpiece control	Establishment of stable fulcrum	Use either external or internal fulcrum (wide fulcrum = increased stability).
		Never use fulcrum on loose teeth.
	Use of lowest possible speed to reduce frictional heat	Use light, steady pressure on rheostat to produce even, low speed.
Rubber cup/abrasive	Gentle activation of rubber cup in polishing agent	Adequately fill rubber cup with polishing paste.
	Dipping into polishing agent to fill rubber cup	Refill rubber cup after completion of every two to three teeth; use adequate amount.
Systematic approach	Polishing of all exposed tooth surfaces	Place lip of cup slightly subgingivally and into interproximal spaces; rubber cup is usually adequate for occlusal surfaces. (A brush may be used for heavily stained occlusal surfaces.)

TABLE 32-9

Engine-driven polishing: procedures control

Polishing considerations	Concerns	Recommended actions
Polishing agent	An empty cup generates more heat.	One rubber cupful of polishing agent should be used to polish only one to two teeth.
Pressure	Moderate intermittent pressure is preferred; heavy pressure creates more heat and more abrasive action.	Intermittent pressure permits heat dissipation.
Engine speed	Speed used should be the lowest possible handpiece speed that will move cup or brush against tooth without stalling; consistent, low speed is recommended.	Observe whine of engine; usually 20 PSI is adequate.
Abrasion control	Increased time spent polishing a tooth surface increases abrasive effect.	Polish approximately 3 to 5 seconds per tooth, usually adequate to remove stain and soft deposit; reinstrumentation may be necessary to remove residual stains or deposit.

Precautions and Safety Issues

Several fundamental principles are important in rubber-cup polishing (Box 32-1). Cosmetic polishing with the rubber cup immediately following scaling and root planing on patients with deep periodontal pockets is contraindicated and should be scheduled for a separate appointment. The polishing agent may be pushed into the pocket and result in increased gingival inflammation.

Air-Powder Polishing

Air-powder polishing is a mechanism for polishing the teeth that propels a slurry of water and sodium bicarbonate under air and water pressure. The pounds of pressure per square inch depend on the type of *air-powder polisher*

being used. In most units, the water temperature is warm and thermostatically controlled. The handpiece has a nozzle through which the slurry is propelled when a foot control is activated. Air-powder polishers are manufactured handpiece units that attach directly to the air/water connector on the dental unit (Fig. 32-22), as separate units, or in combination with an ultrasonic scaler (Fig. 32-23).

Indications for Use

The air-powder polisher has been shown to be a safe, efficient, and effective means of removing extrinsic stain and plaque from tooth surfaces.[8,9] The air-powder polisher was reported to remove plaque and stain as effectively as a rubber cup and does so in less time.[71] It has also shown equal effectiveness in decreasing root surface roughness

BOX 32-1

Principles for Rubber-Cup Polishing

- Review medical history and treatment plan for any possible contraindications to the procedure.
- Determine whether the patient has a history of allergy or toxic reaction to fluoride or latex and adjust equipment (prophy cup or paste) as necessary.
- Use a stable fulcrum (absolutely essential) to provide the patient with a sense of confidence in the technique and avoid slippage and possible damage to the tissues.
- Use intermittent pressure against the tooth in a gentle patting or sweeping motion.
- Apply even pressure when polishing cemental surfaces to prevent ditching.
- Maintain a slow, consistent engine speed (desirable at approximately 20 PSI).
- Keep the rubber cup filled with abrasive to prevent frictional heat build-up in the tooth.
- Use brush attachments on occlusal surfaces *only.*
- Start with the least abrasive agent to prevent unnecessary removal of tooth structure, moving to the next abrasive if the first fails to remove the stain.
- Do not use pumice slurry on primary dentition because of the resulting abrasion.[27]

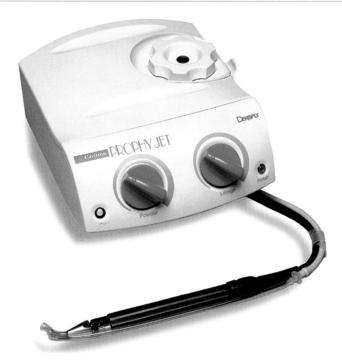

FIG. 32-23 Prophy-jet/ultrasonic scaler combination. (Courtesy Dentsply Professional, York, Pa.)

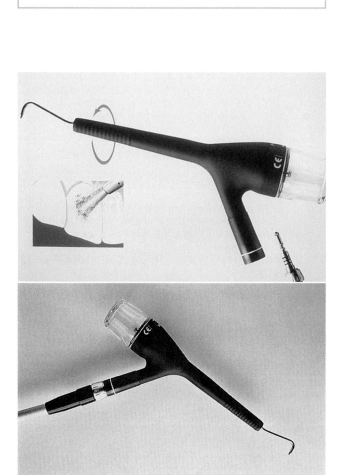

FIG. 32-22 Prophyflex unit. (Courtesy KaVo America, Lake Zurich, Ill.)

after instrumentation.[34] However, it may not prevent plaque reaccumulation as effectively as a rubber cup.[3] Exposed cementum and dentin structures are more vulnerable to abrasion and the loss of these structures due to air-powder polishing has been reported in the literature,[9,19,31] but these same reports indicate no negative effect from using the air-powder polisher on intact enamel surfaces. A summary of indications is found in Table 32-10.

Some patients exhibit extensive staining on root structures, particularly at the cementoenamel junction or on areas with extensive recession. If these stains are removed with a curet, the root structure will be reduced over the years, particularly if those patients are on a short recall interval. One option for stained root surfaces that present no aesthetic concern is to leave the stain on the exposed surface and explain to the patient that stain will not harm the teeth or gingiva and is not related to oral disease. For instances when stain removal is necessary for aesthetic concerns, the air-powder polisher is preferable to the curet. The air-powder polisher has been shown to remove less root structure than the curet in simulated 3-month recalls for 3 years. In addition, stain was removed more than three times faster with the air-powder polisher.[8] Caution is recommended whenever root surface polishing is necessary. Any method capable of removing stain from the root surface will also remove cementum and dentin. Manufacturers and researchers agree that prolonged use of the air-powder polisher on these surfaces is not advised.[9,19]

The air-powder polisher has also been used for debridement of Class V abraded areas before placement of glass ionomer cements. A comparison of the enamel-cement interface of a glass ionomer cement placed in Class V abrasions cleaned by a rubber-cup polish and an air-powder polisher was conducted. Results indicated the air-polished

TABLE 32-10

Air-powder polishing: indications for use

Procedure	Advantages	Disadvantages
Plaque and stain removal	Works as well as rubber cup but in less time Decreases root surface roughness after instrumentation Produces no negative effect on intact enamel surfaces	May not prevent plaque reaccumulation better than rubber cup Reports of loss of exposed cementum and dentin in literature
Class V restorations preparation	Produces less microleakage at enamel/bonding interface	
Sealant preparation	Produces deeper resin penetration into enamel Increases sealant bond strength	Can abrade existing sealants
Orthodontics	Polishes more efficiently than rubber cup Increases bonding strength if used before bonding Not contraindicated on orthodontic bracket adhesive systems	

TABLE 32-11

Air-powder polishing: patient considerations

Polishing considerations	Concerns	Recommended actions
Health history review	Review for contraindications	*Health contraindications:* sodium-restricted diet, respiratory illness, hypertension, infectious diseases *Dental contraindications:* composite or aesthetic restorations, crown margins, existing sealants, minimal abrasive effects on porcelain or gold
Patient preparation	Thorough explanation of procedure	Ask patient to remove contact lenses. Prerinse with antimicrobial agent. Apply lubricant to lips.
Aerosol protection	Both patient and operator protected from aerosol	*Patient:* safety glasses and/or drape over nose and eyes, drape over clothing, preprocedural mouthrinse *Operator:* PPE, face shield, well-fitting high-filtration mask

PPE, Personal protective equipment.

tooth had less microleakage around the enamel-cement interface than the tooth prepared with the rubber-cup polisher.[12] Similar results were noted when using the air-powder polisher before sealant application. The air-powder polisher was reported to be superior to rubber-cup polishing in preparing enamel for etching and sealants.[20,60] Deeper resin penetration into enamel and increased sealant bond strength was also reported in comparison with traditional polishing with pumice and water.[10,54]

Many operators prefer using the air-powder polisher on orthodontic patients, and researchers support this application. Air-powder polishing has been found to be more efficient than rubber-cup polishing and appears to be the most effective method of plaque removal for treating orthodontic patients.[9,21] Also, no contraindications exist on orthodontic bracket adhesive systems with the air-powder polisher. The guidelines for air-powder polishing include patient selection and preparation, unit and operator preparation, and actual clinical technique.

Patient Selection and Preparation
Because of the various indications and contraindications for air-powder use, patient selection and treatment planning are critical. Patient selection should include a thorough health history review to screen out patients on sodium-restricted diets, respiratory illnesses, hypertension, and certain infectious or systemic diseases. Caution or complete avoidance of the air-powder polisher is also advised on patients with composite or cosmetic restorations. (Extensive discussion on maintaining aesthetic restorations is discussed later in this chapter.)

Patient preparation should include a thorough explanation of the procedure, removal of contact lenses, antimicrobial prerinse, and application of a lubricant to the lips. A damp gauze pad may be placed on the patient's tongue to help absorb the powder that accumulates in the patient's mouth. Because of the excessive aerosols produced, additional patient preparation includes protective apparel such as safety glasses or a drape over the nose and eyes and placement of a plastic or disposable drape over the patient's clothing. Patient considerations for air-powder polishing are summarized in Table 32-11.

Unit and Operator Preparation
Unit preparation includes obtaining all the necessary equipment: air-polisher, abrasive powder, floss, disclosing

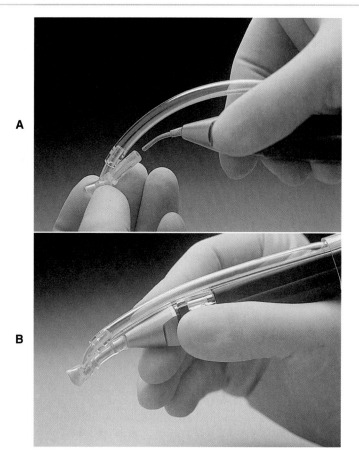

A

B

FIG. 32-24 A, Jet shield assembly. **B,** Jet shield. (Courtesy Dentsply Professional, York, Pa.)

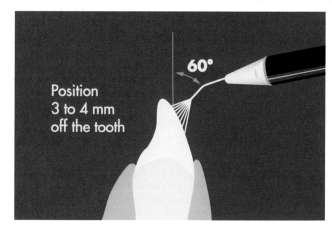

FIG. 32-25 Air-powder polishing anterior 60-degree angle. (Courtesy Dentsply Professional, York, Pa.)

solution, high-speed evacuation system, and preprocedural antimicrobial rinse. Ideally, the unit should be placed on the opposite side of the dental chair within comfortable reach of the clinician. Waterlines should be flushed before use, according to the recommendations of the Centers for Disease Control and Prevention (CDC). The handpiece nozzle is prepared according to manufacturer's suggestions and the powder compartment filled with abrasive suggested for the machine being used. Because of the excessive aerosols produced, operators are advised to add a face shield and a well-fitting mask with high-filtration capabilities[43] to their already existing personal protective equipment. An aerosol-reduction device that connects the suction to the air-polisher handpiece has been shown to be effective in controlling and reducing air-powder aerosols, thus decreasing the potential for disease transmission[44] (Fig. 32-24).

Clinical Technique
Positioning of the patient and operator are basically unchanged, although direct vision and access become elementally important when the polisher is active. Raising the back on the patient's chair up to a 45-degree angle may provide a better field of vision and increase patient comfort. The rheostat has two compression levels. Full compression releases the aerosol powder-abrasive from the tip. Pressing the foot pedal halfway produces a stream of

water useful for rinsing and cleaning. The clinician should check the amount of water and powder coming from the unit before activation in patients' mouths to test the sensitivity of the alternating cycles and confirm the powder/water ratio. The procedure requires adequate evacuation, and use of a high-speed suction with an assistant is optimal. When the clinician is performing air-polishing without the aid of a dental assistant, the use of a saliva ejector and/or an aerosol-reduction device is suggested.

The patient's head is turned slightly toward the clinician, who uses direct vision as much as possible. An external soft tissue fulcrum is established and a modified pen grasp is used with the handpiece and cord resting gently on the hand. Properly managed, the cord supports the necessary light grasp and instrument balance.

The nozzle should be held 3 to 4 mm from the tooth surface. Holding the nozzle farther from the tooth surface minimizes the abrasive action and increases the aerosol. The tip should be angled diagonally, with the spray directed toward the middle one third of the exposed tooth, using a constant circular motion, interproximal to interproximal (sweeping or paintbrush motion). A systematic approach ensures all tooth surfaces are adequately polished. The clinician should alternate cycles of full-compression powder-spray and half-compression rinse every two or three teeth to increase efficiency and patient comfort. For anterior teeth, the tip should be directed at a 60-degree angle to the tooth (Fig. 32-25), for posterior teeth an 80-degree angle (Fig. 32-26), and for occlusal surfaces a 90-degree angle (Fig. 32-27). The stream should *not* be aimed at the soft tissue but toward the occlusal or incisal surfaces. Using correct angulation of the handpiece nozzle reduces the amount of aerosolized spray.[6] The suction device should be held as close as possible to the tip of water/powder, following the tip as it moves in a rapid, sweeping motion from surface to surface. The clinician should use the hand and the patient's cheeks or lips to help contain aerosols. When an aerosol reduction device is used with the air-powder polisher, the clinician should follow the manufacturer's recommendations for variations to adaptation and angulation.

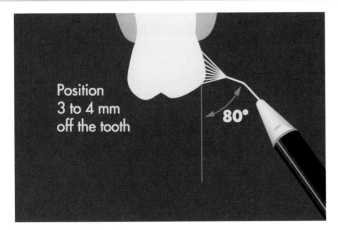

FIG. 32-26 Air-powder polishing posterior 80-degree angle. (Courtesy Dentsply Professional, York, Pa.)

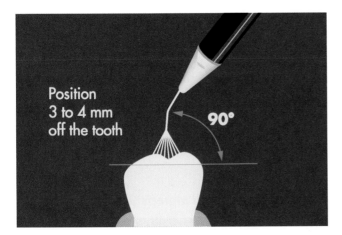

FIG. 32-27 Air-powder polishing occlusal 90-degree angle. (Courtesy Dentsply Professional, York, Pa.)

Clinicians should rinse excessive slurry from the patient's mouth often. In the case of normal soft deposit and stain debridement, the tip should be kept in constant circular motion with an exposure time of ½ to 1 second on each surface.[1,66] Approximately 5 seconds or less on each tooth is generally more than adequate to remove even the most difficult stains. Root surfaces abrade more quickly than enamel surfaces, and less time should be used in these areas. Technique recommendations for the air-powder polisher are summarized in Box 32-2.

The finishing steps that were mentioned with the engine polishing, such as rinsing, flossing, and inspection for remaining stain, should be accomplished at the completion of the air-powder polishing procedure. Thorough rinsing is essential after air-powder polishing because of the basic nature of the sodium bicarbonate. Additional steps, such as allowing the patient to help wipe away the debris from the face with a moist towel and offering lip balm, are often appreciated by the patient (Table 32-12).

BOX 32-2

Equipment and Actions Associated with Air-Powder Polishing

Armamentarium
Air-powder polishing unit
Handpiece/nozzle or necessary attachments
Abrasive powder
Evacuation system/high or low speed
Aerosol reduction device (optional)
Air/water syringe
Floss
Disclosing solution
Preprocedural antimicrobial rinse

Aerosol-Reduction Strategies
Use hand and patients cheeks or lips to contain aerosols.
Hold nozzle 3 to 4 mm from tooth surface.
Use proper tip angles for various areas of mouth.
Angle nozzle diagonally toward incisal to middle one third of tooth.
Use constant circular motion.
Hold suction device as close as possible to movement of working tip.
Use aerosol-reduction device.

Nozzle Angulation
Posterior: 80 degrees
Anterior: 60 degrees
Occlusal: 90 degrees

Sequence
Follow systematic approach.
Keep tip in constant circular motion.
Maintain sweeping motion from interproximal to interproximal.
Allow ½ to 1 full second on each tooth surface.
Alternate cycles of full compression powder spray and half-compression rinsing every 1 to 3 teeth or 1 to 3 seconds.
Rinse excessive slurry from patient's mouth thoroughly and often.
Finishing steps similar to engine-driven polishing.
Perform additional rinsing and provide patients with wipes to help them clean up after procedure.

Considerations
Transient soft tissue abrasion should heal with no long-term effects.
Bacteremia may be created when gingival inflammation present (similar to rubber-cup polishing).
The serum pH can rise; therefore air-powder polishing is contraindicated on patients with sodium-restricted diets, hypertension, or respiratory or infectious diseases.

Precautions and Safety Issues
When the clinician performs air-powder polishing, aerosols of microorganisms that contaminate surfaces several feet from the operative site have been reported.[23] Gloves; masks; protective lenses for patient, operator, and assistants; high-volume evacuation; and a laminar airflow to reduce airborne bacteria are important to minimize this problem. Some researchers suggest using a preprocedural rinse with 0.2% chlorhexidine for 2 minutes helped reduce

TABLE 32-12
Finishing and evaluating the polishing procedure

Polishing considerations	Concerns	Recommended actions
Finishing steps	Thorough removal of remaining interproximal stain	Wipe polishing paste on floss before flossing.
	Flossing of interproximal surfaces	Remove interproximal stains; use fine sandpaper strips to help remove interproximal stains.
	Flossing of surfaces adjacent to edentulous areas	Use regular floss or dental tape.
Follow-up evaluation	Use of disclosing solution, compressed air, and light	If plaque or calculus is still present, reinstrument.
		If stain is still present, reinstrument and/or repolish.

bacterial counts in aerosols,[73] and others have reported no significant reduction of bacteria-laden aerosols with pre-rinsing.[7] Use of an aerosol-reduction device is also suggested. Surface areas require thorough disinfection after this procedure.

Systemic concerns exist when using the air-powder polisher. Blood sample analysis of one patient before and after treatment with an air-powder polisher demonstrated that serum pH rose to a marginally alkaline state; this situation normally resolves in a day or two.[50] Because of these and other concerns it has been suggested that use of the air-powder polisher should be avoided on patients with respiratory or infectious diseases and patients on sodium-restricted diets or hypertension.[6] Some soft tissue abrasion of a transient nature can be expected when using the air-powder polisher. Small blood clots at the margin of the gingiva immediately after use of the air-powder polisher have been noted, with no signs of abrasion or long-term irritation.[32,41] Another study compared the development of bacteremia in subjects receiving a rubber-cup polish and those who were air-powder–polished. Although not statistically significant, more subjects receiving a rubber-cup polish developed bacteremias than those who were air-powder polished. If gingivitis is not present, the likelihood of a patient developing a bacteremia from air-powder polishing is no greater than if he/she were to receive a rubber-cup polish.[29]

MAINTAINING AESTHETIC RESTORATIONS

Aesthetic dentistry has become an integral part of today's dental practice. Patients have crown and bridge restorations and are having cosmetic resin, composite, bonding, and veneers placed to enhance their smile. Because improper oral care can quickly destroy many of these types of restorations, dental hygienists must understand maintenance requirements associated with aesthetic dentistry.

Coarse polishing paste, air-powder polishers,[51] use of acidulated phosphate fluorides,[13,24] and even hard tooth brushing with abrasive toothpaste[61] have been shown to be abrasive and destructive to the surface characteristics of restorative material. One study demonstrated that polishing pastes roughen the surface of composite resins; thus their use should be avoided at those sites.[55] Another

short-term study demonstrated that polishing after root planing improved the smoothness of the marginal portion of cast gold crowns more than simple root planing alone.[74]

Application of the air-powder polisher on most restorative materials should be carefully managed. Aesthetic restorations (composites, veneers, porcelain) have exhibited wear and surface roughness when exposed to the air-powder polisher,[5,11,36,51] although in 1984 Patterson and McLundie reported minimal *in vitro* effects on porcelain and hard gold alloy.[48] Care is recommended around crown margins as cement may be eroded[5] and loss of marginal integrity on porcelain restorations has been identified.[18,67] Air-powder polishing also has been shown to abrade dental sealants.[28]

Polishing Restorative Materials

Basic guidelines for aesthetic dentistry start with careful instrumentation with a curet to debride around the restoration. Scalers and/or powered scalers (sonic or ultrasonic) should not be used because they can scratch the surface and break down the filler particles.[77] The next step is to apply a diamond, aluminum oxide, or low-abrasive toothpaste directly to the restoration and then polish thoroughly using a rubber cup for 30 seconds. Diamond-polishing paste is suggested when only porcelain is exposed. Aluminum oxide paste is recommended for use on highly filled hybrid composites[30] and resin or porcelain restorations when resin cement or cementum is exposed.[38,40] It has also been suggested that a low abrasive toothpaste also may be used for the polishing agent, but no research has been done to document this suggestion.

Clinicians should floss while the paste is still on the restoration to carry the paste interproximally. When all surfaces have been polished, the restoration is rinsed and inspected for further stain.[38,40] If stain remains after initial polishing procedures, aluminum oxide discs, points, and strips of varying *grits* may be used. These steps are followed by aluminum oxide polishing paste to leave an aesthetic, final polish.[45] Aesthetic and porcelain restorations should always be polished first, following the guidelines mentioned above. The remaining teeth may then be polished using the appropriate methods for the clinical situ-

TABLE 32-13

Guidelines used to maintain aesthetic restorations

Polishing considerations	Concerns	Recommended actions
Instrumentation	Improper instrumentation can scratch surface and break down filler particles.	Carefully debride area with curet (scalers and/or powered scalers contraindicated).
Thorough polishing with rubber cup	Diamond-polishing paste should be used when only porcelain is exposed. Aluminum oxide should be used for highly filled hybrid composites, resin, or porcelain restorations when resin cements or cementum is exposed.	Apply a diamond, aluminum oxide, or low-abrasive toothpaste directly to restoration.
Floss	Proximal stain should be thoroughly removed.	Perform while paste is still on restoration to carry paste interproximally.
Rinsing/evaluation	Remaining pumice particles should be thoroughly removed.	If stain remains, use aluminum oxide discs, points, and strips of varying grits from coarse to fine; follow with aluminum oxide–polishing paste for final polish.

Remember to *always* polish aesthetic and porcelain restorations *first;* then polish the remaining teeth using appropriate methods indicated by the clinical situation and treatment plan.

ation. This is to reduce the possibility of having a coarse abrasive (that can scratch the aesthetic surface) remain in the rubber cup or the mouth when aesthetic maintenance is being rendered.

Implant Polishing

In 1989 a team of researchers noted that most professional mechanical cleaning methods cause abrasion to various implant materials[63]; however, use of the air-powder polishing on implant surfaces is controversial. Current literature suggests minimal alteration or damage to implant surfaces from air-powder polishing, which leaves the surfaces smooth and bacteria-free.[2,4,25] In another study, the air-powder polisher was found to remove the surface titanium, replacing the oxide layer with sodium bicarbonate particles that may increase surface corrosion.[49] Many implants have fixed porcelain crowns or bridges with limited access to the actual titanium implant. Professional, clinical decision-making skills are necessary in these situations to achieve the desired clinical outcome. Guidelines used to maintain aesthetic restorations are found in Table 32-13.

THERAPEUTIC POLISHING

Therapeutic polishing is the removal of toxins from the unexposed root surfaces, which results in a decrease in disease parameters. It is possible to polish root surfaces with both the rubber-cup or air-powder polisher; however, the evidence indicates the use of the air-powder polisher for this purpose. The rationale for this selection may be due to the effectiveness and efficiency of this device. Root sur-

faces also may be polished with an air-powder polisher when exposed during a surgical procedure.

The air-powder polisher works well in removing plaque, endotoxins, and stain from root concavities and furcations as an adjunct to periodontal surgery,[26] but it may offer no measurable benefit beyond ultrasonic debridement.[33] One in vitro study suggests that using an ultrasonic scaler followed by air-powder polishing creates an environment in which fibroblast growth and vitality is greater than for either teeth that were ultrasonically scaled without polishing or control teeth with remaining calculus.[22] Whether used as a follow-up to ultrasonic scaling or on calculus-free root surfaces, the air-powder polisher may play a significant role in the future in the removal of endotoxins on exposed root surfaces during surgery.

When polishing for therapeutic benefits with the air-powder polisher, the hygienist should follow the precautions and considerations presented previously. Most importantly, the clinician should take care to direct the air-powder spray against the root surface not the exposed soft tissues.

ROLE OF POLISHING IN DENTAL HYGIENE CARE

Professionals should consider all of the options available in treatment planning the polishing procedure. As with any other procedure, clinicians must consider aesthetic, therapeutic, and patient goals to design the treatment plan that meets each patient's specific needs. Applying these concepts allows the hygienist to accomplish a safe, effective, and thorough polishing procedure for cosmetic and therapeutic treatment.

CRITICAL THINKING ACTIVITIES

1. Develop a treatment plan for Mr. Smith, whose case was presented at the beginning of the chapter. Determine which polishing procedure or combination of procedures would best meet Mr. Smith's clinical and therapeutic goals. Discuss the rationale for each procedure and the specific factors that need to be addressed.

2. Avoid brushing your teeth for one morning. Rinse your mouth with grape juice, then swallow or expectorate. Describe how your mouth feels and the appearance of your teeth and deposits. Which deposits do you think are stained? How do you think this relates to not brushing after meals and eating colored foods? Why do you "feel" the grape juice remaining in your mouth? Evaluate the ease of removing the stained deposits.

3. Examine several student partners. If intrinsic stains are found, try to relate them to childhood diseases, medications, fluorides, restorative materials, or other sources. If extrinsic stains are found, try to identify whether they can be related to tea, coffee, and/or tobacco consumption.

4. Polish stain from a partner's teeth using a porte polisher, engine polisher, and air-powder polisher. Compare the results, the effort and time involved, and your partner's preference.

5. Examine the variety of tips available for use in the porte and engine polishers.

6. Perform routine maintenance on the handpiece and autoclavable prophylaxis angle used for engine polishing in your clinic.

7. Given a nonfunctioning engine polisher, determine why it is not working and correct the problem.

8. Evaluate the effectiveness and quality of disposable prophylaxis angles after clinical application of each.

9. Use the air-powder polisher to polish a quadrant of teeth that are heavily stained. Polish a second quadrant with an engine-driven rubber cup. Compare the results in terms of (1) cleanliness of the teeth, (2) time, (3) patient acceptance, and (4) amount of recurrent stain remaining after polishing and/or at the recall visit.

10. Take two pennies and draw a line to divide each in half. On one half apply dry pumice with a rubber cup. On the other half apply dry chalk with a second rubber cup. Examine each for scratches. On the second penny, apply a slurry of pumice with a rubber cup to one half and a slurry of chalk with a new rubber cup to the other half. Examine each for differences in smoothness and luster. The same exercise can be performed with any abrasive or polishing method.

REVIEW QUESTIONS

Questions 1 through 3 refer to the case study presented at the beginning of the chapter.

1. Which of the following polishing procedures is/are indicated in the polishing of Mr. Smith's teeth?
   a. Air-powder polisher
   b. Coarse prophylaxis paste with engine polisher
   c. Diamond-polishing paste
   d. All the above

2. Which of the following polishing procedures should be performed first on Mr. Smith?
   a. Use of an air-powder polisher
   b. Coarse prophylaxis paste with engine polisher
   c. Use of a diamond-polishing paste

3. Which of the following phrases describes Mr. Smith's stain classification?
   a. Environmental exogenous
   b. Environmental endogenous
   c. Developmental endogenous

4. Which of the following health concerns contraindicates use of air-powder polishing?
   a. Diabetes
   b. Mitral valve prolapse
   c. Asthma
   d. Chronic migraines

5. Which of the following is the stain classification for a green stain?
   a. Exogenous, extrinsic
   b. Endogenous, intrinsic
   c. Endogenous, extrinsic
   d. Exogenous, intrinsic

6. Which of the following factors affect the abrasiveness of a polishing agent?
   a. Particle size and shape
   b. Particle hardness and concentration
   c. Amount of water and fluoride
   d. *a* and *b*
   e. *a* and *c*

7. Through which of the following methods can frictional heat be minimized during engine polishing?
   a. Increase the engine speed
   b. Reduce the engine speed
   c. Decrease amount of paste or abrasive
   d. Increase the amount of time spent on each surface

8. Which of the following is considered a disadvantage of the porte polisher?
   a. Portability of unit
   b. Generation of minimal frictional heat
   c. Slow, tedious process
   d. Minimal aerosols produced

9. Which of the following effects does polishing of unexposed root surfaces during a surgical procedure have on disease?
   a. Cosmetic effect
   b. Therapeutic effect
   c. Placebo effect

SUGGESTED AGENCIES AND WEB SITES

Because of the ever-changing nature of the Internet, some of the web sites listed here may have changed since publication. Please refer to Mosby's Evolve web site for the most current information.

Academy of Dental Materials:
http://www.academydentalmaterials.org

American Academy of Cosmetic Dentistry: http://www.aacd.com

 ADDITIONAL READINGS AND RESOURCES

Barnes CM: The management of aerosols with airpolishing delivery systems, *J Dent Hyg* 65(6):280-2, 1991.

Brothwell DJ, Jutai DKG, Hawkins RJ: An update of mechanical oral hygiene practices: Evidence based recommendations for disease prevention, *J Can Dent Assoc* 64(4):295-306, 1998.

Gutman ME: Airpolishing: A comprehensive review of the literature, *J Dent Hyg* 72(3):47-56, 1998.

McGuire MK, Miller LM: Maintaining esthetic restorations in the periodontal practice, *Intl J Periodont Restor Dent* 16(3):230-9, 1996.

Primosch RE: Rubber cup prophylaxis: A re-evaluation of its use in pediatric dental patients, *J Dent Hyg* 11:525-7, 1980.

 REFERENCES

1. Atkinson DR, Cobb CM, Killoy WJ: The effect of an airpowder abrasive system on in vitro root surfaces, *J Periodontol* 55(1):13-8, 1984.
2. Augthun M, Tinschert J, Huber A: In vitro studies on the effect of cleaning methods on different implant surfaces, *J Periodontol* 69(8):857-64, 1998.
3. Baker DJ: Effects of rubber cup polishing and an air abrasive system on plaque accumulation, *Dent Hyg* 62:55, 1988 (abstract).
4. Barnes CM, Fleming LS, Meuninghoff LA: An SEM evaluation of the in-vitro effects of an air-abrasive system on various implant surfaces, *Int J Oral Maxillofac Implants* 6:463-9, 1991.
5. Barnes CM, Hayes EF, Leinfelder KF: Effects of an airabrasive polishing system on restored surfaces, *Gen Dent* 35(3):186-9, 1987.
6. Barnes CM: The management of aerosols with airpolishing delivery systems, *J Dent Hyg* 65(6):280-2, 1991.
7. Bay NL et al: Effectiveness of antimicrobial mouthrinses on aerosols produced by an air polisher, *J Dent Hyg* 67:312-7, 1993.
8. Berkstein S et al: Supragingival root surface removal during maintenance procedures utilizing an air-powder abrasive system or hand scaling, *J Periodontol* 58:327-330, 1987.
9. Boyde A: Airpolishing effects on enamel, dentine and cementum, *Br Dent J* 55:486-8, 1984.
10. Brocklehurst PR, Joshi RI, Northeast SE: The effect of airpolishing occlusal surfaces on the penetration of fissures by a sealant, *Intl J Ped Dent* 2:157-2, 1992.
11. Cooley RL, Lubow RM, Atrissi GA: The effect of an airpowder abrasive instrument on composite resin, *J Am Dent Assoc* 112(3):362-4, 1986.
12. Cooley RL, Lubow RM, Patrissi GA: The effect of an air-powder abrasive on glass ionomer microleakage, *Gen Dent* 37(1):16-8, 1989.
13. Council on Dental Materials, Instruments and Equipment, Status report: Effect of acidulated phosphate fluoride on porcelain and composite restorations, *J Am Dent Assoc* 116:115, 1988.
14. Davis WR: Cleaning, polishing and abrasion of teeth by dental products, *Cosmet Sci* 1:38, 1978.
15. Dean MC, Douglas MB, Blank LW: A comparison of two prophylaxis angles; disposable and autoclavable, *J Am Dent Assoc* 128(4);444-2, 1997.
16. Dunipace AJ et al: An in situ interproximal model for studying the effect of fluoride on enamel, *Caries Res* 31(1):60-70, 1997.
17. Featherstone JD: Prevention and reversal of dental caries: role of low level fluoride, *Community Dent Oral Epidemiol* 27(1):31-40, 1999.
18. Felton DA et al: Effect of air-powder abrasives on marginal configurations of porcelain-fused-to-metal alloys: An SEM analysis, *J Prosth Dent* 65:38-43, 1991.
19. Galloway SE, Pashley DH: Rate of removal of root structure by the use of the prophy-jet device, *J Periodontol* 58(7):464-9, 1987.
20. Garcia-Godoy F, Medlock JW: An SEM study of the effects of air-polishing on fissure surfaces, *Quint Int* 7:465-7, 1988.
21. Gerbo LR, Barnes CM, Leinfelder KF: Applications of the air-powder polisher in clinical orthodontics, *Am J Ortho Dentofac Ortho* 103:71-3, 1993.
22. Gilman RS, Maxey BR: The effect of root detoxification on human gingival fibroblasts, *J Periodontol* 57(7):436-40, 1986.
23. Glenwright HD, Knibbs PJ, Burdon DW: Atmospheric contamination during use of an air polisher, *Br Dent J* 159(9):294-7, 1985.
24. Gonzalez E, et al: Decrease in reflectance of porcelains treated with APF gels, *Dent Mater* 4(5):289-95, 1988.
25. Homiak AW, Cook PA, DeBoer J: Effect of hygiene instrumentation on titanium abutments; A scanning electron microscopy study, *J Prosth Dent* 67:364-9, 1992.
26. Horning GM, Cobb CM, Killoy WI: Effect of an air-powder abrasive system on root surfaces in periodontal surgery, *J Clin Periodontol* 14(4):213-20, 1987.
27. Hosoya Y, Johnston JW: Evaluation of various cleaning and polishing methods on primary enamel, *J Pedodont* 13(3):253-69, 1989.
28. Huennekens SC, Daniel SC, Bayne SC: Effects of air polishing on the abrasion of occlusal sealants, *Quint Int* 22(7):581-5, 1991.
29. Hunter KM. Et al: Ferguson MM: Bacteraemia and tissue damage resulting from air polishing, *Br Dent J* 167(8):275-8, 1989.
30. Jefferies SR: The art and science of abrasive finishing and polishing in restorative dentistry, *Dent Clin North Am* 42(4):613-27, 1998.
31. Kee A, Allen DS: Effects of air and rubber cup polishing on enamel abrasion, (abstract), *Dent Hyg* 62:55, 1988.

Continued

32. Konturri-Nahri V, Markkanen S, Markkanen H: Gingival effects of dental airpolishing as evaluated by scanning electron microscopy, *J Periodontol* 60:19-22, 1989.

33. Krupa CM et al: In vitro evaluation of air-powder polishing as an adjunct to ultrasonic scaling on periodontally involved root surfaces, *Dent Hyg* 62:55, 1988.

34. Leknes KN, Lie T: Influence of polishing procedures on sonic scaling root surface roughness, *J Periodontol* 62:659-62, 1991.

35. Lobene RR: Effects of dentifrices on tooth stains with controlled brushing, *J Am Dent Assoc* 77(4):849-55, 1968.

36. Lubow RM, Cooley RL: Effect of air-powder abrasive instrument on restorative materials, *J Prosthet Dent* 55(4):462-5, 1986.

37. Marinelli CB et al: An in vitro comparison of three fluoride regimens on enamel remineralization, *Caries Res* 31(6):418-22, 1997.

38. McGuire MK, Miller LM: Maintaining esthetic restorations in the periodontal practice, *Intl J Periodont Restor Dent* 16(3):230-9, 1996.

39. Mellberg JR: Enamel fluoride and its anti-caries effects, *J Prev Dent* 4(1):8-20, 1977.

40. Miller LM: Porcelain veneer protection plan: maintenance procedures for all porcelain restorations, *J Esthetic Dent* 2(3):63-6, 1990.

41. Mishkin DJ et al: A clinical comparison of the effect on the gingiva of the Prophy-Jet and the rubber cup and paste techniques, *J Periodontol* 57(3):151-4, 1986.

42. Moffitt JM et al: Prediction of tetracycline-induced tooth discoloration, *J Am Dent Assoc* 88(3):547-52, 1974.

43. Molinari JA: Face masks: effective personal protection, *Compend Cont Educ Dent* 17(9):818-21, 1996.

44. Muzzin KB, King TB, Berry CW: Assessing the clinical effectiveness of an aerosol reduction device for the air polisher, *J Am Dent Assoc* 130(9):1354-9, 1999.

45. Nash LB: Maximizing aesthetic restorations: the hygienist's role, *Pract Periodont Aesthet Dent* 3(3):17-8, 1991.

46. Ness L, Rosekrans DL, Welford JF: An epidemiologic study of factors affecting extrinsic staining of teeth in an English population, *Community Dent Oral Epidemiol* 5(1):55-60, 1977.

47. O'Brien W, Ryge G: *An outline of dental materials and their selection*, Philadelphia, 1978, WB Saunders.

48. Patterson CJ, McLundie AC: A comparison of the effects of two different prophylaxis regimes in vitro on some restorative dental materials: a preliminary SEM study, *Br Dent J* 157(5):166-70, 1984.

49. Rapley JW et al: The surface characteristics produced by various oral hygiene instruments and materials on titanium implant abutments, *Int J Oral Maxillofac Implants* 5(1):47-52, 1990.

50. Rawson RD et al: Alkalosis as a potential complication of air polishing systems. A pilot study, *Dent Hyg* 59(11):500-3, 1985.

51. Reel DC et al: Effect of a hydraulic jet prophylaxis system on composites, *J Prosthet Dent* 61(4):441-5, 1989.

52. Reid JS, Beeley JA, MacDonald DG: Investigation into black extrinsic tooth stain, *J Dent Res* 56(8):895-9, 1977.

53. Retief DH et al: In vitro fluoride uptake distribution and retention by human enamel after 1- and 24-hour application of various topical fluoride agents, *J Dent Res* 59(3):573-82, 1980.

54. Scott L, Greer D: The effect of an airpolishing device on sealant bond strength, *J Prosthet Dent* 58:384-387, 1987.

55. Serio FG et al: The effect of polishing pastes on composite resin surfaces; a SEM study, *J Periodontol* 59(12):837-40, 1988.

56. Shaw L, Murray JJ: A new index for measuring extrinsic stain in clinical trials, community, *Dent Oral Epidemiol* 5(3):116-20, 1977.

57. Solheim H, Eriksen HM, Nordbo H: Chemical plaque control and extrinsic discoloration of teeth, *Acta Odontol Scand* 38(5):303-9, 1980.

58. Spierings TA, Peters MC, Plasschaert AJ: Thermal trauma to teeth, *Endodont Dent Traumatol* 1(4):123-9, 1985.

59. Steele RC et al: The effect of tooth cleaning procedures on fluoride uptake in enamel, *Pediatr Dent* 4(3):228-33, 1982.

60. Strand GV, Raadel M: The efficiency of cleaning fissures with an air-polishing instrument, *Acta Odontol Scand* 46:113-7, 1988.

61. Strassler HE, Moffitt W: The surface texture of composite resin after polishing with commercially available toothpastes, *Compend Cont Educ Dent* 8826-30, 1987.

62. Thompson RE, Way DC: Enamel loss due to prophylaxis and multiple bonding debonding of orthodontic attachments, *Am J Orthod* 79(3):282-95, 1981.

63. Thompson-Neal D, Evans GH, Meffert RM: Effects of various prophylactic treatments on titanium, sapphire, and hydroxyapatite-coated implants: an SEM study, *Int J Periodont Restor Dent* 9(4):300-11, 1989.

64. Tilliss TS, Hicks MJ: Enamel surface morphology comparison. Polishing with a toothpaste and a prophylaxis paste, *Dent Hyg* 61(3):112-5, 1987.

65. Tinanoff N et al: Effect of a pumice prophylaxis on fluorite uptake in tooth enamel, *J Am Dent Assoc* 88(2):384-9, 1974.

66. Toevs SE: Root topography following instrumentation, *J Dent Hyg* 59(8):350-4, 1985.

67. Vermilyea SG, Prasanna MK, Agar JR: Effect of ultrasonic cleaning and air polishing on porcelain labial margin restorations, *J Prosth Dent* 71:447-52, 1994.

68. Vogel RJ: Intrinsic and extrinsic discoloration of the dentition; (a literature review), *J Oral Med* 30(4):99, 1975.

69. Walsh MM et al: Effect of a rubber cup polish after scaling, *J Dent Hyg* 59(11):494-8, 1985.

70. Waring MB et al: A comparison of engine polishing and toothbrushing in minimizing dental plaque reaccumulation, *J Dent Hyg* 56(12):25-30, 1982.

71. Weaks LM et al: Clinical evaluation of the prophy-jet as an instrument for routine removal of tooth stain and plaque, *J Periodontol* 55:486-8, 1984.

72. White DJ, Chen WC, Nancollas GH: Kinetics and physical aspects of enamel remineralization—A constant composition study, *Caries Res* 22:11-9, 1988.

73. Worral SF, Knibbs PJ, Gelenwrikght HD: Methods of reducing bacterial contamination of the atmosphere arising from use of an air-polisher, *Br Dent J* 163:118-9, 1987.

74. Yagi H et al: Effects of repeated hand instrumentation on the marginal portion of a cast gold crown, *J Periodontol* 69(1):41-6, 1998.

75. Yankell S, Emling RC: Understanding dental products; what you should know and what your patient should know, *Cont Dent Educ* 1:7, 1978.

76. Yankell SL et al: Effects of chlorhexidine and four antimicrobial compounds on plaque, gingivitis, and staining in beagle dogs, *J Dent Res* 61(9):1089-93, 1982.

77. Zitterbart PA: Effectiveness of ultrasonic scalers: a literature review, *Gen Dent* 35(4):295-7, 1987.

CHAPTER 33

Periodontal Dressings *and* Suturing

Katherine Karpinia

Chapter Outline

Suture Materials
Case Studies: Suturing—Three Specific Procedures
Suture Needles
Suture Size
Suture Packaging
Suturing Techniques
   Interrupted sutures
   Continuous sutures

Sling sutures
Mattress sutures
Periosteal sutures
Suture Removal
Periodontal Dressings

Key Terms

Asbestosis
Debride
Free soft tissue graft
Frenectomy

Full-thickness periodontal flap
   (mucoperiosteal flap)
Mesothelioma
Monofilament

Multifilament
Osseous
Osseous surgery
Periodontal dressing (PAK)

Periodontal flap
Periodontal surgery
Surgical flap
Suture material

Learning Outcomes

1. Understand the basic concepts of suture materials, suture design, and suturing techniques.
2. List the available periodontal dressings and state the rationale for their use.
3. Describe the characteristics of the ideal suture material and the ideal periodontal dressing.

4. Discuss the uses, advantages, and limitations of suture materials and periodontal dressings.
5. Assist healthcare professionals in the selection, use, and removal of periodontal sutures and dressings and explain the use of these materials to patients.

After periodontal surgery, periodontal sutures are used to approximate, or bring together, soft tissues and to stabilize the closure. Clinicians use a surgical needle to guide *suture material* through oral soft tissues, thereby approximating a *surgical flap* and increasing the chances of optimal healing. Suture materials vary widely in composition and type and are selected according to the preference of the clinician and the requirements of the procedure. Ideally, sutures function as passive tools; they exert no active control over a *periodontal flap.*

In most cases traumatized tissues have a higher risk of compromised wound healing;[5] therefore the surgical technique is a more important factor than the type of suture selected. A flap that is designed accurately, handled gently,

and positioned carefully will keep its position independent of the suture material or suturing technique. The dental suture and suture knots should be positioned to prevent irritation and should be tied snugly, not tightly, to ensure minimal tissue tension.

SUTURE MATERIALS

Suture materials are classified as absorbable or nonabsorbable, natural, or synthetic (Box 33-1). Absorbable sutures often are selected when suture removal is uncertain or undesirable (e.g., as with small children, a sensitive area, or placement beneath an external flap) or when the difficulty of suture removal outweighs the advantage (e.g.,

33-A

Suturing—Three Specific Procedures

Case 1: Aesthetic Treatment for a Lost Tooth

Henry Augsberger, a 21-year-old male patient, came to the clinic seeking aesthetic treatment for a lost tooth. At age 8 he experienced trauma to the anterior maxilla while playing baseball. Subsequently, the maxillary left central incisor was lost and the underlying bone resorbed, leaving an obvious concavity. Mr. Augsberger requested aesthetic recontouring of the facial maxilla adjacent to the tooth loss site. After considering the treatment options, he chose a *free soft tissue graft* procedure.

Black silk sutures (size 4-0) were used for the procedure. The graft was stabilized with interrupted sutures at the inferior lateral borders, and overlapping figure-X periosteal sutures were placed across the graft's surface (Fig. 33-1). A surgical dressing was not used after suturing was completed.

Case 2: Suturing for a Periodontal Flap Procedure

A periodontal flap procedure and *osseous surgery* were performed on a systemically healthy 58-year-old female patient, Marti Martinez, after completion of initial periodontal therapy. The goals of surgical treatment were to reduce the pocket depth, *debride* root surfaces, and recontour *osseous* defects, thereby improving the long-term prognosis for tooth retention. A *full-thickness periodontal flap (mucoperiosteal flap)* procedure was the surgical method chosen.

A continuous interlocking suture technique was used to approximate facial and lingual soft tissue flaps. The continuous interlocking suture also was used to obtain primary flap closure over the mesial and distal edentulous ridge adjacent to the remaining molar tooth (Fig. 33-2). The entire surgical area was covered with a *periodontal dressing (PAK)* after the procedure.

Case 3: Suturing after Frenum Removal

Before orthodontic closure of a diastema between the maxillary central incisor teeth, a 33-year-old male patient, Cary Fienstra, was advised to have a large maxillary anterior frenum (Fig. 33-3) surgically removed. Excessive musculature and interproximal penetration of the frenum inhibited mesial tooth movement and would have impaired long-term retention after orthodontic treatment. A *frenectomy* was the surgical treatment selected.

Simple interrupted sutures of 4-0 chromic gut were used to approximate the soft tissue borders (Fig. 33-4). A periodontal dressing was not used after the procedure.

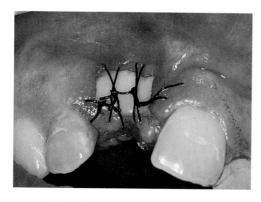

FIG. 33-1 Periosteal suture (silk) secures a free soft tissue graft.

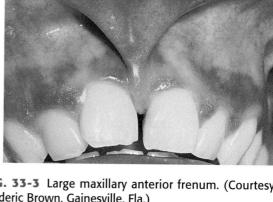

FIG. 33-3 Large maxillary anterior frenum. (Courtesy Dr. Frederic Brown, Gainesville, Fla.)

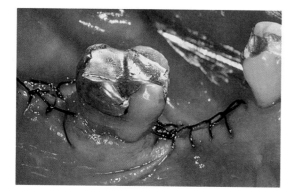

FIG. 33-2 Continuous locking suture (silk) approximates a facial and a lingual periodontal flap.

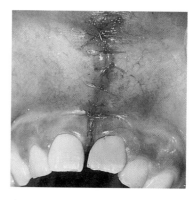

FIG. 33-4 After a frenectomy is performed, simple interrupted sutures (chromic gut) approximate the soft tissue borders. (Courtesy of Dr. Frederic Brown, Gainesville, Fla.)

with limited access, patient anxiety, or postoperative discomfort). Absorbable sutures are manufactured from the collagen of healthy mammals or from synthetic polymers. Absorbable types of suture include plain gut, chromic gut, catgut, polyglycolic acid (Dexon), polyglactin 910 (coated Vicryl), and poliglecaprone 25 (Monocryl; Figs. 33-5, 33-6, and 33-7).

Nonabsorbable sutures improve suture retention over a long period. This type characteristically retains its tensile strength longer, giving the wound sufficient time to heal. Nonabsorbable sutures are especially useful in implant and regenerative procedures. Types of nonabsorbable sutures include silk, plain and chromic collagen, polypropylene, polyester, nylon (Ethilon), and polytetrafluoroethylene (Gore; Fig. 33-8).

The suture material most often used in dentistry is silk.[4] However, no single suture material is recommended by every surgeon within a specialty. Silk sutures are specially processed to provide optimal handling and knot security without excessive capillarity. *Multifilament* sutures, especially silk, have exceptional handling characteristics: flexibility, pliability, ease of manipulation, and superior knot holding. *Monofilament* sutures (i.e., nylon, polypropylene, and gut) generally are stronger and more durable than multifilament sutures and cause less tissue inflammation. However, monofilament sutures are more difficult to manipulate and have inferior knot security. When the

Absorbable Sutures		
Type	Size	Needle
Chromic gut	3-0	⅜ Circle, reverse-cutting
Chromic gut	4-0	⅜ Circle, reverse-cutting
Chromic gut	5-0	⅜ Circle, reverse-cutting
Chromic gut	6-0	⅜ Circle, reverse-cutting

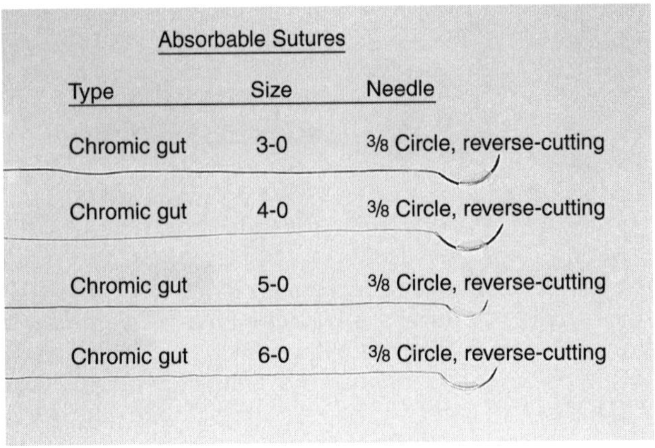

FIG. 33-6 Chromic gut sutures.

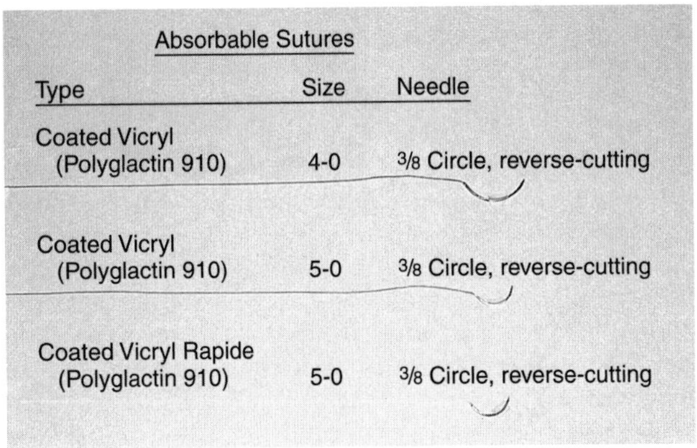

BOX 33-1

Common Suture Materials

Nonabsorbable Sutures
Natural material
Silk
Plain collagen
Chromic collagen
Synthetic material
Polypropylene
Polyester
Nylon
Polytetrafluoroethylene (PTFE)
Absorbable Sutures
Natural material
Plain gut
Chromic gut
Cat gut
Synthetic material
Polyglycolic acid
Polyglactin 910
Poliglecaprone 25

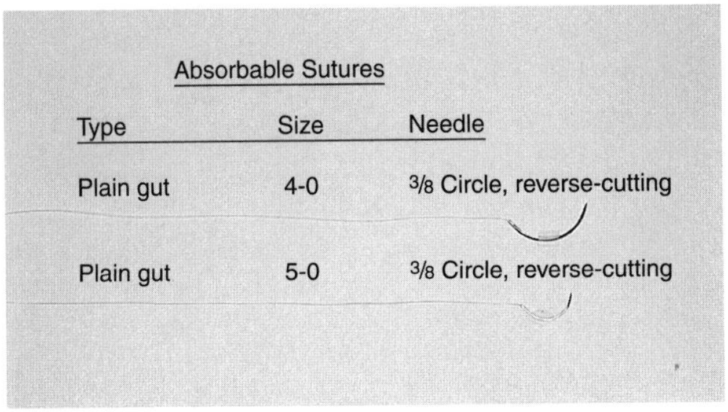

Absorbable Sutures		
Type	Size	Needle
Coated Vicryl (Polyglactin 910)	4-0	⅜ Circle, reverse-cutting
Coated Vicryl (Polyglactin 910)	5-0	⅜ Circle, reverse-cutting
Coated Vicryl Rapide (Polyglactin 910)	5-0	⅜ Circle, reverse-cutting

FIG. 33-7 Examples of absorbable suture materials.

Absorbable Sutures		
Type	Size	Needle
Plain gut	4-0	⅜ Circle, reverse-cutting
Plain gut	5-0	⅜ Circle, reverse-cutting

FIG. 33-5 Plain gut sutures.

Nonabsorbable Sutures		
Type	Size	Needle
Silk	3-0	⅜ Circle, reverse-cutting
Silk	4-0	⅜ Circle, reverse-cutting
Silk	5-0	⅜ Circle, reverse-cutting
Polypropylene	5-0	⅜ Circle, reverse-cutting
Polyviolene	5-0	⅜ Circle, reverse-cutting

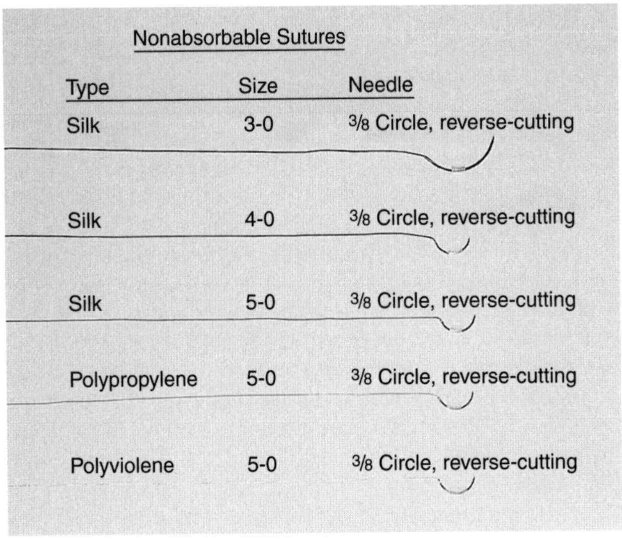

FIG. 33-8 Examples of nonabsorbable suture materials.

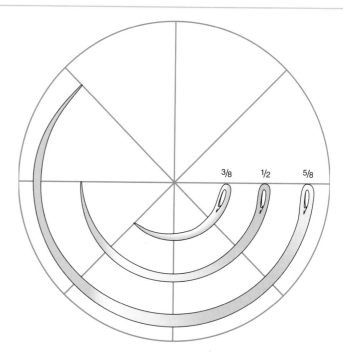

FIG. 33-9 Suture needles are measured as a portion of a complete circle.

reactions of oral tissues to polytetrafluoroethylene (PTFE) suture and silk suture were compared, inflammatory infiltrate increased over a 7-day period for both types of suture. The inflammation appeared more intense with the silk suture.[6] In a comparison of silk, chromic gut, PTFE, and polyglactin 910 suture materials, silk sutures seemed to allow the greatest bacterial migration.[9] PTFE sutures appeared to be the most tissue-friendly.

Unfortunately, the ideal suture material does not exist. However, many types of suture material offer outstanding characteristics and are relatively close to the ideal (Box 33-2).

Natural absorbable sutures (gut) are digested by body enzymes and macrophages. These sutures are made of highly purified collagen from sheep, cattle, or feline intestines. Synthetic absorbable sutures are hydrophobic and eventually are broken down by hydrolysis, a process in which water penetrates the suture material and breaks down its polymer chain. This process correlates with a leukocytic cellular response that removes suture material and cellular debris from the wound area. Some absorbable sutures are chemically structured or manipulated to lengthen the absorption time. For example, chromic gut suture is treated with a chromium salt solution that enhances its resistance to proteolytic enzymes.[4]

SUTURE NEEDLES

Because of the restricted access in the oral cavity, suture needles have a rounded shape. The needle is composed of a point, a body, and an attachment end for the suture material. Most attachment ends are swaged; that is, the suture material is press-fit, or fused to, the metal needle, resulting in less tissue trauma when the needle pulls the suture through tissue. The needle's point generally is sharp and may be standard or taper-cut. Standard points are sharp at the tip, with the cutting ability blending with the needle body as it is engaged. Taper-cut points extend farther along the needle body and offer a more tapered, sharp, and delicate penetration through the tissue. They commonly are used for mucogingival procedures.

The body of the needle is measured in metric units or inches as a portion of a complete circle. The more commonly used needles measure ⅜ inch, ½ inch, or ⅝ inch (Fig. 33-9).[5]

The three types of suture needles are conventional cutting suture needles, reverse cutting suture needles, and taper-cut suture needles. A reverse cutting suture needle is triangular in cross-section (similar to a sickle scaler), has three cutting edges, and is drawn through the tissue with the base of the triangle facing the coronal aspect of the soft tissue. The broad triangular base creates a wide area of enhanced tissue resistance, reducing the risk of the suture material tearing soft tissue as pressure is applied to move and tie the suture. Conversely, conventional cutting suture needles are passed through the soft tissue with the base of the triangular needle facing the apical aspect of the soft tissue. As a result, a narrow V is created at the point where the greatest pressure is exerted when the suture is pulled and tied; this configuration poses a greater risk of tissue tearing and suture loss (Fig. 33-10).

SUTURE SIZE

Suture size is classified by the diameter of the suture's surface material and is stated numerically by the number of zeros. Size is measured in decreasing diameter from 1-0 (pronounced *one-oh*), the largest, to 11-0, the smallest. For example, 5-0 (00000) suture is smaller in diameter than 4-0 (0000) suture. The smaller the suture size, the less tensile strength the suture material has. The suture size most commonly used in dentistry is 4-0, although 5-0 suture often is used for mucogingival procedures (see Figs. 33-5 through 33-8).

SUTURE PACKAGING

When packaging sutures, manufacturers provide an outer, nonsterile covering and an inner, sterile cover that holds the suture needle and material (Fig. 33-11). This packaging technique makes it easier to maintain a sterile surgical field. Nonsterile hands may grasp the outer covering and carefully open the package, allowing the inside sterile package to contact (drop into) the surgical instrument field (Fig. 33-12). Dual packaging is convenient and helps prevent cross-contamination.

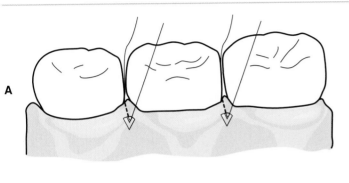

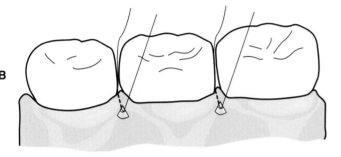

A

B

FIG. 33-10 Triangular cross-section of a needle. **A,** Reverse cutting needle with a broad triangular base facing the coronal aspect of the soft tissue. **B,** Conventional cutting needle with a narrow V facing the coronal aspect of the soft tissue.

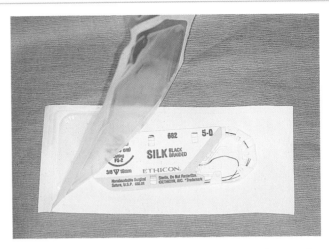

FIG. 33-12 The outer, nonsterile suture wrapping can be opened and the inner, sterile package allowed to drop onto the surgical instrument tray.

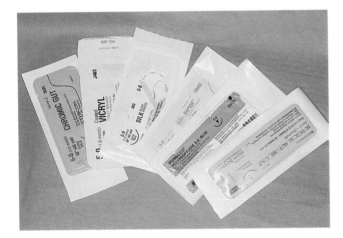

FIG. 33-11 Suture packaging made up of a sterile inner package and a nonsterile outer wrapping.

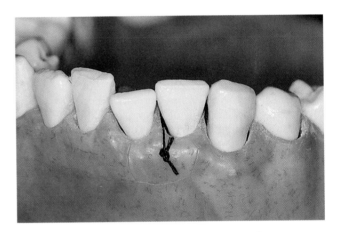

FIG. 33-13 Simple interrupted loop suture (facial view).

SUTURING TECHNIQUES

When suturing periodontal flaps, the clinician inserts the needle through the soft tissue flap approximately 3 mm from the gingival margin. Care must be taken not to drag the suture material through the flap or exert excessive pressure on the wound edge, thereby injuring the flap or tearing through the wound margin. Once the suture has been tied, suture scissors are used to cut the ends to a comfortable length, leaving approximately 2 mm of free suture adjacent to the knot.

Several different techniques can be used to place sutures. Some commonly used suturing techniques are described in the following sections.

INTERRUPTED SUTURES

The simple interrupted loop suture technique and the simple interrupted figure-eight modification of that technique are the methods most commonly used to close flaps. For a simple interrupted loop pattern, the needle enters through the facial flap from the outer epithelial surface toward the underlying bone, passes through the interdental area, penetrates the lingual flap from its inner osseous undersurface, and exits the outer epithelial surface. The clinician ends the loop by passing the needle back through the interdental area and tying a knot on the facial surface (Figs. 33-13 and 33-14), creating a suture circle, or loop. In Case #3, a simple interrupted loop suture technique was used to approximate the wound margins after removal of the maxillary anterior frenum.

For the figure-eight modification of the simple interrupted loop suture pattern, the steps are the same as those

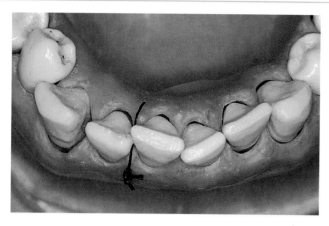

FIG. 33-14 Simple interrupted loop suture (incisal view).

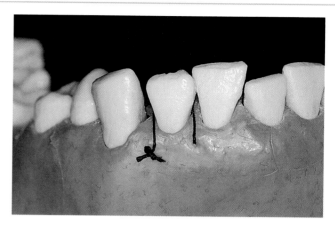

FIG. 33-15 Single interproximal sling suture (facial view).

for the simple loop pattern with one exception: the needle penetrates the lingual flap from its outer epithelial surface and exits the flap's inner osseous surface before being returned to the facial area to be tied. Completion of the suture knot creates the figure-eight form.

CONTINUOUS SUTURES

Continuous sutures join multiple papillae on one flap to an adjacent flap in an uninterrupted fashion, or they allow independent suturing of a periodontal flap. The continuous simple loop suture pattern may be extended to include many adjacent interdental spaces. The needle penetrates the facial flap and passes through the lingual flap, and the pattern continues in this manner until a knot is tied at the termination of the suture. The continuous locking suture technique uses a single interrupted suture first. Subsequently the needle is passed through the outer surface of the facial flap and the inner surface of the lingual flap, forming a loop. The needle then is passed through the loop, and the suture is pulled snugly. This pattern of locking each loop is continued until a knot is tied at the termination of the suture.

 Case #2 Application
The continuous interlocking suture technique was used to secure Mrs. Martinez's facial and lingual flaps over an edentulous osseous ridge.

SLING SUTURES

The single interproximal sling suture technique is used to secure a facial or lingual flap and involves only two papillae. The needle penetrates the outer surface of the distal papilla, passes under the distal contact area, goes around the tooth and under the distal contact area, captures the mesial papilla, and returns by the aforementioned route; the suture then is tied on the facial surface (Figs. 33-15 and 33-16). The continuous independent sling suture technique, which is used for a facial or lingual flap, functions in a similar manner. It captures the adjacent facial or lingual papilla, respectively, as it "slings" individual teeth until the suture is knotted at its termination (Figs. 33-17 and 33-18). The continuous double sling suture

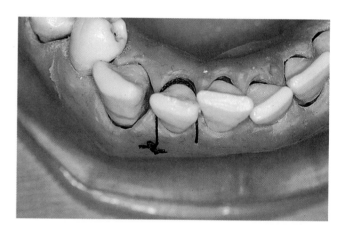

FIG. 33-16 Single interproximal sling suture (incisal view).

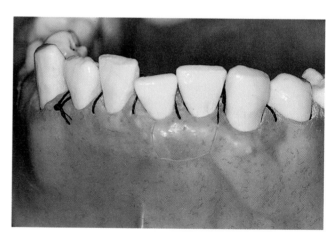

FIG. 33-17 Continuous independent sling suture (facial view).

technique involves both a facial and a lingual flap. One of the flaps, either the facial or the lingual one, is secured first. The opposite flap then is sutured identically (Figs. 33-19, 33-20, and 33-21). The continuous double sling suture requires two knots—the initial loop and the final tie. Both knots usually are located near the original insertion.

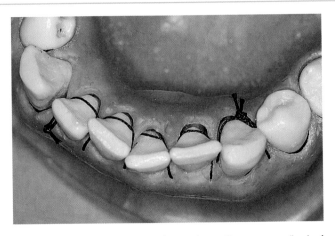

FIG. 33-18 Continuous independent sling suture (incisal view).

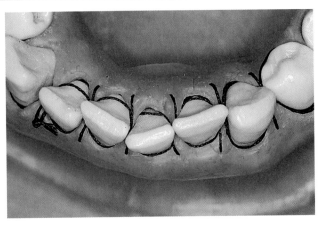

FIG. 33-20 Continuous double sling suture (incisal view).

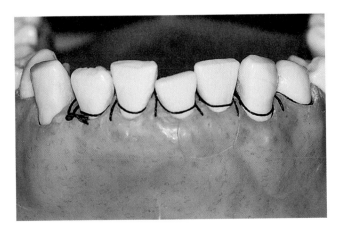

FIG. 33-19 Continuous double sling suture (facial view).

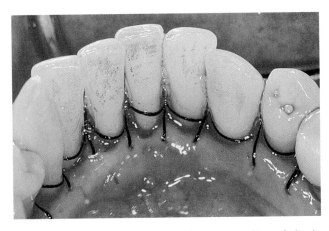

FIG. 33-21 Continuous double sling suture (lingual view).

The continuous double sling suture allows a facial flap to be positioned independently of a lingual flap.

MATTRESS SUTURES

The vertical mattress and horizontal mattress suture techniques permit precise flap placement, adapt flaps to underlying bone, resist muscle pull, and aid adaptation of wound margins. For the vertical mattress suture pattern, the first puncture is placed more apically, and the suture emerges more coronally. The suture is passed through the interproximal area, and a similar technique is used in the opposing flap. The suture is knotted near its origin (Figs. 33-22 and 33-23). The horizontal mattress suture pattern is similar except that the suture runs beneath the flap in a horizontal direction, and the emerging parallel strands cross over the interdental papillae (Figs. 33-24 and 33-25). Both techniques provide unequivocal flap control.

PERIOSTEAL SUTURES

The periosteal suture technique permits involvement of the periosteum and superficial bony surface as an option to soft tissue suturing. The needle penetrates the periosteal

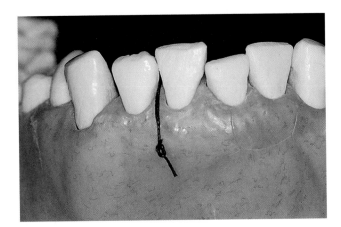

FIG. 33-22 Vertical mattress suture (facial view).

surface at a 90-degree angle and, under gentle pressure, glides along the surface of the bone. It exits the periosteum without having elevated or torn the structure. In Case #1, a periosteal suture was used to secure placement of a free soft tissue graft.

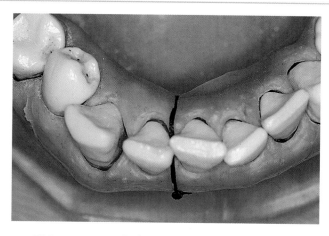

FIG. 33-23 Vertical mattress suture (incisal view).

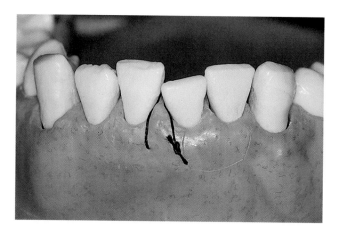

FIG. 33-24 Horizontal mattress suture (facial view).

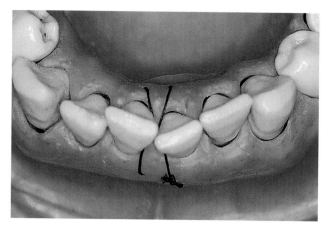

FIG. 33-25 Horizontal mattress suture (incisal view).

 SUTURE REMOVAL

33-B Suture materials become contaminated as they pass through the periodontal flap during initial placement and while they remain in the oral environment. Before sutures are removed, the surgical site should be irrigated with an antimicrobial solution, such as chlorhexidine

gluconate. If a periodontal dressing was used, the remaining dressing should be removed carefully so that healing gingival tissues are not disrupted. Suture knots are lifted carefully, and the suture strand is cut close to the gingival soft tissue. When continuous sutures are removed, each section should be cut individually to prevent the dragging of lengthy, contaminated sutures through healing flaps. Each knot is carefully secured and gently pulled away from the surgical flap, allowing short segments of suture to be guided from the surgical site with minimal discomfort to the patient. As each knot is removed, it should be placed on gauze, and all knots should be counted to ensure complete removal of the suture material. Most sutures are removed 7 to 10 days after placement.

PERIODONTAL DRESSINGS

Periodontal dressings first were introduced in 1923 by Dr. A.W. Ward.[8] Dr. Ward's Wondr-Pak consisted of zinc oxide–eugenol (ZOE) mixed with pine oil, asbestos, and alcohol.

The use of periodontal dressings arose from a desire to protect surgical sites from trauma, which also increased the patient's comfort, prevented wound contamination by oral debris, stabilized periodontal flaps, and immobilized soft tissue grafts. Other advantages included tooth desensitization, tooth splinting, and attempts to prevent excessive proliferation of granulation tissues. Tannic acid was added to periodontal dressings to facilitate hemostasis[3] but later was removed because of the possible risk of liver damage if it were absorbed systemically. Asbestos was removed because of the risk of *asbestosis*, lung cancer, and *mesothelioma.*

ZOE dressings contain approximately 40% to 50% eugenol and in the past were popular because of their anodyne effects on sensitive dentin and gingival soft tissues.[10] However, eugenol, which increases in amount as zinc eugenate decomposes, has been shown to contribute to delayed healing, inflammatory or allergic reactions, and tissue necrosis.[8,10] When set, eugenol dressings have a hard, brittle consistency, with sharp edges and minimal flexibility. Most modern periodontal dressings are formulated without eugenol.[7]

The characteristics of an ideal periodontal dressing are as follows (Box 33-3):
- Set slowly enough to allow adequate manipulation yet be firm enough to maintain the desired shape
- Have smooth, nonirritating surfaces
- Maintain its flexibility to withstand distortion and displacement without fracturing
- Hold its dimensional stability to prevent leakage and the accumulation of debris.[10]
- Be nonallergenic
- Inhibit bacterial growth
- Have an acceptable taste

Some widely used dressings that do not contain eugenol are Coe-Pak Periodontal Dressing (GC America, Inc., Alsip, Ill.; Fig. 33-26), Zone Periodontal Pak (Cadco Dental Products, Oxnard, Calif.; Fig. 33-27), Periocare Periodontal Dressing (Pulpdent Corp., Watertown, Mass.) Peripac Periodontal Pac (Dentsply Preventive Care, York, Pa.), and Barricaid Visible-Light-Cure Periodontal Dress-

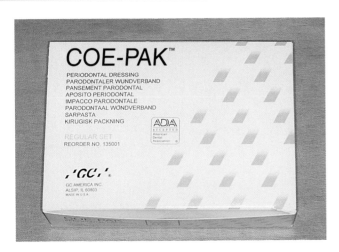

FIG. 33-26 Coe-Pak Periodontal Dressing (GC America, Inc., Alsip, Ill.).

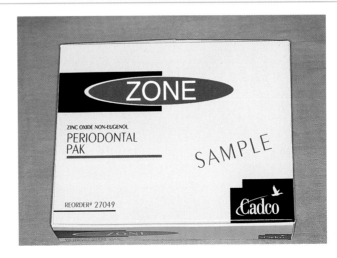

FIG. 33-27 Zone Periodontal Pak (Cadco Dental Products, Oxnard, Calif.).

BOX 33-3

Ideal Properties of a Periodontal Dressing

Able to set slowly enough to allow adequate manipulation

Firm enough to maintain the required shape

Smooth, nonirritating surfaces

Able to maintain its flexibility to withstand distortion and displacement without fracturing

Able to hold its dimensional stability to prevent leakage and the accumulation of debris

Able to inhibit bacterial growth

Nonallergenic

Acceptable taste

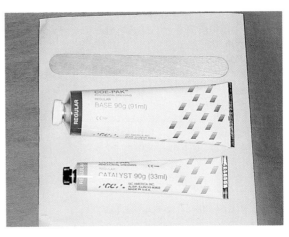

FIG. 33-28 Coe-Pak Periodontal Dressing tubes separate the base *(top)* and the catalyst *(bottom)* before a periodontal dressing is mixed.

ing (Dentsply Preventive Care, York, Pa.). Zone Periodontal Pak, Coe-Pak, and Periocare are prepared for oral use as equal lengths of a paste (catalyst) and a gel (base) are extruded from individual tubes (Figs. 33-28 and 33-29). The extruded materials are thoroughly spatulated on a special mixing pad, and the cohesive product is shaped into a cylindrical rope or log form and carefully molded to fit the surgical site (Figs. 33-30 and 33-31). Peripac is distributed in a ready-to-use form that does not require mixing before placement. Barricaid is a single-component, light-activated periodontal dressing supplied in a syringe that can be used outside the mouth as a wound dressing or as a disposable dispenser for intraoral application of material directly onto the wound site.

During placement of any periodontal dressing, care should be taken to prevent the dressing from extending onto occlusal or incisal surfaces (interfering with occlusion) or from projecting apically, past the mucogingival junction, possibly leading to mucosal irritation. Periodontal dressings become semirigid after setting and can withstand some chewing forces without fracturing. Patients should be instructed to eat semisolid foods (e.g., cooked

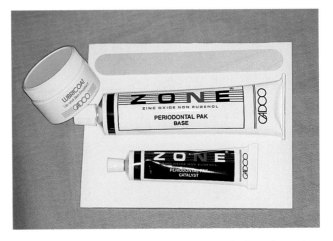

FIG. 33-29 The Zone Periodontal Pak includes a base *(top tube),* a catalyst *(bottom tube),* and a lip and skin emollient *(jar at left).*

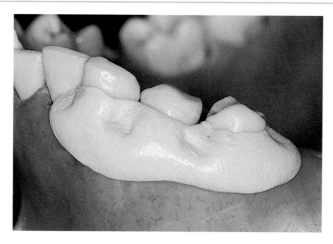

FIG. 33-30 Intraoral placement of a Coe-Pak Periodontal Dressing.

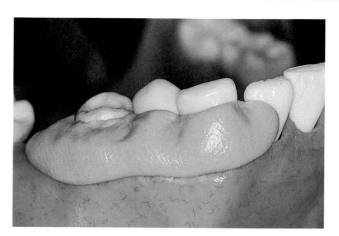

FIG. 33-31 Intraoral placement of a Zone Periodontal Pak.

vegetables, pasta, soft meats, and fish) and generally to avoid eating or tooth brushing on the side where the dressing is located. Many clinicians prescribe an antimicrobial rinse (chlorhexidine gluconate) for the patient to use while the dressing is in place.

Whether to use a dressing after ***periodontal surgery*** is a choice made by the individual clinician.[1,2]

 Case Application
No periodontal dressings were used for either Mr. Augsberger or Mr. Fienstra. However, a surgical dressing was placed on Mrs. Martinez after the procedure.

Most periodontal dressings are removed from the oral cavity within 5 to 10 days of placement. When periodontal dressings are removed, clinician gently dislodges the dressing from the surgical area with a sterile instrument, such as a cotton forceps, taking care to ensure that the sutures themselves are not caught within the dressing. The surgical site should be clean, and the dressing should come off neatly in one large piece or in large individual sections. After the dressing has been removed, the sutures are removed (see the previous section on suture removal), and the postoperative care instructions to be followed at home are explained to the patient.

 RITICAL THINKING ACTIVITIES

1. Manipulate several different types of suture materials and compare their characteristics, sizes, and handling abilities.
2. Visit a periodontal office and observe periodontal suture and dressing placement and removal.
3. Practice placing and removing various periodontal sutures and dressings using a model, an animal jaw (e.g., pig), or another object (e.g., hot dog).
4. Discuss the knowledge you acquired in this chapter with fellow students and paraphrase or restate in your own words the information that is critical to your own practice philosophy.
5. Make up several types of cases and compare the advantages and disadvantages of different suture materials and periodontal dressings under each set of circumstances.

 REVIEW QUESTIONS

Question 2 and 7 refer to the case studies presented at the beginning of the chapter.

1. Which of the following is an example of an absorbable suture material?
   a. Silk
   b. Polypropylene
   c. Nylon
   d. Gut

2. Which suture material was used to support Mr. Augsberger's soft tissue graft?
   a. Chromic gut
   b. Plain gut
   c. Silk
   d. Nylon

REVIEW QUESTIONS—cont'd

3. Which is the most commonly used suture material in dentistry?
   a. Chromic gut
   b. Silk
   c. Plain gut
   d. Polyester
4. Which of the following are characteristics of an ideal suture material?
   a. Inhibits bacterial growth
   b. Has a small diameter but great strength
   c. Is comfortable to use and easy to manipulate
   d. Is sterile and conveniently packaged
   e. All the above
5. Are modern periodontal dressings usually formulated without eugenol?
   a. Yes
   b. No

6. Which of the following are characteristics of the ideal periodontal dressing?
   a. Sets slowly enough to allow easy manipulation
   b. Maintains it flexibility to prevent easy fracture and withstand distortion
   c. Has an acceptable taste
   d. All of the above
7. Which of the following types of suturing technique was used in for Mrs. Martinez?
   a. Continuous interlocking suture
   b. Simple interrupted loop suture
   c. Continuous double sling suture
   d. Periosteal suture

SUGGESTED AGENCIES AND WEB SITES

Because of the ever-changing nature of the Internet, the web site listed here may have changed since publication. Please refer to Mosby's Evolve web site for the most current information.

North Carolina State University ("Biomedical applications of textiles; Sutures"): http://www.bae.ncsu.edu

ADDITIONAL READINGS AND RESOURCES

American Academy of Periodontology: *Annals of periodontology,* 1996 World Workshop in Periodontics, Chicago, The Academy.

Newman MG, Carranza FA, Takei HH: *Clinical periodontology,* ed 9, Philadelphia, 2002, WB Saunders.

REFERENCES

1. Allen D, Caffesse R: Comparison of results following modified Widman flap surgery with and without surgical dressing, *J Periodontol* 54:470, 1983.
2. Jones D, Cassingham R: Comparison of healing following periodontal surgery with and without dressings in humans, *J Periodontol* 50:387, 1979.
3. Levin M: Periodontal suture materials and surgical dressings, *Dent Clin North Am* 24:767, 1980.
4. Lilly G: Reaction of oral tissues to suture materials, *Oral Surg Oral Med Oral Pathol* 26:128, 1968.
5. Meyer R, Antonini C: A review of suture materials, *Compend Cont Dent Educ* (part I) 1:260, 1989; (part II) 10:360, 1989.
6. Rivera-Hildago F et al: Tissue reaction to silk and Gore-Tex sutures in dogs, *J Periodontal Res* 70:508, 1991.
7. Rubinoff CH, Greener EH, Robinson PJ: Physical properties of periodontal dressing materials, *J Oral Rehabil* 13:575, 1986.
8. Sachs H et al: Current status of periodontal dressings, *J Periodontol* 55:689, 1984.
9. Selvig D et al: Oral tissue reactions to suture materials, *Int J Periodontol Rest Dent* 18:474, 1998.
10. von Fraunhofer J, Argyropoulos D: Properties of periodontal dressings, *Dent Mater* 6:51, 1990.

PART VII

Chapter 34
Anxiety Control

Chapter 35
Chemistry and Pharmacology of Anesthetics

Chapter 36
Local Anesthetics: Injectable and Topical

Chapter 37
Nitrous Oxide/Oxygen Sedation

Competency Statements

The learner is expected to possess knowledge, skills, judgments, values, and attitudes to develop the listed competencies.

Core Competencies
- Apply a professional code of ethics in all endeavors.
- Adhere to state and federal laws, recommendations, and regulations in the provision of dental hygiene care.
- Provide dental hygiene care to promote patient health and wellness using critical thinking and problem solving in the provision of evidence-based practice.
- Assume responsibility for dental hygiene actions and care based on accepted scientific theories and research as well as the accepted standard of care.
- Continuously perform self-assessment for life-long learning and professional growth.
- Provide quality assurance mechanisms for health services.
- Communicate effectively with individuals and groups from diverse populations both verbally and in writing.
- Provide accurate, consistent, and complete documentation for assessment, diagnosis, planning, implementation, and evaluation of dental hygiene services.
- Provide care to all patients using an individualized approach that is humane, empathetic, and caring.

Courtesy American Dental Education Association, Washington, DC.

Anxiety
and Pain Control

Health Promotion and Disease Prevention
- Respect the goals, values, beliefs, and preferences of the patient while promoting optimal oral and general health.
- Refer patients who may have a physiologic, psychological, and/or social problem for comprehensive patient evaluation.
- Identify individual and population risk factors and develop strategies that promote health related quality of life.
- Evaluate and utilize methods to ensure the health and safety of the patient and the dental hygienist in the delivery of dental hygiene.

Patient Care
- Select, obtain, and interpret diagnostic information recognizing its advantages and limitations.
- Recognize predisposing and etiologic risk factors that require intervention to prevent disease.
- Obtain, review, and update a complete medical, family, social, and dental history.
- Recognize health conditions and medications that impact overall patient care.
- Identify patients at risk for a medical emergency and manage the patient care in a manner that prevents an emergency.
- Perform a comprehensive examination using clinical, radiographic, periodontal, dental charting, and other data collection procedures to assess the patient's needs.
- Use assessment findings, etiological factors, and clinical data in determining a dental hygiene diagnosis.
- Identify patient needs and significant findings that impact the delivery of dental hygiene services.

- Obtain consultations as indicated.
- Prioritize the care plan based on the health status and the actual and potential problems of the individual to facilitate optimal oral health.
- Establish a planned sequence of care (education, clinical, and evaluation) based on the dental hygiene diagnosis; identified oral conditions; potential problems; etiologic and risk factors; and available treatment modalities.
- Establish a collaborative relationship with the patient in the planned care to include etiology, prognosis, and treatment alternatives.
- Make referrals to other healthcare professionals.
- Obtain the patient's informed consent based on a thorough case presentation.
- Control pain and anxiety during treatment through the use of accepted clinical and behavioral techniques.
- Provide life support measures to manage medical and dental emergencies in the patient care environment.
- Determine the outcomes of dental hygiene interventions using indices, instruments, examination techniques, and patient self-report.
- Evaluate the patient's satisfaction with the oral healthcare received and the oral healthcare status achieved.
- Provide subsequent treatment or referrals based on evaluation findings.
- Develop and maintain a health maintenance program.

Professional Growth and Development
- Access professional and social networks and resources to assist entrepreneurial initiatives.

CHAPTER 34

Anxiety Control

Darnyl King

Chapter Outline

Definition
Case Study: Identification and Management of
  Dental Anxiety
Etiology
Anxiety Related to Dental Hygiene Care
  Assessment
  Care planning
  Creating a positive relationship

Psychological Management
  Patient education
  Patient control
  Behavioral management
Management of Fearful Children

Key Terms

Anxiety
Biofeedback
Distraction

Fear
Hypnosis

Pain
Phobia

Relaxation
Systemic desensitization

Learning Outcomes

1. Differentiate the terms *phobia, fear,* and *anxiety.*
2. Analyze patient responses to questions in the dental history designed to detect anxiety about treatment.
3. Identify the origin of a patient's anxiety through questioning during the initial interview.
4. Identify and evaluate fear-provoking situations with a patient.
5. Recognize the signs and behaviors that indicate dental fear.
6. Evaluate the reliability of tools used to assess dental anxiety.
7. Compare psychological and behavioral strategies for managing dental anxiety.
8. Formulate a personalized treatment plan for a fearful patient, using anxiety-reducing techniques.
9. Use nonpharmacological strategies to promote patient relaxation.

Dental *anxiety* is a problem that affects many individuals. Studies indicate that 10% to 20% of the population in the United States has a moderate to high level of dental *fear.*[19,35] Treating fearful patients can be stressful,[6,9,56] challenging, and problematic for the dental care team.[10] Poor oral health, either real[14] or imagined,[26,35] has been associated with a high level of dental anxiety. Individuals with dental fear or anxiety have fewer dental appointments[22,26,31] and only sporadic checkups.[13,14,60] Individuals who experience dental anxiety more often cancel or fail to show up for appointments,[35] and when they do keep an appointment, they require more time for treatment than individuals who do

not have dental anxiety.[16] Dental school patients with a high level of dental anxiety more often did not complete planned treatment.[52]

Problem behaviors can affect the interpersonal relationship between the patient and the practitioner, the quality of care, and the probability of retaining a patient in the practice.[10] For some patients, dental anxiety presents a significant obstacle to routine care, and the consequence is poor oral health. Dental hygiene practitioners who are skilled in managing anxiety can enhance the oral care experience for such patients and increase the likelihood that treatment will be successful and that patients will comply with supportive care recommendations. Ultimately, the dental hygienist can help anxious patients achieve and maintain optimal oral health for a lifetime.

Pharmacological and nonpharmacological therapies can be used to manage anxious patients during oral care. In this chapter nonpharmacological methods, specifically psychological and behavioral strategies, are the primary focus.

DEFINITION

Anxiety, fear, and *phobia* are related terms but are conceptually different.[17,57] All generate cognitive and physiologic changes in the body, including emotional upset with catastrophic feelings, tachycardia, perspiration, muscle tension, gastrointestinal upset, and shaking. However, fear is the body's response to an immediate threat, whereas anxiety is the body's response to a threat that is not immediate. For example, anxiety is the patient's reaction when thinking about having the teeth probed; fear is the patient's reaction actually to having the teeth probed. Fear or anxiety that is irrational, persistent, and unreasonable in relation to the actual threat is a phobia. In such cases the fear or anxiety is so extreme it causes a person to completely avoid the particular object or situation, thereby interfering with normal daily functioning. In most cases phobic individuals and others with psychological problems require referral to appropriate mental health professionals before undergoing oral care.

ETIOLOGY

Past unpleasant dental experiences are cited most often as the causative factor in anxiety about and avoidance of oral care. For many anxious individuals, this fear originated from traumatic dental experiences in childhood.[28] Individuals who are not anxious or fearful about dental care seldom report having had painful or distressing dental experiences.[11] Fearful individuals avoid visits to the dental office for preventive care and seek care only for emergencies or immediate pain relief.[36] Under these circumstances, care rarely is a positive experience; it often is invasive, painful, and costly, which intensifies the patient's anxiety and avoidance behaviors. This establishes a negative cyclical pattern that is difficult to reverse[43,58] (Fig. 34-1).

Patients also often report feelings of helplessness and lack of control as sources of fear and anxiety. This viewpoint is not surprising, considering the nature of oral care. During treatment patients are reclined in the dental chair so that the head is lower than the feet. Sharp instruments and suction in the oral cavity make it difficult if not impossible for patients to communicate. Thus the patients feel as if they are in a precarious and vulnerable position.

However, some individuals who have never received dental care also show fear. Vicarious learning or stimulus generalization could explain this phenomenon. Vicarious learning occurs when anxiety is acquired by watching, listening to, or reading about the experiences of others. The most common link in vicarious fear development probably is parents to children.[37] Research has shown that many

 Case Study

Identification and Management of Dental Anxiety

A 47-year-old female patient, Sasha Uri, has arrived for a dental hygiene appointment. This is her second scheduled visit; an hour before her first appointment, she phoned to cancel. During the initial conversation, Ms. Uri seems to the hygienist to be aloof, distracted, and in a hurry. The hygienist attempts to build a rapport with Ms. Uri, but most of her questions are met with a curt *yes* or *no*. The dental history shows that the last dental visit was about 2 years ago, for extraction of an abscessed tooth. Ms. Uri could not recall the date of her last prophylaxis appointment, only that "It was several years ago." Questions related to previous unpleasant dental experiences and anxiety about dental care elicit *yes* responses.

With sensitivity and concern, the hygienist inquires about the circumstances of the patient's anxiety. Visibly relieved to be broaching the subject, Ms. Uri reveals that unpleasant childhood dental experiences have left her fearful of oral care. She says that she must force herself to go to the dental office and usually goes only for immediate *pain* relief. The inherently unpleasant nature of emergency treatment has further reinforced her aversion to dental care. Because of this her oral health has deteriorated, resulting in missing teeth, unrestored carious lesions, and early periodontal disease. Ms. Uri wants to achieve good dental health, but she is anxious and unsure whether she will be able to tolerate or follow through with treatment recommendations. How can the hygienist help this patient successfully manage her anxiety and fear allowing for a positive oral care experience?

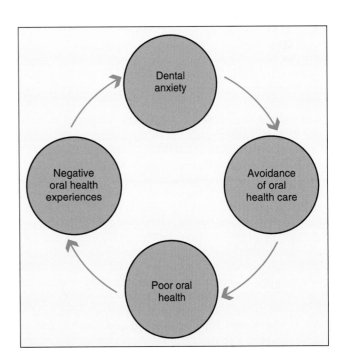

FIG. 34-1 Negative cyclical pattern of dental anxiety. (Modified from Ronis DL: Updating a measure of dental anxiety: reliability, validity, and norms. *J Dent Hyg* 68:228-33, 1994.)

fearful children have fearful parents. The mass media, with its negative portrayal of dentistry in movies, television, and print, could be responsible for the acquisition and perpetuation of dental fear in some individuals.[29] In stimulus generalization, a person who has been conditioned to respond negatively in one situation responds negatively in similar situations. "White coat syndrome" is a classic example, in which fear of the medical profession is generalized to include dental professionals who wear the same uniform.

 Case Application

From Ms. Uri's presentation, can you determine whether she is experiencing anxiety or fear or is dentally phobic? What do you suspect is the etiology of her condition?

ANXIETY RELATED TO DENTAL HYGIENE CARE

Patients report that actual pain and expected pain are major anxiety-provoking factors during care performed by dental hygienists. De Jongh and Stouthard[12] found that treatment performed by hygienists provoked as much and sometimes more anxiety than treatment performed by a dentist. Generally, low levels of pain were associated with dental hygiene treatment; however, during probing and scaling, 25% of patients reported moderate to severe pain.[55] Individuals who focused excessively on pain sensations *(catastrophizing)* were found to experience more pain during dental hygiene treatment than noncatastrophizers.[53,55] For many individuals, dental hygiene care can be a distressing event that elicits varying degrees of pain and anxiety.

ASSESSMENT

Initially, front-office employees should screen for anxiety-related behaviors (e.g., pacing, frequent changes in sitting position, or repetitious hand or leg movements) while the patient is in the reception area (Box 34-1).[38,56,57] If any of these behaviors are noted, the hygienist should be informed that the patient may have dental anxiety. The patient should complete a comprehensive dental history that includes questions designed to identify anxiety, and the hygienist should thoroughly review the history (Box 34-2). However, the hygienist must keep in mind that, possibly because of embarrassment or denial, not all patients are candid in their answers.

At this juncture, patients known or thought to be anxious should be given a dental anxiety questionnaire to determine the degree of anxiety. One of the more popular and widely used instruments is Corah's *Dental Anxiety Scale (DAS),*[7] which consists of four multiple-choice questions related to dental treatment scenarios. Points are given to correspond with the response selected. For example, one point is given for selecting a response to question #1, two points for a response to question #2, and so on. A patient's cumulative DAS score, which can range from 4 (no anxiety) to 20 (high anxiety), represents anticipatory anxiety before treatment. A modification of the DAS, called the *Dental Anxiety Scale–Revised (DAS-R),* has eliminated gender-specific terminology and recognizes dental hygienists, as well as dentists, as oral care providers (Fig. 34-2).[43]

BOX 34-1

Anxious Behaviors in the Reception Area

Fidgeting
Repetitious hand or leg movements
Sitting on the edge of the chair
Pacing
Frequent changes in sitting position
Frequent visits to the rest room
Rapid turning of magazine pages
Startled reaction to office noises

BOX 34-2

Sample Dental History Questions Designed to Identify Anxiety

1. Did your parents have a positive attitude about dental care?
2. Do you recall any past unpleasant dental experiences?
3. Do you have your teeth cleaned at least once a year?
4. How long has it been since your last dental visit?
5. What kind of treatment did you receive? How did it feel?
6. Do you have concerns about your oral health or about receiving treatment?
7. Have you been satisfied with your dental providers?
8. Have you been satisfied with previous dental work?
9. What dental procedures have you received in the past?
10. Are you anxious about receiving care? If so, what is your level of anxiety?

During the initial interview with the patient, the hygienist should sensitively ask questions directed toward discovering the circumstances of the patient's anxiety and determining which strategies might be helpful in reducing that discomfort (Box 34-3).[57] The hygienist should take notes while the patient is talking to demonstrate interest and concern. The hygienist then summarizes and reflects what the patient has said, giving the individual the opportunity to correct any misinterpretations. At this point the hygienist should reassure the patient that his or her concerns are being taken seriously, that dealing with dental anxiety is an element of providing care, and that the hygienist is trained in anxiety management techniques. The purpose of the initial interview is threefold: to build rapport and trust, to gather additional pertinent information, and to reduce fear.

Physiological and behavioral indicators can reveal anxiety in patients during treatment (Box 34-4). However, after commencing therapy is not the ideal time for hygienists to discover that they are working with a fearful patient. Knowing about the patient's condition beforehand allows the hygienist to incorporate anxiety-reducing strategies into the care plan.

Item 1

If you had to go to the dentist tomorrow for a checkup, how would you feel about it?

1. I would look forward to it as a reasonably enjoyable experience.

2. I wouldn't care one way or the other.

3. I would be a little uneasy about it.

4. I would be afraid that it would be unpleasant and painful.

5. I would be very frightened of what the dentist would do.

Item 2

When you are waiting in the dentist's office for your turn in the chair, how do you feel?

1. Relaxed

2. A little uneasy

3. Tense

4. Anxious

5. So anxious that I sometimes break out in a sweat or almost feel physically sick

Item 3

When you are in the dentist's chair waiting while the dentist gets the drill ready to begin working on your teeth, how do you feel?

1. Relaxed

2. A little uneasy

3. Tense

4. Anxious

5. So anxious that I sometimes break out in a sweat or almost feel physically sick

Item 4

Imagine that you are in the dentist's chair to have your teeth cleaned. While you are waiting and the dentist or hygienist is getting out the instruments that will be used to scrape your teeth around the gums how do you feel?

1. Relaxed

2. A little uneasy

3. Tense

4. Anxious

5. So anxious that I sometimes break out in a sweat or almost feel physically sick

FIG. 34-2 Dental Anxiety Scale–Revised (DAS-R). (From Ronis DL: Updating a measure of dental anxiety: reliability, validity, and norms, *J Dent Hyg* 68:228-33, 1994.)

CARE PLANNING

Constructing a care plan that gives the hygienist maximum control over the patient's treatment experience is crucial to a successful outcome. Dental anxiety has been likened to other medical conditions that require modification of the course of treatment. Less difficult and intensive treatments should be performed first, because this increases the patient's tolerance and trust. The care plan should include pharmacological and nonpharmacological therapies, alone or in combination, to alleviate pain and anxiety. If discomfort is expected during periodontal debridement procedures, both topical and local forms of

BOX 34-3

Sample Initial Interview Questions Related to Dental Anxiety

1. Did your previous hygienist cause you anxiety? If so, what did the hygienist do that made you anxious?
2. What dental hygiene procedures make you feel anxious?
3. What could I do as a hygienist to ease your anxiety?
4. What coping techniques have previously helped you feel more relaxed?
5. Are you currently anxious?

BOX 34-4

Signs Associated with Fear during Care

Feet hanging off the side of the dental chair
Fidgeting or constant movement
Continuous turning of the head away from clinician in the headrest
Gripping of the armrests
Folding of the arms across the chest
Excessive talking or remaining silent
Needing to expectorate often
Sighing
Taut lips and cheeks
Perspiration
Rapid breathing
Increased heart rate

anesthesia should be used. Depending on the invasiveness of the treatment and the patient's pain threshold and level of anxiety, the dentist may prescribe other pharmacological agents, such as sedatives, nitrous oxide–oxygen analgesia, and oral analgesics. These pharmaceuticals are discussed in other chapters.

Pharmacological agents are required for painful procedures; however, a purely pharmacological approach may not help patients overcome their anxiety. They may credit the drug, rather than their own coping mechanisms, with enabling them to tolerate treatment. A nonpharmacological approach may be a more effective long-term strategy because it addresses the psychological aspects of patients' anxiety.*

Case Application

Determine the type of care modifications that may need to be made in the therapeutic strategy for Ms. Uri.

Dental hygienists are ideal for introducing anxiety-reducing strategies, because dental hygiene usually is the first phase of treatment in a comprehensive care plan. Patients who have a successful dental hygiene experience may be more inclined to return for restorative services and supportive care.

CREATING A POSITIVE RELATIONSHIP

The clinician's interpersonal relationship with patients influences the way patients perceive their dental experience and their satisfaction with the experience.[37,57] Effective two-way communication is the key to earning patients' trust and building a rapport with them. With anxious patients it is extremely important that the clinician assume a calm, confident demeanor and not appear hurried. The dental hygienist should show care, concern, and respect during all interactions. Words should be chosen carefully so as not to belittle, embarrass, or criticize patients. Pat responses such as "Don't worry; everything will be all right" should not be used, because patients may interpret them as denying, minimizing, or ignoring their

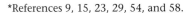
*References 9, 15, 23, 29, 54, and 58.

concerns. If a hygienist fails to establish a positive interpersonal relationship with a patient, the result may be mistrust, anger, increased anxiety, and avoidance. (See Chapter 4 for additional information on effective communication and building a rapport.)

PSYCHOLOGICAL MANAGEMENT

PATIENT EDUCATION

An important step in preparing anxious patients for dental care is explaining the proposed treatment. For most patients, knowing what to expect during care helps reduce fear. Children who received sensory information about the dental experience showed fewer disruptive behaviors, were more cooperative, were rated as less anxious and distressed, and had lower posttreatment pulse rates than children in a control group.[47] The dental hygienist should describe the various sensations the patient can expect: feelings, smells, sounds, and sights. For example, during ultrasonic scaling the patient feels vibrations on the tooth and water spray on the face and hears a high-pitched noise. Clinicians should choose their words carefully to avoid terms that provoke anxiety and dental jargon that the patient might not understand. The hygienist's explanation should help the patient expect a positive experience, thereby countering negative expectations that may have resulted from past dental visits or from information provided by alternative sources.

PATIENT CONTROL

Control is the power that an individual has to exercise direction in a situation.[37] To lessen anxiety, patients must believe that they have control over the activities in their mouth, even though in reality they possess only limited control. The following technique can help the hygienist enhance a patient's sense of control. After explaining the procedure and specifying the amount of time it will require, the hygienist obtains the patient's permission to start. Before beginning, however, the clinician and patient agree on a "stop" signal the patient can use when feeling uncomfortable or needing a rest. Early on, patients may interrupt frequently, but as trust increases, interruptions decline. The hygienist continually offers encouragement and praise, letting the patient know that his or her cooperation has helped achieve a successful treatment outcome.

BEHAVIORAL MANAGEMENT

Research suggests that behavioral strategies, such as relaxation and modeling, can be used to manage patient anxiety.[24,49] A 4-hour course in behavioral techniques taught to a class of dental hygiene students was found to be a significant factor in the reduction of their patient's anxiety levels.[40] Behavioral management techniques can be learned and applied relatively effortlessly in the practice of dental hygiene, to the benefit of anxious patients.

Modeling

Modeling is observation of a peer undergoing a dental treatment, either in person or on videotape, so that aspects of the procedure and sensations that can be expected can be observed. Because children learn much of their behavior by observation and imitation,[2] modeling techniques ideally can be used to alleviate children's dental fear and anxiety. Children who observed a peer modeling appropriate behavior during oral care had lower anxiety levels.[34] The benefit of modeling is twofold: it provides information about the procedure, and it allows the patient observe the model, receiving positive reinforcement for appropriate behavior.

Distraction

Distraction mitigates the patient's anxiety by means of preoccupation. The most basic form of distraction is engaging the patient in positive and interesting conversation. Other distraction techniques include virtual vision glasses, television, video games, and audiotapes. In one study, patients who used an audiovisual device that provided virtual vision reported less anxiety.[45] Researchers found that a video comedy and a video game were nearly equivalent in reducing patient stress, whereas an audio comedy, which demanded the least attention, did not reduce stress significantly better than in controls.[46] Both adults and children can benefit from distraction interventions,[51] even though some of these techniques may not be practical for every procedure because of the possibility of excessive movement. Headsets and a wide selection of audiotapes could be provided for patient use, or patients can be encouraged to bring their own equipment and favorite selections.

Relaxation

Relaxation techniques, such as diaphragmatic and rhythmic breathing, paced respiration, guided imagery, the bensonian relaxation response, and the Wolpe muscle relaxation technique are useful for reducing anxiety. Relaxation techniques are effective because a person cannot be relaxed and anxious at the same time.[8] By monitoring the patient's heart rate, the clinician can determine whether relaxation strategies have been effective.

Diaphragmatic breathing consists of having the patient take deep, slow breaths in a rhythmic pattern that elicits a response from the parasympathetic nervous system.[29] Slow-paced respiration was associated with a decrease in anxiety.[5] The reduction in anxiety was thought to occur because subjects expected to feel less stress, based on their belief that slower-paced respiration resulted in relaxation. For this technique the hygienist has the patient take a deep breath to a slow count of five, hold the breath for 1 second, and then exhale slowly.

For the Bensonian relaxation response,[3] which is similar to meditation, the patient repeats a word or phrase while adopting a passive attitude to bring forth his or her innate ability to relax. The Wolpe technique,[59] a modification of Jacobson's technique,[25] is a process of systematically tensing and relaxing muscles to produce overall body relaxation. Muscle tension, the body's response to anxiety-provoking thoughts, increases a person's subjective experience of anxiety. The Wolpe technique is based on the incompatibility between muscle relaxation and anxiety. Relaxation instructions provided by audiotape[10] or videotape[4,18,41] also have proved effective in reducing patient anxiety.

BOX 34-5

Systematic Desensitization Hierarchy for Tooth Probing

Patient thinks about having the teeth probed.
Patient feels the probe on a finger.
Patient watches a videotape of a person having teeth probed.
Patient watches in a mirror while the hygienist probes a tooth.
Hygienist probes one quadrant.
Hygienist probes entire dentition.

Guided imagery involves the patient's imagination in developing an image of a pleasant environment, thereby facilitating relaxation.[29] Patients should be encouraged to visualize and describe a favorite place while engaging all their senses.

Systematic Desensitization

Systematic desensitization involves the creation of a hierarchy of fear-producing situations related to the specific fear (Box 34-5). Starting with the least feared stimulus, the patient gradually progresses through all situations in the hierarchy while maintaining a relaxed state. Because a relaxation response has replaced the anxiety response, patients can cope with the previously feared situations.

Biofeedback

Biofeedback uses sophisticated monitoring equipment to measure physiological changes in the body during exposure to stressful stimuli. These changes are signaled by a flashing light or a sound. The signal helps an individual to become aware of the body's response, thereby helping that person to eventually achieve relaxation during stressful situations. The goal of this technique is to enable a person to develop control over involuntary bodily functions, such as pulse and blood pressure.

Hypnosis

Hypnosis is an altered state of mind in which suggestions are accepted more readily and acted on more powerfully than in the fully conscious state.[33] Hypnosis has been used successfully in the management of anxious patients.* The technique has not become widely used because it requires an experienced clinician[20]; a considerable amount of time is needed to induce a useful trance; and public misconceptions about hypnosis have made some people reluctant to enter a trance state.[1,50]

 Case Application
Which of the psychological management techniques do you believe would be effective for Ms. Uri?

---

*References 1, 21, 27, 30, 32, 39, 42, 44, 48.

MANAGEMENT OF FEARFUL CHILDREN

Strategies that are effective with adults may not always be helpful with children.[37] Distraction, rational discussion, and detailed explanations do not work with children under 5 years of age. Neither coercion nor coaxing can achieve a positive outcome. Modeling and the "tell, show, do" approach are two commonly used strategies that have proved useful. To encourage cooperative behavior, the clinician should give children specific directions and specific feedback (e.g., "You are doing a great job of holding your head still"). Positive suggestions and praise are important. The hygienist also can foster a sense of control in children by allowing some degree of participation (e.g., letting patients hold the saliva ejector) and by telling them how long the procedure will take.

 RITICAL THINKING ACTIVITIES

1. Invite a guest speaker to discuss and demonstrate hypnosis.
2. Develop videotapes for different age groups to be used for modeling purposes.
3. Use distraction methods by encouraging patients to bring in headsets and audiotapes.
4. Produce a relaxation audiotape for use with clinic patients.
5. Use other relaxation techniques with clinic patients.
6. Practice relaxation techniques to help yourself manage the stress in your life.
7. Through discussion, attempt to identify the origin of a patient's anxiety.
8. Create a stimulus hierarchy for nonsurgical periodontal therapy.
9. With a fellow student, role-play the treatment of an anxious patient. Focus on interpersonal characteristics, communication, and enhancing patient control.
10. Using the DAS-R, identify the number of anxious patients treated in a given month.

 REVIEW QUESTIONS

Questions 1 and 2 refer to the case study presented at the beginning of the chapter.

1. Which of the following behaviors suggest that Ms. Uri is anxious about oral care?
   a. Previous cancellation
   b. Aloofness
   c. Lack of preventive care
   d. Poor oral health
   e. All the above
2. Which of the following interventions should be provided first for Ms. Uri?
   a. Guided use of a muscle relaxation technique
   b. An explanation of the procedure
   c. Administration of an anxiety questionnaire
   d. Referral to a mental health professional
3. Which of the following strategies probably would be most successful for anxious 3- to 5-year-old children?
   a. Modeling
   b. Detailed explanations
   c. Coaxing
   d. Paced breathing
4. Which of the following techniques requires the creation of a hierarchy of fear-producing situations?
   a. Hypnosis
   b. Systematic desensitization
   c. Biofeedback
   d. Progressive muscle relaxation
5. Which of the following factors has the greatest influence on the patient's perception of the oral care experience?
   a. Achievement of complete relaxation
   b. Detailed information about the proposed treatment
   c. The interpersonal relationship between the patient and the care provider
   d. Quality care delivered in an efficient manner

 SUGGESTED AGENCIES AND WEB SITES

Because of the ever-changing nature of the Internet, some of the web sites listed here may have changed since publication. Please refer to Mosby's Evolve web site for the most current information.

American Dental Association, video news releases ("Overcoming dental anxiety"): http://www.ada.org
Ronald B. Baran, DDS, PC ("Dental anxiety"): http://mycroft.net
CBS Healthwatch: ("Ways to relieve dental anxiety" from Powell, DR for the American Institute for Preventive Medicine, 1999): http://cbs.medscape.com
DAPA International (The Dental Anxiety & Phobia Association): http://www.healthyteeth.com

Dental Cyberweb, with Marvin Mansky, DDS ("A simple five minute cure for dental anxiety"): http://www.dentalcyberweb.com
Dental Zone online store ("Conquer your fear of the dentist"): http://www.saveyoursmile.com
Stuart M. Ellis, BDS, DPDS, MFGPD ("Dental phobia & anxiety"): http://www.dentalfear.org

SUGGESTED AGENCIES AND WEB SITES—cont'd

Goodteeth.com, with Joel Goodman, DDS ("Coping with dental anxiety"): http://www.goodteeth.com
Institute for Dental Wellness ("Self-reliance: dental anxiety, fears, and phobias"): http://www.dentalwellness.net
Loyola University Health System ("The truth behind dental anxiety: why people are so fearful of dentists, Loyola psychologist explains"): http://www.luhs.org
Odontologia.com ("Dental anxiety"): http://www.odontologia.com
P&G Dental ResourceNet ("The prevalence of dental anxiety in children from low-income families and its relationship to personality traits"): http://www.dentalcare.com

Don R. Powell, PhD, for the American Institute for Preventive Medicine ("336 Ways to relieve dental anxiety"): http://www.health4india.com
Teeth Canada ("Dental anxiety"): http://www.teethcanada.com
ThirdAge Media, Inc. daily newsletter ("Online help for dental anxiety"): http://www.thirdage.com
University of Michigan, Department of Psychiatry: ("Factors associated with dental anxiety"): http://informatics.dent.umich.edu
University of Nottingham ("Dental anxiety"): http://omni.ac.uk
Wellness Wire, with Bruce A. Sims, DMD, PC ("Fear not: put an end to dental anxiety!"): http://homerun.com

ADDITIONAL READINGS AND RESOURCES

Benson H: *The relaxation response,* New York, 1975, William Morrow.
Bouffard C: Controlling pain and anxiety, *Access* 4:14-8, 1999.
Foreman PA: Practical patient management: the integrated approach, *Anesth Prog* 35:19-25, 1988.
Hoewisch C: Relaxation and imagery for the fearful patient, *Access* 1:29-32, 1993.
King LJ: Treating the anxious patient, *Access* 9/10:10-3, 1991.
Locker D et al: Age of onset of dental anxiety, *J Dent Res* 78:790-6, 1999.

Milgrom P, Weinstein P, Getz T: *Treating fearful dental patients,* ed 2, Seattle, 1995, University of Washington Press.
Pawlicki R: Psychological-behavioral techniques in managing pain and anxiety in the dental patient, *Anesth Prog* 38(4-5):120-7, 1991.
Weiner AA: *The difficult patient: a guide to understanding and managing anxiety,* ed 2, Cambridge, Mass, 1994, Reniew.

REFERENCES

1. Baker SR, Boaz D: The partial reformulation of a traumatic memory of a dental phobic during trance: a case study, *Int J Clin Exp Hypn* 31:14-8, 1983.
2. Bandura A: *Principles of behavior modification,* New York, 1969, Holt, Rinehart & Winston.
3. Benson H: *The relaxation response,* New York, 1975, William Morrow.
4. Carpenter DJ, Gatchel RJ, Hasegawa T: Effectiveness of a videotaped behavioral intervention for dental anxiety: the role of gender and the need for information, *Behav Med* 20:123-32, 1994.
5. Clark M, Hirschman R: Effects of paced respiration on affective responses during dental stress, *J Dent Res* 59:1533, 1980.
6. Corah NL: Dental anxiety: assessment, reduction, and increasing patient satisfaction, *Dentistry* 10:5-9, 23-5, 1990.
7. Corah NL: Development of a dental anxiety scale, *J Dent Res* 48:596, 1969.
8. Corah NL et al: Relaxation and musical programming as means of reducing psychological stress during dental procedures, *J Am Dent Assoc* 103:232-4, 1981.
9. Corah NL, O'Shea RM, Ayer WA: Dentists' management of patients' fear and anxiety, *J Am Dent Assoc* 110:734-6, 1985.
10. Corah NL, O'Shea RM, Skeels DK: Dentists' perceptions of problem behaviors in patients, *J Am Dent Assoc* 104:829-33, 1982.
11. Davey G: Dental phobias and anxieties: evidence for conditioning processes in the acquisition and modulation of a learned fear, *Behav Res Ther* 27:51-8, 1989.
12. De Jongh A, Stouthard M: Anxiety about dental hygienist treatment, *Community Dent Oral Epidemiol* 21:91-5, 1993.

13. Doer PA et al: Factors associated with dental anxiety, *J Am Dent Assoc* 129:1111-9, 1998.
14. Elter JR, Strauss RP, Beck JD: Assessing dental anxiety, dental care use, and oral status in older adults, *J Am Dent Assoc* 128:591-7, 1997.
15. Enneking D et al: Treatment outcomes for specific subtypes of dental fear: preliminary clinical findings, *Spec Care Dent* 12:214-8, 1992.
16. Filewich RJ, Jackson E, Shore H. In Moretti R, Ayer AW, editors: The president's conference on the dentist-patient relationship and the management of fear, anxiety and pain (convened by Robert H. Griffiths), Chicago, 1983, American Dental Association.
17. Gadbury-Amyot CC: Assessing and managing patients with dental fears, *Compend Cont Educ Oral Hyg* 2:3-10, 1995.
18. Gatchel RJ: Impact of a videotaped dental fear–reduction program on people who avoid dental treatment, *J Am Dent Assoc* 112:218-21, 1986.
19. Gatchel RJ: The prevalence of dental fear and avoidance: expanded adult and recent adolescent surveys, *J Am Dent Assoc* 118:591-3, 1989.
20. Gatchel RJ: Managing anxiety and pain during dental treatment, *J Am Dent Assoc* 123:37-41, 1992.
21. Golan HP: Control of fear reaction in dental patients by hypnosis: three case reports, *Am J Clin Hypn* 13:279-84, 1971.
22. Gordon S, Dionne R, Snyder J: Dental fear and anxiety as a barrier to accessing oral health care among patients with special health care needs, *Spec Care Dent* 18:88-92, 1998.
23. Hakeberg M et al: Long-term effects on dental care behavior and dental health after treatments for dental fear, *Anesth Prog* 40:72-7, 1993.

Continued

24. Hammarstrand G, Berggren U, Hakeberg M: Psychophysiological therapy versus hypnotherapy in the treatment of patients with dental phobia, *Eur J Oral Sci* 103:399-404, 1995.

25. Jacobsen E: *Progressive relaxation,* Chicago, 1938, University of Chicago Press.

26. Kaako T et al: Dental fear among university employees: implications for dental education, *J Dent Educ* 62:415-20, 1998.

27. Kleinhauz M, Eli L: When pharmacologic anesthesia is precluded: the value of hypnosis as a sole anesthetic agent in dentistry, *Spec Care Dent* 13:15-8, 1993.

28. Klesges RC, Malott JM: The effects of graded exposure and parental modeling on the dental phobias of a four-year-old girl and her mother, *J Behav Ther Exp Psychiatry* 15:164, 1984.

29. Krochak M, Rubin JG: An overview of the treatment of anxious and phobic dental patients, *Compend Cont Educ Dent* 14:604-15, 1993.

30. Lewis RS: Hypnosis provides therapeutic tool for patient management, *J Mass Dent Soc* 45:2023, 1996.

31. Locker D, Liddell A, Burman D: Dental fear and anxiety in an older adult population, *Community Dent Oral Epidemiol* 19:120-4, 1991.

32. Lu DP, Lu GP: Hypnosis and pharmacological sedation for medically compromised patients, *Compendium* 1732-40, 1996.

33. Meechan JG, Robb ND, Seymour RA: *Pain and anxiety control for the conscious dental patient,* Oxford, 1998, Oxford University Press.

34. Melamed B et al: Reduction of fear-related dental management problems with use of filmed modeling, *J Am Dent Assoc* 90:822-6, 1975.

35. Milgrom P et al: The prevalence and practice management consequences of dental fear in a major U.S. city, *J Am Dent Assoc* 116:641-7, 1988.

36. Milgrom P, Weinstein P: Dental fears in general practice: new guidelines for assessment and treatment, *Int Dent J* 43:288-93, 1993.

37. Milgrom P, Weinstein P, Getz T: *Treating fearful dental patients,* ed 2, Seattle, 1995, University of Washington Press.

38. Millar K et al: Helping anxious adult patients, *Dent Update* 18:18, 20-2, 24-5, 1991.

39. Moore R, Abrahamsen R, Brodsgaard I: Hypnosis compared with group therapy and individual desensitization for dental anxiety, *Eur J Oral Sci* 104:612-8, 1996.

40. Peretz B, Kaplan R, Stabholtz A: The influence of a patient-management course for dental hygiene students on the dental anxiety of their patients, *J Dent Educ* 61:368-73, 1997.

41. Robertson C, Gatchel RJ, Fowler C: Effectiveness of a video-taped behavioral intervention in reducing anxiety in emergency oral surgery patients, *Behav Med* 7(2):77-85, 1991.

42. Rodolfa E, Kraft W, Reilley R: Etiology and treatment of dental anxiety and phobia, *Am J Clin Hypn* 33:22-9, 1990.

43. Ronis DL: Updating a measure of dental anxiety: reliability, validity, and norms, *J Dent Hyg* 68:228-33, 1994.

44. Rustvold S: Hypnotherapy for treatment of dental phobia in children, *Gen Dent* 42:346-8, 1994.

45. Satoh Y et al: Relaxation effect of an audiovisual system on dental patients. II. Palus-amplitude, *J Nihon Univ Sch Dent* 37:138-45, 1995.

46. Seyrek SK, Corah NL, Pace L: Comparison of three distraction techniques, *J Am Dent Assoc* 108:327-29, 1984.

47. Siegel LJ, Peterson L: Stress reduction in young dental patients through coping and sensory information, *J Consult Clin Psychol* 48:785-7, 1980.

48. Sklar B: Hypnosis as an alternative in dentistry, *Access* 1:34-5, 1993.

49. Smith TA: Evaluating a behavioral method to manage dental fear: a two-year study of dental practices, *J Am Dent Assoc* 121:525-30, 1990.

50. Sokol D, Sokol S, Sokol C: A review of nonintrusive therapies used to deal with anxiety and pain in the dental office, *J Am Dent Assoc* 110:217-22, 1985.

51. Stark L et al: Distraction: its utilization and efficacy with children undergoing dental treatment, *J Appl Behav Anal* 22:297-307, 1989.

52. Stewart JE et al: Comprehensive treatment among dental school patients with high and low dental anxiety, *J Dent Educ* 58:697-700, 1994.

53. Sullivan MJ, Neish NR: Catastrophizing anxiety and pain during dental hygiene treatment, *Community Dent Oral Epidemiol* 26:344-9, 1998.

54. Tay K et al: The effect of instruction on dentists' motivation to manage fearful patients, *J Dent Educ* 57:444-8, 1993.

55. Tripp DA, Neish NR, Sullivan MJ: What hurts during dental hygiene treatment? *J Dent Hyg* 72:25-30, 1998.

56. Weiner AA: Dental anxiety: differentiation, identification, and behavioral management, *J Can Dent Assoc* 58:580-5, 1992.

57. Weiner AA: *The difficult patient: a guide to understanding and managing anxiety,* ed 2, Cambridge, Mass, 1994, Reniew.

58. Weinstein P: Breaking the worldwide cycle of pain, fear and avoidance: uncovering risk factors and promoting prevention for children, *Ann Behav Med* 12:141-7, 1990.

59. Wolpe J: Behavior therapy in complex neurotic states, *Br J Psychiatry* 110:28-34, 1964.

60. Woolfolk MW et al: Determining dental checkup frequency, *J Am Dent Assoc* 130:715-723, 1999.

CHAPTER 35

Chemistry *and* Pharmacology *of* Anesthetics

Peggy W. Coleman

Chapter Outline

Case Study: Considerations in the Selection
  of Dental Anesthetic
History of Anesthetics
Physiology of Nerve Conduction
  Resting membrane potential
  Action potential
Mechanism of Action
Chemistry
  Hydrophobic group
  Hydrophilic group
Ionization Factors
Pharmacokinetics
  Absorption
  Distribution
  Metabolism
  Excretion

Systemic Actions of Local Anesthetics
  Peripheral nerve conduction
  Central nervous system
  Cardiovascular system
  Local tissue toxicity
  Neuromuscular blockade
  Drug interactions
Vasoconstrictors in Anesthetic Solutions
Clinical Action of Specific Local Anesthetic Agents
  Amides
  Esters
  Other local anesthetic agents

Key Terms

Action potential	Cocaine	Ketone	Procaine
Amidases	Dyclonine	Lidocaine	Pseudocholinesterase
Amides	Enzyme inhibitor	Mepivacaine	Sympathetic nervous system
Anions	Epinephrine	Methemoglobinemia	Tertiary amine
Articaine	Esters	Nonionized	Tetracaine
Benzonatate	Hydrophilic	Norepinephrine	Toluidine
Bupivacaine	Hydrophobic	Paraaminobenzoic acid	Vasoconstrictor
Cations	Ionized	(PABA)	Xylidine

 ## *Learning Outcomes*

1. Describe the uses of local anesthetics in the practice of
dental hygiene.
2. Name the first local anesthetic and explain why it is no
longer the drug of choice.
3. Describe the chemical classes of local anesthetics.
4. Describe the physiology and chemistry of local
anesthetics.

5. Discuss the purpose of a vasoconstrictor in a local
anesthetic.
6. Describe the clinical action of specific local anesthetics.
7. Evaluate current literature on types of anesthetics.

Local anesthetics cause a loss of sensation in a circumscribed area of the body. When applied to the nerve, they reversibly block impulse conduction along nerve axons. In dentistry, local anesthetics are used primarily to alleviate pain. Local anesthesia may be required if the dental hygiene supportive care plan includes therapeutic scaling and root planing or if the patient's soft tissue or teeth are unduly sensitive. Also, the dentist may ask the hygienist to anesthetize a patient in preparation for restorative therapy or surgery. The great advantage of local anesthesia is that pain is suppressed without generalized depression of the entire nervous system. Local anesthetics allow dental procedures to be performed with much less risk than is associated with general anesthesia or administration of nitrous oxide.[9,14,15]

HISTORY OF ANESTHETICS

Even before the Incas arrived, the ancient inhabitants of the highlands of Peru chewed or sucked the leaves of the coca plant, a shrub that grows in the Andes 1000 to 3000 meters above sea level, for the sense of well-being the leaves produced. When the Spanish conquistadors arrived in 1532, they restricted the chewing of the leaves to the Incan aristocracy for use only during religious ceremonies. However, shortly after the Spanish conquest, the peasants resumed chewing the leaves, which blunted their hunger, allowed them to endure long hours of forced labor in the mines, and erased the sense of humiliation arising from their defeat by the Spanish.

Cocaine was extracted from the coca leaf in 1860 by Albert Niemann, who noted that it had a peculiar effect on the tongue, leaving it numb and almost devoid of sensation. In 1884 Karl Koller discovered cocaine's potent local anesthetic effects on the eye. It was immediately adopted for use in eye surgery because for the first time, operations could be performed on the eye while the patient was fully conscious. In 1884 Hall introduced the use of local anesthesia into dentistry, and in 1885 Halsted used cocaine as a nerve block for general surgery. During this time Sigmund Freud was experimenting with cocaine and its effects on the central nervous system.[9,10]

The realization that cocaine was addictive and toxic prompted a search for more acceptable local anesthetics. In 1905 Alfred Einhorn synthesized *procaine,* which became the prototype for local anesthetic drugs for nearly 50 years. *Lidocaine* became available in 1952 and mepivacaine in 1960. Although many local anesthetics are now available for dental use, the search for the ideal local anesthetic continues.

PHYSIOLOGY OF NERVE CONDUCTION

To understand the way in which a local anesthetic works, the dental hygienist must be familiar with the physiology of nerve conduction.

Except for water, the major chemical substances in the extracellular fluid are sodium and chloride ions; the intracellular fluid contains high concentrations of potassium ions and *ionized,* nondiffusible proteins with negatively charged side chains and phosphate compounds.

Because of these differences in ion concentrations across the plasma membrane, all cells under resting con-

Considerations in the Selection of Dental Anesthetic

Patricia Macklin, age 57, required local anesthesia for root planing of the mandibular right quadrant, a procedure that was estimated to take 30 to 60 minutes. Mrs. Macklin's medical history showed mild hypertension, which was controlled with a daily dose of captopril (Capoten), a converting **enzyme inhibitor.** Her blood pressure was 126/80. Mrs. Macklin had had a hysterectomy 10 years ago, for which she had undergone general anesthesia and had been given succinylcholine. A deficiency of **pseudocholinesterase** had been discovered at that time. Mrs. Macklin said that she once had fainted after injection of a local anesthetic many years ago. Since that time she has received local anesthetic injections for dental procedures without any problems.

Mepivacaine with 2% **epinephrine** was selected as the local anesthetic for Mrs. Macklin. As a precaution, a low concentration of **vasoconstrictor** was selected. About 2 minutes after the injection, Mrs. Macklin said that she felt faint. She was placed in a supine position with her legs elevated. Her symptoms quickly disappeared, and she said that she felt better. When it was apparent that the nerve block had been successful, the debridement procedure was completed.

ditions have a potential difference across the membrane, orientated with the inside of the cell negatively charged with respect to the outside. The resting membrane potential and the magnitude of the membrane potential are determined primarily by a difference in specific ion concentrations in the intracellular and extracellular fluid compartments and differences in membrane permeability to the different ions.

RESTING MEMBRANE POTENTIAL

The resting membrane potential exists because there is a small excess of negative ions *(anions)* inside the cell and a small excess of positive ions *(cations)* outside the cell (Fig. 35-1). The excess positive charges outside the cell are attracted to the excess negative charges inside the cell and vice versa. The potential difference across the membrane varies from about -5 to -100 microvolts (mV), depending on the cell type. In most neurons the resting membrane potential ranges from -40 to -75 mV. The excess charged ions collect in a thin shell at the inner and outer surfaces of the plasma membrane, whereas the bulk of the intracellular and extracellular fluid are neutral. This polarization caused by unequal distribution of the charged particles across the cell membrane plays a significant role in nerve conduction (see Fig. 35-1).

The distribution of ions inside and outside cell membranes is determined partly by the presence of *channels,* or small pores in the membranes. Some channels are always open, and others can be opened or closed. Some channels are very selective, allowing only one kind of ion to pass through.

The membrane is *selectively permeable,* meaning that it allows a single type of ion to diffuse through the mem-

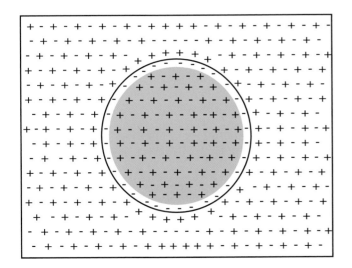

FIG. 35-1 A small excess of positive charges on the extracellular side and a small excess of negative charges on the intracellular side create the membrane potential.

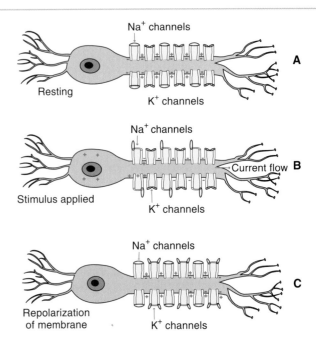

FIG. 35-2 A, Resting nerve cell with sodium ion (Na^+) channels and potassium ion (K^+) channels closed. **B,** Na^+ channels open, allowing an inward flux of sodium, which changes the action potential from -90 mV to $+10$ mV. The current flows in one direction. **C,** Na^+ channels close, K^+ channels open, and the cell repolarizes.

brane pores. In the resting (unexcited) state, the membrane is highly permeable to potassium ions and virtually impermeable to sodium ions. The concentration of potassium ions inside the cell is greater than that outside the cell, and because of the large concentration gradient from inside to outside, the positively charged potassium ions tend to diffuse outward. This carries positive charges to the outside, and the inside becomes negative in relation to the outside. The positive charge outside the cell repels further outward movement of the positively charged potassium ions. At rest the cell membrane is relatively impermeable to sodium ions, and these positively charged ions are prevented from entering the cell (Fig. 35-2, *A*).

The sensations of pain, temperature, touch, pressure, proprioception, and skeletal muscle tone depend on a rapid, complex flow of information between the nervous system and the rest of the body. In the nervous system, a signal is carried over long distances by a rapid change in membrane potential, known as an *action potential.*

ACTION POTENTIAL

The action potential results from rapid, transient change in membrane ion permeability, which permits selected ions to move down their concentration gradients. When opened, protein channels permit sodium ions to enter the cell, which causes a rapid change in permeability. In the resting state, the plasma membrane of neurons is predominantly permeable to potassium ions, and very few sodium ion channels are open. During an action potential, however, the membrane permeability to sodium and potassium ions changes.

During the depolarizing phase of the action potential, the sodium channels open; permeability to sodium in-

creases; and sodium ions are able to move into the cell. More positive charge enters the cell in the form of sodium ions than leaves in the form of potassium ions, and the cell becomes positively charged inside with respect to the outside (see Fig. 35-2, *B*).

Once a stimulus, such as pain or touch, has generated an action potential in a nerve, a local current is produced. This current is the stimulus that depolarizes the adjacent membrane, producing an action potential at the next site, and thus the action potential is propagated along the length of the membrane to the central nervous system (CNS).

Action potentials in nerve cells last about 1 millisecond (ms). The membrane potential rapidly returns to its resting level for two reasons: (1) the sodium channels that opened during depolarization close, and (2) more potassium channels open. The additional flow of potassium out of the cell helps to return the membrane potential quickly to its resting level (see Fig. 35-2, *C*).

The number of sodium ions that enters a cell during an action potential and the number of potassium ions that leave are quiet small in comparison with the total number of ions in the cell. However, if these tiny numbers of ions crossing the membrane with each action potential were not eventually moved back across the membrane, the concentration gradients would disappear, and the action potential could no longer be generated. Accumulation of cellular sodium and potassium loss is prevented by the continuous action of the sodium-potassium adenosine triphosphatase (Na,K^+-ATPase) pump in the cell membrane. The Na,K^+-ATPase pumps move sodium from the inside of the cell to the outside of the cell and return potassium to the inside.[8,17,19]

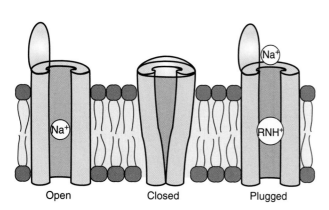

FIG. 35-3 The left channel is open, allowing sodium ions (Na^+) to enter. The middle channel is a closed sodium channel in the resting stage. The right channel is plugged by a local anesthetic, which prevents the influx of Na^+ and generation of an action potential.

MECHANISM OF ACTION

Local anesthetics block conduction of the nerve impulse by diminishing or preventing the transient increase in permeability to sodium ions. Local anesthetics bind to specific receptors on the sodium channels in the nerve membrane. Once the local anesthetic binds to the receptor on the sodium channel, permeability to sodium ions is diminished or prevented. Diminishing or preventing the influx of sodium prevents propagation of action potentials, and nerve conduction fails (Fig. 35-3).[3,16]

CHEMISTRY

Most local anesthetics used in oral health care today fall into one of two chemical groups—*esters* or *amides.* A few other anesthetic agents belong to other chemical classes. It is important for the clinician to know in which chemical division a local anesthetic belongs; a patient who is allergic to a drug in a particular chemical group is very likely to be allergic to other agents in that group. Fig. 35-4 illustrates the structural formulas with representative local anesthetics.

All local anesthetics have a *hydrophilic* amino group and a *hydrophobic* component separated by an intermediate hydrocarbon chain that contains either an ester or an amide linkage (see Fig. 35-4).

HYDROPHOBIC GROUP

The hydrophobic group, which has an aromatic nucleus, allows the anesthetic to penetrate the lipid membrane, where the receptor sites for these drugs are located. The more hydrophobic a local anesthetic, the more potent the drug and the longer the duration of action. The hydrophilic component makes the local anesthetic water soluble, which allows the drug to diffuse through the extracellular fluid and come in contact with the nerve.

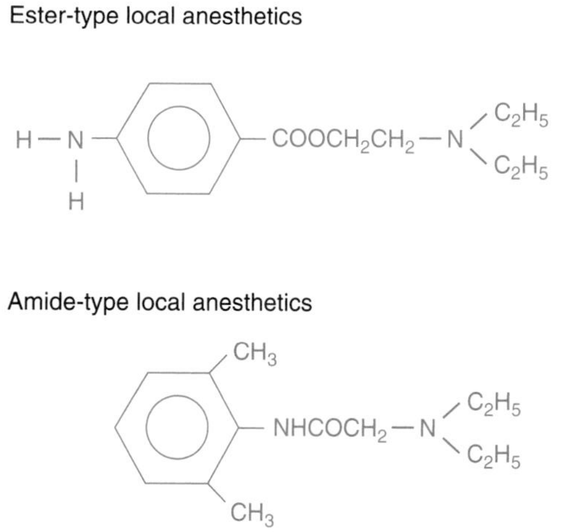

Ester-type local anesthetics

Amide-type local anesthetics

FIG. 35-4 Chemical composition of ester and amide types of local anesthetics.

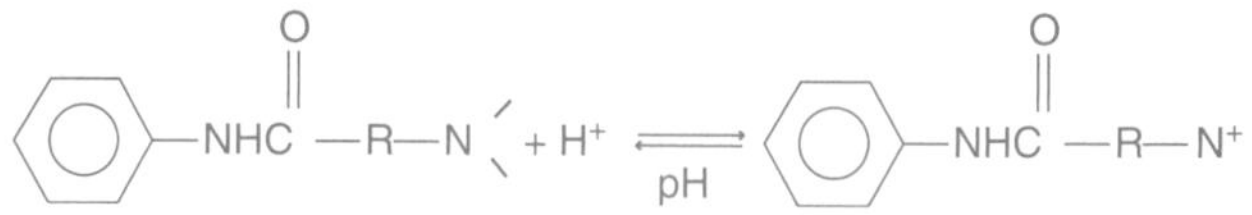

or written simply as

$$RN + H^+ \rightleftharpoons RNH^+$$
Base   Salt

FIG. 35-5 Chemical properties of base and salt forms of local anesthetics.

HYDROPHILIC GROUP

The hydrophilic component usually is a *tertiary amine,* such as lidocaine or *tetracaine.* Prilocaine is a secondary amine. This component allows the anesthetic to diffuse through the extracellular fluid. Local anesthetics without a hydrophilic component, such as benzocaine, cannot be injected but can be used for topical anesthesia.

Except for cocaine, all local anesthetics are synthetic. The synthetic drugs are weak bases, are fat soluble, are viscous liquids or solids, and are unstable on exposure to air.[18] To be clinically useful, these fat-soluble bases must be combined with acids to form salts. In this form the local anesthetic is water-soluble and relatively stable on exposure to air. Solutions for injection can be prepared by dissolving the local anesthetic salt either in saline or in sterile water (Fig. 35-5).

IONIZATION FACTORS

The hydrogen ion concentration (pH) of a local anesthetic solution and of the tissue into which it is injected determines how much of the drug is in the ionized form and how much in the free base, or effective, form *(nonionized).* The local anesthetic must be in the free base form to have nerve-blocking effects. The lower the pH (i.e., the more acidic the solution), the greater the proportion of drug in the ionized form. Local anesthetic solutions avail-

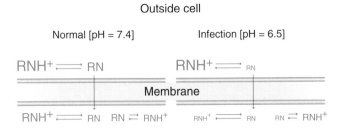

FIG. 35-6 Effect of hydrogen ion concentration (pH) on ionization of local anesthetics.

able for injection have a pH of 5 to 6, and most of the drug is in the ionized form. The pH of normal tissue is 7.4, and once the anesthetic has been injected, the amount of drug in the free base form increases. Infection or inflammation produces an acidic environment, and the pH of an inflamed area (usually below 6) reduces the amount of drug in the free base form. This is one reason it is more difficult to obtain local anesthesia in areas of the oral cavity that are inflamed or infected (Fig. 35-6).

PHARMACOKINETICS

ABSORPTION

The onset of local anesthesia is determined primarily by the molecular properties of the anesthetic. When the anesthetic is injected into the tissues or applied topically, it must diffuse from its site of administration to its sites of action inside the axonal membrane. Anesthetics that have a low molecular weight and a high lipid solubility and that are in the nonionized form cross the nerve axon membrane with ease. Anesthetics that have a high molecular weight and a low lipid solubility and are ionized penetrate the axon slowly and have a slow onset of action.

The duration of action of a local anesthetic agent will last as long as the agent is in contact with the nerve. Although administered for local effects, local anesthetics are absorbed into the systemic blood stream and distributed to all parts of the body. The rate at which the local anesthetic agent is removed from the site of action and anesthesia terminated is determined primarily by the blood flow to the site of administration. Local anesthesia is terminated when the molecules of anesthetic diffuse out of the axon and are carried away in the blood stream. In areas where blood flow is high, anesthetic is rapidly absorbed into the systemic circulation and anesthesia terminated. Local anesthetics with vasodilating properties increase the systemic absorption of the drug, resulting in a reduced period of time of anesthesia. Procaine dilates blood vessels and increases its own absorption, whereas cocaine constricts blood vessels and prevents its absorption. Any procedure that keeps the drug at the axon prolongs the duration of anesthesia. Heat, massage, and inflammation greatly increase systemic absorption of the local anesthetic and hasten termination of local anesthesia.

DISTRIBUTION

After absorption into the blood stream, local anesthetics are distributed throughout the body to all tissues. Local anesthetics' lipid solubility allows them easily to cross the blood-brain barrier and the placenta. The possible toxicity of a local anesthetic depends on the level of the drug in certain organs.

METABOLISM

The toxic effects of local anesthetics depend on the balance between the rates of absorption and elimination. The metabolism of these drugs varies greatly and is a major factor in determining the safety of each anesthetic agent. The two major classes of local anesthetics, the amides and esters, are metabolized differently.

The ester local anesthetics are primarily hydrolyzed and inactivated by plasma pseudocholinesterases.[11] Liver esterases also participate in the hydrolysis of ester local anesthetics. *Paraaminobenzoic acid (PABA)* is the major metabolic by-product of ester hydrolysis and is excreted in the urine. Most allergic reactions after administration of an ester local anesthetic occur in response to PABA and not to the parent drug.

Approximately 1 in 2800 individuals has an atypical form of pseudocholinesterase and cannot hydrolyze ester local anesthetics and other chemically related drugs.[5] This results in higher blood levels in these patients and increases the probability of toxicity.

The metabolism of amide local anesthetics is more complex than that of esters. In general, the amide local anesthetics are metabolized in the liver by microsomal enzymes.[1] Individuals who suffer from alcoholism and patients with severe liver disease may accumulate amide local anesthetics, resulting in systemic toxicity.

Biotransformation of certain amide local anesthetics produces compounds capable of having clinical activity if excessive amounts accumulate in the blood. The amides *articaine* and prilocaine can cause *methemoglobinemia*.[4]

EXCRETION

The kidneys excrete the metabolic by-products of both esters and amides. A very small amount of the local anesthetic is excreted unchanged in the urine. Only small amounts of esters appear unchanged in the urine, because they are almost completely metabolized in the blood. Because the metabolism of amides is more complex, more of the unchanged drug is excreted than with esters. In renal failure both metabolites and free drug can accumulate.

SYSTEMIC ACTIONS OF LOCAL ANESTHETICS

All organs with excitable membranes are affected by local anesthetics, including the cardiovascular system, CNS, autonomic ganglia, neuromuscular junction, and all types of muscle. Action potentials in the nervous system and the cardiovascular system are readily blocked by these agents.

PERIPHERAL NERVE CONDUCTION

The primary clinical function of local anesthetics is reversible blockade of peripheral nerve conduction. Local anesthetics are nonselective and can block the conduction of action potentials in all neurons to which they gain access. These agents can inhibit the conduction of impulses in motor neurons, at sensory endings, and at synapses. Although action potentials can be blocked in all types of neurons, some neurons are blocked more readily than others. The loss of nerve function is related to the anesthetic's ability to penetrate the nerve fiber. As a general rule, local anesthetics block the conduction of action potentials in small, nonmyelinated neurons first.[6] These drugs do not penetrate myelin, and large, heavily myelinated neurons, such as motor neurons, are affected last.

The loss of sensory functions of most nerves is predictable from the rate of block exhibited by the nerve fibers. The sensation of pain usually is lost first, followed by the sensations of cold, warmth, touch, deep pressure, proprioception, and motor function. Nerve function returns in reverse order.

CENTRAL NERVOUS SYSTEM

Local anesthetics are lipid-soluble and can cross the blood-brain barrier with ease. At therapeutic blood levels, the CNS effects are not significant. The earliest signs and symptoms of clinical toxicity are CNS in nature. When absorbed in toxic amounts, local anesthetics cause central nervous system excitation and then CNS depression. Convulsions may occur during the excitation phase. Some anesthetics have demonstrated anticonvulsant effects at plasma levels close to the cardiotherapeutic range and below the toxic level.[2] CNS depression can range from drowsiness to unconsciousness.

Selectivity is achieved by delivering the anesthetic to a limited area. Adverse reactions are proportional to the plasma concentration; the higher the plasma level, the greater the danger of adverse effects.

CARDIOVASCULAR SYSTEM

After absorption into the systemic circulation, local anesthetics act on the cardiovascular system. The primary site of action is the myocardium, where the local anesthetic reduces the force of contraction, electrical excitability, and the conduction rate. In addition, most local anesthetics cause peripheral vasodilation. Normally, high systemic concentrations are necessary to produce the cardiovascular effects. However, cardiovascular collapse and death have been reported with lower doses.[7]

LOCAL TISSUE TOXICITY

Intramuscular and intraoral injections of local anesthetics can cause localized skeletal muscle changes. Longer-acting local anesthetics cause more skeletal muscle damage than do shorter-acting drugs. The damage is reversible, and muscle regeneration is complete within 2 weeks.[13]

NEUROMUSCULAR BLOCKADE

Many local anesthetics can block the sodium channels in motor nerves, producing neuromuscular blockade, although this effect normally is slight and usually clinically insignificant. Administration of a local anesthetic with a depolarizing or nondepolarizing muscle relaxant may lead to prolonged periods of muscle paralysis.

DRUG INTERACTIONS

The CNS depressant effects of local anesthetics is additive with other CNS depressants, such as antianxiety drugs, barbiturates, ethanol, and opioids.

Drugs that induce the hepatic microsomal enzymes may increase the rate at which amide local anesthetics are metabolized.

VASOCONSTRICTORS IN ANESTHETIC SOLUTIONS

Local anesthetics produce an effect only for the period they are in contact with the nerve. Cocaine constricts blood vessels and prevents its own reabsorption. However, most local anesthetics currently used in clinical practice produce some degree of vasodilation. The increased blood flow to the site of injection increases the rate of absorption of the local anesthetic and removes it from the nerve. Absorption of the anesthetic shortens the duration of action and decreases the depth of anesthesia. The extent of vasodilation varies from considerable to minimal. Procaine produces significant vasodilation, whereas mepivacaine has minimal vasodilating activity.

Any procedure that prevents absorption of the drug prolongs the duration of anesthesia by keeping the anesthetic in contact with the nerve for a longer period. In dentistry, local anesthetics frequently are combined with a vasoconstrictor to reduce absorption. The decrease in blood flow to the area produced by the vasoconstrictor reduces systemic absorption of the drug. By slowing the rate of absorption of the local anesthetic into the blood stream, it remains at the injection site longer and the duration of action is prolonged. The vasoconstrictor also reduces the risks of systemic toxicity from the local anesthetic and of bleeding at the site of injection.

The vasoconstrictors used in local anesthetic solutions are identical or similar to the neurotransmitters (epinephrine and *norepinephrine)* released by the *sympathetic nervous system.* Three vasoconstrictors are available in local anesthetic solutions in the United States: epinephrine, levonordefrin, and norepinephrine. Epinephrine is the vasoconstrictor most often used and the standard to which other vasoconstrictors are compared.[12]

The concentration of vasoconstrictor in the local anesthetic solution is expressed as a ratio (e.g., 1 to 1000 is written 1:1000); 1:1000 means that 1 g (1000 mg) of vasoconstrictor dissolved in 1000 ml of anesthetic solution. Local anesthetic solutions used in dentistry are more dilute but quite effective. The most commonly used concentrations are epinephrine 1:100,000 (0.01 mg/ml) and epinephrine 1:200,000 (0.005 mg/ml). Norepinephrine has approximately 25% the vasopressor activity of epinephrine and is included with local anesthetic in a 1:30,000 dilution. Levonordefrin is 15% as effective as epinephrine and is included in a 1:20,000 dilution.

Vasoconstrictors are not ideal drugs. Epinephrine, levonordefrin, and norepinephrine stimulate beta-1 receptors of the myocardium, resulting in an increase in the force of contraction and an increased heart rate. The overall action is direct stimulation with increased systolic and diastolic pressures, increased cardiac output and stroke volume, increased heart rate, increased strength of contraction, and increased myocardial oxygen consumption. The risks and benefits of using a vasoconstrictor must be assessed for each patient.[9,12]

CLINICAL ACTION OF SPECIFIC LOCAL ANESTHETIC AGENTS

5-A

Many local anesthetics are available; however, only a few are used in dentistry. Table 35-1 lists a few local anesthetic combinations currently available in dental cartridges. In the following sections, the amide local anesthetics lidocaine, mepivacaine, prilocaine, and *bupivacaine* are discussed, as are the ester local anesthetics cocaine, tetracaine, propoxycaine, and procaine. Local anesthetics available for topical application also are described.

AMIDES

Lidocaine

Lidocaine (Xylocaine, Octocaine) became available for clinical use in 1948 and within a few years replaced procaine (Novocain) as the drug of choice for pain control in dentistry and medicine. Lidocaine is the most commonly used local anesthetic in dentistry, and all new anesthetics are compared to it. Lidocaine also is used as an antiarrhythmic agent. It is absorbed rapidly after parenteral administration, producing a rapid onset of action.

Use of 2% lidocaine causes vasodilation, which limits

its duration of action. Although lidocaine 2% is effective when used without a vasoconstrictor, adding epinephrine reduces blood flow into the area of injection and therefore reduces the rate of absorption, thus prolonging the duration of action. In dentistry, lidocaine 2% with 1:100,000 epinephrine is used for block and infiltration anesthesia. Lidocaine with epinephrine 1:100,000 provides pulpal anesthesia for approximately 1 hour and soft tissue anesthesia for 3 to 5 hours.

Lidocaine is an effective topical anesthetic as a 5% ointment, a 10% spray, or a 2% viscous solution. When used topically, the onset of anesthesia occurs within 2 to 3 minutes.

For hemostasis during surgical procedures, 2% lidocaine with 1:50,000 epinephrine is recommended. Rebound vasodilation occurs.

Signs of lidocaine toxicity include hypotension, shivering, and drowsiness, leading to a loss of consciousness and respiratory arrest. Cross-allergenicity between the amide lidocaine and other available amides or esters has not been documented.

Mepivacaine

Mepivacaine (Carbocaine, Isocaine), introduced in 1960, is an amide derivative of *xylidine.* Its onset of action, duration, potency, and toxicity are similar to those of lidocaine. Mepivacaine is not effective as a topical anesthetic; however, it is used for infiltration, block, spinal, caudal, and epidural anesthesia.

Mepivacaine produces only slight vasodilation. A 3% solution without a vasoconstrictor can be used in patients for whom a vasoconstrictor is contraindicated and for short dental procedures. In a typical dental patient, 2% mepivacaine with a vasoconstrictor provides adequate depth and duration of pain control for most dental procedures.

Allergic reactions to mepivacaine have not been documented, and the drug shows no cross-allergenicity with the currently available amides.[14]

Prilocaine

Prilocaine (Citanest, Citanest Forte) is a secondary amide derivative of *toluidine.* Its pharmacological profile is similar to that of lidocaine. The primary differences are that it produces less vasodilation than lidocaine and can be used without a vasoconstrictor if desired. Prilocaine is less potent and less toxic than lidocaine.

Several cases of methemoglobinemia have been reported after use of prilocaine (Citanest). This effect is a consequence of the metabolism of the aromatic ring in prilocaine to *o*-toluidine. The development of methemoglobinemia depends on the total dose administered, and the small doses used in dentistry are not likely to present a problem in healthy adults. Prilocaine consistently reduces the blood's oxygen-carrying capacity and should not be administered to patients with any condition in which problems of oxygenation may be critical. Acetaminophen and phenacetin both increase methemoglobin levels. Prilocaine is relatively contraindicated in patients taking these medications.

TABLE 35-1			
Local anesthetic combinations available in dental cartridges			
Generic and trade names	**Percentage (%)**	**Vasoconstrictor**	**Concentration**
Lidocaine			
(Xylocaine,	2	Epinephrine	1:50,000
Octocaine)	2	Epinephrine	1:100,000
Mepivacaine			
(Carbocaine)	3	Mepivacaine plain	–
(Isocaine)	2	Levonordefrin	1:20,000
Prilocaine			
(Citanest)	4	Prilocaine plain	–
(Citanest Forte)	4	Epinephrine	1:200,000
Bupivacaine			
(Marcaine)	0.5	Epinephrine	1:200,000

Prilocaine plain produces anesthesia equal in duration to that obtained from lidocaine or mepivacaine with or without a vasoconstrictor.

The concentration of epinephrine in prilocaine (1:200,000) is lower than in other local anesthetic amide combinations. Patients receiving prilocaine with epinephrine are exposed to half the amount of epinephrine as with lidocaine with epinephrine 1:100,000.

Bupivacaine

Bupivacaine (Marcaine) is a widely used amide local anesthetic. It is structurally related to lidocaine and mepivacaine. It is more potent than the other amides but less toxic. Bupivacaine can produce prolonged anesthesia and is available in dental cartridges as a 0.5% solution with 1:200,000 epinephrine. It is used in lengthy dental procedures when pulpal anesthesia for longer than 90 minutes is required and in the management of the postoperative pain expected after endodontic or periodontal surgery.

Bupivacaine is metabolized in the liver by *amidases* and excreted via the kidneys. Its vasodilating properties are significant; it produces more vasodilation than prilocaine, lidocaine, or mepivacaine.

ESTERS

Cocaine

As explained previously, cocaine occurs naturally in the leaves of the coca shrub. An ester of benzoic acid, it is a white, crystalline solid that is highly water-soluble. It is metabolized by the liver, and unchanged cocaine can be found in the urine.

Cocaine is used exclusively as a topical anesthetic. It has a rapid onset of action, and the duration of anesthesia may be as long as 2 hours. Cocaine produces local vasoconstriction secondary to inhibition of local norepinephrine reuptake. The clinical uses of cocaine are limited by its toxicity and potential for abuse. Cocaine is listed as a schedule II drug by the U.S. Drug Enforcement Agency (DEA). Cocaine currently is used primarily to provide topical anesthesia of the upper respiratory tract when local anesthesia and shrinkage of the mucosa by a single agent are desired. Its use as a topical anesthetic in dentistry is not recommended.

Procaine

Procaine (Novocain), an ester of PABA, was the first injectable local anesthetic, and it quickly replaced cocaine in both medicine and dentistry.

Procaine has a slow onset of action and is about half as toxic and as potent as lidocaine. It causes vasodilation and is quickly removed from the injection site into the systemic circulation. It has a relatively short duration of action unless a vasoconstrictor is added.

Procaine is no longer available as a sole agent in dental cartridges, and it is not effective topically. It currently is used only for infiltration anesthesia and as an antiarrhythmic agent.

Tetracaine

Tetracaine (Pontocaine), another ester of PABA, was introduced in 1932. It can be injected or applied topically. Tetracaine has a slow onset but a long duration of action. It is 10 times more potent than procaine and also is more toxic than procaine because it is metabolized more slowly.

Tetracaine is rapidly absorbed from the mucous membranes. If it is used for topical anesthesia, it should be applied to small areas to prevent rapid absorption. It is available as a 2% solution for topical application and as a 0.15% solution for injection. Currently tetracaine is widely used for spinal anesthesia when a long duration of action is required.

Propoxycaine

The PABA ester propoxycaine (Ravocaine) is more toxic and more potent than procaine. It has a rapid onset and a long duration action but lacks topical activity.

OTHER LOCAL ANESTHETIC AGENTS

Dyclonine

Dyclonine (Dyclone) is a *ketone* topical local anesthetic. Cross-sensitivity with other local anesthetics does not occur, because dyclonine is chemically different from the ester and amide local anesthetics. It may be used in patients who have a history of allergic or adverse reactions to other chemical groups.

Dyclonine has a slow onset of action, requiring up to 10 minutes, but the duration of anesthesia may be as long as 1 hour. Systemic toxicity is low, because the drug is water insoluble and is not absorbed into the extracellular fluid.

Dyclonine is available as a 0.5% solution for use in dentistry. It is not indicated for use by injection or infiltration.

Benzonatate

Benzonatate (Tessalon) is a topical anesthetic that acts on the stretch receptors in the respiratory passages, lungs, and pleura, depressing the cough reflex. It is used for symptomatic relief of coughing. In recommended doses the drug has no effect on the respiratory center.

Because of the depressed cough and gag reflexes that result from this drug, care must be taken to prevent foreign particles from entering the throat. Side effects of benzonatate include nasal congestion, sedation, headache, dizziness, rash, and gastrointestinal upset.

RITICAL THINKING ACTIVITIES

1. Select an anesthetic and review the literature for the following:
   a. Allergic reactions
   b. Preservatives and reactions
   c. Duration of anesthesia
   d. Dosages available
   e. Other properties
2. Apply a topical anesthetic to a cotton-tipped applicator. Place it on the floor of a fellow student's mouth for 10 seconds (providing no medical contraindications exist) and then remove it. Determine the amount of time required for the anesthetic effect to subside.
3. Review the dental records of three patients who were given a local anesthetic for dental procedures. Record the information the same way the dosage notations were made in the record.

REVIEW QUESTIONS

The following questions refer to the case study presented at the beginning of this chapter.

1. An ester-type local anesthetic is contraindicated for Mrs. Macklin because of which of the following conditions?
   a. History of hypertension
   b. Hysterectomy
   c. Pseudocholinesterase deficiency
   d. Current medication
2. A local anesthetic with a low concentration of vasoconstrictor was selected for Mrs. Macklin because of which of the following conditions?
   a. History of hypertension
   b. Hysterectomy
   c. Pseudocholinesterase deficiency
   d. Current medication
3. Which of the following factors bests explains why Mrs. Macklin felt faint 2 minutes after injection of the local anesthetic?
   a. History of hypertension
   b. Hysterectomy
   c. Pseudocholinesterase deficiency
   d. Anxiety

4. Mepivacaine with 2% epinephrine was selected for Mrs. Macklin. Which of the following options describes the function of epinephrine in this solution?
   a. To prolong the depth of anesthesia
   b. To increase the toxicity of the drug
   c. To alter the pH of the injection area
   d. To reduce the patient's anxiety
5. In Mrs. Macklin's case, the effectiveness of the local anesthetic may be reduced for which of the following reasons?
   a. The low pH of the infected area may reduce the formation of free base.
   b. The low pH of the infected area may reduce the formation of salt from the free base.
   c. The high pH of the infected area may reduce the formation of free base.
   d. The high pH of the infected area may reduce the formation of salt from the free base.

SUGGESTED AGENCIES AND WEB SITES

Because of the ever-changing nature of the Internet, some of the web sites listed here may have changed since publication. Please refer to Mosby's Evolve web site for the most current information.

CAI2000 Pharmacology teaching web site ("Local anesthetics side effects/toxicities"): http://www.pharmacology2000.com
Dentistry: http://www.dentistry.about.com

University of Florida College of Medicine, Department of Anesthesiology housestaff manual ("Regional anesthesia [REG]; FSC regional anesthesia [FSCR]"): http://msquared.anest.ufl.edu

ADDITIONAL READINGS AND RESOURCES

Holroyd SV, Wynn RL, Requa-Clark B: *Clinical pharmacology in dental practice,* ed 4, St Louis, 1988, Mosby.
Lehne RA: *Pharmacology for nursing care,* ed 4, Philadelphia, 2001, WB Saunders.
Malamed SF: *Handbook of local anesthesia,* ed 4, St Louis, 1997, Mosby.

Requa-Clark B: *Applied pharmacology for the dental hygienist,* ed 4, St Louis, 2000, Mosby.
Vander AJ, Sherman JH, Luciano DS: *Human physiology: the mechanisms of body functions,* ed 8, New York, 2001, McGraw-Hill.

REFERENCES

1. Arthur GR: Pharmacokinetics of local anesthetics. In Strichartz GR, editor: *Local anesthetics: handbook of experimental pharmacology,* vol 81, Berlin, 1987, Springer-Verlag.

2. Bernhard CG, Bohm E: Local anesthetics as anticonvulsants: a study on experimental and clinical epilepsy. Stockholm, 1965, Almqvist & Wiksell.

3. Butterworth JF IV, Strichartz GR: Molecular mechanisms of local anesthesia: a review, *Anesthesiology* 72:711-34, 1990.

4. Daly DJ, Davenport J, Newland MC: Methemoglobinemia following the use of prilocaine, *Br J Anaesth* 36:737-9, 1964.

5. Foldes FF et al: The relation between plasma cholinesterase and prolonged apnea caused by pseudocholinesterase, *Anesthesiology* 24:208-16, 1963.

6. Gasser HS, Erlander J: The role of fiber size in the establishment of a nerve block by pressure or cocaine, *Am J Physiol* 88:581-91, 1929.

7. Gettes LS: Physiology and pharmacology of antiarrhythmic drugs, *Hosp Pract* 16:89, 1981.

8. Guyton AC, Hall JE: *Textbook of medical physiology,* ed 10, Philadelphia, 2000, WB Saunders.

9. Hardman JG et al, editors: *Goodman and Gilman's the pharmacological basis of therapeutics,* ed 9, New York, 1996, McGraw-Hill.

10. Holroyd SV, Wynn RL, Requa-Clark B: *Clinical pharmacology in dental practice,* ed 4, St Louis, 1988, Mosby.

11. Kalow W: Hydrolysis of local anesthetics by human serum cholinesterase, *J Pharmacol Exp Ther* 104: 122-34, 1952.

12. Lehne RA: *Pharmacology for nursing care,* ed 4, Philadelphia, 2001, WB Saunders.

13. Libelius R et al: Denervation-like changes in skeletal muscle after treatment with a local anesthetic (Marcaine), *J Anat* 106:297, 1970.

14. Malamed SF: *Handbook of local anesthesia,* ed 4, St Louis, 1997, Mosby.

15. Requa-Clark B: *Applied pharmacology for the dental hygienist,* ed 4, St Louis, 2000, Mosby.

16. Ritchie JM: Mechanism of action of local anesthetic agents and biotoxins, *Br J Anaesth* 47:191-8, 1975.

17. Schauf CL, Moffett DF, Moffett SB: *Human physiology: foundations and frontiers,* St Louis, 1990, Mosby.

18. Setnikar I et al: Ionization of bases with limited solubility: investigation of substances with local anesthetic activity, *J Pharm Sci* 55:1190-5, 1990.

19. Vander AJ, Sherman JH, Luciano DS: *Human physiology: the mechanisms of body functions,* ed 6, New York, 1994, McGraw-Hill.

CHAPTER 36

Local Anesthetics: Injectable *and* Topical

Mary Ann Haisch, Nora L. Cromley, Jill Mason

Chapter Outline

Case Study: Administering Local and Topical
  Anesthetic Agents
Equipment
  Needles
  Cartridges
  Syringes
  Safety and handling
Topical Anesthetics
  Benzocaine
  Cocaine hydrochloride
  Dyclonine hydrochloride
  Lidocaine
  Application

Local Anesthesia Techniques
  Guidelines
  Chart entry
Myths about Injection Techniques
  Myth #1: Needle should touch bone
  Myth #2: Bevel of needle must be toward bone
  Myth #3: Rapid injection is better (causes less
    pain)
  Myth #4: Local anesthetic agents should be kept
    in warming device

Key Terms

Anterior superior
  alveolar (ASA)
Aspirating syringe
Aspiration
Gauge
Gow-Gates (G-G)

Greater palatine (GP)
Incisive (I)
Inferior alveolar/lingual (IA)
Infiltration
Infraorbital (IO)
Local infiltration (inf)

Local injectable
  anesthesia
Long buccal (LB)
Mental (M)
Middle superior
  alveolar (MSA)

Nasopalatine (NP)
Nerve block
Posterior superior alveolar
  (PSA)
Scoop technique
Topical anesthetic

Learning Outcomes

1. Discuss the inclusion of local anesthetic injections in dental hygiene practice.
2. Explain how individual state dental practice acts regulate the administration of anesthetic agents.
3. Select the correct armamentarium for individual injections.
4. Prepare the site of injection.
5. Understand the general principles of technique and safety.

6. Recognize the anatomical landmarks associated with the common local anesthetic injections.
7. Describe all major maxillary and mandibular injection techniques used in dental hygiene practice.
8. Understand the myths surrounding injectable local anesthetic administration.
9. Record appropriate chart notations when anesthesia has been administered.

*L*ocal injectable anesthetics are a critical component in providing adequate pain management and hemostasis for dental hygiene care. More than half the state dental practice acts in the United States allow dental hygienists to administer *local injectable anesthesia,* although the level of dental supervision varies among the states. In states that do not allow dental hygienists to administer injectable anesthetics, the dentist must administer anesthesia when necessary, or the patient must do without pain management. When the dentist takes time to anesthetize the hygienist's patients, the productivity of both providers can be adversely affected. A dental hygienist who is educated to administer injectable anesthesia, however, can increase the dentist's productivity by providing that service for the dentist's patients.

Dental hygienists must be familiar with the state practice acts in their specific practice locations because many states do not allow dental hygienists to administer local injectable anesthetic agents. When the dentist administers anesthetic for dental hygiene services, the hygienist is often responsible for the preliminary evaluations of medical histories and the drug reactions and interactions of the selected injectable agent.

EQUIPMENT

The safe and effective administration of regional or local anesthesia partly depends on the equipment used for injections. The use of the single-dose anesthetic cartridge, disposable needle, and sterile *aspirating syringe* ensures accurate placement of the local anesthetic solution without risk to the patient of cross-contamination or intravascular injection. The dental hygienist should be aware of Occupational Safety and Health Administration (OSHA) regulations and work practice controls for standard safety precautions and procedures when using anesthetic equipment. Knowledge of head and neck anatomy, familiarity with injection techniques, and confidence in the use of anesthetic equipment are essential to successful regional or local anesthesia for dental hygiene services.

NEEDLES

Dental hygienists and dentists routinely administer injections with minimal consideration given to the needle used. Safety and sterility of needles are taken for granted. Since its invention in 1853, the hypodermic needle has undergone numerous changes. Research and manufacturing advances have produced a needle that is strong yet flexible, sharp, sterile, and most importantly, designed for single-patient use. Disposable stainless steel needles have a multilevel point designed to produce an efficient puncture with minimal trauma to the mucosa and subcutaneous tissue. Needles are described by length and diameter (gauge), which must be considered for individual injections.

The content of this chapter should not be considered the primary resource for the teaching of local anesthesia. For a more comprehensive text, the reader should refer to *Handbook of Local Anesthesia* by Stanley F. Malamed (ed 4, St Louis, 1997, Mosby), to whom these authors have referred numerous times and wish to thank for the use of photographs and illustrations.

Case Study

Administering Local and Topical Anesthetic Agents

Mr. Brian Shoeman is a 42-year-old computer programmer and a reliable historian. He is 6 feet tall and weighs 238 pounds, has high blood pressure controlled with enalapril (Vasotec, 5 mg/day), and takes loratadine (Claritin) for seasonal allergies. He presents with a blood pressure of 142/93 mm Hg, respiration rate of 17 beats per minute, and heart rate of 102 beats per minute.

Mr. Shoeman's dental issues include generalized aggressive periodontitis. He has had a dental examination and prophylaxis annually; all 32 teeth are present; and no dental restorations or dental caries are evident. Oral findings include generalized subgingival deposits of calculus and plaque, gingival bleeding in all quadrants, supragingival calculus and stain on the linguals of sextant 5.

Mr. Shoeman is scheduled for four 1-hour appointments for quadrant debridement. He indicates that he has many sensitive teeth, and his "gums" hurt when he has his teeth cleaned. Mr. Shoeman has never had local injectable anesthetic and does not like needles.

Length

Needle length varies slightly among manufacturers, but typically a long needle is 1⅝ inches (40 mm) and a short needle approximately 1 inch (25 mm). The type of injection, *infiltration* versus *nerve block,* and individual preference will determine whether a long or short needle is used. Short needles should be used for injections that do not require significant depth of penetration, such as posterior superior alveolar (PSA), middle superior alveolar (MSA), anterior superior alveolar (ASA), long buccal, and mental nerve blocks (see Table 36-3 later in this chapter). Long needles should be used for all major nerve blocks: inferior alveolar, maxillary, Gow-Gates (G-G), and infraorbital (see Table 36-4 later in this chapter). Regardless of the type of injection, no needle should be inserted in soft tissue to its hub. Breakage, although rare, may occur at the hub and is usually the result of lateral pressure exerted against the shank.[5] *The clinician should not attempt to change the direction of a needle when it is embedded in tissue. If the needle must be redirected, it should be withdrawn from the tissue first and then redirected.*[6]

Gauge

The *gauge* of the needle refers to the diameter (width) of the lumen. The most common gauges for regional anesthesia of the oral cavity are 25, 27, and 30; the higher the number, the smaller the opening. Current popularity of the smaller gauge needles (27 and 30) stems from the belief that such needles cause less discomfort during insertion. However, comparisons and clinical studies have shown that a 25-gauge needle can be used as painlessly as a 27- or 30-gauge needle and with more safety.[3,6] The larger gauge needles have two advantages over the smaller gauge needle: less deflection (thus greater accuracy) and ease of positive *aspiration* of blood. The 25-gauge needle is preferred for all injections posing a high risk of positive aspiration, including inferior alveolar, infraorbital, posterior superior alveolar, and Gow-Gates.

CARTRIDGES

Commercial introduction of the disposable glass cartridge for the administration of injectable anesthetics represented a major advance in regional anesthesia of the oral cavity. The convenient dosage form provides for purity and sterility of the anesthetic solution and permits observation of aspirated blood. The dental cartridge is often called a "carpule," which is a trademark name (Carpule is to cartridge as Kleenex is to tissue).

Each year, millions of anesthetic cartridges are used, and the sterility and purity of contents are taken for granted. The proven reliability of cartridges from major pharmaceutical companies is based on a complicated manufacturing process that involves many steps and quality control checks. Cartridges are inspected before shipment, and control samples of each production are set aside for 6 months for continued evaluation.

Although damage to cartridges is rare, it usually occurs during shipment. Before patient use, the cartridges should be visually inspected for (1) signs of breakage (chips, cracks); (2) pea-sized or larger bubbles, which may indicate freezing (as may an extruded plunger); and (3) altered appearance of the anesthetic solution (cloudiness, sediment). Cartridges have a shelf life of 18 months to 5 years depending on the type of anesthetic, vasoconstrictors, and other chemicals used. Expiration dates are clearly printed on each cartridge and on the side and bottom of each container. Any anesthetic solution that has passed the expiration date should not be used.

The contents of each anesthetic cartridge are identified by labeling on the glass tube and include the volume of solution, trade and generic name, concentration of local anesthetic, name and concentration of vasoconstrictors, name and address of supplier, manufacturer's lot number, and expiration date. The dental hygienist should check each cartridge before an injection to guarantee that the desired anesthetic and vasoconstrictors are being administered.

SYRINGES

Several different types of syringes are used in the dental office. The most common types are the metallic cartridge aspirating syringe and the plastic disposable or reusable aspirating syringe.[9] Again, personal preference will determine which type of syringe is used. Regardless of preference, a syringe should meet the American Dental Association (ADA) standards (Box 36-1).[6]

The most satisfactory and widely used syringe for intraoral anesthesia is the metallic cartridge-type syringe, originally introduced in 1921 and modified for aspiration in 1957. One of the hazards of intraoral anesthesia is the inadvertent intravascular injection. The aspirating syringe allows the practitioner to check for this problem by creating negative pressure in the cartridge and visually checking for any signs of blood or discoloration in the cartridge.

BOX 36-1

American Dental Association Standards for Syringes

Syringe should be durable and able to withstand repeated sterilizations without damage. (If disposable, syringe should be packaged in a sterile container.)

Syringe should accommodate a variety of cartridges and needles of different manufacturers and permit repeated use.

Syringe should be inexpensive, self-contained, lightweight, and simple to use with one hand.

Syringe should provide for effective aspiration and should be constructed so that blood may be easily observed in the cartridge.

The plunger on an aspirating syringe engages the rubber stopper with a harpoon or hook and allows the clinician to pull back on the stopper, creating negative pressure inside the cartridge. The incidence of positive aspiration may be as high as 10% to 15% in some injection techniques.[6] The dental hygienist must purposefully conduct an aspiration test (pull back on the plunger) once the injection site has been reached and before administration of the agent. The gauge of the needle also influences the practitioner's ability to aspirate; the 25-gauge needle is the choice for accurate aspiration tests. A self-aspirating syringe was introduced almost 20 years ago, but the initial popularity disappeared because the technique was cumbersome and awkward.

Periodically, new techniques and equipment are introduced for the administration of local anesthetic agents. The computer-controlled and electronic induction techniques have received recent attention. Clinical research studies indicate that these devices are not likely to replace the standard aspirating syringe.[2,4,10]

SAFETY AND HANDLING

Recapping needles has been a risk for infectious disease transmission to healthcare workers. In recent years, health professionals have been at risk for contracting hepatitis B and acquired immunodeficiency syndrome (AIDS) through inadvertent needle sticks after an intraoral injection. When using traditional dental syringe and needles, used needles must never be recapped or otherwise manipulated using both hands.

Needle guards fit on the needle cap and are effective but somewhat cumbersome to use. If a needle is recapped incorrectly when using the needle guard, the tip of the needle will contact the hard paper guard rather than the operator's finger. The *scoop technique* is often recommended by state safety and health agencies.[6] This technique requires that the operator slide the uncapped needle into the needle cap (sheath) while it is lying on the instrument tray or table.

Needle holders are also available for placement of the needle and syringe after use. The needle is covered, protecting the dental healthcare worker. Used recapped needles should be removed from the nondisposable syringe and placed in a sharps container. Disposable syringes may also be placed in the sharps container. Both safety devices and the scoop technique are effective, and the dental hygienist should determine which method is most appropriate for the office circumstances. OSHA has stated recently that "needle guards" are not approved for recapping techniques.

TOPICAL ANESTHETICS

The use of a topically applied local anesthetic is the first step in the process of administering atraumatic local injectable agents. *Topical anesthetic* penetrates any mucous membrane approximately 2 to 3 mm. Deep tissues in the area of application are poorly anesthetized but sufficiently affected to allow painless needle penetration in the mucous membrane.[6]

The concentration of the topical local anesthetic is typically greater than the same agent administered by injection. The higher concentration facilitates diffusion of the drug through the mucous membrane. Higher concentration also leads to a greater potential toxicity, both locally to the tissues and systemically.[1] Because topical anesthetics do not contain vasoconstrictors, and because anesthetics are inherently vasodilating agents, vascular absorption of some topical formulations is rapid, and levels in the blood may soon reach those achieved by direct intravenous administration.[8]

BENZOCAINE

Benzocaine topical anesthetics are the most frequently used topical agents (Table 36-1). Benzocaine is insoluble in water but is soluble in alcohol, propylene glycol, and polyethylene glycol, which are suitable for surface application. Benzocaine is an ester local anesthetic; it is poorly absorbed into the cardiovascular system. Systemic toxic reactions are virtually unknown. Benzocaine remains at the site of application longer than other agents, providing a prolonged duration of action. It is not suitable for injection. Occasionally a localized allergic reaction may occur after prolonged or repeated use.[6]

COCAINE HYDROCHLORIDE

Cocaine hydrochloride is a very effective topical anesthetic. Because of extreme abuse potential, however, cocaine's use as a topical anesthetic in dentistry is not recommended.

DYCLONINE HYDROCHLORIDE

Dyclonine hydrochloride is a unique form of topical local anesthetic because it is a ketone and may be used in patients with sensitivity to other chemical groups. It is commercially available as Dyclone B solution (0.5% dyclonine hydrochloride).

LIDOCAINE

Lidocaine is available in two forms. *Lidocaine base* is poorly soluble in water in a 5% concentration for use on oral abraded or lacerated tissue. *Lidocaine hydrochloride* is water soluble and available in a 2% concentration. Lidocaine is an amide with an exceptionally low incidence of allergic reaction (Table 36-2).

TABLE 36-1		
Common forms of benzocaine		
Trade name	**Form**	**Active ingredient (% benzocaine)**
Cetacaine B (Cycylite Industries)	Liquid, gel	14
Gingicaine (Belport)	Liquid, gel	20
Healthco (Healthco)	Gel	20
Hurricaine (Beutlich)	Liquid, gel, spray	20
Nephron B (Nephron)	Ointment	18
Novol (Novocol Chemical)	Solution	20
Oradent B (Oradent Chemical)	Topical anesthetic	16
Pennwhite B (S.S. White Retail)	Liquid, ointment	20
Preject B (Hoyt Laboratories)	Gel	20
Topex B (Sultan Chemists)	Metered spray	20
Topicale B (Premier Dental Products)	Gel, liquid, ointment	18

TABLE 36-2		
Common forms of lidocaine		
Trade name	**Form**	**Active ingredient (% lidocaine)**
Alphacaine B (Carlisle Laboratories, Rockville Center, N.Y.)	Ointment	5
Lidocaine B (Premier Dental Products, King of Prussia, Pa.)	Gel	5
Lidocaine B (Graham Chemical, Barrington, Ill.)	Liquid (flavored)	5
Lidocaine B (Graham Chemical, Barrington, Ill.)	Ointment	5
Xylocaine B (Astra Pharmaceutical Products, Wilmington, Del.)	Liquid B (flavored)	5
Xylocaine B (Astra Pharmaceutical Products, Wilmington, Del.)	Ointment (flavored)	5
Xylocaine B (Astra Pharmaceutical Products, Wilmington, Del.)	Aerosol	10
Dent. Patch (Noven Pharmaceutical, Miami, Fla.)	Transmucosal patch	20

APPLICATION

After selection of an appropriate topical anesthetic and after use of a topical antiseptic (optional), a small quantity of anesthetic is applied only to the injection site. The use of too much material can lead to adverse effects, unpleasant taste, and anesthesia of the soft palate, pharynx, or tongue. Most importantly, some topical anesthetics can be rapidly absorbed into the cardiovascular system.

The procedure is most efficiently accomplished by placement of a small quantity of topical anesthetic on the tip of a cotton applicator stick, with application directly to the dried injection site for at least 1 minute and preferably 2 minutes before the injection is performed (Fig. 36-1).[6]

Topical anesthesia also may be used for light anesthesia of a small area of gingiva to control discomfort caused by scaling procedures. The area needs to be dry, and the selection of topical anesthesia should provide a relatively long anesthetic effect with low toxicity (e.g., benzocaine product, dyclonine). The clinician should avoid swabbing topical anesthetic throughout the mouth instead of using injections. Swabbing does not provide profound anesthesia, and more importantly, dosage cannot be documented well.[1]

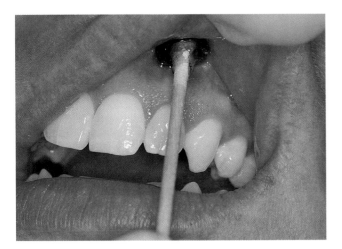

FIG. 36-1 A small quantity of topical anesthetic is placed at the site of needle penetration and permitted to remain for at least 1 minute.

LOCAL ANESTHESIA TECHNIQUES

36-A

It is always important to provide local anesthesia in a safe, aseptic manner to avoid possible complications during the procedure. Safe administration includes a thorough health history review for possible drug interactions or systemic disease that may require special attention (see Chapter 10). Safe technique includes stable fulcrums, slow speed of injection, aspiration, and good personal and patient protection from contamination or injury. Patient observation and good communication techniques are critical during local anesthesia administration.

GUIDELINES

Basic atraumatic injection technique may be used for any injection (Box 36-2). Table 36-3 (Figs. 36-2 through 36-7) and Table 36-4 (Figs. 36-8 through 36-11) outline specific techniques for maxillary and mandibular injections, respectively. The suggested amounts of solution for each injection are for routine closed periodontal scaling procedures, which are usually less than the amount needed for

Text continued on p. 606

BOX 36-2

Guidelines for Successful Injections

1. *Select needle.* Needle length and gauge are based on type of injection. For deeper block injections, such as an infraorbital (IO), inferior alveolar (IA), second division (V_2), or Gow-Gates (G-G), a long needle is recommended. For all other injections, a short needle is adequate and provides an opportunity for a more stable fulcrum, particularly for small hands. The American Dental Association (ADA) standard of care is 25 gauge, but a 27-gauge needle is frequently used in clinical practice.[3] For local infiltrations, a 30-gauge needle may also be used.

2. *Warm anesthetic and syringe.* It is not necessary to warm the solution before injection. Room temperature up to body temperature is sufficient. If the anesthetic has been stored in refrigeration to prolong shelf life and has just been removed, warming the solution may be advised.[7]

3. *Check flow.* After loading the syringe, check to make sure the anesthetic is flowing properly to avoid having to withdraw the needle after insertion to establish the flow.

4. *Position patient.* Position the patient in a supine position.

5. *Dry the tissue.* Dry the site of injection before placing topical anesthetic so that the topical anesthetic will remain in the location of the insertion and will not be flushed away by saliva.

6. *Apply topical antiseptic* (optional). This attempt to disinfect the site before injection is not usually done in practice.

7. *Apply topical anesthetic.* Apply a small amount of the topical anesthetic of choice to the site. A large amount is not necessary and may combine with saliva and may be swallowed by the patient. A numb throat may be an unwelcome feeling for a patient. Allow 1 to 2 minutes for maximum effect before continuing with the insertion.

Continued

BOX 36-2

Guidelines for Successful Injections—cont'd

8. *Communicate with patient.* At all times during the procedure, observe the patient and keep the patient informed to the extent desired. Communicate that you intend to go as slowly as possible to provide the anesthesia as comfortably as possible. Do not promise there will be no pain or discomfort; each patient differs in perception of pain or discomfort, and the interpretation cannot be anticipated. Allow the patient to inform you if discomfort occurs. Address this painful situation by slowing down or withdrawing the needle slightly to alleviate the discomfort.

9. *Use fulcrum.* A stable fulcrum is essential in case of patient movement and to ensure that the needle tip remains at the target while aspirating, while the plunger is advanced, during deposit of solution, and when withdrawing the needle. For people with small hands who cannot reach the face or chin with a fulcrum finger, keeping an elbow against the side of the body may provide stability.

10. *Pull tissue taut.* Taut tissue at the injection site allows easier penetration and can be less traumatic. There is no need to "jiggle" the lip during penetration, a diversion technique used to distract patients. New students of anesthesia may have difficulty jiggling one hand and not the other.

11. *Keep syringe out of sight.* Holding the syringe below the patient's line of sight may reduce anxiety.

12. *Insert needle slowly.* Slow, gentle insertion and expressing a *tiny* amount of anesthetic at a couple of points during insertion can reduce discomfort significantly. It is not necessary to aspirate before each drop that may be expressed during insertion.

13. *Monitor patient.* Monitor the patient's status during the injection, adjusting flow rate as necessary to provide a comfortable dental experience. Allow the patient to signal you by slightly raising the hand away from you if there is discomfort. By allowing the patient some control over the process, you will have a more relaxed patient, and you will be able to deliver a better injection.

14. Slowly *advance the needle to the target.* It cannot be overemphasized that a slow injection is a more comfortable injection. Frequently, injections are the prime cause for anxiety in the dental chair. By learning atrau-

matic techniques in administering anesthesia, you can reduce much of that anxiety.

15. *Deposit a few drops at the periosteum.* The periosteum is extremely sensitive, and many injections require that you inject at or near the periosteum. A couple of drops of anesthetic administered just before reaching the periosteum can avoid the sharp sensation in many injections.

16. *Aspirate.* Before depositing the bolus of anesthetic solution at the target site, aspirate by drawing back on the plunger firmly to ensure that the needle tip is not in a blood vessel. If the needle is in a vessel, blood will be drawn into the cartridge. This *positive aspiration* requires repositioning of the needle tip so that it is not in the vessel. Some authors advocate aspiration on two planes to make sure that the lumen of the needle is not against a vessel wall, thus not providing positive aspiration even though the needle is actually in a vessel.[6] This is a critical step in the injection procedure because injection into a vessel and speed of injection are two common causes of complications from an injection, and both can be prevented by following this technique.

17. Slowly *deposit solution.* Slow depositing of the solution reduces patient discomfort both during and after the injection and helps reduce complications associated with rapid injections.

18. *Continue to communicate with patient.* Again, as a reminder, communication with the patient throughout the injection can allay fears and provide necessary feedback to the dental hygienist.

19. *Slowly withdraw needle.* After slowly withdrawing the needle, recap it by using a one-handed technique for "scooping" up the needle sheath with the syringe hand. Do *not* grasp the needle sheath with your free hand and place it over the needle. OSHA does not allow this practice, which also does not protect the provider from needle sticks.

20. *Observe patient.* Unexpected complications may not occur immediately during or after the injection but may occur a few minutes later. Do not leave the patient unattended once the injection has been completed. Complete the entry in the chart while you observe the patient for a few minutes.

21. *Record injection in chart.*

TABLE 36-3

Technique guide for maxillary injections

Nerve block	Insertion point	Angles	Needle size, depth of insertion	Target	Dose, areas anesthetized
Posterior superior alveolar (PSA)	Height of mucobuccal fold above second molar	Needle directed 45 degrees medially, 45 from long axis of tooth, and 45 from occlusal plane; bevel toward bone	25/27 gauge short. *Depth:* ≥4 mm of needle visible	Slightly above and distal to distobuccal root of last molar, second or third if present (see Fig. 36-2)	0.9-1.8 ml *Teeth anesthetized:* maxillary molars except mesiobuccal root of first molar *Periodontal tissues:* facial to affected teeth
Middle superior alveolar (MSA)	Height of mucobuccal fold above second premolar	Needle directed 20 degrees medially; bevel toward bone	25/27 gauge short; needle inserted until needle tip is above apex of second premolar	Above apex of second premolar (see Fig. 36-3)	0.9-1.2 ml *Teeth anesthetized:* maxillary premolars and mesiofacial root of first molar *Periodontal tissues:* facial to affected teeth
Anterior superior alveolar (ASA)	Height of mucobuccal fold above canine	Needle directed 25 degrees medially; bevel toward bone	25/27 gauge short; needle inserted until needle tip is above apex of canine	Slightly mesial to and above apex of canine (see Fig. 36-4)	0.9-1.2 ml *Teeth anesthetized:* canine, lateral, central *Periodontal tissues:* facial to affected teeth
Nasopalatine (NP)	*Infiltration:* just lateral to incisive papilla *Block:* center of papilla on midline	*Infiltration:* 45 degrees toward incisive papilla *Block:* parallel with long axis of centrals; bevel toward palate	25/27 gauge short *Infiltration:* 3-5 mm *Block:* 6-10 mm	Incisive foramen beneath incisive papilla (see Fig. 36-5)	≤0.45 ml *Periodontal tissues:* palatal to incisors and canines
Greater palatine (GP)	Over palatine foramen at junction of palatine bone and alveolar process above and lingual to second molar	From opposite side of mouth at right angle to target area; bevel toward palate	25/27 gauge short *Depth:* 4-6 mm (<10 mm)	Greater palatine foramen (see Fig. 36-6)	0.4-0.6 ml *Periodontal tissues:* palatal tissues to posterior teeth
Infraorbital (IO)	Height of mucobuccal folder over first premolar	Needle parallel to long axis of tooth; bevel toward bone	25/27 gauge long; half the length of needle	Infraorbital foramen (see Fig. 36-7)	0.9-1.2 ml *Teeth anesthetized:* premolar/incisors *Periodontal tissues:* facial to affected teeth

Modified from Malamed SF: *Handbook of local anesthesia,* ed 4, St Louis, 1996, Mosby.

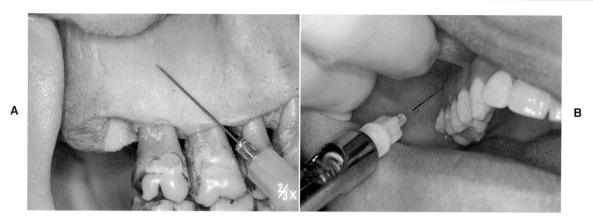

FIG. 36-2   A, Posterior superior alveolar (PSA) injection target. **B,** PSA injection site. (See Table 36-3.) (Courtesy OHSU Department of Dental Hygiene, Portland, Ore.)

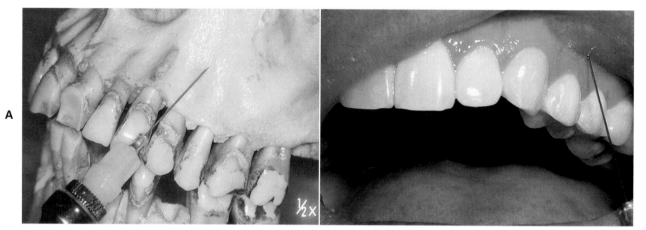

FIG. 36-3   A, Middle superior alveolar (MSA) injection target. **B,** MSA injection site. (See Table 36-3.) (Courtesy OHSU Department of Dental Hygiene, Portland, Ore.)

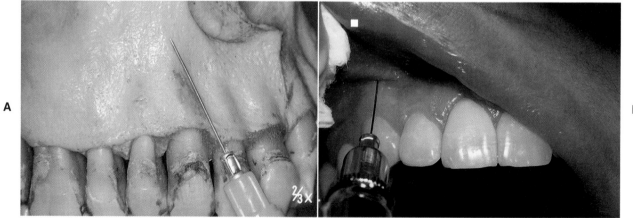

FIG. 36-4   A, Anterior superior alveolar (ASA) injection target. **B,** ASA injection site. (See Table 36-3.) (Courtesy OHSU Department of Dental Hygiene, Portland, Ore.)

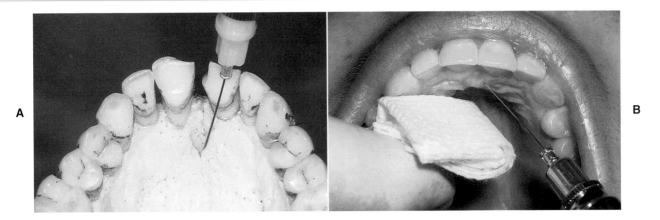

FIG. 36-5 A, Nasopalatine (NP) injection target. **B,** NP injection site. (See Table 36-3.) (Courtesy OHSU Department of Dental Hygiene, Portland, Ore.)

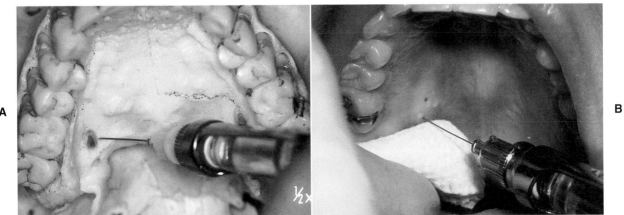

FIG. 36-6 A, Greater palatine (GP) injection target. **B,** GP injection site. (See Table 36-3.) (Courtesy OHSU Department of Dental Hygiene, Portland, Ore.)

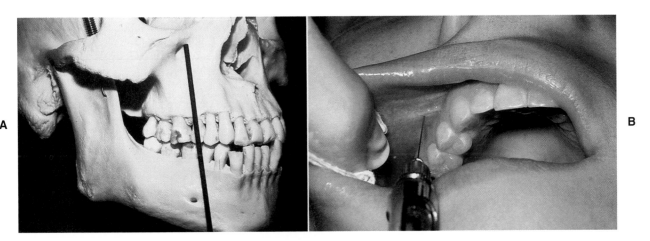

FIG. 36-7 A, Infraorbital (IO) injection target. **B,** IO injection site. (See Table 36-3.) (Courtesy OHSU Department of Dental Hygiene, Portland, Ore.)

TABLE 36-4

Technique guide for mandibular injections

Nerve block	Insertion point	Angles	Needle size, depth of insertion	Target	Dose, areas anesthetized
Inferior alveolar/ lingual (IA)	Midway between maxillary and mandibular molar occlusal plane, lateral to pterygomandibular raphe and medial to internal oblique ridge	Barrel of syringe in corner of mouth on opposite side	25/27 gauge long *Depth:* ⅔ to ¾ length of needle; contact with bone; bevel toward bone	On ramus slightly superior to mandibular foramen (see Fig. 36-8)	1.5-1.8 ml Teeth, periodontal tissues, and tongue in quadrant
Long buccal (LB)	Mucous membrane distal and buccal to most posterior molar	Syringe parallel to occlusal plane but lateral to teeth; bevel facing down toward bone	25/27 gauge long (short also acceptable) *Depth:* ≤4 mm; bevel under tissue	Supraperiosteal, distal, and buccal to most posterior molar (see Fig. 36-9)	0.2-0.3 ml (width of rubber stopper) Soft tissue and periosteum facial to molars
Mental (M)	Mucobuccal fold at or just anterior to mental foramen	Approximately 20 degrees from long axis of premolars Bevel toward bone	25/27 gauge short *Depth:* 5-6 mm	Mental nerve as it exits foramen (see Fig. 36-10)	0.6 ml Soft tissue and periosteum from premolars to midline
Incisive (I)	Mucobuccal fold at or just anterior to mental foramen	Approximately 20 degrees from long axis of premolars; bevel toward bone	25/27 gauge short *Depth:* 5-6 mm	Mental foramen; pressure applied for 2 minutes after injection (see Fig. 36-10)	0.6 ml. Soft tissue, periosteum, and teeth from premolars to midline
Local infiltration (inf)	Mucobuccal fold labial to tooth in question	Needle directed toward apex of tooth	27/30 gauge short *Depth:* 3-5 mm	Apex of tooth	0.6 ml Tooth and soft tissue at site
Gow-Gates (G-G)	Distal to maxillary second molar at height of mesiolingual cusp	Barrel of syringe in corner of mouth on opposite side. Proceed on a line from corner of mouth to tragus	25 gauge long *Depth:* ½ length of needle; contact with bone	Lateral side of condylar neck (see Fig. 36-11)	1.8 ml Teeth, soft tissues, and bone in mandibular quadrant

Modified from Malamed SF: *Handbook of local anesthesia*, ed 4, St Louis, 1996, Mosby.)

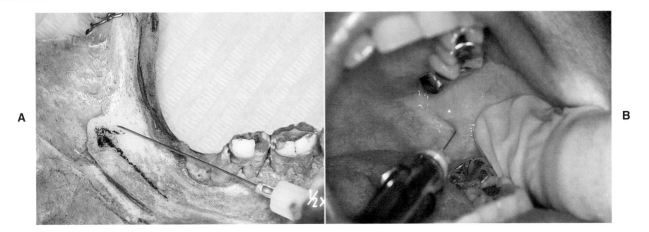

FIG. 36-8 A, Inferior alveolar (IA) injection target. **B,** IA injection site. (See Table 36-4.) (Courtesy OHSU Department of Dental Hygiene, Portland, Ore.)

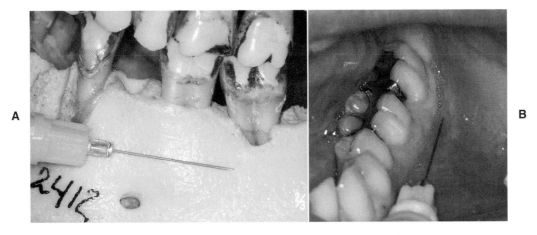

FIG. 36-9 A, Long buccal (LB) injection target. **B,** LB injection site. (See Table 36-4.) (Courtesy OHSU Department of Dental Hygiene, Portland, Ore.)

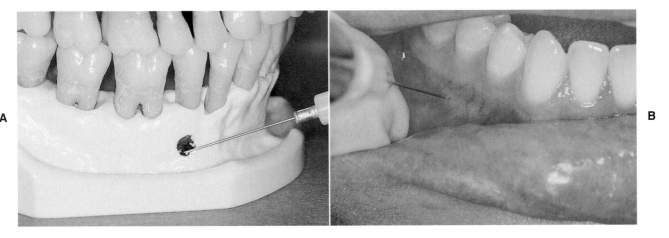

FIG. 36-10 A, Mental/incisive (M/I) injection target. **B,** M/I injection site. (See Table 36-4.)

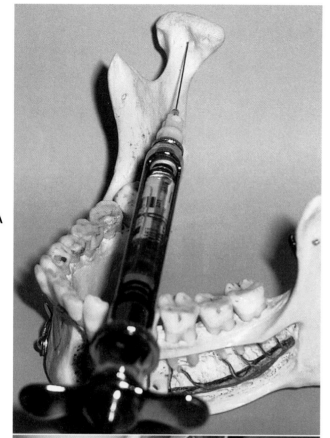

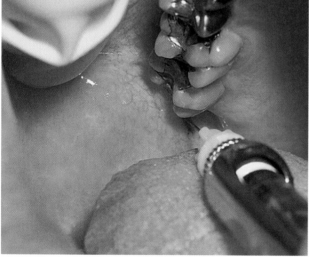

FIG. 36-11 A, Gow-Gates (GG) injection target. **B,** GG injection site. (See Table 36-4.) (Courtesy OHSU Department of Dental Hygiene, Portland, Ore.)

the profound pulpal anesthesia in restorative or surgical procedures.

CHART ENTRY

No anesthesia administration is complete without an appropriate chart entry. Specific information must be documented with administration of injectable or topical anesthetics (Box 36-3).

BOX 36-3

Chart Entry for Local Anesthesia

1. Date
2. Amount of anesthetic administered (e.g., ml/mg/cartridges)
3. Type and concentration of anesthetic (e.g., 3% Carbocaine)
4. Type and concentration of vasoconstrictor (e.g., 1:100,000 epinephrine, 1:20,000 levonordefrin)
5. Type of injection
   Abbreviations: right *(Rt)*, left *(Lt)*, anterior superior alveolar *(ASA)*, middle superior alveolar *(MSA)*, posterior superior alveolar *(PSA)*, inferior alveolar *(IA)*, long buccal *(LB)*, mental *(M)*, incisive *(I)*, nasopalatine *(NP)*, Gow-Gates *(G-G)*, greater palatine *(GP)*, infraorbital *(IO)*, second division *(V₂)*
6. Reactions
7. Name of dental practitioner administering the anesthetic
   Example
   10/10/99: 3.6 ml 2% Xylocaine with 1:100,000 epi, Rt PSA, MSA, GP (no reactions); G. Gardener, RDH

MYTHS ABOUT INJECTION TECHNIQUES

Once the basics are mastered, dental hygienists will develop their own particular techniques and strategies for giving a painless injection. During the learning phase, hygiene students may hear reference to the following myths about injection techniques.

MYTH #1: NEEDLE SHOULD TOUCH BONE

It is not necessary or desirable to have the tip of the needle touch the bone or periosteum. This technique is often mentioned in reference to the mandibular nerve block and locating the medial aspect of the mandible. This suggestion is made to ensure needle placement in the correct anatomical position. The periosteum is sensitive, however, and it is painful when the needle touches the bone. In addition, barbs may be created on the tip of the needle by hitting the bone and may cause *trismus* (muscle soreness) or *paresthesia* (prolonged anesthesia).[11]

MYTH #2: BEVEL OF NEEDLE MUST BE TOWARD BONE

Although it may be desirable to have the bevel toward the bone for reasons of patient comfort during the injection, it is not essential for success of the anesthesia. Placement of the needle bevel toward the bone may result in more anesthetic solution being deposited at the target site. However, clinical studies have shown that three major factors affect the correct deposition of solution: speed of injection, flexibility (lumen size) of needle, and type of bevel. The practitioner should concentrate on the position of the needle in relation to the anatomical structure and a controlled technique rather than focusing on whether the bevel is toward or away from the bone.

MYTH #3: RAPID INJECTION IS BETTER (CAUSES LESS PAIN)

A rapid injection may result in less operator anxiety but not less patient pain. A slow injection is less painful and safer for the patient. It should take a minimum of 1 minute (full 60 seconds) to inject a standard cartridge containing 1.8 ml of anesthetic solution. For the beginning student, 1 minute may seem like an eternity; however, this period allows the operator time to complete several aspiration checks and results in less discomfort for the patient. Injecting a solution into a patient's soft tissue means that a space is created for the fluid. This sensation may be interpreted as pain or pressure by the patient. A slow injection minimizes this sensation.

MYTH #4: LOCAL ANESTHETIC AGENTS SHOUD BE KEPT IN WARMING DEVICE

No significant difference exists in patient acceptance of anesthetic solution at room temperature versus solution maintained in warming equipment. Many dentists consider warming the anesthetic solution before injection to be beneficial, but clinical studies have shown no significant difference between the solution at room temperature and warmed solution. If the anesthetic solution has been refrigerated for storage, the solution should be brought to room temperature before use.[2,7]

RITICAL THINKING ACTIVITIES

1. Inject an anesthetic solution into a cup of water colored with red dye (such as a disclosing solution) and aspirate. This helps in understanding pressure, technique, and positive aspiration.
2. Illustrate needle length, lumen, and bevel using graph paper. This helps in comparing and contrasting sizes and shapes.
3. Using different materials (e.g., tomatoes, hot dogs, fabric, meat), penetrate each with a loaded syringe and needle. Feel the resistance of different surfaces and "tissues."
4. Working in pairs, perform a clinical experiment to determine the differences among 25-, 27-, and 30-gauge needles.
   a. Dry the buccal mucosa in the vestibular area of maxillary arch; do not use topical anesthetic.
   b. Hold mucosa taut.
   c. Gently penetrate the mucosa with each needle size at different sites.
   d. Question the patient (partner) as to which size needle was felt the most or least.

Questions 5 through 13 refer to the case study presented at the beginning of the chapter.
5. How would you proceed on the first appointment of the prescribed treatment for Mr. Shoeman?
6. Which factors will determine the need for the use of local anesthetic?
7. How would you reduce Mr. Shoeman's apprehension?
8. Are there any contraindications to using local anesthetic?
9. Which type of anesthetic would you use? Why?
10. Which injections would you use to begin treatment on quadrant 1?
11. Which are the appropriate length and gauge of the needle for these injections?
12. Which type of topical anesthetic would be most appropriate?
13. With Mr. Shoeman's medical history, which medical complication might occur?

REVIEW QUESTIONS

The following questions refer to the case study presented at the beginning of the chapter.

1. To anesthetize all the hard and adjacent soft tissue indicated for root planing on Mr. Shoeman's quadrant 2, which of the following injections is needed?
   a. Rt G-G; Lt PSA, MSA
   b. Lt PSA, MSA, GP, ASA, NP
   c. Lt PSA, ASA, Rt M
   d. Rt PSA, MSA, GP; Lt PSA, GP
   e. Rt M/I, Lt G-G
2. For PSA injection, the correct needle would have which of the following gauges?
   a. 30 long
   b. 27 short
   c. 30 short
   d. 25 long
   e. 27 long

3. Mr. Shoeman calls the dental office and complains of sloughing of mucosal tissue in his mouth on the treated side. Which of the following is the most likely cause?
   a. Gauze square was used to dry the injection sites.
   b. Local anesthetic solution dripped on the oral tissues.
   c. Patient used too much salt in the saltwater solution used to rinse.
   d. Topical anesthetic gel was in contact with a large area of mucosal tissue.
   e. Patient started home care too soon after root-planing procedure.

Continued

REVIEW QUESTIONS—cont'd

4. Which of the following would be an appropriate local anesthesia chart entry for the appointment to scale Mr. Shoeman's mandibular right quadrant?
   a. 10/21/2002, 2 cartridges of 2% lidocaine with 1:100,000 epinephrine, no reactions; G. Gardener, RDH
   b. 2 cartridges of 2% Xylocaine with 1:100,000 epinephrine, Rt IA, LB. Patient stated he felt his heart "racing" at first, but it returned to normal in approximately 3 minutes; G. Gardener, RDH
   c. 72 mg of 2% lidocaine with 1:100,000 epinephrine, IA, LB; G. Gardener, RDH
   d. 10/21/2002, 2 cartridges of 2% Xylocaine with 1:100,000 epinephrine, Rt IA, LB, no reactions; G. Gardener, RDH
   e. 10/21/2002, 2 cartridges of 2% lidocaine with 1:100,000 epinephrine, I, LB, no reactions

5. To reassure Mr. Shoeman before the administration of the local anesthetic, which of the following techniques might be most effective?
   a. Tell him that many people receive local anesthetic every day for dental treatment, and most state that the injection causes little discomfort.
   b. Explain the entire procedure, indicating what will be done to make it as comfortable as possible.
   c. Show him all the equipment, explain the tract of the needle, and indicate which anatomical structures are pierced.
   d. Premedicate him with a barbiturate compound to calm him down.
   e. Begin the treatment, and demonstrate how uncomfortable the procedure can be to encourage him to try the anesthetic.

6. Mr. Shoeman complains of his heart rate increasing after injection of the 2% lidocaine solution. Which of the following could have caused this increase?
   a. He was very anxious and his heart just beat faster.
   b. The heart rate naturally goes up when local anesthetic is injected.
   c. The local anesthetic solution contains epinephrine.
   d. The solution was injected into a blood vessel.
   e. All the above

 SUGGESTED AGENCIES AND WEB SITES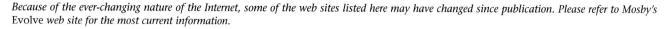

Because of the ever-changing nature of the Internet, some of the web sites listed here may have changed since publication. Please refer to Mosby's Evolve *web site for the most current information.*

About.com ("New advances in dental anesthesia"): anesthesiology.about.com
Academy of General Dentistry ("Consumer information: anesthesia"): http://www.agd.org
American Dental Association ("Oral health topic: anesthesia"): http://www.ada.org
Mobile Anesthesia Medical Group, Inc. ("Candidates for dental anesthesia"): http://www.dental-anesthesia.com
Mobile Anesthesia Medical Group, Inc. ("Dental anesthesia questions and answers for patients"): http://www.dental-anesthesia.com

University of Washington faculty site ("Electronic dental anesthesia"): http://faculty.washington.edu
UTHealth.com (Utah's local health source: "Dental anesthesia on the Web"): http://www.uthealth.com
Web crawler ("Dental anesthesia," web sites): http://www.webcrawler.com

 ADDITIONAL READINGS AND RESOURCES

Jastak JT, Yagiela JA, Donaldson D: *Local anesthesia of the oral cavity,* Philadelphia, 1995, WB Saunders.
Malamed SF: *Medical emergencies in the dental office,* ed 5, St Louis, 2000, Mosby.
Peretz B, Bimstein E: The use of imagery suggestions during administration of local anesthetic in pediatric dental patients, *ASDC J Dent Child* 67(4):263-7, 2000.
Yagiela JA, Neidle EA, Dowd FJ: *Pharmacology and therapeutics for dentistry,* ed 4, St Louis, 1998, Mosby.

REFERENCES

1. Adriani J, Campbell D: Fatalities following topical application of local anesthetics to mucous membranes, *JAMA* 162:1527, 1956.

2. Burke FJ: Dentist and patient evaluation of an electronic dental analgesia system for controlling discomfort of injections, *Dent Update* 24(4):154-7, 1997.

3. Farsakian LR, Weine FS: The significance of needle gauge in dental injections, *Compend Cont Educ Dent Pract* 12(4):262-8 1991.

4. Friedman MJ, Hochman MN: A 21st century computerized injection system for local pain control, *Compend Cont Educ Dent Pract* 18(10):995-1000, 1997.

5. Jastak JT, Yagelia JA: *Regional anesthesia of the oral cavity,* St Louis, 1981, Mosby.

6. Lieberman WH: The wand, *Pediatr Dent* 21(2):124, 1999.

7. Malamed SF: *Handbook of local anesthesia,* ed 4, St Louis, 1997, Mosby.

8. Meechan JG, McCabe JF: Effect of different storage methods on the performance of dental local anesthetic cartridges, *J Dent* 20(1):38-42, 1992.

9. Patterson RP, Anderson J: Allergic reactions to drugs and biologic agents, *JAMA* 248:2637-45, 1982.

10. Piesold J, Muller W, Dreissig J: An experimental study of the aspirating reliability of different types of injection syringes with regard to the formation of punch cylinders, *Br J Oral Maxillofac Surg* 36(1):39-43, 1998.

11. Rowson JE, Preshaw PM: The use of lidocaine in dental practice, *J Dent* 25(5):431-3, 1997.

CHAPTER 37

Nitrous Oxide/Oxygen Sedation

Ann L. Brunick

Chapter Outline

Case Study: Administration of Nitrous
   Oxide/Oxygen Sedation
Analgesic and Other Effects
Pharmacology
Indications
Relative Contraindications
Equipment
Administration
   Stages of anesthesia
   Oversedation
   Technique

Recovery
   Diffusion hypoxia
   Vital signs
   Psychomotor assessment
   Record keeping
Biological Effects and Issues
   Exposure levels
   Trace contamination

Key Terms

Amnesia
Analgesia
Analgesic
Anesthesia
Anesthetic
Anxiety

Anxiolytic
Biovariability
Conscious
Diffusion hypoxia
Gag reflex
Informed consent

Oversedation
Pain
Pharmacologic sedation
Pulse oximeter
Scavenge

Scavenging devices
Tidal volume
Titration
Unconscious

Learning Outcomes

1. Appreciate the history of N_2O use and its association with the dental profession.
2. Identify the effects of N_2O on pain, anxiety, and the body's systems.
3. Understand the properties of N_2O.
4. Explain indications and relative contraindications for the use of N_2O/O_2 sedation.
5. Identify equipment associated with N_2O/O_2 sedation.
6. Describe the appropriate technique for N_2O/O_2 administration.

7. Recognize signs and symptoms of ideal sedation and oversedation.
8. Recognize appropriate recovery from N_2O/O_2 sedation.
9. Separate facts from fallacies associated with chronic exposure to N_2O.
10. Describe methods for detection, assessment and minimization of trace levels of N_2O in the dental setting.

Nitrous oxide/oxygen (N_2O/O_2) sedation has enjoyed a long and successful history as an effective method for the management of **pain** and **anxiety.** In millions of cases documented in the literature, N_2O has been used with no adverse effects.[2,11,15] Thus the safety of the drug is without question. To illustrate its safety further, there has never been a documented allergy to N_2O. Few drugs can replicate these statistics.

Horace Wells, a Connecticut dentist, discovered in 1844 that N_2O has **anesthetic** and **analgesic** effects. He used N_2O to anesthetize patients before tooth extractions and other procedures. He taught the technique to medical and dental professionals in the United States and Europe. The American Dental Association (ADA), American Medical Association (AMA), and several other professional societies posthumously recognized him as the "discoverer of *anesthesia.*"[9] While other anesthetic agents (e.g., ether, cyclopropane) were being introduced in the late 1800s and early 1900s, N_2O kept a low profile. Its use began to increase again, however, when dental schools began teaching nitrous anesthesia as part of their curricula. Currently, as many as 88% of pediatric dentists use N_2O/O_2, as do most other specialists within dentistry, including dental hygiene.[6] Several states allow dental hygienists to administer and monitor N_2O/O_2 sedation after appropriate education. It is anticipated that many other states will allow this expanded function in the future.

As a discipline, dentistry has historically been a primary user of this type of pain and anxiety management. However, many other professions have taken advantage of its effectiveness. Nitrous oxide/oxygen has been used in emergency medicine and for labor and delivery. The disciplines of podiatry, dermatology, endoscopy, and radiology have cited its use for several procedures. With increased outpatient procedures, use of N_2O/O_2 sedation will probably increase as well.

Nitrous oxide/oxygen sedation is a safe and effective method to assist patients in managing the pain and anxiety associated with many clinical situations. When the educated professional uses the appropriate equipment and techniques for administration and scavenging, N_2O/O_2 sedation offers many advantages for both patient and operator.

ANALGESIC AND OTHER EFFECTS

Nitrous oxide has the ability to produce varying degrees of *analgesia* (pain control). The degree of pain reduction depends on a number of factors. Individuals perceive and react to pain differently, and pain is even tolerated differently within the same individual during a variety of different occasions. Stress, age, fatigue, and cultural background are all factors that may influence how a person reacts to pain.

Nitrous oxide has been shown to obtund mild to severe pain.[3] Patients often associate anxiety with pain; when anxiety is present, typically the patient will not tolerate pain as well. Nitrous oxide is a central nervous system (CNS) depressant that provides a level of sedation in which the patient becomes relaxed and comfortable. This sense of well-being allows the patient to better tolerate the stressful situation and raises the patient's pain threshold.

Patients often indicate slight *amnesia* associated with N_2O/O_2 use. Their perception of time passage may be altered slightly. Patients often think their office visit was shorter than the actual time elapsed.

Nitrous oxide/oxygen may be used successfully in combination with other sedation methods and drugs. Effects may be enhanced when words are spoken slowly and soothingly. Nitrous oxide should not be used as a substitute for local anesthesia when the latter is indicated. Rather, the combination offers excellent results.

Edmond Eger II, a prominent anesthesiologist and "adversary-turned-advocate" of N_2O, tested previously reported biologic effects. His research showed no evidence that N_2O was dangerous to a patient having elective surgery.[7] Eger reports that N_2O does not significantly affect the body's systems or adversely affect respiratory, circulatory, cardiovascular, hepatic, or hematopoietic function.

PHARMACOLOGY

Nitrous oxide is manufactured when the raw ingredient, ammonium nitrate (NH_4NO_3), is heated to approximately 250° C. Ammonium nitrate decomposes into N_2O, water, and negligible contaminant compounds. The water and contaminants are removed, and the remaining N_2O gas is compressed into a liquid state. The product is refrigerated and stored until transferred to a hospital or distributing center. All manufacturers must comply with the U.S. Food and Drug Administration (FDA) rules and regulations and meet the specifications of the *U.S. Pharmacopeia.*

Nitrous oxide itself is not flammable; however, it does support combustion. If the gas comes in contact with a substance or flame of 1200° F, it will decompose. If the decomposition occurs under pressure, such as in a high-pressure pipeline or within a cylinder, a violent explosion will occur. A similar reaction will occur if N_2O comes in contact with a hydrocarbon substance, such as lubricant, grease, or oil. In this scenario the temperature of N_2O is critical. A rapid rise in gas temperature combined with

Case Study   Administration of Nitrous Oxide/Oxygen Sedation

Jacob Gruenwald is a 45-year-old construction worker. Significant items on his health history include a family history of hypertension and cancer. He had arthroscopic knee surgery after a sports-related injury. Although he has no medication allergies, he is allergic to dust and has seasonal pollen allergies. He uses prescription antihistamines and decongestants as needed. He carries an inhaler with a bronchodilating drug during "peak season" because he occasionally wheezes on exertion.

Mr. Gruenwald's dental visits have been inconsistent as an adult. He remembers many childhood visits that resulted in at least one restoration. He indicates it "wasn't his favorite place to go." He wants to avoid radiographic procedures (x-rays) because of his intense gag reflex. Tooth brushing and the taste of toothpaste often cause him to gag. His chief complaint at this visit is a lower right molar that throbs at night and has been sensitive to hot, cold, and pressure for several months. He has received no dental care for at least 8 years, and he has made this appointment because he cannot stand the pain any longer.

Mr. Gruenwald has agreed to try N_2O/O_2 sedation while the radiographs are being taken. The dental hygienist has titrated the N_2O to an appropriate level, and Mr. Gruenwald is relaxed and comfortable.

pressure when opening cylinder valves ignites any hydrocarbon contaminant and causes an immediate chemical reaction, resulting in an explosion.

Nitrous oxide is 1½ times heavier than air. Its molecular weight is 44. As a gas, N_2O is slightly sweet smelling and colorless. It is a relatively insoluble drug. N_2O remains unchanged in the blood; the molecule does not break down. The body absorbs limited amounts of the drug. Because of this property, only small quantities of N_2O are required to reach the required blood concentration levels. Clinical action occurs quickly, usually in 3 to 5 minutes.

Nitrous oxide will rapidly replace any nitrogen (N_2) molecule in the body because of a major difference in their pressure gradients. Nitrogen occupies all air-filled cavities and can be found in areas with rigid or nonrigid boundaries. Pressure may increase temporarily in bony areas such as sinuses and middle ear complexes, and volume may increase in nonrigid areas such as the bowel or pleural cavity. Therefore in some clinical situations, N_2O/O_2 sedation may be postponed.

Nitrous oxide is not stored in the body for any significant time. It is not metabolized in the liver at all. A minuscule amount is metabolized in the gastrointestinal tract by specific bacteria. When N_2O flow to a patient is terminated, the molecules exit very quickly back through the respiratory tract. Recovery is as rapid as induction.

INDICATIONS

Use of N_2O/O_2 sedation is appropriate in many clinical situations in various health disciplines. It has been used in obstetrics and emergency medicine in Great Britain for decades. Podiatrists use N_2O/O_2 for outpatient surgeries; it is also used in dermatological, radiological, and endoscopic procedures. N_2O/O_2 sedation has been widely used throughout dentistry. Procedures performed in periodontics, prosthodontics, orthodontics, dental hygiene, restorative dentistry, oral and maxillofacial surgery, endodontics, and especially pediatric dentistry have been assisted by N_2O/O_2 sedation.

Nitrous oxide has *anxiolytic* and analgesic properties. Patients who are mildly anxious for any reason will greatly benefit from this type of sedation. N_2O has the ability to "calm the nerves" or "take the edge off." It produces a relaxed, comfortable feeling. N_2O also has beneficial pain management properties; as fear and anxiety decrease, the pain threshold increases.

Nitrous oxide/oxygen sedation has a tremendous calming effect on the *gag reflex.* Patients who have difficulty with radiographic procedures, rubber dam impressions, and other use of instrumentation are candidates for N_2O/O_2 sedation.

Case Application

Mr. Gruenwald, the patient in this chapter's case study, would benefit from N_2O/O_2 sedation not only for pain and anxiety assistance, but also for management of his hypersensitive gag reflex during radiography.

Nitrous oxide is safe to use in most situations because it does not interact with medications, is not allergenic, and does not significantly affect body systems. If uncertain about a particular condition, the clinician should consult with a professional who is knowledgeable about N_2O or contact the patient's physician before initiating the procedure.

RELATIVE CONTRAINDICATIONS

No absolute contraindications exist for N_2O/O_2 sedation. In some situations, however, use of N_2O/O_2 should be postponed or avoided.

Patients who are severely phobic or who have strong, controlling personalities generally do not benefit from this procedure. The situation may worsen as the patient resists the drug's calming effects.

If a patient is inebriated or "high" on drugs, it is wise to postpone all treatment and avoid N_2O/O_2. Discretion is key in decisions on use of N_2O/O_2 for a recovering alcoholic or drug addict. The experience may simulate physical and mental sensations previously associated with the disease.

Individuals under psychiatric or psychologic care should be carefully evaluated before sedation. Negative aspects of mental disorders could be exacerbated while using N_2O.

Persons who do not possess the mental capability of understanding the drug's effects or who cannot communicate signs and symptoms to the operator should not be exposed to N_2O/O_2 sedation. Effective communication is essential to the operator for assessment and monitoring purposes.

It is always recommended to avoid drug administration for a woman in the first trimester of pregnancy because organogenesis during this time is critical. When delivered appropriately, N_2O should not physiologically threaten the fetus; as with radiation, however, the psychologically disturbed mother might blame N_2O unfairly if a birth defect occurs. The dental practitioner should consult with the patient's physician and discuss all options before using N_2O/O_2 in any stage of pregnancy.

Nitrous oxide/oxygen sedation should be postponed for patients with a cold, sinus infection, allergy-related symptoms, or other respiratory condition that affects airflow through the nasal and bronchial passages. Incomplete or inadequate sedation is likely in these patients.

Patients who are chronically debilitated and on hypoxic drive because of a respiratory condition should be evaluated before use of N_2O/O_2. The concern here is with the delivery of supplemental O_2 rather than the N_2O. In these patients, O_2 is the stimulus for their respiration instead of carbon dioxide. A significant increase in O_2 administration may affect their breathing, and hypoxia could result. Usually these patients are not ambulatory and are not treated in a traditional dental office. Otherwise, however, medical consultation is recommended when a practitioner is unsure of the severity of the patient's condition.

Pressure increases in the middle ear complex as N_2O infiltrates this nitrogen-filled cavity. The clinician should obtain medical consultation before sedation of patients who have recently undergone tympanic membrane surgery or grafting. The pressure increase may affect the surgical results.

EQUIPMENT

Nitrous oxide/oxygen used in the dental office is stored in metal cylinders (Fig. 37-1). The cylinders are typically dis-

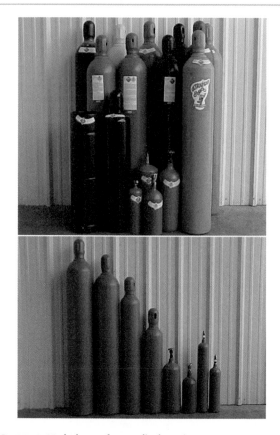

FIG. 37-1 Variations of gas cylinders. (Courtesy Scott Heppel, nexAir LLC, Memphis, Tenn.)

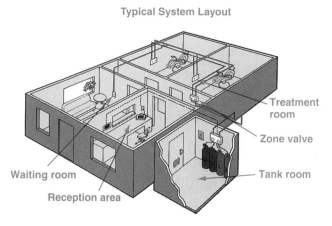

FIG. 37-2 Centralized nitrous oxide/oxygen sedation unit. (From Clark MS, Brunick AL: *Handbook of nitrous oxide and oxygen sedation,* St Louis, 1999, Mosby.)

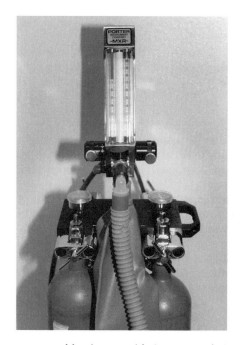

FIG. 37-3 Portable nitrous oxide/oxygen sedation unit.

tributed and exchanged periodically by a distribution company contracted by the office. Depending on the type of N_2O/O_2 sedation system used by the office, the cylinders may be small (*E* size) or larger (*G* and *H* sizes). The cylinders are inspected regularly by the company or distributor to ensure their integrity.

Cylinders are color-coded for correct gas identification. In the United States, N_2O is packaged in blue and O_2 is packaged in green cylinders.

Specific configurations of the cylinder valve stem offer another safety measure to ensure correct gas identification and use. Small tanks use a pin index system. Small holes are drilled into the stem in configurations unique to a particular gas. In order for tanks to be attached correctly, the holes must match small pins on the machine. This system ensures the correct gas tank is attached to the correct side of the system, preventing the accidental delivery of 100% N_2O. Larger tanks have a similar type of safety mechanism within the valve stem.

A full cylinder of N_2O contains approximately 95% liquid and 5% vapor. When N_2O is being used, ambient air vaporizes the liquid to a gas. The outside of the tank will be cool to the touch during this process. The pressure gauge on the N_2O tank will not drop until most of the liquid is gone.

Oxygen is compressed into a cylinder as a gas. As O_2 is used, the pressure gauge drops proportionally and accurately reflects the amount of gas available in the tank. All machines used in dental offices must have a fail-safe mechanism. The presence of such a mechanism means

the machine is driven by O_2 flow. If the O_2 tank is depleted during the procedure, the N_2O flow is terminated. It is important to have additional O_2 available at all times to prevent the interruption of ideal sedation.

Nitrous oxide/oxygen can be delivered in a dental office through two types of systems. A *centralized system* uses a mechanism called a *manifold* to connect several large tanks together (Fig. 37-2). The manifold will automatically activate a full container when one becomes low. This system delivers gas through copper piping to individual treatment rooms and is economically advantageous over a portable system for an office that frequently uses N_2O/O_2 sedation. A *portable system* can also deliver N_2O/O_2 sedation (Fig. 37-3). The unit houses smaller cylinders and may be easily moved from one treatment area to another. This type of system may be preferred in offices where N_2O/O_2 sedation is used infrequently.

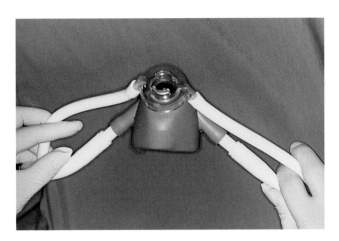

FIG. 37-4 Scavenging nasal hood.

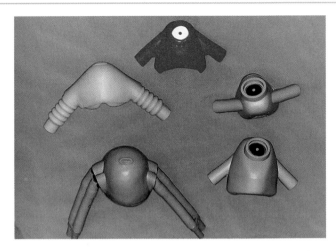

FIG. 37-5 Variations of scavenging nasal hoods. (From Clark MS, Brunick AL: *Handbook of nitrous oxide and oxygen sedation,* St Louis, 1999, Mosby.)

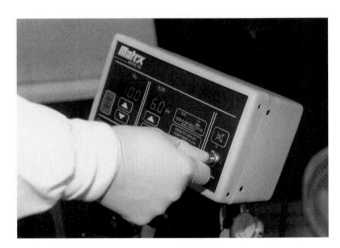

FIG. 37-6 Variation of flowmeter with lighted electronic display and key lock.

Both systems have regulators that reduce gas pressure from the tank. Low pressure is necessary for delivery to a patient. Both systems also have a *flowmeter,* which delivers N_2O/O_2. The amount of each gas being delivered must be visibly monitored on the flowmeter. Knobs, levers, or buttons are used to adjust the gas flow.

A *reservoir bag* hangs in front of the flowmeter. This bag is used as an extra supply of gas if the patient should need more than that being delivered. The bag is also used to monitor the patient's respiration; it slightly inflates and then deflates concomitantly with inhalation and exhalation. In addition, the reservoir bag can be used in an emergency situation as a source of positive-pressure O_2.

The *conduction tubing* and *nasal hood* are the parts of the unit that bring gas to the patient. All units currently used must have *scavenging capabilities,* which means the devices must have an exhaust to vent exhaled gas out of the building. To do this, one hose on the end of the conduction tubing must be inserted into the evacuation system. The nasal hood must have both delivery and scavenging hoses attached to it (Fig. 37-4). One or more hoses deliver fresh gas to the patient while other hoses *scavenge* the exhaled gas. Using equipment without these capabilities is practicing below the accepted standard of care for sedated patient, placing the office and practitioners in legal jeopardy or U.S. Occupational Safety and Health Administration (OSHA) noncompliance.

Nasal hoods are available in a variety of sizes, both scented and unscented (Fig. 37-5). Newer products are designed for single-patient use; however, autoclavable models are still available. Many products are now latex-free.

All units currently manufactured are designed to deliver a minimum of 30% O_2 at all times. This level ensures that the patient is breathing at least the amount of O_2 in ambient air (21%). The equipment is also designed to limit the amount of N_2O that can be delivered to a patient. No more than 70% N_2O can be delivered to a patient when using analgesia/sedation equipment. It is unlikely that N_2O concentrations higher than 70% will be used in the dental setting.

Unit features vary according to manufacturer. Some units have lighted electronic displays (LEDs), locks, and audiovisual alarms that indicate low O_2 levels (Fig. 37-6). Ergonomics, infection control, ease of portability, and space-saving qualities are manufacturing design considerations.

ADMINISTRATION

The success of the N_2O/O_2 experience for both operator and patient largely depends on the technique of administration. Accurate monitoring of the patient for appropriate signs and symptoms of sedation is essential. Healthcare providers must understand the significance of sedation levels and the critical importance of vigilant patient monitoring.

STAGES OF ANESTHESIA

Levels of anesthesia described in the literature primarily pertain to anesthesiologists inducing general anesthesia in an operating room. These levels or stages of anesthesia describe various physical and physiological effects that occur when the CNS is depressed. Consciousness and cognitive awareness leads to unconsciousness, loss of reflexes, and eventually, loss of organ/system function. During N_2O/O_2 sedation in an ambulatory setting, the patient remains in the beginning stage of this progression. A patient also may become ***unconscious*** when N_2O/O_2 is used. Knowing the appropriate signs and symptoms of each stage is critical for patient comfort and safety.

In the first stage the patient is relaxed, comfortable, and aware of the surroundings. The patient is always ***conscious*** in this stage and has complete control of gag and cough reflexes. However, patients may experience a variety of other signs and symptoms when appropriately sedated. For example, the patient may feel a slight tingling sensation in the extremities or near the mouth. The patient may also sense increased but not uncomfortable body warmth. Some patients feel as if their body has become heavier; some feel lighter.

All patients do not experience the same effects, however, and practitioners must not rely on the presence of these signs and symptoms as indicators of appropriate sedation. With practice the operator will be able to use body language, facial expression, and eye movement to assist the assessment of an appropriate sedation level. In ideal sedation the operator may notice that the patient's body is not as rigid. The patient may also take deeper and slower respirations. In most instances the patient's eyes are good indicators of sedation levels. Active blinking and rapid eye movement may suggest the patient is not completely relaxed. When eye movement slows and the patient has a "glazed" look, the sedation level may be more appropriate. Smiles come easily to an ideally sedated patient.

OVERSEDATION

Oversedation is most often a result of operator error. Generally the oversedated patient is uncomfortable. The patient may enter the second stage of CNS depression rapidly and exhibit only subtle signs. The operator must be cognizant of the signs and symptoms associated with oversedation. Patients should never be left alone when receiving N_2O/O_2 sedation.

If oversedated, the individual may become detached from the environment and indicate an out-of-body or floating experience. Some patients indicate an inability to move or communicate. Some may enter a dreamlike state, whereas others hallucinate. Generally these feelings are not pleasant, and patients do not want to repeat the experience. Other signs and symptoms of oversedation include drowsiness, dizziness, nausea, or an uncomfortably warm body temperature. When oversedated, the patient may be sluggish, may delay responses, may slur words, and may not make verbal sense. The patient may begin to laugh uncontrollably or may become agitated, violent, or even combative.

Vomiting is associated with oversedation. This is an especially serious problem if a practitioner is not closely monitoring the patient. *Silent regurgitation* may occur, in which the patient vomits to a point where aspiration of vomitus occurs. This presents a life-threatening situation that may happen quietly and quickly. Vomiting is also very embarrassing for a patient. Most likely, if vomiting occurs during N_2O/O_2 sedation, the patient was oversedated by the operator.

It is possible for an unconscious patient on N_2O/O_2 se-

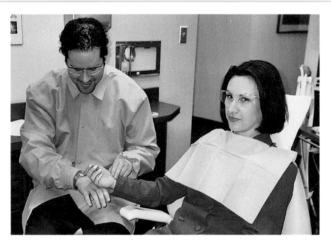

FIG. 37-7 Preoperative vital signs taken for baseline values.

dation to enter the third stage of anesthesia. At this stage, surgical procedures are performed in an operating room. The patient has inactive laryngeal and pharyngeal reflexes and cannot breathe independently. The depth of anesthesia required for actual surgery most likely cannot be adequately achieved with N_2O alone; however, the practitioner can oversedate the patient to unconsciousness by using N_2O in the ambulatory setting.

TECHNIQUE

A major advantages of N_2O/O_2 sedation is that the exact amount of drug may be used to achieve the desired level of sedation. This concept is called ***titration.*** Most methods of ***pharmacologic sedation*** do not allow for titration. By titrating N_2O in increments, operator can (1) achieve the desired level of sedation, (2) assess the current level of sedation, (3) maintain and adjust the level during the appointment, and (4) terminate the procedure at any point.

To begin administering N_2O/O_2 sedation, the operator must first have the equipment ready. Machines must be turned on, tanks opened, and ***scavenging devices*** checked for proper operation.

Informed consent must be obtained before any type of drug is administered for patient treatment. The patient must have a clear understanding of the procedure and its associated effects. If the patient is mentally incapable of understanding this information or communicating during the procedure, N_2O/O_2 sedation is not recommended.

At each visit the patient's health history should be updated. Vital signs such as blood pressure, pulse, and respiration should be obtained and recorded as baseline values (Fig. 37-7).

The appropriate size and type of nasal hood are selected for the patient. Nasal hood size is important because it facilitates gas flow; a poorly fitting hood may block gas flow to the patient or may allow excess gas to contaminate the surrounding air. The clinician secures the hood to the conduction tubing and begins the O_2 flow to the unit, establishing the appropriate flow in liters per minute (L/min). The amount of flow needed largely depends on the patient's ***tidal volume,*** or amount of gas inspired into the lungs. Larger bodies and more physically fit individuals

TABLE 37-1

Nitrous oxide/oxygen percentage chart

Liters per minute nitrous oxide	LITERS PER MINUTE OXYGEN									
	1	2	3	4	5	6	7	8	9	10
1	50	33	25	20	17	14	13	11	10	9
2	67	50	40	33	29	25	22	20	18	17
3	75*	60	50	43	38	33	30	27	25	23
4	80*	67	57	50	44	40	36	33	31	29
5	83*	71	63	56	50	45	42	38	36	33
6	86*	75*	67	60	55	50	46	43	40	38
7	88*	78*	70	64	58	54	50	47	44	41
8	89*	80*	73	67	62	57	53	50	47	44
9	90*	82*	75*	69	64	60	56	53	50	47
10	91*	83*	77*	71	67	63	59	56	53	50

From Clark MS, Brunick AL: *Handbook of nitrous oxide and oxygen sedation,* St Louis, 1999, Mosby.
*Percentage exceeds maximum amount of N_2O needed for effective pain/anxiety management in an ambulatory setting and exceeds amounts able to be delivered by analgesia machines.

have a greater tidal volume than smaller or more physically challenged persons. The amount of gas inspired into the lungs per minute is called *minute ventilation*. By multiplying the tidal volume by the person's respiration rate, the operator can determine the appropriate L/min. On average, 500 ml (tidal volume) × 12 to 15 respirations per minute = approximately 6 to7 L/min. Initially the operator may want to set the O_2 flow slightly higher than this level. Increasing the flow of O_2 at this point eliminates the suffocating or claustrophobic feeling that some patients may experience on initial placement of the nasal hood. Flow may be decreased when the patient has acclimated to the hood.

The operator can confirm the appropriate amount of total gas flow by observing the reservoir bag. If the bag is collapsing as the patient is breathing, he or she is demanding more flow than is being provided. The operator should increase L/min until the bag remains two-thirds full during patient respiration. Conversely, if the bag has overinflated, the amount of O_2 should be decreased because the patient is not using as much as is being delivered. It is important to monitor the reservoir bag constantly for changes in flow amount as required by the patient.

Once the patient is comfortable with the amount of flow being delivered, the operator may begin titrating N_2O. It is important to know the type of delivery system. Some machines have separate controls that independently regulate the flow of each gas. As N_2O is added, O_2 flow must be decreased proportionally to maintain the established L/min flow. For example, if the patient required a total of 8 L/min, the addition of 0.5 L N_2O would mean that the O_2 level must be reduced by 0.5 L to 7.5 L. The combined total would then remain at 8 L/min because of the addition of 0.5 L with the reduction to 7.5 L. The separate control system requires adjustment of both gases each time N_2O is added.

Other machines automatically adjust the O_2 flow as N_2O is titrated. In this case the established L/min flow re-

mains constant. No need exists to adjust the O_2 level manually with these machines.

The levels of gas depicted by the floating balls or flashing lights do *not* represent the actual percentage of N_2O being delivered, which is calculated by dividing the N_2O L/min by the total L/min (Table 37-1).

Some machines display the amount of O_2 being delivered. When N_2O is added, it is necessary to subtract that amount from the amount of O_2. For example, if 70% O_2 is being displayed on a dial or LED, the N_2O percentage being delivered would be 30%.

Nitrous oxide must be titrated to the patient slowly and in small amounts. The dental hygienist should begin by administering 10% N_2O and then proceed in increments of 5% N_2O. Slow titration allows for maximum clinical effects to occur before additional drug is given. At least 60 seconds should elapse before more N_2O is added.

N_2O delivery or adjustment mandates careful patient monitoring for signs and symptoms. The patient should be asked to breathe through the nose and should refrain from talking to allow maximum drug effect and to reduce the amount of contaminating trace gas dispersed into the air. Patient talking is one of the primary sources of trace gas contamination of the air. The patient is watched for signs and symptoms of ideal sedation. The patient should be relaxed and comfortable; the patient should *never* be uncomfortable. If the patient is dizzy, excessively warm, nauseous, or blacking out or does not respond to inquiries, the amount of N_2O is *immediately* decreased and the amount of O_2 is subsequently increased. The patient should breathe deeply and understand that the uncomfortable feeling will soon disappear. It is better to make the patient comfortable as soon as possible and begin the process again rather than leaving the patient uncomfortable by insufficient reduction of N_2O. These uncomfortable feelings often explain why patients do not choose N_2O again.

Uncomfortable feelings indicate that the patient was oversedated. The operator must use the appropriate ad-

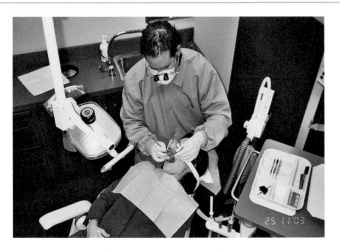

FIG. 37-8 Operative treatment with patient receiving nitrous oxide/oxygen sedation.

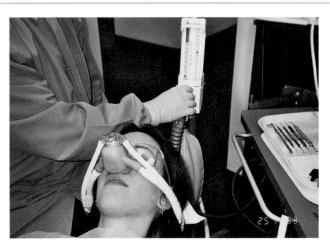

FIG. 37-9 Postoperative oxygenation.

ministration technique, constantly monitoring the patient's status. No preset, ideal, or average percentage of N_2O will achieve optimal sedation. Each individual is unique and requires a different percentage. The N_2O amount used at one visit does not predict the amount needed for the next visit. *Using a prescribed level of N_2O or an amount based on a previous visit does not reflect the current standard of care for N_2O/O_2 administration.* Oversedation and the resultant negative patient experience are likely when using this approach. Again, oversedation is caused by operator error.

Sedation levels may be adjusted intraoperatively when using N_2O and O_2. Adjustments may be made to increase the level of sedation during difficult or uncomfortable procedures or to reduce the sedation level for finishing or less uncomfortable procedures. This flexibility is one of the many advantages associated with N_2O/O_2 sedation (Fig. 37-8).

RECOVERY

Providing the patient with postoperative O_2 is the final step in the sedation process (Fig. 37-9). As procedures are being completed, N_2O flow may be terminated to begin the required time of postoperative O_2. Nitrous oxide exits the body unchanged through the lungs. Approximately 5 minutes of 100% O_2 is considered the minimum time necessary for the patient to recover completely. However, recovery must be assessed before the O_2 is removed from the patient. The patient should be asked how he or she feels. If the patient does not feel completely normal, 100% O_2 is continued incrementally every 3 to 5 minutes. It may be appropriate to oxygenate some patients for 15 or more minutes.

DIFFUSION HYPOXIA

Historically associated with N_2O/O_2 sedation, *diffusion hypoxia* is defined as the process by which N_2O exits faster than the N_2 that replaces it. Oxygen is slightly diluted and serum O_2 saturation decreased. These levels return to normal in a short period. This phenomenon has

proved to be clinically insignificant.[13] The symptoms of postoperative headache, lethargy, and lightheadedness have been previously associated with diffusion hypoxia. Generally, adequate postoperative O_2 eliminates these symptoms for most patients.

VITAL SIGNS

Postoperative vital signs are an objective measure of recovery. Blood pressure, pulse, and respiration rates should be within a reasonably comparable range of preoperative values. A *pulse oximeter* may be used to monitor serum O_2 saturation levels during N_2O/O_2 administration. Some devices simultaneously record blood pressure and pulse, and postoperative vital signs are already calculated. A printout of these values recorded before, during, and after procedures can be placed in the patient's file.

PSYCHOMOTOR ASSESSMENT

Psychomotor assessments have been made after N_2O/O_2 administration. Jastak and Orendurff[10] evaluated participants for driving errors and concluded that patients could safely operate motor vehicles after N_2O/O_2 sedation. This study has been the foundation for practitioners dismissing patients without an escort. However, the practitioner is always responsible for ensuring adequate recovery before patient dismissal.

RECORD KEEPING

It is always important to maintain complete and accurate records of patient/operator interactions and procedures. The same is true when using N_2O/O_2 sedation. Several items require documentation after the procedure. Notes can be directly entered on a service record in the patient's chart or on a separate sedation record kept in the chart. If a separate sheet is used, the patient's name and date must be included. It would be appropriate to include the reason for using this type of sedation. For example, notes would indicate that N_2O/O_2 was used for anxiety or to calm a hypersensitive gag reflex.

N₂O/O₂ SEDATION RECORD

Date:_____   Patient:_____Age:_____

Informed consent: Patient/parent signature:_____

ASA classification: I   II   III   IV
Med consult needed: Yes / No   Operative procedure:_____

Procedural data: **Preoperative**   **Postoperative**

   BP   _____   _____
   Pulse   _____   _____
   Respiration   _____   _____

   N₂O total time: _____min
   Postoperative O₂:_____min

   Titrated % of N₂O:_____
   (for documentation purposes only)

Comments:

Clinician signature:_____

FIG. 37-10 Example of nitrous oxide/oxygen sedation record. *ASA,* American Society of Anesthesiologists.

Similar to other clinical situations, medical consultation with a physician or other healthcare provider should be documented in the patient's record. This serves as legal documentation as well as a source of information for future practitioners.

Preoperative and postoperative vital signs should be recorded. This documents prudent recovery assessment. The patient's tidal volume or the required L/min flow is an optional item. Generally the amount of gas (N_2O and O_2) delivered will not change between visits unless the patient has lost significant weight or has significantly increased physical fitness status. This number might be used as a reference point for the next visit.

The N_2O percentage used during a patient visit should not be used as a reference for the next visit, and the operator should decide whether this number should be included in the patient record. As mentioned, because of individual *biovariability*, the N_2O percentage used in one situation will not be the same on a different occasion. Again, it is inappropriate to begin N_2O/O_2 administration at a fixed point or to assume the percentage will be the same from a previous visit.

The operator should record the amount of postoperative oxygenation time (in minutes) required for patient recovery to document an accurate assessment of recovery. Any negative or adverse reaction to the N_2O/O_2 sedation experience should be noted in the patient record to provide other practitioners a history of patient experiences (Fig. 37-10).

BIOLOGICAL EFFECTS AND ISSUES

Since the late 1960s, many references in the literature have implicated N_2O as the causative agent for significant health problems in healthcare personnel chronically exposed to the drug. Nitrous oxide has been the common gas delivered by anesthesiologists for most surgical procedures and therefore was initially singled out as the etiological agent for reproductive problems, spontaneous abortions, cancer, and other conditions. Most research in the 1970s and early 1980s reported similar results. The majority of this research was done with a retrospective survey design, which is not proven reliable or valid. From more than 800 articles written on the subject until 1995, fewer than 25 were shown to merit reliability and validity.[4] These biological effects sensationalized in the literature were noted when high levels of unscavenged trace N_2O amounts were measured.

Since those early studies, equipment and delivery methods have improved tremendously. It is now considered standard of care to use equipment with the capability of scavenging trace gas from the patient. The manufacturers of N_2O/O_2 delivery equipment are continually improving their products and conducting research to ascertain new methods for scavenging trace gas.

The most significant biological effect linked to N_2O exposure is its ability to inactivate vitamin B_{12}. This inactivation affects the enzyme methionine synthetase, which is essential for deoxyribonucleic acid (DNA) production. Fetal abnormalities in animals and reproductive problems in humans were linked to this DNA effect with chronic exposure to high levels of unscavenged N_2O.[5,8] Chronic exposure to N_2O has also resulted in neurological signs and symptoms. Individuals acknowledging misuse of N_2O for purposes other than patient treatment have experienced numbness, tingling, and paresthesia in their limbs. They also report impaired dexterity, clumsiness, and a slow or shuffled gait. Some individuals indicate gradual improvement of these symptoms when the abuse is terminated, whereas others note permanent neural injury.[12]

It is important to recognize that no evidence to date indicates a direct causal relationship between reproductive health

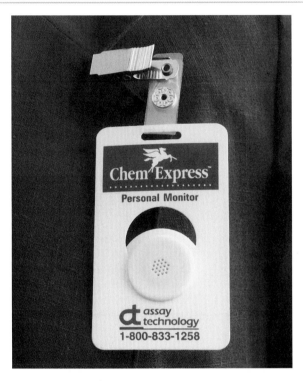

FIG. 37-11 Nitrous oxide personal monitoring device. (Courtesy Assay Technology, Pleasanton, Calif.)

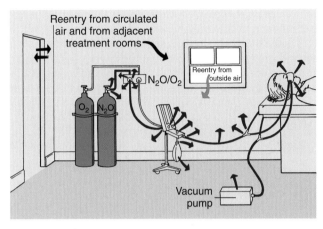

→ = Leak sources

FIG. 37-12 Sources of potential nitrous oxide leaks. (From Clark MS, Brunick AL: *Handbook of nitrous oxide and oxygen sedation*, St Louis, 1999, Mosby.)

and scavenged low levels of N₂O for persons chronically exposed to the gas.[14] *Also, no adverse biological effect has been reported in patients receiving N₂O/O₂ sedation for pain and anxiety management in a dental office.*

EXPOSURE LEVELS

The National Institute for Occupational Safety and Health (NIOSH) and the American Conference of Governmental Industrial Hygienists (ACGIH) established exposure recommendations during administration of N_2O/O_2 over an 8-hour period.[1] These levels, established in 1977, were based on unfounded research and inadequate equipment. It is required that the level of N_2O/O_2 not exceed 50 parts per million (ppm) in a dental office. OSHA still requires that these values be upheld, although at present these limits are being challenged with new research. It is anticipated that soon these agencies will recommend new, accurate, and obtainable limits.

To determine the level of trace N_2O in a dental office, the operator must use a measuring device that detects atmospheric N_2O, such as an infrared spectrophotometer. These machines may be purchased or rented for periodic evaluation. A wall-mounted device offers a continuous reading that may be advantageous for offices using N_2O frequently.

Health practitioners can also determine the amount of their N_2O exposure over a specific period. A personal monitoring device similar to a radiation dosimetry badge can be worn (Fig. 37-11). The time-weighted average (TWA) device contains an absorbent material that collects N_2O. The device is returned to the company for analysis. The company returns a written report to the individual that details exposure levels.

TRACE CONTAMINATION

Dental personnel should use all measures available to minimize the amount of trace N_2O contamination in the office. Potential sources for trace gas leakage exist (Fig. 37-12), and several methods are available to scavenge contaminant.

Baseline values of N_2O contamination should be established for offices that use N_2O/O_2 sedation. A baseline figure documents the amount of trace N_2O in the office when using current equipment and procedures. From that point a comparison can be made when additional scavenging methods are employed. TWA dosimetry devices may be used if desired.

All equipment must have the capability to scavenge exhaled gas from the patient's mask into the evacuation system. If this type of equipment is not being used, the practitioner is practicing below the standard of care and may be subject to legal repercussions. Gas can leak from any portion of a central piping system or through any point of connection with cylinders or valves. A common soap and water test can assess the adequacy of fittings and connections. The flowmeter itself can leak. Manufacturers recommend periodic evaluation and routine maintenance of equipment. A maximum of 2 years has been suggested for the time period between equipment evaluations. Conduction tubing and reservoir bags should be routinely inspected for cracks and tears. The soap and water test can be used for these items as well.

It is important to ensure the adequacy of the existing evacuation system. The system must have sufficient force to evacuate scavenged gas from the nasal hood and must possess properly venting pumps. Office ventilation and air exchange in the ambulatory setting is an area currently being investigated for ways to improve the removal of waste N_2O. Air conditioners typically recirculate ambient air rather than provide an air exchange. In this case, N_2O could be circulated throughout the office rather than being removed. Fresh-air vents should be located near the ceiling, whereas exhaust outlets should be near the floor. In addition, open windows are suggested as a method for removing waste gas. Oscillating room fans can assist the gas movement toward an open window or exhaust vent.

The health and safety of the professional dental team is second only to patient safety. All members should be educated on the potential biological effects and issues associated with chronic exposure to N_2O. Personnel should use all available measures to reduce or minimize trace gas contamination. Proper equipment and administration procedures are mandatory. Dental professionals must keep abreast of new technology and reputable research. It is also important to participate in continuing education programs that provide the latest recommendations or guidelines.

RITICAL THINKING ACTIVITIES

1. Investigate the status of N_2O/O_2 administration by hygienists in your state's dental practice act. Determine the requirements (e.g., number of course hours, supervision levels, fees) for practicing this skill in your state.
2. Debate the pros and cons of using N_2O/O_2 sedation in dental hygiene care.
3. Develop a persuasive paper on the use of N_2O/O_2 sedation in dental hygiene care.
4. Visit dental offices and identify the type of N_2O/O_2 equipment used.
5. Check with supply houses as to the cost of various tank sizes of N_2O and O_2.

REVIEW QUESTIONS

Questions 3 through 6 refer to the case study presented at the beginning of the chapter.

1. A dental hygienist using a scavenging nasal hood is assured this device will prevent waste gas from being eliminated through the patient's mouth.
   a. True
   b. False
2. Which of the following is major source of trace N_2O that contaminates the ambient air in a dental office?
   a. Patient talking
   b. Cracked reservoir bag
   c. Leaking valve stems on cylinder
   d. Improperly soldered central piping
3. Mr. Gruenwald heard that a person with allergies or asthma should not use N_2O/O_2 sedation, and he is concerned because he has some allergies. Your response could be any of the following *except* which one?
   a. Nitrous oxide is nonirritating to mucosa in the respiratory system.
   b. There has been no documented allergy to N_2O in more than 150 years.
   c. Occasionally, asthma attacks occur in nervous or anxious people, so N_2O/O_2 sedation is beneficial for these patients.
   d. N_2O can initiate an asthmatic attack because it irritates bronchial tissues.
4. During Mr. Gruenwald's care experience with N_2O/O_2 sedation, the dental hygienist can monitor his respiration by which of the following?
   a. Adjusting the N_2O amount being delivered
   b. Checking the pressure gauges on the equipment
   c. Observing the movement of the reservoir bag
   d. Watching the floating balls in the flowmeter tubes
5. Mr. Gruenwald has had a positive experience with N_2O/O_2 sedation and is ready to be dismissed. He is wondering how long the N_2O stays in his system. You assure him that N_2O is eliminated quickly by which of the following?
   a. Kidneys
   b. Skin
   c. Lungs
   d. Liver
   e. Urine
6. As you assess Mr. Gruenwald's recovery from N_2O/O_2 sedation, which of the following would indicate that his recovery may not yet be complete?
   a. You have administered 5 minutes of 100% oxygen postoperatively, and he is feeling normal.
   b. His postoperative vital signs are within close range of his preoperative values.
   c. He says that it seems like his appointment went quickly and that it did not feel like he was at the office very long.
   d. He says he feels groggy and still "out of it."
7. Providing N_2O/O_2 sedation for patients is an important part of your office philosophy. It is also important that the office staff follow an established routine for checking the equipment and making sure all scavenging devices are working appropriately. You follow the guideline set by the manufacturers and send the flowmeters back to the company for evaluation over which period?
   a. 6 months
   b. 1 year
   c. 2 years
   d. 5 years
8. Scavenging trace gas from the dental office can be accomplished in all the following ways *except* which one?
   a. Adequate suction system that vents to an outside source
   b. Recirculating exhaust ventilation system
   c. Oscillating floor fans directed away from the operator
   d. Regular inspection of equipment for leakage
   e. Use of scavenging mask and nasal hood

SUGGESTED AGENCIES AND WEB SITES

Nitrous Oxide/Oxygen Equipment Manufacturers

Accutron, 2020 West Melinda Lane, Phoenix, AZ 85027; (800) 531-2221 (phone); (602) 780-0444 (fax)

MDS Matrx Medical, 145 Med County Dr, Orchard Park, NY 14127; (800) 847-1000 (phone); (716) 662-7130 (fax)

Porter Instrument, 245 Township Line Rd, Box 907, Hatfield, PA 19440-0907; (800) 457-2001 (phone); (215) 723-2199 (fax)

Personal Monitoring Devices

Advance Chemical Sensors, 350 Oaks Lane, Pompano Beach, FL 33069; (305) 979-0658

Assay Technology, 1070 East Meadow Circle, Palo Alto, CA 94303; (800) 833-1258

Health Career Learning Systems, 37557 Schoolcraft Rd, Livonia, MI 48150; (800) 829-4257

Kem Medical Products, 14 Engineers Lane, Farmingdale, NY 11735; (800) 553-0300.

Landauer, 2 Science Rd, Glenwood, IL 60425-1586; (708) 755-7000 (phone); (708) 755-7016 (fax)

Nevin, 5000 South Halsted St, Chicago, IL 60609; (800) 544-5337

Infrared Spectrophotometry

Foxboro, 600 N Bedford St, Box 500, East Bridgewater, MA 02333; (800) 321-0322 (phone); (508) 378-5505 (fax)

Related Organizations

American Dental Society of Anesthesiologists, 211 East Chicago Ave, Suite 780, Chicago, IL 60611; (800) 722-7788 (phone); (312) 642-9713 (fax)

American Society of Anesthesiologists, 520 N Northwest Hwy, Park Ridge, IL 60068-2573; (847) 825-5586 (phone); (847) 825-1692 (fax)

Compressed Gas Association, 1725 Jefferson Davis Hwy, Suite 1004, Arlington, VA 22202-4102; (703) 412-0900 (phone); (703) 412-0128 (fax)

National Institute for Occupational Safety and Health (NIOSH), 4676 Columbia Parkway, Cincinnati, OH 45226; (800) 356-4674 (phone); (513) 533-8573 (fax)

National Welding Supply Association, 1900 Arch St, Philadelphia, PA 19103; (215) 584-3484 (phone); (215) 584-2175 (fax)

Nellcor Puritan Bennett, 9101 Bond St, Overland Park, KS 66214; (913) 495-3606 (phone); (913) 495-3698 (fax)

Occupational Safety and Health Administration (OSHA), Health Standards Programs, US Department of Labor, 200 Constitution Ave NW, Washington, DC 20210; (202) 219-7075

 ## ADDITIONAL READINGS AND RESOURCES

Clark MS, Brunick A: *Handbook of nitrous oxide and oxygen sedation,* St Louis, 1999, Mosby.

Malamed SF: *Sedation: a guide to patient management,* ed 4, St Louis, (in press), Mosby.

 ## REFERENCES

1. Bruce DL, Bach MJ: *Trace effects of anesthetic gases on behavioral performance of operating room personnel,* HEW Pub no (NIOSH) 76-169, Cincinnati, 1976, US Department of Health, Education, and Welfare.
2. Chancellor JW: Dr. Wells' impact on dentistry and medicine, *J Am Dent Assoc* 125:1585-9, 1994.
3. Chapman WP, Arrowood JG, Beecher HK: The analgesic effects of low concentrations of nitrous oxide compared in man with morphine sulfate, *J Clin Invest* 22:871-5, 1943.
4. Clark MS, Renehan BW, Jeffers BW: Clinical use and potential biohazards of nitrous oxide/oxygen, *Gen Dent* 45:486-91, 1997.
5. Cohen EN et al: Occupational disease in dentistry and chronic exposure to trace anesthetic gases, *J Am Dent Assoc* 101:21-31, 1980.
6. Davis MJ: Conscious sedation practices in pediatric dentistry: a survey of members of the American Board of Pediatric Dentistry College of Diplomates, *Pediatr Dent* 10:328-9, 1988.
7. Eger E II et al: Clinical pharmacology of nitrous oxide: an argument for its continued use, *Anesth Analg* 71:575-85, 1990.
8. Fujinagra M, Baden JM, Mazze RI: Susceptible period of nitrous oxide teratogenicity in Sprague-Dawley rats, *Teratology* 40:439-44, 1989.
9. Jacobsohn PH: What others said about Wells, *J Am Dent Assoc* 125:1583-4, 1994.
10. Jastak JT, Orendurff D: Recovery from nitrous sedation, *Anesth Prog* 22:113-6, 1975.
11. Jorgensen NB: *Sedation, local and general anesthesia in dentistry,* ed 2, Philadelphia, 1985, Lea & Febiger.
12. Layzer RB: Myeloneuropathy after prolonged exposure to nitrous oxide, *Lancet* 2:1227-30, 1978.
13. Papageorge MB, Noonan LW Jr, Rosenberg M: Diffusion hypoxia: another view, *Anesth Pain Control Dent* 2:143-9, 1993.
14. Rowland AS et al: Reduced fertility among women employed as dental assistants exposed to high levels of nitrous oxide, *N Engl J Med* 327:993-7, 1992.
15. Ruben H: Nitrous oxide analgesia in dentistry, *Br Dent J* 132:195-6, 1972.

PART VIII

Chapter 38
Operative Procedures

Chapter 39
Cosmetic Whitening

Competency Statements

The learner is expected to possess knowledge, skills, judgments, values, and attitudes to develop the listed competencies.

Core Competencies
- Apply a professional code of ethics in all endeavors.
- Adhere to state and federal laws, recommendations, and regulations in the provision of dental hygiene care.
- Provide dental hygiene care to promote patient health and wellness using critical thinking and problem solving in the provision of evidence-based practice.
- Use evidence-based decision making to evaluate and incorporate emerging treatment modalities.
- Assume responsibility for dental hygiene actions and care based on accepted scientific theories and research as well as the accepted standard of care.
- Provide accurate, consistent, and complete documentation for assessment, diagnosis, planning, implementation, and evaluation of dental hygiene services.
- Provide care to all patients using an individualized approach that is humane, empathetic, and caring.

Health Promotion and Disease Prevention
- Respect the goals, values, beliefs, and preferences of the patient while promoting optimal oral and general health.

Courtesy American Dental Education Association, Washington, DC.

Operative Therapies

- Refer patients who may have a physiologic, psychological, and/or social problem for comprehensive patient evaluation.
- Identify individual and population risk factors and develop strategies that promote health related quality of life.
- Evaluate factors that can be used to promote patient adherence to disease prevention and/or health maintenance strategies.
- Evaluate and utilize methods to ensure the health and safety of the patient and the dental hygienist in the delivery of dental hygiene.

Community Involvement
- Evaluate reimbursement mechanisms and their impact on patients'/client's access to oral health care.

Patient Care
- Select, obtain, and interpret diagnostic information recognizing its advantages and limitations.
- Recognize predisposing and etiologic risk factors that require intervention to prevent disease.
- Obtain, review, and update a complete medical, family, social, and dental history.
- Recognize health conditions and medications that impact overall patient care.
- Perform a comprehensive examination using clinical, radiographic, periodontal, dental charting, and other data collection procedures to assess the patient's needs.
- Determine a dental hygiene diagnosis.
- Identify patient needs and significant findings that impact the delivery of dental hygiene services.

- Obtain consultations as indicated.
- Prioritize the care plan based on the health status and the actual and potential problems of the individual to facilitate optimal oral health.
- Establish a planned sequence of care (educational, clinical, and evaluation) based on the dental hygiene diagnosis; identified oral conditions; potential problems; etiologic and risk factors; and available treatment modalities.
- Establish a collaborative relationship with the patient in the planned care to include etiology, prognosis, and treatment alternatives.
- Make referrals to other healthcare professionals.
- Perform dental hygiene interventions to eliminate and/or control local etiologic factors to prevent and control caries, periodontal disease, and other oral conditions.
- Control pain and anxiety during treatment through the use of accepted clinical and behavioral techniques.
- Determine the outcomes of dental hygiene interventions using indices, instruments, examination techniques, and patient self-report.
- Evaluate the patient's satisfaction with the oral healthcare received and the oral healthcare status achieved.
- Provide subsequent treatment or referrals based on evaluation findings.

Professional Growth and Development
- Access professional and social networks and resources to assist entrepreneurial initiatives.

CHAPTER 38

Operative Procedures

Peter T. Triolo Jr., William Patrick Kelsey III, Eric E. Spohn, Thomas G. Berry

Chapter Outline

Case Study: Application of Operative Therapies
Classification and Nomenclature
    Black's restorative lesion classification
    Black's principles for surgical repair of a
      diseased tooth
    Components of prepared cavities
    Class I cavity preparations
    Class II cavity preparations
    Class III cavity preparations
    Class IV cavity preparations
    Class V cavity preparations
Minimally Invasive Dentistry
    Amalgam-sealant combinations
Aesthetic Dentistry
Isolation of Teeth
    Armamentarium
    Preparation of patient
    Examination of mouth

Selection of clamp
Placement of clamp
Preparation of rubber dam
Placement of rubber dam and frame
Application of gingival retractor clamp
Removal of rubber dam
Evaluation Criteria
    Application of rubber dam
    Removal of rubber dam
Restorative Materials
    Amalgam
    Cavity sealers, liners, and bases
Restorative Procedures
    Amalgam placement techniques
    Direct resin composite restorations
    Placement of composite restorations
    Finishing of composite restorations

Key Terms

Amalgam
Cavity base
Cavity liner
Cavity sealer
Cavosurface
Composite
Convenience form

Corrosion
"Extension for prevention"
Galvanic reaction
Glass ionomer
Line angle
Marginal breakdown

Microleakage
Outline form
Point angle
Polymerization shrinkage
Resistance form
Retention form

Rubber dam
Rubber dam clamp
Submargination
Tofflemire universal matrix system
Wall

 ## *Learning Outcomes*

1. Assess patient needs for operative dental treatment and the rationale for treatment planning procedures.
2. Describe the characteristics of Class I through VI cavity preparations, identifying walls, cavosurfaces, line angles, and point angles.
3. Discuss the rationale for minimally invasive treatment.
4. Know the rationale and describe proper technique for placement of a rubber dam.

5. Discuss the advances in aesthetic materials and techniques.
6. Discuss the rationale for use of bases and liners.
7. Compare the advantages and disadvantages of various restorative materials.
8. Describe the function and placement of a matrix.

The dental hygienist serves as an important member of the oral healthcare team, evaluating all surfaces of teeth in the patient's oral cavity with both visual and tactile senses. For many patients the dental hygienist is their most regular healthcare provider. The dentist relies on the hygienist to provide important assessment information in order to develop proper preventive and therapeutic strategies. Because the dental hygienist frequently observes the patient's condition before the dentist does, mental and written documentation of findings is important to assist in the subsequent care.

Operative dentistry is defined as the diagnosis, prevention, and treatment of diseases, developmental defects, and traumatic injuries of hard tissues of individual teeth.[15,16] To ensure proper treatment of an individual tooth, the correct diagnosis must be made. The first step in the diagnosis of a patient is a proper medical and dental history (see Chapter 10). Prevention has both primary and secondary components. *Primary prevention* is to prevent the disease before evidence of its occurrence. *Secondary prevention* is to prevent a recurrence of the disease or an incipient case from progressing to a more severe state.

CLASSIFICATION AND NOMENCLATURE

38-A BLACK'S RESTORATIVE LESION CLASSIFICATION

Until recently, most dental restorations were based on the designs of G.V. Black,[5] often referred to as the "father of modern restorative dentistry." Dr. Black's classifications and principles were based on the restorative materials of his time, which were primarily dental *amalgam* and gold.

Black did not have the benefit of modern bonding systems and restorative materials. His initial classifications are as follows:

Class I lesion occurs in pits and fissures of a tooth (Fig. 38-1).

Class II lesion occurs on the proximal surface of a posterior tooth (Fig. 38-2).

Class III lesion occurs on the proximal surface of an anterior tooth (Fig. 38-3).

Class IV lesion occurs on the proximal surface of an anterior tooth from which the incisal angle is missing (Fig. 38-4).

Class V lesion occurs on the gingival third of the labial, buccal, or lingual smooth surfaces of the tooth (Fig. 38-5).

Eventually a sixth category was added, although not by Dr. Black, as follows:

Class VI lesion occurs on the tips of the cusps or the biting surfaces of the incisors (Fig. 38-6).

BLACK'S PRINCIPLES FOR SURGICAL REPAIR OF A DISEASED TOOTH

Black also developed a series of principles to be followed when surgically repairing a diseased tooth.

Outline Form

This process involves placement of the cavity margins (cavosurface) in the position on the tooth that they will occupy in the completed restoration. The *outline form* should encompass the carious lesion and may include portions of caries-susceptible areas on the tooth being restored. The outline form should follow a gentle sweeping curve, especially on the occlusal surface. Clinicians should visualize

---

Case Study **Application of Operative Therapies**

You greet a 53-year-old female, Mrs. Daniella Dixon, in the waiting room. She is 10 to 20 pounds overweight and well dressed. She is married and has two children. When you call her name, Mrs. Dixon responds immediately by standing and beginning to smile but not broadly. She moves quickly and follows you into the treatment room.

A review of Mrs. Dixon's medical history reveals the following:

Age 15: Hospitalized after severe automobile accident; thrown into dash/windshield; spent 2 days in hospital with moderate head injuries, including concussion; lost consciousness for a few minutes after accident.

Age 27: Gave birth to female.

Age 30: Gave birth to male.

Age 50: Postmenopausal; prescribed hormone supplement. No other significant medical problems.

Social history: Mrs. Dixon is somewhat reserved and rarely smiles. Both children have finished college, have good jobs, and live away from home. Her husband has a management position with a successful company and has just been transferred to your city. Mrs. Dixon drinks both coffee and tea throughout the day. She generally drinks wine with her dinner.

Dental status: Interproximal enamel lesions, root caries, Class V lesions, restored anterior teeth, and multiple posterior restorations.

Periodontal disease: Gingival recession, increased probing depths with spontaneous bleeding, marginal inflammation and edematous gingival tissue.

Missing teeth: All third molars were extracted at age 21. All other teeth are intact and are moderately stained.

Oral soft tissues
- Palate: presence of small (3-mm) ulcerated areas just palatal to the maxillary incisors.
- Lips: 3-mm raised vesicles on lower lip near the right angular border.

General comments: Mrs. Dixon states that she brushes twice a day. She normally uses Crest toothpaste but may buy the product on sale if she has seen it advertised on TV. She flosses a couple of times a week. She generally goes to the dentist once a year, although because of the recent move and her son finishing college, she has not been to a dentist in more than 2 years.

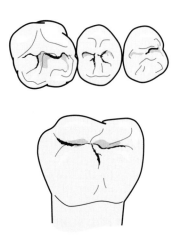

FIG. 38-1 Class I lesion.

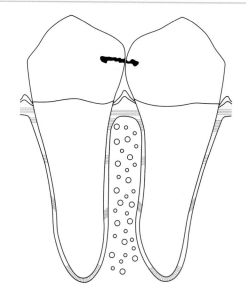

FIG. 38-2 Class II lesion.

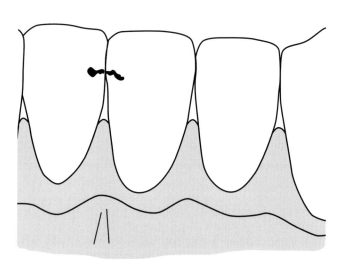

FIG. 38-3 Class III lesion.

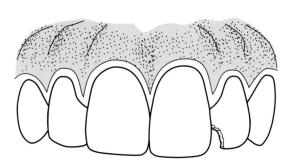

FIG. 38-4 Class IV lesion.

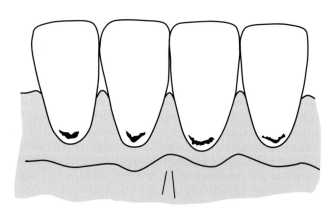

FIG. 38-5 Class V lesion.

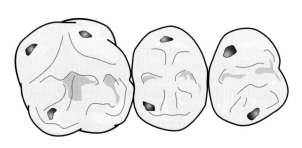

FIG. 38-6 Class VI lesion.

this form before any tooth reduction occurs to prevent overcutting of tissue. Outline form is determined by many factors, including location and size of the lesion, anatomy of the tooth, type of restorative material, aesthetic requirements of the situation, relative position of adjacent structures, functional requirements, and retentive factors. Black proposed two general principles to guide the establishment of outline form: (1) removal of all enamel not supported by dentin *(undermined enamel)* and (2) placement of margins in areas of low caries susceptibility, often referred to as *"extension for prevention."*

Resistance Form

Resistance form is the design and position of the cavity walls that best enable the tooth and the restoration to withstand forces and avoid fracture or breakage. Fundamental principles of resistance form include (1) flat floors prepared at right angles to the forces of mastication, (2) restriction of preparation extensions to allow strong cuspal and marginal ridges, (3) removal of weakened tooth tissue in the preparation design to prevent future tooth fracture, and (4) consideration of the properties of the restorative materials.

Retention Form

Retention form is that shape of the cavity preparation that permits the restoration to resist displacement (or dislodgment) through sliding, tipping, or lifting forces. Factors that enhance retention form include "dovetails," converging walls, (relatively) sharp internal line angles, grooves, pins, frictional resistance of walls, and acid etching (with bonded materials).

Convenience Form

Convenience form is that shape of the preparation that allows adequate observation, accessibility, and ease of operation during the preparation and restorative phases of treatment. Inadequate convenience form prevents proper instrumentation of the cavity preparation. Factors that enhance convenience form include extension of the cavity preparation (taking care to limit excessive extension due to its negative effect on resistance form), a change in the line of approach, and a change in the operating instrument.

Removal of Remaining Carious Dentin

This process involves the excavation of any infectious material remaining after the basic cavity design has been completed. *Incipient lesions,* which penetrate the dentinoenamel junction (DEJ) no more than 0.5 mm, are generally removed at the completion of outline, resistance, retention, and convenience form sequence. *Extensive lesions,* which penetrate the DEJ more than 0.5 mm, will be subjected to further surgical extension until all diseased tissue is removed (or medicated).

Finishing of Enamel Walls

The finishing process involves the smoothing or refinement of the walls of the cavity preparation and cavosurface angles. This step helps to (1) create an optimal marginal seal between the restorative material and the tooth, (2) allow for optimal marginal adaptation (which is less noticeable to the patient and is less plaque-retentive), and (3) provide maximum strength to the restorative material and to the tooth at the margin.

Cleansing and Medicating of Preparation

This process includes removal of all debris, drying of the preparation (preparation is left slightly damp for increased bonding strength with current systems[10]), inspection for decay and unsound tooth tissue, and placement of medication if indicated.

COMPONENTS OF PREPARED CAVITIES

Prepared cavities have walls, line angles, and point angles **38-B** just as the crown of the tooth has surfaces, line angles, and point angles. The nomenclature involved is quite similar in both cases. Most cavity preparations are considered to have a "box" form, and these components are most easily visualized in this form.

Wall

A vertical or horizontal surface within the cavity preparation is called a *wall* and is named according to the closest external surface (e.g., facial, mesial, or lingual wall), for the structure that it approximates (e.g., pulpal wall), or for its relationship to the long axis of the tooth (e.g., axial wall).

Cavosurface

The uncut tooth tissue adjacent to the cavity preparation is the *cavosurface.*

Line Angle

A *line angle* is formed along the junctions of two walls or the junction of one wall and the cavosurface *(cavosurface margin).* Line angles are named according to the walls and surfaces involved.

Point Angle

A *point angle* is formed by the junction of three walls within a cavity preparation and is named according to the walls involved.

CLASS I CAVITY PREPARATIONS

A Class I cavity preparation on a molar is used to illustrate the derivation of the nomenclature (Fig. 38-7).

Walls

A Class I molar preparation normally has curving walls along the facial and lingual sides that blend with the mesial and distal walls. These vertical walls end at a horizontal wall called the *pulpal wall* or *pulpal floor.* Fig. 38-8 presents the preparation as a box to assist the dental hygienist in learning the nomenclature.

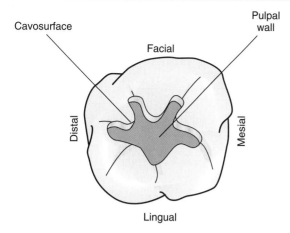

FIG. 38-7 Class I cavity preparation. Outer surfaces of tooth are designated mesial, lingual, distal, and facial. Wall at the bottom of the cavity is the *pulpal wall.* Unprepared external surface of the tooth adjacent to the preparation is the *cavosurface.*

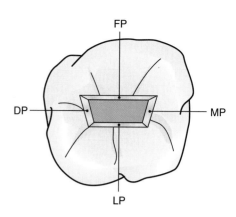

FIG. 38-9 The four line angles formed at the intersections of the vertical walls with the pulpal wall are the mesiopulpal *(MP),* lingopulpal *(LP),* distopulpal *(DP),* and faciopulpal *(FP).*

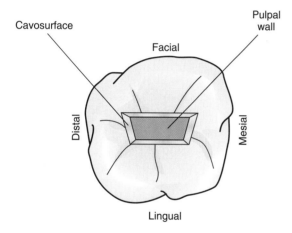

FIG. 38-8 Compare with Fig. 38-7. Preparation is a "box" with four walls and bottom. Walls of the preparation are named for external surfaces to which they are adjacent; the bottom is called the "pulpal wall" because of its proximity to the pulp.

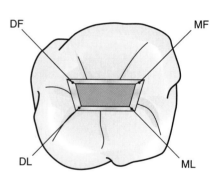

FIG. 38-10 The four line angles formed where the vertical walls intersect one another are the mesiolingual *(ML),* distolingual *(DL),* distofacial *(DF),* and mesiofacial *(MF).*

Line Angles

The three sets of line angles in the Class I preparation are named according to the walls involved (Figs. 38-9, 38-10, and 38-11).

Rule 1

When the name of a line angle or point angle is being developed, the *al* should be dropped and *o* substituted at the end of all words in the name except the last one (e.g., the line angle formed by the facial wall intersecting the pulpal wall is the *faciopulpal* line angle). Fig. 38-9 shows the remaining line angles formed by the pulpal wall. These line angles are not straight but follow the outline form of the preparation. Fig. 38-10 shows the line angles formed by the intersection of one vertical wall with another. In the actual cavity preparation these are not sharp corners but curves. Fig. 38-11 illustrates the four line angles formed by the intersection of the vertical walls with the cavosurface.

Rule 2

When "cavosurface" is one of the words used in the description of a line angle, it is placed last (e.g., the intersection of the facial wall with the cavosurface is the *faciocavosurface* line angle). The other three cavosurface line angles are named in a similar manner.

Point Angles

Four internal point angles constitute a Class I occlusal preparation (Fig. 38-12). The name of each is derived by combining the names of the involved walls using rule 1.

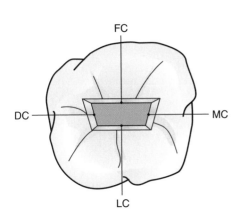

FIG. 38-11 The four cavosurface line angles formed where the vertical walls intersect the uncut tooth surface are the mesiocavosurface *(MC)*, linguocavosurface *(LC)*, distocavosurface *(DC)*, and faciocavosurface *(FC)*.

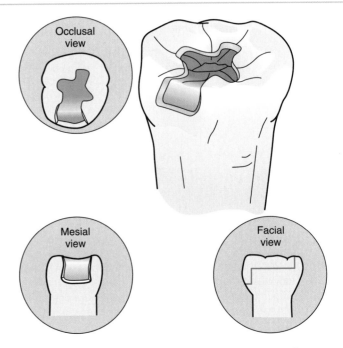

FIG. 38-13 Class II mesioocclusal cavity preparation on tooth #19. Compare with the occlusal view in Fig. 38-7.

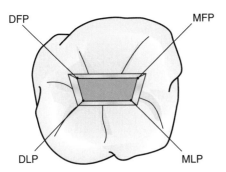

FIG. 38-12 The four *point* angles formed at the intersection of three internal walls. Intersection of three walls at lower left, for example, is the mesiolinguopulpal *(MLP)* point angle. *DLP,* Distolinguopulpa; *DFP,* distofaciopulpal; *MFP,* mesiofaciopulpal.

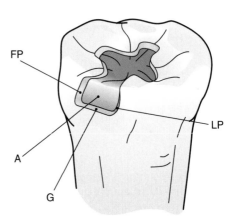

FIG. 38-14 The walls of the proximal portion of the preparation are the gingival *(G)*, linguproximal *(LP)*, axial *(A)*, and facioproximal *(FP)*.

CLASS II CAVITY PREPARATIONS

The Class II cavity preparation removes the proximal surface (Fig. 38-13). The occlusal portion is prepared similar to a Class I preparation, but the marginal ridge is involved to allow access to the proximal surface. A Class II preparation is an extension of the Class I into the proximal area.

Walls and Cavosurface

The occlusal walls are identical to those of the Class I preparation. The proximal portion includes an axial wall parallel to the long axis of the tooth and a gingival wall (floor) adjacent to the gingival tissues (Fig. 38-14). The facial and lingual walls of the proximal portion are termed the *facioproximal* and *linguoproximal* walls.

Line Angles

In the proximal portion the *internal* line angles are (1) axiopulpal, (2) axiogingival, (3) axiolinguoproximal, (4) axiofacioproximal, (5) gingivolinguoproximal, and (6) gin-

givofacioproximal (Fig. 38-15). In the proximal portion the *external* line angles are (1) linguoproximocavosurface, (2) facioproximocavosurface, and (3) gingivocavosurface (Fig. 38-16).

Point Angles

The intersection of the gingival and axial walls with each of the proximal walls forms two point angles, axiogingivolin*guo*proximal and axiogingivo*facio*proximal (Fig. 38-17).

CLASS III CAVITY PREPARATIONS

Dental caries on the proximal surface of anterior teeth may be removed by either a facial or a lingual approach.

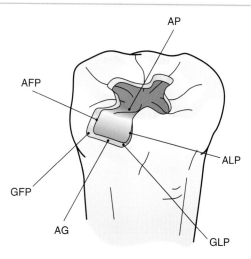

FIG. 38-15 The line angles of the proximal portion of Class II mesioocclusal preparation are the gingivolinguoproximal *(GLP)*, axiolinguoproximal *(ALP)*, axiopulpal *(AP)*, axiogingival *(AG)*, axiofacioproximal *(AFP)*, and gingivofacioproximal *(GFP)*.

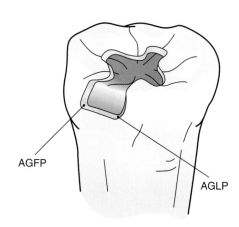

FIG. 38-17 The internal *point* angles of the mesioproximal portion of Class II mesioocclusal preparation are the axiogingivolinguoproximal *(AGLP)* and axiogingivofacioproximal *(AGFP)*.

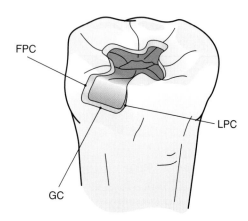

FIG. 38-16 The cavosurface line angles of the proximal portion of Class II preparation are the gingivocavosurface *(GC)*, linguoproximocavosurface *(LPC)*, and facioproximocavosurface *(FPC)*.

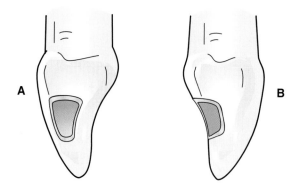

FIG. 38-18 Walls of Class III cavity preparation. **A,** Labial access. **B,** Lingual slot access.

Fig. 38-18 illustrates the cavity outlines resulting from each approach as well as the walls resulting from the preparations. The dental practitioner can identify line angles and point angles for each of the preparations.

CLASS IV CAVITY PREPARATIONS

Fig. 38-19 is a proximal view of a Class IV restoration to help develop the nomenclature for this preparation.

CLASS V CAVITY PREPARATIONS

The Class V preparation is similar to a Class I preparation except for its location in the gingival one third of the facial or lingual surface. Class V also may be viewed as a box with four sides and a bottom (Fig. 38-20). On an anterior tooth the occlusal wall is called the *incisal wall*.

MINIMALLY INVASIVE DENTISTRY

The traditional treatment for the carious lesion has remained essentially the same since Black introduced his principles more than a century ago. As stated, "extension for prevention" had become an important tenet for every dentist educated in the twentieth century, although there were some challenges to Black's ideas. Bronner[6] and Markley[11] published works on more conservative cavity design in the first half of the twentieth century. Osborne and colleagues[13] and Sigurjons[18] addressed these issues in the 1970s and 1980s.

AMALGAM-SEALANT COMBINATIONS

The advent of adhesive dentistry began in the 1950s when Buonocore[7] discovered that acid etching of tooth

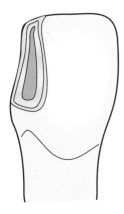

FIG. 38-19 Proximal view of Class IV cavity preparation walls.

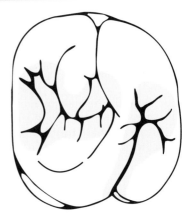

FIG. 38-21 Occlusal view of molar for sealant application. Shaded area is etched, and a pit fissure sealant or flowable resin composite is bonded in place.

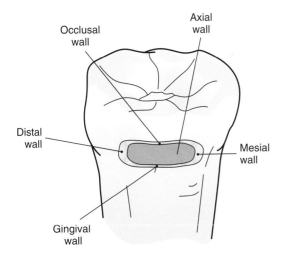

Occlusal wall

Axial wall

Distal wall

Mesial wall

Gingival wall

FIG. 38-20 Walls of Class V cavity preparation on posterior tooth.

enamel increased the retention of restorative materials. With subsequent advances in bonding systems[20] and resin *composite* materials, prevention of caries and greater conservation of tooth structure became possible. These advances initiated the era of minimally invasive dentistry.

A 10-year clinical study by Mertz-Fairhurst and colleagues[12] compared traditional Class I amalgam restorations to Class I amalgams placed only in areas of the fissure systems where actual caries had been diagnosed. In the latter group the fissures remaining after the placement of those smaller restorations were sealed with a resin fissure sealant. At 10 years, seven of the 79 traditional amalgam restorations had failed, and only one of the 77 amalgam-sealant combination restorations had failed. This definitive study provided excellent support for dentists limiting the size of cavity preparation to the decayed area and addressing "extension for prevention" with materials such as fissure sealants.

The establishment of outline form using these parameters may be accomplished simply by removal of carious dentin and the overlying unsupported enamel. Osborne and Summitt[14] state that this allows for conservation and maintenance of tooth structure and leaves more occlusal enamel, which is better suited for occlusal function and resistance to occlusal wear than restorative materials. These concepts, along with surgical treatment of only active caries observed radiographically to have penetrated the dentin and with use of all available means to stop and reverse caries, represent truly minimal intervention and the current state of the art in operative dentistry.

With the advent of adhesive dentistry, prevention of caries and greater conservation of tooth structure are possible. In addition, evidence indicates a possible shift in philosophy from the traditional surgical model of excision to a more modern medical model of treatment.[2,8] Hume[9] stated that dentists should modify their 200-year-old philosophy of treating caries like gangrene by extracting or excavating and filling. He advocated a treatment approach based on the structure and behavior of the lesion. Carious lesions in dentin and cementum are reversible to some degree, and Hume further recommended that clinicians consider including nonsurgical healing of these lesions in the treatment plan.

Case Application

Mrs. Dixon's treatment plan called for a number of small occlusal restorations, which would be opportune situations for minimally invasive procedures. Rather than the standard Black-style outline form on the occlusal surface of her mandibular molar, the outline could be confined to the area of localized caries in the central pit. The caries would be surgically excised in this area only, and a small aesthetic composite (or small amalgam) suitable for the posterior teeth could be bonded in place. The adjacent grooves could then be treated with a fissure sealant (Fig. 38-21). In essence, Black's "extension for prevention" would be obtained not by the outline of the preparation, but rather by the conservative treatment of the adjacent fissures with proven sealants.

AESTHETIC DENTISTRY

Since the introduction of the acid-etch technique,[7] dental manufacturers have developed numerous generations of restorative tooth-colored materials. Patients are becoming more informed on the availability of these aesthetic materials and are demanding their use by the dental profession. Many are aware of the option of treating stained teeth with a bleaching or whitening technique (see Chapter 39) or coverage by direct or indirect resin composite or porcelain veneers and crowns. Patients may also have spaces *(diastemata)* that can be closed with the same materials. Some patients, however, are not educated about the availability of these products and techniques.

The patient's personality change after aesthetic treatment is one of the most rewarding accomplishments for the dental team. Many new materials have been developed and many traditional ones substantially improved to add to the dental team's armamentarium for the treatment of these cases.

 Case Application

Mrs. Dixon does not smile often primarily because she is self-conscious about the discoloration of her maxillary anterior teeth. With proper education from the dental team, she can be made aware of aesthetic interventions for the treatment of her dentition.

ISOLATION OF TEETH

A proper operating field is necessary to perform operative procedures with optimal results. Isolating the field (1) prevents moisture contamination, (2) retracts and controls the soft tissues, (3) protects the patient against aspiration of instruments and materials, and (4) provides optimal visibility of the operating site. While isolating the operative field, the clinician should not interfere with visual or mechanical access to the operating site, injure soft or hard tissues, or cause discomfort.

The type of isolation required depends on the duration of the procedure and the degree of dryness necessary. For some procedures, *cotton roll isolation* can be accomplished with a saliva ejector and a high-volume oral evacuation system. Cotton roll holders can be used in the mandibular arch. Absorbent triangles over the parotid duct can be used with cotton rolls for increased moisture control. Cotton roll isolation offers ease and speed of application. However, risks include contamination of the operating field, limited retraction of soft tissues, and no protection against the patient aspirating debris or objects.

The *rubber dam* meets the criteria listed for isolation. Disadvantages are that the clamp can irritate the gingiva, placement of the dam can be time-consuming for the beginning clinician, and some patients are sensitive to the latex of the rubber dam. Overall, however, the advantages of using a rubber dam outweigh the disadvantages.

ARMAMENTARIUM

Fig. 38-22 illustrates the necessary armamentarium for rubber dam placement. The *Young's frame* is a common type of rubber dam holder. This metal or plastic U-shaped frame holds the dam away from the patient's face. The

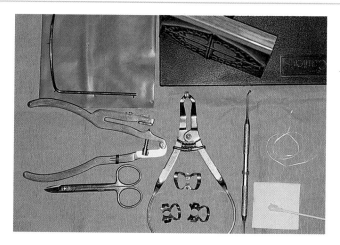

FIG. 38-22 Tray set-up for rubber dam application.

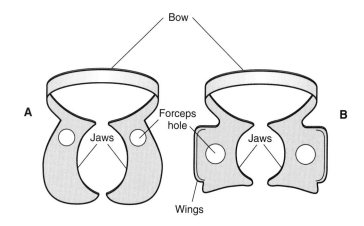

FIG. 38-23 Rubber dam clamps. **A,** Wingless. **B,** Winged.

Woodbury holder is an elastic band that fits around the back of the patient's head and is attached to the sides of the dam with three clips on each side. It provides excellent lip and cheek retraction.

The *rubber dam clamp* anchors the dam to the tooth (Fig. 38-23). Therefore this tooth is referred to as the *anchor tooth*. Clamps may be winged or wingless. The jaws of the winged clamp have small projections *(wings)* that allow the clamp to be mounted on the dam before it is placed on the teeth. The dental chart is helpful in the determination of which clamps are most likely to fit particular teeth (Fig. 38-24).

The dam material is available in several weights (thicknesses) and in various colors. Heavier material is typically used for restorative procedures because the added weight provides better retraction of the gingivae, lips, and cheeks and because the material does not tear easily. Lightweight material is used more often during endodontic procedures because only one tooth is isolated; tearing is less of a problem; and the lighter material is easier to manipulate.

PREPARATION OF PATIENT

If the patient has never experienced placement of a rubber dam, the clinician should explain the benefits, such as

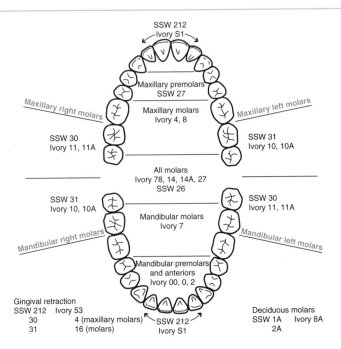

FIG. 38-24 Chart of suggested clamps to be used in various areas of mouth.

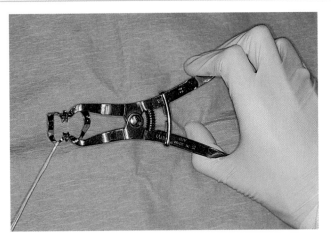

FIG. 38-25 The locking ring is engaged by pointing forceps upward, then squeezing and releasing (see Box 38-1).

elimination of debris in the mouth and prevention of a contaminated restorative site. The procedure also should be explained briefly so that the patient knows what to expect. Because the patient will not be able to talk with the dam in place, the clinician may suggest signals to be used if the patient should need to communicate.

EXAMINATION OF MOUTH

The clinician should examine the site where the dam is to be placed and floss the teeth to determine whether passing the dam between any of the teeth will be difficult. If floss cannot be passed through the contact, the reason should be determined. Calculus, restoration overhangs, and rough proximal surfaces should be removed. Teeth with very tight contacts may need to be wedged apart before dam placement. If needed, a wooden wedge may be placed into the involved proximal space for 1 to 2 minutes, then the contact checked again with dental floss. The clinician also must check the patient's occlusion to determine whether any unusual anatomical parts may interfere with the restoration. The shape and size of the arch, position of the teeth, edentulous spaces, and fixed prostheses must be noted. This information will be needed to punch the rubber dam holes correctly.

SELECTION OF CLAMP

The rubber dam clamp is selected on the basis of the anatomy of the anchor tooth (see Fig. 38-24). The location and number of the involved teeth will determine which teeth are to be isolated. Minimal access is obtained by isolation of one tooth distal and two teeth mesial to the teeth being restored. The most distal tooth in the quadrant should be clamped and isolation extended to the opposite lateral incisor to obtain (1) greater access, (2)

> ### BOX 38-1
>
> #### Steps for Clamp Placement
> 1. Determine the anchor tooth and select the appropriate clamp.
> 2. Tie floss around the bow of the clamp to permit retrieval if the clamp slips off the tooth.
> 3. Place the clamp on the forceps.
> 4. Squeeze the handles together to open the jaws of the clamp.
> 5. With the tips of the forceps upward, the locking ring will slide towards the handle of the forceps holding the jaws of the clamp open (see Fig. 38-25).
> 6. Position the clamp over the tooth.
> 7. Rotate it lingually to seat the lingual jaw first because vision is more restricted in this area.
> 8. Rotate the clamp facially to seat the facial jaw. Be certain that the jaws do not drag across the tooth, scarring the cementum.
> 9. Squeeze the handles of the forceps to release the locking ring and allow the jaws of the clamp to engage the tooth.

maximum retraction of the lips, cheeks, and tongue, and (3) more teeth for a finger rest. If only the anterior teeth are involved, the clinician may isolate from the first premolar to the contralateral first premolar. Both premolars may be clamped or ligated with dental floss or a small piece of rubber dam used to wedge the dam in the interproximal areas.

PLACEMENT OF CLAMP

Box 38-1 provides a list of steps used to place the clamp. When properly placed, all four prongs should contact the tooth near its line angles at a position cervical to the height of contour (Figs. 38-25 and 38-26). The clamp should be stable when rocked gently from side to side with light finger pressure and should not impinge on the soft tissue. If these criteria are not met, the clamp should be repositioned or, if necessary, another clamp selected. If

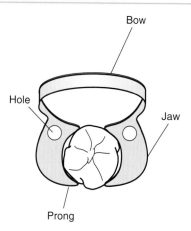

FIG. 38-26 All four prongs of clamps should be in contact with tooth.

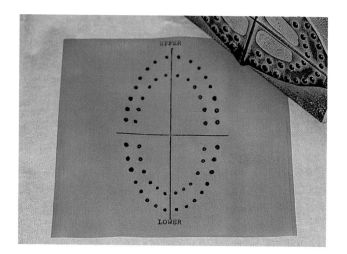

FIG. 38-27 Rubber dam stamp.

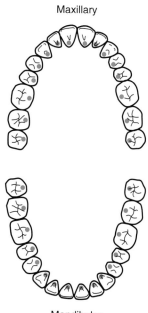

FIG. 38-28 For the average-sized arch, punch the central incisors approximately 1½ inches from the edge of the dam near the midline. Punch additional holes using guidelines in text.

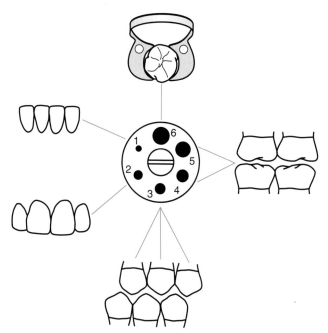

FIG. 38-29 Suggested sizes of holes to be punched in dam for various teeth.

the clamp rotates or slides off the tooth or rests on the papilla, it is too large. If the clamp does not fit over the height of contour or pops off the tooth, it is too small. Because the prongs are pointed and can cut the gingiva or gouge the root surface, forceps should always be used to disengage or reposition the clamp.

PREPARATION OF RUBBER DAM

The rubber dam is punched to suit each clinical situation. The number, size, and location of the holes are determined by (1) the location and size of the teeth to be isolated, (2) the shape and size of the arch, (3) the position and spacing of the teeth, and (4) the type of preparation. A template or rubber dam stamp can be used as a guide to mark the location of the holes to be punched (Fig. 38-27). If this is not available, the dam can be punched according to a mandibular and maxillary chart (Fig. 38-28).

The clinician should mark the central incisors near the midline of the dam, allowing 4 mm of rubber between anterior holes and 5 mm of rubber between posterior holes. The holes for Class V restorations should be marked 1 mm to the facial side for facial lesions or 1 mm to the lingual side for lingual lesions. An additional 1 mm of rubber be-

tween adjacent teeth should be allotted for the gingival retraction needed for access to the Class V lesion.

The size of the hole to be punched depends on the size of the tooth. For a six-hole punch, the smaller size-2 hole is used for all mandibular incisors and maxillary lateral incisors; the medium size-3 hole for premolars, canines, and maxillary central incisors; the size-5 hole for molars; and the size-6 hole for the anchor tooth and clamp (Fig. 38-29).

As the hole is punched, the clinician should pull dam up the punch spike to be certain it has cut completely through the dam.

PLACEMENT OF RUBBER DAM AND FRAME

Before rubber dam placement, preparatory steps are as follows:
1. Lubricate the patient's lips with petroleum jelly to protect them against dryness and irritation from the dam.
2. Place the powdered side of the dam facing you to reduce light reflection.
3. Choose one of two alternative methods of placing the clamp and dam on the tooth based on the clinical situation, clinician's preference, and availability of clamps.
4. If a wingless clamp is used, place the clamp on the tooth and recheck its stability.
5. Orient the rubber dam, and place the index finger of each hand on opposing sides of the hole to be placed over the clamped tooth.
6. Stretch the dam to enlarge the hole, and slide the dam over the bow and under each of the jaws.
7. When the tooth and clamp are fully exposed with the rubber dam against the gingiva, use a T-ball burnisher blade to pull the floss tied to the clamp through the hole.

The dam may also be placed on the bow of the wingless clamp before placement on the tooth, which may be easier for the inexperienced clinician. This allows maximum access and visibility while applying the clamp. Care must be exercised to avoid placement of excess pressure on the clamp, thus traumatizing the tooth or surrounding gingiva as the dam is seated.

To use a winged clamp, the clinician should orient it to the correct hole in the dam, and proceed as follows:
1. Lubricate the patient's lips with petroleum jelly to protect them against dryness and irritation from the dam.
2. Place the powdered side of the dam facing you to reduce light reflection.
3. Engage the clamp onto the forceps.
4. Slide one wing into the hole, then stretch the dam toward and over the opposite wing (Fig. 38-30). The dam may be placed on the frame at this stage if desired.
5. Place the clamp on the anchor tooth as described previously, looking through the opening and under the dam to check the position of the clamp relative to the gingiva before releasing the forceps.
6. Pull the rubber dam off the wings, and allow it to slide against the tooth and rest under the clamp. Vision is more limited with this method, but placement is faster because the clamp, dam, and frame are placed simultaneously. After the clamp and approximating dam are positioned properly, isolate the most anterior tooth. Then place the frame, if not already carried into position with the clamp, to hold the dam away from the patient's face and to provide access to the working area.
7. Position the base of the U-shaped frame downward, with the concave side of the frame toward the patient.
8. Gently pull the rubber dam over the small metal protrusions on the frame to hold the dam in place.
9. Stretch the dam to open the holes over the remaining teeth, one at a time.

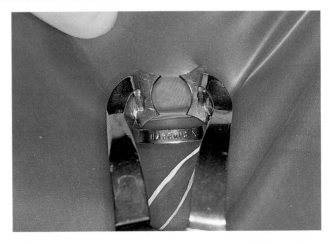

FIG. 38-30 Winged clamp being held by dam before placement on tooth.

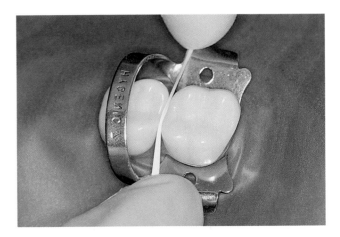

FIG. 38-31 When necessary, push the interseptal rubber through the contacts with dental floss.

10. Pass the dam through the contact areas. This is more easily done with an assistant, who stretches the dam over each contact area.
11. Push the rubber through the contact areas by using waxed floss or tape to engage the leading edge of the rubber and carrying it first against one proximal surface and then the other (Fig. 38-31). Do not try to force the whole width of the septum through at once; this is difficult to accomplish and may result in tearing of the dam. If the dam is not fully through the contact areas, it will be difficult to tuck it into the facial and lingual sulci. Repeat the flossing procedure if needed.
12. After the dam is through the contact areas, readjust the frame to hold the dam more tightly.
13. Center the frame to avoid endangering the patient (i.e., the ends of the frame should be away from the patient's eyes).
14. Tie the floss attached to the clamp to the frame so that it is out of the operating field.
15. Tuck (invert) the dam into the sulcus around each tooth to prevent seepage of sulcular fluid and saliva. Starting at the distal, position the blade of a plastic

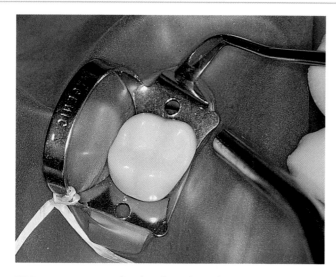

FIG. 38-32 Invert the dam into the sulcus using a thin (not sharp) blade. Air helps to dry the tooth and dam and creates a seal.

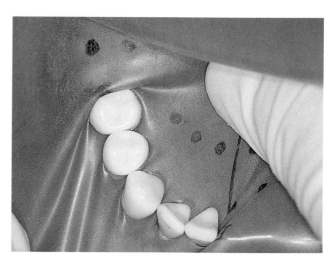

FIG. 38-34 Stretch the piece of rubber dam, and push it into the contact area.

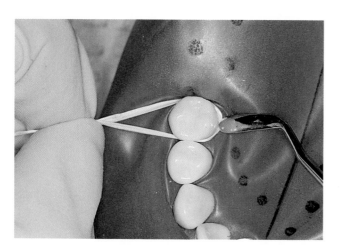

FIG. 38-33 Push the loop of ligature below the cingulum with the blade while pulling the ends in an apical direction.

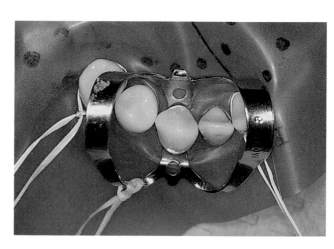

FIG. 38-35 Isolation achieved through properly mounted rubber dam.

instrument or T-ball burnisher parallel to the distofacial line angle of the tooth, directed slightly into the sulcus. Slide it to the mesial line angle, using the edge of the blade to push the rubber into the gingival sulcus (Fig. 38-32). Simultaneously, direct a stream of air into the sulcus to dry the tooth, rubber dam, and soft tissue to prevent the rubber dam from sliding back out of the sulcus. Repeat this step for each tooth on both the facial and the lingual surfaces.

16. Stabilize the rubber dam by ligating a piece of dental floss around the most anterior tooth (Fig. 38-33) or by wedging a small piece of rubber into the embrasure between the last exposed tooth and the rubber dam (Fig. 38-34). For dam applications isolating the teeth from first premolar to first premolar, the ligature or rubber dam wedge method of stabilization may be used instead of clamps.

17. After the dam is correctly placed, insert a saliva ejector under the rubber dam onto the floor of the mouth.

A properly applied rubber dam (1) should isolate the working area with no moisture present, (2) should expose the teeth to be treated and provide sufficient visual access and finger rests for the clinician, (3) should be stable and secure with no potential damage to the hard and soft tissues, (4) should be inverted into the gingival sulcus, and (5) should be comfortable (Fig. 38-35).

APPLICATION OF GINGIVAL RETRACTOR CLAMP

The gingival retractor clamp pushes the gingival tissue and rubber dam material away from the site of the Class V preparation (Box 38-2). This retractor has two jaws, with prongs, two bows, and notches for the clamp forceps. The bows have different lengths, which provides this clamp

BOX 38-2

Steps for Application of Gingival Retractor Clamp for Class V Restorations

1. Insert the forceps into the notches and expand the jaws of the retractor. For greater access and visibility, seat the lingual jaw first.
2. Slide it gently against the lingual surface until it is apical to the height of contour and flush with, but not impinging on, the gingival tissue.
3. Use the opposite hand to stabilize the lingual jaw.
4. At the same time rotate the forceps to move the facial jaw apically along the facial surface until the facial jaw is apical to the height of contour and contacts the dam overlying the gingiva.
5. Using the jaws of the clamp, gently retract the gingiva and dam to expose the gingival extent of the carious lesion.
6. Spread the jaws wide enough to avoid scraping against the tooth as the jaws are seated. This would scar the tooth, making it more susceptible to plaque accumulation and caries. If possible, retract the gingiva until it is at least 0.5 to 1.0 mm apical to the gingival margin of the lesion. The bows of the clamp should be parallel to the tooth's occlusal plane to ensure even retraction of the gingiva.
7. Remove the forceps from the retractor while continuing to support the lingual and facial aspects of the retractor with the other hand.
8. Continue the support until dental compound has been placed under the bows and onto the occlusal/incisal surfaces of the surrounding teeth (see Fig. 38-37). Dental compound stabilizes the gingival retractor to avoid slippage during the procedure. Trauma to tooth structure and the preparation or restorative material may occur if the clamp slips.
9. Warm the compound stick over a flame until the end begins to sag.
10. Temper it in warm water until the material is warm and malleable but not hot.
11. Mold the compound over the top of one retractor bow and the occlusal/incisal surface.
12. Continue molding the compound until it fills the space between the bow and the tooth. Repeat procedure for the other bow.
13. Check the retractor with light finger pressure to make sure that it resists movement, is stable, and evenly retracts the gingiva and rubber dam.

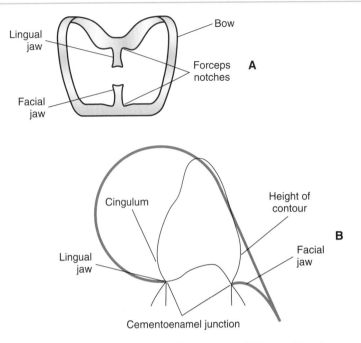

FIG. 38-36 A, Parts of gingival retractor. **B,** Relationship of gingival retractor jaws to landmarks on anterior tooth.

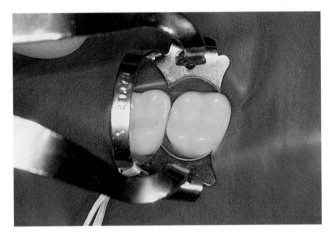

FIG. 38-37 Mounting and placement of gingival retractor (see Box 38-2).

with specific lingual and facial sides (Fig. 38-36). When the retractor is oriented to the tooth, the flat portion of the bow will be to the facial lesion side of the tooth. The gingival retractor clamp should be stabilized with compound (Fig. 38-37).

REMOVAL OF RUBBER DAM

Before removing the dam, high-volume evacuation should be used to remove all debris from the operating field. If a gingival retractor has been used, the clinician should remove it first and apply the forceps in an occlusolingual direction to break the compound off the teeth. The retractor then is removed carefully in an occlusal direction without touching the newly placed restoration or the tooth surface. The clinician then must remove any remaining compound with a sharp instrument and remove the ligature or rubber dam wedge from the most anterior tooth. The dam should be stretched to the facial side, away from the teeth, and one finger placed under the stretched dam to protect the patient's lips and cheeks while the interdental areas of the dam are cut (Fig. 38-38). The clinician should cut the entire septum with one stroke from the facial aspect and pull the dam in a lingual direction.

Pulling an uncut dam up through the contacts or snipping the interproximal areas in stages may cause thin

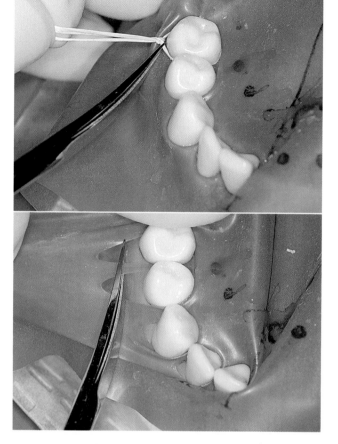

FIG. 38-38 Rubber dam removal. The tip of the lower scissors blade extends well beyond the rubber to ensure complete cutting of the septum each time.

pieces of dam to tear or remain around the tooth. A ring of rubber dam material remaining around a tooth would tend to migrate apically because the apex is the most constricted area of the tooth. This could cause a gingival abscess, bone destruction, or even loss of the tooth.[1]

The clinician must remove the clamp, dam, and frame at the same time, laying the dam on a light-colored surface and checking to ensure that no small pieces of rubber are missing and still in the patient's mouth. Except for the severed interdental pieces, the dam should appear as it did before placement (Fig. 38-39). Any piece that is left in the mouth should be removed with dental floss or an explorer.

The clinician then must rinse and evacuate the oral cavity, examining the soft tissue for any trauma. The patient should be informed that some discomfort may occur after the anesthetic wears off.

EVALUATION CRITERIA

APPLICATION OF RUBBER DAM

1. Isolated area is clean and dry.
2. Number of teeth exposed provides visual access and finger rests.
3. Clamp is stable and secure and does not impinge on gingiva.

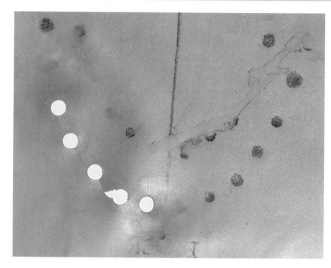

FIG. 38-39 Clamp, dam, and frame removal. A piece of rubber dam is missing next to the fourth hole from the bottom.

4. Dam is held securely by ligature or wedges.
5. Dam is inverted into the gingival sulcus.
6. Patient is comfortable.
7. If used, gingival retractor is stable and retracts the gingiva and dam.

REMOVAL OF RUBBER DAM

1. All rubber dam material, ligatures, and other debris have been removed.
2. No significant soft tissue injury is present.

RESTORATIVE MATERIALS

Four primary materials are used in the restoration of teeth: (1) dental amalgam and (2) resin composite or *glass ionomers* and combinations or modifications, (3) gold or other precious or nonprecious metals, and (4) porcelain or other ceramic materials. Dental amalgam, resin composite, and gold foil materials can be placed *directly* in one appointment. Laboratory-processed resin composite, cast gold, and porcelain are generally considered *indirect* restorative materials and are placed in two separate dental appointments. This discussion focuses on the directly placed materials.

AMALGAM

Amalgam by definition is an alloy of mercury with any other metal. *Dental amalgam* is made by vigorously mixing mercury with a silver-tin alloy for a few seconds. The plastic mass is then placed into a cavity preparation, with the mixture compressed *(condensation)* to remove the excess mercury-rich phase. The hardening mass is then carved and finished to restore tooth form and function.

Advantages

1. *Durable.* When properly placed under ideal conditions (dry field) and in conservative cavity preparations, amalgam has a long service life.

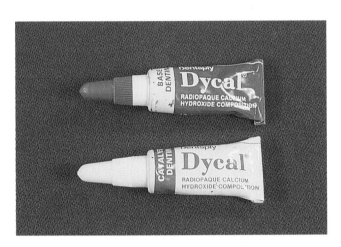

FIG. 38-40 Calcium hydroxide liner.

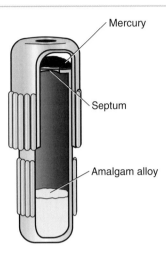

FIG. 38-41 Preproportioned capsule showing mercury and powder separated by septum that must be perforated before mixing.

2. *Economic.* Amalgam is the least expensive of the restorative materials and usually can be placed in the least amount of time.
3. *Low technique sensitivity.* Amalgam is less affected by clinician error and nonideal placement conditions.
4. *Broad applicability.* Amalgam can be used routinely in Class I, II, V, and VI lesions and also in certain Class III situations.
5. *Easy.* Amalgam is easily manipulated.
6. *Quick.* Amalgam requires less placement time.
7. *Sealant capability.* **Corrosion** products seal the tooth-restoration interface, which can reduce **microleakage.**
8. *Direct placement.* Amalgam is placed in a single appointment, although certain physical properties may be improved by polishing, which would be accomplished at a subsequent appointment. No interim restoration is normally required.

Disadvantages

1. **Marginal breakdown.** Amalgam is a brittle material with poor edge strength.
2. *Nonaesthetic.* Amalgam has a silver-gray shade.
3. *Potential* **galvanic reaction.** If it comes into contact with dissimilar metals, amalgam may cause the patient to experience a tingling or shocklike feeling.
4. *Public perception.* The general public has a poor perception of mercury toxicity.

CAVITY SEALERS, LINERS, AND BASES

After a cavity preparation has been completed, it is recommended that the cut tooth surface be treated before the placement of the amalgam restoration. The three principal options are cavity sealers, liners, and bases. *Cavity sealers* include (1) resins dissolved in a volatile solvent that leaves a resin layer after evaporation that is 2 to 5 microns thick and (2) resin bonding agents. *Cavity liners* are thin (less than 1 mm) resin or cement coating materials used to provide a barrier for protection of the pulp from restoration by-products and oral fluids. Liners can also be used to provide a therapeutic effect. *Cavity bases* are thicker (greater than 1 mm) cement filler materials used to provide ther-

mal protection for the pulp or replacement material for missing dentinal tooth structure (Fig. 38-40).

RESTORATIVE PROCEDURES

AMALGAM PLACEMENT TECHNIQUES

Class I, V, and VI Preparations

Once the tooth has been prepared and the freshly exposed surface has been treated with a cavity sealer, liner, or base, the clinician can begin placing the restorative material. Most amalgam delivery systems are *capsule*-based. Some require activation of the capsule before mixing. *Activating* is essentially breaking the barrier that exists in the capsule that prevents the mixing of the silver-tin alloy with the mercury during storage (Fig. 38-41). Usually this procedure consists of pressing the two halves of the capsule together or twisting them in opposite directions. This will vary according to manufacturer.

The clinician should set the controls on the *amalgamator* to the manufacturer's recommended settings, place the activated capsule in the *triturator*, and turn it on. When it shuts off, the capsule may be removed. With some products the recommendation may be to remove the pestle from the capsule and triturate again for a short time. This process is known as *mulling* and may improve the plasticity of the mix.

Once mixed, the amalgam must be placed (Figs. 38-42 and 38-43), condensed, and carved in a limited period. This "working time" varies by manufacturer and product (Box 38-3).

The three objectives of condensation are (1) removal of excess mercury from the mix to obtain minimal mercury in the final restoration, (2) compaction of the plastic mass to increase the density of the restoration by reducing voids, and (3) adaptation of the amalgam as closely as possible to the preparation walls and angles. A *condenser* should be selected that will fit all areas of the preparation. A small *nib* imparts more pressure than a larger nib, assuming that a constant load is applied. The technique for

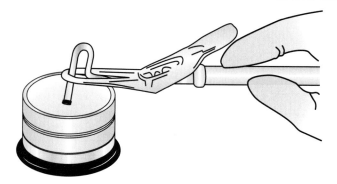

FIG. 38-42 An amalgam well is used to hold the amalgam after trituration (see Box 38-3).

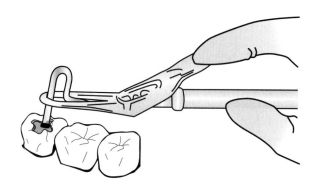

FIG. 38-43 Amalgam is transported from the amalgam well to the cavity preparation with an amalgam carrier (see Box 38-3).

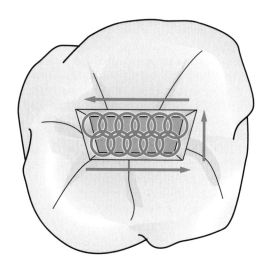

FIG. 38-44 The pattern of condensation should be continuous overlapping strokes.

condensation of the amalgam should be in an orderly, stepwise, and overlapping pattern (Fig. 38-44).

Multiple increments of amalgam are almost always required to restore a tooth. In these cases it is best to use a series of smaller mixes rather than one large mix, because the last portion of a large mix has often lost much of its plasticity and will not be able to be condensed and carved properly. Each individual placement of the amalgam must

---

> ### BOX 38-3
>
> **Amalgam Placement for Class I, V, and VI Preparations**
>
> 1. Place the mixed amalgam into an amalgam well (see Fig. 38-42).
> 2. Load the amalgam carrier and transport the amalgam to the tooth with this instrument (see Fig. 38-43).
> 3. Express the contents of the carrier into the preparation.
> 4. The objective is to condense the amalgam before it loses its plasticity. If too much time is taken to condense the amalgam, the condensation process becomes more difficult, the mercury is not expressed as readily, and the possibility of creating voids in the material increases. If a dual-cured bonding agent is used as the sealer for the restoration, the amalgam must be condensed before the bonding agent has polymerized in order to improve the adaptation of the materials to the tooth and to avoid marginal discrepancies.

be completely condensed before an additional increment is placed. *Do not fill cavity with multiple increments of amalgam and then condense all at one time.* The clinician should continue filling and condensing the cavity incrementally until it is moderately overfilled. This is done to ensure that (1) the mercury-rich surface layer is removed from the area that will become the surface of the restoration and (2) all cavosurface margins are covered with the restorative material.

Once the cavity has been overfilled and condensed, limited time is available to carve the restoration. The objective of carving the amalgam is to reproduce the desired anatomy and thus ensure a proper harmony of form and function. Carving should be performed with sharp instruments to eliminate thin overextensions of material beyond the preparation margins. These overextensions, termed *flash,* are very thin and brittle, which makes them susceptible to fracture, resulting in rough or open margins. The initial phase of *carving,* or formation of the restoration anatomy and contours, should be accomplished before the amalgam has reached its initial set.

For the *Class I* and *Class VI* restorations, the clinician should begin carving by using an instrument such as a Walls, Hollenback, or cleoid-discoid carver or a large burnisher to remove the excess amalgam and to locate the restoration margins. An amalgam carver of choice is used to remove the remainder of the excess by placement of the carver on the tooth surface and carving parallel to the located margin (Fig. 38-45). Correct carving technique for placement of tooth anatomy requires carving from the tooth surface to the amalgam. Carving from amalgam to tooth can result in gouging or ditching the restoration at its margin. The clinician should place cuspal inclines by carving perpendicular to the margins, with a portion of the blade resting on sound tooth structure (Fig. 38-46). If the blade of the carver is not resting on the tooth *(free-floating),* it can easily overcarve or gouge the restoration (Fig. 38-47). Care must be taken to avoid carving grooves that are too deep and that tend to leave thin margins susceptible to fracture. These deep grooves may expose preparation

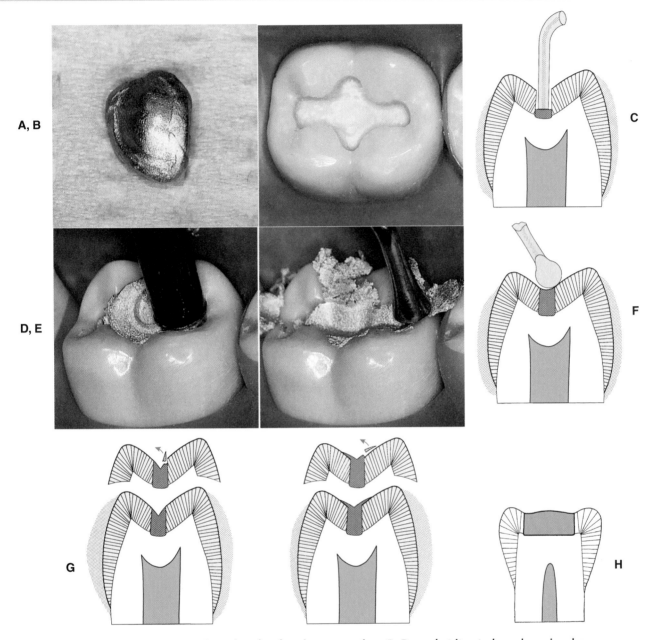

FIG. 38-45 Restoration of occlusal cavity preparation. **A,** Properly triturated amalgam is a homogenous mass with slightly reflective surface. It flattens slightly if dropped on a tabletop. **B,** Clinician should have a mental image of outline form of preparation before condensing amalgam to assist in locating cavosurface margins during carving procedure. **C,** Amalgam should be inserted incrementally and condensed with overlapping strokes. **D,** Cavity preparation should be overpacked to ensure well-condensed marginal amalgam that is not mercury-rich. **E,** Before carving procedure, burnishing with a large burnisher is a form of condensation. **F,** Carver should rest partially on external tooth surface adjacent to margins to prevent overcarving. **G,** Deep occlusal grooves invite chipping of amalgam at margins. Thin portions of amalgam left on external surfaces soon break away, giving the appearance that amalgam has grown out of cavity. **H,** Carve fossae slightly deeper than proximal marginal ridges. (From Roberson TM, Heymann HO, Swift EJ Jr: *Sturdevant's art and science of operative dentistry,* ed 4, St Louis, 2001, Mosby.)

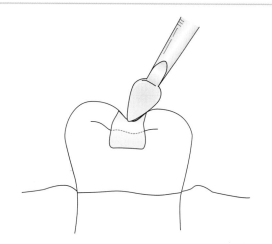

FIG. 38-46 Correct vertical angulation of cleoid carver.

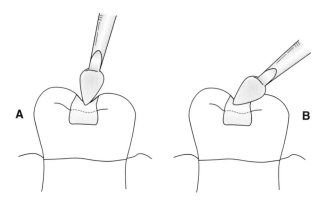

FIG. 38-47 A, Vertical angulation of cleoid is too steep. **B,** Vertical angulation of cleoid is too flat, and tip is displaced too far toward the opposite cavosurface margin.

walls as the clinician removes amalgam from the cavosurface margin while attempting to form cuspal anatomy in harmony with the deep grooves. Deep grooves are also more difficult to polish during finishing procedures.

The *Class V* restoration is a much easier restoration to carve. An explorer or other instrument of choice is generally used to remove the excess amalgam and to obtain the proper inciso(occluso)gingival and mesiodistal contours of the tooth (Fig. 38-48). It is also essential to allow part of the instrument tip to remain on the tooth structure (as with the Class I) so that the restoration borders are not submarginated or gouged. *Submargination* is the exposure of a portion the prepared cavity wall caused by underfilling the preparation with the restorative material or by removal of the restorative material from the cavity wall during the carving procedure.

After the appropriate anatomy and contours have been created and the restoration has reached its initial set, the final step of carving, known as *burnishing,* can be performed. Burnishing is a process of smoothing or polishing and is accomplished by lightly rubbing the surface of the amalgam after it has reached its initial set. This process affects only the surface, not the amalgam in the deeper aspects of the restoration. Burnishing removes pits and scratches left by the carving process, improves margins by

increasing the density of the restorative material, and expresses more free mercury to make the surface of the restoration stronger. Burnishing should not produce an exceptionally shiny surface. If it does, it has been overburnished. Overburnishing increases the risk of surface corrosion because an excessive amount of mercury was brought to the surface, where it oxidizes and corrodes.

When the clinician finishes the procedure, any residual amalgam should be expressed from the amalgam carrier. This residue and all amalgam remaining in the well, as well as any scraps remaining from the carving process, should be placed into containers designated for this purpose.

Class II Preparations

Included in Mrs. Jones' treatment plan was the need to replace one of the existing Class II amalgam restorations on tooth #19. Class II preparations present an additional challenge in restorations because they are missing one of the confining walls that exist in a Class I, V, or VI preparation. A Class II lesion, by definition, extends onto either the mesial or distal (or both) surface(s) (see Fig. 38-13). Placement and condensation of amalgam into such a cavity preparation will result in the restorative material being expressed out of the cavity because of the missing wall.

To compensate for this lack of natural confinement, a *matrix system* is used. This system provides a temporary surface to confine the placement and condensation of amalgam. Desirable characteristics of a matrix system include ease of application, convenience of use, easy removal, sufficient rigidity to withstand condensation forces, sufficient versatility to accommodate differently sized and shaped teeth, proper height so as not to obstruct the clinician's view, and ability to contour to replicate natural tooth structure.

No matrix system meets all required criteria for all needs. The most popular system is the **Tofflemire universal matrix system** (Fig. 38-49). This system is composed of two major components: (1) a *retainer,* which holds the band in close approximation to the tooth, and (2) a *band,* which supplies the missing wall. The Tofflemire retainer is versatile in that it can be placed on either the facial or the lingual side of the tooth to be restored. The retainer and band are generally stable when placed properly. The retainer is easily separated from the band when finished. Bands with varying occlusogingival widths are available, although they are flat and need to be individually contoured. The band is placed on a paper pad (or other resilient surface) and burnished to achieve the desired contour. If a bonding system is to be used as the cavity sealer, a light coating of wax or petroleum jelly is necessary to reduce adhesion of the amalgam to the matrix band.

Placement of Matrix

When using the Tofflemire system, the clinician should place the band into the retainer so that the narrow end of the formed loop is directed toward the gingiva (Fig. 38-50). The slot openings in the retainer also must be directed toward the gingiva. This will allow for easy removal of the retainer after the placement process. In most cases the retainer will be placed on the facial side of the tooth. If lingual placement is required, a contraangled retainer is recommended. For facial placement, the proper orientation of the band (when the retainer is sitting on the counter

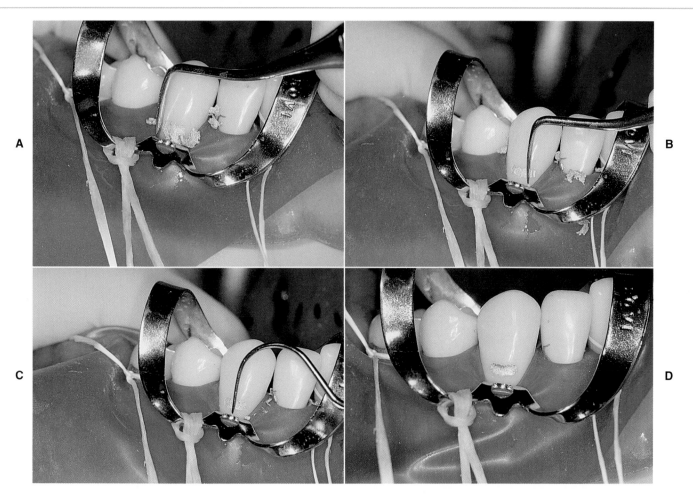

FIG. 38-48 Carving and contouring of restoration. **A,** Begin carving procedure by removing excess and locating incisal margin. **B** and **C,** Use explorer to remove excess and locate mesial and distal margins. **D,** Finally, remove excess and locate gingival margin.

with the slot opening downward in the gingival direction) will have it exiting the end of the retainer to the *left* for placement in the mandibular left and maxillary right quadrants and exiting to the *right* for the mandibular right and maxillary left quadrants.

The clinician places the two ends of the band into the retainer's angled slit and tightens the outer knurled knob. The band then is slipped over the tooth and pushed gently into place. The clinician should inspect for correct placement. The band should extend beyond the gingival seat. No rubber dam material should be caught between the band and the tooth. The cavosurface margin also must be inspected to ensure that all enamel is sound and intact. The band should extend slightly above the occlusal border of the preparation. The clinician tightens the band by turning the long inner knurled knob.

The band should be sealed at the gingival margin by the use of a wooden *wedge*. The wedge will adapt the band against the tooth to prevent any amalgam from being condensed out of the preparation into the gingival sulcus, creating an "overhang" of amalgam. Such an overhang can have deleterious effects on the health of the periodontal tissue.[1] The wedge also provides some separation of the teeth, which will help to compensate for the thickness of the matrix band so that proximal contact can be properly restored when the band is removed. Placement

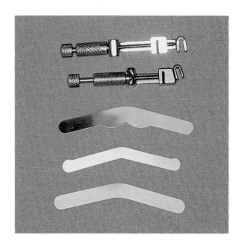

FIG. 38-49 Straight-angled and contraangled universal (Tofflemire) retainers. Bands are available with varying occlusogingival measurements.

of the wedge creates gingival tissue retraction, which will assist the clinician in exposing, visualizing, and carving the amalgam in the area of the gingival seat when the matrix is removed. Wedge placement will also aid in the development of the proximal contour and will prevent or di-

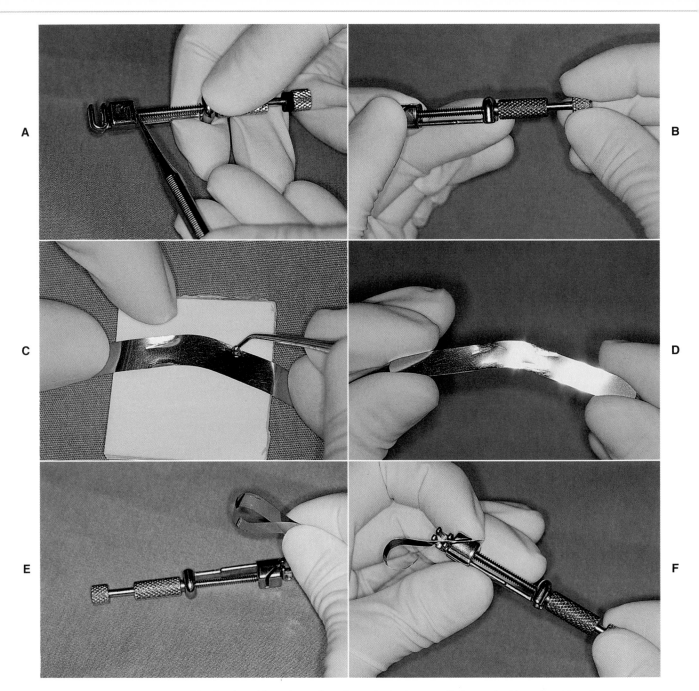

FIG. 38-50 Positioning band in universal retainer. **A,** Explorer pointing to locking vise. View is showing gingival side of vise. **B,** Pointed spindle is released from locking vise by turning small knurled nut counterclockwise. **C,** Contour band with egg-shaped burnisher. **D,** Contoured band. **E,** Fold band to form loop and position in retainer, with occlusal edge of band first. **F,** Tighten spindle against band in locking vise.

minish seepage of fluid at the gingival margin of the preparation.

Placement of Wedge

The clinician should select a wedge of the proper height, width, and contour. If the wedges available are not the proper size, they can be modified with a sharp blade. The wedge should be placed from the embrasure that allows the closest adaptation of the band to the tooth, usually into the embrasure from the side opposite the retainer. Most of the wedge should be located gingival to the gingival cavosurface margin of the preparation (Fig. 38-51). After insertion, the clinician applies moderate pressure with an amalgam condenser, the handle of a mirror, or the handle of cotton pliers to drive the wedge into the gingival embrasure and create tight adaptation of the band and slight separation of the teeth. The position of the wedge should be checked routinely because the rubber dam

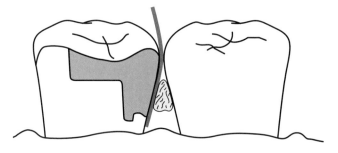

FIG. 38-51 Wedge placement.

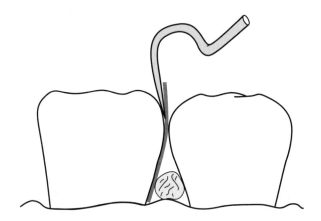

FIG. 38-52 Carve excess amalgam to free the matrix band and form the occlusal embrasure. This reduces the risk of an amalgam fracture in the area of the marginal ridge during matrix band removal (see Box 38-4).

tends to push the wedge out of the embrasure. The clinician reapplies pressure as needed to reinsert the wedge.

The technique for placement of amalgam into a Class II preparation is similar to that for the Class I, with additional consideration to the proximal box (Fig. 38-52). The amalgam is triturated and carried to the preparation in the manner described previously (Box 38-4).

DIRECT RESIN COMPOSITE RESTORATIONS

The term *composite* refers to the fact that an inorganic filler has been added to an organic resin matrix. Modern dental resin composites have been designed for use in all areas of the dentition, with anterior composites, posterior composites, universal composites, and composites specially designed to imitate multiple shades and opacities of enamel and dentin. Each of these various types of composite has its own peculiar advantages and disadvantages.[15]

Advantages

1. *Aesthetic.* Resin composites are much more natural appearing than metals.
2. *Economic.* Composites are slightly more expensive than amalgam but are less expensive than ceramics or metals.
3. *Broad applicability.*
4. *Direct placement.* Resin composite restorations can be applied in a single appointment.

BOX 38-4

Amalgam Placement for Class II Preparations

1. In a Class II situation, the initial placement of amalgam should be on the gingival floor of the proximal box. In order to obtain proper adaptation to the gingival floor, the small end of the amalgam carrier and the small amalgam condenser should be used.
2. Condense the amalgam first into the proximal point and line angles.
3. Use lateral condensation against the matrix band and against the proximal walls.
4. Continue to add amalgam and to condense into the proximal box until the axiopulpal line angle is reached.
5. At this point, add and condense amalgam to the occlusal and proximal portions of the preparation concurrently until a moderate overfill condition exists.
6. Carve back to locate margins as in the Class I situation.
7. Free the occlusal surface of the band in the area of the marginal ridge by carving the occlusal embrasure with the tip of an explorer (see Fig. 38-52). This will allow smooth removal of the band without fracturing the amalgam in the proximal box.
8. Remove the wedge with cotton pliers. Stabilize the matrix band and amalgam with an index finger.
9. Loosen both nuts on the retainer and remove it from the band.
10. Remove the band from the uninvolved contact (if only one proximal surface is being restored) while stabilizing the restoration with the index finger.
11. Remove the band from between the restoration and adjacent tooth by gently pulling in an oblique direction (45 degrees occlusofacially).
12. Carve the gingival seat area with an interproximal carver or explorer and then carve the proximal margin walls before finishing the occlusal carving as described earlier.
13. Check proximal contour and contact.

---

5. *Sets on demand.* Resins are light-polymerized, so material sets only when exposed to a particular type of light.
6. *Low marginal leakage on enamel.* When placed properly, margins are bonded.
7. *No galvanic response.* Resins are nonmetallic.
8. *No mercury.* Public perceptions are positive regarding composite restorations.

Disadvantages

1. ***Polymerization shrinkage.*** Material shrinks as it polymerizes.
2. *Durability.* "Life expectancy" is less than for amalgam, metal, or ceramic. Wear is greater.
3. *High technique sensitivity.* As a bonded restoration, appropriate isolation and tooth conditioning are vital.
4. *Variable handling.* Products vary as to stiffness, slumping, and packing. New "packable" composites do not handle as well as amalgam.
5. *Time requirements.* Generally, resin takes more time to set than amalgam.

PLACEMENT OF COMPOSITE RESTORATIONS

All composite restorations must have the tooth surface *acid-conditioned* or *acid-etched* before placement of the restoration. The use of 30% to 40% phosphoric acid has been the material of choice in most cases of resin composite bonding. Recently, some manufacturers have introduced bonding systems with self-etching primers.[3,22]

Case Application

Mrs. Dixon also has Class III and Class V restorations included in her treatment plan.

The use of acid to etch the tooth decalcifies the enamel, leaving microscopic irregularities that increase the surface area and provide for mechanical interlocking of the resin with the tooth. Acid also cleans the surface, which decreases the contact angle between the enamel and the adhesive and permits increased wetting of the surface. The etched enamel has a very high surface energy, more than twice that of untreated enamel. This causes a low-viscosity resin to be drawn into these surface irregularities by capillary action, resulting in improved adaptation to the tooth and thus improved marginal seal of the restoration.

Shade must be obtained before the placement of the rubber dam. After rubber dam placement, the teeth reversibly dehydrate, which causes them temporarily to appear lighter. If obtained at this time, the shade will not match that obtained after the rubber dam is removed and the teeth rehydrate to their normal state; the new restoration will appear lighter.

Next, the rubber dam should be placed. After the dentist has prepared the cavity, the clinician should apply the phosphoric acid etchant to the tooth for 10 to 30 seconds[4] and rinse thoroughly with water for at least 10 seconds. Many bonding systems have different application procedures. The clinician must follow each system's requirements precisely. The steps that can be used with one system cannot be used with another. Currently, products are available from six generations of development. These systems may vary from one to eight different components in a kit but generally include a primer (sometimes provided in two bottles to be mixed immediately before use) and a relatively low-viscosity resin as the bonding agent.

Class III Preparations

A Class III preparation poses a similar problem to the Class II preparation in that a proximal wall is missing to confine the restorative material. The same solution, the matrix band, is used. Because composites are light-polymerized materials, a clear Mylar matrix band without a retainer is generally used. After preparation the clear matrix is placed between the preparation and the adjacent tooth. A wedge is placed in a manner similar to the Class II situation. The matrix should extend beyond the gingival wall and beyond the incisal wall of the preparation. It should be long enough to wrap around the tooth so that it can be grasped with the fingers and adapted to the surface of the tooth being restored.

The clinician must place bonding agent as directed by the manufacturer, limiting its placement to those areas in need of restoration. Excess bonding agent smeared beyond the extent of etching will not bond to the tooth and may entrap oral fluids, which will lead to staining. After placement of the bonding agent, light polymerization should be performed as recommended by the manufacturer. The clinician should ensure that the polymerization unit is in proper working order and check it regularly with a radiometer to ensure that it has sufficient output (300 mW/cm^2).[17,19]

The composite of choice then should be placed into the preparation and pushed into position. Resin composite handles much differently than amalgam. It cannot be condensed with much pressure; because the composite is essentially a liquid, attempts to do so will result in the condenser being pushed through it. Composites also cannot be carved in the same way, so little need exists to overfill. The clinician must take care to adapt the composite to the walls and especially into retention divots or grooves to improve retention. Increments should not be greater than 2 mm thick because evidence indicates that such thickness may not be adequately polymerized internally.[16]

After slightly overfilling the preparation, the clinician may sculpt the material to proper form. The matrix band then is pulled around the tooth to condense the composite, and the material is polymerized. All margin seals should be checked, and no voids, pits, or submarginal areas should exist. If such defects occur, material can be added at this time if the surface has remained uncontaminated.

Class I, II, and VI Preparations

The Class I, II, or VI composite restoration is placed similar to the amalgam restorations of the same class. The major difference is in the handling characteristics of the materials. The Class II posterior composite restoration must use a matrix band, which can be of the Tofflemire style or a system designed specifically for use with resin composite.

FINISHING OF COMPOSITE RESTORATIONS

The primary objective of finishing the composite restoration is to obtain the smoothest surface possible. The smoother the surface, the lower is the possibility of plaque accumulation and staining and the greater is the possibility of an acceptable aesthetic result. The smoothest surface is that obtained by the tight adaptation of a matrix band to the restorative material.[21] Therefore the clinician should attempt to use only the amount of material necessary to fill the cavity. Any excess needs to be removed, which will necessitate additional finishing and polishing procedures and will reduce the smoothness of the surface.

It is extremely difficult to gauge the precise amount of restorative material needed to fill the preparation exactly so that no finishing is necessary. Therefore the removal of excess material is almost always required, as is the need to modify restoration contours so that they are compatible with tooth form. In short, composite resin finishing procedures are typically required.

All contouring, finishing, and polishing techniques and associated systems use the principle of *sequential removal* of various amounts of material. These techniques

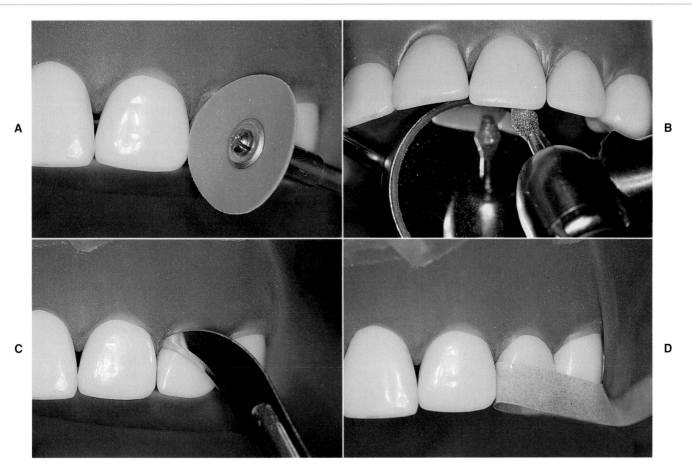

FIG. 38-53 Finishing composites. **A,** Abrasive disc mounted on mandrel can be used for finishing when access permits. **B,** Round carbide finishing bur is well suited for finishing lingual surfaces. **C,** No. 2 surgical blade in Bard-Parker handle can be used for removing interproximal excess. **D,** Abrasive strip should be curved over area to be finished.

begin with the coarsest abrasive necessary to accomplish removal of the defect, followed by the use of finer abrasives until the required surface smoothness is obtained. This process is begun by removal of the gross excess material at the gingival margin with a sharp blade (no. 12 scalpel, composite blade, or gold knife). Carbide or diamond composite finishing burs then are used to contour surfaces and refine marginal areas. Abrasive impregnated disks are available in various thicknesses and grits for facial, lingual, incisal, and some proximal areas. Composite finishing strips can be used in areas where the discs are not accessible. Final polishing can be accomplished with the use of fine abrasive rubber rotary instruments and polishing pastes (Fig. 38-53; see also Chapter 32).

 RITICAL THINKING ACTIVITIES

1. Form a study group and research the differences in the practice patterns of operative therapies among the various states.
2. Discuss the differences in practice patterns with your instructors, especially those who have practiced in various states.
3. Conduct a panel discussion with hygienists who practice in both traditional and expanded-function settings to learn about the associated challenges.
4. Obtain prepared dentoforms.
    a. Identify cavosurface margins, point angles, line angles, walls, and floors.
    b. Practice the placement of various matrix systems.
    c. Practice the placement of the rubber dam in various areas of the dentoform.
    d. Practice the placement and finishing of various restorative materials.
5. Evaluate a classmate's restorations and request that he or she critique your restorations.

REVIEW QUESTIONS

1. Which of the following statements best describes the differences between a Class I cavity preparation and a Class II cavity preparation?
   a. Class II includes the extension of a Class I into the incisal edge of an anterior tooth.
   b. Class II includes the extension of a Class I into the facial or lingual gingival margin area.
   c. Class II includes the extension of a Class I into the proximal area over the marginal ridge.
   d. Class II includes the extension of a Class I and is located on a cusp tip.

2. All the following are advantages to minimally invasive dentistry *except* which one?
   a. Preserves tooth structure
   b. Increases tooth resistance to further breakdown
   c. Requires extension of preparation for prevention
   d. Uses less amalgam

3. Which of the following lists describes the major components found in dental amalgam?
   a. Silver, tin, mercury
   b. Silver, nickel, tin
   c. Silver, copper, zinc
   d. Silver, mercury, gold

4. Resin composite is a tooth-colored restoration resulting in less marginal leakage than amalgam.
   a. Both the first and the second parts of the statement are true.
   b. The first part of the statement is true, and the second part is false.
   c. The first part of the statement is false, and the second part is true.
   d. Both the first and the second parts of the statement are false.

5. Which of the following reasons best describes why a dental practitioner would use a wooden wedge?
   a. Increases setting time and hardness of amalgam
   b. Prevents overhang and allows for easier removal of the matrix band
   c. Decreases amalgam setting time and assists with occlusal adjustment
   d. Increases amalgam setting time and prevents overhang

 SUGGESTED AGENCIES AND WEB SITES

Because of the ever-changing nature of the Internet, some of the web sites listed here may have changed since publication. Please refer to Mosby's Evolve web site for the most current information.

American Dental Association: http://www.ada.org
American Dental Hygienists' Association: http://www.adha.org
Creighton University Dental School:
   http://cudental.creighton.edu/indexreal.htm
Dental Town: http://www.DentalTown.com
Dentsply Dental Products: http://www.dentsply.com
Espe Dental: http://www.espe.com
Ivoclar North America: http://www.ivoclarna.com

Journal of Operative Dentistry: http://www.jopdent.org
Kerr Dental Products: http://www.Kerrdental.com
Pulpdent Corporation: http://www.pulpdent.com
3M Dental Products: http://www.3M.com/dental
Ultradent Dental Products: http://www.ultradent.com
University of Texas–Houston Dental Branch:
   http://www.db.uth.tmc.edu

 ADDITIONAL READINGS AND RESOURCES

Baum L, Phillips RW, Lund MR: *Textbook of operative dentistry,* ed 3, Philadelphia, 1995, WB Saunders.
Clinical Research Associates Newsletter, Salt Lake City, Utah (monthly issues).
Cochran MA: *Operative Dentistry,* the Journal of the Academy of Operative Dentistry, Indianapolis, Ind.
Craig RG, Powers JM, Wataha JC: *Dental materials: properties and manipulation,* ed 7, St Louis, 2000, Mosby.

Farrah J, Powers J: *The Dental Advisor,* Ann Arbor, Mich (monthly issues).
Miller M: *Reality,* vol 14, Houston, 2000, Reality Publishing.
Schwartz RS, Summitt JB, Robbins JW: *Fundamentals of operative dentistry: a contemporary approach,* Chicago, 1996, Quintessence.

 REFERENCES

1. Abrams H et al: Gingival sequelae from a retained piece of rubber dam: a report of a case, *J Ky Dent Assoc* 30:21, 1978.
2. Anderson MH, Bales DJ, Omnell K: Modern management of dental caries: the cutting edge is not the dental bur, *J Am Dent Assoc* 124:37-44, 1993.
3. Barkmeier WW, Shaffer SE, Gwinnett AJ: Effects of 15 vs 60 second enamel acid conditioning on adhesion and morphology, *Oper Dent* 11:111-16, 1986.
4. Barkmeier WW, Los SA, Triolo PT: Bond strengths and SEM evaluation of Clearfil Liner Bond 2, *Am J Dent* 8:289-93, 1995.

5. Black GV: *The technical procedures in filling teeth,* Chicago, 1903, Blakely Printing.

6. Bronner FJ: Engineering principles applied to Class II cavities, *J Dent Res* 10:115-19, 1930.

7. Buonocore MG: A simple method of increasing the adhesion of acrylic filling materials to enamel surfaces, *J Dent Res* 34:849-53, 1955.

8. Elderton RJ: Variability on the decision-making process and implications for change toward a preventive philosophy. In *Quality evaluation of dental restorations: criteria for placement and replacement,* Chicago, 1989, Quintessence.

9. Hume WR: Need for change in standards of caries diagnosis: perspective based on the structure and behavior of the caries lesion, *J Dent Educ* 57:439-43, 1993.

10. Kanca J III: Effects of resin primer solvents and surface wetness on resin composite bond strength to dentin, *Am J Dent* 5:213-15, 1992.

11. Markley M: Restorations of silver amalgam, *J Am Dent Assoc* 43:133-46, 1951.

12. Mertz-Fairhurst EJ et al: Ultraconservative and cariostatic sealed restorations: results at year 10, *J Am Dent Assoc* 128:55-66, 1998.

13. Osborne JW, Hoffman R, Ferguson GW: Conservation of tooth structure, *J Ala Dent Assoc* 56:24-6, 1972.

14. Osborne JW, Summit JB: Extension for prevention: is it relevant today? *Am J Dent* 11:189-96, 1998.

15. Roberson TM, Heymann HO, Swift EJ Jr: *Sturdevant's art and science of operative dentistry,* ed 4, St Louis, 2001, Mosby.

16. Rueggeberg FA, Caughman WF, Curtis JW Jr: Factors affecting cure at depths within light-activated composite resins, *Am J Dent* 6:91-5, 1993.

17. Rueggeberg FA, Caughman WF, Curtis JW Jr: Effect of light intensity and exposure duration on cure of resin composite, *Oper Dent* 6:91-5, 1994.

18. Sigurjons H: Extension for prevention: historical development and current status of G.V. Black's concept, *Oper Dent* 8:57-63, 1983.

19. Tate WH, Porter KH, Dosch RO: Successful photocuring: don't restore without it, *Oper Dent* 24:109-14, 1999.

20. Triolo PT, Swift EJ, Barkmeier WW: Shear bond strengths of composite to dentin using six dental adhesive systems, *Oper Dent* 20: 46-50, 1995.

21. Trushowsky RD: Use of a clear matrix to minimize finishing of a posterior composite, *Am J Dent* 10:111, 1997.

22. Vargas MA, Cobb DS, Denehy GE: Evaluation of adhesive systems using acidic primers, *Am J Dent* 10:219-23, 1997.

CHAPTER 39

Cosmetic Whitening

Marie A. Collins

Chapter Outline

Case Studies: Cosmetic Whitening
Evolution of Bleaching
Dental Bleaching Agents: Composition and Mode of Action
Patient Selection: Indications and Contraindications
Data Collection: The Clinical Examination
Patient Instructions

Modes of Delivery: Bleaching Techniques
   In-office bleaching
   Laser bleaching
   Dentist-prescribed, home-applied bleaching
Side Effects of Bleaching
Role of the Dental Hygienist

Key Terms

Carbamide peroxide
Crest Whitestrips
Extrinsic stain

Fluorosis
Hydrogen peroxide

Minocycline
Nightguard vital bleaching (NVB)

Potassium nitrate
Tetracycline

Learning Outcomes

1. Discuss the validation of the psychological and sociological effects of physical attractiveness on human self-esteem.
2. Recognize common side effects of dental whitening and their contributing factors including the tolerability of peroxide-containing whitening agents.
3. List the common side effects of dental whitening and their contributing factors.
4. Explain the importance of dentist-patient communication throughout the bleaching process and the role of the dental hygienist in dental-whitening therapy.
5. Demonstrate and describe the clinical techniques used for fabrication of a nightguard.

6. Compare and contrast the whitening effect of in-office and home-applied vital tooth bleaching and how these two systems might be used in conjunction with one another.
7. Discuss the effects of whitening agents on enamel, dentin, pulp, and restorative materials.
8. Investigate products currently available for cosmetic whitening, including professional, over-the-counter, in-office, and home-applied whiteners.
9. Describe the role of dental hygienists in planning, implementing, and evaluating cosmetic-whitening procedures.

Case Study **Cosmetic Whitening**

Case 1: Cosmetic Whitening for Fluorosis

Patient profile: Jimmy Rogers, a 13-year-old boy, has relocated to the Southeast after living in Colorado since birth. He is healthy and participates in sports.

Chief complaint: Jimmy exhibits brown discoloration on the right central incisor (Figs. 39-1 and 39-2). Etiology is unknown.

Health history: Within normal limits (WNL)

Dental history: There are no significant findings. Jimmy has maintained routine dental treatment on a 6-month basis since age 3. The brown discoloration has been present since eruption, and no evidence of similar discoloration is noted on other teeth. Neither the patient nor his parents mentioned any history of trauma to the primary and permanent teeth. Generalized hypocalcification is present.

Case 2: Cosmetic Whitening for Tetracycline Stain

Patient profile: Kathleen O'Bryan is a 43-year-old Caucasian woman, 5 feet 8 inches, 145 pounds. She works in manufacturing and currently lives in the southeastern portion of the United States. Ms. O'Bryan's family relocated from Denver 5 years ago. She is married and has two children, ages 21 and 17.

Chief complaint: Ms. O'Bryan states that she never smiles open enough to show her teeth in a photograph because of the color of her teeth. She has not previously had any treatment for the discoloration except for a whitening dentifrice.

Health history: The patient's mother has insulin-dependent diabetes. Ms. O'Bryan was tested for diabetes 10 years ago, and normal blood sugar levels were found. She reports allergies to sulfonamides and aspirin. She also reports frequent headaches (1-2 times a week). She took tetracycline as a young child but cannot recall her exact age at the time.

Dental history: Ms. O'Bryan has a history of trauma to the maxillary left central tooth #9, which was subsequently treated endodontically. An incisal chip was repaired with a mesioincisal (MI) composite.

Radiographic findings: Radiographs of anterior teeth revealed a periapical lesion on her mandibular left lateral tooth #23. The maxillary left central tooth #9 requires restorative treatment (Fig. 39-3).

Diagnosis: Ms. O'Bryan has experienced moderate tetracycline staining and requires restoration (Figs. 39-4 through 39-8).

Case 3: Cosmetic Whitening for Yellowing

Patient profile: Margo Randall is a 29-year-old singer who belongs to a local repertory theater. Ms. Randall is currently in a production of the musical *Carousel.* Because of her full-time employment as a medical receptionist to support her husband through law school and her busy rehearsal schedule for the upcoming production, Ms. Randall says she feels that she has little time for herself.

Chief complaint: Ms. Randall has noticed a slight yellow cast to her teeth and wonders whether she could do something to make her smile brighter (Fig. 39-9).

Health history: Noncontributory

Dental history: Ms. Randall has received regular, routine dental care since early childhood. Her oral hygiene is remarkable, with no bleeding on probing at any previous dental examination. She has benefited from a fluoridated water supply and fluoridated dentifrice all her life. Except for the slight yellow color apparent in her anterior teeth, she is not experiencing any dental problems at this time.

Extraoral findings: A round 3- × -3-mm elevated, pigmented nevus is evident on her left cheek, just inferior to the zygoma.

Diagnosis: No restorative needs; cosmetic need for whiter teeth (Fig. 39-10).

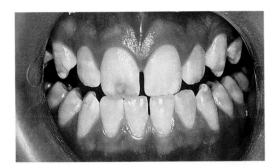

FIG. 39-1 Case #1 intraoral photograph: the right central incisor of 13-year-old Jimmy Rogers exhibits brown discoloration of unknown etiology. (From Haywood VB, Leonard RH: Nightguard vital bleaching removes brown discoloration for 7 years: a case report, *Quint Int* 29(7):450-1, 1998.)

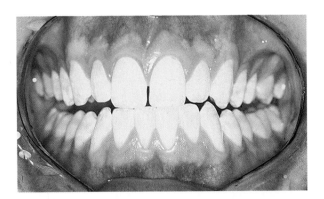

FIG. 39-2 Case #1 intraoral photograph: at the 7-year recall appointment, with no interim treatment, Jimmy Rogers' brown discoloration has not returned. (From Haywood VB, Leonard RH: Nightguard vital bleaching removes brown discoloration for 7 years: a case report, *Quint Int* 29(7):450-1, 1998.)

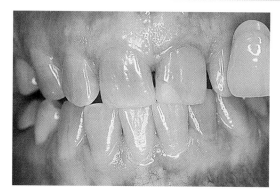

FIG. 39-3 Case #2 intraoral photograph of 43-year-old Kathleen O'Bryan: moderate tetracycline stain. Maxillary left central incisor has undergone endodontic therapy. (From Haywood VB: *Contemp Esthet and Restor Pract* 15, 1997.)

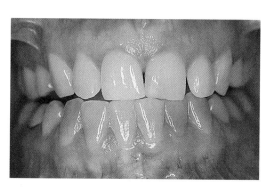

FIG. 39-4 Case #2 intraoral photograph of Kathleen O'Bryan: 12-month bleaching recall. Maxillary left central incisor retained discoloration. (From Haywood VB: *Contemp Esthet and Restor Pract* 16, 1997.)

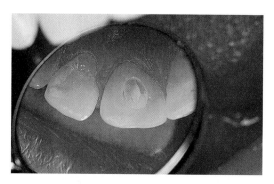

FIG. 39-5 Case #2 intraoral photograph of Kathleen O'Bryan: the old discolored composite is removed from the nonvital maxillary left central incisor. (From Haywood VB: *Contemp Esthet and Restor Pract* 17, 1997.)

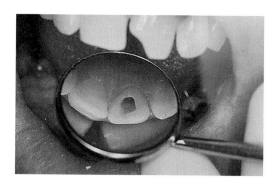

FIG. 39-6 Case #2 intraoral photograph of Kathleen O'Bryan: results following an in-office application of 35% hydrogen peroxide. (From Haywood VB: *Contemp Esthet and Restor Pract* 17, 1997.)

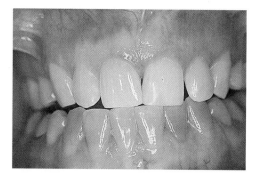

FIG. 39-7 Case #2 intraoral photograph of Kathleen O'Bryan: results following restorative placement of white composite core in pulp chamber. (From Haywood VB: *Contemp Esthet and Restor Pract* 17, 1997.)

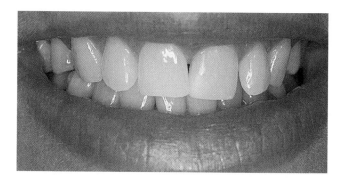

FIG. 39-8 Case #2 intraoral photograph of Kathleen O'Bryan: 13-month recall. Whitening effects were successfully achieved. (From Haywood VB: *Contemp Esthet and Restor Pract* 17, 1997.)

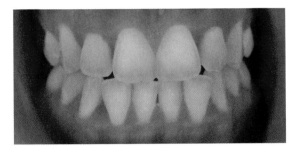

FIG. 39-9 Case #3 intraoral photograph of Margo Randall: before tooth-whitening procedures. (From Sagel PA et al: Vital tooth whitening with a novel hydrogen peroxide strip system: design, kinetics, and clinical response, *Compend Contin Educ Dent* 21(suppl 29):S15, 2000.)

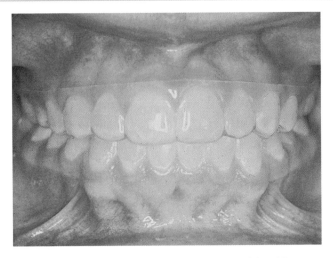

FIG. 39-11 Nonscalloped and nonreservoir bleaching tray design. (Courtesy Van B. Haywood, DMD, Augusta, Ga.)

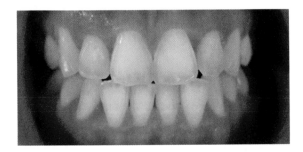

FIG. 39-10 Case #3: 2-week results of simultaneous treatment of the maxillary and mandibular arches. (From Sagel PA et al: Vital tooth whitening with a novel hydrogen peroxide strip system: design, kinetics, and clinical response, *Compend Contin Educ Dent* 21(suppl 29):S15, 2000.)

EVOLUTION OF BLEACHING

"His eyes will be darker than wine, his teeth whiter than milk."[3] This biblical reference illustrates the idea that teeth should be at their whitest. Then and now, the whiteness of teeth is equated to success and beauty. As time goes on, the appearance of teeth will have a continued impact on the psychological and sociological aspects of physical attractiveness.

To appreciate research contributions, it is important to understand the evolution of dental-bleaching practices. One hundred years ago the literature reported tooth bleaching as an aesthetic treatment option.[5] However, it was not until 1937 that conventional bleaching of vital teeth with heat and strong chemical oxidizing agents was introduced.[2] Many subtle improvements occurred in the basic bleaching procedures throughout the following decades. The most notable improvement in dental bleaching occurred in the 1970s and was made by Klusmier, an orthodontist, and Wagner, a periodontist. Klusmier and Wagner independently used Proxigel, an over-the-counter (OTC) 10% carbamide peroxide solution indicated for the healing of canker sores and wounds. In addition to promoting wound healing, they also noticed that the material lightened the color of the teeth. With favorable results, Klusmier and Wagner continued to use Proxigel as a bleaching agent.[13]

In 1988 Haywood and Heymann conducted a formal clinical and laboratory bleaching study. Their research led to the first published article in dental literature that detailed the bleaching procedure now known as ***nightguard vital bleaching (NVB).***[14] NVB involves the fabrication of a custom-fitted tray in which the bleaching solution is applied. The patient shown in Fig. 39-11 is wearing a custom-fitted maxillary tray. The introduction of bleaching raised concerns about the efficacy and safety of bleaching ingredients. The Food and Drug Administration (FDA) and the American Dental Association (ADA) addressed these concerns.[6,12] NVB has since been widely accepted by dental groups and practitioners, particularly in the United States. Ongoing research is being conducted on the technique, ingredients, efficacy, and safety, but since the early 1990s tooth bleaching has generally been regarded as one of the safest procedures a dentist can provide to patients.

Haywood reported a success rate up to 97% for NVB with a 6-week application on patients with non–tetracycline-type stains.[17] In this particular study, the NVB tray was worn for an average of approximately 7 hours per night. Teeth stained by ***tetracycline*** showed a 75% success rate. The study reported the duration of the bleaching effects to last 1 to 3 years with 62% of respondents noting no perceivable loss of color lightening after 3 years.[17] However, some reports have shown bleaching effects to last for up to 7 years.[16] It is important, however, to identify what each individual patient envisions as a satisfactory result. For example, some patients may approach treatment with the ideal of obtaining "Hollywood-style white teeth," whereas others may just want to lighten their teeth by a few shades. Determining the patient's expectations will assist the clinician with appropriate patient education.[19]

In 2000 a novel trayless delivery system—*Crest Whitestrips*—was introduced to dental professionals. This product, shown in Fig. 39-12, consists of a thin, flexible polyethylene strip coated with an adhesive gel that contains ***hydrogen peroxide.*** The strips offer a more convenient, easy-to-use bleaching regimen for many patients relative to the NVB trays.[24] Because the strips contain a

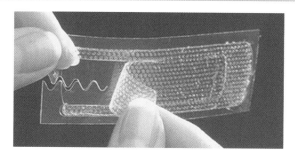

FIG. 39-12 Crest Whitestrips. (Courtesy The Procter & Gamble Company, Cincinnati, Ohio.)

relatively low dose of hydrogen peroxide, they are generally well-tolerated by patients.[9]

DENTAL BLEACHING AGENTS: COMPOSITION AND MODE OF ACTION

Carbamide peroxide has been the active ingredient most widely used for NVB. The solution is available in concentrations that range from 5% to 40%. In saliva, carbamide peroxide converts to hydrogen peroxide, the active bleaching agent, and urea. A general rule is that a carbamide peroxide concentration is equivalent to approximately three times the comparable hydrogen peroxide concentration. Therefore a 10% carbamide peroxide gel is roughly equivalent to a 3% hydrogen peroxide gel. Other possible ingredients of tooth-bleaching gels are glycerin, carbopol (slow oxygen releasing), sodium hydroxide, flavors, and fluoride.

Most bleaching products are categorized by their chemical composition and presence or absence of carbopol rather than by their pH. Oxygen-release rates determine the replenishment of bleaching solutions. Products with slow release rates, such as carbopol, have a greater substantivity and retention rates. Therefore to obtain full oxygen release, 2 to 3 hours of tray wear is recommended for bleaching gels that contain carbopol.[15] Solutions that do not contain carbopol typically maximize the oxygen release in less than 1 hour, thus frequent replenishment is required.

Although the exact mechanisms of the dental bleaching process are still being studied, oxidation is believed to be primarily responsible for the observed whitening. During oxidation, the active bleaching ingredient, hydrogen peroxide, typically generates short-lived oxygen intermediates, such as the hydroxyl radical, that enter the enamel or dentin of the discolored teeth and diffuse to areas containing the discoloration. The hydroxyl radicals then break down some of the double bonds in the discolored or stained compounds, which results in a whitened appearance. For vital teeth, stains can be attacked only from the surface. Oxidizing agents typically have poor substantivity; therefore glycerin has been added as a thickening agent to several bleaching products. Glycerin keeps the carbamide peroxide localized to the area of treatment.

When proper application techniques are followed, nonresolving detrimental effects have been reported neither on teeth, existing restorations, or oral tissues nor systemically. One study researched the use of a 10% carbamide peroxide solution worn for 8 hours a day. After 2 weeks, he found no detrimental effects on oral tissues.[8]

Another researcher used confocal laser scanning microscopy to show that even in exaggerated usage conditions, bleaching with hydrogen peroxide or carbamide peroxide gels results in no changes to the enamel or dentin ultrastructure.[26] However, continual research is being conducted, particularly on the response of acrylic composite restorative materials to bleaching agents.

OTC Proxigel was the first solution used to establish the efficacy of dental bleaching. Because of its fluidlike consistency, Proxigel provided poor substantivity or retention in bleaching trays as a result of its rapid oxygen release. Proxigel requires constant replenishing for bleaching to occur. Dental product manufacturers addressed this issue with the creation of more viscous solutions specifically for dental bleaching. The ADA has given its Seal of Acceptance to a number of dental-bleaching products. (To inquire whether a product has received the ADA's Seal of Acceptance, send an electronic message to adaseal@ada.org.)

Several OTC dental-bleaching systems using the tray method are available and may contain ingredients similar to professional bleaching products. However, at the time of this publication, the ADA has not approved any of these systems. These OTC systems mimic the procedures for professional dental bleaching (i.e., use of tray with solution). Dental professionals should inform patients that these systems typically lack efficacy, have not been researched for safety, and may contribute to the unhealthy side effects explained later in this chapter.[17]

In contrast, Crest Whitestrips have been well researched, and their efficacy and safety results are well documented. Both professionally dispensed Whitestripes (Crest Whitestrips Supreme 14% hydrogen peroxide and Crest Whitestrips Professional 6.5% hydrogen peroxide) and the OTC version (6.0% hydrogen peroxide) have been shown to provide comparable efficacy to the tray-based dentist-dispensed carbamide peroxide systems.

In several clinical studies, NVB was proven just as safe as any other routine dental procedure. Although some have questioned the carcinogenicity (cancer-causing) and genotoxicity (gene-altering) of peroxides, none have found any statistically significant links.[28] Furthermore, the research that first raised this as an issue was flawed because the animals used in the study did not have the critical enzyme that humans possess for the breakdown of peroxides. During the past decade, the issues of carcinogenicity and genotoxicity of hydrogen peroxide when used in bleaching products has essentially been put to rest.

When compared with nonbleached teeth, the amount of enamel removed using a 10% carbamide peroxide solution is equivalent to that lost during a 2.5-minute exposure to a cola beverage.[20] Bleaching agents have also been shown to have no or minimal effect on the surface texture, hardness, and wear resistance of enamel. Various studies have shown no indication of either etching or significant changes in the surface morphology of enamel when evaluated under a scanning electron microscope.[15] The aforementioned confocal laser scanning microscopy study showed that bleached teeth had no micromorphological changes in the subsurface enamel, dentinoenamel junction, or dentin.[26]

In 1972 a research team studied the effects of the penetration of bleaching solution into the pulp chamber and canals. It was found that penetrating solution created the potential for irreversible pulp damage—but only in the presence of excessive heat or trauma. The passage of some of the bleaching material to the pulp occurs within 15 minutes.[7] No difference was found in the pulpal reading before the bleaching process or at any point during the study. Pulpal necrosis occurred during conventional bleaching only when excessive heat or trauma existed. It should be noted that the relationship between exposure time and pulpal necrosis has not been substantiated.[25]

Bleaching agents can also permeate nonvital teeth that have lost their nutrient supply as a result of damage (trauma) or removal of the pulp (endodontic therapy). Over time, the loss of nutrients will result in a darkened tooth. In contrast to vital bleaching, which works through the outer surface of the tooth and is heat–technique-sensitive, nonvital bleaching is either applied within the pulp chamber or applied to the tooth surface without concern for damaging the pulp. Traditionally, treatment options for nonvital teeth sacrificed tooth structure (e.g., crowns, veneers, bonding). An alternative for such teeth is nonvital bleaching, which is a more conservative treatment option.

 Case #2 Application

Ms. O'Bryan had an endodontically treated maxillary left incisor before completing cosmetic whitening. Nonvital bleaching was indicated for her (see Figs. 39-3 through 39-8). Accelerated in-office bleaching supplemented by dentist-prescribed, home-applied whitening is a treatment option for her.

PATIENT SELECTION: INDICATIONS AND CONTRAINDICATIONS

In any discussion of the patient selection criteria for potential bleaching therapy, it is important to begin with a thorough diagnosis, which has been described as "the single most important determinant of the success of bleaching for any discoloration."[10] Components of this phase include a thorough medical-dental history and clinical examination. Pertinent medical history questions should address systemic medications, such as tetracycline, minocycline, and fluoride, that cause intrinsic tooth discoloration. Although rare, other conditions, such as jaundice and *amelogenesis imperfecta*, may also contribute to tooth discoloration. Dental conditions such as caries or faulty restorations may contribute to tooth discolorations and should be identified before bleaching therapy is prescribed. Conditions such as erosion, large pulp chambers, exposed root surfaces, hypersensitivity, white or opaque spots, dark stains, and aesthetic restorations should be considered for dentist-supervised NVB.

A thorough health history would reveal previous ingestion of tetracycline or a derivative of tetracycline. For example, the patient may have cystic fibrosis and use tetracycline, a common treatment for this disease. Teeth are most susceptible to tetracycline discolorations during formation, beginning the second trimester in utero and continuing to approximately 8 years of age.

 Case #2 Application

Ms. O'Bryan's case illustrates tetracycline staining (see Fig. 39-3).

It is believed that tetracycline particles incorporate in the dentin during calcification of the teeth through chelation with calcium, which forms tetracycline orthophosphate.[21] The result is the discoloration of the dentin. The process, displays itself as a result from exposure to sunlight. Because the labial surfaces of the incisors are more prone to sunlight exposure, they tend to darken faster and more intensely than their molar counterparts.

The dentist should identify the severity and type of discoloration. Some patients respond favorably to the bleaching process, whereas others do not. Tetracycline stains have four degrees. The first degree is a light-yellow–light-gray stain that is uniformly distributed in localized areas and is amenable to bleaching techniques. The second degree is a darker and more extensive yellow-gray hue. This degree is also amenable to the bleaching techniques. Third and fourth degrees are more intense dark gray-blue, banding stains. Favorable results have been achieved with third-degree stains by lengthening the bleaching duration. Fourth-degree stains are too dark for successful vital bleaching.[10]

A derivative of tetracycline is **minocycline,** which is a routine prescription for adolescent and adult treatment of acne and a variety of other infections. This medication may cause a sudden appearance of a ringlike stain. Although tetracycline use results in dentin discoloration during calcification of the teeth, minocycline use leads to discolorations in already erupted and formed teeth. Unfortunately, adults are also at risk for this stain because minocycline is absorbed in the gastrointestinal tract. The tooth pigmentation results from minocycline's ability to chelate with iron and form insoluble complexes. Like tetracycline staining, minocycline stains have degrees of severity and distribution. The mild cases are amenable to bleaching, whereas more severe cases (heavier banding) may require porcelain lamination.[4,10]

The medical-dental history may also reveal whether fluoride has been ingested. An excessive amount of fluoride ingestion results in *fluorosis.* The fluorosis stain exhibits itself as brown or flat gray pigmentation on smooth enamel, or white spots.[27] The teeth most commonly affected are the maxillary premolar and molar regions. The bleaching process does not remove the white spots; however, it lightens the background crown area, creating less contrast. Bleaching is contraindicated for fluorosis conditions with severe enamel loss.

Age is another factor that affects the coloration of teeth. Studies have confirmed that teeth darken and become more yellow as age increases.[23] With age, teeth may appear darker as a result of lifelong consumption of chromogenic foods. For example, years of coffee drinking and smoking can have a cumulative and drastic effect on the appearance of the teeth. These stains readily adhere to tiny cracks and fractures on the enamel surface. Fortunately, these types of stains respond favorably to bleaching.

Dental implications of aging include a gradual thinning of enamel that is caused by natural occlusal forces. As a response to these forces, reparative or secondary dentin forms, a natural protective mechanism of the tooth. This secondary dentin is more translucent and appears darker in color. Unfortunately, this natural occurrence is more difficult to bleach. Other conditions that should be considered for dentist-supervised NVB patient selection include erosion, large pulp chambers, exposed root surfaces, hypersensitivity, white or opaque spots, dark stains, and aesthetic restorations.

Although the success of bleaching has been widely documented, some patients may not benefit from the bleaching process. Therefore it is important not to encourage unrealistic expectations. A thorough clinical examination can be helpful in the determination of the appropriateness of bleaching and in the projection of realistic bleaching outcomes.

DATA COLLECTION: THE CLINICAL EXAMINATION

The clinical examination should include a thorough periodontal debridement, radiographs, and dental and periodontal charting. Periodontal debridement is crucial to the beginning phases of bleaching treatment. The air polisher is ideal for removing *extrinsic stain* from smooth and fissured enamel surfaces. Following periodontal debridement, some patients may be satisfied with the appearance of their teeth. Therefore the need for bleaching may be eliminated.

A radiographic evaluation rules out potential acute problems such as abscesses, internal resorption, and caries. These problems should be treated before bleaching. Radiographs are also used to assess the pulp size. Enlarged pulp chambers may increase the potential for hypersensitivity.

Dental and periodontal charting are other components of the clinical examination needed before bleaching. The dental charting exhibits caries, faulty restorations, and other restorative needs. The periodontal charting records areas of attachment loss (gingiva or bone). Specific teeth may require pulp vitality and transillumination testing. Additional information such as the patient's history of bruxism, sensitivity, and dental injuries should be collected. Before initiating bleaching, the dentist should address and treat all of these potential problems. The data-collection phase helps inform the patient of bleaching modalities, time commitment, potential side effects, anticipated cost, and predicted outcomes.

After the clinical examination, the dentist can then develop a treatment plan and present options to the patient. It should be stressed that the bleaching process may involve periodic reevaluations to monitor progress.

PATIENT INSTRUCTIONS

Specific patient instructions should be given to the patient both orally and in writing. Dental providers should advise patients to refrain from smoking during bleaching. It is important, as with any dental procedure, to provide the patient with written instructions. These instructions should detail application technique, side effects, care of the mouthguard and solution (if NVB is being used), and procedures to report uncommon or extreme reactions.[13,19] Many ADA-approved bleaching systems have the appropriate patient education instructions in the kit.

MODES OF DELIVERY: BLEACHING TECHNIQUES

IN-OFFICE BLEACHING

In-office bleaching, also known as *power bleaching,* is a technique used by dentists. This application technique uses a higher concentration of hydrogen peroxide than NVB (typically 35% or greater). This system requires precision isolation and close patient monitoring throughout the procedure. Local anesthetics are contraindicated because they hinder patient communication about procedural discomforts (e.g., gingival burning, improper rubber dam clamp placement). This system is ideal for patients who need quick results or for those who have stubborn unresolved stains. Various heat-activated light systems are on the market.

In-office bleaching has advantages and disadvantages. It may consist of only one or several office visits in conjunction with home administration. The procedure may also be costly. Most insurance policies do not cover bleaching administered solely for aesthetic purposes.

LASER BLEACHING

Lasers are also used within the clinical setting for dental bleaching. The laser generates heat that increases the resorption rate of the hydrogen peroxide. This process is time-consuming, but it may produce quicker results. However, the cost is four to seven times higher than NVB.[1] Safety and efficacy issues are currently under investigation, and the ADA has not approved laser use in dentistry.

DENTIST-PRESCRIBED, HOME-APPLIED BLEACHING

Tray Method

NVB is one the "dentist-prescribed, home-applied" methods. This technique is initiated in the dental office after the data-collection phase has been completed and informed consent has been obtained. The first step is to replicate the patient's oral cavity (alginate impression) to form a study cast. From the study cast, a custom-fit plastic nightguard (bleaching tray) is fabricated with a vacuum-forming machine. The tray is then trimmed. Tray design is dependent on the viscosity of the bleaching material and the individual manufacturer suggestions.[11]

Tray design and fabrication options include soft or rigid, reservoir or nonreservoir, and scalloped or nonscalloped trays. Soft trays are now preferred to the original rigid trays for ease of fabrication and patient comfort. Reservoirs are used with the more highly viscous bleaching materials. The reservoirs are formed with the addition of 0.5 mm of light-cured resin or spacer on the facial aspect of each tooth on the dental cast. Scalloped trays are trimmed after the tooth is contoured at the gingival-tooth interface, as illustrated in Fig. 39-13. A nonscalloped tray, pictured in Fig. 39-11, is evenly trimmed approximately 2 mm from the gingival crest onto the gingival tissue.

Case #2 Application

Tray designs can vary depending on individual patient indications. For example, a scalloped reservoir tray was used initially for Ms. O'Bryan. However, when she returned 7 months later, a nonscalloped, nonreservoir tray was indicated (see Fig. 39-11) because it can seal the environment and hold the bleaching agent against the neck of the tooth. This second tray provided the supply of material needed to whiten the challenging gingival third of the tooth.

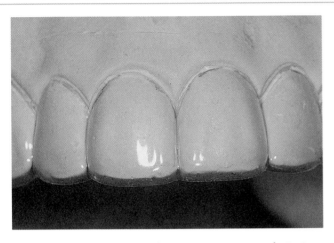

FIG. 39-13 Scalloped tray design. (From Haywood VB: *Contemp Esthet and Restor Pract* 9, 1999.)

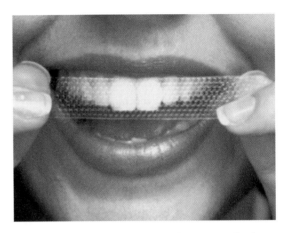

FIG. 39-14 Aligning the maxillary whitening strip. (Courtesy The Procter & Gamble Company, Cincinnati, Ohio.)

The self-applied bleaching process usually takes 2 to 6 weeks. Additional time may be indicated for slow-responding discolorations such as tetracycline, brown fluorosis, or inherent discolorations. Although retreatment is typically not indicated for several years, patients are told to expect stable results for 1 to 3 years with cosmetic whitening. Some color changes may be permanent or longer-lasting.

Case #1 Application

Jimmy showed stabilization for 7 years without requiring interim or touch-up bleaching treatments. The posttreatment photograph is shown in Fig. 39-2.

The patient should wear the nightguard for 2 to 6 hours a day. Initially, when NVB was first introduced, treatments were scheduled for 1 to 2 hours. It has been suggested though that more than 60% of the peroxide remains active in the tray—even after 4 hours of use. Therefore patients may obtain better whitening results with a specified amount of gel if they can wear the tray overnight.[22] Thus nighttime bleaching is the method most often preferred.

Patients should be informed that the teeth may appear "splotchy" during the early stages of bleaching treatment. This is a result of the individual tooth's response or is caused by the varying amounts of bleaching agent on the tooth. It is important to reassure patients that a more homogeneous appearance can be expected with continued treatment.

Whitestrips Method

Another dentist-prescribed home-applied bleaching technique uses a trayless method. The dentist prescribed Crest Whitestrips Supreme (14% hydrogen peroxide) and the Crest Whitestrips Professional (6.5% hydrogen peroxide) contains a 3-week supply of strips. The OTC Crest Whitestrips contain a concentration of 6.0% hydrogen peroxide and the kit contains a 2-week supply. Alignment of the maxillary and mandibular strips are shown in Fig. 39-14 and Fig. 39-15, respectively. When using either form of Whitestrips, the patient should be aware of the inherent advantages (convenience, ease of use, tolerability, cost)

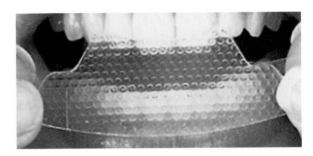

FIG. 39-15 Aligning the mandibular whitening strip. (Courtesy The Procter & Gamble Company, Cincinnati, Ohio.)

and disadvantages (less tooth coverage, potential difficulty in keeping strips in place) of the strip system relative to the tray method. (See Fig. 39-16).

Case #3 Application

Given Ms. Randall's lack of personal time and her desire for a whiter-appearing smile, she is an excellent candidate for Whitestrips technology (see Figs. 39-9 and 39-10).

Brush-Applied Method

OTC brush-applied peroxide whitening systems are available, simple to use and produce whiter teeth. Colgate Simply White is 18% carbamide peroxide liquid in an applicator bottle and Colgate Simply White Night contains a 6.7% hydrogen peroxide solution for overnight use. Dual polymers in the gel allow it to adhere to the teeth and penetrate the enamel to remove both extrinsic and intrinsic stains. Crest Night Effects is a 19% sodium percarbonate peroxide in a silicone polymer based suspension and is packaged in unit dose sachets, painted on the teeth and dries to form an adherent film. Both brush-applied methods are more effective when used with whitening toothpaste.

SIDE EFFECTS OF BLEACHING

In one clinical study, 66% of patients reported occasional short-duration side effects of thermal tooth sensitivity and/or gingival irritation when using a tray system.[17] Thermal sensitivity is thought to be a result of the permeation of peroxide into dentin tubules. This is especially a concern for patients with exposed root surfaces and a history of hypersensitivity. Sensitivity can have various manifestations. Some patients report sensitivity while wearing the tray, yet others report a residual sensitivity an hour after removing the loaded tray. To reduce sensitivity while wearing the tray, the practitioner may recommend decreasing the wear time, decreasing the solution concentration, or alternating the use of the bleaching solution with **potassium nitrate** (a desensitizing dentifrice) or fluoride. Some bleaching kits include a desensitization product.

Chronic sensitivity may occur immediately following the removal of the loaded tray or after completing the process. This type of sensitivity is attributed to the freely diffusible nature of the peroxide gel rather than the pH and may be treated with the desensitization techniques previously described. Clinical studies have confirmed that discontinuing the bleaching process will stop sensitivity. Haywood showed that an average duration of the side effects was 4.8 days during 42 days of 7-hour treatments.[17] Potential sensitivity issues should be disclosed to the patient before the bleaching process is begun. Initial disclosure prepares the patient for any negative side effects and helps ensure overall compliance.

Another reported side effect is gingival irritation. Gingival irritation could be a result of contact with the bleaching solution or an ill-fitting bleaching tray. Various adjustment appointments may be necessary to trim the tray for a better fit. This is yet another reason why OTC tray bleaching systems are not recommended. Although these systems can be readily found in the market, the trays are usually ill-fitting to the gingiva, and the bleaching solution may contain high concentrations of peroxide. Gingival examination and tray adjustment by a dental professional are crucial to successful and healthy dental bleaching when using a tray system.

With the trayless bleaching method, the issue of ill-fitting trays is avoided. Therefore some patients who have difficulty tolerating trays because of gingival irritation may find that they are more comfortable with the whitening strips. Also, with regard to sensitivity, because the strips only cover the six to eight teeth in the front, there is little to no peroxide exposure to the molars, where sensitivity can often occur. Therefore whitening strips may also be an option for patients who experience sensitivity with the tray systems.

General indications for nonvital tooth bleaching techniques are similar to vital bleaching. Patient preference, cost, compliance, and level of difficulty in the removal of certain discolorations dictate the choice of treatment or treatment combinations. Not all treatment successes are equal, nor is one technique more effective in a given situation than another. Offering a combination of costs (in-office treatments as the most expensive to whitening strips as the least expensive) and prescribed home-applied techniques with varying concentrations of

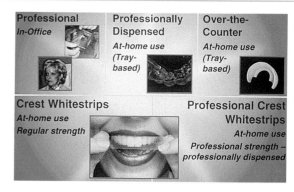

FIG. 39-17 Methods of vital tooth bleaching. (Courtesy The Procter & Gamble Company, Cincinnati, Ohio.)

bleaching formulas is an excellent way for the dental professional to meet the variety of needs for a large number of patients.

ROLE OF THE DENTAL HYGIENIST

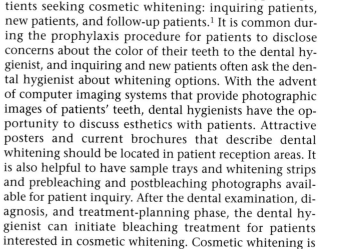

The dental hygienist will encounter three types of patients seeking cosmetic whitening: inquiring patients, new patients, and follow-up patients.[1] It is common during the prophylaxis procedure for patients to disclose concerns about the color of their teeth to the dental hygienist, and inquiring and new patients often ask the dental hygienist about whitening options. With the advent of computer imaging systems that provide photographic images of patients' teeth, dental hygienists have the opportunity to discuss esthetics with patients. Attractive posters and current brochures that describe dental whitening should be located in patient reception areas. It is also helpful to have sample trays and whitening strips and prebleaching and postbleaching photographs available for patient inquiry. After the dental examination, diagnosis, and treatment-planning phase, the dental hygienist can initiate bleaching treatment for patients interested in cosmetic whitening. Cosmetic whitening is a service that brings great pleasure, boosts confidence, and improves the quality of patients' lives. At the same time, knowledge of cosmetic-whitening procedures can make the dental hygienist a more effective team member in the changing dental care environment. Fig. 39-17 summarizes the currently available methods of vital tooth bleaching.

Marketing of dental whitening products is broadening as many dentifrices now include whitening agents. More recently, whitening floss has been researched and marketed. A study of this novel whitening dental tape and floss concluded that it was more effective in removing extrinsic stain in comparison with a control product.[18] Most importantly, as new whitening products are introduced, the dental hygienist should critically review evidence-based research that evaluates the safety and efficacy of each product.

CRITICAL THINKING ACTIVITIES

1. With the help of a classmate, obtain, pour, and trim alginate impression.
2. Fabricate an NVB tray for the maxillary arch with the following specifications:
   Right quadrant: nonreservoir, nonscalloped
   Left quadrant: reservoir, scalloped
3. Evaluate a patient's health history and clinical assessment to determine whether cosmetic whitening is warranted.
4. Debate the advantages and disadvantages of tray (NVB) versus trayless (whitening strips) bleaching systems.
5. With the use of a tooth shade guide system, evaluate the clinical results of cosmetic whitening on a patient who has completed the procedure.
6. Peruse the Internet (http://www.dentalcare.com) for consumer and professional education on Professional and OTC Crest Whitestrips.

REVIEW QUESTIONS

Questions 11 and 12 refer to Case #1, 13 through 16 refer to Case #2, and 17 refers to Case #3.

1. Which of the following home-applied bleaching concentrations is safe and effective, as determined by the ADA?
   a. 5% Hydrogen peroxide
   b. 10% Carbamide peroxide
   c. 15% Carbamide peroxide
   d. 10% to 15% Hydrogen peroxide
2. Which of the following tray designs is recommended for patients who experience gingival irritation from the bleaching gel?
   a. Reservoir
   b. Scalloped
   c. Nonreservoir
   d. Rigid
3. In-office bleaching offers which of the following advantages?
   a. Less monitoring during the procedure
   b. Faster whitening results
   c. Lower concentration of hydrogen peroxide
   d. All the above
4. In saliva, carbamide peroxide is converted into which of the following substances?
   a. Urea
   b. Glycerin
   c. Carbopol
   d. Hydrogen peroxide
5. Which of the following is a disadvantage of the use of whitening strips for vital tooth bleaching?
   a. Less tooth coverage
   b. Cost
   c. Difficulty in use
   d. Uncomfortable tray
6. Proxigel was first used for dental bleaching but because of its _____; it was replaced by _____ gels specific for dental bleaching.
   a. Poor substantivity; less viscous
   b. High concentration; more fluidlike
   c. Poor substantivity; more viscous
   d. High concentration; less fluidlike

7. Deleterious effects of cosmetic whitening include which of the following?
   a. Carcinogenicity
   b. Genotoxicity
   c. Pulpal necrosis
   d. Gingival irritation
8. Optimally, when should patient education occur in relation to cosmetic whitening so that realistic expectations of treatment are communicated?
   a. Before treatment
   b. After treatment is completed
   c. Before and after treatment
   d. Before, during, and after treatment
9. Tooth sensitivity associated with dentist-prescribed, home-applied bleaching can be controlled and reduced through which of the following methods?
   a. Reducing the frequency of bleaching
   b. Reducing bleaching time
   c. Using a lower concentration of carbamide peroxide
   d. All the above
10. Safety concerns regarding at-home bleaching agents have been raised because they contain which of the following ingredients?
    a. Peroxide compounds
    b. Glycerin
    c. Carbopol
    d. Fluoride
11. Which of the following is the *most likely* etiology for the brown discoloration noted on Jimmy's maxillary incisor?
    a. Disturbance in enamel-dentin matrix
    b. Ingestion of high levels of fluoride
    c. History of trauma
    d. Interruption of permanent tooth formation
12. Which of the following tray designs would be indicated for Jimmy?
    a. Scalloped, reservoir
    b. Scalloped, nonreservoir
    c. Nonscalloped, reservoir
    d. Nonscalloped, nonreservoir

Continued

REVIEW QUESTIONS—cont'd

13. Which of the following degrees of tetracycline stain does Ms. O'Bryan most likely exhibit?
    a. First
    b. Second
    c. Third
    d. Fourth

14. The tray design was changed at Ms. O'Bryan's 7-month recall for which of the following reasons?
    a. To obtain cervical third coverage
    b. Because Ms. O'Bryan misplaced her original tray
    c. Because the original tray was ill-fitting
    d. Because the bleaching material was changed

15. After successful bleaching therapy, which of the following best represents the next phase of treatment?
    a. Routine prophylaxis
    b. Bleaching therapy on mandibular arch

    c. Composite on maxillary left incisor
    d. 6-Month recall

16. Bleaching Ms. O'Bryan's tetracycline-stained teeth with 10% carbamide peroxide resulted in which of the following outcomes?
    a. Highly sensitive teeth
    b. Noticeable results with long-term bleaching
    c. Excellent short-term whitening results
    d. No whitening effect

17. Given her lack of personal time and desire for whiter teeth, which of the following tooth-whitening systems would you recommend for Ms. Randall?
    a. Tray bleaching
    b. Professional Crest Whitestrips
    c. Whitening dentifrice
    d. Laser whitening

SUGGESTED AGENCIES AND WEB SITES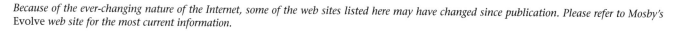

Because of the ever-changing nature of the Internet, some of the web sites listed here may have changed since publication. Please refer to Mosby's Evolve web site for the most current information.

Dentist-Prescribed, Home-Applied Professional Whitening Products with the ADA Seal
Colgate Oral Pharmaceutical, Inc. (Colgate Platinum Daytime professional tooth whitening system): http://www.colgateprofessional.com
Crest Whitestrips (Procter & Gamble): http://www.dentalcare.com
Den-Mat Corporation (Rembrandt Lighten gel): http://www.denmat.com

Discus Dental, Inc. (Nite White whitening gel): http://www.discusdental.com
Patterson Dental Company (Patterson Brand tooth-whitening gel): http://www.pattersondental.com
Ultradent Products, Inc. (Opalescence Whitening Gel): http://www.ultradent.com

ADDITIONAL READINGS AND RESOURCES

Blankenau R, Goldstein RE, Haywood VB: The current status of vital tooth whitening techniques, *Compendium* 20(8):781, 1999.

Compend Cont Educ Dent 21(suppl 29), 2000 (entire issue).

Haywood VB: Are reservoirs necessary? *J Esthet Dent* 11(4):175-6, 1999.

Haywood VB et al: Tray delivery of potassium nitrate-fluoride to reduce bleaching sensitivity, *Quint Int* 32:105-9, 2001.

Dentist-Prescribed, Office-Applied Professional Whitening Products with the ADA Seal
Spectrum Dental, Inc.: *Starbrite In-Office Bleaching Gel:* 8554 Hayden Place, Culver City, CA 90232; (800) 556-7606

Personal References
Robert W. Gerlach, DDS, MPH, Principal Scientist, The Procter & Gamble Company, 2 Procter & Gamble Plaza, Mason, Ohio 45202-3314; gerlach.rw@pg.com

Van B. Haywood, DMD, Professor, Medical College of Georgia, School of Dentistry, Department of Oral Rehabilitation, 1120 15th Street, AD3144, Augusta, GA 30912-0200; vhaywood @mail.mcg.edu.

REFERENCES

1. Adams M: Patient education: from the hygienist's perspective, *Contemp Esthet and Restor Pract* 3(suppl 1):10, 1999.
2. Ames G: Removing stains from mottled enamel, *J Am Dent Assoc Dent Cosmos* 24:1674-7, 1937.
3. Barker et al, editors: *The NIV study bible,* Genesis 49:12, Grand Rapids, 1995, Zondervan Publishing.
4. Bowles WH, Bokemeyer TJ: Staining of adult teeth by minocycline by specific proteins, *J Esthet Dent* 9(1):30-4, 1997.

5. Burchard HH: *A textbook of dental pathology and therapeutics,* Philadelphia, 1898, Lea & Febiger.

6. Burrell KH: ADA supports vital tooth bleaching—but look for the seal, *J Am Dent Assoc* 128(suppl):3S-5S, 1997.

7. Cooper JS, Bokmeyer TJ, Bowles WH: Penetration of the pulp chamber by carbamide peroxide bleaching agents, *J Endod* 18(7):315-7, 1992.

8. Curtis JW et al: Assessing the effects of 10% carbamide peroxide on oral soft tissue, *J Am Dent Assoc* 127(8):1218-23, 1996.

9. Gerlach RW et al: A randomized clinical trial comparing a novel 5.3% hydrogen peroxide whitening strip to 10%, 15% and 20% carbamide peroxide tray-based bleaching systems, *Compend Cont Educ Dent,* 29(suppl):S22-28, 2000.

10. Goldstein RE et al: Bleaching of vital and pulpless teeth. In *Pathways of the pulp,* ed 6, St Louis, 1994, Mosby.

11. Haywood VB: Nightguard vital bleaching: current concepts and research, *J Am Dent Assoc* 128(suppl):19-25, 1997.

12. Haywood VB: The Food and Drug Administration and its influence on home bleaching, *Curr Opin Cosmet Dent* pp. 12-8, 1993.

13. Haywood VB: Nightguard vital bleaching: a history and products update: part 1, *Esthet Dent Update* 2(4):63-6, 1991.

14. Haywood VB, Heymann HO: Nightguard vital bleaching, *Quint Int* 20(3):173-6, 1989.

15. Haywood VB, Houck VM, Heymann HO: Nightguard vital bleaching: effects of varying pH solutions on enamel surface texture and color change, *Quint Int* 22(7):775-82, 1991.

16. Haywood VB, Leonard RH: Nightguard vital bleaching removes brown discoloration for 7 years: a case report, *Quint Int* 29(7):450-1, 1998.

17. Haywood VB et al: Effectiveness, side effects, and long-term status of nightguard vital bleaching, *J Am Dent Assoc* 125(9):1219-26, 1994.

18. Holland JP et al: Effectiveness of novel floss products in reducing extrinsic stain, 2000, unpublished time of printing.

19. Jay AT: Tooth whitening: the financial rewards, *Dent Manag* December 30(12)28-31, 1990.

20. McCracken MS, Haywood VB: Demineralization effects of 10 percent carbamide peroxide, *J Dent* 24(6):395-8, 1996.

21. Mello HS: The mechanism of tetracycline staining in primary and permanent teeth, *J Dent Child* 34(6):478-87, 1967.

22. Nathoo SA et al: Kinetics of carbamide peroxide degradation in bleaching trays, *J Dent Res* 75(2149):286, 1996 (IADR abstracts).

23. Odioso LL et al: Impact of demographic, behavioral, and dental care utilization parameters on tooth color and personal satisfaction, *Compend Cont Educ Dent* 29(suppl):S35-41, 2000.

24. Sagel PA et al: Vital tooth whitening with a novel hydrogen peroxide strip system: design, kinetics, and clinical response, *Compend Cont Educ Dent,* 29(suppl):S10-15, 2000.

25. Schulte JR et al: The effects of bleaching application time on the dental pulp, *J Am Dent Assoc* 125(10):1330-5, 1994.

26. White DJ et al: Effects of tooth whitening gels on enamel and dentin ultrastructure: a confocal laser scanning microscopy pilot study, *Compend Cont Educ Dent* 29(suppl):S29-34, 2000.

27. Wilkins EM: *Clinical practice of the dental hygienist,* ed 8, Philadelphia, 1999, Lippincott Williams & Wilkins.

28. Yiming L: Tooth bleaching using peroxide-containing agents: current status of safety issues, *Compend Cont Educ Dent* 19(8):783-94, 1998.

PART IX

Chapter 40
Salivary Dysfunction

Chapter 41
Neurological and Sensory Impairment

Chapter 42
Hormonal Imbalances

Chapter 43
Mental and Emotional Disturbances

Chapter 44
Immune System Dysfunction

Chapter 45
Head and Neck Cancer and Radiation

Competency Statements

The learner is expected to possess knowledge, skills, judgments, values, and attitudes to develop the listed competencies.

Core Competencies
- Apply a professional code of ethics in all endeavors.
- Adhere to state and federal laws, recommendations, and regulations in the provision of dental hygiene care.
- Provide dental hygiene care to promote patient health and wellness using critical thinking and problem solving in the provision of evidence-based practice.
- Use evidence-based decision making to evaluate and incorporate emerging treatment modalities.
- Assume responsibility for dental hygiene actions and care based on accepted scientific theories and research as well as the accepted standard of care.
- Continuously perform self-assessment for life-long learning and professional growth.
- Promote the profession through service activities and affiliations with professional organizations.
- Provide quality assurance mechanisms for health services.
- Communicate effectively with individuals and groups from diverse populations both verbally and in writing.
- Provide accurate, consistent, and complete documentation for assessment, diagnosis, planning, implementation, and evaluation of dental hygiene services.
- Provide care to all patients using an individualized approach that is humane, empathetic, and caring.

Health Promotion and Disease Prevention
- Promote the values of oral and general health and wellness to the public and organizations within and outside the profession.

Courtesy American Dental Education Association, Washington, DC.

Care Modifications
for Special Needs Patients

- Respect the goals, values, beliefs, and preferences of the patient while promoting optimal oral and general health.
- Refer patients who may have a physiologic, psychological, and/or social problem for comprehensive patient evaluation.
- Identify individual and population risk factors and develop strategies that promote health related quality of life.
- Evaluate factors that can be used to promote patient adherence to disease prevention and/or health maintenance strategies.
- Evaluate and utilize methods to ensure the health and safety of the patient and the dental hygienist in the delivery of dental hygiene.

Community Involvement
- Provide screening, referral, and educational services that allow clients to access the resources of the health care system.
- Facilitate client access to oral health services by influencing individuals and/or organizations for the provision of oral health care.

Patient Care
- Select, obtain, and interpret diagnostic information recognizing its advantages and limitations.
- Recognize predisposing and etiologic risk factors that require intervention to prevent disease.
- Obtain, review, and update a complete medical, family, social, and dental history.
- Recognize health conditions and medications that impact overall patient care.
- Identify patients at risk for a medical or dental emergency and manage the patient care in a manner that prevents an emergency.
- Perform a comprehensive examination using clinical, radiographic, periodontal, dental charting, and other data collection procedures to assess the patient's needs.
- Determine a dental hygiene diagnosis.

- Identify patient needs and significant findings that impact the delivery of dental hygiene services.
- Obtain consultations as indicated.
- Prioritize the care plan based on the health status and the actual and potential problems of the individual to facilitate optimal oral health.
- Establish a planned sequence of care (education, clinical, and evaluation) based on the dental hygiene diagnosis; identified oral conditions; potential problems; etiologic and risk factors; and available treatment modalities.
- Establish a collaborative relationship with the patient in the planned care to include etiology, prognosis, and treatment alternatives.
- Make referrals to other healthcare professionals.
- Perform dental hygiene interventions to eliminate and/or control local etiologic factors to prevent and control caries, periodontal disease, and other oral conditions.
- Control pain and anxiety during treatment through the use of accepted clinical and behavioral techniques.
- Determine the outcomes of dental hygiene interventions using indices, instruments, examination techniques, and patient self-report.
- Evaluate the patient's satisfaction with the oral healthcare received and the oral healthcare status achieved.
- Provide subsequent treatment or referrals based on evaluation findings.
- Develop and maintain a health maintenance program.

Professional Growth and Development
- Identify alternative career options within healthcare, industry, education, and research and evaluate the feasibility of pursuing dental hygiene opportunities.
- Access professional and social networks and resources to assist entrepreneurial initiatives.

CHAPTER 40

Salivary Dysfunction

Mary R. Pfeifer, George M. Taybos

Chapter Outline

Development of Salivary Glands
Classification of Salivary Glands
Case Study: Dental Management of Salivary Gland
  Dysfunction
Salivary Gland Dysfunction
  Medications
  Radiation therapy
  Sjögren's syndrome

Dental Management of Salivary Gland Dysfunction
  Caries
  Oral candidiasis
  Xerostomia
  Sjögren's syndrome
Clues to Determine the Presence of Xerostomia

Key Terms

Candidiasis
Cevimeline (Evoxac)
Dysphagia
Exocrine glands

Glossitis
Glossodynia
Keratoconjunctivitis sicca
Mucositis

Pilocarpine (Salagen)
Radiation caries
Radiation osteomyelitis/osteonecrosis

Salivary gland acini
Sjögren's syndrome (SS)
Xerostomia

Learning Outcomes

1. Know the classification of the salivary glands according to their type of secretion.
2. Recognize information in a patient's health history that may be related to salivary gland dysfunction.
3. Identify patients with decreased salivary function by (1) asking specific questions, (2) assessing their subjective complaints, and (3) evaluating abnormal intraoral findings that are consistent with decreased salivary gland function.

4. Manage the oral health problems directly caused by salivary gland dysfunction.
5. Make an overall positive impact in the life of a patient with xerostomia (dry mouth).
6. Become familiar with salivary substitution products available in your area.

The salivary glands are important structures in the oral cavity that produce saliva. Saliva is needed for normal speaking, tasting, chewing, swallowing, and digesting. In addition, saliva has numerous protective properties, including lubrication, maintenance of pH and tooth integrity, antimicrobial activity, debridement, and maintenance of healthy mucous membranes of the oral flora.

DEVELOPMENT OF SALIVARY GLANDS

The parotid glands are formed by the sixth week of prenatal life, the submandibular glands at the end of the

sixth week and beginning of the seventh week, the sublingual glands by the eighth week, and the minor salivary glands after the twelfth week.[2,5] Salivary glands are *exocrine glands,* which have ducts that transport the secretion (saliva) from the glands.

CLASSIFICATION OF SALIVARY GLANDS

The salivary glands are divided into major glands and minor glands.[2,5] The major salivary glands are the parotid, submandibular, and sublingual glands. These glands are responsible for most of the 0.5 to 0.75 liters of daily saliva production. The minor salivary glands are found throughout the oral cavity and are named according to where they are located (i.e., labial minor, buccal minor, palatal). The salivary glands may also be classified according to their type of secretion: serous, mucus, or mixed. The serous salivary secretion is composed of water, some enzymes (amylase and maltose), salts, and organic ions. The mucous secretion is composed of mucin, which is a lubricating material that aids in chewing, swallowing, and digesting.

Table 40-1 illustrates the three major salivary glands. The *parotid gland,* the largest of the three glands, contributes approximately 25% of the total salivary secretions, produces a serous secretion, and is innervated by the glossopharyngeal nerve (cranial nerve IX). The *submandibular gland,* intermediate in size, contributes approximately 60% of the total salivary secretions, produces a mixed secretion that is predominantly serous, and is innervated by the chorda tympani of the facial nerve (cra-

nial nerve VII). The *sublingual gland,* the smallest of the major salivary glands, contributes only 5% of the salivary secretions, produces a mixed secretion that is predominantly mucus, and is innervated by the chorda tympani of the facial nerve (cranial nerve VII).

The minor salivary glands can also be classified by the type of secretion. Mucous secretion is found in the glossopalatine, palatine, and posterior lingual minor salivary glands; serous secretion is found only in von Ebner's glands, located on the circumvallate papillae of the tongue; mixed secretion glands that are predominantly mucus are found on the anterior tongue, buccal mucosa, and labial mucosa. The minor salivary glands collectively contribute 5%-10% of the total salivary secretion.

SALIVARY GLAND DYSFUNCTION

The two most common dental complaints from patients **40-A** are vague tooth pains and dry-mouth problems. It is often difficult and sometimes frustrating to determine the underlying cause of the complaints. The most common form of salivary gland dysfunction is **xerostomia.** Xerostomia by definition is "a dryness of the mouth from a lack of normal salivary gland secretion." Dry mouth is often a subjective complaint by the patient and cannot be correlated to any actual salivary gland dysfunction.[1] In a healthy individual, the saliva lubricates and protects the oral mucosa, aids in cleaning the mouth, regulates the acidity (pH), maintains the integrity of the dentition, and destroys bacteria.[12] Therefore when there is a decrease in salivary function, there will be predictable sequelae in the oral cavity. The changes in the oral mucosa can range from a dry, smooth appearing mucosa to ulcerations with secondary infections such as **candidiasis.**[14] The decreased salivary function increases the susceptibility of the dentition to caries.[6,8] The patient also may report an altered taste, **glossodynia** or **glossitis,** and difficulty in chewing and swallowing.

The most common causes of xerostomia are (1) medications, (2) radiation therapy for head and neck cancers, and (3) immunological disease, particularly Sjögren's syndrome.

MEDICATIONS

Xerostomia can occur in any age group but is a common complaint in older adults. A long-held belief was that salivary function decreased with age; however, this was proven as incorrect.[3,4] There does, however, appear to be a decreased stimulated saliva rate in individuals who take medications.[3,15] Therefore medications—not increasing age—affect the salivary function. In one study, a review of the drug intake for a population revealed that 22% take antihypertensive drugs, 20% consume alcohol, 14% take mood-altering drugs, 9% take antihistamines, and 7% take decongestants.[9] Of the 200 most-prescribed medications in 1998, 55 list xerostomia as an expected adverse effect (Boxes 40-1 and 40-2).[17] If age groups are correlated to the use of drugs that can cause xerostomia, the findings reveal a prevalence of xerostomia in 27% of the 18-34 age group, 35% of the 35-54 age group, and 60% of the 55-and-older age group.[13] This clearly shows that patients of all ages can experience xerostomia from use of medications.

TABLE 40-1

Major salivary glands: amounts and types of secretions and innervations

Salivary gland	Amount and type of secretion*	Innervations
Parotid gland	25%; serous secretion	Glossopharyngeal nerve (cranial nerve IX)
Submandibular gland	60%; mixed secretion but mostly serous	Chorda tympani of the facial nerve (cranial nerve VII)
Sublingual gland	5%; mixed secretion but mostly mucus	Chorda tympani of the facial nerve (cranial nerve VII)

*Minor salivary glands produce approximately 5% to 10% of the saliva.

Case Study

Dental Management of Salivary Gland Dysfunction

Martha Anthony is a 52-year-old Caucasian woman. She has not had a supportive dental care visit in more than a year. At this visit she seems to be blinking her eyes frequently, and when she speaks it sounds as if her mouth is dry. You question Ms. Anthony about your observations, and she says her eyes have been dry for several months. She purchased some artificial tears from the pharmacy, which work most of the time but only for a few hours. Ms. Anthony did not use the artificial tears this morning because she was in a hurry and did not want to be late for the appointment. She also reports that her mouth has also seemed dry during the last several months and that she constantly sips water. These two findings are of concern to you as a dental hygienist because you suspect that Ms. Anthony may have a serious underlying disease. The resulting dry mouth could cause additional oral disease, especially where she has recession.

Oral Signs and Symptoms of Adverse Drug Reactions

Angioedema
Candidiasis
Cough
Dysgeusia
Erythema multiforme
Gingival bleeding
Gingival hyperplasia
Glossodynia/glossitis
Increased gag reflex
Lichenoid drug reaction
Mouth ulcerations/stomatitis
Mouth/jaw discomfort
Oral paresthesia
Pharyngitis
Reflux/hyperacidity
Tooth disorder
Vomiting
Xerostomia

Drug Categories that Cause Xerostomia

Amphetamines: dextroamphetamine and amphetamine (Adderall)
Analgesic agents: nonsteroidal antiinflammatory drugs, narcotics
Antianxiety agents: benzodiazepines
Anticonvulsant drugs: gabapentin (Neurontin)
Antidepressant agents: selective serotonin reuptake inhibitors, tricyclics
Antihistamines
Antimicrobial agents: ciprofloxacin (Cipro)
Antipsychotic agents: risperidone (Risperdal)
Asthma drugs
Cardiovascular agents: ACE inhibitors, calcium channel blockers, alpha-1 blockers
Decongestants
Gastric acid secretion inhibitors: omeprazole (Prilosec)
Prokinetic gastrointestinal tract agents
Skeletal muscle relaxants: cyclobenzaprine
Tobacco-cessation drugs: bupropion (Zyban)

SURGERY AND RADIATION THERAPY

In 2001 it was estimated that 30,100 individuals would be diagnosed with cancer of the oral cavity and pharynx. The treatments for head and neck cancer are surgery, radiation therapy, chemotherapy, or a combination of the three modalities. Each modality by itself is wrought with adverse effects. The surgical approach can result in loss of function and disfigurement. Chemotherapy can result in alopecia (hair loss), anorexia, nausea, and immunosuppression with its increased risk for infection. Though chemotherapy can cause a transient salivary gland dysfunction, xerostomia is not generally associated with the chemotherapeutic and surgical modalities. This unfortunately is not the case with radiation therapy.

The direct effects of radiation therapy to the oral structures are *mucositis,* difficulty in swallowing *(dysphagia),* xerostomia, candidiasis, *radiation caries,* and *radiation osteomyelitis/osteonecrosis.* The patient undergoing radiation therapy will report decreased saliva almost immediately (during the first week of therapy), whereas mucositis generally becomes noticeable after 2 weeks of therapy. Indirect effects of radiation therapy are caused by irreversible changes in the vascular tissue and bone. The most dramatic and dose-limiting effect during radiation therapy is mucositis, which begins in the second week of therapy and then increases in severity as the treatment progresses. Mucositis may become so severe that a nasogastric tube is inserted for feeding and the radiation therapy regimen is interrupted until the oral signs and symptoms improve. After the radiation therapy is completed, the atrophy and degeneration of the irradiated salivary glands results in little or no salivary gland secretions.

SJÖGREN'S SYNDROME

Sjögren's syndrome (SS) (pronounced *show-grens*) is an autoimmune disorder characterized by a classic triad of clinical conditions: (1) *keratoconjunctivitis sicca* (dry eyes), (2) xerostomia, and (3) connective tissue disease. SS can occur in two ways: primary and secondary. The primary form of SS is characterized by the presence of only dry eyes and xerostomia. The secondary form is characterized by dry eyes, xerostomia, and the presence of a systemic connective tissue disorder, such as rheumatoid arthritis (30%-50%), systemic lupus erythematosus (5%), progressive systemic sclerosis (5%), polymyositis (4%), or mixed connective disease (3%). The prevalence of SS is unknown; however, it is estimated to occur in 0.5% of the population, with 80% to 90% of those affecting middle-aged women. The salivary gland dysfunction that occurs with SS is a direct result of the autoimmune lymphocytic infiltration of the salivary gland tissue that destroys the saliva-producing component of the gland. Some evidence exists that viral infections, heredity, and hormones may in some way contribute to SS. Most patients with SS have a reduced resting and stimulated salivary flow rate.[11] Patients with SS may have an increased risk for lymphoma (non-Hodgkin's β cell)—up to 40 times greater than the normal population.[10]

DENTAL MANAGEMENT OF SALIVARY GLAND DYSFUNCTION

The patient with decreased salivary production creates a unique and oftentimes frustrating management problem for the dental hygienist and dentist because no cure is available.

CARIES

Because of the marked reduction in salivary gland function, the patient is at greater risk for caries activity regardless of age. This requires the patient to have a more serious and meticulous approach to oral hygiene procedures. Patients with salivary gland dysfunction should be treated more frequently, such as every 3 months. The increased caries activity can be controlled if the patient improves home care, implements daily use of a focused custom fluoride tray, and rinses with chlorhexidine so that organisms responsible for caries are reduced.

ORAL CANDIDIASIS

The increased risk for developing oral candidiasis (erythematous type) is directly related to the decreased salivary function. For the patient who develops candidiasis, antifungal agents should be prescribed to treat the infection. Oral nystatin preparations can be a problem for the patient with xerostomia. The lozenge and pastilles contain large quantities of sugar, and the suspension may require 2-minute rinses four times a day for 30 days or more. The patient may be better managed with a systemic antifungal agent such as ketoconazole or fluconazole.

Throughout the chapter, *Rx* is the prescription; *Disp* is to dispense; and *Sig* is the dosing direction.

Rx: Ketoconazole (Nizoral) 200 mg tablets
Disp: Tablets No. 15
Sig: Take two tablets on first day at mealtime, then one tablet each day at mealtime, until gone.

NOTE: Ketoconazole is taken at mealtime because the active antifungal drug requires low gastric pH for maximum systemic absorption.

Rx: Fluconazole (Diflucan) 100 mg tablets
Disp: Tablets No. 15
Sig: Take two tablets on first day at mealtime, then one tablet each day at mealtime until gone.

XEROSTOMIA

When evaluating the patient's xerostomia problem, the patient's complaint and the hygienist's concern may be different. Remember to always listen to what patients describe; that will be their priority. The dental hygienist may focus on the potential for increased caries activity, whereas the patient's main concern is the oral dryness that results in difficulty in chewing and swallowing food and even in speaking. The patient's concern is directly related to a decrease in both quantity and quality of the saliva. Relief may be found by treating symptoms with over-the-counter pain relievers, artificial tears, ointments, and saliva substitutes. If the patient's xerostomia is caused by medications, the management is limited to keeping the mouth moist with plain water and/or artificial saliva substitutes such as Oral Balance (Laclede, Inc., Rancho Dominguez, Calif.) and Salivart (Gebauer Co., Cleveland, Ohio).

If, however, xerostomia is the result of head and neck radiation therapy, oral *pilocarpine (Salagen),* a prescription medication approved by the Food and Drug Administration (FDA), can be used for treatment. For pilocarpine to have a positive effect, there must be some residual active salivary gland tissue present. The suggested regimen is for the patient to take a 5-mg tablet 30-45 minutes before each meal and, if desired, at bedtime. The most frequently noted adverse effect from pilocarpine is perspiration.[16] Evidence exists that use of oral pilocarpine during radiation therapy will decrease the severity of salivary gland atrophy and degeneration and also decrease the ex-

tent and severity of predictable mucositis. If oral pilocarpine is suggested for a patient who is to undergo radiation therapy, a dose of pilocarpine must be taken 1 hour before the radiation treatment. This action results in the degranulation of the secretory granules in the *salivary gland acini.* One of the mechanisms of salivary gland destruction during radiation therapy is the interaction of the ionizing radiation with the granules, which results in the production of destructive free radicals.

SJÖGREN'S SYNDROME

For patients with SS, the use of pilocarpine and *cevimeline (Evoxac)* is FDA-approved and can be used in the same regimen as with postradiation xerostomia.

Management of the SS patient should also include care by an ophthalmologist for the dry eyes and by a rheumatologist if arthritis or a connective tissue disorder is present.

Rx: Cevimeline HCl (Evoxac) 30 mg
Disp: Caps No. 120
Sig: Take one capsule 60 to 90 minutes before meals and a bedtime.
Refills: 6 (This is a 6-month supply.)

Rx: Oral pilocarpine (Salagen) 5 mg tablets
Disp: Tablets No. 120
Sig: Take one tablet 30-45 minutes before meals and at bedtime.
Refills: 6 (This is a 6-month supply.)

NOTE: The patient is directed to take oral pilocarpine 30 to 45 minutes before meals. For most individuals, ingestion of the oral tablet will result in maximum salivary gland stimulation within 45 to 60 minutes. This ensures that saliva is present at mealtime. For the patient who takes oral pilocarpine during head and neck radiation therapy, one tablet must be taken 1 hour before the radiation treatment. To obtain the same results with cevimeline the medication is taken 60 to 90 minutes before meals.

CLUES TO DETERMINE THE PRESENCE OF XEROSTOMIA

To assist the dental hygienist in identifying a patient with decreased salivary function, Fox[7] has developed the questions listed in Box 40-3. Box 40-4 indicates conditions to look for in a medical history that could be related to salivary gland dysfunction. Subjective complaints that may be related to salivary gland dysfunction are listed in Box 40-5. Intraoral findings might also indicate decreased salivary function (Box 40-6).

BOX 40-4

Medical History Items that May Be Related to Salivary Gland Dysfunction

Atrophic vaginitis
Chronic sinusitis (antihistamines)
Current chemotherapy
Depression (xerostomia-causing medications)
Diabetes
Dry eyes or corneal ulcers and photosensitivity
History of head and neck radiation
Hypertension (xerostomia-causing medications)
Lupus/mixed connective tissue disorders (secondary Sjögren's Syndrome)

Recurrent oral candidiasis
Rheumatoid arthritis (secondary Sjögren's Syndrome)
Sore muscles/sore joints (analgesic medications)
Other medical conditions involving the heart, lungs, liver, and digestive and gynecological systems
Other mixed connective tissue disorders (polymyositis, scleroderma, sclerosis)
Hormonal imbalance (menopause)

BOX 40-5

Subjective Complaints that May Be Related to Decreased Salivary Gland Function

Sore or burning sensation in the mouth
Dry, itchy, or tired eyes or feeling of sand in eyes
Continuous cold hands and feet (Raynaud's phenomenon)
General achy muscles and fatigue
History of dry, atrophic vaginitis
Need to suck on candies (e.g., lemon drops) to assist in the lubrication of mouth throughout the day (this also increases the risk of dental decay)

Need to sip on water throughout the day and night
Difficulty speaking for more than 10 minutes without drinking water
Difficulty swallowing food at mealtime and need to often drink water to swallow food

BOX 40-6

Intraoral Findings that May Be Related to Decreased Salivary Gland Function

Atrophic buccal mucosa
Atypical increased activity in dental decay (especially cervical and incisal teeth)
Boggy, smooth, and glassy appearance of the gingival margin (if the gingival sulcus is air-dried, decreased, or no gingival crevicular fluid fills the area and the sulcus stays dry and open)

Dental mirror 'sticks' to the patient's buccal mucosa
Frothy saliva (thick and bubbly but little or no serous component)
No pooling of saliva in the anterior floor of the mouth
Oral candidiasis
Decreased filiform papilla (glossitis)

 RITICAL THINKING ACTIVITIES

1. Visit five pharmacies. Determine the type of salivary substitutes each one stocks.
2. Ask the pharmacist at each of pharmacies visited what advice is provided to patients who have problems with xerostomia or dry mouth.
3. Develop an educational pamphlet outlining the signs and symptoms indicative of xerostomia. Provide oral self-care recommendations for the xerostomic patient.
4. Ask your personal dentist or dental hygienist whether their practice treats any patients with SS and if so, how that patient is managed.

REVIEW QUESTIONS

1. Saliva is needed for all of the following functions *except* which one?
   a. Digesting
   b. Tasting
   c. Swallowing
   d. Sensing
   e. Speaking

2. Properties of saliva include all the following *except* which one?
   a. Lubrication of the tissues
   b. Mastication
   c. Antimicrobial activity
   d. Oral pH regulation
   e. Debridement

3. The parotid gland is the largest of the major salivary glands. Which of the following is *not* a characteristics of the parotid gland?
   a. 25% of total daily secretion
   b. Innervated by cranial nerve IX (glossopharyngeal nerve)
   c. Salivary secretion predominately mucus
   d. Salivary secretion predominately serous

4. Which of the following chief complaints would you be *least* likely to hear from a patient with xerostomia?
   a. "My tongue feels like it is burning."
   b. "I have to sip water all day long."
   c. "Spicy food makes my mouth feel better."
   d. "Food doesn't taste good."
   e. "I have a hard time talking for more than 10 minutes."

5. Which of the following dental management methods is best for patients with decreased salivary production?
   a. 1-Year dental hygiene recall program
   b. Dietary management
   c. Aerobic exercise
   d. 3-Month dental hygiene supportive care interval
   e. Use of electric toothbrush

6. Of the 200 most-prescribed medications in the United States in 1998, how many list xerostomia as an adverse effect?
   a. More than 50
   b. 25
   c. 100
   d. 75

 # SUGGESTED AGENCIES AND WEB SITES

Because of the ever-changing nature of the Internet, some of the web sites listed here may have changed since publication. Please refer to Mosby's Evolve web site for the most current information.

American Academy of Oral Medicine, 2910 Lightfoot Drive, Baltimore, MD 21209-1452; (410) 602-8585: http://www.aaom.com

American Fibromyalgia Syndrome Association, Inc., 6380 East Tanque Verde, Suite D, Tucson, AZ 85715; (520) 733-1570: http://www.afsafund.org

Chronic Fatigue Syndrome: http://www.chronicillnet.org

Fibromyalgia Network, P.O. Box 31750, Tucson, AZ 85751-1752; (800) 853-2929: http://www.fmnetnews.com

[The] International Association for the Study of Pain: http://www.iasp-pain.org

Missouri Arthritis Rehabilitation Research and Training Center: http://www.hsc.missouri.edu

National Arthritis Foundation, P.O. Box 19000, Atlanta, GA 30326; (404) 872-7100 or (800) 283-7800: http://www.arthritis.org (Contact the local state chapter of the Arthritis Foundation for more information on Sjögren's syndrome and local support meetings.)

National Institute of Musculoskeletal and Skin Disease: NIMAS Information Clearinghouse, Box AMS, Bethesda, MD 20892; (301) 495-4484

[The] Oregon Fibromyalgia Foundation: http://www.myalgia.com

Sjögren's Syndrome Foundation, 8120 Woodmont Ave., Suite 530, Bethesda, MD 20814; (800) 475-6473: http://www.sjogrens.org

Dry Eyes–Ocular Disease

American Academy of Ophthalmology, P.O. Box 7424, San Francisco, CA 94120; (415) 561-8500: http://www.aao.org

National Eye Institute, 2020 Vision Place, Bethesda, MD 20892-3655; (301) 496-5248: http://www.nei.nih.gov

Emotional Support

American Psychological Association, 750 First Street NE, Washington, D.C. 20002-4242; (202) 336-5500: http://www.apa.org

GriefNet: http://rivendell.org

National Organization for Rare Disorders, Inc., P.O. Box 8923, New Fairfield, CT 06812-8923: http://www.rarediseases.org

Finding a Physician

University of Kansas Medical Center Physician Referral Directory, (913) 588-1227 or (800) 332-6048: http://www.kumc.edu

U.S. News & World Report, Inc. ("America's best hospitals"): http://www.usnews.com

General Health Information

Medscape, Inc.: http://www.medscape.com

National Health Information Center (NHIC): http://nhic-nt.health.org

National Institutes of Health (NIH), Bethesda, MD 20892: www.nih.gov

Products for Dry Mouth

Biosonics, Inc. (Salitron), 185 Commerce Drive, Suite 103, Fort Washington, PA 19034-2503; (800) 547-4357: http://www. biosonics.com.

Block Drug Company (Division of GlaxoSmithKline Consumer Healthcare), 257 Cornelison Ave., Jersey City, NJ 07302-3198105; Oral Care Division; (800) 652-5625: http://www. blockdrug.com

Conair Corporation for Advanced Oral Care Systems, 150 Milford Road, East Windsor, NJ 08520; (800) 355-5391: http://www. conair.com

Continued

SUGGESTED AGENCIES AND WEB SITES—cont'd

Daiichi Pharmaceutical Corporation (Evoxac), 11 Philips Parkway, Montvale, NJ 07645-1810; (877) 324-4244: http://www.daiichius.com

Gebauer Company, 9410 Saint Catherine Avenue, Cleveland, OH 44104; (800) 321-9348: http://www.gebauerco.com

Johnson & Johnson, 199 Grandview Road, Stillman, NJ 08558; (800) 526-3967: http://www.jnj.com

Kingswood Laboratories, Inc., 10375 Hague Road, Indianapolis, IN 46256; (800) 968-7772

Laclede, Inc. (Biotene, Oral Balance), Medical Products Division, Rancho Dominguez, CA 90220; (800) 922-5856: http://www.laclede.com

MGI Pharma, Inc. (Salagen), 6300 West Old Shakapee Road, Suite 110, Bloomington, MN 55438-2318; (800) 562-5580: http://www.mgipharma.com

Omnii Oral Pharmaceuticals Online, 1500 North Florida Mango Road, Suite 1, West Palm Beach, FL 33409; (800) 445-3386: http://www.omniiproducts.com

Oral-B Laboratories, 600 Clipper Road, Belmont, CA 94002; (800) 446-7252: http://www.oralb.com

Proctor & Gamble, P.O. Box 429553, Cincinnati, OH 45242; (800) 543-2577: http://www.dentalcare.com

Roxane Laboratories, Inc., P.O. Box 16532, Columbus, OH 43216; (800) 520-1631: http://www.roxane.com

Support Groups

American Society for Quality, Health Care Division: http://www.healthcare.org

National Osteoporosis Foundation, 1232 22nd Street NW, Washington, DC 20037-1292; (202) 223-2226: http://www.nof.org

WebMD Corporation: http://my.webmd.com

 ## REFERENCES

1. Atkinson JC, Wu AJ: Salivary gland dysfunction: causes and symptoms, treatment, *J Am Dent Assoc* 125:409-15, 1994.
2. Avery JK: *Oral development and histology,* ed 3, New York, 2000, Thieme Medical.
3. Baum BJ: Evaluation of stimulated parotid saliva flow rate in different age groups, *J Dent Res* 60(7):1292-6, 1981.
4. Ben-Aryeh H et al: The salivary flow rate and composition of whole and parotid resting and stimulated saliva in young and old healthy subjects, *Biochem Med Metabol Biol* 36:260-5, 1986.
5. Bhaskar SN: *Orban's oral histology and embryology,* ed 11, St Louis, 1991, Mosby.
6. Burnett GW: The microbiology of dental infections, *Dent Clin N Am* 14(4):681-95, 1970.
7. Fox PC et al: Sjögren's Syndrome: a model for dental care in the 21st century, *J Am Dent Assoc* 129:719-28, 1998.
8. Mandel ID: The role of saliva in maintaining oral homeostasis, *J Am Dent Assoc* 199:298-394, 1989.
9. Meurmen JH, Rantonen P: Salivary flow rate, buffering capacity and yeast counts in 187 consecutive adult patients from Kuopio, Finland, *Scand J Dent Res* 102(4):229-34, 1994.
10. Neville BW et al: *Oral and maxillofacial pathology,* ed 2, Philadelphia, 2002, WB Saunders.
11. Rhodus NL: Oral pilocarpine HCL stimulates labial (minor) salivary gland flow in patients with Sjögren's Syndrome, *Oral Dis* 3:93-8, 1997.
12. Rhodus NL: Xerostomia: an increasingly significant dental management challenge, *NW Dent* 4:14-8, 1997.
13. Sreebny LM, Valdini A, Yu A: Xerostomia, part II: relationship to nonoral symptoms, drugs and disease, *Oral Surg* 68(4):419-27, 1989.
14. Wolff A et al: Oral mucosal status and major salivary gland function, *Oral Surg* 70:49-54, 1990.
15. Wu AJ, Ship JA: *Characterization of major salivary gland flow rates in the presence of medication and systemic diseases,* American Academy of Oral Medicine Annual Meeting, 1993 (abstract).
16. Wynn RL: Oral pilocarpine (Salagen): a recently approved salivary stimulant, *Gen Dent* 44(1):22-32, 1996.
17. Zoeller J: The top 200 drugs, *Am Druggist* February: 41-48, 1999.

CHAPTER 41

Neurological *and* Sensory Impairment

Kim Curbow Wilcox, Robert A. DeVille

Chapter Outline

Case Study: Supportive Care Challenges in the
   Treatment of the Quadriplegic Patient
Selected Conditions
   Stroke
   Brain injury
   Cerebral palsy
   Parkinson's disease
   Spinal injury
   Spina bifida
   Multiple sclerosis
   Amyotrophic lateral sclerosis
   Hydrocephalus
   Alzheimer's disease
   Bell's palsy

Muscular dystrophy
Autism
Impairments, Level of Severity, and Effect on
   Dental Care
   Neuromuscular deficits
   Musculoskeletal deficits
   Respiratory deficits
   Bowel and bladder dysfunction
   Integumentary deficits
   Cognitive and perceptual deficits
   Visual deficits
   Communication deficits
   Mobility deficits

Key Terms

Alzheimer's disease (AD)
Amyotrophic lateral sclerosis (ALS)
Arteriovenous malformation (AVM)
Ataxic cerebral palsy
Athetoid cerebral palsy
Autism
Bell's palsy

Brain injury (BI)
Cerebral palsy (CP)
Cognition
Hemorrhagic
Hydrocephalus
Infarction
Ischemic

Lou Gehrig's disease (also *ALS*)
Mobility
Multiple sclerosis (MS)
Muscle tone
Muscular dystrophy (MD)
Musculoskeletal

Parkinson's disease
Respiratory
Spastic cerebral palsy
Spina bifida
Spinal cord injury (SCI)
Visual deficits

Learning Outcomes

1. Describe the prevalence, incidence, and distribution of selected neurological and sensory impairments in specific populations.
2. Describe some of the more common causal agents that lead to neurological and sensory impairment(s).
3. Demonstrate a basic understanding of the pathophysiology that leads to selected impairment(s).
4. List and describe the specific impairments that are characteristic of each neurological and sensory disorder.

5. Demonstrate a basic understanding of the classifications of severity for selected impairments.
6. Describe the conventional treatment modalities for each selected condition, including surgical and nonsurgical approaches such as pharmacological, behavioral, dietary, interventional, and the use of assistive devices and special accommodations.
7. Determine which impairments would most likely impinge on the delivery of oral care.

Continued

Learning Outcomes—cont'd

8. Determine the appropriate modification(s) necessary in dental care delivery to accommodate the patient's needs.

9. Determine the most appropriate method of interacting with a patient who demonstrates a disability.

10. Know how to access further information on specific disorders.

11. Demonstrate a basic understanding of the major legal implications for the provider in the delivery of healthcare services.

Supportive Care Challenges in the Treatment of the Quadriplegic Patient

Leo Crosswell is a 53-year-old Caucasian man with quadriplegia caused by a high level **spinal cord injury (SCI).** In 1979 his cervical spine was fractured with resulting spinal cord damage as a result of a swimming pool diving accident in Central America. Because of political unrest and a military revolution in the country at the time, his transport to medical attention was delayed for approximately 1 week.

This injury to the cervical vertebrae C-2 and C-3 left Mr. Crosswell paralyzed below the neck, although basic breathing function remains. He is fitted with an internal urinary catheter with a leg bag and regulates bowel functions with dietary control and assistance. A caregiver helps him with transportation needs and personal hygiene needs, including feeding, dressing, shaving, tooth brushing, and flossing.

Mr. Crosswell is independently mobile with the assistance of a battery-powered wheelchair, which he controls with oral "sip and puff" tubes that control the wheelchair's steering and speed mechanisms (Fig. 41-1). His torso and extremities rest in custom-fitted cushioned areas and are secured with Velcro straps. He travels to work in a specially modified side-lift van

and has a full-time job with a government wildlife and fisheries agency. Mr. Crosswell operates his telephone and computer with the assistance of a custom-fitted "mouthstick," which is designed to minimize occlusal trauma (Fig. 41-2).

On awakening, or after prolonged reclining, Mr. Crosswell's weakened respiratory condition requires initial ventilation with an Ambu bag to reduce the likelihood of orthostatic hypotension. Occasionally, he experiences mild to moderately severe muscle spasms, generally in his extremities, that last from a few seconds to a few minutes. His vital signs fall within normal ranges.

Mr. Crosswell's dental history is unremarkable. He understands the special importance of his teeth, given his dependence on his mouthstick. Accordingly, he brushes twice a day and flosses once a day with caregiver assistance. He has used a variety of manual and electric toothbrushes. Mr. Crosswell uses a fluoridated toothpaste and over-the-counter mouthrinses, some with fluoride. He exhibits good gingival health but has mild recession and mild toothbrush abrasion resulting from bruxism and mouthstick use.

---

*W*ith increasing life spans, higher standards of living, and complex lifestyles, the morbidity and morality of disease processes and accidents have dramatically changed in the past century. The impairments that often result from disease or accidents may severely restrict a person's ability to participate in a full, productive, and healthy life. Historically, one of the most significant restrictions has been the lack of adequate health care for those with impairments and disabilities.[36] This is especially regrettable because those with debilitating conditions often need far more health care than those in the unimpaired population.

Throughout the 1900s, strides in medicine, public attitudes, and law have dramatically shifted the focus of health care in the United States away from treatment and more toward rehabilitation, delivery systems, costs, and healthcare access. Strides and measures in these areas are well documented in the literature.[27,32,34]

Until recently, little attention has been given to the modifications that healthcare providers must make to deliver routine services to those with physical or mental impairments. All too often a general practitioner would refer a special-needs patient to a "specialist," which results in increased costs and decreased access to routine services.

The purpose of this chapter is to introduce the reader to a selected variety of common conditions that may impact the provider's ability to effectively deliver routine dental care. The chapter will also review some specific techniques and measures that may be used in the care of patients with physical or mental impairments. Although not all conditions are covered here, the case presented for illustration and the impairments reviewed were chosen to provide the reader with a basic resource database that, with modification and adaptation where appropriate, will allow the reader to further research a wider range of impairments and deficits.

SELECTED CONDITIONS

STROKE

41-A

Stroke, also called cerebrovascular accident (CVA) or acute brain attack (ABA), is defined as an interruption of the cerebral circulation, resulting in neurological disability.[25] Strokes, categorized according to the nature of the circulatory disturbance, consist of four general types: *arteriovenous malformation (AVM), ischemic, hemorrhagic,* and *infarction.*[7,25] The primary risk factors for stroke in-

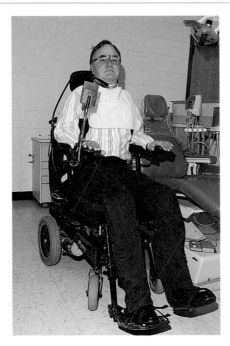

FIG. 41-1 Oral "sip-and-puff" controlled self-powered wheelchair for patients with quadriplegia.

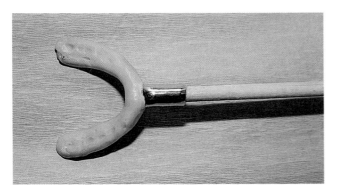

FIG. 41-2 Custom-fabricated mouthstick for patients with quadriplegia.

clude chronic hypertension (HTN), atherosclerosis, smoking, tobacco use, heart disease, and diabetes.[10,25] Secondary risk factors include elevated cholesterol and lipid levels, alcohol use, obesity, and inactivity.[10] Many of the risk factors may be controlled through medical intervention and pharmacological measures.

Stroke is the third leading cause of death and one of the leading causes of disability in the United States. Approximately 730,000 new or recurrent strokes occur each year, which result in 160,000 deaths. Currently more than 4 million people in the United States have survived a stroke and deal with varying degrees of impairment. The risk of stroke increases with age, with more than two thirds of all strokes occurring in persons more than 65 years of age. Additionally, stroke occurs more often in African Americans and women.[21]

A patient who has experienced a stroke may exhibit an especially wide variety of neuromuscular, musculoskeletal, bowel and bladder, integumentary, cognitive, perceptual, visual, behavioral, and communication deficits. The general neuromuscular deficits include impairments of motor control such as hemiparesis (or hemiparalysis), dysarthria, and dysphagia. An increase or decrease in *muscle tone* of the affected side, contractures, edema, decreased tactile and proprioceptive sensations, bowel and bladder dysfunction, and reduced coordination may also be demonstrated. The patient may complain of pain, primarily of the affected shoulder. These impairments combine to produce deficits in *mobility* including the ability to perform bed mobility, transfers, wheelchair propulsion, balance in sitting and standing, and ambulation. Typical cognitive deficits include confusion; lack of orientation to person, place or time; decreased attention span; inability to process information; and a decrease in memory abilities. Patients who have experienced a stroke may also demonstrate perceptual deficits, including unilateral neglect or inattention, distorted body image, or visuospatial distortions. Visual disturbances may include field cuts or problems with depth perception. Many patients who have had a stroke demonstrate changes in behavior including emotional lability and depression. Communication deficits are common when the dominant cerebral hemisphere is involved. These deficits may include expressive or receptive communication and word-finding problems.[23,25,29]

BRAIN INJURY

Brain injury (BI) is defined as damage to the brain caused by a primary insult such as trauma or a secondary insult such as metabolic and physiological events that occur following the primary damage.[25,28] A BI, often called a traumatic brain injury (TBI) or acquired brain injury (ABI), is caused by an external force to the head that results in damage to the brain.[6]

BIs result in more than 50,000 deaths each year.[6] Yearly, more than 1 million people experience a brain injury, resulting in long-term disability for 80,000 people.[6] BIs occur most often in men between the ages of 15 and 24, with 50% of injuries caused by motor vehicle accidents, 21% by falls, 12% by violence, and 10% by recreational activities.[6,23]

Patients with BI may exhibit many of the same characteristics as patients with stroke, including neuromuscular, musculoskeletal, cognitive, perceptual, visual, behavioral, and communication deficits. The patient may experience unilateral or bilateral paresis or paralysis in addition to changes in muscle tone, sensation, bowel and bladder control, edema, and coordination. The patient may develop contractures, which further hinder mobility activities. Depending on the location of the brain damage, the patient may experience respiratory difficulty. Cognitive, perceptual, and visual disturbances may be present along with behavioral and communication deficits. The patient may experience memory loss and difficulty processing information or concentrating on a task. In addition, the patient may experience seizures, headache, or emotional disturbances. The Rancho Los Amigos Levels of Cognitive Functioning, a 7-point scale that describes the cognitive and behavioral recovery sequence, is often used to provide a general description of the patient's abilities.[6,23,25,28]

CEREBRAL PALSY

The term *cerebral palsy (CP)* is used to describe a variety of nonprogressive motor disturbances that result from prenatal development of abnormalities or perinatal/postnatal damage to the central nervous system before 5 years of age.[9,25] Possible causes of CP include in utero disorders, birth trauma, or neonatal asphyxia.[25] CP is characterized by involuntary muscular movement, which shows varying degrees of involvement. In addition, many people with CP also may demonstrate varying levels of cognitive involvement.

More than 5000 infants and an additional 1200 to 1500 school-age children are diagnosed with CP each year. The United Cerebral Palsy Association estimates that approximately 500,000 children and adults live with the effects of CP.[38]

CP has three broad categories: *spastic cerebral palsy, athetoid cerebral palsy,* and *ataxic cerebral palsy.*

Spastic Cerebral Palsy

Spastic CP, caused by damage to upper motor neurons, is the most common form and is evident in 70% of those diagnosed with CP.[9,25] Spastic CP, characterized by stiffness or rigidity of the muscles, directly affects motor function and the ability to perform mobility and activities of daily living (ADLs). Involvement may be categorized as *hemiplegia* in which one side of the body is affected, *paraplegia,* in which the lower extremities are affected, or *diplegia,* in which all four limbs are affected with the lower extremities demonstrating a higher degree of involvement.

Athetoid Cerebral Palsy

Athetoid CP, which affects 20% of those diagnosed, is caused by damage to the basal gangila.[25] This type of CP is characterized by low muscle tone (hypotonia) in early childhood with the development of involuntary muscle contractions and contorted movement (athetoid movement) in late childhood.[9,25] The patient may demonstrate communication deficits including dysarthria and may require an augmentative communication device such as a picture board or letter board. The patient's level of intelligence may be affected, resulting in learning deficits.

Ataxic Cerebral Palsy

Ataxic CP, the final category, affects 10% of those diagnosed and is caused by involvement of the cerebellum.[9] Patients with ataxic CP demonstrate a wide-based, unsteady gait with balance, coordination, and speech deficits. Ataxic CP is often associated with epilepsy and the presence of intention tremors.[9,25]

Patients with CP may demonstrate difficulty with control of oral musculature, resulting in speech involvement, lack of control of secretions, and difficulty with chewing and swallowing. A hyperactive bite reflex and irregular movements of the head and body may be present. Lack of coordination and lack of control of the extremities produce difficulties in performing daily activities, including wheelchair mobility, ambulating, grooming, dressing, and eating. CP may produce a variety of secondary problems including learning and perceptual disorders, changes in muscle tone, sensory deficits, range-of-motion limitations (including contractures), respiratory inefficiency, and growth disturbances.[22,25]

PARKINSON'S DISEASE

Parkinson's disease is a chronic neurological condition that results in a gradual deterioration of motor control. This slowly progressing disease affects the substantia nigra or basal ganglia. It may be seen clinically as changes in movement and functional capabilities caused by a reduction in the production of dopamine. The specific cause of the reduction in dopamine is unknown. Although Parkinson's disease has not been shown to be genetically transmitted, there is an increased incidence of the disease in some families. There are no known preventative measures or cures for Parkinson's disease.[19,25]

Parkinson's disease affects more than 1.5 million Americans. Although the diagnosis is usually made after the age of 50, earlier onset is not uncommon.[19,25]

Patients diagnosed with Parkinson's disease may exhibit a wide range of symptoms, including neuromuscular, musculoskeletal, and communication deficits. The patient may experience bradykinesia, rigidity, or a unilateral resting tremor of the upper or lower extremities, all of which severely impair function. As the disease progresses, the patient may exhibit difficulty maintaining balance during gait and functional activities. The patient with Parkinson's disease may also exhibit an increase in flexion of the neck, trunk, and lower extremities. The facial muscles may be affected, resulting in an inability to show facial expressions. The patient may demonstrate dysphagia, dysarthria, or a reduced speaking volume. A festinating gait, "freezing" in place of movements, and postural ability changes may also be apparent and increase the risk of falls.[14,19,25]

SPINAL INJURY

Injury to the spinal cord results in a partial or complete loss of neurological function distal to the level of the injury. The classification of complete spinal cord injury (SCI) indicates a total loss of motor and sensory functions distal to the injury. In comparison, an incomplete SCI, which includes the diagnoses of Brown-Sequard, anterior cord syndrome, posterior cord syndrome, and central cord syndrome, indicates that some motor and sensory function has been retained distal to the level of injury. In the United States approximately 54% of all SCIs are classified as incomplete.[34]

More than 7800 spinal injuries occur in the United States each year, with 250,000 to 400,000 people living with the effects of the injury. Of SCIs, 80% occur in people less than 40 years of age, with the highest occurrence between the ages of 16 and 30. Single men are more likely to sustain an SCI than women, and the incidence among the unemployed is higher than in the employed population. More than 44% of all SCIs are caused by motor vehicle accidents, with 24% resulting from violence, 22% from falls, and 8% from sports activities.[20]

A spinal injury may result in paraplegia or quadriplegia. Paraplegia indicates that the injury occurred in the thoracic, lumbar, or sacral regions of the spine. This results in paresis or paralysis and sensory changes of the trunk and lower extremities. Quadriplegia indicates injury in the cervical region of the spine with motor and sensory changes in the upper extremities, trunk, and lower extremities. Patients with quadriplegia or quadriparesis may also demonstrate impairment of the respiratory muscles. Depending on the location of the spinal injury, the patient may demonstrate motor and sensory impairments, altered temperature control, impaired respiration, bowel and bladder dysfunction, and changes in muscle tone.[25,30,34] Secondary problems may include contractures, heterotopic ossification, postural hypotension, decubitus ulcers, and deep vein thrombosus.[30,34] Patients may also experience autonomic dysreflexia, which is exhibited as disorientation, facial and body flush, perspiration, and significantly increased blood pressure. Autonomic dysreflexia, caused by a noxious stimulus such as pain or urinary backflow, is usually resolved when the noxious stimulus is removed.[4,25,34] Autonomic dysreflexia is more common in persons with quadriplegia.

SPINA BIFIDA

Spina bifida is defined as defective closure of the vertebral column that usually occurs in the lower thoracic, lumbar, or sacral regions.[9,25] The defect typically involves three to six vertebral segments and is usually associated with spinal deformities such as scoliosis.[25] The severity of spina bifida ranges from a completely open spine (rachischisis or spina bifida aperta), which usually results in severe neurological disturbances and death, to spina bifida occulta, in which an abnormality exists but results in mild neurological involvement.[7,25] The defect may include only the sac containing the meninges (meningocele), only the spinal cord (myelocele), or both the meninges and the spinal cord (myelomeningocele).[7,9,31] The cause of spinal bifida is questionable, with many experts attributing the disorder to environmental factors and maternal vitamin deficiency, specifically folic acid.[9,25] Spina bifida may occur in conjunction with other congenital defects, such as hydrocephalus.[9]

Approximately 1 of every 1000 newborns is diagnosed with spina bifida.[35] The effects of spina bifida include neuromuscular involvement such as paralysis or paresis below the level of the lesion, changes in muscle tone, and sensory deficits. Musculoskeletal complications include scoliosis and other bony deformities as a result of muscle imbalances and changes in muscle tone. The spinal and bony deformities often limit the patient's ability to sit correctly or ambulate and, if severe, may result in respiratory insufficiency. In addition, the sphincters of the bladder and rectum are usually affected, resulting in incontinence or requiring the use of internal or external catheters. The patient's risk of pressure areas and skin breakdown is increased when the musculoskeletal deformities are combined with sensory deficits and bowel and bladder incontinence. Secondary complications of spina bifida include hip dislocation or subluxation and osteoporosis. Each of these deficits contributes to the patient's difficulty in performing mobility activities and ADLs. Because the lesion is typically in the lower one-third to one-half of the spinal column, the upper extremities are usually not affected. The patient also typically does not exhibit communication, cognitive, or perceptual deficits if spinal bifida is the only diagnosis.[9,25,31]

MULTIPLE SCLEROSIS

Multiple sclerosis (MS) is a chronic degeneration of the myelin in the brain and spinal cord.[9] Patients diagnosed with MS demonstrate deficits in both motor and sensory functioning.

The onset of MS typically occurs between the ages of 20 and 40, with an increased incidence in women and Caucasians.[18,25] Although the reason is unknown, the incidence of MS increases as the distance from the equator increases. The cause of MS is largely unknown; however, many theories have been offered. These include the presence of a slowly progressing virus, an abnormal immunological event, a chronic lack of essential fatty acids, and environmental factors. The course of MS is usually exhibited as periods of exacerbation and remission of varying lengths of time.[8,9,25]

Patients with MS demonstrate varying symptoms depending on the location and severity of the demyelination. Symptoms typically include fatigue; visual disturbances; bladder and bowel dysfunction; weakness of facial, oral, and body musculature; changes in muscle tone; and deficits in the performance of mobility activities and ADLs. Additionally, the patient may demonstrate sensory deficits, speech involvement, movement disorders, and reduced respiratory capacity. Secondary complications include osteoporosis, heterotrophic classification, and pressure sores as a result of inactivity and poor positioning. In the most advanced stages of MS, the patient may demonstrate a reduction in cognitive functioning; however, this area is usually not affected in the earlier stages.[8,9,25]

AMYOTROPHIC LATERAL SCLEROSIS

Amyotrophic lateral sclerosis (ALS), also called **Lou Gehrig's disease,** is characterized by degeneration of the cells in the motor neurons of the spinal cord and cerebral cortex. This includes the degeneration of the corticospinal tract and/or the bulbar motor nuclei and/or the anterior horn cells. The cell degeneration leads to progressive muscle atrophy and eventually to death as a result of respiratory failure. The cause of ALS is unknown; however, research is currently directed toward the investigation of gene abnormalities.[2,25]

More than 5000 people are diagnosed with ALS yearly with no trends in racial or ethnic characteristics noted. ALS affects men more often than women and is generally diagnosed after 55 years of age. Death within 3 to 5 years, usually from respiratory failure, occurs in approximately 50% of patients with ALS.[2,25]

ALS affects both upper motor neurons and lower motor neurons. Initial symptoms of ALS include muscle cramping, weakness, and atrophy that begins in the small muscles of the hand and forearm. The patient eventually demonstrates dysphagia, dysarthria, muscle atrophy, and paralysis with changes in muscle tone as a result of the progressive deterioration of the motor neurons. The patient retains all sensory modalities and cognitive capabilities as well as volitional eye movement and control of the urinary sphincter even during the final stages of ALS.[25]

HYDROCEPHALUS

Hydrocephalus is a condition that occurs when the amount of cerebrospinal fluid (CSF) produced by the body is greater than that absorbed.[7,9] This produces a dilation of the ventricles of the brain, which results in an increase in intracranial pressure and may result in enlargement of the cranium if not addressed.[7,9,37] A valve or shunt may be placed to control the excessive fluid and resulting increased pressure by diverting the fluid to the peritoneum or atrium.[9,37] The shunt may be observed just under the skin behind one or both ears, depending on specific medical considerations. Because patients with hydrocephalus exhibit an excessive level of CSF protein and an increased risk for bacterial colonization, the shunt must be consistently maintained to prevent blockage.[9] Signs of shunt malformation may include a change in appetite, lethargy, vomiting, seizures, reduced sensory and motor function, and memory deficits.[25]

Hydrocephalus may be congenital or acquired and may be classified as *communicating* or *noncommunicating*. In communicating hydrocephalus, the CSF is not adequately absorbed, but there is no obstruction between the ventricles. In comparison, noncommunicating, or obstructive, hydrocephalus is caused by a blockage of the ventricular pathways.[37]

With proper treatment, patients with hydrocephalus live productive lives with a normal life span and activities. The most common complication of hydrocephalus is learning disability; however, difficulty with visual and motor skills may also be evident. Hydrocephalus may accompany other diagnoses, which increases the deficits present.[25,37]

ALZHEIMER'S DISEASE

Alzheimer's disease (AD) is a progressive deterioration of the cerebral cortex and other areas of the brain.[25] Although the progression is not predictable and varies considerably, the advanced stage of AD may be reached in as little as 2 to 3 years following the initial diagnosis.[9,25] Although the exact cause of AD is not known, the degeneration of the brain cells may be caused by an abnormality of Chromosome 21, or there may be a genetic predisposition to the development of the disease. The risk of AD increases with increasing age and family history.[1,25]

More than 4 million Americans have been diagnosed with AD. With an increased incidence with aging, 10% of those more than 65 year of age and 50% of those more than 85 years of age will be diagnosed with this progressive disease.[1]

Memory loss is the most common initial symptom of AD. As the brain deterioration increases, symptoms progress to multiple medical and motor problems, including deficits in planning motor activities, balance and coordination deficits, difficulty in performing mobility activities and ADLs, and a progressive inability to use assistive devices such as canes and hearing aids.[25] The patient also begins to show cognitive deterioration, including reductions in safety awareness, lack of orientation to place and time, inability to learn or reason, and progressive memory deficits. Secondary problems associated with AD include alterations in sleep patterns, reduction in bowel and bladder control, depression, and oral motor dysfunction that leads to oral neglect.[25]

BELL'S PALSY

Bell's palsy is a peripheral lesion of cranial nerve VII that produces unilateral facial weakness or paralysis. Bilateral involvement may occur but is not common. Cranial nerve VII, the facial nerve, innervates the muscles of facial expression. The patient typically experiences sensory changes followed by motor deficits. The cause of Bell's palsy is inflammation of the cranial nerve caused by a variety of reasons, including infection of the middle ear, immune disease, and herpes zoster or herpes simplex type 1 of the geniculate ganglion.[7,17,25]

Bell's palsy affects 4 out of 10,000 people, with no age or race characteristics noted. Between 15 and 40 new cases are diagnosed each year nationwide. The incidence of Bell's palsy increases during pregnancy and with increasing age. Of those diagnosed with the palsy, 50% show spontaneous recovery without medical intervention; 20% recover within 1 to 3 months; and 10% recover within 4 to 6 months.[17]

Patients with Bell's palsy initially complain of pain posterior to one ear. This is later followed by a unilateral facial paralysis, a reduction in the sense of taste, and possibly the inability to blink or close the unilateral eye. The facial paralysis affects the patient's oral motor control, resulting in dysarthria, unilateral drooping of the mouth, difficulty controlling secretions, and an increase in salivation. The patient may also complain of tearing or dryness of the eye along with asymmetrical facial expressions.[17,25]

MUSCULAR DYSTROPHY

Muscular dystrophy (MD) is a genetic condition that results in a progressive degeneration of skeletal muscle.[9] The major forms of MD include Duchenne (most common in children), Becker, limb-girdle, distal, facioscapulohumeral, and myotonic (most common in adults). The cause is believed to be an X-linked recessive gene that is transmitted by the mother.[16,25]

MD is usually diagnosed in boys between the ages of 3 and 7. The children typically exhibit a gradual decline in functional abilities, leading to full-time wheelchair use by the age of 10 to 12. Death before the age of 20, caused by respiratory complications, is not unusual.[16,25]

Depending on the type of MD, patients may exhibit proximal muscle weakness, atrophy, and imbalances that progress to the distal musculature. The typical progression is from the pelvic girdle muscles to the shoulder girdle muscles followed by the trunk and extremities, respectively. The patient with Duchenne's MD demonstrates hypertrophied calf muscles that affect the ability to ambulate and perform other functional activities throughout the day. The patient may demonstrate a toe-walking or waddling gait, difficulty negotiating stairs, and recurring falls. As a result of the progressive loss of trunk and cervical muscle control, the patient may demonstrate a reduction in head control and oral motor control, which may result in dysphagia and dysarthria. Additional secondary complications include contractures and spinal deformities that may result in skin breakdown. During the later stages of MD, the patient may demonstrate difficulty with opening the mouth. The cranial nerves are not involved in MD.[9,16,25]

AUTISM

Autism is described as an emotional disturbance demonstrated through a lack of social interaction and developmental deficits in language, communication, and social skills.[7] Children diagnosed with autism typically do not have any significant medical problems and may demonstrate normal to superior intelligence.[9] Physical deformities are rare unless there is a concurrent medical diagnosis.

Autism affects 1 child in 500 with more than 500,000 patients diagnosed in the United States. Males are more often affected than females. There are no common racial, ethnic, or educational characteristics of those diagnosed.[3]

Patients with autism demonstrate an inability to interact with others, which includes a delay in speech development and language skills. The patient may exhibit resistive behaviors, including holding food in the mouth and refusing all but soft, easily chewed foods. In addition, the patient may demonstrate learning disabilities and self-stimulation behaviors, such as head banging, rocking, or repeated body movements. The patient may also complain of or demonstrate sensitivity to light, sounds, smells, touch, or taste.[3]

IMPAIRMENTS, LEVEL OF SEVERITY, AND EFFECT ON DENTAL CARE

41-B

Table 41-1 lists a number of impairments and disabilities and their associated effects on the body.

NEUROMUSCULAR DEFICITS

Motor Control (Oral Motor, Dysphagia, Dysarthria)

Definition

Motor control is defined as the interaction of neuromuscular, musculoskeletal, cognitive, perceptual, and sensory components to produce functional movement.[23] Deficits in motor control of the trunk, extremities, and/or orofacial musculature are common in patients with the diagnoses of stroke, brain injury, CP, Parkinson's disease, SCI, spina bifida, MS, ALS, hydrocephalus, AD (late stage), Bell's palsy, and MD. These patients may demonstrate difficulty in planning, controlling, and/or sequencing muscle movements required for efficient functioning.

Deficits in motor control may be exhibited as hemiparesis, paraplegia, diplegia, dysarthria, or dysphagia. The patient may also exhibit ataxia of the trunk or extremities or a resting or intention tremor.

Level of Severity

The level of motor control impairment is determined through a wide range of examination tools. The measures include examination of the patient's range of motion, muscle tone, and muscle strength because impairment in these areas will affect motor control. Motor control examination generally includes observation of movement and performance of functional activities.

Treatment Modalities

Patients with motor control deficits may participate in physical therapy, occupational therapy, speech and language therapy, and therapeutic recreation to improve function. The focus of the therapeutic intervention is the improvement of planning, controlling, and sequencing muscle movement.

Delivery of Dental Care

Loss of muscle sequencing and control generally does not significantly restrict the delivery of most dental services. It does, however, often require certain accommodations on the part of the provider. Neuromuscular deficits may interfere with the patient's ambulatory abilities, thus making it more difficult to access a dental office and seat oneself in a dental chair. Fortunately, the Americans with Disabilities Act of 1990 (ADA) mandated the removal of many of the physical barriers to access. For example, the

TABLE 41-1

Neurological and sensory impairments and disabilities

Impairment/ disability	Neuro- muscular	Musculo- skeletal	Respiratory	Bowel/ bladder dysfunction	Integu- mentary	Cognitive/ perceptual	Visual	Communi- cation	Mobility
Stroke	X	X		X	X	X	X	X	X
Brain injury	X	X	X	X	X	X	X	X	X
Cerebral palsy	X	X		X	X	X		X	X
Parkinson's disease	X	X	X		X			X	X
Spinal injury	X	X	X	X	X				X
Spina bifida	X	X	X	X	X				X
Multiple sclerosis	X	X	X	X	X	X (late-stage)	X	X	X
Amyotrophic lateral sclerosis	X	X	X		X			X	X
Hydrocephalus	X					X	X		
Alzheimer's disease	X	X	X	X	X	X		X	X
Bell's palsy	X						X	X	
Muscular dystrophy	X	X	X		X			X	X
Autism						X		X	

addition of handicap parking spaces, handicap access ramps, wider doorways, and handicap accessible restrooms have made most offices reasonably accessible.

Ambulatory problems resulting from neuromuscular deficits may range from dependency on an assistive device such as a cane, crutches, walker, or wheelchair to simply requiring more time to accomplish a specific motor task. In many cases the provider simply needs to ensure that the office complies with ADA requirements and to allow sufficient time to get the patient into the office and chair as well as out of the chair and office after treatment has been completed. In most cases, the actual treatment time needs little or no adjustment.

Case Application

Mr. Crosswell was transported to the dental office with the assistance of his part-time driver/caregiver, who drives a specially equipped van. He moves his battery-powered wheelchair into the dental operatory using a series of "sip and puff" switches that control the speed and direction of the chair as well as recline it (see Fig. 41-1). Once in the treatment room Mr. Crosswell may be transferred to the dental chair using a standard one- or two-person patient transfer technique. If a transfer is made, care must be exercised to ensure that any urinary catheter or leg bag remains uncompromised and that gravitational forces are not "working against" normal urinary drainage forces while the patient is positioned in a supine position during lengthy appointments.

However, for patients such as Mr. Crosswell, a transfer is usually not necessary because the patient may be treated in his own chair, which is equipped with a headrest and reclines much like a dental chair.

Many wheelchair manufacturers offer both manual and powered wheelchairs that can be tilted and/or reclined to a variety of positions. Equally crucial to the ability to treat patients in their own chairs is the ability of dental equipment to reach patients. Some equipment delivery systems work exceedingly well, whereas others do not (Figs. 41-3 and 41-4). Some manufacturers offer optional air/water/suction/light extensions that are useful when treating patients in wheelchairs.

Meriting special consideration is the patient with dysphagia. Here, special care must be taken to maintain a patent airway. Fortunately, modern high volume evacuation (HVE) is almost universally available and is invaluable in the rapid removal of saliva, other fluids, and debris from the oral cavity. Use of the rubber dam where possible may prevent accidental aspiration of foreign objects or dropped items. Unfortunately, some patients report increased problems with swallowing while the rubber dam is in place.

When dysphagia is exacerbated by conditions such as rhinitis or upper respiratory tract infections, a simple rescheduling of the appointment may be sufficient. If not, the patient may better tolerate the appointment in an erect or semierect position.

Another condition meriting special attention is the patient with hemiparesis in which the ability to close one eyelid on the deficit side is impaired. This is common in the patient with Bell's palsy. When this condition occurs, the patient's eye must be protected from both drying and from aerosols and debris. This can be accomplished with the

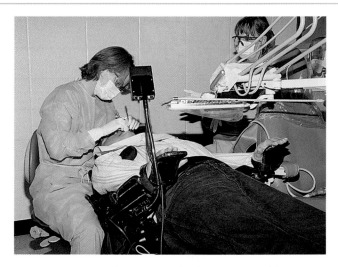

FIG. 41-3 Patient being treated in his own wheelchair. Note self-contained headrest.

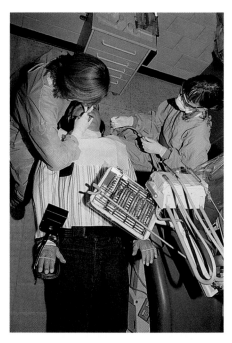

FIG. 41-4 Over-the-patient delivery system by A-DEC (A-DEC, Inc., Newbury, Ore.)

placement of a damp gauze over the open eye, using care to not touch the eyeball itself. The patient may also have his or her own eyedrops or ointment to keep the eye moistened.

When movement of other structures such as the tongue, lips, or jaw is a problem, various devices are available to keep the dental arches open and steady. Bite blocks, or mouth props, or tongue and cheek protectors may be helpful.

Muscle Tone

Abnormal changes in muscle tone contribute to deficits in motor control. Muscle tone may be increased (hypotonia) or decreased (hypertonia) beyond what is considered normal. An increase in muscle tone with a corresponding increase in reflexes and a velocity-dependent resistance to passive stretch is often referred to clinically as *spasticity*.[7,23] The type and degree of abnormal muscle tone varies widely among patients with neurological deficits; however, functional activities are consistently affected by any abnormal changes in tone.

MUSCULOSKELETAL DEFICITS

Definition

Musculoskeletal refers to the interaction of the muscular and skeletal systems of the body.[7] Because these two systems are intimately related, a deficit or problem in one system directly affects the functioning of the other system. For example, an imbalance in the tone or strength of antagonistic muscles may produce range-of-motion deficits. Musculoskeletal deficits in patients with neurological diagnoses may be exhibited in a variety of forms, including decreased flexibility, soft tissue contractures, joint contractures, and skeletal deformities such as scoliosis.

Any deficit in the musculoskeletal system affects the ability of the patient to move efficiently and to perform functional activities. A skeletal deficit may also contribute to integumentary complications caused by excessive pressure on the bony prominences as a result of poor positioning or poor posture in the bed or wheelchair.

Deficits in the musculoskeletal system may be observed in patients with the diagnoses of stroke, brain injury, CP, Parkinson's disease, SCI, spina bifida, MS, ALS, AD (late-stage), and MD.

Level of Severity

The level of severity of musculoskeletal dysfunction is assessed through range-of-motion measurements, flexibility tests, radiographs, postural observation, muscle tone evaluation, muscle strength tests, sensory tests, reflex tests, and observation of functional activities.[23,25]

Treatment Modalities

Deficits in the musculoskeletal system may be addressed through therapeutic and medical measures, depending on the specific cause of the problem. For example, an increase in muscle tone as a result of upper motor neuron or lower motor neuron damage may be addressed through medication, range-of-motion exercises, and appropriate positioning.

Delivery of Dental Care

Musculoskeletal impairments may occur in such a variety of forms that the dental clinician must carefully assess each patient on an individual basis. In mild cases, the orofacial area may be totally unaffected, in which case the clinician may only need to be cognizant of a patient's other concerns, such as ambulation or the existence of any pressure points.

In cases where the orofacial area is moderately affected, numerous bite blocks, props, and positioning devices are available to maintain the jaws in an open and steady posi-

tion while reducing fatigue of the patient's muscles of mastication. Where muscle spasticity is a concern, aspiration devices and retractors are available to protect the patient's tongue, cheeks, and other soft tissues from sharp dental instruments. In more severe cases, in which the spasticity is pronounced and constant, a consultation with the patient's physician is needed to determine which, if any, pharmacological agents (e.g., muscle relaxants) might be safely administered along with their appropriate dosages and sequence.

 Case Application

Mr. Crosswell occasionally experiences muscle spasms in his extremities. These spasms usually last from a few seconds to approximately a minute. He reports that this usually occurs when his dietary intake has been altered and his electrolyte balance has been disrupted. The spasms are sometimes sufficient to vibrate his oral cavity area. Whenever this occurs during a dental appointment, a pause in treatment is usually adequate.

RESPIRATORY DEFICITS

Definition

Respiration is defined as the process of inspiration, where oxygen is taken into the lungs, and expiration, where carbon dioxide and water is expelled from the lungs. In humans, the **respiratory** process is controlled through the diaphragm, which is innervated by cervical spinal segments C3 to C5. Although the diaphragm is the primary respiratory muscle, the abdominal, intercostal, and other accessory muscles also assist in this function.[7,23,34]

Level of Severity

Respiratory function is evaluated through pulmonary function tests such as tidal volume, inspiratory reserve volume, and vital capacity. In addition, evaluation of range of motion, muscle strength (especially of the respiratory muscles), posture, and exercise tolerance may be conducted.[23,25]

A wide range of diagnoses may affect the respiratory function of a patient, including brain injury, Parkinson's disease, SCI, spina bifida, MS, ALS, AD (late stage), and MD. For example, a patient with a spinal cord lesion above the level of C4 requires the use of mechanical assistance to breathe.

The presence of any respiratory difficulty adversely affects the patient's ability to perform mobility and ADLs. The patient may exhibit shortness of breath, decreased endurance, excessive fatigue, or difficulty with verbal communication. In addition, the patient may complain of difficulty with sleeping, concentrating, or participating in routine activities.[23,25]

Treatment Modalities

Respiratory disorders may be addressed through pharmacological measures, respiratory therapy, or a combination of both. The diagnoses and the prognosis for recovery determine the treatment of choice. Depending on the diagnosis, the need for continued respiratory care may gradually decline as the patient improves.[23]

Delivery of Dental Care

Respiratory problems are common in the dental setting. Even patients with ideal health often experience breathing difficulties that stem from dental anxiety. Elevated respiratory rates, hyperventilation, and other physiological changes may affect almost anyone. However, this respiratory difficulty may become critical in the patient with existing respiratory problems.

Fortunately, nitrous oxide (oxygen analgesia) and sedation calm the anxious patient, and most modern nitrous systems also deliver a minimum of 30% oxygen (compared with only approximately 21% oxygen in ambient air). This, along with the sedative effect of nitrous oxide, reduces the oxygen demand on the patient and reduces the respiratory rate. Whether coupled with nitrous oxide or not, an emergency oxygen-delivery system should be available in any dental office. An *E*-size cylinder is recommended. It provides 30 minutes of oxygen and is portable.[13] An Ambu bag with a clear mouth and nose mask and linkage to pure oxygen is also recommended.

If anesthetic is to be injected in the course of treatment, the clinician should always use care to avoid an intravascular injection and carefully consider the possible consequences of agent or vasoconstrictor overdose. For most patients with respiratory problems, however, the use of a vasoconstrictor is not an absolute contraindication.

If the level of respiratory difficulty is sufficient to require a respirator, a medical consultation is indicated before the selection and use of a local anesthetic. Some respirator manufacturers supply equipment that is sufficiently portable to allow the patient a fair degree of mobility, in which case the patient may be treated in the dental office. In cases where the respirator is not portable, several dental specialty companies manufacture dental delivery systems and radiograph equipment that is portable, thus allowing for home or institutional treatment of the patient.[15]

Case Application

Mr. Crosswell initially depended on a respirator. Over time, and with respiratory therapy and determination, he was able to "wean off" of the respirator. Currently, his only assistive respiration requirement is to have his primary caregiver use an Ambu bag to initiate air exchange each morning before the patient arises into a sitting position and is transferred to his wheelchair. This is necessary to avoid orthostatic hypotension or a feeling of "light-headedness." If dental procedures are prolonged, a change in position is appropriate every 20 to 30 minutes.

BOWEL AND BLADDER DYSFUNCTION

Definition

Problems with control of the bladder or bowel are most often referred to as *incontinence,* which is defined as the inability to prevent leakage or excretion of body fluids.[7] Incontinence, although a significant inconvenience that may produce psychosocial disturbances for patients, may also result in serious medical problems. Kidney damage, decubitus ulcers, and autonomic dysreflexia (in persons with spinal cord injuries) may result from incontinence.[34]

Level of Severity

The level of severity for bladder or bowel dysfunction may be described in several ways. The number of episodes of urinary or bowel incontinence per day or per hour may be recorded. This documentation allows the patient or caregiver to monitor changes in patient status.

Urinary incontinence may be classified as stress incontinence, urge incontinence, overflow incontinence, or mixed incontinence. Stress incontinence occurs with an increase in intraabdominal pressures such as coughing or laughing, whereas urge incontinence is a strong desire to urinate combined with an uncontrolled release of urine. Overflow incontinence is caused by an overly distended bladder and an inability to prevent urine leakage. Mixed incontinence is a combination of any of the types described.

Treatment Modalities

Deficits in bowel and bladder control may be exhibited in patients with the diagnoses of spina bifida, stroke, brain injury, CP, SCI, MS, and AD. Patients are given many options for the control of bladder or bowel incontinence. Patients with bladder incontinence may use intermittent catheterization, external catheters, training programs, or, as a last resort, padding to prevent medical complications. Patients with bowel dysfunction may use a bowel management program, digital stimulation, and diet to prevent medical complications. Medications are available to assist in these areas but are usually used when no other means of control has been effective.[12,34]

Delivery of Dental Care

A wide variety of conditions may lead to problems with bladder and bowel continence. In more severe cases the patient may be outfitted with a urinary tract catheter and collection device (usually a leg bag) and/or a colostomy and collection device. In less severe cases, simple absorbent liners within undergarments may suffice. In either case, the patient can generally be treated fairly routinely with attention to a few "common sense" guidelines.

Because bowel and bladder continence problems are often considered somewhat delicate subjects, the provider must approach the subject professionally and maintain a sense of confidentiality. Once a problem is apparent, the provider should determine factors such as the appropriate treatment interval, time of day for the appointment, dietary precautions, and any precipitating factors that could trigger an episode of incontinence. During ambulation or transport, the patient equipped with any collection device or catheter must be kept free of snagging or kinking of lines or tubes.

Furthermore, any collection bags or devices should not be allowed to get into any position (e.g., a leg bag higher than the bladder) that would impede gravitational drainage of urine. This becomes more obvious when—for ergonomic reasons pertaining to the clinician—modern dental treatment often places the patient's head at or even slightly lower than the body and feet (similar to the Trendelenburg position).

Incontinence is surprisingly common among small children who are unimpaired; thus a vinyl type of chair covering is usually preferred to fabric. If fabric is the only material available, a plastic or vinyl sheet may be placed over the chair before seating the patient. Similarly the operatory should have noncarpeted floors for ease in cleaning and overall sanitation and disinfection.

Case Application

Mr. Crosswell wears an internal urinary catheter and a leg bag for collection. Bowel incontinence is almost never a problem. By maintaining the leg bag in a slightly lower position than the bladder and monitoring its contents and collection capacity, routine care is relatively simple. A simple valve allows for draining of the bag. Careful attention is given so that the tubes leading to the bag remain free from any snagging or crimps that would impede drainage.

INTEGUMENTARY DEFICITS

Definition

The *integumentary* system functions in the protection of the body, primarily to preserve the necessary fluids required for efficient cellular activity and to protect from the environment. In addition, the skin serves as an organ of excretion through the sebaceous and sweat glands and also assists with temperature regulation and sensation.[7] A lack of skin integrity, also referred to as *skin breakdown,* is a complication of a wide range of diagnoses, including those presented in this chapter.

Level of Severity

A deficit in the integumentary system may be exhibited in a range from a small laceration to a decubitus ulcer. A decubitus ulcer, often called a *pressure sore* or *bedsore,* may be defined as one of four stages or grades. Grade 1 indicates superficial damage to the epidermis and dermal layers, whereas Grade 4 refers to damage of the soft tissue to the depth of the bone (Box 41-1).[25]

Because a pressure sore can begin within only a few minutes but requires an extensive amount of time to heal, it is important to avoid prolonged pressure on any bony prominence. The patient is at greater risk of developing a decubitus ulcer if there is an absence or impairment of tactile, proprioceptive, and pressure sensations. A reduction in activity and mobility skills and cognitive impairment may also contribute to decubitus ulcer development.[23,25,34]

BOX 41-1

Grades of Skin Breakdown

Grade I: Superficial damage to epidermal and dermal layers

Grade 2: Damage to epidermal and dermal layers, adipose tissue

Grade 3: Damage to epidermal and dermal layers, adipose tissue and muscle

Grade 4: Damage to soft tissues to depth of bone, may include bone

---

Treatment Modalities

The most effective method to treat any deficit in skin integrity is prevention. Prevention may be accomplished through daily, even hourly, skin checks for redness, bruises, or lacerations and through appropriate patient positioning in the bed or wheelchair. Pressure relief, also called *raises,* should be performed every 30 to 60 minutes if the patient is sitting to allow the blood to flow to those areas with increased pressure. Treatment following the development of a reduction in skin integrity may include hydrotherapy with wound care, electrical stimulation, or the administration of hyperbaric oxygen. All effective treatment programs include prevention and positioning.[23,25,34]

Delivery of Dental Care

Patients who are confined to a bed or wheelchair are at risk for developing bedsores. The practitioner should keep this in mind because recent dental trends are toward longer dental procedures. Additionally, when treating patients with multiple problems, including difficulty in getting to a dental office, the provider may feel a sense of urgency to accomplish a lot during the patient's scheduled appointment, thus extending the appointment duration. The provider could thus unwittingly exacerbate an existing or prior condition or even initiate a new one. The patient may be aware of existing pressure point areas that are problematic and thus can inform the provider of positions to avoid.

Treatment is generally practiced through accommodation with special pillows, blankets, or other supports along with frequent position changes (raises) as needed. Occasionally, a patient may require treatment in the semi-supine or fully upright position (e.g., some cases of spina bifida). Treatment considerations such as protection of the constantly open eye have been addressed in this chapter's section on neuromuscular deficits.

COGNITIVE AND PERCEPTUAL DEFICITS

Definition

Cognition is defined as the thinking, learning, and memory processes required for knowledge, whereas perception is defined as the ability to recognize and interpret an object. Patients with cognitive or perceptual deficits may have diagnoses such as stroke, brain injury, CP, MS (late-stage), hydrocephalus, AD, or autism.[7,23]

Patients with cognitive deficits may exhibit confusion; lack of orientation to person, place, or time; and decreased attention span. The patient may also demonstrate difficulty in processing information, which may be further complicated by impaired memory.[5,23,25,33]

Patients with impaired perception may exhibit unilateral neglect or inattention to one side of the body. Deficits in body image and visuospatial orientation are also common, including deficits in right-left discrimination, vertical disorientation, somatagnosia, or ideomotor apraxia.[5,23,,25,33]

Level of Severity

The severity of cognitive or perceptual deficits is usually determined through an evaluation by an occupational therapist, speech-language pathologist, or neuropsychologist. The evaluation includes multiple extensive tests to determine the extent of the deficits and how the deficits affect daily functioning. The dental hygienist, however, may perform general testing to determine the patient's short-term memory, attention span, and basic perceptions (Box 41-2).

Treatment Modalities

Treatment of cognitive and perceptual deficits may be conducted by occupational therapists, speech-language pathologists, or neuropsychologists, among others.

Delivery of Dental Care

Cognitive and perceptual deficits are relatively common in the dental setting. Such deficits may range from the more rare cases of severe disorders to the more common cases of patients not being able to accommodate the clinician by complying with simple requests such as "open" and "close" or by confusing "left" and "right."

In instances where minor problems are evident, patience and empathy on the part of the provider may be all that is required. In severe cases, a consultation with an occupational therapist, speech-language therapist, and/or the patient's neuropsychologist may be necessary.

 Case Application

Mr. Crosswell did not exhibit any cognitive or perceptual deficits.

VISUAL DEFICITS

Definition

Visual deficits may be caused by damage to the eye, to the pathways from the eye, or to the brain resulting in difficulties in the reception, transmission, and interpretation of the array. Visual deficits may include visual field cuts (i.e., one area of the visual field is no longer seen or

recognized), diplopia, double vision, and poor visual acuity (secondary to a reduction in oculomotor control).[23]

Level of Severity

The severity of visual deficits is usually determined through an examination by an occupational therapist or ophthalmologist.

Treatment Modalities

The wide variety of patients with visual deficits occurring in the dental setting dictates a wide variety of treatment considerations. Partially sighted or unsighted patients may require differing levels of assistance in getting to and around the office and in being seated.

Delivery of Dental Care

Once treatment has begun, care should be used to avoid any further damage by the high-intensity dental light as it is focused and directed in the facial area. Care must also be used to shield the eyes of both the clinician and patient from the dental "curing light" if sealants, composites, bonding agents, or certain liners and bases are used. This light is not only extremely high in intensity but also has a characteristic wavelength that must be filtered with an amber-colored translucent shield to prevent retinal damage.

If dental radiographs are to be taken, extra care should be used to shield the lens of the eye because it is radiosensitive and cataract formation is linked to radiograph exposure.[11] This can be accomplished with careful placement of the beam (central ray) and adequate collimation (elimination of any part of the beam with undesired direction) through lead-lined "collimators." This should be a matter of routine for all patients, but it bears special mention because the patient with visual deficits is so dependent on the remaining level of sight.

The clinician should also establish whether the visual deficit involves any special problems such as diplopia, field cuts, or loss of eye movement. This is important for two reasons. First, the clinician must accommodate certain visual handicaps whenever a demonstration or "show, tell, do" is involved. Second, home-care instructions may have to be modified so the patient can adequately administer and modify the home care.

The patient with visual deficits may also require slightly more time for explanations. In instances where a cosmetic component of the procedure is to be highlighted, the opinion of a trusted primary caregiver may be highly valuable.

COMMUNICATION DEFICITS

Definition

Communication is defined as "an exchange of information between individuals using symbol systems such as spoken language or writing."[7] Communication may be accomplished through verbal or written means or through gestures and augmentative communication devices.

A deficit in communication may occur in diagnoses such as stroke, brain injury, CP, Parkinson's disease, MS, ALS, AD, Bell's palsy, MD, or autism. When there is dam-

---

BOX 41-2

General Testing for Cognitive and Perceptual Impairments

Level of alertness: Does patient observe or interact with the environment or other people?
Is patient lethargic or agitated?
Level of attention: How long does patient attend to an activity without being easily distracted?
Does patient attend to some activities and not to others?
Level of memory: Does patient respond appropriately to biographical questions?
Is patient able to recall the steps to a specific activity, such as preparing to brush the teeth?
Level of perception: Does patient ignore one side of the body or any part of the body?
Does patient demonstrate awkwardness when performing an activity of which he or she is capable?
Does patient confuse directions, such as *left* and *right* or *up* and *down*?

age to the central nervous system (CNS), the difficulty in communication is caused by brain damage. This may result in expressive aphasia, receptive aphasia, global aphasia, word-finding deficits, and an overall reduction in language skills. The patient may also demonstrate difficulty with communication caused by oral-motor deficits resulting in dysarthria. Although the mechanism of the deficit varies among the diagnoses, the results are similar. The patient demonstrates difficulty or an inability to understand written or spoken language and is unable to make desires and needs known to others.[14,23]

Level of Severity

The severity of communication deficits is determined through an extensive evaluation by a speech-language pathologist.

Treatment Modalities

Treating a patient with communicative deficits can be challenging. Hopefully, a primary caregiver will be able to provide the clinician with an overview of the nature of the deficit and coping modalities that work best.

Delivery of Dental Care

If the problem focuses more on dysarthria (impaired ability to articulate clearly), the use of pencil and paper, a letter (or picture) board, or a primary caregiver (who is more accustomed to the individual's speech) may be all that is necessary. If, however, the deficit relates to an inability of the patient to receive communication input (e.g., deafness, blindness), more extensive strategies may need to be used. In these more complex situations, the assistance of the primary caregiver, family, or friends may again prove invaluable. These persons may have developed or have access to someone with special communication skills (e.g., "signing"). Consulting with a speech-language pathologist may also be required.

Case Application

Mr. Crosswell has no difficulty with normal verbal communication, although he pauses often to breathe. He signs papers, such as consent forms, with an ordinary ballpoint pen held between his teeth (Fig. 41-5). Plastic pens are preferable to metal ones because they presumably cause less occlusal (and subsequent periodontal) trauma in the anterior region of the mouth and are easy to sanitize. The patient is able to communicate with others through the telephone and computer with the use of a custom-fitted mouthstick.

MOBILITY DEFICITS

Definition

Mobility may be defined as functional activities that are used throughout the course of the day. These activities include bed mobility, transfers to all surfaces, wheelchair propulsion, ambulation, and balance in both sitting and standing. Bed mobility includes the ability to roll to either side, come to a sitting position, return to a supine or side-lying position, and assume the prone position. Transfers to the bed, chair, wheelchair, bathtub, toilet, or car may be

accomplished through a stand pivot, sit pivot, sliding board, or mechanical lift transfer. A patient with a neurological deficit may use a wheelchair for mobility within the home or community or may be able to ambulate with or without an assistive device. Regardless of the mode of transportation, the patient must be able to negotiate level and unlevel surfaces to be functional. Balance in both the sitting and standing positions is required for safe and efficient performance of ADLs.[23-26,34]

Level of Severity

The level of severity or level of assistance required during mobility activities may be specified on a scale of 1 to 7, ranging from total dependence to total independence. Level 1, total dependence, indicates that the patient requires the assistance of another person to perform mobility activities. Level 7, total independence, indicates that the patient does not require the use of another person nor an assistive device for safe and efficient performance of mobility activities. Each of the levels in between refers to the level of assistance required based on the amount of effort expended by the patient and the caregiver.

Treatment Modalities

The physical therapist and occupational therapist address deficits in mobility activities through functional activity.

Delivery of Dental Care

Mobility deficits have been considered throughout this chapter. This impairment has been addressed from the broadest approach possible, such as transport to and from the dental office, to mobility issues of getting in and out of the dental chair.

Case Application

Mr. Crosswell is an example of a level 1 (totally dependent) mobility deficit. He requires assistance for essentially all functions. Despite these obstacles, his case demonstrates that routine in-office dental care and home hygiene are possible with minimal accommodation on the part of the provider.

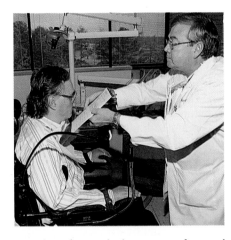

FIG. 41-5 Patient shown signing consent form using plastic pen held between teeth.

CRITICAL THINKING ACTIVITIES

1. Discuss the advantages and disadvantages of a custom-fitted mouthstick for a quadriplegic patient (as opposed to a "stock" flat, plastic wafer type of mouthstick).
2. Working in small groups of two to five, devise a hypothetical treatment plan to deliver dental hygiene supportive care services to patients with selected impairments with differing levels of severity. Have each group present its case and plan to the other groups for critique. Use either the specific disorders discussed in the chapter (e.g., stroke, autism) or the manifestations of such disorders (e.g., neuromuscular, respiratory) to guide your selection.
3. Arrange to visit a special needs patient care facility such as a nursing home, special needs day-care facility, or behavioral healthcare facility to observe the techniques used in transportation and patient care. If this is not possible, ask a professional staff member to address the class.
4. Work in pairs (one student as the provider, one as the patient) and role-play selected scenarios in a preclinical setting. The impairment selected for each student should be researched and presented by the student to the class before the preclinical exercise.

REVIEW QUESTIONS

1. Your patient had a stroke 4 years ago and is stable but has difficulty keeping her mouth open for more than a few seconds at a time. Additionally, her mandible occasionally moves involuntarily. Which of the following presents your best first option to address these problems?
   a. Consider administering muscle relaxants to the patient
   b. Refer the patient to a specialist
   c. Obtain a medical consult
   d. Use a mouth prop
   e. Shorten the visit
2. A patient with severe scoliosis related to spina bifida has scheduled a supportive care appointment. The receptionist noted that when the patient made the appointment, she reported that she had recently developed difficulties with decubitus ulcers. Which of the following actions should you perform during this patient's appointment to prevent decubitus ulcers?
   a. Minimize the time the patient is seated in the treatment room chair
   b. Ensure that the patient will freely communicate any positioning discomfort
   c. Alter the patient's position to another comfortable position at least every 30 to 60 minutes
   d. All the above
   e. None of the above
3. You are about to treat a patient with a high level (C-5) spinal cord injury who has difficulty breathing freely. This condition is aggravated from a long history of heavy smoking before his injury and a resulting nagging and persistent cough. Your treatment calls for radiographs, debridement, polishing, and a periodic examination. Which of the following treatments is relatively *contraindicated*?
   a. Topical fluoride
   b. Rubber cup prophylaxis
   c. Air polishing
   d. Subgingival irrigation
   e. Any of these treatments is acceptable.

4. You are planning to debride a patient's maxillary right quadrant. Because of the heavy deposits, patient sensitivity, and length of the last visit to treat another quadrant (more than 2 hours), local anesthesia will be used. The patient has an in-dwelling catheter and leg bag and takes "fluid pills" that his physician gives him for mild hypertension. Which of the following precautions might you wish to exercise?
   a. Reposition the patient every 15 to 20 minutes
   b. Check the leg bag every 15 to 20 minutes
   c. Reschedule the patient for two shorter appointments.
   d. Avoid elevating the leg bag higher than the hips and watch for kinks in the drain line kink
   e. Treat the patient in an upright position
5. You are disappointed that your older adult patient is not keeping up with her oral self-care, specifically her daily brushing and flossing. She reports that she "forgets a lot." Which of the following options should you choose?
   a. Include a primary caregiver (such as a spouse or family member if possible) in the case and especially in the self-care instructions
   b. Repeat the instructions several times
   c. Ask the patient to repeat the instructions to you
   d. Schedule the patient for bimonthly recalls
   e. All the above
6. A patient mentions that she has had several operations, procedures, and medications prescribed in the past few years for cataract formations. Which of the following dental procedures call for special precautions?
   a. Radiograph exposure
   b. Administration of local anesthesia with vasoconstrictor
   c. Full-mouth probing
   d. Air polishing
   e. Use of latex gloves

REVIEW QUESTIONS—cont'd

7. As you introduce yourself to a new patient and review his patient registration and health history, you become convinced that he suffers from dysarthria, possibly related to the loss of orofacial muscle coordination that you observe. The patient reports having a serious automobile accident with brain damage and significant facial asymmetry and scarring. Which of the following actions should you perform as a first step in effectively communicating with this patient?
   a. Ask questions that can be responded to with a simple "yes" or "no"
   b. Give the patient a pencil and notepad
   c. Speak clearly and allow the patient more time to respond
   d. None of the above
   e. *a* and *b*
8. You are assisting a dentist in designing and setting up a new dental practice that is located in a retirement community in your area. Features that you should stress include which of the following?
   a. Access ramps for assistive devices such as wheelchairs and walkers
   b. Wider doors
   c. Handicap-designated parking spaces
   d. Dental chairs and delivery systems that allow for treatment of selected patients in their own wheelchairs
   e. All the above

 SUGGESTED AGENCIES AND WEB SITES

Because of the ever-changing nature of the Internet, some of the web sites listed here may have changed since publication. Please refer to Mosby's Evolve web site for the most current information.

Alzheimer's Association: http://www.alz.org
American Heart Association, 77320 Greenville Avenue, Dallas, TX 75231: http://www.americanheart.org
Amyotrophic Lateral Sclerosis Association: http://www.alsa.org
Association for Spinal Bifida and Hydrocephalus: http://www.asbah.org
Autism Society of America: http://www.autism-society.org
Brain Injury Association, Inc: http://www.biausa.org
Centers for Disease Control and Prevention: http://www.cdc.gov
The Hydrocephalus Foundation, Inc.: http://www.hydrocephalus.org
Muscular Dystrophy Association of America: http://www.mdausa.org

National Centers for Facial Paralysis, Inc: http://www.bellspalsy.com
National Institute of Neurological Disorders and Stroke (includes information on stroke and epilepsy): http://www.ninds.nih.gov
National Institutes of Health, 900 Rockville Pike, Bethesda, MD 20892: http://www.nih.gov
National Multiple Sclerosis Society: http://www.nmss.org
National Parkinson Foundation, Inc.: http://www.parkinson.org
National Spinal Cord Injury Association: http://www.spinalcord.org
National Stroke Association, 9707 Easter Lane, Englewood, CO 80112: http://www.stroke.org
Spina Bifida Association of America: http://www.sbaa.org
United Cerebral Palsy Association: http://www.ucpa.org

 ADDITIONAL READINGS AND RESOURCES

Grundy MC, Shaw L, Hamilton DV: *An illustrated guide to dental care for the medically compromised patient,* St Louis, 1993, Mosby.

Wilkins EM: *Clinical practice of the dental hygienist,* ed 8, Philadelphia, 1999, Lippincott Williams & Wilkins.

 REFERENCES

1. Alzheimer's Association: [Internet], Chicago, 1999, The Association [http://www.alz.org].
2. Amyotrophic Lateral Sclerosis Association: [Internet], Calabasas Hills, Calif, 1999, The Association [http://www.alsa.org].
3. Autism Society of America: [Internet], Bethesda, Md, 1999, The Society [http://www.autism-society.org].
4. Bloch R: Autonomic dysfunction. In Bloch R, Basbaum M, editors: *Management of spinal cord injuries,* Baltimore, 1986, Williams & Wilkins.
5. Bouska MJ, Kauffman NA, Marcus SE: Disorders of the visual perceptual system. In Umphred DA: *Neurological rehabilitation,* ed 3, St Louis, 1995, Mosby.
6. Brain Injury Association, Inc.: [Internet], Alexandria, Va, 1999, The Association [http://www.biausa.org].
7. Dirckx JH, editor: *Stedman's concise medical dictionary for the health professions,* ed 3, Baltimore, 1997, Williams & Wilkins.
8. Frankel D: Multiple sclerosis. In Umphred DA: *Neurological rehabilitation,* ed 3, St Louis, 1995, Mosby.
9. Grundy MC, Shaw L, Hamilton DV: *An illustrated guide to dental care for the medically compromised patient,* Aylesbury, England, 1993, Wolfe Publishing.
10. Hollinshead WH: *Textbook of anatomy,* ed 3, Philadelphia, 1974, Harper & Row.

Continued

11. Johnson ON: *Essentials of dental radiography for dental assistants and hygienists,* ed 6, Stamford, Conn, 1999, Appleton & Lange.

12. Kraft C: Bladder and bowel management. In Buchanan LE, Nawoczenski DA, editors: *Spinal cord injury: concepts and management approaches,* Baltimore, 1987, Williams & Wilkins.

13. Malamed SF: *Medical emergencies in the dental office,* ed 5, St Louis, 2000, Mosby.

14. Melnick ME: Basal ganglia disorders: metabolic, hereditary, and genetic disorders in adults. In Umphred DA: *Neurological rehabilitation,* ed 3, St Louis, 1995, Mosby.

15. Murphy JE: *Mobile dentistry,* Tulsa, Okla, 1996, PennWell.

16. Muscular Dystrophy Association of America: [Internet], Tucson, Ariz, 1999, The Association [http://www.mdausa.org].

17. National Centers for Facial Paralysis: [Internet], 1999, The Centers [http://www.bellspalsy.com].

18. National Multiple Sclerosis Society: [Internet], New York, NY, 1999, The Society [http://www.nmss.org].

19. National Parkinson Foundation, Inc: [Internet], Miami, Fla, 1999, The Foundation [http://www.parkinson.org].

20. National Spinal Cord Injury Association: [Internet], Bethesda, Md, 1999, The Association [http://www.spinalcord.org].

21. National Stroke Association: [Internet], Englewood, Colo, 1999, The Association [http://www.stroke.org].

22. Nelson CA: Cerebral palsy. In Umphred DA: *Neurological rehabilitation,* ed 3, St Louis, 1995, Mosby.

23. O'Sullivan SB, Schmitz TJ: *Physical rehabilitation: assessment and treatment,* ed 3, Philadelphia, 2001, FA Davis.

24. Palmer ML, Toms JE: *Manual for functional training,* Philadelphia, 1992, FA Davis.

25. Pauls JA, Reed KL: *Quick reference to physical therapy,* Gaithersburg, Md, 1996, Aspen.

26. Pierson FM: *Principles and techniques of patient care,* Philadelphia, 1994, WB Saunders Company.

27. Roemer MI: *Comparative national policies on health care,* New York, 1997, Marcel Dekker.

28. Rosenthal M et al: *Rehabilitation of the head injured adult,* Philadelphia, 1985, FA Davis Company.

29. Ryerson SJ: *Hemiplegia resulting from vascular insult or disease.* In Umphred DA: *Neurological rehabilitation,* ed 3, St Louis, 1995, Mosby.

30. Schneider FJ: Traumatic spinal cord injury. In Umphred DA: *Neurological rehabilitation,* ed 3, St Louis, 1995, Mosby.

31. Schneider JW: Congential spinal cord injury. In Umphred DA: *Neurological rehabilitation,* ed 3, St Louis, 1995, Mosby.

32. Shi LDA, Singh DA: *Delivering health care in America: a systems approach,* ed 2, Gaithersburg, Md, 2001, Aspen.

33. Simmons NN: Disorders in oral, speech, and language function. In Umphred DA: *Neurological rehabilitation,* ed 3, St Louis, 1995, Mosby.

34. Somers MF: *Spinal cord injury: functional rehabilitation,* Upper Saddle River, NJ, 2001, Prentice Hall.

35. Spina Bifida Association of America: [Internet], Washington, DC, 1999, The Association [http://www.sbaa.org].

36. Sultz HA, Young KM: *Health Care USA: understanding its organization and delivery,* ed 2, Gaithersburg, Md, 1999, Aspen.

37. The Hydrocephalus Foundation, Inc: [Internet], Sangus, Mass, 1999, The Foundation [http://www.hydrocephalus.org].

38. United Cerebral Palsy Association: [Internet], Washington, DC, 1999, The Association [http://www.ucpa.org]

CHAPTER 42

Hormonal Imbalances

Michelle G. Klenk

Chapter Outline

Case Studies: Hormonal Considerations
   in the Female Dental Patient
Female Sex Hormones
   Estrogen and progesterone
   Effects on oral flora
Clinical Manifestations
   Puberty
   Menstruation

Pregnancy
Oral contraceptives
Menopause
Hormone Replacement Therapy
Osteoporosis
Dental Hygiene Supportive Care Plan

Key Terms

Burning mouth syndrome
Estrogen
Hormone replacement
  therapy (HRT)

Menopause
Oral contraceptives (OCs)
Osteoporosis
Perimenopause

Postmenopause
Pregnancy
Pregnancy gingivitis

Progesterone
Puberty
Puberty gingivitis

Learning Outcomes

1. Appreciate the role of hormones in the oral health of the female patient.
2. Describe physiological actions of estrogen and progesterone.
3. Relate systemic effects of hormones to oral health.

4. Identify clinical manifestations of female hormonal changes.
5. Develop appropriate preventive and therapeutic dental hygiene care plans for female patients.
6. Relate female life stages to clinical oral manifestations.

The influence of sex hormones on the oral health of the female has been recognized for many years. Early studies on the effects of hormones on gingivitis during puberty and pregnancy showed an exacerbated gingival response in the presence of bacterial plaque. The role of the dental hygienist in treatment of the female patient is important in recognizing hormonal effects and educating the patient regarding management of clinical manifestations related to hormonal release or hormonal therapies in the form of oral contraceptives or hormone replacement therapy.[3,13,17]

As the age of puberty onset in females decreases and as the number of postmenopausal women increases, the dental hygienist will treat an increasing number of patients who may be influenced by hormonal imbalances.

FEMALE SEX HORMONES

Girls begin to develop reproductive organs and secondary 42-A sex characteristics during *puberty*, usually between ages 9 and 16, and start to ovulate and develop a regular menstrual cycle. The menstrual cycle is controlled by the release of female sex hormones. These hormones regulate the release of the ovum from the ovaries and prepare the uterus for implantation of a fertilized ovum. If fertilization does not occur, the hormones cause a shedding of the uterine lining, which is the *menses*. This cycle lasts 28 days, with variation from 22 to 34 days (Fig. 42-1).

Hormonal imbalances may alter the female patient's established menstrual cycle. *Pregnancy* may be the most common condition associated with hormonal imbalances.

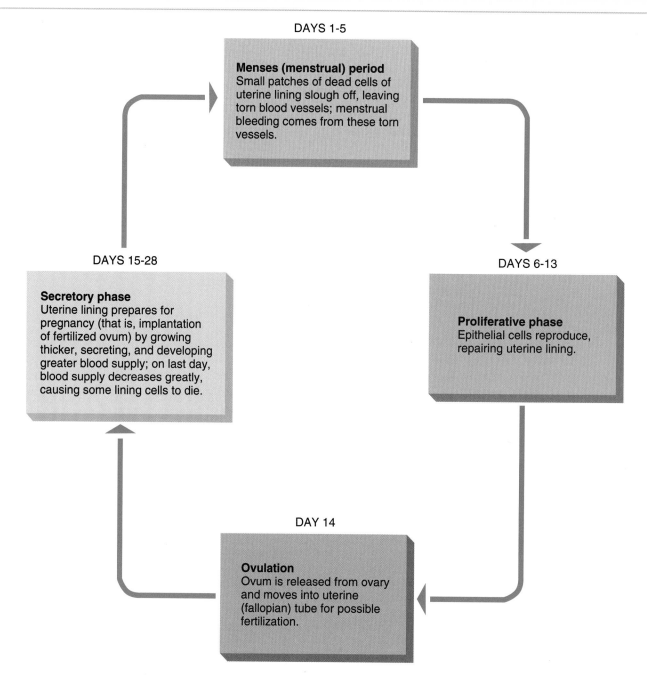

FIG. 42-1 The 28-day menstrual cycle. (Modified from Thibodeau GA, Patton KT: *The human body in health and disease,* ed 3, St Louis, 2002, Mosby.)

Hormonal Considerations in the Female Dental Patient

Case 1: Supportive Care and the Menopausal Patient

Your 10 AM appointment is Theda Ledbetter, a 51-year-old female patient who works at the local college as an academic administrator. She presents for a 6-month supportive care appointment. Ms. Ledbetter reports no changes in her health history but warns you that she may "heat up your chair" during treatment. She has an appointment with her gynecologist next week to discuss hormone replacement therapies. Her oral examination reveals no abnormal findings.

Case 2: Supportive Care and the Pregnant Patient

Roxy Novatna, a 23-year-old female patient, presents for a 6-month supportive care appointment and reports that she is 4 months pregnant. She says that she is feeling well and is pleased that her morning sickness has subsided. Ms. Novatna admits that her normally meticulous oral hygiene has been poor for the past few months because she has had difficulty getting her toothbrush into the posterior portions of her mouth without gagging. An oral examination reveals red, edematous, bleeding gingiva in the posterior sextants.

The female body undergoes many changes during pregnancy that result in significant systemic and oral effects. The woman who uses *oral contraceptives (OCs)* will experience hormonal imbalances similar to those in pregnancy. The hormones contained in OCs act to inhibit the release of the ovum from the ovary, thereby preventing fertilization.

As females approach midlife, hormonal imbalances become evident in the cessation of menstruation and presentation of various symptoms indicative of the changing hormone levels during perimenopause and menopause. Some females choose **hormone replacement therapy (HRT)** to control symptoms such as vaginal dryness, hot flashes, and increased urinary frequency and urgency.

ESTROGEN AND PROGESTERONE

Female sex hormones include **estrogen** and **progesterone.** Estrogens are responsible for cyclical changes in the vaginal epithelium and endometrium of the uterus and for the development of female sex characteristics. Hormonal fluctuations are evident at the onset of puberty or adolescence, when the girl begins to develop sex organs and secondary sex characteristics and begins menstruating and ovulating. A natural pattern of estrogen and progesterone levels occurs throughout the woman's reproductive life (Fig. 42-2).[25]

During the menstrual cycle, estrogen levels peak at ovulation and decrease during the second half of the cycle. Progesterone is responsible for changes in the endometrium in preparation for implantation of the fertilized egg and development of the placenta and mammary glands. Progesterone levels remain stable until after ovulation occurs.[20]

As women approach ages 35 to 58, hormonal changes become evident as estrogen and progesterone levels decrease. When low hormone levels result in a cessation of menstruation, the woman is in **menopause.** The period before complete cessation of menstruation is termed **perimenopause.** During this time, approximately between ages 31 and 44, many females experience symptoms of hormonal imbalance, including irregular menstrual cycles and decreased bleeding. **Postmenopause** is the period when the woman has reached the end of her reproductive cycle.[13]

EFFECTS ON ORAL FLORA

Hormonal imbalances affect the oral cavity by changing the microflora of the gingival sulcus and altering the types of bacteria that grow in plaque. These changes result in plaque that is more likely to produce gingival disease.[9,18] Effects of the female sex hormones on the oral microflora include dilated capillaries, regulated cellular proliferation, decreased keratinization, increased vascular permeability, and increased production of gingival crevicular fluid.[6,15] These changes result in clinical manifestations of increased bleeding response and gingivitis in the absence of large amounts of bacterial plaque.

The inflammatory response is further affected through an increase in the periodontal pathogens *Porphyromonas gingivalis* and *Actinobacillus actinomycetemcomitans.* An increase in prostaglandin E also serves as a mediator for inflammation.[15] Progesterone and estrogen have also been shown to influence the immune system by depressing neutrophil chemotaxis and phagocytosis as well as antibody and T-cell responses.[11] Progesterone alters both the rate and the pattern of collagen production in the gingiva, resulting in a reduced ability to repair and maintain the structure of the gingiva.[26]

Microbes that are allowed to multiply as a result of this effect include gram negative anaerobes such as *Prevotella intermedia,* which has the ability to substitute estrogen and progesterone for vitamin K, thereby affecting the individual's blood-clotting ability.[23] An increase in gram-negative *Capnocytophaga* has been documented along with *P. intermedia* as increasing the bleeding tendency during puberty.[6]

CLINICAL MANIFESTATIONS

42-B

PUBERTY

The hormonal imbalances evident during puberty result in an increased incidence of gingivitis. Bacteria in the gingival sulcus act to increase the bleeding tendency and result in an exaggerated response to apparently minor local irritants. **Puberty gingivitis** decreases in severity over time but does not disappear until local irritants are removed. Clinically the gingival tissues appear enlarged, bluish-red, and bulbous (Fig. 42-3).[15]

MENSTRUATION

During the menstrual cycle the level and types of hormones released influence the oral cavity, as evidenced by erythematous swollen gingival tissues, herpes labialis, aphthous ulcers, prolonged hemorrhage after oral surgery, and swollen salivary glands.[16] Patients may not be aware of the correlation between the menstrual cycle and their periodic episodes of these manifestations.

PREGNANCY

Gingivitis has been reported in 30% to 100% of all pregnant women, frequently in the range of 60% to 75%.[4,7] As in gingivitis associated with hormonal imbalances in puberty, **pregnancy gingivitis** manifests in the presence of local irritants with an exaggerated response. During pregnancy, as levels of estrogen and progesterone increase, the periodontal *P. intermedia* bacteria also increase.[9] Gingival changes are most evident between the second and eighth month. Clinically the gingival tissues appear bright red and edematous at the marginal gingiva and interdental papilla, with an increased bleeding tendency.

Some women develop a pyogenic granuloma during pregnancy (Fig. 42-4). This benign lesion sometimes is referred to as a *pregnancy tumor* and should be removed surgically so that the tissue can return to health.

Pregnancy gingivitis decreases in severity after childbirth. However, gingival inflammation remains until irritants are removed.

ORAL CONTRACEPTIVES

Oral contraceptives contain estrogen and progesterone to alter the physiological functioning of the ovaries and

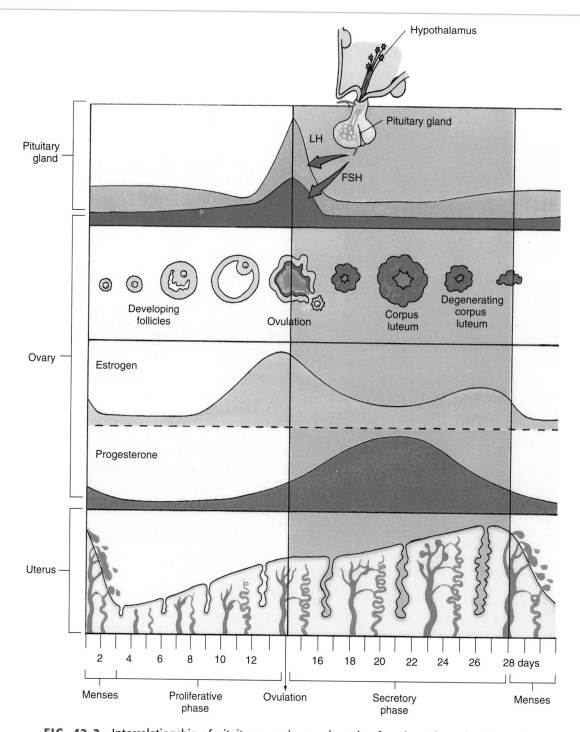

FIG. 42-2 Interrelationship of pituitary, ovarian, and uterine functions throughout a typical 28-day menstrual cycle. Sharp increase in luteinizing hormone *(LH)* causes ovulation, whereas menstruation is initiated by lower levels of progesterone. *FSH,* Follicle-stimulating hormone. (From Thibodeau GA, Patton KT: *The human body in health and disease,* ed 3, St Louis, 2002, Mosby.)

uterus. The oral effects of these hormones, taken as OCs, include two distinct areas of concern. The most common effect is an increase in *gingival inflammation,* similar to that seen in puberty and pregnancy gingivitis. OCs are available in a wide range of formulations combining the two hormones. No correlation exists between the type of progesterone or estrogen used and the level of inflammation. However, the degree of inflammation may be associated with the duration of HRT, with more periodontal destruction evident if OCs are taken longer than 1½ years.[1,8]

The second effect of OC use is an increased incidence of localized *osteitis* after extraction of mandibular third molars.[16] This is attributed to the effects of estrogen on blood-clotting factors. Therefore it is recommended that extractions be performed between days 23 and 28 of the OC cycle because of the lack of estrogen delivered during this time.[19]

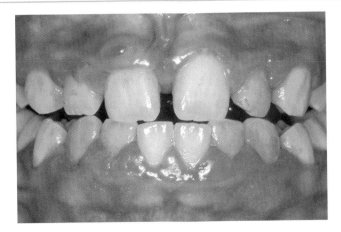

FIG. 42-3 Puberty gingivitis.

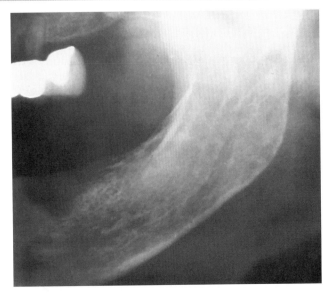

FIG. 42-5 Osteoporosis of the mandible. (From White SC, Pharoah MJ: *Oral radiology: principles and interpretation*, ed 4, St Louis, 2000, Mosby.)

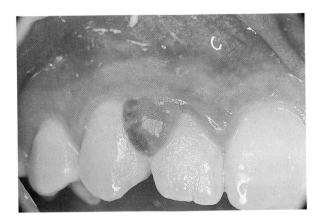

FIG. 42-4 Pyogenic granuloma, also known as a *pregnancy tumor*.

MENOPAUSE

Oral effects of hormonal imbalances associated with menopause may include burning mouth syndrome, dry mouth, menopausal gingivostomatitis, altered taste sensation (salty, peppery, or sour), bone loss, tissue atrophy, pain, and sensitivity to hot and cold.[13,26] A combination of these symptoms has been reported in 20% to 90% of menopausal and postmenopausal women. The use of estrogen replacement therapies appears to alleviate most symptoms.[16,24]

HORMONE REPLACEMENT THERAPY

As the life expectancy of women increases, the number of women living in a postmenopausal state is growing. During this time the decreased amount of estrogen released by the ovaries puts the individual at risk for osteoporosis and cardiovascular disease. HRT has been used to decrease these risks.

Hormone replacement therapy is prescribed in two forms: estrogen replacement therapy and combined HRT. *Estrogen* replacement therapy, although more effective in preventing cardiovascular disease, is prescribed only for women who have had their uterus removed because estrogen alone causes hyperplasia of the uterine lining, leading to endometrial cancer. *Combined* HRT includes both estrogen and progesterone and mimics the normal release of hormones.

OSTEOPOROSIS

Osteoporosis is defined as a reduction in bone mass associated with deformity, fractures, and at times pain. Osteoporosis affects an estimated 25 to 28 million Americans, 80% of whom are women.[14] The effects of hormonal imbalances associated with the menopausal or postmenopausal female focus on the osteoporotic effect on maxillary and mandibular bone.

A correlation exists between systemic osteoporosis and loss of attachment and eventual tooth loss.[5,10,12,22] Estrogen replacement therapy has been shown to protect against osteoporosis and maintain bone density (Fig. 42-5).

DENTAL HYGIENE SUPPORTIVE CARE PLAN

Given the documented effects of hormonal imbalances on the oral cavity of female patients, the dental hygienist must be prepared to develop effective care plans to meet these special needs. In general the hygienist must assess for an exaggerated response to local irritants with resulting gingivitis. This may occur in association with puberty, menstruation, pregnancy, and OC use. A thorough periodontal examination must be completed, including gingival assessment, evaluation of bleeding response, and periodontal probing. The patient should be informed of possible symptoms and the role of hormones in the disease process.

The scheduling of oral surgery procedures is important to consider for the patient taking OCs as well as during certain times in the menstrual cycle. It is recommended that the patient schedule surgical procedures during the nonestrogen days of the cycle or days 23 to 28 of OC use to avoid possible osteitis.

The symptoms associated with a decrease in or the absence of estrogen in menopause present unique treatment planning challenges. The patient reporting altered taste sensations, burning mouth syndrome, dry mouth, or tissue atrophy may require a variety of treatment modalities. Saliva substitutes may be prescribed for the dry mouth symptoms and zinc supplements for taste alterations.

Burning mouth syndrome occurs in a number of patients and presents one of a major treatment challenge. The patient may experience a burning sensation on the tongue or other oral tissues with no clinically evident changes to these tissues. Other contributing factors may include vitamin deficiencies, dentures, candidiasis, and psychological conditions.[2] Spontaneous remission occurs in about half of patients after several years.[21]

With periodontal disease or tooth loss associated with systemic osteoporosis, the dental hygienist must recognize the systemic condition and educate the patient about its oral effects. The patient may not make the connection between the systemic diagnosis and the gradual loss of periodontal attachment.

Dry mouth and tissue atrophy also pose a challenge for the patient with removable prostheses. Attention must be given to proper fit and prevention of sore spots as the oral conditions change over time.

Awareness of the influence hormones have on the oral cavity is essential in identifying causative factors for a wide range of oral manifestations. The dental hygienist must identify these factors and educate the female patient regarding prevention and treatment of oral manifestations.

 CRITICAL THINKING ACTIVITIES

1. Compile a list of common hormone replacement medications and oral contraceptives, and review drug information sheets for oral effects.
2. Interview obstetric/gynecologic physicians and nurses regarding patient education on oral effects of hormonal imbalances.

3. Prepare a dental health education program for a prenatal class related to hormonal imbalances and effects on the oral cavity during pregnancy.

 REVIEW QUESTIONS

1. Which of the following female sex hormones is responsible for changes in the endometrium during the second half of the menstrual cycle?
   a. Estrogen
   b. Progesterone
2. Progesterone affects the health of gingival tissues in which of the following ways?
   a. Dilation of capillaries
   b. Decrease in keratinization
   c. Increase in vascular permeability
   d. Alterations in collagen production
3. Which of the following is characterized by enlarged, bluish red, and bulbous tissue?
   a. Puberty gingivitis
   b. Pregnancy gingivitis

   c. Gingivitis associated with oral contraceptive use
   d. Menopausal gingivostomatitis
4. Which of the following hormone replacement formulations is recommended for women who have had hysterectomies?
   a. Estrogen replacement therapy
   b. Combined hormone replacement therapy
5. Oral surgery procedures should be scheduled during which days of the oral contraceptive cycle?
   a. 7 to 12
   b. 13 to 18
   c. 19 to 22
   d. 23 to 28

 SUGGESTED AGENCIES AND WEB SITES

Because of the ever-changing nature of the Internet, some of the web sites listed here may have changed since publication. Please refer to Mosby's Evolve *web site for the most current information.*

American Academy of Periodontology: http://www.perio.org
American Dental Association: http://www.ada.org
International Association for Dental Research/American Association for Dental Research: http://www.iadr.com

National Institutes of Health: http://www.nih.gov
Society for Women's Health Research:
   http://www.womens-health.org
Women's Oral Health: http://www.womensoralhealth.org

ADDITIONAL READINGS AND RESOURCES

American Dental Association: *Women's oral health issues,* Chicago, 1995, The Association.

American Dental Association: *Women and periodontal disease* [brochure], Chicago, The Association.

Hatch JP et al: Is the use of exogenous estrogen associated with temporomandibular signs and symptoms? *J Am Dent Assoc* 132(3):319-26, 2001.

Shrout M et al: Comparison of morphological measurements extracted from digitized dental radiographs with lumbar and femoral bone mineral density measurements in postmenopausal women, *J Periodontol* 71(3):335-40, 2000.

Tezal M et al: The relationship between bone mineral density and periodontitis in postmenopausal women, *J Periodontol* 71(9): 1492-8, 2000.

REFERENCES

1. Amar S, Chung KM: Influence of hormonal variation on the periodontium of women, *Periodontol* 6:79-87, 1994.
2. Bogetto F et al: Psychiatric comorbidity in patients with burning mouth syndrome, *Psychosom Med* 60(3):378-85, 1998.
3. Cohen LK: Women's health: implications for an agenda for oral health research and education, *J Dent Educ* 57:736-7, 1993.
4. Ferris GM: Alteration in female sex hormones their effect on oral tissues and dental treatment, *Compend Cont Educ Dent* 14(12):1558-70, 1993.
5. Grodstein F et al: Post-menopausal hormone use and tooth loss: a prospective study, *J Am Dent Assoc* 127(3): 370-7, 1996.
6. Gusberti F et al: Changes in subgingival micriobiota during puberty, *J Clin Periodontol* 17:685-92, 1990.
7. Jensen J, Lilijmack W, Bloomquist C: The effect of female sex hormones on subgingival plaque, *J Periodontol* 52:599-602, 1981.
8. Knight GM, Wade AB: The effects of hormonal contraceptives on human periodontium, *J Periodontal Res* 9:18, 1974.
9. Kornman K, Loesche W: The subgingival microflora during pregnancy, *J Periodontal Res* 15:111-22, 1980.
10. Kribbs PJ: Two-year changes in mandibular bone mass in an osteoporotic population, *J Prosthet Dent* 67(5):653-5, 1992.
11. Lopatin DE, Kornman KS, Loesche WJ: Modulation of immunoreactivity to periodontal disease–associated microorganisms during pregnancy, *Infect Immun* 28:713-8, 1980.
12. Mohammad AR et al: The strength of association between systemic postmenopausal osteoporosis and periodontal disease, *Int J Prosthodont* 9(5):479-83, 1996.
13. Murray D, Fried J: Dental hygienists' knowledge of menopause and its potential oral manifestations, *J Dent Hyg* 73: 22-8. 1999.
14. National Institute of Dental Research: *Advances in women's health research,* Bethesda, Md, Society for Women's Health Research.
15. Newman MG, Takei HH, Carranza FA: *Carranza's clinical periodontology,* ed 9, Philadelphia, 2001, WB Saunders.
16. Rose LF: Sex hormonal imbalances, oral manifestations, and dental treatment. In Genco RJ, Goldman HM, Cohen DW, editors: *Contemporary periodontics,* St Louis, 1990, Mosby.
17. Silverton S et al: *Women's health in the dental school curriculum: report of a survey recommendation,* Washington, DC, 1999, Department of Health and Human Services, National Institutes of Health.
18. Soorlyamoorthy M, Gower DB: Hormonal influences on gingival tissue: relationship to periodontal disease, *J Clin Periodontol* 16:201-8, 1989.
19. Sweet JB, Butler DP: Increased incidence of postoperative localized osteitis in mandibular third molar surgery associated with patients using oral contraceptives, *Am J Obstet Gynecol* 127:518, 1977.
20. Thomas CL, editor: *Taber's cyclopedic medical dictionary,* Philadelphia, 1997, FA Davis.
21. Trikkas G et al: Glossodynia: personality characteristics and psychopathology, *Psychother Psychosom* 65(3):163-8, 1996.
22. VanWowern N, Kausen B, Kollerup G: Osteoporosis: a risk factor in periodontal disease, *J Periodontol* 65:1134-8, 1994.
23. Vitlek J et al: Specific estrogen receptors in human gingiva, *J Clin Endocrinol Metab* 54:608-12, 1982.
24. Wardrop RW et al: Oral discomfort at menopause, *Oral Surg Oral Med Oral Pathol* 67:535-40, 1989.
25. Wilkins EM: *Clinical practice of the dental hygienist,* ed 8, Philadelphia, 1999, Lippincott/Williams & Wilkins.
26. Zachariasen R: Oral manifestations of menopause, *Compend Cont Educ Dent* 14:1584-91, 1993.

CHAPTER 43

Mental *and* Emotional Disturbances

Victoria C. Vick

Chapter Outline

Case Study: Fear and Anxiety in the Dental Patient
Definitions and Classification
Anxiety Disorders
    Etiology
    Panic attack
    Panic disorder
    Phobic disorder
    Agoraphobia
    Social phobia
    Specific ("simple") phobias
    Generalized anxiety disorder
    Obsessive-compulsive disorder
    Posttraumatic stress disorder
    Treatment
    Dental considerations
Mood Disorders
    Major depressive disorder
    Bipolar disorder
Personality Disorders
    Cluster A: disorders of "odd" or "eccentric" behavior

Cluster B: disorders of dramatic, emotional, or erratic behavior
Cluster C: disorders involving anxiety and fearfulness
    Treatment
Eating Disorders
    Anorexia nervosa
    Bulimia nervosa
    Dental considerations
Schizophrenia
    Types and onset
    Delusions
    Hallucinations
    Disorganized thinking
    Grossly disorganized behavior
    Catatonic behavior
    Treatment
    Dental considerations

Key Terms

Agoraphobia
Anorexia nervosa
Antisocial personality disorder
Anxiety
Anxiety disorder
Avoidant personality disorder
Bipolar disorder
Bulimia nervosa
Catatonic behavior
Delusions

Dependent personality disorder
Depression
Disorganized thinking
Fear
Generalized anxiety disorder (GAD)
Hallucination
Histrionic personality disorder
Hypomania
Major depression
Mania

Narcissistic personality disorder
Neuroleptic
Obsessions
Obsessive-compulsive disorder (OCD)
Obsessive-compulsive personality disorder
Panic attack
Paranoid personality disorder
Personality disorder
Phobia

Posttraumatic stress disorder (PTSD)
Process schizophrenia
Reactive schizophrenia
Schizoid personality disorder
Schizotypal personality disorder
Social phobia
Stimulus generalization
Worry

Learning Outcomes

1. Recognize certain behaviors associated with mental and emotional disorders.
2. Identify patients who may be at risk of hurting themselves.
3. Learn appropriate ways of relating to individuals with mental and emotional disturbances.
4. Know where to obtain additional information and make appropriate referrals.

5. Identify specific mental disorders and their relevance to oral care.
6. Develop treatment plans that include a mental health assessment.
7. Identify the potential oral side effects of the major neuroleptic medications.
8. Identify distinctive modifications to care based on the type of mental or emotional disorder.

 Case Study   **Fear and Anxiety in the Dental Patient**

The young patient in the reception area, 11-year-old Cissy Holstrom, appears so anxious that you wonder if she might leave before her appointment. Her mother is completing Cissy's health history form and is aggravated at or disinterested in her daughter's anxious state. She gives the form to the receptionist and says that this is the third office they have tried in the past year because "Cissy has just not liked any of the others, and she is afraid of everything. I just hope you can do something with her because this is a real problem taking her to all these appointments." The mother is irritated by the inconvenience to *her*. She says that she has another appointment and will be back to pick up Cissy.

When you take Cissy into the treatment room, she is very quiet, almost tearful. She approaches the room cautiously but is trying to cooperate. When she is seated, you realize that your time with her may be best spent trying to gain the girl's confidence, even if no actual procedures are accomplished. You would prefer the mother had stayed so that you could explain your rationale for proceeding slowly to develop the trust lacking in her daughter. You realize that you will have to intervene to ensure that Cissy is not blamed for another "inconvenience" and that the mother understands the importance of your building trust and Cissy overcoming fear for a successful long-term outcome in dental treatment.

You begin asking Cissy general questions to find a non-threatening area of interest. Such a topic will allow her to feel some control and self-confidence, which are lacking in any anxiety-provoking situation. Once Cissy begins to understand that you are interested in her as a person and that she has some control, she will likely begin to relax. She may say, "This isn't so bad after all" or "I think I'm going to like it here" or "Nobody has ever listened to me before."

Now you both are in a better position to plan appropriate interventions. You later explain to Cissy's mother your approach to forming a therapeutic alliance with her daughter. You state that Cissy was *very* cooperative and an *excellent* patient. It is important to reiterate Cissy's cooperation with both Cissy and her mother present so that they hear the same information. Cissy's positive attitude regarding her appointment and her eagerness to return for her next appointment pleasantly surprise her mother.

At her next appointment, Cissy may again appear hesitant. It is important to reinforce what occurred at the previous appointment. The patient needs time and the practitioner needs patience to help the anxious dental patient overcome the fear and anxiety that have developed over time. It is rewarding to see a patient overcome dental fears and anxiety.

$\mathcal{T}$he dental hygienist must understand the relationship between mental disorders and oral health. Psychological problems are common today; almost one third of the U.S. population will experience at least one psychiatric disorder in their lifetime. In addition, it has been stated that "dental disease and psychiatric disorders are the most prevalent health problems in the United States."[48] This extremely powerful statement should alert dental professionals to the likelihood that they will encounter many psychiatrically troubled individuals and must be knowledgeable and well prepared to treat this segment of the population.

Life actually has two different dimensions. *Quantity* of life relates to the life expectancy in terms of years, whereas *quality* of life is a more subjective evaluation of life in general. Assessment of the quality of life should include (1) physical functioning, (2) disease- and treatment-related physical symptoms, (3) psychological functioning, and (4) social functioning. Mental health is integrated into all four of these domains because it can significantly affect a person's quality of life as defined by these domains. *Mental health* in fact may be the common criterion that allows an individual to live a happy and meaningful life, almost regardless of life circumstances.[33]

BOX 43-1

DSM-IV-TR **Multiaxial Classification**

Axis I: Clinical disorders, other conditions of clinical interest
Axis II: Personality disorders, mental retardation

Axis III: General medical conditions
Axis IV: Psychosocial and environmental problems
Axis V: Global assessment of functioning

Modified from *Diagnostic and statistical manual of mental disorders,* ed 4 (text revision), Washington, DC, 2000, American Psychiatric Association.

BOX 43-2

DSM-IV-TR **Axis I: Clinical Disorders**

Delirium, dementia, amnestic, other cognitive disorders
Mental disorders caused by general medical condition
Substance-related disorders
Schizophrenia and other psychotic disorders
Mood disorders
Anxiety disorders
Somatoform disorders

Factitious disorders
Dissociative disorders
Sexual and gender identity disorders
Eating disorders
Sleep disorders
Impulse control disorders not classified elsewhere
Adjustment disorders
Other conditions of clinical interest

Modified from *Diagnostic and statistical manual of mental disorders,* ed 4 (text revision), Washington, DC, 2000, American Psychiatric Association.
NOTE: Disorders usually are first diagnosed in infancy, childhood, or adolescence.

BOX 43-3

DSM-IV-TR **Axis II: Personality Disorders and Mental Retardation**

Paranoid personality disorder
Schizoid personality disorder
Schizotypal personality disorder
Antisocial personality disorder
Borderline personality disorder
Histrionic personality disorder

Narcissistic personality disorder
Avoidant personality disorder
Dependent personality disorder
Obsessive-compulsive personality disorder
Personality disorder not otherwise specified
Mental retardation

Modified from *Diagnostic and statistical manual of mental disorders,* ed 4 (text revision), Washington, DC, 2000, American Psychiatric Association.

DEFINITIONS AND CLASSIFICATION

43-A The American Psychiatric Association (APA) defines mental disorders as "clusters of persistent, maladaptive behaviors that are associated with personal distress, such as anxiety or depression, or with an impairment in social functioning, such as job performance or personal relationships."[9] The etiology of these disorders is multifactorial, including biological, psychological, genetic, physical, and neurobiological imbalances.[11,26,37]

A major challenge to mental health professionals has been to develop a medical classification system for abnormal behavior. Many systems have been developed over the years, but professionals in the United States now classify and diagnose abnormal behavior according to one accepted system. The APA system is published as the *Diagnostic and Statistical Manual of Mental Disorders.* The text revision of the fourth edition (*DSM-IV-TR*) provides comprehensive definitions of more than 200 diagnostic categories for identifying and classifying abnormal behavior.

DSM-IV-TR provides a guide to clinical practice for all mental health professionals, facilitates research and education, and improves communication between clinicians and researchers. Psychologists, social workers, and psychiatrists use it for diagnostic purposes and for filing insurance coverage claims.

In *DSM-IV-TR,* each disorder is identified as a clinically significant behavioral or psychological pattern and is associated with current life problems. *DSM-IV-TR* uses a framework that identifies five separate categories, or *axes,* each referring to a specific set of information (Box 43-1). The first three axes are designed to assess the patient's primary disorder, developmental problems in children and adolescents, and physical illnesses (Boxes 43-2 to 43-4). The last two axes focus on the severity of environmental stressors and the general level of functioning in the past year in social relationships, work, and leisure activities (Box 43-5). The assessment of a person's level of functioning represented on axis V is accomplished using the *global assessment of functioning* (GAF, Table 43-1). The GAF scale has 10

BOX 43-4

DSM-IV-TR **Axis III: General Medical Conditions**

Infectious and parasitic diseases
Neoplasms
Endocrine, nutritional, and metabolic diseases and immunity disorders
Diseases of blood and blood-forming organs
Diseases of nervous system and sense organs
Diseases of respiratory system
Diseases of digestive system
Diseases of genitourinary system

Complications of pregnancy, childbirth, and puerperium
Diseases of skin and subcutaneous tissue
Diseases of musculoskeletal system and connective tissue
Congenital anomalies
Certain conditions originating in perinatal period
Symptoms, signs, and poorly defined conditions
Injury and poisoning

Modified from *Diagnostic and statistical manual of mental disorders,* ed 4 (text revision), Washington, DC, 2000, American Psychiatric Association.

BOX 43-5

DSM-IV-TR **Axis IV: Psychosocial and Environmental Problems**

Problems with primary support group
Problems related to social environment
Educational problems
Occupational problems
Housing problems

Economic problems
Problems with access to healthcare services
Legal problems
Other psychosocial or environmental problems

Modified from *Diagnostic and statistical manual of mental disorders,* ed 4 (text revision), Washington, DC, 2000, American Psychiatric Association.

TABLE 43-1

Global assessment of functioning (GAF) scale

Score	Functional capacity	Examples
100	Superior functioning in wide range of activities, life's problems never seem to get out of hand, sought out by others because of positive qualities	No symptoms
90	Good functioning in all areas, generally satisfied with all areas of life, normal life concerns	Mild anxiety before exam Occasional argument with family members
80	If symptoms present, in response to psychosocial stressors or slight, temporary impairment in social, occupational, or school functioning	Difficulty concentrating after family argument Temporarily falling behind in schoolwork
70	Some difficulty with social, occupational, or school functioning, but generally functioning at an adequate level; has some interpersonal relationships	Depressed mood and mild insomnia Occasional truancy or theft within household
60	Moderate difficulty with social, occupational, or school functioning	Flat affect and circumstantial speech, occasional panic attacks Few friends, conflicts with peers or co-workers
50	Serious difficulty with social, occupational, or school functioning	Suicidal ideation, severe obsessional rituals, frequent shoplifting No friends, unable to keep a job
40	Some impairment in reality testing or communication *or* Major impairment in several areas, such as work, school, family relations, judgment, thinking, and mood	Speech at times illogical, obscure, or irrelevant *or* *Adult:* avoid social contact, neglect family, unable to work *Child:* frequently beats up younger children, is defiant at home, failing at school
30	Behavior considerably influenced by delusions or hallucinations or serious impairment in communication or judgment *or* Inability to function in almost all areas	Sometimes incoherent, actions grossly inappropriately, suicidal preoccupation *or* Stays in bed all day; no job, home, or friends

Modified from *Diagnostic and statistical manual of mental disorders,* ed 4 (text revision), Washington, DC, 2000, American Psychiatric Association.

Continued

TABLE 43-1

Global assessment of functioning (GAF) scale—cont'd

Score	Functional capacity	Examples
20	Some danger of hurting self or others *or* Occasionally fails to maintain minimal personal hygiene *or* Gross impairment in communication	Suicide attempts without clear expectation of death, frequently violent, manic excitement *or* Smears feces *or* Largely incoherent or mute Recurrent violence to self or others
10	Persistent danger of hurting self or others *or* Persistent inability to maintain minimal personal hygiene *or* Serious suicidal acts with clear expectation of death	

Modified from *Diagnostic and statistical manual of mental disorders,* ed 4 (text revision), Washington, DC, 2000, American Psychiatric Association.

BOX 43-6

DSM-IV-TR **Classification**

Disorders usually first diagnosed in infancy, childhood, or adolescence
Delirium, dementia, amnestic, and other cognitive disorders
Mental disorders caused by general medical condition not classified elsewhere
Substance-related disorders
Schizophrenia and other psychotic disorders
Mood disorders
    Major depressive disorder
    Bipolar disorders
Anxiety disorders
    Panic disorder
    Agoraphobia
    Specific phobia
    Social phobia
Obsessive-compulsive disorder
Posttraumatic stress disorder
Acute stress disorder
Generalized anxiety disorder
Somatoform disorders
Factitious disorders
Dissociative disorders
Sexual and gender identity
Eating disorders
    Anorexia nervosa
    Bulimia nervosa
Sleep disorders
Impulse control disorders not classified elsewhere
Adjustment disorders
Personality disorders
Other

Modified from *Diagnostic and statistical manual of mental disorders,* ed 4 (text revision), Washington, DC, 2000, American Psychiatric Association.

divisions of functioning. The GAF assessment is a single number (on a scale of 0 to 100) that the clinician uses to reflect the patient's level of psychological, social, and occupational functioning[9] (see the additional readings and resources at the end of this chapter for full description).

This chapter addresses the classification and description of mental disorders, symptoms, diagnostic criteria, and treatment strategies, including the implications for treating patients in the dental setting (Box 43-6). Recognition of these disorders by clinicians helps in understanding patients' behavior, motivation, and response to needed and recommended dental treatment.

ANXIETY DISORDERS

Anxiety disorders have been identified as early as the fourth century BC in the writings of Hippocrates. With the interest in the nineteenth century primarily on psychotic disorders, the study of anxiety disorders was left to internal medicine specialists such as Freud. It was not recognized until the last half of the twentieth century that anxiety disorders could be effectively treated pharmacologically, as well as psychologically.

Anxiety is an irrational emotional response to an imagined threat. Rather than focusing on current circumstances, anxiety focuses on *anticipated* outcomes of future events, or "worrying about worry." *Worry,* as related to the person with an anxiety disorder, can be defined as "a relatively uncontrollable sequence of negative, emotional thoughts and images that are concerned with possible future threats or danger."[9] *Fear,* on the other hand, is a rational response to a real threat that helps to prepare the person to respond to immediate danger.[9,26,37]

All persons experience anxiety, or a feeling of apprehension, as a reaction to stressful situations. However, some people experience anxiety when there is no identifiable external cause. The anxious person is hypervigilant and displays high levels of diffuse negative emotion, a sense of be-

DSM-IV-TR Anxiety Disorders

Panic disorder
Agoraphobia
Specific phobia
Social phobia
Obsessive-compulsive disorder
Posttraumatic stress disorder
Acute stress disorder
Generalized anxiety disorder
Anxiety disorder caused by general medical condition
Substance-induced anxiety disorder*
Anxiety disorder not otherwise specified*

Modified from *Diagnostic and statistical manual of mental disorders,*
ed 4 (text revision), Washington, DC, 2000, American Psychiatric
Association.
*Indicates topics not discussed in text.

ing out of control, and a state of self-preoccupation relative
to what they perceive as a threat. If this anxiety occurs
without justification and begins to impair the person's ability to function at a normal level, it is considered a psychological problem known as an **anxiety disorder.** Along with
the feeling of apprehension, the individual may experience
predictable physiological changes, such as increased muscle
tension, shallow rapid breathing, increased perspiration,
and dry mouth. Anxiety provokes two levels of reaction:
subjective feelings (e.g., fear or dread) and physiological responses (e.g., rapid breathing).[9,11,26,37]

Some anxiety can be an adaptive response because it
helps to provide motivation to be prepared to meet an upcoming event (e.g., anxiety before exams), thus providing
the initiative and focus to perform well. The other extreme is a prolonged level of high anxiety, not directed at
any known upcoming event, which impairs concentration
and performance. Prolonged anxiety is nearly an intolerable experience and likely explains why antianxiety medications have become the most popular prescription medications ever developed.[11,32,37]

The Epidemiologic Catchment Area (ECA) study examined the frequency of specific types of anxiety disorders
and found that anxiety disorders are more common than
any other form of mental disorder. The National Institute
of Mental Health (NIMH) reported that within a 6-month
period, 7% to 15% of the population may be diagnosed
with one or more of the several anxiety diagnoses (3 to 42
million people). Others have suggested an even higher
prevalence of 20%, or about 56 million people. One national study found that 17% of U.S. adults have at least
one type of anxiety disorder in any given year. These
numbers represent a significant portion of the U.S. population, suggesting the enormity of the problem.[40] The major symptom of all 10 anxiety disorders defined by APA is
avoidance behavior, or the attempt to avoid the situation
that causes or produces the anxiety (Box 43-7).[9]

ETIOLOGY

The etiologic basis for anxiety disorders includes stressful
life events and biological components. Neurotransmitters

such as serotonin are involved in the etiology of both anxiety disorders and mood disorders (e.g., depression). Similar symptoms in anxiety disorders and mood disorders
include guilt, worry, panic, avoidance, and anger, which
can lead to a dual diagnosis.[7,9,26,32,37]

The intuitive relationship between stressful life events
and onset of anxiety is supported by several studies.[5,35]
These studies demonstrate that patients with anxiety disorders are more likely than control subjects to have experienced a negative life event in the months preceding
the initial onset of symptoms. The quality or nature of the
stressful event may also be important in influencing the
type of problem.

In one study, researchers interviewed women attending a general medical clinic to track relative negative life
events to specific psychological outcomes. This study included women who were depressed, those with anxiety
disorders, and women who met dual diagnostic criteria.
During the year preceding the onset of symptoms, 82% of
the depressed women and 93% of the anxious/depressed
women reported at least one severe negative life event.
Only 34% of the control group reported a similar event.
Women with anxiety symptoms were much more likely
to have experienced an event that involved danger,
whereas the women who were depressed were more likely
to have experienced a severe loss. The women who presented with mixed symptoms often reported experiencing
both types of events. Therefore the type of environmental
stress can influence the type of psychological response the
patient may exhibit.[12]

PANIC ATTACK

Panic attacks can occur alone or with other anxiety disorders, mental disorders, or general medical conditions.
Panic attacks are experienced as the sudden onset of intense apprehension, often with symptoms such as shortness of breath, palpitations, chest pain, and the sense of
losing control. The attack has a sudden onset, usually
reaching its peak for fear and apprehension within 10 minutes or less, with the person experiencing a sense of impending doom and the urgent need to flee. To meet diagnostic criteria, at least 4 of 13 symptoms must be present
(Box 43-8). The anxiety characteristic of this disorder can
be distinguished from generalized anxiety because the anxiety is of greater severity and occurs intermittently. Panic
attacks can also occur concurrently with a variety of the
other anxiety disorders (e.g., specific, social, posttraumatic
stress syndrome, acute stress disorder). The three types of
panic attacks are (1) unexpected (*uncued*), (2) situationally
bound (*cued*), and (3) situationally predisposed. The unexpected attacks happen "out of the blue," whereas situationally bound attacks occur on exposure to or expectation
of the situational *cue,* such as speaking in public.[9,11,26,37]

The occurrence of panic attacks is required for a diagnosis of panic disorder (with or without agoraphobia).[9]

PANIC DISORDER

To meet the *DSM-IV-TR* diagnostic criteria for panic disorder, a patient must (1) experience recurrent unexpected
panic attacks, followed by at least 1 month of persistent
concern about having another panic attack, (2) worry
about implications or consequences of the panic attacks,

BOX 43-8

DSM-IV-TR Diagnostic Criteria for Panic Attack

Discrete period of intense fear or discomfort, in which four or more of the following symptoms developed abruptly and reached a peak within 10 minutes:
1. Palpitations, pounding heart, or accelerated heart rate
2. Sweating
3. Trembling or shaking
4. Sensations of shortness of breath or smothering
5. Feeling of choking
6. Chest pain or discomfort
7. Nausea or abdominal distress
8. Feeling dizzy, unsteady, lightheaded, or faint
9. Derealization (feelings of unreality) or depersonalization (being detached from oneself)
10. Fear of losing control or going crazy
11. Fear of dying
12. Paresthesias (numbing or tingling sensations)
13. Chills or hot flashes

Modified from *Diagnostic and statistical manual of mental disorders,* ed 4 (text revision), Washington, DC, 2000, American Psychiatric Association.

BOX 43-9

DSM-IV-TR Diagnostic Criteria for Panic Disorder

1. Both 1 and 2 are present, as follows:
   a. Recurrent unexpected panic attacks
   b. At least one of the attacks followed by at least 1 month of one or more of the following:
      1) Persistent concern about having additional attacks
      2) Worry about the implications of the attack or its consequences (e.g., losing control, having a heart attack, "going crazy")
      3) Significant change in behavior related to attacks
2. Panic attacks not caused by direct physiological effects of a substance (e.g., drug abuse, medication) or a general medical condition (e.g., hyperthyroidism)
3. Panic attacks not better accounted for by another mental disorder (e.g., social phobia, specific phobia, obsessive-compulsive disorder, posttraumatic stress disorder)

Modified from *Diagnostic and statistical manual of mental disorders,* ed 4 (text revision), Washington, DC, 2000, American Psychiatric Association.

---

or (3) exhibit a significant behavioral change related to the attacks (Box 43-9).

Coexistence of a mood disorder such as major depression ranges from 10% to 65% in patients with panic disorder. Comorbid anxiety disorders may be seen. The age of onset varies considerably, but most attacks occur in late adolescence and into the early 30s. Some patients may have no symptoms for years. Most often the condition is chronic, with periods of latency and activity. First-degree relatives are 20 times more likely to experience panic disorder if onset was before age 20. Twin studies have found a genetic component in the development of panic disorder.[9,11,26]

PHOBIC DISORDER

A *phobia* is defined as "an irrational fear or an obsessive dread."[9] People with a phobic disorder exhibit a fear that is unreasonable, exaggerated, or inappropriate and that leads them to avoid that object, activity, or situation. This avoidance is significant enough that the fear and the response are disruptive to the individual's life. The three basic types of phobias are (1) agoraphobia, (2) social, and (3) specific. Phobias are common and occur in children and adults of either gender, although they are more frequently diagnosed in women. People may be "closet phobics," keeping their fears hidden from others and only pretending to feel better.[26,37]

Many causal factors can lead a person to have irrational fears such as those found in phobic disorders. Many theorists believe that these fears are conditioned emotional responses to specific circumstances. A classic experiment by John Watson provides an example of the development of a fear based on exposure to a frightening experience. Albert, a toddler, was shown a white rat and expressed no fear of the rat. Then a loud sound was generated behind Albert while he was in the presence of the rat. The loud noise frightened Albert, producing a *startle response,* and the child began to cry. After that experience, when exposed to the rat, Albert would cry and try to avoid it. Albert had acquired a fear of the rat he initially did not have through exposure to a loud and frightening noise, thus developing a *conditioned* fear of the rat. Applying this experiment to common fears, one can see that exposure to a bad experience, whether an object or a situation, can lead to the development of excessive fear. For example, if a child is mocked during a grade-school presentation, he or she is likely to carry that experience into adulthood and continue to fear speaking in public. Likewise, a person who has a negative dental experience may become a "dental-fears patient."[10]

Watson also discovered that objects similar to the conditioned fear (the white rat), such as Santa Claus, a white rabbit, or crumpled white terrycloth towel, also produced fear in Albert. This *stimulus generalization* is a tendency to display a learned response to situations or objects that are similar to the original feared object or situation. Importantly, parents with irrational fears can "infect" their children with a tendency to develop similar behavioral patterns.[49]

AGORAPHOBIA

Agoraphobia means "fear of open places" and is characterized by a group of related fears: being alone, public places, and traveling away from home, where the person may be unable to escape from an unpleasant or embarrassing situation. The individual with this disorder may avoid stores, crowds, restaurants, and social events; in extreme cases the person becomes housebound, never traveling far from the known safe environment.[9,37]

SOCIAL PHOBIA

Social phobia is a "marked and persistent fear of social or performance situations in which embarrassment may occur."[9] Social phobia affects 3% to 13% of the U.S. popula-

Frequently Reported Specific Phobias

Acrophobia: fear of heights
Algophobia: fear of pain
Astraphobia: fear of thunder, lightning, winds, and heavy rain
Claustrophobia: fear of confinement or closed areas
Cynophobia: fear of dogs
Demophobia: fear of crowds
Hyptephobia: fear of being touched
Monophobia: fear of being alone
Mysophobia: fear of germs
Nyctophobia: fear of darkness or night
Pathophobia: fear of disease
Pyrophobia: fear of fire
Zoophobia: fear of animals

tion. Patients experience an immediate anxious response to particular social interactions, which often leads to avoidance of the situation or anticipation with a sense of dread. Common features associated include hypersensitivity to criticism, negative evaluation, or rejection; difficulty being assertive; and low self-esteem. Examples of social phobia include (1) fear of public speaking, (2) fear of meeting strangers, (3) hesitation to accept invitations to social functions, (4) embarrassment when eating in public, and (5) fear of maintaining conversations or eye contact with others in social situations. The diagnosis is made, however, only if the anxiety response interferes with the person's occupational functioning or social life or if the person is significantly distressed about the condition.[9,37]

Adults with social phobia are aware that their fear is excessive. Children, however, may not be aware of the excessive nature of their fears. The onset of social phobia usually is in midadolescence, often following a childhood history of shyness. Onset of the condition may immediately follow a stressful or humiliating event. Unlike adults, children are less likely to have the option of avoiding the feared situations or to understand the nature of their intense fear.[9,37]

SPECIFIC ("SIMPLE") PHOBIAS

In specific, formerly "simple," phobias the source of fear can be readily identified. The fear is persistent and excessive or unreasonable, cued by the presence or anticipation of a specific object or situation (e.g., flying, heights, animals, dental treatment). Exposure to the phobic cue almost invariably provokes an immediate anxiety response. The phobic situation(s) is either avoided or endured with intense anxiety or distress. The avoidance, anxious anticipation, or distress in the feared situation(s) interferes significantly with the person's normal routine, occupational (or academic) functioning, social activities, or relationships. The person may be greatly distressed about having the phobia.[9,37] These phobias are "simple" only in that the sense that the source of the fear is not complex (Box 43-10).[9]

GENERALIZED ANXIETY DISORDER

Generalized anxiety disorder (GAD) is defined in terms of excessive anxiety and worry that the person finds difficult to control and that leads to significant distress or impairment in occupational or social functioning. Symptoms that are often associated with the anxiety are restlessness, feeling on edge, easy fatigue, difficulty concentrating, irritability, muscle tension, and sleep difficulties. The intensity, duration, and frequency of the anxiety are greatly exaggerated relative to the likely outcome of the feared situation. The person finds that the thoughts are intrusive and that they interfere with normal functioning. Adults with GAD often worry about routine daily responsibilities related to job, finances, or minor activities (e.g., household chores, car repairs). Children with GAD tend to worry about school or athletic performance.[9,37]

Many people with GAD also experience cold and clammy hands, dry mouth, sweating, nausea, trouble swallowing, and an exaggerated startle response. Depression often occurs with GAD, as may other mood disorders. Many people with GAD say that they have been anxious all their lives, but the condition may begins after age 20. The course is chronic and often worsens during or after stressful life events.[9,11,26,37]

OBSESSIVE-COMPULSIVE DISORDER

Obsessive-compulsive disorder (OCD) may be seen as three disorders: (1) a compulsive disorder, (2) an obsessive disorder, and (3) a combination obsessive-compulsive disorder. Patients are plagued with unwanted thoughts (obsessions) and feel that they must take some action (compulsion) that they are not able to control. OCD affects an estimated 1 in 200 teenagers.[9,37]

OCD is characterized by recurrent *obsessions,* ideas or thoughts that constantly and involuntarily intrude into awareness. These thoughts are generally of a pointless nature, such as continually washing one's hands or checking to make certain the door is locked, over and over again. The person with OCD realizes that these compulsive actions serve no useful purpose but cannot stop them. Theoretically, these obsessive and compulsive actions may be used to prevent other anxiety-producing behaviors or thoughts.[9,37]

POSTTRAUMATIC STRESS DISORDER

The onset of *posttraumatic stress disorder (PTSD)* is preceded by exposure to an extreme traumatic stressor and followed by the development of characteristic symptoms. This stressful event is "outside the normal human experience" or threatens one's basic held values and beliefs. Of those who experience a severely traumatic event, about 15% will exhibit symptoms of PTSD. The traumatic event is reexperienced in many ways.

DSM-IV-TR diagnostic criteria include (1) recurrent and intrusive recollections of the event, (2) recurrent distressing dreams, (3) acting or feeling as if the traumatic event were recurring, (4) intense psychological distress on exposure to internal or external cues that symbolize or resemble the traumatic event, and (5) physiological reactions to these cues. The reexperiencing of the event is often accompanied by persistent avoidance of stimuli associated with the trauma and numbing of general responsiveness (not present before the trauma). The person may make efforts to avoid thoughts, feelings, or conversations associated with the trauma or avoid activities, places, or people that arouse recollections of the trauma. Patients with

PTSD may have greatly diminished interest or participation in significant activities, a feeling of detachment or estrangement from others, and a restricted range of affect. They may sense a "foreshortened future." These patients also often experience persistent symptoms of increased arousal, such as difficulty falling or staying asleep, irritability or outbursts of anger, difficulty concentrating, hypervigilance, or exaggerated startle response.[9,37]

PTSD can occur at any age. The onset of symptoms usually occurs within 3 months of the trauma, although symptoms have not appeared until many months or years after the trauma in some cases. The symptoms of the disorder and the level of reexperiencing, avoidance, and hyperarousal symptoms may vary over time. The severity, duration, and proximity of the individual to the event are important in influencing the likelihood of developing PTSD. This disorder can develop in individuals who have no predisposing conditions, especially if the stressor is extreme. Recovery from PTSD is often determined by other complicating factors (e.g., alcoholism, drug abuse, depression), whether the person experienced psychological problems before the onset of PSTD, and the social support system in place for the patient.[9,37]

TREATMENT

Treatment of anxiety disorders can be approached psychologically, pharmacologically, or often with both therapies. Of the various psychological treatment strategies, a cognitive-behavioral approach for phobic disorders, OCD, and PTSD is appropriate.

Pharmacologically these disorders are usually treated with antianxiety medications (Table 43-2). These medications reduce many of the symptoms of anxiety disorders, such as muscle tension, increased vigilance, increased perspiration, palpitations, and gastrointestinal distress. They do, however, have several side effects, including daytime sedation, dry mouth, slight impairment in the ability to concentrate, constipation, and with specific drugs, blurred vision. Withdrawal from these medications can be problematic if the patient has been using the drug for some time, as the original symptoms often return (known as *rebound anxiety*). Equally if not more important than the difficulty patients encounter when they discontinue use of benzodiazepines is their potential for addiction.[6,7,32,37]

TABLE 43-2
Common benzodiazepines* used in treatment of anxiety disorders

Generic name	Trade name
Alprazolam	Xanax
Diazepam	Valium
Lorazepam	Ativan
Temazepam	Restoril
Triazolam	Halcion

Modified from Gage TW, Pickett FA: *Mosby's dental drug reference,* ed 5, St Louis, 2001, Mosby.
*All central nervous system (CNS) depressants.

DENTAL CONSIDERATIONS

Patients presenting in the dental office with an anxiety disorder may or may not exhibit signs of the disorder. Given the prevalence of anxiety disorders, many patients are likely to be affected, and the healthcare professional will need to assess the patient's current status at the beginning of the appointment. A sensitive approach enables the dental practitioner to form a clinical judgment as to the patient's mental health status. This assessment is critical to the delivery of care. A calm, quiet approach should be taken so that the patient is not exposed to stimuli that might trigger the onset of a panic attack or undue anxiety. Patients with social phobia should have limited interactions during treatment and should receive positive reassurance. If the patient presents in a state of high anxiety, medical consultation with his or her psychiatrist or other medical professional may be necessary to determine whether the patient's current condition is stable enough to continue with the dental appointment.*

Patients with anxiety disorders are often taking benzodiazepines or newer medications. The benzodiazepines are known to cause *xerostomia* (dry mouth), which can exacerbate preexisting periodontal conditions and increase dental caries. Patients may suck hard candy and increase their consumption of cariogenic beverages to alleviate the dry mouth. This can also lead to an increase in dental caries and dental plaque in general. The patient should be advised of the potential danger of relying on these methods to alleviate dry mouth. Xerostomia reduces the self-cleansing nature of the oral cavity and often leads to increased levels of plaque with no change in brushing habits.

It is important to explain the implications of xerostomic changes to patients and inform them of actions to reduce the risks of dental disease. Mouthrinses that contain high levels of alcohol should be avoided because they can cause oral ulcerations to dry mucosal surfaces. Patients should be advised to rinse with water often during the day and to be careful not to brush aggressively if they find their oral tissues are tender and dry from the xerostomia. Vigorous brushing under these conditions can lead to gingival tissue abrasion. Patients with excellent oral hygiene may have difficulty in maintaining their previous level of plaque control. Supportive interventions include use of sugarless gum and lozenges to increase salivary flow and help restore the natural cleansing provided by saliva. These patients must understand the reason for their increased plaque accumulation so as not to worsen their anxiety.†

Appointments should be scheduled for the morning, and these patients should not have to wait. Length of appointment and amount of work should be minimized to prevent a stressful experience. With a dental-fears patient or a patient diagnosed with an anxiety disorder, it is important to maintain a calm environment and to explain treatment procedures carefully so that the patient is informed and comfortable.[46,47]

*References 15, 16, 22, 32, 43, 52.
†References 7, 10, 13, 15, 16, 22, 23, 28, 32.

MOOD DISORDERS

Everyone has "bad days," when they feel sad and depressed. Some people, however, experience these "mood swings" for long periods so severely that it significantly interferes with the person's ability to function at acceptable levels. Everyone has experienced one or more significant disappointment in life and the resulting sadness. This reflects a normal period of mourning during which some level of *depression* is to be expected. People who suffer from *major depression* have similar feelings but of much greater severity and duration.

The etiology of mood disorders is controversial. Psychoanalytic theory states that depression results from turning one's anger inward and feeling responsible for all the "bad things." As Maslow suggests, persons might become depressed because they are not able to experience *self-actualization,* the ability to optimize their talents and potential. Others have found convincing evidence that both major depression and *bipolar disorder* are biological in origin, resulting from an imbalance of neurotransmitters in the brain caused by a genetic predisposition or unusually severe stressors. A cognitive approach to causation suggests that depression is *learned helplessness;* people experience stress as inescapable and intolerable. Although no single cause of depression exists, depression clearly results from complex interactions among multiple variables, including biochemical influences, situational stress, and learned experiences.[9,37]

MAJOR DEPRESSIVE DISORDER

Queen Victoria, Lincoln, Moses, and Freud all are thought to have suffered from major depression. Intelligent people who engage in too much self-analysis and self-criticism often experience depression. Although depression receives much publicity when experienced by famous people, many ordinary people suffer from the same condition. Major depression is characterized by at least 2 weeks of depressed mood or loss of interest in otherwise pleasurable activities. At least four additional symptoms must exist (Box 43-11). These symptoms must also be accompanied by impairment in social, occupational, or educational functioning.[9,37]

The incidence of unipolar mood disorder in the U.S. population is 6% to 10%. The cost of depression to society is an astounding $44 billion a year.[27] Women are twice as likely to experience a major depressive episode as men, with 25% of all women likely to have major depression at some point in their lives. Research shows an increase in depression worldwide, as well as earlier onset. Episodes tend to recur in 50% to 80% of patients with a diagnosis of a major depressive disorder. An episode can last from several months to more than a year, depending on availability of treatment and the patient's support structure.[11,37]

Major stressful life events increase the likelihood of a person developing clinical depression. The events most often associated with increased risk for depression are "major life changes" involving losses of important people or roles.[37]

People experience major depressive episodes in different ways. Patients with major depression find that once-pleasurable activities no longer are important. Families often notice social withdrawal, although depressed individuals may deny feeling sad. *Insomnia* is the most common sleep disturbance associated with clinical depression. Insomnia can be characterized as *initial* (difficulty falling asleep), *middle* (waking up in the middle of the night and having difficulty falling back to sleep), or *terminal* (waking up early and not being able to go back to sleep).[9,37]

Depressed adults lack motivation, find work and social interactions difficult and exhausting, have marked weight loss or gain, have difficulty sleeping or sleep too much, have a general negative outlook or hopelessness, and possess a sense of worthlessness. The sense of worthlessness or guilt is often exaggerated as trivial day-to-day events are taken as evidence of personal weakness. Many individuals report an impaired ability to think and concentrate and may complain of memory loss. They often blame themselves for being ill and failing to meet interpersonal or occupational responsibilities. Thoughts of death and suicidal ideation are common, with variable frequency, intensity, and lethality.[9,37]

Children and adolescents may manifest an *irritable mood* rather than a sad or depressed mood. For children, depression can interfere with the development of close relationships and interests in learning and in play. Children and adolescents may exhibit a drop in school achieve-

---

BOX 43-11	
***DSM-IV-TR* Diagnostic Criteria for Major Depressive Episode**	
At least one of the symptoms is either (1) depressed mood or (2) loss of interest or pleasure that represents a change from previous functioning for 2 weeks, plus five of the following: 1. Depressed mood 2. Loss of interest or pleasure 3. Significant (5% of body weight in a month) weight gain or loss, or change in appetite 4. Insomnia or excessive sleep 5. Psychomotor agitation or retardation	6. Fatigue, loss of energy 7. Feelings of worthlessness or excessive guilt 8. Diminished ability to think or concentrate or indecisiveness 9. Recurring thoughts of death or suicidal ideas or attempt The following criteria also apply: The mood disorder is not caused by bereavement, medical disease, or substance abuse. The symptoms cause distress or impair functioning.

Modified from *Diagnostic and statistical manual of mental disorders (DSM-IV),* ed 4, (text revision), Washington, DC, 2000, American Psychiatric Association.

ment as a result of a reduced ability to concentrate. In children, other mental disorders frequently occur in conjunction with a major depressive episode, especially disruptive behavior disorder, attention deficit disorder, and anxiety disorders. In adolescents, disruptive behavior disorders, attention deficit disorder, anxiety disorders, substance-related disorders, and eating disorders are frequently associated with a major depressive disorder.[9,30,37]

Treatment

As with most other mental disorders, treatment of major depressive disorder can be psychological, pharmacological, or combination therapy. Research has shown conflicting results in regard to the most effective therapeutic intervention. Most evidence supports a combination of psychotherapeutic and pharmacologic interventions. The two therapies complement each other; one addresses the ability to cope with life events while the other addresses a change in levels of neurotransmitters that control mood.[11,32,37,44]

The first "antidepressant" was a drug originally developed to treat tuberculosis and had side effects of greater optimism and happiness in treated patients. This drug was found to cause irreversible liver damage and was removed from the market, but its introduction dramatically changed the way clinicians viewed treatment of depression. Currently a number of medications are used to treat depression, including monoamine oxidase inhibitors (MAOIs), tricyclics, tetracyclics, selective serotonin reuptake inhibitors (SSRIs), and atypical antidepressants (Table 43-3).[7,25,32,37,53]

Hospitalization is warranted when the patient may be a danger to self or others. Forced hospitalization of a patient jeopardizes the psychotherapeutic relationship and should be done only when no other choice exists.[11,26,37]

Dental Considerations

A patient with a major depressive episode may present with feelings of sadness, loss, and rejection. Patients often lose interest and motivation for self-care and may not maintain their previous level of oral hygiene. For these patients it is important to take care in minimizing stressful aspects of the appointment. If the patient appears significantly distraught, a consultation with the patient's psychiatrist, psychologist, or primary care physician should precede any significant treatment. The clinician should ensure that the patient receives positive feedback and support relative to oral hygiene habits; patients view negative comments as further example of their worthlessness. It is important to be respectful of these patients and their emotional pain and to demonstrate sincere interest in their well-being.*

SSRIs, such as fluoxetine, fenfluramine, and dexfenfluramine, are frequently used in the treatment of depression. A common side effect of these medications is xerostomia (see earlier discussion). Preventive dietary and dental hygiene guidance is appropriate for this patient population.†

BIPOLAR DISORDER

Bipolar disorder, formerly "manic-depressive illness," is a common, recurrent, and severe psychiatric illness that affects 1% to 3% of the U.S. population. The illness is characterized by episodes of mania, depression, and mixed states (simultaneous manic and depressive symptoms). Bipolar disorder frequently goes unnoticed and untreated for years. The typical onset of a bipolar disorder is between ages 28 and 33 years, with the first set of symptoms equally as likely as manic or depressive. The average manic episode lasts 2 to 3 months; the depressive episode lasts somewhat longer. The long-term outcome of bipolar disorder is mixed, with the majority of individuals experiencing multiple episodes over a lifetime. Both genetic and early environmental factors are associated with the course of bipolar disorder.[9,37]

During their manic episodes, patients display inflated self-esteem, grandiosity, excessive speech, racing and rapidly changing ideas, excessive participation in pleasurable activities, and a decreased need for sleep. *Mania* cannot be maintained for long periods because it is exhausting. Some patients experience increased activity that cannot be considered a full-blown manic episode; this is known as *hypomania.* Hypomanic and manic episodes differ in duration and severity. The hypomanic episode is noticeable to others and lasts at least 4 days (versus 1 week for a full manic episode), without impairment to social or occupational functioning.[9,37]

Treatment

Although psychotherapy is helpful to patients with bipolar disorder, medication is necessary for a successful out-

TABLE 43-3 Antidepressants	
Generic name	**Trade name**
Atypical	
Bupropion	Wellbutrin
Nefazodone	Serzone
Trazodone	Desyrel
Venlafaxine	Effexor
MAOIs	
Phenelzine	Mardil
Tranylcypromine	Parnate
SSRIs	
Fluoxetine	Prozac
Fluvoxamine	Luvox
Paroxetine	Paxil
Sertraline	Zoloft
Tetracyclics	
Maprotiline	Ludiomil
Mirtazapine	Remeron
Tricyclics	
Amitriptyline	Elavil
Amoxapine	Asendin
Clomipramine	Anafranil
Imipramine	Tofranil

MAOIs, Monoamine oxidase inhibitors; *SSRIs,* selective serotonin reuptake inhibitors.

---

*References 2, 14, 18, 19, 21, 32.
†References 2, 4, 7, 13, 18, 19, 21, 24, 28, 32, 39, 42, 45, 52, 53.

come. The three phases of bipolar disorder need to be addressed in developing a treatment strategy. Active therapies need to be developed for the depressive and manic phases and a maintenance strategy for long-term support. Bipolar disorder can lead to serious personal, interpersonal, and social problems, often accompanied by violence, alcoholism, and sometimes suicide.[37]

Discovered by an Australian psychiatrist, *lithium* has proved to be an excellent treatment for bipolar patients formerly resistant to treatment. Lithium reduces the recurrence of bipolar disorder when used as a maintenance therapy. The side effect profile includes gastrointestinal irritation, hand tremor, thirst, and muscular weakness. As with any long-term drug therapy, frequent monitoring is required.[14,37]

Carbamazepine and valproate are alternatives to lithium in the treatment of bipolar disorder. Topiramate, a new antiepileptic agent, appears to have efficacy for manic and mixed manic and depressive phases of bipolar disorder. One approach to treatment-resistant patients is to use a combination of mood stabilizers, but this demands a knowledge of pharmacokinetic interactions. Other novel approaches for treatment resistant bipolar disorder include high-dose thyroid hormones, calcium channel blockers, and electroconvulsive therapy. The effectiveness of psychosocial strategies is under investigation. The current use of psychological intervention primarily involves identification of stress factors and early signs of recurrence. As with all mental disorders, the patient's social support system is invaluable in the long-term prognosis.[11,37]

Dental Considerations

The dental patient with bipolar disorder in its manic phase may present for dental treatment with active symptomatology, including restlessness, aggressiveness, argumentativeness, and irritability. These patients may rapidly switch thought patterns, may be unable to concentrate or focus on topics, and may react unpredictably if pressured.

As with other patients who have anxiety disorders, bipolar patients require a quiet and nonstressful clinical environment. The clinician must approach each procedure carefully, using clear, concise explanations and a calm but firm approach to maintain a controlled setting. These patients are often restless and may not react positively to long discussions of oral health strategies. At times the patient may not be receptive even to brief comments because of the many factors that are hallmarks of bipolar disorder.[32]

PERSONALITY DISORDERS

A *personality disorder* is an "enduring pattern of inner experience that deviates markedly from the expectations of the individual's culture, is pervasive and inflexible, has an onset in adolescence or early adulthood, is stable over time, and leads to distress or impairment."[9] The personality traits that make up these disorders must be present separate from any situational stressor (see Box 43-3).[9,37]

Personality disorders are divided into three clusters in the *DSM-IV-TR* based on descriptive similarities. *Cluster A* includes the paranoid, schizoid, and schizotypal personality disorders. Individuals with these disorders often appear "odd" or "eccentric." *Cluster B* includes the antisocial, borderline, histrionic, and narcissistic personality disorders. These individuals often appear dramatic, emotional, or erratic. *Cluster C* includes the avoidant, dependent, and obsessive-compulsive personalities. These patients exhibit fear and anxiety.

Individuals with personality disorders do not see their behavior as problematic because of the minimal personal distress associated with the disorder. Many lead normal lives but encounter problems when the personality traits "just below the surface" begin to emerge.

CLUSTER A: DISORDERS OF "ODD" OR "ECCENTRIC" BEHAVIOR

Paranoid Personality Disorder

People with *paranoid personality disorder* exhibit unwarranted sensitivity, suspiciousness, envy, and mistrust of others. They show a limited range of emotions and avoid intimacy in interpersonal relationships. These people rarely seek help because of their suspicious nature and thoughts that others' motives are malevolent.[9,37]

Schizoid Personality Disorder

Persons with *schizoid personality disorder* display a marked indifference to the development of interpersonal relationships. They are rarely involved in social events and appear aloof and disinterested in others (a "loner").[9,37]

Schizotypal Personality Disorder

A person with *schizotypal personality disorder* exhibits acute discomfort in close interpersonal relationships and behaves in an eccentric manner.[9,37]

CLUSTER B: DISORDERS OF DRAMATIC, EMOTIONAL, OR ERRATIC BEHAVIOR

Antisocial Personality Disorder

People with *antisocial personality disorder* usually have a history of lying, fighting, stealing, and irresponsibility. They demonstrate a pattern of disregard for the rights of others and manifest impulsive tendencies with little concern of the consequences. These patients seldom seek treatment unless forced to do so, often through the court system, and treatment is often unsuccessful.[9,11,26,37]

Histrionic Personality Disorder

Patients with *histrionic personality disorder* tend to be overdramatic and want to draw attention to themselves and be the center of attention. They have difficulty forming intimate interpersonal relationships but tend to be dependent on others. They often overreact to small matters and seek excitement.[9,11,26,37]

Narcissistic Personality Disorder

People with *narcissistic personality disorder* exhibit a sense of grandiosity and consistent need for admiration.

BOX 43-12

DSM-IV-TR **Diagnostic Criteria for Narcissistic Personality Disorder**

A pervasive pattern of grandiosity (in fantasy or behavior), need for admiration, and lack of empathy, beginning in early adulthood and present in a variety of contexts, as indicated by five or more of the following:
1. Grandiose sense of self-importance
2. Preoccupation with fantasies of unlimited success, power, brilliance, beauty, or ideal love
3. Belief that he or she is "special" and unique and can only be understood by, or should associate with, other "special" or high-status people (or institutions)
4. Need for excessive admiration
5. Sense of entitlement
6. Interpersonally exploitative
7. Lack of empathy
8. Arrogant, haughty behaviors or attitudes

Modified from *Diagnostic and statistical manual of mental disorders,* ed 4 (text revision), Washington, DC, 2000, American Psychiatric Association.

They believe they are superior or unique and are entitled to special treatment, and they expect others to recognize this "status." They often believe that they should associate only with people of this same status. Their self-esteem is very fragile, and they are preoccupied with how others view them. They often display great charm and the desire to be pampered. Narcissistic individuals become furious when they do not receive this expected attention. They typically exploit others and display a lack of sensitivity to the needs of others. Those who try to develop close interpersonal relationships with these narcissistic persons are often met with emotional coldness and a lack of reciprocal interest. Disordered narcissists believe that others are envious of them and commonly display arrogant and haughty behaviors (Box 43-12).

Narcissistic traits during adolescence are not necessarily predictive of later narcissistic personality disorder. Men represent 50% to 75% of those diagnosed with this disorder, and less than 1% of the general population is affected. Many highly successful people exhibit narcissistic personality traits, but the diagnosis of narcissistic personality disorder is made only when these traits are inflexible and cause significant impairment or distress.[9,11,26,37]

CLUSTER C: DISORDERS INVOLVING ANXIETY AND FEARFULNESS

Avoidant Personality Disorder

Patients with *avoidant personality disorder* exhibit a pattern of social inhibition and lack self-esteem. They are afraid that others will criticize their performance or person. These traits are present by early adulthood and cause problems in various situations (Box 43-13). Unlike the schizoid personality, the avoidant personality does *not* want to be alone and wants to enter into social relationships but avoids them because of the fear of failure.[9,11,26,37]

BOX 43-13

DSM-IV-TR **Diagnostic Criteria for Avoidant Personality Disorder**

A pervasive pattern of social inhibition, feelings of inadequacy, and hypersensitivity to negative evaluation, characterized by four more of the following:
1. Avoids occupational activities that involve significant interpersonal contact because of fears of criticism, disapproval, or rejection
2. Is unwilling to become involved with people unless certain of being liked
3. Shows restraint within intimate relationships because of fear of being shamed or ridiculed
4. Is preoccupied with being criticized or rejected in social situations
5. Inhibited in new interpersonal situations because of feelings of inadequacy
6. Views self as socially inept, personally unappealing, or inferior to others
7. Is unusually reluctant to take personal risks or to engage in any new activities because they may prove embarrassing

---

Modified from *Diagnostic and statistical manual of mental disorders,* ed 4 (text revision), Washington, DC, 2000, American Psychiatric Association.

Dependent Personality Disorder

Persons with *dependent personality disorder* display a "pervasive and excessive need to be taken care of that leads to submission and clinging behavior and fears of separation."[9]

Anger at those they depend on for support is not expressed because of their extreme fear of alienating them. Individuals with this disorder often belittle themselves and their abilities and take criticism as proof of their worthlessness. The initiation of a project is unthinkable because of their lack of self-confidence, and they often present themselves as incompetent. They will make extraordinary self-sacrifices or tolerate verbal, physical, or sexual abuse to maintain an important relationship (Box 43-14).[9,11,26,37]

Cultural factors should be considered because some cultures emphasize passivity, politeness, and respectfulness, which may be misinterpreted as traits of dependent personality disorder.

Obsessive-Compulsive Personality Disorder

Persons with *obsessive-compulsive personality disorder* display "a preoccupation with orderliness, perfectionism, and mental and interpersonal control, at the expense of flexibility, openness, and efficiency."[9] Estimates put the prevalence of obsessive-compulsive personality disorder at about 1% of the U.S. population.

People with obsessive-compulsive personality disorder have a need to control and will do so through inordinate attention to details, procedures, lists, or rules to the extent that an important project may never be completed (Box 43-15). They check repeatedly for mistakes, then check again. Perfectionism causes these individuals great distress

BOX 43-14

DSM-IV-TR Diagnostic Criteria for Dependent Personality Disorder

Dependent personality disorder is a persuasive and excessive need to be taken care of, beginning in early adulthood and indicated by five or more of the following:
1. Has difficulty making everyday decisions without excessive advice from others
2. Needs others to assume responsibility for most major areas of life
3. Has difficulty expressing disagreement with others due to fear of loss of approval
4. Has difficulty initiating projects or doing things on own
5. Goes to excessive lengths to obtain nurturance and support from others
6. Feels uncomfortable when alone due to fear of being unable to care for self
7. Urgently seeks another relationship as source of support when a close relationship ends
8. Unrealistically preoccupied with fears of being left to care for self

Modified from *Diagnostic and statistical manual of mental disorders,* ed 4 (text revision), Washington, DC, 2000, American Psychiatric Association.

BOX 43-15

DSM-IV-TR Diagnostic Criteria for Obsessive-Compulsive Personality Disorder

Obsessive-compulsive personality disorder is a pervasive pattern of preoccupation with orderliness, perfectionism, and mental and interpersonal control, beginning by early adulthood and indicated by four or more of the following:
1. Preoccupation with details, rules, lists, order, organizations, or schedules to the extent that the major point of the activity is lost
2. Perfectionism that interferes with task completion
3. Excessive devotion to work and productivity to the exclusion of leisure activities and friendships
4. Over-conscientiousness, scrupulousness, and inflexibility about matters of morality, ethics, or values
5. Inability to discard worn-out or worthless objects even when they have no sentimental value
6. Reluctance to delegate tasks or to work with others unless they submit to his or her rules
7. Adoption of a miserly spending style toward self and others; money hoarded for future catastrophes
8. Rigidity and stubbornness

Modified from *Diagnostic and statistical manual of mental disorders,* ed 4 (text revision), Washington, DC, 2000, American Psychiatric Association.

because they can never attain their unreasonably high standards.[9,11,26,37]

TREATMENT

Personality disorders are one of the more perplexing groups of mental disorders to treat. These patients rarely appear for treatment of their own volition and are unable to form long-term, stable relationships, such as that needed for successful psychotherapy. They tend to be unaware of their problem. These patients also usually have a coexisting axis I disorder, making it difficult to separate the two in terms of treatment planning.[11,26,37]

EATING DISORDERS

Dieting is an American obsession, with more than 90 million people in the United States striving to reach their "ideal" weight. About one third of the U.S. population (and increasing) is obese, but these individuals choose weight loss measures that can be life-threatening. Eating disorders, or their recognition, is a rather recent concern, with few references in the literature before 1960. The increased prevalence of eating disorders in recent decades may be explained by beauty being increasingly equated with thinness, particularly in Western cultures. These disorders are most common in the United States, Canada, Europe, Australia, Japan, New Zealand, and South Africa. In third-world countries, larger body size is seen as beauty and a sign of success.[9,37]

Only anorexia nervosa and bulimia are designated in the *DSM-IV-TR*. However, *binge eating* is included in "eating disorders otherwise not determined," a classification that includes a number of proposed new categories and disorders.

The cause of eating disorders is not clear but is likely the result of a combination of biological, psychological, and societal factors. Some suspect a physiological cause such as a chemical imbalance in the hypothalamus or pituitary gland. Psychologists hypothesize that causes include the societal value on thinness and a negative view of obesity. Others maintain that overly critical parents and the demand of perfectionism in many performance areas lead to eating disorders.[9,11,26,37]

ANOREXIA NERVOSA

Persons with **anorexia nervosa** refuse to maintain a minimal normal weight for their age and height. Anorexia can lead to a life-threatening medical condition. Patients are obsessively concerned with being thin, are intensely afraid of gaining weight, and have a distorted perception of the size and shape of their body (Box 43-16). This disorder is found primarily in females (90%) between the ages of 12 and 40. It is estimated that 15% to 20% of anorexic persons literally starve themselves to death. Death occurs most often from starvation, suicide, or electrolyte imbalance.[9,11,31,36,37]

Weight loss is attained primarily through the reduction of food intake, with persons initially excluding foods that they consider to be highly caloric. As they lose weight, the fear of weight gain often intensifies. Their self-esteem is highly dependent on their perception of body size and shape. Weight loss is seen as a significant achievement and weight gain as failure. Individuals with this disorder seldom seek treatment because they lack insight or practice denial. Many exhibit coexisting symptoms of OCD and are often preoccupied with thoughts of food. Many individuals with

DSM-IV-TR Diagnostic Criteria for and Types of Anorexia Nervosa

Criteria
1. Refusal to maintain body weight at or above a minimally normal weight for age and height
2. Intense fear of gaining weight or becoming fat, even though underweight
3. Disturbance in how body weight or shape is experienced, undue influence of body weight or shape on self-evaluation, or denial of the seriousness of the current low body weight
4. In females, absence of at least three consecutive menstrual cycles.

Types
Restricting: During current episode the person has not regularly engaged in binge eating/purging behavior.
Binge eating/purging: During current episode the person has regularly engaged in binge eating or purging.

Modified from *Diagnostic and statistical manual of mental disorders,* ed 4 (text revision), Washington, DC, 2000, American Psychiatric Association.

DSM-IV-TR Diagnostic Criteria for Bulimia Nervosa

1. Recurrent episodes of binge eating, as evidenced by the following:
   a. Eating an amount of food that is definitely larger than most people would eat during a similar period under similar circumstances
   b. Lacking a sense of control over eating during the episode
2. Recurrent inappropriate compensatory behavior to prevent weight gain, such as self-induced vomiting, misuse of laxatives, diuretics, enemas, fasting, or excessive exercising
3. Binge eating and inappropriate compensatory behaviors at least twice a week for 3 months on average
4. Self-evaluation unduly influenced by body shape and weight
5. Disturbance not occurring exclusively during episodes of anorexia nervosa

Modified from *Diagnostic and statistical manual of mental disorders,* ed 4 (text revision), Washington, DC, 2000, American Psychiatric Association.

anorexia nervosa exhibit depressive symptoms (e.g., social withdrawal, insomnia, depressed mood) that may meet the diagnostic criteria for "major depressive disorder." Other features include a strong need to control one's environment, perfectionism, restrained emotional affect, concerns about eating in public, and inflexible thinking.[9,11,26,37]

During an episode of anorexia nervosa, one of two subtypes can be used in the development of an appropriate treatment plan (see Box 43-16). The *restricting type* describes weight loss accomplished primarily through dieting, fasting, or excessive exercise; in the current episode the patient has not regularly engaged in binge eating or purging. The *binge eating/purging type* describes the individual who regularly engages in binge eating, purging, or both. Most bingers with anorexia practice self-induced vomiting and misuse laxatives or diuretics. Recovering from anorexia nervosa is possible, but some individuals struggle with their fluctuating weight and the resulting deterioration of their health over the course of many years.

BULIMIA NERVOSA

Bulimia nervosa is an eating disorder characterized by repeated episodes of eating abnormally large amounts of food in a short period, often followed by purging. Similar to anorexia nervosa, individuals diagnosed with bulimia nervosa are typically within the normal weight/height range for their age group. This problem usually develops in adolescence or early adulthood. In contrast to the anorexic person, who takes pride in demonstrating self-control, a person who suffers from bulimia feels out of control and ashamed. Bulimia nervosa occurs rarely among moderately or morbidly obese individuals. With both disorders, patients place extraordinary emphasis on body shape and size to determine self-worth and self-esteem.[9,37]

Bulimia is characterized by repeated binge eating episodes followed by extreme efforts to avoid weight gain (Box 43-17). A *binge* is defined as "eating in a discrete period of time an amount of food that is definitely larger than most individuals would eat under similar circumstances."[9] A gallon of ice cream or a whole pie may be consumed at one time, followed by feelings of guilt and depression. Binge eating usually takes place in secrecy, is characterized by rapid consumption, and may or may not be planned. Binge eating episodes are usually triggered by some interpersonal stressor, hunger after a period of fasting, a depressed mood, or unresolved conflicts about body shape, weight, and shape. Bulimic persons may then induce vomiting or take laxatives to rid themselves of the food, a behavior known as *purging.* Vomiting is the most common method used, as practiced by 80% to 90% of bulimic individuals. They use a number of different methods to induce vomiting, such as fingers or instruments to induce their gag reflex. Over time they are able to vomit at will.[9,11,26,37]

The cause of bulimia appears to be both biological and psychological. Biologically, a chemical imbalance may exist in the hypothalamus or pituitary gland. Bulimic persons may not feel "full" after they have eaten or even binged, which results from a low level of specific hormones that control the feeling of satiety. Psychologically, societal pressures value slenderness, and a negative stigma is associated with obesity. A separate hypothesis suggests that both anorexia nervosa and bulimia are the result of a rigid, rule-governed parental style. Bulimic patients have often experienced an unreasonable amount of rejection and blame during childhood and an inordinate need to strive for perfection to gain positive regard from important figures in their lives.[9,11,26,37]

Bulimia nervosa is distinguished by two subtypes.

Characteristically, the patient with the *purging subtype* is described as "an individual that engages in self-induced vomiting and/or the misuse of laxatives, diuretics, or enemas during the current episode."[9] The *nonpurging subtype* describes the person who uses other methods of inappropriate compensation for the act of overeating; a passive example is fasting, whereas an aggressive method is excessive exercising. Individuals with purging bulimia are more likely to exhibit symptoms of depression and greater preoccupation with body shape and size than individuals with nonpurging bulimia.[9,37]

Individuals with bulimia exhibit an increased frequency of depression and lack of self-esteem. Anxiety disorders are likely to coexist, and at least 30% of these individuals experience a substance-abuse problem. Substance abuse usually stems from initial use of stimulants to control appetite.

DENTAL CONSIDERATIONS

The oral health of patients with bulimia is known to be at risk from the damaging effect on the enamel structure from the intensified acid challenge from regurgitation of gastric contents.

Low, unstimulated salivary flow rates and very high counts of mutans streptococci and lactobacilli lead to higher susceptibility to both dental caries and enamel erosion in patients with diagnosed eating disorders. A significant correlation exists between parotid enlargement and enamel erosion in bulimic patients. Painless enlargement of the parotid salivary glands is common with chronic vomiting. Salivary gland impairment, poor oral hygiene, and poor diet adversely affect dental health.[29,31,36,41,51]

Often, generalized destruction of tooth structure directly results from highly acidic stomach contents on the patient's dentition. The damage that follows the binge-purge episodes is reduced by meticulous oral hygiene measures, including regular use of fluoride products.

The dental professional is in a unique position among healthcare professionals in helping to identify patients with eating disorders. Questions regarding diet, eating habits, and exercise may help uncover patterns indicative of some aspect of an eating disorder.

If the patient is younger than 18 years of age, the matter can become a legal and ethical one. In such cases the dental professional becomes responsible for cautiously advising the parent or legal guardian of the suspected problem. Because eating disorders have long-term health effects and can be life-threatening, the manner in which these matters are handled can make a significant difference in its outcome. The dental professional who approaches the situation with great sensitivity for the patient and recognizes that intervention is in that patient's best interest can help enable the patient to get the necessary help.

SCHIZOPHRENIA

People with schizophrenia make up most of the patients hospitalized for a mental disorder. A patient with schizophrenia has a mixed set of characteristic symptoms, such as delusions, hallucinations, and thought disturbances

---

BOX 43-18

***DSM-IV-TR* Diagnostic Criteria for Schizophrenia**

1. Two or more of the following symptoms for at least 1 month:
   a. Delusions
   b. Hallucinations
   c. Disorganized speech
   d. Grossly disorganized or catatonic behavior
   e. Negative symptoms (e.g., flattened affect, reduced speech)
2. Duration
   Patient has shown evidence of the disorder for at least 6 months.
3. Social/occupational dysfunction
   Patient has significantly impaired ability to work, study, socialize, or provide self-care.
4. Substance abuse or general medical condition exclusion
5. Schizoaffective or mood disorder exclusion
6. Relationship to a developmental order exclusion

Modified from *Diagnostic and statistical manual of mental disorders*, ed 4 (text revision), Washington, DC, 2000, American Psychiatric Association.

(Box 43-18). These distortions in thinking, perception, and emotion are often accompanied by social withdrawal and bizarre behavior. Schizophrenia involves a reduced level of functioning in one or more major areas of life, such as work, interpersonal relations, education, and self-care. Probably the most distressing symptom of the disorder is the person's feeling of being out of control regarding thoughts and actions. Along with the dramatic *(positive)* symptoms are the less dramatic *(negative)* symptoms, including a flattened affect or apparent absence of emotional expression. Individuals with schizophrenia have poor insight into their illness, which itself is a manifestation of the disorder.[9,11,26,37]

TYPES AND ONSET

The five types of schizophrenia are catatonic, disorganized, paranoid, undifferentiated, and residual (Table 43-4).[9]

Two primary time frames exist for the onset of schizophrenia. In *process schizophrenia* the symptoms begin to develop early in life, with subtle changes becoming more pronounced over time. In *reactive schizophrenia* the onset is dramatic and sudden. Reactive schizophrenia has been shown to respond to treatment more favorably and with a better long-term prognosis than process schizophrenia.[11,26,37,38]

The pattern to the onset of schizophrenia is (1) predromal, (2) active, and (3) residual. The *predromal* stage is evidenced by social isolation or withdrawal, marked impairment in role functioning, very peculiar behavior, blunted affect, lack of initiative or interests, and impairment in personal hygiene or inappropriate dress (e.g., wearing multiple layers of winter clothing on an extremely hot day). The *active* phase is characterized by either positive or negative symptoms. Positive symptoms

TABLE 43-4

Major types of schizophrenia

Type	Symptoms
Disorganized	Inappropriate laughter and giggling
	Silliness
	Incoherent speech
	Infantile behavior
	Strange and sometimes obscene behavior
Paranoid	Delusions and hallucinations of persecution or of greatness
	Loss of judgment
	Erratic and unpredictable behavior
Catatonic	Major disturbances in movement
	In some phases, loss of all motion, with patient frozen in a single position and remaining that way for hours or even days
	In other phases, hyperactivity and wild, sometimes violent, movement
Undifferentiated	Variable mixture of major symptoms of schizophrenia
	Classification used for patients who cannot be typed into any of the more specific categories
Residual	Minor signs of schizophrenia after more serious episode

Modified from Feldman RS: *Understanding psychology,* New York, 1996, McGraw-Hill.

include delusions, hallucinations, disorganized speech, catatonia, and disorganized or bizarre behavior. Negative symptoms include flattened or blunted emotions, lack of initiative toward goal-directed behaviors, limited or no verbal communication, and no satisfaction from previously pleasurable activities. The negative symptoms are often difficult to judge because they occur on a continuum and can be attributed to many other factors (e.g., side effect of medication, depression, situational stress).[9,11,26,37]

Schizophrenia is also "categorized" into positive and negative symptoms. *Negative symptom schizophrenia* is characterized by a significant reduction in level of functioning, social withdrawal, and a flattened emotional affect. The patient with *positive symptom schizophrenia* presents with delusions, hallucinations, and extremes in emotional display.[9,37]

The schizophrenic patient demonstrates an obvious deterioration of functioning in the student, employee, or parent/homemaker role. Disturbances of thought and language are also noted.[9,37]

DELUSIONS

Delusions are bizarre beliefs in spite of their preposterous nature. These patients hold strongly to their beliefs even when presented with overwhelming evidence to the contrary. They are preoccupied with thoughts about their delusional beliefs during the active phase of the condition. Common delusions include belief that thoughts are being inserted into one's mind, people are reading the patient's

mind, and external forces are exerting control over thoughts and actions.[9,37]

HALLUCINATIONS

Hallucination is defined as "false sensory perception in the absence of an actual external stimulus."[9] Auditory hallucinations are the most common and are most often experienced as voices giving instructions or commenting on behavior. Although these experiences are often frightening to the patient, they may also provide a sense of security and comfort. Hallucinations are very real to the person and persist over time despite having no basis in reality.[9,37]

DISORGANIZED THINKING

The characteristic of *disorganized thinking* may be the most important diagnostic criterion for schizophrenia. It involves the tendency of a person to say things that make no sense or that are so incoherent that they are regarded as "word salad." Patients with disorganized thinking also tend to answer questions in a very tangential manner and frequently and abruptly shift topics, referred to as "derailment" or "loose associations."[9,37]

GROSSLY DISORGANIZED BEHAVIOR

Individuals with schizophrenia may have difficulty in daily living activities, such as preparing meals or attending to personal hygiene. They may dress inappropriately for the weather. Aggressive behaviors such as shouting and swearing often occur without external stimulus.[9,37]

CATATONIC BEHAVIOR

Catatonic behavior is seen as an extreme degree of maintaining a rigid posture and resisting efforts to be moved. The other extreme is seen as excessive activity. Catatonic behavior is not specific to schizophrenia and may be seen with other mental disorders.[9,37]

TREATMENT

Neuroleptic Drugs

The most troublesome side effects are called *extrapyramidal symptoms,* including muscular rigidity, tremors, restlessness/agitation, and peculiar postures. Long-term treatment with *neuroleptic* drugs often leads to the development of *tardive dyskinesia* (TD), which is characterized by involuntary, grotesque movements of the mouth as well as spasmodic movements of the extremities. This distressing problem is frequently irreversible even after discontinuation of the medication. The incidence of TD increases with length of time taking the medication, with 25% of patients developing the syndrome within 3 months of treatment.[1]

If medication is not continued after recovery from the acute psychotic episode, as many as 75% of patients will experience another psychotic episode within the first year. Although the continued use of the neuroleptic medication cannot prevent a relapse, it can reduce the recurrence by about 60%. Some patients can function at least as well without medication as when taking medication. The difficulty is an inability to distinguish those who *do* from those who *do not* need the continued pharmacological treatment. Some clinicians choose to prescribe lower doses of neuroleptics to patients with schizophrenia to minimize the potential side effects. Positive aspects of this approach include less blunted affect, better social psychosocial functioning, and less unusual movement or motor behavior.[37]

Newer forms of antipsychotic medications, known as *atypical antipsychotics,* do not produce extrapyramidal symptoms or TD. These drugs have also proven especially useful for patients who do not respond to the classic neuroleptics, with up to 60% of previous nonresponders showing improvement.

In addition to pharmacological therapy, *psychosocial treatments* have been developed for individuals with schizophrenia, including family-oriented aftercare, social skills training, and institutional programs. The aftercare focuses on improving the family's coping skills. Education is probably most important aspect; the family is informed about what to expect and educated about the nature of the disease. This enables the patient to remain in the home on an outpatient basis and may reduce relapse rates to about 20%, compared with 40% of patients not receiving family-oriented aftercare.

Many patients continue to have impaired social and interpersonal skills even when receiving medication. To address these problems, social skills training focuses on role playing, role modeling, and reinforcement or social reinforcement for appropriate behaviors. Few data demonstrate improved social adjustment with this approach. Besides outpatient programs, various types of institutional care continue to be important for the patient with schizophrenia. Most patients experience recurrent phases of the disorder, and brief periods of hospitalization are often beneficial. Some individuals, however, are significantly disturbed and require long-term institutionalized care. Programs are available that reward patients for demonstrating desired behaviors (e.g., grooming, general social courtesies) in an effort to decrease undesirable behaviors (e.g., violence). These positive behaviors are then rewarded with "tokens," which can be exchanged for food or privileges. Positive behaviors are rewarded, but inappropriate behaviors are largely ignored. This aspect of treatment has shown outstanding results.[11,26,37]

Schizophrenia affects many areas of a person's ability to function, including cognitive and perceptual, so a multifaceted approach to treatment is required.

DENTAL CONSIDERATIONS

In providing dental care to schizophrenic patients, the clinician must be aware of the need to alter and adjust treatment approaches for patients who have impaired ability to think logically. The dental practitioner must also consider the side effects of neuroleptics and the potential for adverse interactions between medications for schizophrenia and drugs used in dental treatment. These patients often present with significant oral disease. A reduced ability to perform adequate self-care is often associated schizophrenia, including preventive oral care. The neuroleptic medications used to treat and maintain these patients may cause bizarre body movements, often in the orofacial region. These spasms can cause the dislocation of the temporomandibular joint, cause difficulty in swallowing, dislodge dentures, and interfere with the natural gag reflex.[1,8] The medications to treat schizophrenia also reduce saliva, resulting in xerostomia. This reduced salivary flow increases the risk of periodontal disease and the onset of rapidly progressive caries activity.*

Schizophrenic patients often have hallucinations that are orally fixated. They have reported "hearing voices in fillings" and have tried to rid themselves of these "out-of-control" feelings by cutting out their tongue, performing extractions on themselves, and burning the gingiva with caustic solutions. They may believe that removing the "offending" body part will serve as a means to make up for the "bad" parts of themselves.[20]

In providing dental treatment to schizophrenic patients, preventive health education is extremely important. Many of these patients, however, do not have the inclination or coordination for routine oral hygiene. The use of colorful educational materials and the demonstration of brushing and flossing in front of a mirror may help them to focus on the task at hand. It is helpful for dental professionals to demonstrate on themselves because patients are often unable to follow the most basic verbal instructions without direct demonstration. Communication with these patients at times can be difficult and on rare occasions, dangerous. Caution must be used when the potential exists for a violent outburst by the patient.[17,43]

---

*References 3, 7, 8, 17, 20, 21, 48.

RITICAL THINKING ACTIVITIES

1. Consider how the U.S. culture views women in the popular media (e.g., movies, advertisements, fashion magazines). Do you share those views? What attributes do you include in your attitude about women's appearance?
2. If you had to develop a dental health plan for a mental health hospital, what would be the component elements of that plan? What parts of that plan would differ significantly from what you might expect to do in private practice?
3. Based on your understanding of the oral implications of the use of psychotropic medications, do you think that psychiatrists or general practitioners should inform patients about potential oral health problems and their prevention? If so, what information do you think should be provided? Should dental healthcare professionals alert the medical community about the effects of these medications on oral health?

Continued

CRITICAL THINKING ACTIVITIES—cont'd

4. Considering the prevalence of mental disorders, do you think the development of a mental health "screening" would be of value? What areas would you address, and how would you approach the patient on sensitive issues?

5. If you were to provide information to medical professionals (e.g., psychiatrists, psychiatric nurses, pri-

mary care providers) about oral care and mental health, what means of communication would be best? Given your recommendation, develop an outline of the program or presentation, and review it with a colleague.

 REVIEW QUESTIONS

1. Which of the following antidepressants is a selective serotonin reuptake inhibitor (SSRI)?
   a. Wellbutrin
   b. Serzone
   c. Zoloft
   d. Mardil
   e. Tofranil

2. Which of the following disorders is the fear of germs?
   a. Acrophobia
   b. Claustrophobia
   c. Mysophobia
   d. Demophobia
   e. Hyptephobia

3. If a person had a negative life event beyond normal experience and disruptive of previously held views, which of the following disorders would likely be the primary diagnosis?
   a. Bipolar disorder
   b. Schizophrenia
   c. Obsessive-compulsive disorder
   d. Posttraumatic stress disorder
   e. Major depressive episode

4. An individual who consumes large amounts of food in an almost frenzied state and then uses extraordinary means to prevent weight gain would be suffering from which of the following disorders?
   a. Obsessive-compulsive disorder
   b. Anorexia nervosa
   c. Histrionic personality disorder

   d. Bulimia nervosa
   e. Dissociative disorder

5. A person who hears voices from outer space has which one of the following symptoms?
   a. Delusion
   b. Hallucination
   c. Disorganized speech
   d. Catatonic behavior
   e. Flattened affect

6. Which one of the following is the manual developed by the American Psychiatric Association that names and categorizes over 200 mental disorders?
   a. *DSM-IV-TR*
   b. *ICD-10*
   c. *NIDA*
   d. *NIMH-4*

7. Which of the following drug categories would most likely cause tardive dyskinesia?
   a. Antidepressant
   b. Antianxiety
   c. Antipsychotic
   d. Antimanic

8. Which of the following would *not* be a diagnostic criterion for a major depressive episode?
   a. Loss of interest in previously enjoyable activities
   b. Disruption of normal sleep patterns
   c. Sense of entitlement
   d. Significant increase or decrease in food intake
   e. Feelings of worthlessness or hopelessness

 SUGGESTED AGENCIES AND WEB SITES

Because of the ever-changing nature of the Internet, some of the web sites listed here may have changed since publication. Please refer to Mosby's Evolve web site for the most current information.

American Psychiatric Association, 1400 K St NW, Washington, DC 20005: http://www.psych.org

American Psychological Association, 750 First St NE, Washington, DC 20002-4242; (202) 336-5500: http://www.apa.org

Canadian Mental Health Association, 2160 Yonge, 3rd Floor, Toronto, Ontario M4S 2Z3, Canada; (416) 484-7750: http:// www.ontario.cmha.ca

Center for Mental Health Services Knowledge Exchange Network: http://www.mentalhealth.org

Eating Disorders Awareness and Prevention, Inc. (EDAP): http://www.edap.org

Mental Health Network: http://www.mentalhealthnet.org

Mental health resources: http://www.mentalhealth.miningco.com

SUGGESTED AGENCIES AND WEB SITES—cont'd

National Association of Anorexia Nervosa and Associated Disorders (ANAD): http://www.anad.org

National Association of State and Mental Health Directors: http://www.nasmhpd.org

National Council on Disability ("State mental health agencies"): http://www.ncd.gov

National Institute of Mental Health: 6001 Executive Blvd, Rm 8184, MSC 9663, Bethesda, MD 20892-9663; (301) 443-4513 (telephone); (301) 443-4279 (fax): http://www.nimh.nih.gov

The Substance Abuse and Mental Health Services Administration: http://www.samhsa.gov

U.S. Department of Health and Human Services: 200 Independence Ave SW, Washington, DC 20201; (202) 619-0257 (telephone); (877) 696-6775 (toll free): http://www.hhs.gov

U.S. surgeon general site: http://www.surgeongeneral.gov

World Federation of Mental Health: http://www.wfmh.com

 ADDITIONAL READINGS AND RESOURCES

Brinck VM: Oral health and treatment needs among patients in psychiatric institutions for the elderly, *Community Dent Oral Epidemiol* 21:169-71, 1993.

Dayhoff SA: *Diagonally-parked in a parallel universe: working through social anxiety,* Placitas, NM, 2000, Effectiveness-Plus.

Flach F: *Psychobiology and psychopharmacology,* New York, 1988, Norton.

Freud A: *The ego and the mechanisms of defense,* revised ed, Madison, Conn, 1966, International Universities Press.

Klivington K: *The science of the mind,* Cambridge, Mass, 1989, MIT Press.

Mahrer AR: *Therapeutic experiencing: the process of change,* New York, 1986, Norton.

McWilliams N: *Psychoanalytic diagnosis: understanding personality structure in the clinical process,* New York, 1994, Guilford.

Milosevic A, Brodie DA, Slade PD: Dental erosion, oral hygiene, and nutrition in eating disorders, *Int J Eat Disord* 21(2):195-9, 1997.

Wilcox DT, Karamanoukian HL, Glick PL: Toothbrush ingestion by bulimics may require laparotomy, *J Pediatr Surg* 29(12):1596-8, 1994.

REFERENCES

1. Bassett A, Remick RA, Blasberg B: Tardive dyskinesia: an unrecognized cause of orofacial pain, *Oral Surg Oral Med Oral Pathol* 61:570-2, 1986.
2. Beck FM, Kaul TJ: Recognition and management of the depressed dental patient, *J Am Dent Assoc* 99:967-71, 1979.
3. Ben-Aryeh H et al: Salivary flow-rate and composition in schizophrenic patients on clozapine: subjective reports and laboratory data, *Biol Psychiatry* 39:946-9, 1996.
4. Bertram U, Kragh-Sorensen P, Rafaelsen OJ, Larsen N-E: Saliva secretion following long-term antidepressant treatment with nortriptyline controlled by plasma levels, *Scand J Dent Res* 87:58-64, 1979.
5. Blazer D, Hughes D, George LK: Stressful life events and the onset of a generalized anxiety syndrome, *Am J Psychiatry* 144(9):1178-83, 1987.
6. Bohn DJ et al: Clonazepam in the treatment of social phobia: a pilot study, *J Clin Psychiatry* 51(5):35-40, 1990.
7. Council on Scientific Affairs, Ciancio S, editor: *American Dental Association guide to dental therapeutics,* Chicago, 1998, ADA Publishing.
8. Craig TJ, Richardson MA, Pass R, Haugland G: Impairment of the gag reflex in schizophrenia, *Compr Psychiatry* 24:514-20, 1983.
9. *Diagnostic and statistical manual of mental disorders (DSM-IV),* ed 4, (text revision), Washington, DC, 2000, American Psychiatric Association.
10. Doebling S, Rowe MM: Negative perceptions of dental stimuli and their effects on dental fear, *J Dent Hyg* 74(2):110-16, 2000.
11. Feldman RS: *Understanding psychology,* New York, 1996, McGraw-Hill.
12. Findlay-Jones R, Brown GW: Types of stressful life events and the onset of anxiety and depressive disorder, *Psychol Med* 11(4):803-15, 1981.

13. Fox PC et al: Xerostomia: evaluation of a symptom with increasing significance, *J Am Dent Assoc* 110:519-25, 1985.
14. Friedlander AH, Birch NJ: Dental conditions in patients with bipolar disorder on long-term lithium maintenance therapy, *Spec Care Dentist* 10(5):148-51, 1990.
15. Friedlander AH, Eth S: Dental management considerations in children with obsessive-compulsive disorder, *ASDC J Dent Child* 58(3):217-22, 1991.
16. Friedlander AH, Freymiller EG, Yagiela JA, Eth S: Dental management of the adolescent with panic disorder, *ASDC J Dent Child* 60(4):365-71, 1993.
17. Friedlander AH, Friedlander IK, Eth S, Freymiller EG: Dental management of child and adolescent patients with schizophrenia, *ASDC J Dent Child* 60(4):281-7, 1993.
18. Friedlander AH, Friedlander IK, Yagiela JA, Eth SE: Dental management of the child and adolescent with major depression, *J Dent Child* 60(2):125-31, 1993.
19. Friedlander AH, Kawakami KK, Ganzell S, Fitten IJ: Dental management of the geriatric patient with major depression, *Spec Care Dent* 13(6):249-53, 1993.
20. Friedlander AH, Liberman RP: Oral health care for the patient with schizophrenia, *Spec Care Dentist* 11(5):179-83, 1991.
21. Friedlander AH, Mahler ME: Major depressive disorder: psychopathology, medical management and dental implications, *J Am Dent Assoc* 132(5):629-38, 2001.
22. Friedlander AH, Mills MJ, Wittlin BJ: Dental management considerations for the patients with post-traumatic stress disorder, *Oral Surg Oral Med Oral Pathol* 63(6):669-73, 1987.
23. Friedlander AH, Serafetinides EA: Dental management of the patient with obsessive-compulsive disorder, *Spec Care Dent* 11(6):238-42, 1991.
24. Friedlander AH, West LJ: Dental management of the patient with major depression, *Oral Surg Oral Med Oral Pathol* 71(5):573-8, 1991.

Continued

25. Gage TW, Pickett FA: *Mosby's dental drug reference,* ed 6, St Louis, 2002, Mosby.

26. Gerow JR: *Psychology: an introduction,* ed 3, New York, 1992, HarperCollins.

27. Greenberg PE, Stiglin LE, Finkelstein SN, Berndt ER: Depression: a neglected major illness, *J Clin Psychiatry* 54(11):425-6, 1993.

28. Haverman CW, Redding SW: Dental management and treatment of xerostomic patients, *Tex Dent J* June: 43-56, 1998.

29. Hellstrom L: Oral complications in anorexia nervosa, *Scand J Dent Res* 85(1):71-86, 1977.

30. Hetherington EM, Parke RD: *Child psychology: a contemporary viewpoint,* New York, 1993, McGraw-Hill.

31. Jensen OE, Featherstone JD, Stege P: Chemical and physical oral findings of anorexia nervosa and bulimia, *J Oral Pathol* 16(8):399-402, 1987.

32. Little JW, Falace DA: *Dental management of the medically compromised patient,* ed 6, St Louis, (in press), Mosby.

33. Mauro V, Mendloiwuez MV, Stein MB: Quality of life in individuals with anxiety disorders, *Am J Psychiatry* 157:669-82, 2000.

34. McGrath E, Keita GP, Strickland BR, Russo NF: *Women and depression: risk factors and treatment issues,* Washington, DC, 1990, American Psychological Association.

35. Monroe SM, Simons AD: Diathesis-stress theories in the context of life stress research: implications for depressive disorders, *Psychol Bull* 11(3):406-25, 1991.

36. Ohrn R, Eazeil K, Angmar-Mansson B: Oral status of 81 subjects with eating disorders, *Eur J Oral Sci* 107(3):157-63, 1999.

37. Oltman FO, Emery RE: *Abnormal psychology,* Princeton, NJ, 1995, Prentice Hall.

38. Onstad S, Skre I, Torgersen S, Kringlen E: Subtypes of schizophrenia: evidence from a twin-family study, *Acta Psychiatr Scand* 84(2):203-6, 1991.

39. Peeters FP, deVries MW, Vissink A: Risks for oral health with the use of antidepressants, *Gen Hosp Psychiatry* 20:150-4, 1998.

40. Reiger DA et al: One-month prevalence of mental disorders in the United States, based on five epidemiologic catchment area sites, *Arch Gen Psychiatry* 45(11):977-86, 1988.

41. Roberts MW, Tylenda CA: Dental aspects of anorexia and bulimia nervosa, *Pediatrician* 16:178-84, 1989.

42. Rundegren J, Van Dijken J, Mornstad H, Von Knorring L: Oral conditions in patients receiving long-term treatment with cyclic antidepressant drugs, *Swed Dent J* 9:55-64, 1985.

43. Shuman SK, Bebeau MJ: Ethical and legal issues in special patient care, *Dent Clin N Am* 38(3):553-75, 1994.

44. Simons AD, Gordon JS, Monroe SM, Thase ME: Toward an integration of psychologic, social and biologic factors in depression effects on outcome and course of cognitive therapy, *J Consult Clin Psychol* 63(3):369-77, 1995.

45. Slome BA: Rampant caries: a side effect of tricyclic antidepressant therapy, *Gen Dent,* Nov-Dec 1987, pp 494-6.

46. Sullivan MJ, Neish N: Catastrophic thinking and the experience of pain during dental procedures, *J Ind Dent Assoc* 79(4): 16-19, 2001.

47. Sullivan MJ, Neish NR: Psychological predictors of pain during dental hygiene treatment, *Probe* 31(4):123-6, 1997.

48. Thomas A, Lavrentzou E, Karouzos C, Kontis C: Factors which influence the oral condition of chronic schizophrenia patients, *Spec Care Dent* 15(2):84-86, 1996.

49. Watson JB, Raynor R: Conditioned emotional reactions, *J Exp Psychol* 3:1-14, 1920.

50. Weisman MM: The changing rates of major depression: cross-national comparisons, *JAMA* 268(21):3098-3105, 1992.

51. Wolcott RB, Yager J, Gordon G: Dental sequelae to the binge-purge syndrome (bulimia): report of cases, *J Am Dent Assoc* 109(5):723-5, 1984.

52. Woodall IJ: *Comprehensive dental hygiene care,* ed 4, St Louis, 1993, Mosby.

53. Wynn RL: New antidepressant medications, *Gen Dent* 45(1): 24-8, 1997.

CHAPTER 44

Immune System Dysfunction

Debbie Manne

Chapter Outline

Immune System Function
Immune System Dysfunction
   Aging
   Diabetes
   Autoimmmune diseases
Case Study: Case 1: Oral Care Considerations
  for the Cancer Patient
Cancer
   Incidence and risk factors
   Treatment
   Emotional aspects

Role of the dental hygienist
Oral complications related to chemotherapy
Case Study: Case 2: Oral Care Considerations
  for the HIV-Positive Patient
Acquired Immunodeficiency Syndrome
   Incidence and risk factors
   Treatment
   Role of the dental hygienist
   Oral manifestations
   Associated periodontal diseases

Key Terms

Acquired immunodeficiency
  syndrome (AIDS)
Cancer

Chemotherapy
Human immunodeficiency virus (HIV)

Immune system
Mucositis
NADIR

Neurotoxicity
Xerostomia

Learning Outcomes

1. Compare and contrast two forms of immunity.
2. Describe diseases and conditions from which an acquired immune system dysfunction can result.
3. Become familiar with the pathophysiology of immune system dysfunction.
4. Identify incidence, risk factors, and treatment of cancer.
5. Discuss the oral complications common for a chemotherapy patient, and discuss the prevention and care associated with each complication.
6. Develop a plan of care for a patient undergoing chemotherapy.

7. Distinguish autoimmune disorders and the use of immunosuppressant therapies.
8. Demonstrate the five roles of the dental hygienist in caring for an immunocompromised patient.
9. Identify incidence, etiology, risk factors, and treatment of HIV and AIDS.
10. Compare and contrast the clinical characteristics of HIV and AIDS.
11. Develop a care plan for patients with HIV and AIDS.

IMMUNE SYSTEM FUNCTION

The *immune system* is a complex system that protects the body from potential pathogens. This system is composed of T and B lymphocytes that act together in host defense. Two types of immunity function in this process: *innate* and *adaptive*. Innate immunity is present before any exposure to a pathogen, providing general immunity. Examples of innate immunity in the oral cavity are the oral mucosa and saliva. Salivary enzymes, pH, and normal bacterial flora help resist infection. Adaptive immunity occurs after exposure to a pathogen. After exposure, adaptive immunity works to develop antibodies (B cells) to this foreign body or antigen. The next time the body is exposed to that same antigen, the immune system "remembers" through the action of T cells. The T cells then relay this information to B cells that produce specific antibodies that attack the antigen. The body also learns to recognize the difference between self-antigens and foreign antigens. This is an important function of the immune system.

IMMUNE SYSTEM DYSFUNCTION

Immune system dysfunction results when the immune system does not work properly to protect the body. Congenital, spontaneously acquired, or iatrogenic factors cause immunodeficient syndromes.[4] Inherited immune system dysfunctions include T- and B-cell and phagocytic deficiencies.[4] Of the five types of leukocytes circulating in the blood, B lymphocytes (B cells) and T lymphocytes (T cells) are the most abundant. Each B cell and T cell is specific for a particular antigen. When these cells are defective, they fail to recognize and bind to the particular molecular structure to which they respond, thus disabling the immune system.

Forms of acquired immune dysfunction can result from diabetes, alcoholism, chronic obstructive pulmonary disease (COPD), malnutrition, aging, and acquired immunodeficiency syndrome (AIDS). Chemotherapy, radiation therapy, immunosuppressive therapy, bone marrow/stem cell transplantation, and organ transplantation are viewed as iatrogenic causes of immune deficiency. Although some of these conditions are discussed in other chapters (e.g., aging, diabetes, radiation therapy), this brief overview of the immune system and the impact these acquired immunodeficiencies have on oral heath is warranted. A listing of lesser-known immune system diseases is presented in Box 44-1.

AGING

In the aging population, immune system dysfunction can be influenced by medications or simply by the process of aging. For example, older adults are more likely to develop oral bacterial and fungal infections. They are also more prone to xerostomia, which contributes to a decrease in the natural protective barriers of the oral cavity. When caring for an older adult, a thorough oral examination is essential to ascertain any signs of infection or xerostomia. Suggestions for oral self-care and management of the symptoms of dry mouth for older adult patients are important responsibilities of the oral healthcare team.

BOX 44-1

Lesser-Known Immune System Diseases

Addison's disease
B-cell defects
Multiple sclerosis
Myasthenia gravis
Pernicious anemia
Psoriasis
Rheumatoid arthritis
Scleroderma
System lupus erythematosus
T-cell defects
Thyroid diseases (autoimmune)
  Hashimoto's thyroiditis (hypothyroidism)
  Grave's disease (hyperthyroidism)

DIABETES

Diabetes manifests as two types: insulin-dependent diabetes mellitus (IDDM) and non–insulin-dependent diabetes mellitus (NIDDM). IDDM results when the pancreas does not produce enough insulin. The cause is thought to be because of an autoimmune response (i.e., the body attacks its own cells perceiving them as foreign). Antibodies are believed to be directed against pancreatic islet cells, which are responsible for the production of insulin. IDDM is commonly diagnosed in juveniles and young adults. In NIDDM, the opposite is true. Although the pancreas produces enough insulin, the body is not able to use it. Here, the action of insulin is inefficient at the tissue level. The condition is known as *insulin resistance.*

In both IDDM and NIDDM, an immune system dysfunction is evident. Because of this dysfunction, patients with diabetes are more prone to infections and experience delayed healing times. This may be a result of poor circulation to various tissues because of vascular occlusion. Dental implications for patients with diabetes include greater incidences of periodontal infection and slower healing after surgery or extractions. This also leads to infection from bacteria, such as thrush and bacterial plaque. Chronic oral infections are especially evident in patients with poorly controlled diabetes. Obviously, thorough daily oral self-care is critical to the oral health of patients with diabetes.

AUTOIMMMUNE DISEASES

Autoimmune diseases result when the body begins to recognize self-antigens as foreign antigens. Common autoimmune diseases include rheumatoid arthritis, systemic lupus erythematosus, and IDDM. Some autoimmune diseases have oral manifestations, while others do not.

Rheumatoid Arthritis

The most debilitating form of arthritis is rheumatoid arthritis (RA), which causes aching, throbbing, and deformity in joints. Distinct from osteoarthritis, which results from normal wear and tear on the joints, RA is an inflammatory condition believed to be a result of the immune system attacking the synovium. RA affects approximately 25 million Americans; it is three times more common in women than in men, striking between the ages of 20 and 50.

In RA, the rheumatoid factor (RF), a group of antibody molecules, are incorporated into to the individual's own gamma globulin blood proteins. When circulating, this complex of antibodies and proteins causes tissue inflammation and muscle and bone deformities. Although RA tends to be chronic, it can vary in severity or even come and go. When the disease is active, patients with moderate to severe symptoms report a disruption in normal, routine tasks. This is especially true when RA affects the hands. As a result, tasks such as oral self-care require modifications in both recommended techniques and self-care tools.

Lupus Erythematosus

The term *lupus,* Latin for "wolf," was first used in the eighteenth century to describe the classic facial rash associated with this disease. Lupus is also considered a butterfly rash because of its facial distribution. The etiology of development is not understood. Although the disorder appears to be genetic, most persons with lupus do not have family members with lupus or other autoimmune disease. One explanation for onset of lupus is that the body, once exposed to an infectious agent, attempts to rid the body of this agent by exciting the immune system to action. In this disease, once the immune system has been activated, it is unable to deactivate, and thus the immune system continues to attack normal tissue.

Lupus is actually a broad term that is used to describe several different types of this autoimmune disease.

Discoid Lupus Erythematosus
This form of lupus affects the skin. It appears as a raised rash that can become thick and scaly and can last for days or years. It disappears and reappears but is most often chronic and causes scarring. Some patients with discoid lupus later develop systemic lupus erythematosus (SLE).

Drug-Induced Lupus
Drug-induced lupus causes symptoms similar to those of SLE that disappear once the drug is no longer taken. Drugs associated with drug-induced lupus include hydralazine (Apresoline), procainamide (Procan, Pronestyl), methyldopa (Aldomet), quinidine (Quinaglute), isoniazid (INH), and some antiseizure medications such as phenytoin (Dilantin) and carbamazepine (Tegretol).

Neonatal Lupus
This form of lupus affects newborns of women with SLE or certain other immune system disorders. Infants with neonatal lupus may develop serious heart defects, skin rash, liver abnormalities, or low blood counts.

Systemic Lupus Erythematosus
Systemic lupus erythematosus (SLE) is an autoimmune disease that affects all races, genders, and ages; however, it is three times more common in the African-American population and some Asian populations than in Native Americans and whites and it affects more women than men (8 out of 10 persons affected by SLE are women).

SLE affects the skin, lungs, heart, kidney, brain, and joints and exhibits as a myriad of signs and symptoms that require careful physician follow-up to diagnose. No standard set of symptoms exists for SLE. Patients with SLE have numerous symptoms, including mouth ulcers, extreme fatigue, painful or swollen joints, chest pain, skin rashes, and kidney disease. The treatment depends on the level of disease involvement, and currently there is no cure. SLE is characterized by periods of illness (exacerbation) and wellness (remission).

Patients with lupus tend to have other disorders. As many as one third of lupus patients have Sjögren's syndrome (dry eyes, dry mouth, arthritis). The antibody level in the Sjögren patient is typically elevated, which can cause the blood to thicken and result in mental clouding, confusion, and dizziness. The dental professional is in an ideal position to raise awareness and to assist in the diagnosis of Sjögren's syndrome.

Mucous membrane involvement of the nose or mouth, occurring in 7% to 40% of patients with SLE, can result in painful ulcerations that often make it difficult to swallow. Lesions on the lips may appear fissured and edematous. Intraoral lesions begin as petechia on the buccal mucosa, palate, or gingiva and develop into shallow, painful ulcers that increase to 1 to 2 cm in diameter, are covered with a grayish base, and are surrounded by a halo of erythema.

Treatment of intraoral lesions may be palliative, including a therapeutic gargle of hydrogen peroxide or the application of a dental gel containing steroids (Kenalog in Orabase). Antimalarial agents are useful in healing mucosal lesions. A dentifrice, especially a product that contains a strong flavoring agent, should be avoided. Persons with lupus should use baking soda with a soft toothbrush to clean the teeth. Denture wearers should avoid using denture powders and pastes until the disease is in remission. Other oral problems experienced by the lupus patient are gingivitis and caries, especially in the patient with xerostomia.

The lupus patient needs to pay careful attention to oral self-care and should be instructed to perform an intraoral self-examination on a regular basis to check for red or irritated areas and to bring them to the attention of the dental professional or physician. It may be necessary to recommend the use of an electric toothbrush if joint pain interferes with oral care. The use of a floss-threader may also prove successful in thorough interproximal plaque removal. During periods of lupus flares, dental treatment should be postponed.

Pernicious Anemia

The absorption of dietary vitamin B_{12} occurs in the small intestine and requires a secretion from the stomach known as *intrinsic factor.* If intrinsic factor is deficient, absorption of vitamin B_{12} is severely diminished. Vitamin B_{12} deficiency impairs the body's ability to make blood, accelerates blood cell destruction, and damages the nervous system. The result is pernicious anemia (PA). In the classical definition, PA refers only to vitamin B_{12} deficiency anemia caused by a lack of intrinsic factor.

True PA is probably an autoimmune disease in which the immune system destroys cells in the stomach that secrete intrinsic factor. Less common causes of vitamin B_{12} deficiency include gastrointestinal surgery, pancreatic disease, intestinal parasites, and certain drugs. Pregnancy, hyperthyroidism, and advanced stages of cancer may increase the body's requirement for vitamin B_{12}, which sometimes leads to a deficiency state. Mucosal pallor, angular cheilitis, painful atrophic and erythematosus mucosa all can result from this autoimmune disease. The patient also may experience loss of papillae on the dorsum of the tongue, burning of the tongue, and mucosal irritation. Palliative treatment of painful ulcerations and suggested alternative oral self-care products would be appropriate patients with this disease.

Myasthenia Gravis

Myasthenia gravis is an autoimmune neuromuscular disease that is characterized by muscle weakness that increases during periods of activity and improves after periods of rest. Most facial muscles can be involved, including those that control chewing, talking, and swallowing. Under normal conditions, muscle movement is controlled by neuralgic impulses that travel down the nerve. The nerve endings then release a neurotransmitter substance called *acetylcholine.* In myasthenia gravis, antibodies produced by the body's own immune system block, alter, or destroy acetylcholine receptors.

Dental concerns with a myasthenia gravis patient center around the ability to maintain oral self-care. It may be necessary to modify the type of products used and the technique to accommodate the neuromuscular deficit.

Multiple Sclerosis

In this autoimmune disease, nerve tissues of the central nervous system undergo intermittent attack. Symptoms can be intermittent or the symptoms may become constant, which results in a progressive disease process that may lead to possible blindness, paralysis, and premature death. Multiple sclerosis (MS) is the most common disabling disease of young adults and afflicts 1 in 700 people in this country. Triggers for this disease are not well understood. The patient with MS may need little to no special dental attention with regard to oral self-care recommendations or may be unable to perform oral self-care tasks.

Inflammatory Bowel Diseases

Crohn's disease and ulcerative colitis are two diseases in which the immune system attacks the intestine. These chronic inflammatory conditions primarily affect the small and large intestines but can affect the digestive system anywhere between the oral cavity and the anus. Named after a physician who described the disease in 1932, Crohn's disease affects men and women equally. Once the disease begins, it tends to be a chronic, recurrent condition that enters periods of exacerbation and remission. Although some researchers believe certain bacteria cause the infection, no conclusive evidence has been presented in the literature. Extraintestinal complications can occur to the skin, joints, spine, eyes, liver, and bile ducts. If joint pain is a persistent and severe problem, dental considerations in oral self-care products and regimens need to be carefully planned.

Psoriasis

Psoriasis is an immune system disorder that affects the skin, covering small areas or the entire body. The plaques associated with this disease are not uniform in size, shape, or severity and may be both painful and unattractive. Most treatments focus on a topical application to relieve the symptoms of inflammation, itching, and scaling. For more severe cases, oral medications are used. The dental clinician should exercise caution in stretching any affected skin areas near the mouth.

Scleroderma

Scleroderma is a rare, chronic autoimmune disease that affects an estimated 150,000 to 500,000 Americans, primarily ages 30 to 50. Women are three times more likely to suffer from autoimmune diseases in general. However, with scleroderma, the incidence is more prevalent in men, affecting them at a 4:1 ratio versus women. Two basic forms of the disease exist: *localized* and *systemic.* Localized forms affect only the skin, never an internal organ, and do not impact life expectancy. The systemic form can affect any part of the body.

In scleroderma the immune system sets up an inflammation response that triggers the overproduction of collagen. The systemic form of scleroderma causes fibrosis, the formation of scar tissue around internal organs. The fibrosis eventually immobilizes whatever is in its path and completely shuts down organ function; it can result in death.

Dental symptoms occur in systemic but not localized scleroderma. Noted symptoms include bone resorption, *Candida* overgrowth, caries, periodontal disease, dentinal sensitivity, temporomandibular joint dysfunction (TMD), and xerostomia. Radiographically, collagen deposition can be noted around the periodontal ligament. As the ligament expands, teeth can become loose. The associated xerostomia makes these patients more prone to *Candida* in-

 Case Study

Case 1: Oral Care Considerations for the Cancer Patient

Theodore Jacobsen, a 52-year-old male schoolteacher and periodontal maintenance patient, has missed his regularly scheduled supportive therapy appointment. On follow-up, you learn that he recently had surgery for colon cancer. After surgery, he developed blood clots for which he takes warfarin (Coumadin). He calls your office 3 months later to schedule a supportive care appointment. From the discussion with Mr. Jacobsen, you learn that he is currently receiving chemotherapy and has a portacath in place. You direct the patient to ask his oncologist when would be an appropriate time to schedule a supportive care appointment. In addition, you ask Mr. Jacobsen for the current values of his white blood cell and platelet count. The patient indicates he has symptoms that you associate with mucositis and dry mouth and would like your suggestions to manage these oral side effects of chemotherapy.

fection and dental caries. When scleroderma affects the muscles of the oral cavity, the functions of chewing, brushing, flossing, and having dental work performed may become challenging. Facial exercises are recommended to help maintain muscle flexibility.

Autoimmune Thyroid Diseases

Autoimmune thyroid diseases afflict as many as 4 out of 100 women and are frequently found in families that exhibit other autoimmune diseases. Hashimoto's thyroiditis—the most common form of hypothyroidism—and Grave's disease—the most common form of hyperthyroidism—result from immune system dysfunction. In Hashimoto's thyroiditis, the immune system either destroys thyroid tissue or prevents the secretion of sufficient quantities of thyroid hormone. Symptoms of thyroid hypofunction are typically nonspecific and can develop slowly or may appear suddenly. Symptoms include fatigue, nervousness, cold or heat intolerance, weakness, changes in hair texture or amount, and weight gain or loss. In Grave's disease, the body produces antibodies that overstimulate the production of thyroid hormone. Symptoms of hyperthyroidism include nervousness, irritability, shaky hands, increased perspiration, warm skin, thinning hair, weight loss, decreased menstruation, eye changes, and weak leg muscles. In children, hyperthyroidism can cause premature exfoliation of primary teeth and eruption of permanent teeth. In women, it can cause osteoporosis of the maxilla and mandible and a burning sensation of the tongue.

Addison's Disease

Addison's disease is a rare endocrine and hormonal disorder that affects men and women equally. Addison's disease is usually caused by the gradual destruction of the adrenal cortex (the outer layer of the adrenal glands) by the body's own immune system. In this disease, the adrenal glands do not produce sufficient quantities of the hormone cortisol and occasionally the hormone aldosterone. Cortisol is classified as a glucocorticoid, which affects almost every organ and tissue in the body. The most significant job of this hormone is to help the body respond to stress. The hormone aldosterone belongs to a class of hormones called *mineralocorticoids,* also produced by the adrenal glands. Aldosterone helps balance the water-to-salt ratio and maintains blood pressure, which helps the kidneys retain sodium and excrete potassium. Treatment of Addison's disease involves replacing one or both hormones when deficient. An Addisonian crisis can be life-threatening. It is important for patients with Addison's disease to maintain regular visits with a physician. Patients with Addison's disease may experience brown pigmentation of the skin and melanotic macules on the oral mucosa.

CANCER

Cancer continues to be a significant health concern. It was estimated that 1 million new cases of cancer would be diagnosed in the year 2000.[24] Yet with an increase in prevention, screening, and early detection, cancer-related deaths are on the decline.[24] Cancer treatment affects the ability of a patient to maintain oral health,[38] and dental hygienists are in a unique position to not only provide needed oral care to patients with cancer but also to participate as part of the multidisciplinary team involved in patient care.[5] In private practices, dental hygienists will likely treat more patients with cancer diagnoses than in the past and thus will need to be prepared to meet the challenges presented.[5,6] Box 44-2 provides tips on oral self-care for the cancer patient.

INCIDENCE AND RISK FACTORS

Definitions

Cancer does not have one single definition. The word *cancer* actually defines more than 100 different distinct malignancies. Cancer is described as a group of abnormal cells that ignore the usual controls in place for cell growth and division. As cancer cells continue to grow and multiply, they eventually take over the host organ or tissue and ultimately cause its death.[19] Cancer cells can multiply rapidly

---

BOX 44-2

Oral Self-Care for the Cancer Patient

Three Good Reasons to See a Dentist before Cancer Treatment
1. *Feel better.* Cancer treatment may be easier if the patient works with the dentist and hygienist. The patient should have a pretreatment checkup.
2. *Save teeth and bones.* A dentist can help protect the mouth, teeth, and jaw bones from damage caused by radiation and chemotherapy. Children also need special protection for their growing teeth and facial bones.
3. *Fight cancer.* Physicians may have to delay or stop cancer treatment because of problems in the mouth. To fight cancer best, the cancer care team should include a dentist.

Protecting the Mouth during Cancer Treatment
Brush gently and often
Brush the teeth and tongue gently with an extra-soft toothbrush.
If the mouth is sore, soften the bristles in warm water.
Brush after every meal and at bedtime.
Floss gently every day
Floss once a day to remove plaque.
If the gums bleed and hurt, avoid the areas that bleed or are sore but continue to floss the other teeth.
Keep the mouth moist
Rinse often with water.
Do not use mouthrinses containing alcohol.
Use a saliva substitute to help moisten the mouth.

Modified from National Institute of Dental and Craniofacial Research, Rockville, Md, The Institute.   *Continued*

Oral Self-Care for the Cancer Patient—cont'd

Eat and drink with care
Choose soft, easy-to-chew foods.
Protect the mouth from spicy, sour, or crunchy foods.
Choose lukewarm foods and drinks instead of hot or icy-cold ones.
Avoid alcoholic drinks.
Keep trying to quit using tobacco
Ask the cancer care team to help in efforts to stop smoking or chewing tobacco. (People who quit smoking or chewing tobacco have fewer mouth problems.)
When to Call the Cancer Care Team about Mouth Problems
Take a moment each day to check the mouth visually and feel it. Call the cancer care team if any of the following occurs:
• A mouth problem from the following discussions appears.
• An old problem worsens.
• Any abnormal change occurs.
Tips for Mouth Problems
Sore mouth, sore throat
To help keep the mouth clean, rinse often with ½ tsp of baking soda and ⅛ tsp of salt in 1 cup of warm water. Follow with a plain-water rinse. Ask the cancer care team about medicines that can help alleviate pain.

Dry mouth
Rinse the mouth often with water; use sugar-free gum or candy; talk to the dentist about saliva substitutes.
Infections
Call the cancer care team immediately if a sore, swelling, or bleeding occurs or if a sticky, white film appears in the mouth.
Eating problems
The cancer care team can help by providing medicines to numb the pain from mouth sores and by demonstrating ways to choose foods that are easy to swallow.
Bleeding
If the gums bleed or hurt, avoid flossing the areas that bleed or are sore but continue to floss the other teeth. Soften the bristles of the toothbrush in warm water.
Stiffness in chewing muscles
Open and close the mouth as far as is possible without causing pain 3 times per day. Repeat this procedure 20 times.
Vomiting
Rinse the mouth after vomiting with ¼ tsp of baking soda in 1 cup of warm water.
Cavities
Brush the teeth after meals and before bedtime. The dentist might prescribe nighttime fluoride for the teeth to help prevent cavities.

Modified from National Institute of Dental and Craniofacial Research, Rockville, Md, The Institute.

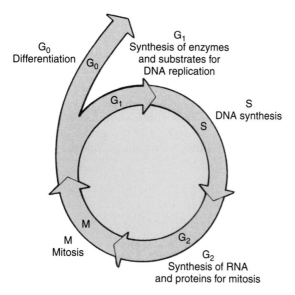

FIG. 44-1 The cell cycle. (From Belcher AE: *Cancer nursing,* St Louis, 1992, Mosby.)

or be somewhat slow in their replication. This growth and replication occurs during the cell cycle (Fig. 44-1). Each phase of the cell cycle is responsible for a different stage of a new cell's reproduction. Chemotherapy drugs are classified according to their activity or nonactivity during a particular phase of the cell cycle.[19,26] The use of chemotherapy drugs is discussed later in this chapter.

Incidence and Prevalence

Annually, the American Cancer Society projects cancer incidences and deaths for the following 12 months. The cancers estimated to have the highest *incidence* in 2000 were as follows: *men*—(1) prostate, (2) lung and bronchus, and (3) colon and rectum; *women*—(1) breast, (2) lung and bronchus, and (3) colon and rectum. The cancers estimated to have the highest *deaths* in 2000 were as follows: *men*—(1) lung and bronchus, (2) prostate, and (3) colon and rectum; *women*—(1) lung and bronchus, (2) breast, and (3) colon and rectum.[16] Although lung cancer surpassed breast cancer in 1987 as the leading cause of cancer deaths in women, in 2000 it was estimated to be the cause of 25% of all cancer deaths.[16]

Risk Factors

Numerous risk factors have been identified and shown to contribute to the development of certain types of cancer (Box 44-3). Tobacco has long been linked to an increased risk for the development of lung and oral cancer. Excessive exposure to sunlight, especially ultraviolet rays, increases the risk for the development of different types of skin and lip cancer. Chronic use of alcohol increases the risk for the development of liver cancer and, when used in combination with tobacco, greatly increases a person's risk for also developing head and neck cancer. The cancer risk for the use of estrogen by postmenopausal women remains controversial. Although the benefits of estrogen replacement therapy (ERT) are widely known, continued use of estrogen by post-menopausal women has been shown to increase their risk for breast cancer.[34,42]

Radiation Exposure as a Risk Factor

Past exposure to radiation is also another risk factor for the development of certain types of cancer. An adult who received radiation treatment as a child for cancer may develop a second primary cancer because of the radiation exposure. Similarly, persons exposed to radiation from nuclear fallout are more prone to developing cancer. For example, the people of Russia and China who lived through the Chernobyl incident are at higher risk for developing cancer. In addition, many years ago some types of skin lesions or acne were treated with radiation or x-ray treatments.[34,42]

Other Risk Factors

Occupational-Related Risks
Occupational and environmental hazards can pose risk factors for the development of cancer. Work sites that are linked with increased cancer risks include uranium and coal mines; steel manufacturing plants; manufacturing plants that handle radon, asbestos, and lead; and oil refineries.

Nutrition
Nutrition can be both a preventive agent and a risk factor for the development of cancer. It has been suggested that a high-fiber, low-fat diet can decrease the risk of colon cancer, and a diet high in fat might increase a woman's risk for breast cancer.

Virus
Viruses have been implicated in the etiology of certain types of cancer (e.g., human papillomavirus increases the risk for cervical cancer; Epstein-Barr virus increases incidences of Burkitt's lymphoma). Viruses are also implicated in the etiology of some types of cancer when no other risk factors can be identified.[34,42]

Ethnic, Socioeconomic, and Educational Factors
Ethnicity is considered a risk factor for developing cancer. African Americans have the highest incidence of cancer and are more likely to die from the disease than any other ethnic group.[24] Along with ethnicity, socioeconomic and educational status play a role in increasing a person's risk for developing cancer. Poor individuals are less likely to participate in cancer screening and early detection tests than are individuals with a higher income; therefore the poor are more likely to be diagnosed with an advanced stage of cancer.[34,42] Most cancer-education materials are written at the twelfth grade level, yet most individuals can only read at the sixth grade level.[42]

TREATMENT

The variety of methods used in the treatment of cancer are shown in Box 44-4. The treatment used depends on several factors: cancer type, tumor location, and treatment goal (curative, palliative, tumor reduction). It should be noted that not all cancers respond to current treatment regimens and thus there are no known effective treatments. Cancer treatments are frequently used in combination to achieve the best results with the fewest side effects for the patient. Surgery is performed to completely remove the tumor, debulk the tumor before or after chemotherapy or radiation therapy, or for palliation. Radiation therapy (see Chapter 45) uses ionizing radiation, either external or internal, to treat many types of slow-growing tumors. Hormone therapy is used both as a prevention and treatment for prostate and breast cancer. Bone marrow/peripheral stem cell transplantation is another cancer treatment that is used after cancer has reoccurred or metastasized to another location in the body.

Chemotherapy

Chemotherapy is a method frequently used to treat many forms of cancer and is the focus of this chapter's discussion on cancer treatments. Chemotherapy involves the use of antineoplastic drugs designed to attack the rapidly dividing cancer cell either at various points during the cell cycle or at any time (cell-cycle specific or nonspecific).[19,26] These agents are categorized according to their action. Alkylating agents are the oldest group of antineoplastic drugs and are most active during the G_0, or resting phase. Plant alkaloids work during the mitosis, or M phase. They also inhibit ribonucleic acid (RNA) synthesis during the G_2 phase and deoxyribonucleic acid (DNA) synthesis during the S phase. Antitumor antineoplastics are both cell-cycle–specific and phase-nonspecific. They work during all phases of the cell cycle with specific action against DNA synthesis. Antimetabolites work during the S phase of the cell cycle.[19,26]

Chemotherapy agents cause immunosuppression of both normal and abnormal rapidly dividing cells.[19,26] The normal cells usually affected are those of the gastrointestinal mucosa, hair follicles, and bone marrow (which include white blood cells [WBC], red blood cells, and platelets). This suppression starts after the first dose of the agent and reaches, on average, its lowest point (or *NADIR*) within 7 to 14 days. After the NADIR is reached, recovery begins.

Patients are most at risk for infection during after NADIR because the immune system is depressed (WBC, red blood cells, and platelets are at their lowest). The development of an infection at this time could be life-threatening. A normal WBC count ranges between 5000 to 10,000 cells/mm^3. An absolute neutrophil count (ANC) is another way to determine a patient's risk for developing infection. It is computed by multiplying a patient's WBC by the percentage of neutrophils (bands + segs).[26] If a patient's ANC is below 1500 cells/mm^3, the patient is at increased risk of developing an infection. To provide oral care, the ANC needs to be at least 1500 cells/mm^3 or higher. Another parameter that impacts the provision of oral care is the platelet count. A normal platelet count ranges from 150,000 to 350,000 cells/mm^3. An increased risk for bleeding begins when the platelet count drops below 50,000 cells/mm^3.[1,9,27,32] Once the count drops below 20,000 cells/mm^3, the risk for bleeding is very high. Dental care cannot be provided unless the platelet count is above 50,000 cells/mm^3.

It is important to know a cancer patient's chemotherapy regimen before providing any dental care to make certain the patient has adequate immune system protection to fight off infection.[5,6,7] Patients can experience hair loss and increased oral and gastrointestinal problems (e.g., mucositis, xerostomia, nausea, vomiting, diarrhea).[20,27] An increase in oral problems has a direct impact on providing any type of oral care.[5,6,7]

Chemotherapy is administrated in pill form, intravenously through a peripheral line or an indwelling central venous catheter, or as an injection.[19,26] When an indwelling catheter has been placed, the patient must be premedicated with antibiotics before receiving dental care.[7] The American Heart Association regimen is typically used; however, consultation with the patient's oncologist is necessary to determine whether a longer course of antibiotics is warranted.

Case #1 Application

Mr. Jacobsen tells you that he is on a yearlong regimen of 5-FU and leucovorin. He receives chemotherapy once a week in 4-week intervals. He is scheduled to receive his next treatment next week. His blood counts (WBC and platelets) are all within normal limits. He has a portacath and a history of a heart murmur for which he has received antibiotic premedication in the past. He no longer takes Coumadin, and his oncologist has stated that this is a good time for him to receive dental care. Mr. Jacobsen tells you he has some oral sores and dry mouth, which the oncologist has said is related

to chemotherapy.[30] Mr. Jacobsen asks for your suggestions on what to do about it.

EMOTIONAL ASPECTS

When presented with a cancer diagnosis, a patient can experience a wide range of emotions (Box 44-5).[5] It is important to remember not to take any emotional response personally as information is obtained from the patient. Be an active listener and let each patient set the pace of the conversation. Remember the patient may not want to talk about cancer, and that is an acceptable option. Also, there may be periods of silence during the conversation. Learn to be comfortable with that silence. Respect for all patients, especially those with personal crisis, is critical to successful outcomes. The patient's emotional state greatly influences the course of oral care.

ROLE OF THE DENTAL HYGIENIST

Five roles have emerged for the dental hygienist in providing care for the patient undergoing cancer therapy (Box 44-6). Each role provides the means to meet the complex needs of this patient population. A discussion of each follows. 44-A

First, the dental hygienist should identify and eliminate oral infection (within the scope of dental hygiene practice). To begin, a thorough health history needs to be gathered. The health history should include the following:

- The type of cancer being treated
- The name of the patient's medical and/or radiation oncologist
- Information regarding any surgery that will be or has already been performed

---

BOX 44-5

Patient Reactions* to Cancer Diagnosis

Shock	Fear	Anxiety	Withdrawal	Bargaining
Anger	Hostility	Denial	Depression	Acceptance

Copyright 1994, Deborah S. Manne, RDH, RN.
*This listing includes emotions that the cancer patient *may* experience.

BOX 44-6

Role of the Dental Hygienist in Cancer Treatment

Identify and eliminate any oral infection (within the scope of dental hygiene practice)
Improve and/or maintain oral hygiene status
Provide symptom management for oral complications that result from chemotherapy and/or head-neck radiation therapy
Provide education to patients and family members regarding the oral effects of cancer therapy
Serve as a liaison between the patient, the oncologist, and the dentist before, during, and after cancer therapy

Copyright 1994, Deborah S. Manne, RDH, RN.

- The chemotherapy regimen—specifically, the drugs being used, the frequency of use, and the route of administration
- If radiation therapy is to be used, the place and time it will be initiated

Next, the dental hygienist should gather an updated dental history in conjunction with a thorough examination of the oral cavity.[23,55,56] The dental hygienist next develops a plan for therapeutic intervention and personalized prevention that includes the assessment, dental hygiene diagnosis, plan of care, implementation or interventions, and evaluation of the care. Finally, the dental hygienist performs the necessary dental hygiene care, which includes full-mouth debridement and appropriate fluoride treatment.

The next role is to improve and/or maintain oral hygiene status. The dental hygienist should evaluate a patient's knowledge and level of preventive oral self-care practices so that information on oral self-care can be provided at the level most appropriate for the patient. Next, the intervention and prevention regimens should be integrated to help the patient reach optimal oral health. Then the dental hygienist should evaluate the oral cavity and oral self-care practices at frequent intervals so reinforcement of information or alternatives can be suggested in a timely manner.

In the third role, the dental hygienist provides symptom management for oral complications that result from cancer therapy.

The fourth role is to educate patients and family members regarding the oral effects of cancer therapy.[5] Numerous resources, many of which are free of charge, are available for providing information and support to patients and their family members.[39,40] (See the suggested agencies and web sites and the additional readings and resources at the end of this chapter.)

Finally, the fifth role is to serve as a liaison between the patient, the oncologist, and the dentist before, during, and after cancer therapy. The role of patient advocate is an important one because it keeps the needs of the patient at the forefront of treatment.

ORAL COMPLICATIONS RELATED TO CHEMOTHERAPY

Oral Mucositis

Oral *mucositis* is characterized as an inflammation of the mucosal lining.[14,41] The cells lining the oral mucosa turn over at a rapid rate—approximately every 10 to 14 days. The administration of a chemotherapeutic agent suppresses the replication of both cancer and healing cells, which results in tissue breakdown.[52] Within the first few days of chemotherapy administration, the initial signs of mucositis can be evident. They appear as an erythema, commonly with patient complaints of a burning sensation. Within days, ulcerations can appear, either localized or generalized (Fig. 44-2). Mucositis is painful, making it difficult for the patient to eat, drink, talk, or practice oral self-care.* Although mucositis resolves within a few weeks

after completion of the chemotherapy, during therapy it can be a very painful side effect.

Oral Management

The patient must be encouraged to keep the oral cavity as clean as possible.[1,8,35] Use a soft-bristle toothbrush with a gentle technique. If the patient reports that the soft toothbrush feels too harsh, an ultra-soft toothbrush can be suggested. A fluoride toothpaste can be continued until sensitivity occurs. Then a paste of baking soda and warm water can be used as an alternative.[7,9] Patients who wear partial or complete dentures need to be instructed to not wear them when sores are present in the mouth. Direct the patient to clean the appliance(s) daily and store them in clean water when not in use. Instruct the patient to stop the use of any oral rinses that contain alcohol because they can have a drying and irritating effect on already sore tissue. The use of hydrogen peroxide as a mouthrinse should be avoided because of its disruptive effect on newly granulating tissue and oral flora. Although chlorhexidine may be prescribed by the patient's oncologist,[1,13,18,46] the alcohol content may be too irritating to the oral mucosa when used as an oral rinse. A cotton swab or toothette may yield better compliance with its use.[44,47]

Pain management is an issue for patients who suffer from generalized mucositis.[15,57] Several topical preparations available over-the-counter can be suggested to provide temporary pain relief. Another option is the preparation of a taffy made with capsaicin, the active ingredient of chili peppers, that when held in the mouth and allowed to dissolve, produces a burn and up to several hours of pain relief.[11] The patient's oncologist also may prescribe a "magic mouthwash" for the patient to use for the relief of severe pain. This concoction, made by a pharmacist, typically contains viscous lidocaine, Benalyn cough syrup, and some type of coating agent (Milk of Magnesia, Kaopectate, or Mylanta).[7,55] Patients are instructed to swish a tablespoon of this mixture in their mouths 30 minutes before eating. Patients need to be aware of the reduced gag reflex that occurs from the lidocaine.

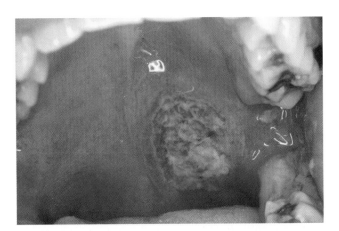

FIG. 44-2 Necrotizing ulcerative mucositis. Large area of soft tissue necrosis of the posterior soft palate on the left side. (From Neville BW et al: *Oral & maxillofacial pathology,* ed 2, St Louis, 2002, WB Saunders.)

*References 1, 5, 6, 7, 20, 27, 31.

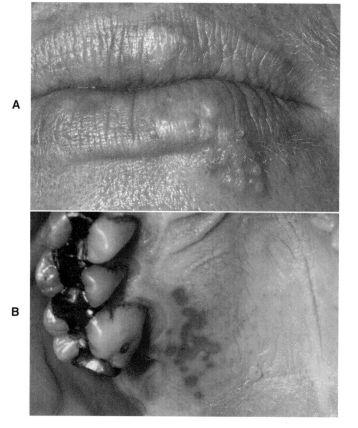

FIG. 44-3 **A,** *Herpes labialis.* Multiple fluid-filled vesicles adjacent to the lip vermilion. **B,** Intraoral recurrent herpetic infection. Multiple coalescing ulcerations on the hard palate. (From Neville BW: *Oral & maxillofacial pathology,* ed 2, St Louis, 2002, WB Saunders.)

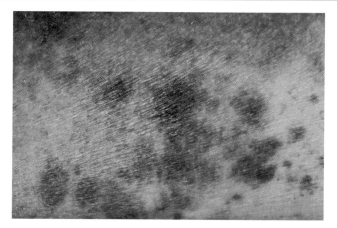

FIG. 44-4 Thrombocytopenia. The bruising (purpura) seen on this patient's forearm is a result of reduced platelet count. (From Neville BW: *Oral & maxillofacial pathology,* ed 2, St Louis, 2002, WB Saunders.)

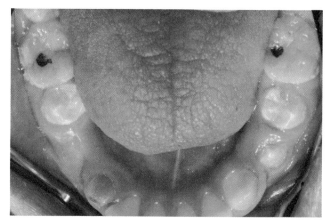

FIG. 44-5 Xerostomia. Dry, leathery tongue in a patient with aplasia of the salivary glands. (From Neville BW: *Oral & maxillofacial pathology,* ed 2, St Louis, 2002, WB Saunders.)

Infection

Because the protective capacity of the oral mucosa is compromised and the immune system is suppressed, the risk for developing an oral infection is greatly increased.[41,59] Patients with a history of oral herpes may experience a reactivation of the herpes virus during chemotherapy.[41,46,48] Typically, the reaction is more severe and can involve the entire oral cavity (Fig. 44-3). Localized or generalized candidiasis can be noted because of the immune system depression and may not present with a typical clinical picture.[41,46] The only indication that an oral infection exists may be the presence of a fever.

Oral Management

For patients with a past history of oral herpes, prophylactic use of an antiviral agent is sometimes used.[32,41,46,49] In the presence of oral fungal infection, nystatin "swish and swallow" mouthrinse is frequently used. There are also troches that can be held in the mouth and allowed to gradually dissolve.[37,41] Any other type of oral infection may require a culture of oral cells to determine the appropriate antibiotic to use.[41,50]

Bleeding

A decrease in the platelet count below the normal range is known as *thrombocytopenia.*[1,31,41] This happens in response to the immunosuppressive effects of the chemotherapy. Recovery happens in a few weeks after chemotherapy has ended.

Oral Management

When the platelet count drops to below 50,000 cells/mm³, flossing should be stopped as a precaution against causing uncontrolled bleeding.[1,31,32,41] Below 20,000 cells/mm³, all oral hygiene care must be stopped because the risk of a spontaneous hemorrhage is too great (Fig. 44-4). Patients should be cautioned to avoid any activities that might cause bleeding. If a spontaneous hemorrhage occurs, a blood transfusion may be required.[32]

Xerostomia

Xerostomia (dry mouth) occurs in varying degrees of severity during chemotherapy (Fig. 44-5). Chemotherapy causes a change in the amount and pH of the saliva, which inhibits its protective capabilities.[29] The saliva becomes more acidic and places the patient at an increased risk for developing caries, especially along cervical areas.

For some patients, the xerostomia is mild, although in others it can be severe. Xerostomia caused by chemotherapy typically resolves after the cessation of chemotherapy. During therapy, however, management is essential for the prevention of further dental disease.

Oral Management

Patients should be encouraged to increase their oral fluid intake. Several commercially available over-the-counter products for dry mouth (saliva substitutes, mouth moisteners, oral lubricants) provide temporary relief. Some patients find relief with the use of a humidifier while sleeping. Patients should be cautioned to avoid tobacco products, alcohol, caffeinated beverages, spicy foods with sharp edges, and salty foods. It may become necessary to prescribe a rinse or gel of a neutral sodium fluoride or unflavored stannous fluoride.[5,7]

Neurotoxicity

Some chemotherapy agents (e.g., plant alkaloids) are toxic to peripheral nerves accumulating in peripheral nerve endings and result in *neurotoxicity.* A patient undergoing a chemotherapy regimen derived from plant alkaloids may have symptoms of bilateral toothaches. The patient may also complain of tingling or numbness in the hands and feet. On examination, typically no indication of the cause is found. The chemotherapy drugs can affect the peripheral nerves of the teeth, causing pain. On completion of chemotherapy, this pain goes away.[15]

Oral Management

Palliative pain management is all that can be done until the chemotherapy has been completed.[15]

Case #1 Application

Develop a plan of care for Mr. Jacobsen that includes the following:

- Antibiotic coverage for his heart murmur and the portacath
- Periodontal prophylaxis
- Oral hygiene instructions with additional information for management of his mucositis and xerostomia
- Follow-up with the patient to assess symptom relief
- 4-Month supportive care appointment

ACQUIRED IMMUNODEFICIENCY SYNDROME

INCIDENCE AND RISK FACTORS

Acquired immunodeficiency syndrome (AIDS) is caused by an infection with one of ten known subtypes of the *human immunodeficiency virus (HIV).*[54] Approximately 30 million people worldwide are living with HIV/AIDS. In the United States alone there were approximately 362,000 deaths from AIDS by the end of 1996.[54] HIV is a retrovirus that has RNA as its genetic material. Enzymes called *reverse transcriptase* cause the RNA to convert into DNA, which is the opposite of normal cell replication.[54,58] HIV attaches itself to CD4+ T-lymphocytes and infects the cell nucleus once inside. Everything replicated after that is considered HIV-infected. CD4+ T-lymphocytes are an important component of a person's immune system. By depleting

Case Study Case 2: Oral Care Considerations for the HIV-Positive Patient

Nicole Bobo, a 52-year-old female former patient, called to schedule a supportive care appointment. Your office has not seen her for more than 2 years. Ms. Bobo asked to speak privately with your periodontist employer. She told him that she has been diagnosed as HIV-positive after being accidentally stuck by a needle of an AIDS patient for whom she was caring for as a volunteer. Ms. Bobo states her condition was discovered when she came down with bacterial endocarditis. Currently, her blood counts are normal, and she takes no medications. The periodontist talked with her about the need for premedication because of the history of bacterial endocarditis, and an appointment was scheduled.

CD4+ T-lymphocytes, a person is unable to mount a normal immune response. This leaves the HIV-infected person at greater susceptibility to developing bacterial, fungal, and viral opportunistic infections.[25,54,58]

Most body fluids have demonstrated detectable levels of HIV. However, the fluids that are the main routes of transmission are blood, semen, vaginal secretions, and breast milk. Although the first documented cases of AIDS in 1981 were among homosexual men, this disease is also found among the heterosexual population and affects men, women, and children.[27]

The course of the HIV infection is monitored by the CD4+ T-lymphocyte count and the number of copies per milliliter of plasma.[54] Antibodies can be detected in the blood from between 1 to 3 months after an exposure. Most HIV-infected patients experience a long period of clinical latency. This could be up to 10 years with no clinical signs of the disease. During this time, CD4+ cells continue to decline, and eventually opportunistic infections are seen. CD4+ counts greater than 500 cells/mm³ are the range for early HIV disease. At between 200 to 500 cells/mm³, the intermediate stage, more signs of opportunistic infection occur. Medications are usually started at this stage. When CD4+ count reaches 50 to 200 cells/mm³, this is called the *late stage,* or full-blown AIDS. It is at this stage that opportunistic infections become more frequent and more severe. Alterations in mental status, wasting syndrome, and neoplasms such as Kaposi's sarcoma frequently occur.

TREATMENT

Although no known cure for HIV or AIDS exists, drug therapy is used to suppress the virus.[54] The first drug approved in 1987 to treat infection was zidovudine, or AZT. Its activity against the virus is through the reverse transcriptase enzyme. Unfortunately, HIV can develop resistance to AZT's effects. AZT therapy has been used with success to reduce the transmission of HIV from an HIV-infected mother to her baby during pregnancy, delivery, and through breastfeeding.

In 1995 the Food and Drug Administration (FDA) approved another HIV inhibitor, lamivudine, or 3TC, for use in combination with AZT. These two drugs work synergistically to help delay development of the virus's resistance to AZT. Protease inhibitors are another type of drug used to attack the HIV. Saquinavir, ritonavir, indinavir, and nelfinavir have FDA approval for the treatment of AIDS. The current best approach is triple-drug therapy. This therapy uses a protease inhibitor, AZT, and lamivudine. It reduces detectable virus to nondetectable levels in the blood plasma. It is also believed that this triple combination will help decrease the ability of the virus to become resistant to all three of the drugs. Unfortunately, the longer a patient is on the drug therapy, the more likely it is for drug resistance by HIV to occur.[54]

Case #2 Application

Ms. Bobo arrives for her appointment, and you confirm that her antibiotic premedication has been taken. Your periodontist employer completes a periodontal examination and notes several areas of periodontal pocketing throughout her mouth. Full-mouth radiographs are taken. Following a review of Ms. Bobo's radiographs, it is determined that she needs full-mouth periodontal debridement. After this therapy is completed and her mouth is reevaluated, Ms. Bobo will be placed on a 3-month supportive care schedule.

ROLE OF THE DENTAL HYGIENIST

When treating the patient with HIV/AIDS, the dental hygienist has five roles and procedures, the same as those discussed for the patient undergoing cancer therapy (see Box 44-4). It is critical to gather as much information as possible about the patient's health history. The dental hygienist then performs a thorough oral assessment each time the patient is seen so that the oral signs of the disease can be identified. Using the same ideals, the hygienist forms intervention and prevention strategies and performs necessary oral care to improve and/or maintain the patient's oral health status. The dental hygienist also educates the patient on the signs and symptoms of oral disease and oral disease prevention, frequently reinforcing good oral hygiene practices, including frequent professional oral prophylaxis. Finally, the dental hygienist should act as a patient advocate among the patient, dentist, and physician to ensure oral needs are met.[43]

ORAL MANIFESTATIONS

Candidiasis

Oral candidiasis is seen in both HIV-positive and AIDS patients.* Its frequency has been associated with CD4+ counts less than 300 cells/mm^3 and with xerostomia. Oral candidiasis manifests in one of three ways: pseudomembranous candidiasis, erythematous candidiasis, and angular cheilitis. Pseudomembranous candidiasis appears as a white, wipeable plaque located in any part of the mouth. Erythematous candidiasis is a red plaque found on mucosal surfaces and the tongue. Angular cheilitis is located in the corners of the mouth.

Oral Management

Oral candidiasis is treated either topically or systemically.[43,51,53,58] Topical preparations include clotrimazole, nystatin, miconazole, or amphotericin. More frequently used are the systemic antifungals fluconazole and ketoconazole. Relapses are common with both topical and systemic antifungals.

Herpes Simplex Viruses

The appearance of oral herpes simplex is typically a reactivation of a dormant herpes simplex virus (HSV).* It can appear anywhere in the oral cavity but more commonly as herpes labialis and palatal herpes. Varicella-zoster, or VSZ infection, is also found among HIV-infected patients as a reactivation of this HSV. Oral lesions are uncommon. Cytomegalovirus (CMV) can contribute to HIV immunosuppression. It is uncommon to see oral lesions with CMV, but when they do occur, they are large and painful. It is believed that the presence of oral CMV indicates disseminated disease. Epstein-Barr virus (EBV) has been implicated in Burkitt's lymphoma and nasopharyngeal carcinoma. It has also been linked to hairy leukoplakia, a common oral occurrence in HIV-infected patients. Hairy leukoplakia is a white patch, usually found on the tongue, that is corrugated.

Oral Management

Oral or systemic acyclovir is used in the treatment of HSV.[17,43,51,58] With CMV, ganciclovir is given either orally or intravenously. Treatment for hairy leukoplakia is rarely needed, but acyclovir and desciclovir have been used successfully.

Neoplasms

Oral cancers are more common in the patient with HIV infection.† The most common neoplasm is Kaposi's sarcoma (KS), which can sometimes be the first sign of HIV infection. KS can be found in any area of the mouth, but more common sites are primarily on the palate and secondly on the gingiva. KS can become widespread throughout the body as the infection progresses from HIV-positive to AIDS, or it can remain localized in the oral cavity. Oral lesions of KS have been treated with radiation therapy. In addition, single or multiple agent chemotherapy and interferon therapy have also been used with mixed results.

Non-Hodgkin's lymphoma (NHL) is the second most common neoplasm of the oral cavity in patients with HIV infection and AIDS. With NHL, combination chemotherapy and radiotherapy are also used. In AIDS patients this neoplasm tends to be more aggressive, with survival rates being poor.

Squamous cell carcinoma (SCC) is another oral neoplasm. It occurs infrequently in younger HIV-infected patients with no other risk factors. SCC is treated by radiation therapy.

---

*References 10, 25, 33, 43, 45, 51, 53, 58.

*References 10, 17, 25, 43, 45, 51, 58.
†References 16, 21, 25, 43, 51, 58.

ASSOCIATED PERIODONTAL DISEASES

Linear Gingival Erythema

When researchers first started noticing gingival changes in patients with HIV infection and AIDS, the condition was called *HIV-associated gingivitis*. In 1994 The American Academy of Periodontology shared in its position paper the latest international classifications of this phenomenon. What was once called HIV-associated gingivitis is now called *linear gingival erythema (LGE)*.[2] Clinically, it appears as a 2- to 3-mm band of erythema along the gingival margin seen around all of the teeth, but it is possible to also see localized areas. Bleeding on probing occurs easily. Treatment involves full-mouth debridement, antimicrobial oral rinse, and plaque control, which results in little improvement.

Necrotizing Ulcerative Gingivitis

Necrotizing ulcerative gingivitis (NUG) in the HIV-positive patient presents a clinical picture similar to NUG seen in the non–HIV-positive population.[12,43,60] The difference lies in its rapid progression and severity. Again, the same treatment is used in the HIV population (full-mouth debridement, plaque control, pain management, antimicrobial mouthrinse, antibiotic therapy); however, little improvement is noted.

Periodontal Disease

The periodontal disease seen in HIV-infected patients is typically severe and rapid in progression and has been called *necrotizing ulcerative periodontitis (NUP)*.* Although

---

*References 2, 3, 12, 22, 28, 36, 43, 58, 60, 61.

clinical similarities do exist between periodontal disease in non–HIV-infected individuals and in NUP in HIV-infected patients, the rapid progression sets them apart. It is not clear what exactly causes this to occur, but rapid, severe loss of clinical attachment levels, loss of alveolar bone, and soft-tissue necrosis make this disease difficult for the patient to manage. Treatment for NUP follows the same procedure stated for NUG: full-mouth debridement, antimicrobial irrigation, plaque control, antibiotic therapy, and home usage of an antimicrobial mouthrinse. The response seen depends on what stage of HIV infection the patient is in, current medication status, and the patient's oral self-care habits. Again, the results will not equal what is usually seen in a patient without HIV/AIDS.

 Case #2 Application

Ms. Bobo returns every 3 months for the next year. At her third visit since being diagnosed, she tells you that her CD4+ count has started to fall and that she started a drug therapy consisting of Viracept and Combivir (AZT and lamivudine). Currently her viral load is nondetectable, but her periodontal condition has started to decline. Probing depths are increasing, and she reports smoking more frequently. After gathering all of this updated information and consulting with your periodontist employer, you develop a plan of care for Ms. Bobo that includes the following:

- Antibiotic coverage for the history of bacterial endocarditis
- Periodontal debridement with selected areas of antimicrobial irrigation
- Review of oral self-care
- Suggestions for the patient to stop or at least reduce her smoking habit
- Referral to a general dentist for extractions and restorative therapy

---

 RITICAL THINKING ACTIVITIES

1. Perform an oral assessment on a patient before, during, and after chemotherapy.
2. Describe the oral complications associated with chemotherapy to a classmate and role-play the interaction between a dental hygienist and an immune-compromised patient. Provide the appropriate symptom management for each oral complication.
3. Visit a dental oncology clinic to observe oral treatment management of chemotherapy patients.
4. Outline an educational program for a group of patients undergoing chemotherapy about the oral complications they might experience.
5. Present an educational program to a group of dental hygienists, dentists, oncologists, or oncology nurses, and outline a team approach to patient care.

6. Contact a medical oncologist to inquire about the types of oral care information given to patients. Offer to provide an educational program, if appropriate.
7. Develop a plan of care for patients experiencing the following conditions:
   a. Rheumatoid arthritis
   b. HIV with low CD4+ counts to AIDS
   c. Oral manifestations associated with chemotherapy
8. Visit a clinic that provides care for HIV/AIDS patients.
9. Present an educational program about oral care to a group of patients with HIV/AIDS.
10. Arrange to perform an oral assessment on a newly diagnosed patient with HIV and one with full-blown AIDS.

REVIEW QUESTIONS

1. Cancer can be defined as which of the following?
   a. A group of normal cells that grow more rapidly than normal
   b. A group of abnormal cells that grow more rapidly and ignore the usual controls that prevent them from going past their intended size
   c. A group of abnormal cells that have no impact on the host organ

2. The American Cancer Society estimated that in the year 2000 the top three cancers to be diagnosed in women would be which of the following?
   a. Breast, lung, and colon and rectum
   b. Breast, ovary, and uterus
   c. Lung, melanoma, and breast

3. Which of the following is the role of the dental hygienist in working with a cancer patient?
   a. Identify and eliminate any oral infection (within the scope of dental hygiene practice)
   b. Improve and/or maintain oral hygiene status
   c. Provide symptom management for oral complications that result from cancer therapy
   d. All the above

4. To safely receive dental care, the absolute neutrophil count should be which of the following?
   a. 500
   b. 750
   c. 1500

5. To safely receive dental care, a platelet count should be at least which of the following?
   a. 1,000
   b. 15,000
   c. 60,000

6. Chemotherapy patients with an indwelling venous catheter require which of the following?
   a. No special precautions before dental hygiene care is given
   b. Antibiotic premedication coverage according to the American Heart Association guidelines for endocarditis prophylaxis
   c. Antibiotic coverage for several days before dental hygiene care is given

7. Which of the following body fluids carry HIV?
   a. Blood, saliva, and sweat
   b. Blood, semen, and sweat
   c. Semen, blood, and breast milk

8. Of the following therapies, which is the most effective way to treat HIV infection and AIDS?
   a. One drug—AZT
   b. Protease inhibitors
   c. A three-drug combination that includes AZT and protease inhibitors

9. Of the following oral manifestations, which might been seen in a patient with HIV?
   a. Candidiasis
   b. Herpes lesions
   c. Kaposi's sarcoma
   d. All the above

10. Periodontal disease in HIV-infected patients is characterized by which of the following?
    a. Much more severe and rapidly progressing
    b. Progresses at approximately the same rate as that seen in non–HIV-infected individuals
    c. Progresses at the same rate in HIV-infected patients as in healthy patients but more slowly than with AIDS patients

SUGGESTED AGENCIES AND WEB SITES

Because of the ever-changing nature of the Internet, some of the web sites listed here may have changed since publication. Please refer to Mosby's Evolve web site for the most current information.

[The] American Foundation for AIDS Research: (800) 39AMFAR
Centers for Disease Control and Prevention: http://www.cdc.gov
General information on AIDS: (800) 342-AIDS
General information for healthcare providers, HIV Telephone Consultation Service: (800) 933-3413
National Association of People with AIDS: 202-898-0414
National Cancer Institute, (800) 4-CANCER: http://www.nci.nih.gov

National Institute of Dental and Craniofacial Research: http:// www.nidr.nih.gov
National Oral Health Information Clearinghouse, (301) 402-7364: http://www.aerie.com
Procter & Gamble, Co., Global Dental Resources: http://www.dentalcare.com

ADDITIONAL READINGS AND RESOURCES

Cancer Fax: 301-402-5874
Colgate (Prevident, Gel Kam, Optimoist, Perioguard): (800) 225-3756
Dental Resources, Inc. (REVIVE Remineralizing Gel): (800) 328-1276
Laclede Professional Products (Biotene, Oral Balance): (800) 922-5856
MGI Pharma, Inc. (Salagen): (800) 562-4531

National Cancer Institute: *Understanding the immune system,* NIH Pub. No. 92-529, Bethesda, Md, 1992, National Institutes of Health.
Oral-B: (800) 446-7252

ADDITIONAL READINGS AND RESOURCES–cont'd

Oral Health in America: *A report of the surgeon general*, NIH Pub. No. 00-4713, Rockville, Md, 2000, U.S. Department of Health and Human Services, National Institute for Dental and Craniofacial Research, National Institutes of Health.

National Institute for Dental and Craniofacial Research: *Oral health, cancer care, & you*, Rockville, Md, 2000, The Institute [folder of printed materials that can be obtained via telephone at (877) 216-1019].

PHB, Inc. (Ultra Suave toothbrush): (800) 553-1440

Sage Products, Inc.: (800) 323-2220

Silverman S: *Color atlas of oral manifestations of AIDS,* ed 2, St Louis, 1996, Mosby.

UNIMED, Inc. (MOUTHKOTE Products): (800) 541-3492

REFERENCES

1. American Academy of Periodontology Position Paper: Periodontal considerations in the management of the cancer patient, *J Periodont* 68(8):791-801, 1997.

2. American Academy of Periodontology Position Paper: Periodontal considerations in the HIV-positive patient, *Committee Res, Sci, Therapy,* 1-9, April 1994.

3. Armitage GC: Systemic factors influencing periodontal diseases. In Perry DA, Biemsterboer PL, Taggart EJ, editors: *Periodontology for the dental hygienist,* Philadelphia, 1996, WB Saunders.

4. Atkinson JL, O'Connell A, Aframian D: Oral manifestations of primary immunological diseases, *J Am Dent Assoc* 131:345-56, 2000.

5. Barker GJ: Dental hygiene care for the individual with cancer. In Darby ML, Walsh MW, editors: *Dental hygiene theory and practice,* Philadelphia, 1995, WB Saunders.

6. Barker G, Barker B: Management of the patient undergoing cancer chemotherapy: the role of the dental hygienist, *J Dent Hyg* 65(4):184-7,1991.

7. Barker GF, Barker BF, Gier RF: *Oral management of the cancer patient: a guide for the health care professional,* Kansas City, Mo, 1996, Biomedical.

8. Bavier AR: *Nursing management of acute oral complications of cancer,* NCI monogr 9, NIH Pub. No. 89-3081, 123-8, Bethesda, Md, 1990, National Cancer Institute.

9. Beck SL: Prevention and management of oral complications in the cancer patient, *Cur Issues Ca Nurs Prac* 1(6):1-12,1992.

10. Begg MD, et al: Oral lesions as markers of severe immunosuppression in HIV-infected homosexual men and injection drug users, *Oral Surg Oral Med Oral Pathol* 73(2):193-200, 1992.

11. Berger AM, et al: Capsaicin for the treatment of oral mucositis pain, *Princ Prac Onc* 9(1):1-11, 1995.

12. Crawford JM: Human immunodeficiency virus–associated periodontal diseases: a review, *J Dent Hyg* 67(4):198-207,1993.

13. Dodd MJ, et al: Randomized clinical trial of chlorhexidine versus placebo for prevention of oral mucositis in patients receiving chemotherapy, *Oncol Nurs Forum* 23(6):921-27, 1996.

14. Dreizen S: *Description and incidence of oral complications,* NCI monogr 9, NIH Pub. No. 89-3081, 11-15, Bethesda, Md, 1990, National Cancer Institute.

15. Epstein JB, Schubert MM: Management of orofacial pain in cancer patients, *Oral Oncol, Bur J Cancer* 29B(4):243-250, 1993.

16. Epstein JB, Silverman S: Head and neck malignancies associated with HIV infection, *Oral Surg Oral Med Oral Pathol* 73(2):193-200, 1992

17. Eversole LR: Viral infections of the head and neck among HIV-positive patients, *Oral Surg Oral Med Oral Pathol* 73(2):155-163,1992.

18. Ferretti GA, et al: *Oral antimicrobial agents—chlorhexidine,* NCI monogr 9, NIH Pub. No. 89-3081, 51-5, Bethesda, Md, 1990, National Cancer Institute.

19. Fischer DS, Knobf MT, Durivage HJ: Cancer chemotherapy and pharmacology. In Fischer DS, Knobf MT, Durivage HJ, editors: *The cancer chemotherapy handbook,* ed 4, St Louis, 1993, Mosby.

20. Fischer DS, Knobf MT, Durivage HJ: Gastrointestinal toxicity. In Fischer DS, Knobf MT, Durivage HJ, editors: *The cancer chemotherapy handbook,* ed 4, St Louis, 1993, Mosby.

21. Flavitz CM, Silverman S: Human immunodeficiency virus (HIV)–associated malignancies. In Silverman S, editor: *Oral cancer,* ed 4, London, 1998, BC Decker, Inc.

22. Friedman RB, et al: Periodontal status of HIV-seropositive and AIDS patients, *J Periodontol* 62(10):623-7, 1991.

23. Graham KM, et al: Reducing the incidence of stomatitis using a quality assessment and improvement approach, *Ca Nurs* 16(2):117-122, 1993.

24. Greenlee RT, et al: Cancer statistics, 2000, *CA Cancer J Clin* 50(1):7-33,2000.

25. Greenspan JS, et al: Oral manifestations of HIV infection, *Oral Surg Oral Med Oral Pathol* 73(2):142-4, 1992.

26. Guy JL, Ingram BA: Medical oncology: the agents. In McCorkle R, Grant M, Frank-Stromborg M, Baird SB, editors: *Cancer nursing: a comprehensive textbook,* ed 2, Philadelphia, 1996, WB Saunders.

27. Iwamoto RR: Alterations in oral status. In McCorkle R, Grant M, Frank-Stromborg M, Baird SB, editors: *Cancer nursing: a comprehensive textbook,* ed 2, Philadelphia, 1996, WB Saunders.

28. Klein RS, Quart AM, Small CB: Periodontal disease in heterosexuals with acquired immunodeficiency syndrome, *J Periodontol* 62(8):535-40,1991.

29. Laine P, et al: Salivary flow and composition in lymphoma patients before, during, and after treatment with cytostatic drugs, *Oral Oncol, Eur J Cancer* 28B(2):125-8, 1992.

30. Loprinzi CL, Dose AM: *Studies on the prevention of 5-fluorouracil–induced oral mucositis,* NCI monogr 9, NIH Pub. No. 89-3081, 93-4, Bethesda, Md, 1990, National Cancer Institute.

31. Madeya M: Oral complications from cancer therapy: Part 1: pathophysiology and secondary complications, *Oncol Nurs Forum* 23(5):801-7, 1996.

32. Madeya M: Oral complications from cancer therapy: Part 2: nursing implications for assessment and treatment, *Oncol Nurs Forum* 23(5):808-21, 1996.

33. McCarthy OM: Host factors associated with HIV-related oral candidiasis, *Oral Surg Oral Med Oral Pathol* 73(2):181-6, 1992.

34. Mettlin C, Michalek: The causes of cancer. In McCorkle R, Grant M, Frank-Stromborg M, Baird SB, editors: *Cancer nursing: a comprehensive textbook,* ed 2, Philadelphia, 1996, WB Saunders.

Continued

35. Miaskowski C: *Management of mucositis during therapy,* NCI monogr 9, NIH Pub. No. 89-3081, 95-8, Bethesda, Md, 1990, National Cancer Institute.

36. Moore LVH, et al: Periodontal microflora of HIV-positive subjects with gingivitis or adult periodontitis, *J Periodontol* 64(1): 48-56, 1993.

37. Muzyka BC, Olick M: A review of oral fungal infections and appropriate therapy, *J Am Dent Assoc* 126(1):63-72,1995.

38. National Cancer Institute: *Consensus development conference on oral complications of cancer therapies: diagnosis, prevention, and treatment,* NCI monogr 9, NIH Pub. No. 89-3081, Bethesda, Md, 1990, National Cancer Institute.

39. National Institute of Dental and Craniofacial Research: *Oral complications of cancer therapy: what the oral health team can do,* NIDCR brochure, NIH Pub. No. 99-4372, 1-7, Rockville, Md, 1999, The Institute.

40. National Institute of Dental and Craniofacial Research: *Chemotherapy and your mouth,* NIDCR pamphlet, NIH Pub. No. 99-4361, 1-11, Rockville, Md, 1999, The Institute.

41. National Institutes of Health Consensus Development Panel: *Consensus statement: oral complications of cancer therapies,* NCI monogr 9, NIH Pub. No. 89-3081, 3-8, Bethesda, Md, 1990, The Institutes.

42. Olsen SJ, Frank-Stromborg M: Cancer screening and early detection. In McCorkle R, Grant M, Frank-Stromborg M, Baird SB, editors: *Cancer nursing: a comprehensive textbook,* ed 2, Philadelphia, 1996, WB Saunders.

43. Perry DA: Dental hygiene care for the individual with HIV infection. In Darby ML, Walsh MW, editors: *Dental hygiene and practice,* Philadelphia, 1995, WB Saunders.

44. Peterson DE: *Pretreatment strategies for infection prevention in chemothrerapy patients,* NCI monogr 9, NIH Pub. No. 89-3081, 61- 71, Bethesda, Md, 1990, National Cancer Institute.

45. Piluso S, et al: Cause of oral ulcers in HIV-infected patients, *Oral Surg Oral Med Oral Pathol Oral Radiol Endod* 82(2):166-72, 1996.

46. Poland J: Prevention and treatment of oral complications in the cancer patient, *Oncology* July 1991.

47. Ransier A, et al: A Combined analysis of a toothbrush, foam brush, and chlorhexidine-soaked foam brush in maintaining oral hygiene, *Ca Nurs* 18(5):393-6, 1995.

48. Redding SW: *Role of herpes simplex virus reactivation in chemotherapy-induced oral mucositis,* NCI monogr 9, NIH Pub. No.89-3081, 103-5, Bethesda, Md, 1990, National Cancer Institute.

49. Saral R: *Management of acute viral infections,* NCI monogr 9, NIH Pub. No. 89-3081, 107-10, Bethesda, Md, 1990, National Cancer Institute.

50. Schimpff SC: *Surveillance cultures,* NCI monogr 9, NIH Pub. No. 89-3081, 37-42, Bethesda, Md, 1990, National Cancer Institute.

51. Scully C, McCarthy G: Management of oral health in persons with HIV infection, *Oral Surg Oral Med Oral Pathol* 73(2):215-25, 1992.

52. Silverman S: *Oral defenses and compromises: an overview,* NCI monogr 9, NIH Pub. No. 89-3081, 17-9, Bethesda, Md, 1990, National Cancer Institute.

53. Silverman S, et al: Clinical characteristics and management responses in 85 HIV-infected patients with oral candidiasis, *Oral Surg Oral Med Oral Pathol Oral Radio Endod* 82(4):402-7, 1996.

54. Slavkin HC: An update on HIV/AIDS, *J Am Dent Assoc* 127: 1401-4,1996.

55. Sonis ST, Woods PD, White HA: *Pretreatment oral assessment,* NCI monogr 9, NIH Pub. No. 89-3081, 29-32, Bethesda, Md, 1990, National Cancer Institute.

56. Stevenson-Moore P: *Essential aspects of a pretreatment oral examination,* NCI monogr 9, NIH Pub. No. 89-3081, 33-6, Bethesda, Md, 1990, National Cancer Institute.

57. Turbal NS, Erdal S, Karacay S: Efficacy of treatment to relieve mucositis-induced discomfort, *Support Care Cancer* 8(1):55-8, 2000.

58. Wilkins EM, Romano JE: Infection control: transmissible diseases. In Wilkins EM, editor: *Clinical practice of the dental hygienist,* ed 8, Philadelphia, 1999, Lippincott Williams & Wilkins.

59. Wingard JR: *Infectious and noninfectious systemic consequences,* NCI monogr 9, NIH Pub. No. 89-3081, 21-6, Bethesda, Md, 1990, National Cancer Institute.

60. Winkler JR, Robertson PH: Periodontal disease associated with HIV infection, *Oral Surg Oral Med Oral Pathol* 73(2):145-50, 1992.

61. Yeung SCH, et al: Progression of periodontal disease in HIV-seropositive patients, *J Periodontol* 64(7):651-7, 1993.

CHAPTER 45

Head *and* Neck Cancer *and* Radiation

Christina B. DeBiase

Chapter Outline

Case Study: Intraoral Considerations in the Dental
    Treatment of a Patient with Head and Neck
    Cancer
Etiology and Contributing Factors
Clinical Diagnosis
Staging
Early Detection

Treatment
    Radiation therapy
    Oral complications
Oral Care Protocol
    Treatment before radiotherapy
    Treatment during radiotherapy
    Treatment after radiotherapy

Key Terms

Benign
Biopsy
Carcinoma
cGy (centigray)
Chemotherapy
Dysgeusia

Dysplasia
Fractionation
Hyperbaric oxygen
In situ
Malignant

Metastasis
Oncology
Palliative
Photodynamic therapy (PDT)
Prognosis

Radiation modifiers
Radiotherapy
Staging
Survival rate
Trismus

 Learning Outcomes

1. Know important statistics and terminology associated with head and neck cancer and radiation therapy.
2. Understand the possible causes of cancers of the head and neck.
3. Identify head and neck cancer by its appearance, symptoms, and location and be able to identify the stage of the disease.
4. Discuss the various methods for evaluating lesions.

5. Explain the types of radiation therapy and the dosage regimens.
6. Describe the types of oral complications associated with radiation therapy and their management.
7. Outline a typical oral care protocol for patients before, during, and after radiation therapy.

More than 1.2 million new cases of cancer were estimated to be diagnosed in the United States in 2001, and approximately 30,000 of those cases involved tumors in the head and neck. Cancers of the head and neck represent only 3% of estimated new cancer cases in male patients, but a significant proportion of those cases now involve female patients; the male-to-female ratio has changed over the past several years from

3:1 to 2:1. Women are developing more head and neck cancers because their use of alcohol and tobacco has increased. The mean age of onset for both genders is 63 years of age.[21]

In India, southeastern Asia, Africa, Brazil, and other developing countries, cancers of the head and neck are much more prevalent. These cancers include *malignant* tumors of the upper aerodigestive tract, the paranasal

Intraoral Considerations in the Dental Treatment of a Patient with Head and Neck Cancer

Dr. Kay Matthews, a dentist, was consulted by a hospital oncologist about a 22-year-old patient, E. Thomas Fitzgibbons, who was diagnosed 5 years ago with nasopharyngeal carcinoma. The tumor was staged according to the tumor, node, metastasis (TNM) system as $T_2N_0M_0$. Mr. Fitzgibbons underwent a 6-week course of radiation therapy in another state. Although he had been scheduled numerous times for medical and dental follow-up, he had left home after turning 18 years of age and had refused further treatment. The only remaining side effect of the treatment was severe xerostomia. Mr. Fitzgibbons had been cancer-free and pain-free until he appeared to begin developing trismus. His mouth opening was becoming progressively smaller, and he had lost 15 pounds in 3 months. These symptoms prompted Mr. Fitzgibbons to seek care.

Extraoral palpation revealed what appeared to be a cervical node about the size of a dime. The oral opening was only 9 mm wide. A cursory assessment of the oral cavity revealed dry, inflamed mucosa and extensive carious lesions. Two premolars and one molar were present in the form of retained root tips.

Medical assessment revealed recurrence of the tumor, and Dr. Matthews advised Mr. Fitzgibbons to undergo another course of radiation therapy as soon as possible. Treating Mr. Fitzgibbons' dental needs was paramount, and radiation therapy could not begin until several extractions and extensive restorative procedures had been performed to eliminate oral infection. Because of Mr. Fitzgibbons' previous exposure to radiation, **hyperbaric oxygen** treatments were scheduled to flood the tissues with oxygen to increase the blood supply, particularly at the extraction sites, to reduce the risk of osteoradionecrosis.

The oncologist, dentist, and dental hygienist spent considerable time explaining to Mr. Fitzgibbons the treatment regimen, and they required a commitment on his part to follow through with dental treatment before, during, and after **radiotherapy** to ensure that the risk of infection would be kept to a minimum.

---

sinuses, the major and minor salivary glands, the parathyroid and thyroid glands, and the skin, soft tissue, bone, and neurovascular structures in the head and neck region. More than 90% of all oral carcinomas are of squamous cell origin.[35]

ETIOLOGY AND CONTRIBUTING FACTORS

The cause of oral cancer is unknown, but several factors have shown a high correlation with the development of this disease. Smoking and other forms of tobacco use usually are associated with oral cancer or cancers of the head and neck. The smoke and heat from cigarettes, cigars, and pipes irritate the oral mucosa, and smokeless tobacco products irritate these membranes through direct contact. Smokeless tobacco products should not be considered a safe alternative to smoking. A dose-response relationship exists between smokeless tobacco and health; the more tobacco used, the greater the risk of cancer. Chewing tobacco may also be related to cancers of the upper digestive tract. Excessive alcohol intake, particularly in combination with smoking, has been associated with most cases of oral squamous cell *carcinoma* (Fig. 45-1).[32,35]

Individuals exposed to sunlight may be at risk for lip cancer. People at increased risk of head and neck carcinomas are those with congenital and acquired defects of the immune system and organ transplant patients. Controversy exists as to whether upper aerodigestive carcinomas become clinically evident only when the immune system is impaired.[26]

New research suggests that viruses also are involved in the development of oral cancers. The human papillomavirus and herpes viruses have been detected in oral cancer biopsies. Kaposi's sarcoma, which is related to acquired immunodeficiency syndrome (AIDS), has a preference for the head and neck area, most commonly causing lesions on the hard palate and gingiva.[20,23]

Other risk factors that have been implicated previously in the development of some types of oral cancer are poor oral hygiene; nutritional deficiencies, particularly diets lacking in fruits and vegetables; heavy exposure to certain materials, such as wood and metal dust; and chronic thermal or physical trauma.[34,39] However,

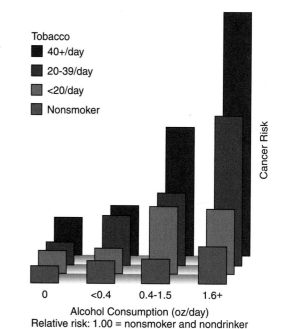

FIG. 45-1 Relative risk of cancer related to alcohol consumption and tobacco use.

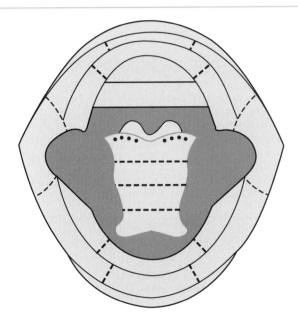

FIG. 45-2 Shaded area shows the location of most oral cancers.

these risk factors currently are acknowledged to have little relevance to the development of oral or oropharyngeal squamous cell carcinoma.[26]

Some supplements and foods seem to reduce the risk of oral cancer. Vitamins and minerals, particularly vitamin E and beta-carotene, appear to have anticarcinogenic properties.[14] The polyphenols in green tea also are believed to have antimutagenic properties, which help lower the incidence of oral and esophageal cancers.

CLINICAL DIAGNOSIS

45-A Carcinomas of the head and neck may appear clinically as red, speckled (mixed red and white), or white lesions that do not rub off. Histologically these lesions may be described as hyperkeratosis, parakeratosis, atypia, *dysplasia*, carcinoma *in situ*, or varying grades of invasive cancer. The malignant potential of "white lesions" (traditionally referred to as *leukoplakias*) may range from 0.1% to 6%, depending on the source.[23,25,26] With "red lesions" *(erythroplakias),* the risk of the lesion developing into an oral carcinoma is three to five times greater than for leukoplakias.

Most early oral cancers are small, asymptomatic, smooth red lesions or speckled, granular red lesions with patchy areas of keratin or normal mucosa within or around the lesion. Approximately 60% of invasive oral carcinomas have a granular texture, whereas an equal percentage of carcinomas in situ are smooth.[25] The patient should be asked how long the lesion has been present, in order to distinguish cancer from an inflammatory lesion, which normally lasts about 10 days to 2 weeks.

The most common sites for oral cancer are the floor of the mouth, the ventrolateral borders of the tongue, and the soft palate, including the uvula, lingual aspect of the retromolar trigone, and the anterior tonsillar pillars (Fig. 45-2).[8] Individuals who use chewing tobacco are more prone to cancer of the buccal mucosa. Histologically, the tissues at high risk are not protected by keratin.

As a tumor enlarges, symptoms often appear. The tumor may ulcerate and bleed. Dysgeusia, ear pain, and difficulty opening the mouth, speaking, chewing, and swallowing may also develop.

STAGING

Head and neck carcinomas are staged to correlate treat- **45-B** ment outcomes with the initial extent of the tumor. The tumor is assessed by inspection, palpation, and histological confirmation of the diagnosis. Carcinoma in situ, as its name implies, is noninvasive but has the strong potential to become invasive if not treated.[27] The diagnosis of invasive squamous cell carcinoma is made when abnormal cells disrupt the basement membrane and extend into the underlying connective tissue. The deeper the primary tumor's invasion, the greater the risk of lymph node involvement and the more adverse the effect on the *prognosis.*[26]

The boundaries of an invasive carcinoma may be graded as G_1 (well-differentiated), G_2 (moderately well-differentiated), G_3 (poorly differentiated), and G_4 (undifferentiated).[2] Well-differentiated tumors usually are considered less aggressive than poorly differentiated ones. However, the degree of differentiation and the biological behavior of a tumor are unpredictable, particularly in patients with an impaired immune response.[26]

The stages of a tumor are defined by the international tumor, node, metastasis (TNM) classification system. *T* refers to the size of the tumor; *N* refers to the extent of lymph node involvement; and *M* indicates whether *metastasis* has occurred[23] (Box 45-1).

EARLY DETECTION

In most patients a primary tumor can be detected by a thorough intraoral and extraoral examination. This involves careful assessment of the skin of the face, scalp, and neck; the regional lymph nodes (Fig. 45-3); the thyroid gland; the salivary glands; the oral cavity; and the oropharynx. Good lighting and radiographs are essential for a complete examination (see Chapters 11 through 17). Delays in diagnosis may be attributed to the patient or the professional, or both. Patients must be taught the importance of oral self-examination, how to perform it, when to perform it, and which findings may warrant a visit to a healthcare provider (Box 45-2).

A knowledge of the common locations and appearance of lesions that have the greatest carcinogenic potential is paramount in detecting cancers early. Unfortunately, many lesions are missed or considered innocuous. Toluidine blue stain can be used to rule out subjective clinical impressions of questionable lesions or as a screening rinse for patients who have high-risk behaviors, such as smoking and drinking. The dye clinically stains malignant lesions; normal mucosa remains unchanged. Although nonmalignant inflammatory areas may also stain, producing a false-positive result, restaining after 2 weeks may clarify the findings, because inflammatory lesions should have resolved by then. The brush biopsy recently has gained acceptance as a screening tool used to identify questionable oral lesions at an early stage. Patients with advanced lesions or those with typical malignant presentations should be referred for diagnosis.

BOX 45-1

International TNM System of Classification and Staging of Oral Carcinomas

T: Size of Tumor

T_{1s}: Carcinoma in situ
T_1: Tumor <2 cm in size
T_2: Tumor <2 cm to >4 cm in size
T_3: Tumor >4 cm in size
T_4: Massive tumor with deep invasion into bone, muscle, skin, etc.

N: Regional Lymph Node Involvement

N_0: No palpable nodes
N_1: Single, homolateral palpable node <3 cm in diameter
N_2: Single, homolateral palpable node 3 to 6 cm
or
Multiple, homolateral nodes, none >6 cm
N_3: Single or multiple homolateral nodes, one >6 cm,
or
Bilateral nodes (stage each side of neck),
or

Contralateral nodes

M: Metastases

M_0: No known distant metastasis
M_1: Distant metastasis
    PUL (pulmonary)
    OSS (osseous)
    HEP (liver)
    BRA (brain)

Stages*

Stage	Classification
I	T_1, N_0, M_0
II	T_2, N_0, M_0
III	T_3, N_0, M_0
	T_1, T_2 *or* T_3, N_1, M_0
	T_4, N_0, N_1, M_0
IV	Any T, N_2, N_3, M_0
	Any T, any N, M_1

N1 <3 cm	N2a <3-6 cm	N2b Multiple nodes	Bilateral N2c *or* Contralateral node(s) <6 cm	N3 >6 cm Single or multiple

Data from Shah JP et al: *Curr Probl Surg* 30:273-344, 1993.
Modified from Beahrs OH et al, editors: *American Joint Committee on Cancer: manual for staging cancer*, ed 4, Philadelphia, 1992, Lippincott.
*In text, these designations are written as $T_1N_0M_0$ or $T_4N_1M_0$, for example.

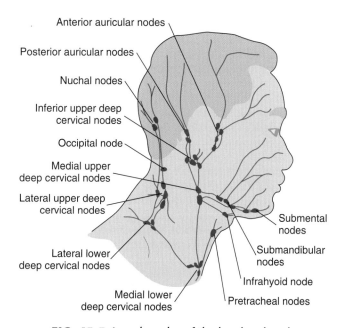

FIG. 45-3 Lymph nodes of the head and neck.

Anterior auricular nodes
Posterior auricular nodes
Nuchal nodes
Inferior upper deep cervical nodes
Occipital node
Medial upper deep cervical nodes
Lateral upper deep cervical nodes
Lateral lower deep cervical nodes
Medial lower deep cervical nodes
Submental nodes
Submandibular nodes
Infrahyoid node
Pretracheal nodes

The final diagnosis for oral lesions can be established only with a biopsy. Incisional ***biopsy*** is the method of choice for microscopic analysis of suspected intraoral carcinoma. Excisional biopsy is recommended when the clinical examination indicates that a lesion most likely is ***benign*** but has the potential for functional impairment or when a malignant lesion is so small that it can be removed completely without compromising function. Biopsy diagnosis is required before the type and extent of therapy can be determined.[11,26]

TREATMENT

Early cancers (stage I or stage II) are highly curable by surgery or radiation therapy. The mode of treatment is dictated by several factors, including the tumor's stage, grade, and location; the patient's age, overall medical status, personal desires, and history of carcinoma and treatment; the anticipated functional and cosmetic results of treatment; socioeconomic issues; and the availability of professional resources. The collaborative efforts of professionals specializing in rehabilitation; preventive, restorative, and prosthetic dentistry; and social services are an integral part of a patient's recovery plan.[18,26,28,41]

BOX 45-2

Self-Exam Procedures for Oral Cancer

Self-examination for oral cancer is an essential procedure for everyone. Oral cancers are painless in their initial stages and often go unnoticed. Take a few minutes and learn this easy three-step self-examination.

Before a well-lighted mirror observe each of the structures discussed below for any swelling, ulceration, or change in color or texture.

Lips

1 Look at your lips with your mouth closed and then opened; feel the lip for any hard swelling by pressing and rolling the lip between your index finger and thumb of the same hand.

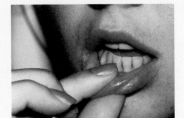

Retract your lips and slide your fingers all the way back, exposing the insides of your cheeks and gums. Observe for any differences in appearance.

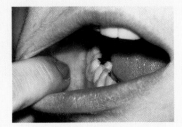

Tongue

2 Stick out your tongue and check for any swelling, ulcers, or changes in size, color, or texture.

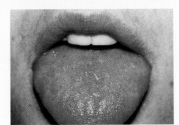

Pull the tip of your tongue to your right with a washcloth as you examine the left side of your tongue. Now examine the opposite side of the tongue by pulling the tip of the tongue to the left.

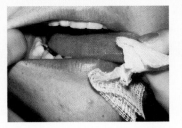

Floor of the Mouth

3 Touch the roof of your mouth with the tip of your tongue, open wide, and look at the bottom surface of the tongue and the floor of the mouth. Veins observed on the underside of the tongue are normal, so don't be alarmed. Notice the flow of saliva from the opening of the duct. It should be free-flowing, watery, and clear.

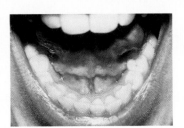

Modified from Bouquot J, DeBiase CB, Graves CE: *Self-exam procedures for oral cancer,* West Virginia University, 1987, Biomedical Communications.

Continued

BOX 45-2

Self-Exam Procedures for Oral Cancer–cont'd

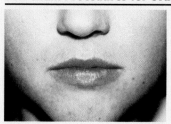

This simple three-step exam could save your life by helping you to find oral cancer early, when it is most treatable.

Oral cancer affects almost 30,000 persons yearly. Approximately one third of these individuals will die. Tobacco usage, excessive consumption of alcohol, and overexposure to the sun increase your chances of developing a cancer of the mouth.

Q *Why should you examine your mouth bimonthly?*
Most people visit their dentist/physician once a year. Because oral cancers found early and treated promptly have a better prognosis, learning how to examine your mouth properly could help save your life. Follow the self-exam procedures shown here.

Q *When is the best time to examine your mouth?*
Every 2 months right after brushing your teeth is the best guide. Following the self-exam procedures regularly will give you peace of mind, and seeing your dentist at least once a year will reassure you that there is nothing wrong.

Q *What should you do if you find a sore, thickening, or lump?*
If a sore, thickening, or lump is discovered during the self-exam procedures, it is important to see your dentist as soon as possible. Don't be frightened. Most changes are not cancer, but only your dentist/physician can make the diagnosis.

Know Oral Cancer's Warning Signals!

1. A sore that does not heal within a 2-week period	2. Unusual bleeding continuing beyond 1 week	3. Thickening or a lump on any oral tissue	4. Indigestion or difficulty swallowing
	5. Obvious change in color or texture of any oral tissues	6. Nagging cough or hoarseness	

These signals may pertain to an oral cancer most often seen as one or more of the following:

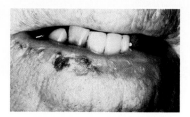

An ulceration of the lower lip

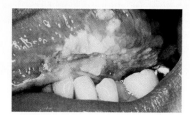

A white area on the side of the tongue

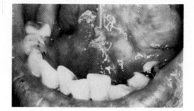

A swelling under the tongue

Modified from Bouquot J, DeBiase CB, Graves CE: *Self-exam procedures for oral cancer,* West Virginia University, 1987, Biomedical Communications.

Combined therapy (surgery and radiation) usually is recommended for stage III and stage IV tumors and for early cancers that have poorly defined margins or a tumor depth greater than 5 mm. The risk of recurrence, particularly second primary tumors of the aerodigestive tract, increases for tumors that have advanced to these levels.

Radiation modifiers or *chemotherapy* combined with surgery or radiation (or both) may be administered to limit local recurrence and distant metastases.[7,15,28]

An antineoplastic drug, 5-fluorouracil, applied topically in combination with laser surgery, has been used to treat carcinoma in situ. *Photodynamic therapy (PDT)* is undergoing evaluation for the treatment of T_1 tumors, Kaposi's sarcoma, carcinoma in situ of the oral cavity, and laryngeal carcinoma.[39]

The prognosis for cancers of the lip and oral cavity varies depending on the tumor's stage and location. Generally, the higher the tumor's stage number, the worse the prognosis. Because cancers of the lip are readily observable, most such lesions are detected and treated early with surgery or radiation. Cure rates generally are 90% to 100%. Other small lesions of the retromolar trigone, hard palate, and gingiva are equally curable by either treatment method. Small cancers of the anterior tongue, the floor of the mouth, and the buccal mucosa have cure rates of about 90% when treated with radiation therapy or surgery.[40]

Moderately advanced lesions without evidence of spread to the cervical lymph nodes usually are curable, with control rates of 90% for the retromolar trigone; 80% for lesions involving the hard palate, gingiva, and buccal mucosa; 70% for the floor of the mouth; and 65% for the anterior tongue.[38,40] Unfortunately, professional consultation often is delayed until the patient has some type of discomfort. By that time, in more than half of these patients the cancer has metastasized to the lymph nodes of the neck or axilla, reducing the 5-year *survival rate* to 30% to 40%.

The most important factor in determining the prognosis for a squamous cell carcinoma of the head and neck is whether metastasis to the lymph nodes has occurred.[37] The cure rate for patients with lymph involvement is half that of an individual without nodal metastasis. The goals of treatment are cure, maintaining quality of life, and preventing subsequent primary lesions.[35]

RADIATION THERAPY

Radiation can be delivered externally through ports (e.g., Cobalt, linear accelerator) or internally by implantation of radioactive materials in tissues or body cavities. Radioactive isotopes may also be administered orally or intravenously or by instillation. These materials are metabolized by the body, and caregivers must use safety precautions to avoid exposure to radioactive materials.

A simulator determines the field of radiation from an external source. The simulator is a diagnostic x-ray unit used to visualize the proposed treatment site. Masks or head holders are used to keep the head stabilized in the same position for all treatments. Field markings are placed on the masks, rather than on the skin, to alleviate the conspicuous facial tattoos once used in the past. Superficial lesions usually are treated through a single field; multiple fields are used for deep and/or large tumors. Multiple fields maximize the amount of radiation to the tumor and reduce the amount of scatter radiation to normal tissues. Lead blocks, also used to protect vital body organs and tissues, are secured to a plastic tray and placed on the head of the treatment machine between the beam and the person receiving treatment.[5]

Ionizing radiation destroys tumor cells by damaging the cell nucleus, preventing the growth and replication of these cells. Radiation can directly damage deoxyribonucleic acid (DNA) or can interact with water and oxygen molecules, producing free radicals that indirectly cause cell death through DNA damage.[23,42] Unfortunately, nor-

TABLE 45-1

Degree of organ radiosensitivity

Organ	Radiosensitivity
Lymph, bone marrow, blood, testes, ovaries, intestines	Very high
Skin, oral cavity, esophagus, rectum, bladder, vagina, cervix, ureters, cornea	High
Stomach, growing cartilage and bone, fine vasculature, optic lens	Moderate
Mature cartilage and bone, salivary glands, kidney, liver, pancreas, respiratory organs, thyroid, adrenals, pituitary gland	Moderately low
Muscle, brain, spinal cord	Low

Modified from Rubin P, Constantine L, Nelson D: Late effects of cancer treatment: radiation and drug toxicity. In: Perez C, Brady LW, editors: *Principles and practice of radiation oncology,* Philadelphia, 1992, Lippincott.

mal tissues also are affected by the radiation, which creates side effects that serve as a dose-limiting gauge for determining tumor destruction and host survival. The frequency, severity, and duration of the damage in the irradiated tissues of the head and neck are a function of this radiobiological effect, the dosing schedule, the type and *fractionation* of the radiation administered, the host response, and the volume and radiosensitivity of the tissues involved. In general, rapidly dividing cells are more sensitive to radiation (Table 45-1).[33] Radiosensitizers are used to sensitize tumor cells to the effects of radiation so that the amount of radiation needed to kill tumor cells can be reduced, thereby limiting radiation injury to normal cells.[23]

Adjuvant radiation therapy can be administered preoperatively or postoperatively. Physicians rarely choose preoperative irradiation because of the dose limitations, impaired oxygenation and healing potential of the intended surgical site, and poor compliance by some patients on following through with surgery after radiation treatment. Postoperative irradiation, on the other hand, is highly recommended. The dose limitation is much higher; the complications associated with wound healing do not exist; and accurate pathologic *staging* of the tumor is possible.

Patients who smoke while undergoing radiation therapy have a diminished healing response and shorter survival duration than those who do not.[4] It is imperative that patients be counseled to stop smoking before therapy. Patients receiving radiation to the neck to kill oral cancer cells that have spread to the lymph nodes are five to six times more likely to have damaged carotid arteries, making them more vulnerable to strokes. These patients often drink or smoke heavily (or both), have hypertension, and have already developed osteoradionecrosis (bony destruction) of the mandible.[13]

Therapeutic dosages of radiation normally range from 5000 to 7000 *cGy (centigray)* over a 6- to 7-week period. Doses usually are fractionated into 150 to 200 cGy on weekdays, leaving the weekends for normal cell repair.

Total body irradiation (TBI) is administered as part of a preparatory regimen for bone marrow transplantation (BMT). TBI (1000 cGy) and cyclophosphamide condition the graft recipient by inducing immunosuppression and killing all malignant cells. BMT is not a suggested treatment for carcinomas of the head and neck.[23]

ORAL COMPLICATIONS

45-C Radiation-induced oral complications can significantly affect morbidity, the patient's ability to tolerate treatment, and overall quality of life.[29] The effects of radiation are cumulative; as the dosage of radiation increases and/or the rate of delivery accelerates, the type and severity of oral complications increase.[10] Oral complications may become apparent as early as the first week of therapy and may continue for a few weeks or months after completion of therapy. The early changes are caused by alterations in cellular division and maturation. They particularly affect epithelial and glandular tissue in the form of mucositis, ulcerations, salivary gland dysfunction, alterations in taste, and dermatitis. Later complications usually are associated with tissues that have slower turnover rates, such as muscle or bone, and result in **trismus** or osteoradionecrosis. Salivary gland damage and vascular or osseous changes from irradiation usually are permanent. The walls of blood vessels thicken, and the lumens narrow, reducing blood flow and oxygenation in the tissues. Consequently, the healing capacity of the tissues or bone is impaired, leading to necrosis in response to trauma or infection.

Mucositis

Inflammation of the oral mucous membranes, with or without oral ulcerations, usually develops about the second week of radiation therapy, primarily on nonkeratinized tissues and the lateral borders of the tongue. Chemotherapy given in conjunction with irradiation can accelerate the onset and increase the severity of mucositis.[3,9,23,29,30,42] Because oral mucosal cells have a life span of only 10 to 14 days, the basal cell layer is destroyed faster than it can reproduce. Consequently, mucositis clinically manifests as edematous, erythematous tissue, followed in more severe cases by the formation of ulcerations and pseudomembranes. Mucositis usually is painful, and the involved mucosa frequently is sensitive to temperature extremes and pressure. A patient with dentures may not be able to tolerate wearing them. An unpleasant odor is common, caused by the sloughing necrotic tissue, bleeding, and plaque accumulation (Fig. 45-4). Breaks in the mucosal integrity caused by mucositis become portals of entry for infection, compromising the patient's overall health. Mucositis may become so severe that radiation therapy is suspended temporarily and the patient is hospitalized for pain and infection control and intravenous fluid and nutritional support.[12] Mucositis usually heals about 6 weeks after therapy is complete. The epithelium never fully recovers and tends to be thin and friable.

Management

Treatment of mucositis is primarily **palliative** Brushing with an ultrasoft toothbrush is recommended. Although tooth swabs or sponges do not remove plaque, they may

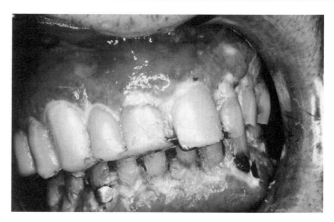

FIG. 45-4 Oral mucositis in a patient receiving radiation therapy for cancer of the head and neck. (Courtesy J.E. Bouquot, DDS, Morgantown, W.V.)

be used to apply rinsing agents to the teeth and sensitive oral tissues. Frequent rinsing with a baking soda solution, alone or with saline, throughout the day followed by a plain water rinse should make the patient more comfortable. Chlorhexidine rinsing reduces inflammation, particularly when mechanical plaque removal is hindered by the pain caused by mucositis. More recently, rinsing of the oral cavity with a povidone-iodine solution has shown some promise in the treatment of mucositis.[1] Commercial mouthwashes with high alcohol content should not be used because of their drying, irritating effects. Hydrogen peroxide should be limited to short-term use and diluted with water in a 1:4 concentration to prevent disruption of the normal flora.

Mucositis may make mastication, swallowing, and speaking painful. Topical anesthetic or antiinflammatory rinses, gels, or ointments such as Orabase or Clark's solution (equal parts diphenhydramine elixir, milk of magnesia, and viscous lidocaine) may be applied before eating or speaking to increase comfort. Systemic pain medications may also become necessary. A soft, bland diet that is low in citric acid and served at room temperature is advised. Alcoholic beverages and smoking must be avoided.

Xerostomia

Radiation may cause permanent damage to the salivary glands if they are in the field of treatment.* Changes occur in the volume of saliva produced and its consistency according to the dosage of radiation, the extent of gland involvement in the field, and the age of the patient. A 50% reduction in saliva may occur in the first week and may progress to a volume depletion of up to 90%. The saliva produced also is more acidic, which increases the risk of enamel demineralization and subsequent dental caries (Fig. 45-5). *Radiation caries* is a term used to describe the rampant caries activity that may result from the reduction in salivary volume and pH and the increase in cariogenic bacteria. Clinically, this form of caries manifests as a circumferential breakdown at the cervical margin of the

---

*References 3, 9, 23, 29, 30, 42.

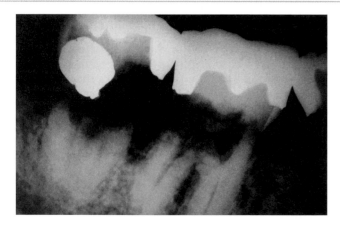

FIG. 45-5 Radiograph showing "radiation caries," the pattern of cervical decay that can develop in a patient with xerostomia that occurs secondary to irradiation of the salivary glands. (Courtesy J.E. Bouquot, DDS, Morgantown, W.V.)

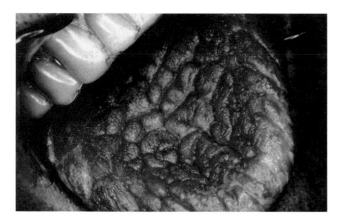

FIG. 45-6 Effects of severe radiation-induced xerostomia on the tongue and other oral soft tissues. (Courtesy J.E. Bouquot, DDS, Morgantown, W.V.)

teeth and may lead to tooth fracture at the gingival line in a matter of weeks or months (a finding consistent with the facts of the case study at the beginning of the chapter). The increased viscosity of the saliva reduces its self-cleansing ability, making the patient more susceptible to periodontal and candidal infections. Dry, friable mucosa may be prone to cracking and bleeding (Fig. 45-6). This creates a portal of entry for infection, which increases the risk of osteoradionecrosis. Denture wearers may not be able to tolerate their prostheses because of reduced surface tension between the dry mucosa and the denture. Oral dryness also can compromise eating, taste, swallowing, and speech.

Management
Strategies for managing xerostomia include oral pilocarpine therapy,[17,22] artificial salivas, sugarless chewing gum, frequent sips of water, ice chips, humidifiers, and a diet of moist foods. Caries, the dental sequela of xerostomia, is best managed by fluoride gel (1.1% neutral sodium fluoride or 0.4% stannous fluoride) applied daily in a custom tray, meticulous plaque control, and a diet low in su-

crose. In addition to fluoride, a calcium phosphate remineralizing gel may be applied with custom trays to manage early enamel breakdown in patients with severe xerostomia.

Infections

Candidiasis is the infection most often seen in patients with oral mucositis and hyposalivation.[3,23,42] These fungal lesions may be classified as pseudomembranous, erythematous, atrophic, or hyperplastic. The most frequently affected oral sites are the tongue, mucosa, and commissures of the lips. Bacterial, mycotic, and viral infections may also result, but these are more often associated with chemotherapy.

Management
Oral candidiasis can be treated effectively with topical antifungals such as nystatin or clotrimazole. Antifungal preparations containing sucrose should be avoided. In more extensive infections, ketoconazole, fluconazole, or amphotericin B may be indicated. The oral soft tissue should be examined frequently to assess for candidiasis. If a prosthesis is worn, it should be soaked in a disposable container with an antimicrobial solution such as chlorhexidine gluconate to prevent reinfection of the mouth.

Secondary infections caused by bacteria or viruses require proper diagnosis and subsequent treatment with organism-specific antibiotics and antivirals.

Dysgeusia

Loss of taste is believed to occur as a result of damage to the microvilli and outer taste cells of the tongue or as a side effect of xerostomia and mucositis.[23,30,42] Dysgeusia may be complete or partial, with bitter or acidic sensations most often affected first. Taste acuity for salt and sweet may be altered as therapy progresses. The symptoms usually appear within the first week of therapy, and the condition resolves 2 to 4 months after radiation is complete, if saliva is adequate. Often *dysgeusia* leads to a loss of appetite.

Management
Food aversions often develop with alterations in taste and smell. Patient education regarding dietary and preparation alternatives and meal planning suggestions are helpful strategies for promoting proper nutrition and minimizing the risks associated with a poor diet. Dietary supplements of zinc have been prescribed to manage chronic taste loss.[36]

Dysphasia

Difficulty swallowing is not uncommon in patients who have received radiation to the head and neck. Videofluoroscopy has revealed prolonged pharyngeal transit times in postirradiation patients.[31] Dysphasia is further complicated by xerostomia and results in eating and speaking difficulties.

Management
Taking small bites of food, eating a soft to semisoft diet, and taking frequent sips of liquids while eating can enhance swallowing.

Nutritional Deficiency

Xerostomia, mucositis, dysgeusia, and dysphasia trigger eating difficulties. Regardless of whether a loss of appetite is caused by a sore mouth or a lack of desire, poor nutritional intake can lead to fatigue, dehydration, and compromised healing.

Management

Nutritional liquid supplements are an ideal means of boosting calories in a patient who for any reason is not eating. Unfortunately, they contain sucrose, and caries assessments should be made frequently. Foods that are easy to chew and swallow include cooked cereals, eggs, mashed potatoes, noodles, pureed meats, fruits and vegetables, milkshakes and puddings, gelatins, ice cream, sherbet, and sorbet.

Osteoradionecrosis

The bone and soft tissue in the field of radiation may become necrotic because irradiation has made it hypovascular, hypocellular, and hypoxic.* The result is a change in the growth and repair potential of the bone and a diminished resistance to infection. Insults in the form of trauma (e.g., extraction or an ill-fitting appliance) or infection (e.g., periodontal disease or a dental abscess) may lead to the development of osteoradionecrosis (ORN). In response to trauma or infection, alveolar destruction may be progressive and extensive. Denture wearers often are advised to leave their prostheses out from the initiation of therapy to 6 months after completion to reduce the risk of ORN. Blood vessels in the periodontium and periosteum are similarly affected, resulting in a widening of the periodontal ligament space.

Symptoms may manifest shortly after radiation therapy or may take years to develop. Osteoradionecrosis has been reported to occur as late as 25 years after radiation therapy. The mandible is more susceptible to ORN because it is denser and less vascular than the maxilla and consequently absorbs more radiation. Patients undergoing radiation doses above 7000 cGy also are at greater risk. As in the case study presented earlier, the greatest risk is to the patient whose mandible has received extensive irradiation and who requires tooth extractions sometime after completion of radiation therapy.

Management

The key to reducing the risk of ORN is prevention. Before radiotherapy begins, a thorough assessment of the hard and soft oral tissues must be made to determine any possible risks of infection or trauma. All hopeless and questionable teeth (e.g., furcation involved; advanced periodontitis; impacted, nonrestorable implants with an uncertain prognosis; root fragments; and any potential soft tissue or bony pathologic condition) should be removed. If extractions are indicated, a minimum a 14 days is required for primary closure of the socket before initiating radiotherapy. Periodontal care and restorations must be completed. A dentulous patient must practice meticulous oral hygiene before, during, and after radiotherapy.

Daily fluoride gel applications using smooth, well-fitting custom fluoride trays are essential throughout the patient's life. Frequent supportive care to eliminate any sources of trauma or infection must be established. New prostheses may need to be fabricated after therapy to ensure smooth edges and a comfortable fit.

Treatment of ORN requires conservative measures to promote healing. A series of hyperbaric oxygen treatments to flood the tissue with oxygen is recommended before any invasive procedure on irradiated tissues. Advanced cases may involve extended antibiotic therapy and surgery for the removal of bony sequestra or a portion of the mandible.

Trismus

Trismus results from fibrosis of the muscles of mastication or the temporomandibular joint when these muscles are in the field of irradiation.[9,23,42] Patients with nasopharyngeal, maxillary sinus, and palatal tumors often develop trismus (as was suspected in the case study). The usual onset of trismus is 3 to 6 months after completion of radiation therapy. Opening the mouth is difficult and often painful.

Management

A mouth block should be placed between the beam and the patient during irradiation to prevent scatter radiation to the muscles of the face. The patient should perform exercises designed to maintain or improve oral range of motion daily. Isometric exercises involve the use of opposing finger pressure on the incisal edges of the mandibular anterior teeth as the patient tries to open the mouth or opening against gentle pressure exerted by placing the fist against the midline of the mandible. Ten repetitions of finger pressure for 30 seconds five to six times daily is advised. The patient also can be given the maximum number of tongue blades that will comfortably stack between the maxillary and mandibular anterior teeth. One additional blade is then slid between the others to stretch the oral opening. Mechanical stretching devices also are available.

Developmental Anomalies

The extent of damage to the developing dentition depends on the total and fractional dose of radiation received and the stage of tooth development at the time of exposure. Irradiation of the developing dentition and facial bones with doses as low as 400 cGy may result in hypocalcification, enamel hypoplasia, delayed or arrested tooth development, premature closure of root apices, microdontia, complete or partial anodontia, micrognathia, retrognathia, and skeletal and dental malocclusion.[6,19,24]

Management

Parents must be alerted to the possible anomalies that may arise when their children receive radiation therapy to the head and neck. Long-term dental follow-up is necessary, and dental professionals should be diligent in observing and rehabilitating the dentition before, during, and after radiotherapy. Before radiotherapy, mobile teeth should be extracted, and gingival opercula and orthodontic bands should be removed if they pose a risk of food entrapment, trauma, or infection. Often several dental specialists are required to restore the dentition. The im-

---

*References 3, 9, 10, 23, 29, 30, 42.

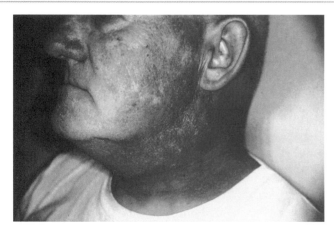

FIG. 45-7 Skin erythema from exposure to therapeutic doses of radiation. (Courtesy J.E. Bouquot, DDS, Morgantown, W.V.)

portance of supervised, meticulous oral hygiene home care cannot be overemphasized. Fluoride therapy must be monitored carefully to prevent fluorosis. Psychosocial issues related to facial deformity and delayed eruption or missing teeth should not be discounted.

Skin Erythema

The skin of the face and neck in the field of irradiation develop erythema as early as the second week of radiotherapy (Fig. 45-7).[8] The skin becomes red, as if sunburned. Desquamation of the skin can occur, causing a breakdown of skin integrity and creating a portal of entry for infection. Radiation treatments may be postponed to allow for healing. In some cases facial hair is lost.

Management

Patients should be instructed to shield the irradiated field from sunlight and ultraviolet rays and not to use soaps or lotions in the area, because they can contribute to necrosis of the skin. The treated area of the face and neck should not be exposed to temperature extremes of hot and cold; this includes heating pads and ice packs.

ORAL CARE PROTOCOL

Each phase of radiation therapy—before treatment, during treatment, and after treatment—must be considered individually.*

TREATMENT BEFORE RADIOTHERAPY

Before radiotherapy begins, the following oral care regimen should be completed:
1. Evaluation of the patient's physical and mental status and the condition of the teeth and associated tissues, including the following:
   a. Panoramic and periapical radiographs as indicated
   b. Intraoral photographs

*References 3, 6, 9, 16, 19, 24, 29, 30, 43.

   c. Palpation of the soft tissues intraorally and extraorally
   d. Visual examination of the teeth and mucosa:
      1) Dental charting (caries, restorations, missing and unerupted teeth, and vitality)
      2) Periodontal charting (probing depths, recession, bleeding index, furcation involvement, description of gingival color and texture, calculus and plaque indices, and amount and consistency of saliva)
   e. Patient's oral health knowledge and motivation
   f. Mouth opening
2. Removal of all hopeless and questionable teeth (see earlier section on osteoradionecrosis)
   Bone contouring, antibiotic coverage (if warranted), and complete surface coverage with soft tissue
3. Denture evaluation, if applicable, and correction of any areas causing irritation
4. Periodontal debridement and selective polishing
5. Restorative dental procedures
6. Oral hygiene education and motivation program:
   a. Tooth brushing, interdental cleaning, and rinses (e.g., antimicrobial rinses and saliva substitutes)
   b. Fabrication of custom fluoride trays and initiation of fluoride gel applications or any patient-applied fluoride agents that ensure compliance
   c. Discussion of possible oral complications and their management
7. Nutritional counseling (diet modifications, elimination of alcoholic beverages and tobacco use)

TREATMENT DURING RADIOTHERAPY

Treatment during the course of radiotherapy includes the following measures:
1. Oral examination and oral hygiene follow-up weekly
2. Prevention and management of oral complications (e.g., daily fluoride applications for xerostomia-induced caries, oral rinses for mucositis, exercises for trismus, removal of dentures to prevent trauma, and drug therapy for infection and pain control)
3. Meal planning, management of dietary concerns or tube feeding issues as applicable
4. Avoidance of invasive procedures (to prevent osteoradionecrosis). For emergencies:
   Antibiotic coverage, hyperbaric oxygen (HBO) therapy to ensure healing, and consideration of more conservative alternatives, such as endodontic therapy

TREATMENT AFTER RADIOTHERAPY

Treatment after radiotherapy consists of the following regimen.
1. Frequent dental examinations coordinated with **oncology** follow-up visits
2. Continuation of meticulous oral hygiene practices
3. Treatment of additional or remaining side effects of irradiation
4. Monitoring of salivary flow and assessment of compliance with fluoride regimen and dietary changes
5. Restorative and prophylactic dental procedures as needed
6. Evaluation of the need for new dentures if applicable
7. Extractions and other surgical procedures, performed with caution (e.g., using HBO and antibiotics)

CRITICAL THINKING ACTIVITIES

1. Perform an oral examination on a patient with cancer of the head and neck area.
2. Visit a hospital radiation therapy department and observe the administration of radiation therapy to a patient with a carcinoma of the head and neck.
3. Perform oral debridement and a polishing procedure on a patient undergoing radiation therapy for a cancer of the head and neck.
4. Observe the oral complications associated with radiation therapy and provide appropriate palliative instructions for managing each of these side effects.
5. Attend a maxillofacial surgical procedure for treatment of a head and neck cancer.
6. Visit a maxillofacial prosthodontist to observe the fabrication of various prostheses used in the management of facial deformities associated with head and neck cancer.
7. Fabricate custom fluoride mouth trays for a patient with radiation-induced xerostomia.

REVIEW QUESTIONS

Questions 2 and 5 refer to the case study presented at the beginning of the chapter.

1. Which of the following is the life span of oral mucosal cells?
   a. 3 to 5 Days
   b. 5 to 10 Days
   c. 10 to 14 Days
   d. 15 to 21 Days
2. Mr. Fitzgibbons is at greatest risk for which of the following side effects of radiation therapy?
   a. Trismus
   b. Mucositis
   c. Osteoradionecrosis
   d. Bleeding
   e. Dysgeusia
3. The risk factor referred to in question #2 would be managed best by administration of which of the following?
   a. Artificial saliva
   b. Hyperbaric oxygen
   c. Chlorhexidine rinse
   d. Zinc supplements
   e. Topical thrombin

4. Which of the following forms of fluoride is not recommended for daily application?
   a. 1.23% Acidulated phosphate fluoride
   b. 0.4% Stannous fluoride
   c. 1.1% Neutral sodium fluoride
   d. None of the above
5. Mr. Fitzgibbons has which of the following stages of carcinoma?
   a. I
   b. II
   c. III
   d. IV
6. Which of the following organs is the least radiosensitive?
   a. Oral cavity
   b. Salivary glands
   c. Bone marrow
   d. Brain

SUGGESTED AGENCIES AND WEB SITES

Because of the ever-changing nature of the Internet, some of the web sites listed here may have changed since publication. Please refer to Mosby's Evolve web site for the most current information.

American Cancer Society: http://www.cancer.org
Cancer Research Foundation of America:
   http://www.preventcancer.org
Medline Plus Health Information: http://www.nlm.nih.gov

National Cancer Institute:
   http://www.graylab.ac.uk/cancernet
Radiation Therapy-Oral Management:
   http://www.dent.ohio-state.edu

ADDITIONAL READINGS AND RESOURCES

Epstein JB et al: Surgical periodontal treatment in the radiotherapy-treated head and neck cancer patient, *Spec Care Dent* 14:182-7, 1994.

Meraw SJ, Reeve CM: Dental considerations and treatment of the oncology patient receiving radiation therapy, *J Am Dent Assoc* 129:201-5, 1998.

Wang RR, Pillai K, Jones PK: In vitro backscattering from implant materials during radiotherapy, *J Prosthet Dent* 75:626-32, 1996.

Whitmeyer CC, Esposito SJ, Terezhalmy GT: Radiotherapy for head and neck neoplasms, *Gen Dent* 45:363-70, 1997.

REFERENCES

1. Adamietz IA et al: Prophylaxis with povidone-iodine against inducing mucositis by radiochemotherapy, *Support Care Cancer* 6:373-7, 1998.
2. Bansberg SF, Olsen KD, Gaffey TA: High grade carcinoma of the oral cavity, *Arch Otolaryngol Head Neck Surg* 100:41-8, 1989.
3. Barker GJ, Barker BF, Gier RE: *Oral management of the cancer patient: a guide for the health care professional,* Kansas City, Mo, 1996, Biomedical Communications.
4. Browman GP et al: Influence of cigarette smoking on the efficacy of radiation therapy in head and neck cancer, *N Engl J Med* 328:159-63, 1993.
5. Bushong SC: *Radiologic science for technologists,* ed 4, St Louis, 1988, Mosby.
6. Chin EA, Hopkins KP, Bowman LC: A brief overview of oral complications in pediatric oncology patients and suggested management strategies, *J Dent Child* 6: 468-73, 1998.
7. Day GL, Blot WJ: Second primary tumors in patients with oral cancer, *Cancer* 70:14-9, 1992.
8. DeBiase CB: *Dental health education: theory and practice,* Philadelphia, 1991, Lea & Febiger.
9. DeBiase CB: The patient with cancer. In Wilkins EM, editor: *Clinical practice of the dental hygienist,* ed 8, Philadelphia, 1999, Lippincott Williams & Wilkins.
10. Epstein JB et al: Surgical periodontal treatment in the radiotherapy-treated head and neck cancer patient, *Spec Care Dent* 14:182-7, 1994.
11. Epstein JB, Scully C: Assessing the patient at risk for oral squamous cell carcinoma, *Spec Care Dent* 17:120-8, 1997.
12. Epstein JB, Van der Meij EH: Complicating mucosal reactions in patients receiving radiation therapy for head and neck cancer, *Spec Care Dent* 17:88-93, 1997.
13. Friedlander AH et al: Detection of radiation-induced accelerated atherosclerosis in patients with osteoradionecrosis by panoramic radiography, *J Maxillofacial Surg* 56:455-9, 1998.
14. Garewall HS: Beta-carotene and vitamin E oral cancer prevention, *J Cell Biochem Suppl* 17(suppl F):262-9, 1993.
15. Hong WK et al: Prevention of second primary tumors with isotretinoin in squamous cell carcinoma of the head and neck, *N Engl J Med* 323:795-801, 1990.
16. Jansma J, Vissink A, Spijkervet FKL: Protocol for the prevention and treatment of sequelae resulting from head and neck radiation therapy, *Cancer* 70:2171-80, 1992.
17. Johnson JT et al: Oral pilocarpine for postirradiation xerostomia in patients with head and neck cancer, *N Engl J Med* 329:390-5,1993.
18. Jones KR et al: Prognostic factors in the recurrence of stage I and II squamous cell cancer of the oral cavity, *Arch Otolaryngol Head Neck Surg* 118:483-5, 1992.
19. Kaste SC, Hopkins KP, Bowman LC: Dental abnormalities in long-term survivors of head and neck rhabdomyosarcoma, *Med Pediatr Oncol* 25:96-101, 1995.
20. Kelloff GJ et al: Progress in applied chemoprevention research, *Semin Oncol* 17:438-455, 1990.
21. Landis SH et al: Cancer statistics, *CA Can J Clin* 51(1):15-36, 2001.
22. LeVeque FG et al: A multicenter, randomized, double-blind, placebo-controlled, dose-titration study of pilocarpine for the treatment of radiation-induced xerostomia in head and neck cancer patients, *J Clin Oncol* 11:1124-31, 1993.
23. Little JW et al: *Dental management of the medically compromised patient,* ed 6, St Louis, (in press), Mosby.
24. Maguire A et al: The long-term effect of treatment on the dental condition of children surviving malignant disease, *Cancer Nurs* 25:70-5, 1987.
25. Mashberg A, Feldman LJ: Clinical criteria for identifying early oral and oropharyngeal carcinoma: erythroplasia revisited, *Am J Surg* 156:273-5, 1988.
26. Mashberg A, Samit A: Early diagnosis of asymptomatic oral and oropharyngeal squamous cancers, *CA Can J Clin* 45:328-351, 1995.
27. Miller BF, Keane CB: *Encyclopedia and dictionary of medicine, nursing, and allied health,* ed 6, Philadelphia, 1997, WB Saunders.
28. Millon RR, Cassisi NJ, editors: *Management of head and neck cancer: a multidisciplinary approach,* St Louis, 1986, Mosby.
29. National Institutes of Health Consensus Development Conference Statements: Oral complications of cancer therapies: diagnosis, prevention, and treatment, *NCI Monogr* 9:3-8, 1990.
30. Peterson DE, D'Ambrosio JA: Nonsurgical management of head and neck cancer patients, *Dent Clin North Am* 38: 425-445, 1994.
31. Rhodus NL, Moller K: Dysphagia in postirradiation therapy head and neck cancer patients, *J Cancer Res Ther Control* 4:49-55, 1994.
32. Rothman K, Keller A: The effect of joint exposure to alcohol and tobacco on risk of cancer of the mouth and pharynx, *J Chron Dis* 25:711-6, 1972.
33. Rubin P, Constantine L, Nelson D: Late effects of cancer treatment: radiation and drug toxicity. In Perez C, Brady LW, editors: *Principles and practice of radiation oncology,* Philadelphia, 1992, JB Lippincott.
34. Shafer WG, Hine MK, Levy BM: *A textbook of oral pathology,* ed 4, Philadelphia, 1983, WB Saunders.
35. Shah JP, Lydiatt W: Treatment of cancer of the head and neck, *CA Can J Clin* 45:352-368, 1995.
36. Silverman S, editor: *Oral cancer,* ed 2, New York, 1985, American Cancer Society.
37. Spiro RH et al: Cervical node metastasis from epidermoid carcinoma of the oral cavity and oropharynx: a critical assessment of current staging, *Am J Surg* 128:562-7, 1974.
38. Takagi M et al: Causes of oral tongue cancer treatment failures: analysis of autopsy cases, *Cancer* 69:1081-7, 1992.
39. United States Department of Health, Education, and Welfare: Management guidelines for head and neck cancer, PHS pub no 80-2037, Washington, DC, 1979, The Department.
40. Wallner PE et al: Patterns of care study: analysis of outcome survey data: anterior two-thirds of the tongue and floor of the mouth, *Am J Clin Oncol* 9:50-7, 1986.
41. Wang CC, editor: *Radiation therapy for head and neck neoplasms: indications, techniques and results,* ed 2, Littleton, Mass, 1990, John Wright-PSG.
42. Whitmeyer CC, Waskowski JC, Iffland HA: Radiotherapy and oral sequelae: prevention and management protocols, *J Dent Hyg* 71:23-9, 1997.
43. Wright WE: Pretreatment oral health care interventions for radiation patients, *NCI Monogr* 9:57-9, 1990.

PART X

Chapter 46
Evaluation and Supportive Care

Chapter 47
Case Development, Documentation, and Presentation

Competency Statements

The learner is expected to possess knowledge, skills, judgments, values, and attitudes to develop the listed competencies.

Core Competencies
- Apply a professional code of ethics in all endeavors.
- Adhere to state and federal laws, recommendations, and regulations in the provision of dental hygiene care.
- Provide dental hygiene care to promote patient health and wellness using critical thinking and problem solving in the provision of evidence-based practice.
- Use evidence-based decision making to evaluate and incorporate emerging treatment modalities.
- Assume responsibility for dental hygiene actions and care based on accepted scientific theories and research as well as the accepted standard of care.
- Continuously perform self-assessment for life-long learning and professional growth.
- Promote the profession through service activities and affiliations with professional organizations.
- Provide quality assurance mechanisms for health services.
- Communicate effectively with individuals and groups from diverse populations both verbally and in writing.
- Provide accurate, consistent, and complete documentation for assessment, diagnosis, planning, implementation, and evaluation of dental hygiene services.
- Provide care to all patients using an individualized approach that is humane, empathetic, and caring.

Health Promotion and Disease Prevention
- Promote the values of oral and general health and wellness to the public and organizations within and outside the profession.

Courtesy American Dental Education Association, Washington, DC.

Evaluation of Care

- Respect the goals, values, beliefs, and preferences of the patient while promoting optimal oral and general health.
- Refer patients who may have a physiologic, psychological, and/or social problem to other healthcare providers for comprehensive patient evaluation.
- Identify individual and population risk factors and develop strategies that promote health related quality of life.
- Evaluate factors that can be used to promote patient adherence to disease prevention and/or health maintenance strategies.
- Evaluate and utilize methods to ensure the health and safety of the patient and the dental hygienist in the delivery of dental hygiene.

Community Involvement

- Provide screening, referral, and educational services that allow clients to access the resources of the healthcare system.
- Provide community oral health services in a variety of settings.
- Facilitate client access to oral health services by influencing individuals and/or organizations for the provision of oral healthcare.

Patient Care

- Select, obtain, and interpret diagnostic information recognizing its advantages and limitations.
- Recognize predisposing and etiologic risk factors that require intervention to prevent disease.
- Obtain, review, and update a complete medical, family, social, and dental history.
- Recognize health conditions and medications that impact overall patient care.
- Identify patients at risk for a medical emergency and manage the patient care in a manner that prevents an emergency.

- Perform a comprehensive examination using clinical, radiographic, periodontal, dental charting, and other data collection procedures to assess the patient's needs.
- Determine a dental hygiene diagnosis.
- Identify patient needs and significant findings that impact the delivery of dental hygiene services.
- Obtain consultations as indicated.
- Prioritize the care plan based on the health status and the actual and potential problems of the individual to facilitate optimal oral health.
- Establish a planned sequence of care (educational, clinical, and evaluation) based on the dental hygiene diagnosis; identified oral conditions; potential problems; etiologic and risk factors; and available treatment modalities.
- Establish a collaborative relationship with the patient in the planned care to include etiology, prognosis, and treatment alternatives.
- Make referrals to other healthcare professionals.
- Perform dental hygiene interventions to eliminate and/or control local etiologic factors to prevent and control caries, periodontal disease, and other oral conditions.
- Determine the outcomes of dental hygiene interventions using indices, instruments, examination techniques, and patient self-report.
- Evaluate the patient's satisfaction with the oral healthcare received and the oral healthcare status achieved.
- Provide subsequent treatment or referrals based on evaluation findings.
- Develop and maintain a health maintenance program.

Professional Growth and Development

- Access professional and social networks and resources to assist entrepreneurial initiatives.

CHAPTER 46

Evaluation and Supportive Care

Katharine R. Stilley

Chapter Outline

Case Study: Evaluating Periodontal Outcomes
Risk Assessment
    Attachment loss
    Age
    Tobacco use
    Abnormal tooth mobility
    Other factors
Rationale for Supportive Care
Patient Compliance
Evaluation of Initial Therapy
Supportive Care Intervals for Periodontal Patients
Review of Patient Record
Elements of the Periodontal Supportive Care
  Appointment
    Review of patient record
    Update of health history
    Subjective assessment: comments, observations,
        or concerns

Extraoral and intraoral examinations
Hard tissue examination
Periodontal examination
Professional's review of personal care,
    behaviors, and attitudes
Debridement as necessary
Deplaquing and polishing as necessary
Scheduling of subsequent periodontal
    supportive care appointments
Responsibility for Periodontal Supportive Care
  Appointments
Supportive Care for Dental Caries and Other
  Chronic Oral Conditions
    Dental caries
    Other chronic oral conditions

Key Terms

Active periodontal
    therapy
Adherence
Compliance

Full-mouth disinfection
Intervals
Periodontal maintenance
    (PM)

Supportive care
Supportive periodontal
    care (SPC)

Supportive periodontal therapy
    (SPT)
Therapeutic alliance

 ## Learning Outcomes

1. Identify patients with oral health risks and problems requiring close intervals for supportive care.
2. Recognize symptoms or conditions that indicate referral and discuss them with the patient.
3. Plan a supportive care program based on the patient's disease control skills and the risk of disease recurrence.

4. Identify successful or reasonable outcomes, which may vary from patient to patient.
5. Document everything.
6. Evaluate current literature on the topic of periodic supportive care intervals.

Case Study

Evaluating Periodontal Outcomes

Mrs. Lucy Lightfoot, age 62, who is one-quarter Native American, completed active periodontal treatment 9 months ago. Mrs. Lightfoot is taking Tolinase (tolazamide) for non–insulin-dependent diabetes mellitus (NIDDM), as well as a diuretic and a calcium channel blocker to control her blood pressure. She is experiencing some osteoarthritis, for which she takes over-the-counter (OTC) naproxen as needed. Mrs. Lightfoot alternates her professional oral care every 3 months between the periodontal and the general dental offices. This is her third 3-month periodontal supportive care visit but the first time you have seen her. She has been faithful in keeping her 3-month **periodontal maintenance (PM)** appointments but appears to be indifferent to the procedures performed during the appointment.

During the periodontal assessment, you notice that the bleeding index has gradually increased; it now is 25%, and you think her plaque control could be improved. Her recession has not increased, but she has five deeper probe measurements, 5 mm in two marginal and three interproximal sites.

As you prepare to ask the receptionist to make Mrs. Lightfoot's next appointment with the periodontist, she informs you that she will be traveling at that time and cannot keep the appointment.

---

*I*mplicit in the title of this chapter is the concept that patients with a persistent problem or chronic disease should receive professional care at regular **intervals.** The most familiar example of regular professional supervision to control and mitigate chronic disease in dentistry is the common 3-month appointment intervals of individuals who have had active, nonsurgical or surgical periodontal therapy. *Active periodontal therapy* includes debridement to reduce initial infection and/or surgical correction of bony and gingival defects. Periodontal supportive care focuses on individuals prone to periodontal diseases. Supportive care is also important for patients with a high caries rate or other less common problems that require closer professional supervision.

The terminology for regular, periodic supervision of individuals with periodontal disease has gone through several transitions. For procedures done after completion of active therapy, the terms *maintenance, therapy, care, recare, recall,* and *treatment* are all found in the literature. In 1989 the Worldwide Workshop in Periodontics adopted the term *supportive periodontal treatment* (SPT) and defined it as the periodic care intervals for periodontal patients.[26] In January 2000 the Board of Trustees of the American Academy of Periodontology approved the term *periodontal maintenance* (PM) to replace **supportive periodontal therapy (SPT).**[7]

In Europe the term **supportive periodontal care (SPC)** refers to three levels of care: preventive, posttreatment, and palliative.[14] The three levels of assessment for periodontal patients are the patient (or systemic level), the tooth, and the site at risk. In this chapter, *periodontal maintenance* refers to the supportive periodontal care for an in-

dividual at risk for various periodontal problems. Supportive care for other chronic oral problems that benefit from regular professional intervention also is discussed.

RISK ASSESSMENT

An individual who has had an infection or disease usually **46-A** is considered at risk for recurrence unless the initial infection was one that could have resulted in immunity. When immunity is conferred, the disease is not chronic, and the patient is then considered *protected* from future disease. However, the most common oral infections (e.g., periodontal diseases, caries, herpetic outbreaks, and certain oral mucosal lesions) are chronic conditions. Therefore a person who has lost clinical attachment, has had carious lesions in the past year, or has had a herpetic lesion ("cold sore,") is at greater risk for future disease than a person who has never had a attachment loss, caries, or an herpetic lesion.

Four important factors can help identify patients at risk for periodontal disease: (1) attachment loss, (2) age, (3) tobacco use, and (4) abnormal tooth mobility.[15]

ATTACHMENT LOSS

Patients at risk for periodontal disease are those who have lost 2 mm or more of periodontal attachment. Although no test or index has been accepted as predictive of attachment loss, the correlation has been shown. (See Chapter 15 for calculation of attachment loss.)

AGE

Older adults (over age 70) may require more intensive supportive periodontal therapy.[19] A decline in general health, increasing cognitive and physical impairments, and an increase in the number of medications taken may impair an older adult's ability for oral self-care.

TOBACCO USE

The oral effects of tobacco use vary. Localized tissue changes are obvious when tobacco is held in direct contact with mucosal and gingival tissues. Smoking is a well-documented risk for periodontal problems. The consequences of smoking include changes in the gingival crevicular fluid and oral microbiology and adverse effects on blood vessels, connective tissue, and the immune response.[6]

ABNORMAL TOOTH MOBILITY

Physiological mobility of 1 mm or less is normal. Teeth affected by periodontal disease, however, are significantly more mobile. Pathologically mobile teeth place stress on a weakened periodontium and may be treated with corrective restorative procedures, orthodontics, periodontal procedures, or all of these.

OTHER FACTORS

Patients who cannot perform oral self-care or who have systemic medical conditions that influence oral health are at greater risk for recurrence of disease.

RATIONALE FOR SUPPORTIVE CARE

Periodic monitoring of a periodontal patient with a chronic condition is important (1) to help the patient achieve a stable dental condition and sometimes even attain a higher level of health; (2) to extend periods of disease remission; and (3) to lessen the extent and severity of acute, episodic flair-ups. For patients susceptible to chronic infections, personal efforts at disease control, alone, are difficult and often inadequate for achieving continued remission.

Bleeding on probing, deeper probe depths, increasing attachment loss, and increasing tooth mobility are clinical indicators that some form of periodontal disease is currently active. These same clinical indicators are the criteria for failure.[5] The goals of periodontal maintenance are to eliminate and prevent or, with some patients, to reduce these negative outcomes. The need for continuing professional care and monitoring to identify signs of the progression or recurrence of disease is part of the supportive care cycle (Fig. 46-1).

Supportive care is recommended to periodontal patients for several reasons, as follows:[3]

- The outcome of periodontal therapy needs to be monitored at frequent intervals because the patient has demonstrated a predilection for periodontal breakdown.
- Periodontal supportive care is also an option for patients who are not candidates for periodontal surgery.[17]
- Surgery may not be possible for patients with general health problems (e.g., poorly controlled diabetes mellitus or immunosuppression) or for adult patients in active orthodontics due to the instability of the periodontal fibers.
- Teeth with a poor surgical prognosis may be improved by periodontal maintenance.
- Some patients may not be able to achieve sufficient plaque control unless they receive more frequent supportive periodontal care.
- A patient may simply refuse surgical correction or augmentation but may agree to supportive periodontal care.
- Reducing the oral bacteria and maintaining a healthy mouth can reduce stress on the immune system in general.[1]

Supportive periodontal care should provide the following:[22]

- Plaque control assistance and stability of the healthy periodontium
- Protection from adverse effects on the periodontium related to systemic conditions
- Lessening of suspected deleterious effects of periodontopathogenic microbes systemically, with particular attention to the possible relationships between periodontal disease and stroke, heart attack, low–birth-weight babies, and diabetes mellitus.

Reevaluation of a patient's periodontal status by the oral healthcare provider at regular intervals is evidenced-based practice. Dental research has shown that the combination of daily personal plaque control efforts and frequent professional care produces the most stable periodontal health.[2] Individuals who receive regular, professional periodontal supportive care have less gingivitis, loss of attachment, and tooth loss compared with individuals who do not receive periodic supportive periodontal care. The shortened intervals of care and the specific periodontal procedures are based on patients who have demonstrated a risk of periodontal disease.[16]

PATIENT COMPLIANCE

One critical factor in the control of chronic infections is patient *compliance.* Haynes[8] defines compliance as "the extent to which a person's behavior coincides with medical or health advice." The terms **adherence** and **therapeutic alliance** are also used to describe the congruence between medical advice and individual behavior.[21] Patient compliance in periodontal disease or caries control is twofold: (1) diligence with daily oral self-care and (2) attendance (showing up) at the dental office for regular professional monitoring of the oral health status.

It is important to impress upon each patient his or her role in oral disease control and that attaining periodontal health requires a daily, lifetime commitment (Box 46-1). It is especially important to stress patient involvement in oral health maintenance from the first appointment through the final phases of periodontal therapy, including each supportive periodontal care appointment. Patients should demonstrate their involvement by learning and practicing oral care techniques, by understanding the purpose and anticipated outcomes of periodontal care, and by learning how to evaluate the health of their own mouths. Currently the single best criterion for patients to use in evaluating their periodontal stability is the absence of bleeding.

Many reasons have been suggested to explain why the average patient with a chronic disease is not particularly

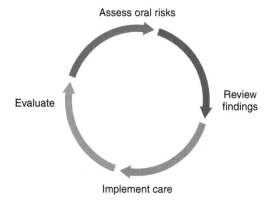

FIG. 46-1 Cyclical nature of supportive care.

BOX 46-1

Suggestions for Improving Patient Compliance

1. Set goals *with* the patient, not for the patient.
2. Write down what you say and what the patient agrees to, possibly using the patient's signature to reinforce the importance of the goals and the patient's understanding of them.
3. Simplify self-care as much as possible.
4. Use positive reinforcement.
5. Involve the entire office in encouraging the patient.
6. Discuss noncompliance with patient and seek remedies.
7. Use appointment reminders.

compliant (Box 46-2). For example, after active therapy, surgery, or emergency treatment, patients often consider themselves healed, or at least improved, and often attribute the change to "seeing the doctor" or to the care the therapist provided. It is incumbent upon the healthcare professional, and in dentistry most often the dental hygienist, to help patients recognize their daily role in maintaining oral health. This is probably the most challenging role in oral care—to impress on patients with chronic disease that they must take responsibility for daily self-care. Patients with periodontal or chronic oral diseases find it difficult to make the adjustments required to perform more frequent and often dexterity-challenging self-care procedures that require more time and special materials or equipment. Often family and friends fail to support the extra time, money, and commitment.

Another impediment to patients with chronic disease is that they may not feel bad when they are symptom-free. Periodontal disease is typically painless. During active periodontal therapy the dental hygienist must stress that healthy tissues do not bleed. The supportive care patient will come to understand that bleeding is a sign of disease. Absence of bleeding is one of the best clinical signs for the patient, whereas the dental hygienist looks for stability of the clinical attachment. When the signs of gingival bleeding cease, patients may become lax in following a demanding oral self-care program.

An attentive, caring, and competent dental hygienist is essential in helping the patient to fight a chronic disease because these patients are particularly vulnerable to discouragement and discomfort. Encouragement, support, external motivation, and advice are part of the dental hygienist's responsibility in patient relations and are essential components of each supportive care appointment.

EVALUATION OF INITIAL THERAPY

When active disease has been reduced, whether through a series of quadrant debridements with anesthesia or through *full-mouth disinfection* (a procedure completed within 24 hours), the results must be evaluated (Box 46-3). The interval for this evaluation usually is 4 to 6 weeks after initial therapy, which is differentiated from the less frequent (typically 3 months) supportive care interval. Tissue response and the patient's personal care effectiveness

are the parameters of evaluation. The response to the initial debridement dictates the choice of further treatment options, which include debridement in areas of continued infection; consideration of antimicrobial use; a 3-month interval of supportive periodontal care; and/or surgical correction of periodontal defects. It has been recommended that surgery not be considered until at least 3 months after the initial debridement. When inflammation and bleeding on probing are absent, the patient typically is placed on a supportive care interval appropriate for the level and type of disease.

When areas of infection persist (i.e., erythema, bleeding, exudate, or no decrease in probe depth), several etiological possibilities can be considered. Minute areas of undisturbed plaque or calculus may be present, which the clinician can redebride where needed. The patient may not have mastered plaque control sufficiently to maintain gingival health; furthermore, conditions in the mouth, such as deep periodontal pockets, misaligned teeth, or poorly contoured margins, may thwart the patient's plaque control efforts. Listening to the patient and watching him or her demonstrate the plaque control techniques used at home are important keys to determining why the patient is not achieving the desired level of plaque control. The clinician must continue to encourage and work with the patient to detect the problems in accessing plaque. Some of these problems may be improved only through surgery, or an underlying systemic problem may be retarding gingival healing. If systemic factors are suspected, the patient should be further evaluated by a physician. When gingival health has improved, the patient might be recommended for periodontal surgery, or the individual may be placed on one 3-month interval to allow for maximum tissue improvement before evaluation for surgery.

Due to either anatomical factors associated with periodontal disease and/or patient compliance, plaque control measures may not be as complete; therefore the hygienist will need to deplaque where the patient has not adequately

---

BOX 46-2

Factors Contributing to Poor Patient Compliance

Symptoms disappear.

Patient feels better.

Self-care regimen is inconvenient, demanding, or too difficult.

Patient is not convinced of the value and efficacy of recommended self-care routines and treatment.

Periodontal maintenance visits are too frequent, too expensive, or too uncomfortable.

Patient is unsure whether periodontist or generalist will handle the periodontal maintenance visit.

Patient exhibits general discouragement (common with chronic conditions).

BOX 46-3

Procedure for Evaluation of Initial or Presurgical Periodontal Debridement*

Review the patient's record.

Greet the patient.

Update the patient's health history.

Obtain the patient's evaluation of the success of the treatment and discuss any problems or complaints.

Recheck any previously identified extraoral and intraoral irregularities that might affect the course of the appointment.

Evaluate the gingival response.

Check the patient's oral hygiene status (level of plaque control, reaccumulation of calculus, presence of stain from chlorhexidine or tobacco).

Observe, adjust, and encourage the patient's plaque control skill if disease is still present.

Debride and polish as necessary.

Assist with determination of referral for surgical therapy or preventive maintenance.

*This evaluation usually is performed 4 to 6 weeks after the debridement procedure.

TABLE 46-1

Treatments for cases of unresolved healing

Problem	Treatment
Incomplete debridement	Debride inflamed areas; consider obtaining a culture specimen to identify the bacteria causing the inflammation.
Poor plaque control	Reassess the patient's skills and attitude; change aids or modify the current procedure; consider irrigation or antimicrobial intervention.
Deep defect	Refer for surgery.
Complicating oral conditions	Refer for correction or improvement of oral conditions.
Complicating systemic conditions	Consider medical and laboratory examinations for possible underlying systemic disease.

BOX 46-4

Factors Affecting the Interval of Supportive Professional Care

Patient's current oral condition and general health status

Risk of reinfection

Clinical evidence that more frequent professional monitoring and intervention result in improved patient health

Patient's compliance or adherence regarding recommended personal oral health regimens

Patient's willingness to return for regular supportive periodontal care appointments

---

disturbed bacterial activity. The hygienist also must determine whether the patient lacks motivation or skill, needs a different self-care device, or should try some type of antimicrobial therapy. Helping the patient learn effective daily plaque control is as essential a service as the finest technical skills the hygienist may possess. Patient education and instruction should never be delivered to place blame on a patient or cause the patient to feel uncomfortable.

Periodontal patients typically have teeth that are more difficult to deplaque because of tooth position and root exposure and usually need to use more than a toothbrush and floss to deplaque the dentition (see Chapter 21). Periodontal patients with chronic disease may benefit from the use of a local or systemic antimicrobial agent. It is appropriate at supportive care appointments to consider the use of an antimicrobial agent if bleeding has not been controlled through mechanical means (see Chapter 24).

Persistent or unresolved periodontal disease may be site-specific or generalized and can be due to several factors (Table 46-1). Incomplete debridement results in incomplete wound healing because sufficient bacteria to cause infection have remained in the periodontal pocket. The host immune response can become overwhelmed and defeated when the bacterial load or pathogenicity of the plaque is too great. In some patients professional and self-care mechanical procedures cannot adequately reach and disrupt periodontal bacterial pathogens, such as in furcations, very deep pockets, or around tooth defects. In these cases the clinician and patient can discuss other options for attaining a healthy periodontium. Historically, periodontal surgery, among other procedures, was used to eliminate deep pockets that act as bacterial reservoirs. However, repeated periodontal surgery may not be desirable. A less invasive and less expensive procedure, such as antimicrobial therapy, should be considered when mechanical debridement and oral self-care are not adequate to maintain gingival health.

SUPPORTIVE CARE INTERVALS FOR PERIODONTAL PATIENTS

Regularly spaced intervals of professional care have proved beneficial for most individuals prone to a chronic disease.[2,11,24] The recommended average interval of support-

ive professional treatment for patients susceptible to periodontal disease is 3 months.[13,22] This interval sometimes can be lengthened or shortened based on a number of individual factors (Box 46-4).

More frequent patient visits allow the oral healthcare professional to monitor for recurrence of infection, to encourage the patient to continue the daily regimen, and to provide preventive procedures if active infection is present.

It should be noted that the typical 3-month periodontal maintenance interval is not the same as the 1- or 2-week appointment interval for up to 6 weeks that is scheduled after surgery. Generally, 1- or 2-week reevaluation appointments after periodontal surgery improve oral health in the healing phase.[20]

REVIEW OF PATIENT RECORD

The 1989 World Workshop in Periodontics stated that regular monitoring at regular intervals should include "treatment of areas of previous attachment loss and areas where clinical signs of inflammation are found."[26] However, just as the patient with blood pressure problems frequently has more difficulty regulating blood pressure, and the insulin-dependent person must take extra care to maintain a stable blood sugar, periodontal patients must work harder to maintain a healthy periodontium. Therefore the prevention and intervention plans must be realistic, and patients should feel that they can achieve the objectives.

To plan an individual prevention program, several questions must be answered:

1. What is the patient's risk level for recurrence of the disease?
2. What are the patient's attitude and psychomotor abilities in controlling the disease?
3. Which kinds of supportive care procedures are best for different patients?
4. Based on the patient's primary problem, what is the optimum interval length for supportive care?

These questions are challenging, and the answers differ from patient to patient. Patients' needs, problems, and general health status are not static; therefore a care plan including goals and evaluation measures is necessary for each supportive care appointment. Specific supportive care procedures require periodic reevaluation.

To focus the supportive care plan, it is important to identify the intended outcomes, the criteria by which patients and clinicians can judge success. Currently the desirable outcome in supportive periodontal therapy is stability; that is, attachment loss is halted. Complete absence of bleeding and exudate are end points of therapy that can be measured by the clinician and observed by the patient. However, these are criteria for judging the *success* of preventive and therapeutic measures; the *prediction* of periodontal disease or periodontal breakdown is considerably less well-defined. It is important to identify the desired outcomes and reinforce the patient's role in therapeutic outcomes. The only successful interventions are those that help achieve those goals.

ELEMENTS OF THE PERIODONTAL SUPPORTIVE CARE APPOINTMENT

The sequencing of the elements that make up the periodontal supportive care appointment is similar to that for the accepted annual examination of a person with no previous periodontal problems. The significant differences are the shortened interval between professional care appointments; the particular time, care, and emphasis on the patient's periodontal status; and the types of interventions that may be necessary. Such interventions may include use of antimicrobial agents, reinstruction or changes in oral hygiene, a shorter interval of care for the next supportive care appointment, or consideration of a return to active therapy.

REVIEW OF PATIENT RECORD

A review of the patient's record, including chartings and radiographs, before the appointment can refresh the clinician's mind as to the patient's general health, the extent of previous periodontal concerns, the type of surgical therapy, the level of stability currently attained, specific problem sites, and the patient's contribution to his or her own periodontal health. A knowledge of the patient's need for anesthesia or antibiotic premedication or preference for a particular debridement and polishing technique and other patient-specific concerns allows the clinician to prepare for a more beneficial and efficient appointment.

UPDATE OF HEALTH HISTORY

Updating the health history as every patient appointment is essential. General health and physiological vigor, specific health problems and recent medical care, the patient's stress level, and medications must be reviewed, because positive responses to some of these questions have a significant impact on periodontal conditions (see Chapters 9, 10, and 14 and all the chapters in Part IX). Research has shown evidence of connections between periodontal disease and systemic risks or problems beyond those of diabetes mellitus or bacterial endocarditis. A thorough familiarity with each patient's health and wellness allows the clinician to modify the care plan and to help determine why, in different patients, the level of plaque evident at a previous supportive care appointment does not result in comparable periodontal health.

SUBJECTIVE ASSESSMENT: COMMENTS, OBSERVATIONS, OR CONCERNS

No one is as familiar with a patient's oral condition as the patient; therefore it makes good sense to listen to the patient's evaluation of how the mouth "feels." Of particular interest to the clinician are comments about any kind of tooth sensitivity; mechanical problems or problems with therapeutic drugs; what does or does not "feel right" in the patient's mouth; and any concerns about changes in oral condition. In accepting the patient as a co-therapist in periodontal care, the value of listening to periodontal concerns cannot be overemphasized.

EXTRAORAL AND INTRAORAL EXAMINATIONS

An extraoral and intraoral examination should be performed.[23] This examination is particularly important in older patients, patients who have had a previous malignancy, and patients with high oral health risk behaviors, such as tobacco and alcohol use.

HARD TISSUE EXAMINATION

Changes in tooth position, extractions, periapical infections, the status of restorative work, and certain conditions all affect the health of the periodontium. The dentition must be examined with attention to the effects on the periodontium, such as plaque retention areas, excessive and destructive occlusal influences, and the anatomical shapes of teeth.

PERIODONTAL EXAMINATION

Thorough attention to the site around each tooth is critical in periodontal maintenance appointments. All the components of the periodontal examination (see Chapter 15) generally are performed at each periodontal supportive care appointment, with particular attention given to any areas of change. A change of 2 mm or more of attachment loss, along with other clinical findings, is a suggested criterion for more aggressive intervention. Two millimeters accounts for the 1 mm accepted variation in probe depth measurements. However, for a patient with significant previous attachment loss, even a 1-mm increase in attachment loss may be an unfavorable clinical sign. Bleeding on probing is an important clinical sign that must be recorded at each supportive care appointment.[10] The absence of bleeding on probing is considered more predictive of periodontal health than the presence of bleeding on probing is predictive of increased attachment loss. A bleeding score of less than 16% should result in no change in the supportive care interval; with a bleeding score of 16% or higher, the interval should be shortened by 1 month.[25] When a patient shows a loss of clinical attachment level, microbial analyses and biochemical assays may provide definitive information that would aid the selection of appropriate interventions.[9,18] Genetic testing is a new tool used to assess periodontal disease and may prove beneficial in the future.[4]

PROFESSIONAL'S REVIEW OF PERSONAL CARE, BEHAVIORS, AND ATTITUDES

Being attuned to the patient's mental and emotional status, attitude toward the mouth, sense of responsibility for the problems in the mouth, and ownership of successes is an important task for the dental hygienist. This type of information about the patient and its influence on his or her periodontal status are assessed from the beginning to the end of therapy. The clinician's and each staff member's genuine attitudes of encouragement throughout the appointment or appointment sequence demonstrate interest and support for the periodontal patient. The best time to review psychomotor skills and have the patient practice in a problem area is after the mouth has been disclosed or before professional debridement. Finally, through effective motivation and encouragement, the dental hygienist, the dentist, and the office staff serve as part of the patient's support group.

DEBRIDEMENT AS NECESSARY

The clinician must concentrate on sites that show *any* undesirable changes, from the most subtle rolled or shiny gingival margin or swollen interdental papilla to frank bleeding or pus-producing areas. These signs are evidence of the body's response to an infection.

New technological advances in dentistry are making it possible to further investigate the actual site of inflammation. The Perioscope (DentalView Co., Irvine, Calif.) provides visualization and magnification within the periodontal pocket, sulci, furcas, and crown margins and is proving indispensable for finding plaque retentive missed, burnished calculus, or rough root surfaces responsible for plaque retention. Debridement disturbs the bacterial matrix, making the plaque less pathogenic. Although calculus deposits usually are not large or tenacious at 3-month intervals, all calculus should be removed because it is a retentive area for bacterial plaque.

DEPLAQUING AND POLISHING AS NECESSARY

Deplaquing is particularly difficult for patients with periodontal problems. Exposed root surfaces, furcations, malpositioned teeth, and complex restorative correction frequently pose difficult challenges in plaque control. Also, the patient's level of plaque control is not always sufficient by itself to halt attachment loss.

Polishing is necessary to remove stains and other heavy plaque at and under the gingival margin. This process is particularly important when gingival disease is present.

SCHEDULING OF SUBSEQUENT PERIODONTAL SUPPORTIVE CARE APPOINTMENTS

Because most periodontal supportive care intervals are established at 3 months, a date for the next appointment often is made before the patient leaves the office. This is a common practice for any appointments that are not 6 months into the future so that the appropriate interval is maintained and the interval is not lengthened through scheduling problems. Attention to maintaining the recommended interval of care is important whether the supportive care appointment is at the same office or alternates between two offices.

One additional element that is vital to the success of periodontal supportive care is allowing for adequate appointment time. In 1981 Schallhorn and Snider[17] conducted a study of the average time required for different components of periodontal maintenance. One hour is the generally accepted minimum for a supportive care appointment, although some patients require more time.

However, 20 years later more activities are required during that hour. For example, the infection control protocol has become more involved, and intraoral preventive options (e.g., antimicrobial therapy and instruction) have increased. Patients who require full-mouth local anesthesia usually are given two appointments so that only the left or right half of the mouth is anesthetized at one visit.

Any treatment plan must include criteria for outcome assessment, which variously can be defined as results, completion, achievement, success, or simply progress (see Chapters 29 and 30). Outcomes goals can vary and may be established as short term or long range, but both patient and clinician must agree to them. Although the goals of therapeutic intervention and prevention strategies are not always the same for therapist and patient, the criteria for a successful outcome from supportive periodontal care appointments should be discussed and agreed upon with the patient.

RESPONSIBILITY FOR PERIODONTAL SUPPORTIVE CARE APPOINTMENTS

The severity of the patient's periodontal condition and the extent of active treatment are the most common determinants by which the professional office should oversee supportive periodontal care. The patient's preference, the distance to the offices, and insurance coverage are other factors.

After the initial periodontal treatment, four courses of action are possible: (1) the patient may be seen in the specialist's office for all supportive care appointments, an arrangement that is preferable for very involved periodontal conditions and medically complex patients[12]; (2) the patient may alternate 3-month visits between the general dental office and the periodontal office; (3) the general dental office may resume responsibility for all patient care, an option that works best in simple periodontal cases with minimal bone loss or for isolated procedures such as crown lengthening or gingival grafts; and (4) the patient may decide not to seek supportive periodontal care despite the clear advice given during the initial periodontal therapy. The periodontist should suggest which of the first three options is best, but the patient ultimately decides the course of action.

SUPPORTIVE CARE FOR DENTAL CARIES AND OTHER CHRONIC ORAL CONDITIONS

46-B

DENTAL CARIES

Developmental pits and fissures at risk for dental decay should be protected with sealants. Patients with active caries or those who are at risk for smooth surface and root caries should be placed on a professionally supervised program of more frequent intervals for several reasons (see Chapters 22 and 26). One is to advise the patient in and monitor the use of multiple forms of fluoride, which assist in remineralization, and other primary preventive agents for controlling and healing the incipient lesion. The clinician may also consider the use of chlorhexidine as an anticarious agent. Frequent appointments for caries control include intensive plaque control instructions and motivation and encouragement of sugar and carbohydrate discipline (see Chapters 18 and 21).

The clinician must first update the caries risk assessment; that is, the hygienist reviews all the caries-producing influences peculiar to the individual patient to determine which risk factors must be reduced or modified. Risk factors may include dietary choices, frequency of eating, types of snacks, degree of exposure to topical fluoride, salivary influences, quality of tooth development, medications, and genetic and social factors. Youth is no longer as strong a risk factor for caries as other considerations. Occlusal caries are developing much later than the historical pattern of early caries formation. Changes in tooth position, root exposure, diet, medication, oral care, and lifestyle influence a person's susceptibility to caries, and these influences occur across the life span. Any patient who has had active caries in the past 12 months should be considered at high risk for the development of new caries and requires close professional supervision and modification of care for caries control.

The extent and effectiveness of patient compliance with the caries control program are assessed at each appointment. *Listening* to patients to determine their self-care regimens, their attitudes and feeling about oral self-care—its value, its success—and how the mouth has been feeling is vital to understanding the level of patient compliance. The dental hygienist also should watch patients perform oral care in areas where they mention having difficulty with plaque removal or fluoride application or where the dental hygienist notes a problem.

Use of fluoride considerably enhances the control of dental decay. The clinician should determine the availability of systemic fluoride for the patient (see Chapter 22). Also, the patient's use of fluoride must be reviewed and reevaluated at each supportive care appointment because exposure to small daily doses of fluoride is considered the best caries-preventive interval. The need for professionally applied topical fluoride, as well as its frequency and type, should be evaluated. For both personal and professional fluoride therapy, changes in application might be suggested based on the progress seen and the current severity of the disease, the patient's acceptance of products, or the availability of a new product. For example, it is widely accepted that fluoride enhances remineralization of enamel and has an effect on exposed dentin. It is also known that chlorhexidine has a deleterious effect on *Streptococcus mutans,* the putative organism in incipient caries. Effective, efficient means of applying chlorhexidine, such as with varnish or spray, are being developed to help retard or prevent caries.

OTHER CHRONIC ORAL CONDITIONS

A few patients have other chronic oral problems, such as dentinal sensitivity, rapid deposit accumulation, herpetic lesions, aphthous ulcers, or the tissue conditions associated with Sjögren's syndrome. A more frequent interval of professional supportive oral care is generally advisable for these patients. The oral healthcare professional can monitor the patient's condition and often ameliorate the severity of the tissue breakdown, with the expected result of improved oral comfort and health for the patient.

At times a chronic condition can, in effect, disappear. For example, dentinal sensitivity may resolve; deposit accumulation may diminish; gingivitis may be eliminated through effective plaque control; tissue health may improve when deleterious habits such as smoking or bruxism are eliminated or controlled; and a reduction in salivary flow or adverse effects on gingival tissue may resolve when medications that cause these problems are withdrawn or replaced. Generally, dentinal sensitivity lessens with time and the use of antisensitivity pastes and treatments. Deposit accumulation may change with the patient's daily care, habits, and salivary status. Bruxism and clenching can be treated or controlled. Sometimes medications can be changed to types that do not contain sugar or contribute to xerostomia.

Changes in mental and emotional status affect health and chronicity, even though their effects are less understood and documented. A patient suffering emotional or mental stress or trauma may precipitate a chronic condition or may cause a chronic condition to become acute. The interrelationship of the physiologic mechanisms, hormonal influences, patient psyche, and attention or skill with at-home care is not completely clear. The oral mucosal tissue is a commonly affected area, and the multifactorial type of chronic problem includes the autoimmune classes of oral mucosal disease.

Chronic, infectious attacks of herpetic origin would not be a reason for more frequent supportive care. For some patients simple manipulation of the oral tissues during a dental appointment causes recurrence of a herpetic lesion. Over-the-counter products for alleviating the symptoms are the best therapy currently available for chronic herpetic lesions.

RITICAL THINKING ACTIVITIES

1. With the emphasis on evidence-based care, some of the same questions regarding the interval of patient care must be periodically reexamined. Search the dental literature for the answers to the following questions:
   a. Is 3 months still the recommended interval for supportive care for patients with periodontal disease?
   b. What are the desired outcomes of successful periodontal maintenance?
   c. How should periodontal supportive care outcomes be determined: clinically, microbially, through diagnostic testing, or by laboratory analyses?
   d. What are the parameters for each type of periodontal supportive care outcome?
   e. According to the dental literature on evidenced-based care, what are the current recommendations on the use of pharmacotherapeutical agents and controlled delivery as supportive adjuncts?

Continued

CRITICAL THINKING ACTIVITIES—cont'd

2. Find the report of the 1994 First European Workshop on Periodontology and study the concept of supportive periodontal care as described in this workshop. What are the parallel descriptions or terms used by the American Association of Periodontology? Refer to the association's web site and read the position paper and parameters of care for maintenance therapy.

3. For periodontal patients whom you see for more than one interval, keep a journal of what appears to motivate each patient. Write down whether patient observations were helpful (or not helpful). Examine your notes to determine if anything appears to be aiding compliance for different patients. Could some aspect of the patient's attitude or some behavior on your part encourage the patient to improve plaque control and adhere to the appropriate interval of care?

4. Role-play the part of a dental hygienist faced with a pleasant but noncompliant patient. Develop the skills of listening to the patient's difficulties, such as plaque control, keeping appointments, finances, time, or dealing with more than one office. Practice responding in a beneficial and positive manner. (Hint for patient role-player: Mention any and all problems, reasons, and excuses you can think of for why you are not responsible for conditions in your mouth.)

REVIEW QUESTIONS

The following questions refer to the case study presented at the beginning of the chapter.

1. Mrs. Lightfoot is taking prescription drugs for her medical problems. For which illness might she be taking medication that could have an adverse effect on her plaque control?
   a. NIDDM
   b. High blood pressure
   c. Osteoarthritis

2. Which of the following would be the least likely reason for the increased bleeding Mrs. Lightfoot shows?
   a. Gingival hyperplasia
   b. Hyperglycemia
   c. Poor plaque control
   d. A change in the diuretic prescribed

3. In Mrs. Lightfoot's case, which of the following is the most likely reason her probe measurements are deeper?
   a. Poor probe technique
   b. An increase in gingival margin height
   c. Apical migration of periodontal attachment
   d. Poor plaque control

4. Based on the information you have on Mrs. Lightfoot, how would you schedule her next supportive periodontal care session?
   a. Schedule her appointment in 2 months.
   b. Recommend that she visit a dental hygienist while she is traveling.
   c. Schedule her next supportive periodontal care appointment for when she returns from her trip.
   d. Wait until she returns from her trip to schedule her appointment.

5. Which of the following do you think is the most serious problem Mrs. Lightfoot faces?
   a. She will be unable to keep her 3-month appointment interval.
   b. Her plaque control is poor.
   c. Her bleeding index is now 25%.
   d. She does not understand her role in controlling periodontal disease.

6. Which of the following illnesses might hamper Mrs. Lightfoot's ability to deplaque her teeth?
   a. NIDDM
   b. High blood pressure
   c. Osteoarthritis

 ## SUGGESTED AGENCIES AND WEB SITES

Because of the ever-changing nature of the Internet, the web site listed here may have changed since publication. Please refer to Mosby's Evolve web site for the most current information.

American Academy of Periodontology: http://www.perio.org

ADDITIONAL READINGS AND RESOURCES

American Academy of Periodontology: Parameters of care, *J Periodontol* 71(5 suppl):i-ii, 847-83, 2000.

Wilson TG Jr: Supportive periodontal treatment and retreatment in periodontitis, *Periodontology 2000* 12:7-140, 1996.

REFERENCES

1. American Academy of Periodontology, Committee on Research, Science, and Therapy: Periodontal disease as a potential risk factor for systemic diseases: a position paper, *J Periodontol* 69:841-50, 1998.
2. Axelsson P, Lindhe J, Nystrom B: On the prevention of caries and periodontal disease: results of a 15-year longitudinal study in adults, *J Clin Periodontol* 18:182-9, 1991.
3. Baehni PC: Supportive care of the periodontal patient, *Curr Opin Periodontol* 4:151-7, 1997.
4. Bowers JE: Genetic testing: one part of periodontal risk assessment, *J Pract Hyg* 8:31-4, 1999.
5. Chace R: Retreatment in periodontal practice, *J Periodontol* 48:410-2, 1977.
6. American Academy of Periodontology Consensus Report, Section 11, Periodontal diseases: pathogenesis and microbial factors, *Ann Periodontol* 1:926-32, 1996.
7. Foreword to the supplement, *J Periodontol* 71:i, 2000.
8. Haynes R: A critical review of the "determinates" of patient compliance with therapeutic regimes. In Sackett D, Haynes R, editors: *Compliance with therapeutic regimes,* Baltimore, 1976, Johns Hopkins University Press.
9. Lamster IB: In-office diagnostic tests and their role in supportive periodontal treatment, *Periodontology 2000* 12:49-55, 1996.
10. Lang NP, Joss A, Tonetti MS: Monitoring disease during supportive periodontal treatment by bleeding on probing, *Periodontology 2000* 12:44-8, 1996.
11. Lindhe J, Nyman S: Long-term maintenance of patients treated for advanced periodontal disease, *J Clin Periodontol* 11:504-14, 1984.
12. Ogilvie AL: Maintenance of the periodontal patient. In Schluger S, Yuodelis RA, Page R, editors: *Periodontal disease,* ed 2, Philadelphia, 1990, Lea & Febiger.
13. American Academy of Periodontology: Parameter on periodontal maintenance, *J Periodontol* 71:849-50, 2000.
14. Lang NP, Karring T, editors: Proceedings of the First European Workshop on Periodontology, London, 1994, Quintessence.
15. Ramfjord SP: Maintenance care and supportive periodontal therapy, *Quintessence International* 24:465-71, 1993.
16. Rosén B et al: Effect of different frequencies of preventive maintenance treatment on periodontal conditions: 5-year observations in general dentistry patients, *J Clin Periodontol* 26:225-33, 1999.
17. Schallhorn RG, Snider LE: Periodontal maintenance therapy, *J Am Dent Assoc* 103:227-31, 1981.
18. Slots J: Microbial analysis in supportive periodontal treatment, *Periodontology 2000* 12:56-9, 1996.
19. Wennström JL: Treatment of periodontal disease in older adults, *Periodontology 2000* 16:106-12, 1998.
20. Westfelt E et al: Significance of frequency of professional tooth cleaning for healing following periodontal surgery, *J Clin Periodontol* 10:148-56, 1983.
21. Wilson TG Jr: Compliance and its role in periodontal therapy, *Periodontology 2000* 12:16-23, 1996.
22. Wilson TG Jr: Supportive periodontal treatment introduction: definition, extent of need, therapeutic objectives, frequency, and efficiency, *Periodontology 2000* 12:11-5, 1996.
23. Wilson TG Jr: A typical supportive periodontal treatment visit for patients with periodontal disease, *Periodontology 2000* 12:24-8, 1996.
24. Wilson TG Jr et al: Tooth loss in maintenance patient in a private periodontal practice, *J Periodontol* 58:231-5, 1987.
25. Wilson TG Jr, Kornman KS: Retreatment, *Periodontology 2000* 12:119-21, 1996.
26. Nevins M, Becker W, Kornman K, editors: Proceedings of the World Workshop, Princeton, NJ, 1989, American Academy of Periodontology.

CHAPTER 47

Case Development, Documentation, *and* Presentation

Bonnie Francis

Chapter Outline

Case Study: Use of Patient Case Documentation for
  Extended Learning
Uses and Applications
  Legal documentation and insurance submission
  Teaching tools and education
Theory
  Case development
  Case documentation

Case content
Case presentation
Example of Case Development and Documentation
  Guidelines
  Purpose
  Audience
  Patient selection guidelines
  Case documentation guidelines

Key Terms

Case documentation
Case development
Case presentation

Learning Outcomes

1. Provide an example for the use of development and documentation of a patient case.
2. Assess the purpose, intended audience, and goal of case development in a given situation.
3. Identify the components that can be developed and documented on a given case.

4. Compile all material necessary to document the therapeutic interventions and strategies of patient care provided in the case being developed.
5. Demonstrate case presentation skills to peers and other professionals in either written or oral format.
6. Document a case.

Case-based instructional methods have been favorably accepted by students and educators alike.* Case-based concepts enhance learning, promote self-directed learning, expand critical thinking, increase clinical reasoning skills and decision making, allow students to solve real-world problems in the safe environment of the classroom, and most importantly, promote life-long learning patterns.† The use of properly designed cases facilitates active learning and enhances higher levels of critical thinking, which requires the learner to integrate knowledge from basic and dental sciences with clinical applications.[2,4,5]

---

*References 3, 8, 10, 11, 13, 14.
†References 1, 3, 6, 7, 9, 11, 13, 14.

USES AND APPLICATIONS

Case representation of patient care can be used in several ways. The first and perhaps most obvious is patient education. "A picture is worth a thousand words" is true when motivating a person to change oral care behavior or to encourage a patient to continue the present course. Documenting the changes or progression of health may motivate the patient and the dental hygienist.

Cases also may be used by the hygienist to review patient outcomes and to determine when goals are met and what adjustments may be needed in either patient self-care habits or the clinician's strategies and/or skills. Reviewing documentation of some patients who exhibit

Case Study

Use of Patient Case Documentation for Extended Learning

Jennifer Shaw, a senior dental hygiene student, has recently received an assignment to prepare a case for her periodontology course. She has thoroughly reviewed the criteria established for the assignment (see the case application later in this chapter) and is aware of the aspects required to complete the task. The patient that was scheduled for Jennifer in today's clinical session, 70-year-old Ann Cronin, appeared to have the necessary elements that would allow her to complete her **case documentation** assignment. Jennifer discussed the prospects with her faculty and then informed Ms. Cronin and gathered the necessary clinical data for **case development** and documentation.

dramatic changes in tissue response and oral self-care is encouraging to the dental hygienist and the patient. Conversely, a patient may demonstrate subtle oral health changes and the process of capturing this information visually may assist in the evaluation of the therapy provided. Case documentation may provide motivation and self-evaluation for both the patient and dental hygienist.

LEGAL DOCUMENTATION AND INSURANCE SUBMISSION

Accurate and thorough records of patient care, which are an essential part of case development, also serve as legal documents and may help form a valuable defense if needed. Additionally, case documentation is required when insurance claims are filed for some procedures. Submitting an organized, thorough, and accurate case documentation with accompanying visual images with an insurance claim form assists in claim reimbursement.

TEACHING TOOLS AND EDUCATION

Case documentation also may be used for teaching in the academic setting and in professional presentations to peers. *Case presentations* are organized presentations of patient care. All components of a case are gathered and presented along with visual images to support objective clinical and radiographic findings. Chartings, radiographs, photographs, study models, and laboratory tests are combined with written documentation to "tell the story" of the patient's care from the initiation of therapy through the post-therapy evaluation.

THEORY

CASE DEVELOPMENT

Case development and documentation require a visual and written representation of a patient's clinical case. Information to be considered in the development of a case may include specifics about the case, visual elements representing the case, and specific details of case management and proceedings.[15] Selection of a case to develop involves three considerations: the *purpose* of developing the case; the *intended audience,* and define the expected outcomes, or *goal.*

Establishing Purpose

First of all, what is the purpose of developing this case? Various reasons for developing a case presentation may differ between clinicians. Case presentations may enhance any variety of learning processes. For example, a case may be developed to demonstrate clinical efficiency of a specific procedure or to showcase unique clinical condition. Determination of the purpose of a specific case development is enhanced by answering the following questions:
1. Why document this case?
2. Why is this case worth sharing?
3. What makes this case different, or unique?
4. What should others learn or see from this case?

 Case Application

When Jennifer realized that Ms. Cronin had specific periodontal challenges, she recognized that the development of this case would satisfy her class assignment and provide an interesting learning experience for her and her classmates.

Considering the Intended Audience

The second issue to consider is the intended audience. Will this case be developed for personal viewing? Will this case be seen and evaluated by instructors, patients, and/or professional colleagues?

 Case Application

Jennifer will be presenting her case to her classmates and faculty advisors. A clear understanding of the intended audience may help identify various components of the case that may need to be addressed more thoroughly, briefly, or not at all.

Defining Expected Outcomes

The overall goal of developing each case should be thoroughly explored. Understanding why this case should be developed and the value of the finished product may stimulate the effort needed for appropriate case selection and review. Developing and documenting a case presentation can be time-consuming and demanding. Ideally, when these three issues are addressed, the resulting information can act as an outline for prompting content organization, thoroughness in the design, and precision and objectivity in the implementation and presentation of the case.

CASE DOCUMENTATION

Because the purpose, audience, and goals of each case are varied and unique, the actual components of each case also vary depending on the issues to be addressed. Each case presentation has a unique flow in response to the issues addressed previously. The following discussion of case development is intended to introduce ideas and options rather than to give specific guidelines. Proper case design and development centers on thorough and accurate documentation.

Definition

According to the *Meriam Webster Online Language Center* (http://www.webster.com), the definition of *documentation* is the act or an instance of furnishing or authenticating with documents. For the purposes of this chapter, documentation refers to the process of recording events, words, and/or images of a case to reflect aspects of preventive and/or therapeutic care. Documentation of procedures performed in the record is only one facet of case development. Cases also may include a record of the patient's present health status, self and family health history, social history, beliefs and practices, extraoral and intraoral observations, charts, and photographic and/or radiographic imaging. Cases may include assessments of self-care and identification of oral risks. Notations of the therapeutic interventions and photographic images taken during the course of treatment also may be included to document the progress toward health. Any aspect of an interesting case, procedure performed, diagnostic aid used, or test result may become components of a case.

CASE CONTENT

Information about each case may include, but would not be limited to, obtaining information for the patient profile, supporting clinical evidence, and case management details.

Patient Profile

The patient profile may include health, medical, dental, and family or social histories. The idea of the patient profile is to provide basic information about the individual, which introduces the patient to the audience. By sharing information such as age, gender, ethnicity, behavior and beliefs, and professional and/or familial roles, the case becomes "real" to the audience. Current and historical background information in health, dental, or personal categories often adds essential insight to the components of the case. These categories in case development provide an opportunity to inform the audience of significant and apparently insignificant information that have affected or may have a future influence on the events and strategies within the case.

Clinical Evidence

Clinical evidence that represents the actual case may include data obtained from the initial clinical assessment. Items such as intraoral and extraoral examination (EIX), periodontal examination, indices (gingival [GI], plaque [PI], and bleeding [BI]), radiographic examination, oral hygiene assessment, caries assessment, risk assessment, and/or nutritional assessment compromise potential clinical assessment data. Clinical representation of the case also may include components such as intraoral photographs or images, radiographs, diagnostic study casts, and/or supplementary diagnostic test results such as salivary tests or results from pulp testing. Because these items represent the patient and must accurately characterize the case in physical absence of the patient, it is important for

them to be clinically accurate and of high diagnostic quality. Accurate, complete, and thorough documentation is essential to show health/disease progress and changes that occurred as therapy progressed.

Case Management

Details of case management and proceedings are represented by the documentation of treatment goals and strategies introduced, implemented, and evaluated. Components presented in this section may include strategies of treatment, instrumentation, oral self-care instruction, patient management, and/or follow-up evaluations. Organization and clinical accuracy of content must be observed.

Depending on the intended audience, this section could focus on specific strategies that were introduced and accepted by the patient, implemented, and then evaluated following therapy. The clinician may detail the discussion during the introduction of the strategy or perhaps revisions to initial strategies implemented during the course of therapy with explanations of when and why strategies needed to be revised. Any of these issues may affect the final outcome or course of the case. By reporting the strategies and variations in treatment, case documentation presents a more realistic case with explanations for and/or observations of the events or changes that occurred.

CASE PRESENTATION

Cases may be presented in a variety of formats. Oral presentations are the most widely used because of the variety of options in presenting and the interactivity between presenter and audience. Written format also may be developed for use in a document, such as a journal article or electronic delivery. Once again, the purpose of the presentation, the intended audience, and the presentation goals must be addressed to determine the appropriate format. A case that has been thoroughly and accurately documented may be easily adapted to fit either of the presentation formats.

Oral

Oral presentations provide an opportunity for interaction between the presenter and the audience. The dialog may guide discussion topics and provide feedback toward specific items that may need clarification and/or further discussion. The purpose of an oral presentation is to verbally address the important issues or elements of the case with the audience. The information may be presented on an individual basis such as clinician to patient, small group such as a gathering of colleagues or patients, or large audience such as professional or public meetings. The composition and size of the audience and the amount of time permitted for discussion determines the content to be delivered and the discussion issues to be addressed. To effectively communicate with a given audience, terminology and professional jargon used need to be appropriate to that audience and correct pronunciation must be rehearsed.[12] The goal of an oral presentation is to provide an accurate representation of the case and to provide opportunities for discussion and learning at a level appropriate for the audience.

Written

Written presentations demand a more organized and thorough presentation of the material to ensure all relevant data is covered. Discussion questions are generally included with the written presentation to provide guided learning opportunities or objectives. The purpose of a written presentation is to distribute a case example that can provide valuable learning opportunities to others. The exact audience may not always be known ahead of time. Because of the nature of publication distribution, the scope of the audience is not always known. Therefore avoiding professional jargon or nomenclature that may be misinterpreted or misunderstood by the general population is critical. Also important is provision of a thorough, accurate representation of the case, along with discussion issues that highlight or affect the learning points of the case. The goal of a written presentation therefore is to distribute a clinically accurate representation of a case that may be reviewed and discussed by anyone.

Developing a case requires attention to detail and organization; it forces the clinician to thoroughly seek and document all relevant information that may affect the case and/or the outcomes of various therapeutic strategies. Paying attention to the details of case development assists the clinician in recognizing the value of thorough accurate record keeping and providing well-constructed strategies for quality patient care. The presentation of a case provides the clinician with an opportunity to design, implement, evaluate, and share the strategies used in the therapeutic management of a particular case. Participating in the audience, a case presentation may provide an opportunity to review, discuss, evaluate, and learn various aspects of patient care directly from the clinician. Case presentation also may assist the audience in recognizing the value of maintenance of high standards of record keeping, therapeutic excellence, and comprehensive quality of oral care. Together, case development, case documentation, and presentation provide an opportunity for dental professionals to share case examples and learn more about the strategies and challenges that arise in the daily clinical practice of their profession.

EXAMPLE OF CASE DEVELOPMENT AND DOCUMENTATION GUIDELINES

47-A
47-B

The following example of case development and documentation guidelines was established for Jennifer's upper-level periodontology course (see case study). The case application to follow outlines Jennifer's completed case documentation.

PURPOSE

The purpose of this periodontal case development and documentation exercise is to provide upper level dental hygiene students the opportunity to select a periodontally involved patient and complete the case documentation, treatment, and posttherapy evaluation for discussion and learning purposes.

AUDIENCE

The audience for the case presentation may be a student's peers and faculty. This exercise also provides students with the opportunity to work through a difficult periodontal case, actually implementing treatment and evaluating the efforts of their treatment. The exercise provides students with the opportunity to share their case, strategies, and ideas with classmates. As a result of this exercise, the overall goal is to provide valuable learning experiences and increase understanding of the variety and complexity of treating periodontal cases. Ideally, this exercise benefits the student developing the case and the students who view the case presentation.

PATIENT SELECTION GUIDELINES

The patient selected must present with active periodontal disease and a plan for periodontal therapy. Ideally, the patient should present with some unique case feature(s), treatment, or outcome aspect that provides learning opportunities. Students need to complete the assessment, planned treatment, and post-therapy evaluation on the patient to complete case documentation and presentation requirements for this course.

CASE DOCUMENTATION GUIDELINES

Section I: Patient Information

This section is intended to introduce the patient to the audience. Thorough summaries of each of these components provide relevant background information that may affect oral health outcomes.

Demographic and Health History Assessment
1. Patient profile: summary of basic information about patient
2. Patient's chief concern (CC): summary of main reason for visit
3. Health history: comprehensive summary of health related findings
4. Dental history: comprehensive summary of dental related findings
5. Medical or dental indications: summary of significant dental or medical interactions with medications and/or health systems.

Section II: Clinical Assessment

Thorough summaries of each of these components provide descriptive information about the case:
1. Extraoral exam: summary
2. Intraoral exam: summary
3. Current dental conditions: summary of existing restorations, occlusal classification, caries activity, or edentulous conditions
4. Radiographic exam: summary of periodontal, restorative, and pathologic findings
5. Periodontal exam: general summary of periodontal status including probe depth, furcation involvement, mobility, clinical attachment loss, gingival description, AAP classification, and/or bleeding index

6. Oral risk assessment: summary
7. Psychosocial observations: summary of behavior, communication abilities, oral health status motivation
8. Current self-care routine: summary
9. Referral needs with rationale

Section III: Planning Phase

Thorough summaries of each of these components provide insight strategies in therapy and patient instruction:
1. Rationale for case selection: summary
2. Treatment goals/desired outcome: summary
3. Initial therapeutic strategy: must accurately reflect patient's chief complaint, treatment needs, psychosocial needs, and/or pain management
4. Preventive education strategy: oral heathcare aids to be introduced (when and why)
5. Instrumentation strategy: must accurately reflect patient's needs and operator skill level
6. Discussion points with patient: possible therapeutic alternatives, potential complications, expected results, patient's responsibility in treatment outcomes, and consequences of no treatment
7. Consent: informed and or written consent of treatment strategies

Section IV: Implementation Phase

Thorough summaries of each of these components provide descriptive information about the actual therapeutic and preventive care of the patient during the implementation phase:
1. Date of appointment and number of appointments in series: necessary to provide information on spacing interval of treatment and timeline of therapy
2. Actual services completed or treatment performed: what was actually accomplished on this date and appointment number
3. Treatment revisions with rationale: identifies changes in treatment plan and discusses reasons why changes to original therapeutic strategies were implemented
4. Patient care: identifies how the patient is responding to care and answer questions such as the following: Is the patient more or less motivated? Is the patient evaluating or noticing his/her own progress and healing? Is the patient having postoperative pain or sensitivity, and is that concern being addressed during the appointment?
5. Self care: summarizes patient's progress with preventive education plan and discusses rationale for home care aids being introduced or changed to meet therapeutic and psychosocial goals

Section V: Case

This section is intended to provide visual representation of the patient's clinical findings. Clinical accuracy and thoroughness provide visual information and clinical data relating directly to the case (see Chapters 9 through 20).
1. Intraoral photographs: includes all photos necessary to adequately provide documentation and visualization of patient's existing gingival and periodontal condition (see Chapter 19)

2. Study models: trimmed and presented according to diagnostic study model guidelines
3. Intraoral radiographs: based on diagnostic need of patient; must be of diagnostic quality and mounted correctly (see Chapter 17)
   a. Current or previous full mouth radiographic series - FMX
   b. Current bitewing series (vertical or horizontal)
4. Complete and accurate dental/periodontal chart
   a. Existing restorations
   b. Existing pathology
   c. Probe depths (PD): initial visit, post-therapy follow-up visit
   d. Clinical attachment loss (CAL)
   e. Gingival recession: draw in gingival margin and identify mucogingival discrepancies when applicable
   f. Furcations: presence, location, and extent properly identified
   g. Mobility: classified as I, II, or III
   h. Bleeding: noted on chart and summarized as % score
   i. Exudate: presence and types determined
   j. Presence and distribution of plaque and calculus: plaque index summarized as a percentage score
   k. Gingival description: color, contour, consistency, location, and extent of involvement (mild, moderate, or severe; see Chapter 15)
5. Oral risk assessment: completed and assessed according to oral risk assessment guidelines; identifies systemic and oral/behavioral risk factors that may contribute to periodontal condition or may influence periodontal therapy (see Chapter 29)

Section VI: Study Questions and Answers

This section is intended to identify discussion topics and items of clinical interest that may be addressed with the case. Evidence-based support for therapeutic strategies may be considered in this section to encourage decision-making skills based on current scientific literature, as follows:
1. Three questions are developed that can be drawn from your case as a learning or discussion point.
2. Answers to questions must be provided.

Section VII: Posttreatment Evaluation (4 to 6 Weeks)

This section is intended to describe the post-therapy clinical evaluation findings of the patient. Thorough summaries of each of these components provide descriptive information about the therapeutic and preventive outcomes and identify future needs of the patient, as follows:
1. Intraoral photographs as indicated
2. Review of chief complaint, health history, extraoral/intraoral exam (EIX): whether completed care addressed goals, risks, and patient concerns; summary of health history update, and changes in EIX noted
3. Periodontal examination: summary of probe depths (PD), bleeding on probing (BOP), plaque index (PI), and gingival description
4. Oral home care outcomes: summary of patient's understanding and effectiveness of oral hygiene, current recommendations based on BI, PI, PD, and gingival description

5. Therapeutic outcomes: summary of effectiveness of previously performed periodontal therapy and assessment of patient's response
6. Discussion points with patient: based on results of exam, status of patient's disease, therapeutic alternatives, potential complications, the expected results, and their responsibilities in treatment; explanation of consequences of no treatment
7. Future care recommendations
   a. Indications for referrals: specify referral protocol
   b. Active therapy continued: possible need for further active therapy, which might include antimicrobial therapy (site-specific or systemic) or further debridement (localized or generalized); specific actions and therapeutic strategy for continued active therapy
   c. Periodontal maintenance therapy: interval recommended for the maintenance of a healthy periodontium

Section VIII: Student Evaluation of Therapeutic and Preventive Outcomes

This section is intended to provide the student an opportunity to discuss planning, implementation, and evaluation of the therapeutic and preventive strategies as applied to the case. Supporting documentation from current scientific literature may be introduced at this time to validate the therapeutic strategies. Thorough summaries of each of these components provide self-evaluation opportunities and appraisal of lessons learned, as follows:

1. What was learned from treating the case: summary
2. Which modifications would enhance treatment outcomes: summary

Case Application

Jennifer's Completed Case Assignment
The following information represents Jennifer's completed case documentation.

PATIENT PROFILE
Ann Cronin, a 70-year-old retired seamstress, is a new patient to the dental practice. She recently has moved and now lives with her daughter, son-in-law, and three grandchildren. She is concerned that her small monthly pension will not cover her financial needs and has asked to delay any major dental treatment. (Ms. Cronin's patient record can be located on this text's accompanying CD-ROM. All forms used to summarize the following information are included in the record.)

CHIEF CONCERN
Ms. Cronin complains that her lower partial denture does not fit. She occasionally has not worn her partial denture for several days at a time.

Of what relevance to the supportive care appointment is Ms. Cronin's chief complaint?

HEALTH HISTORY
Ms. Cronin takes Premarin 1.25 mg once/day and Celebrex 100 mg twice/day for arthritis. She began smoking when she was 16 years old but quit more than 5 years ago.

Which oral considerations or concerns do these medications present?

DENTAL HISTORY
Ms. Cronin says that her teeth are sensitive to cold. She does not add ice to her beverages; she finds that her mouth is quite dry and believes that she needs to sip beverages or suck mints constantly to relieve her "dry throat." This visit is her first dental visit in 3 years. She uses a medium toothbrush with fluoridated toothpaste, brushes once a day, and uses an OTC mouthrinse. Ms. Cronin reports that she has difficulty holding the toothbrush and does not think that she does an adequate job of cleaning her mouth.

Does her dental history support the disease pattern(s) reflected in her dental record?

DIET HISTORY
She sucks on mints throughout the day because of her dry mouth. Her sugar intake is also evident in the four cups of sweetened coffee she consumes during the day. Ms. Cronin enjoys snacking on chips, cookies, and crackers.

Does her diet support oral disease?

HEALTH BELIEFS AND BEHAVIORS
Ms. Cronin says that she believes that she is more likely than most people to have cavities. She feels that she has spent a good deal of her adult life in the dental chair. She also believes in the importance of oral self-care to prevent caries and periodontal disease and says she welcomes recommendations. She does not want to change any current habits and does not believe that she is in control of her oral health.

Ms. Cronin receives a physical examination annually and adheres to her physician's advice but only sometimes changes her health behaviors on the recommendation of a dental professional. She reports that her eating habits are out of control and that she does not exercise or participate in sports or recreational activities.

What concerns do her current health beliefs and behaviors present to health promotion and disease prevention?

EXTRAORAL EXAMINATION
Ms. Cronin has bilateral 5-mm × 4-mm crusted areas at the commissures. Review her patient records for other findings.

INTRAORAL EXAMINATION
Review Ms. Cronin's intraoral photographs (Fig. 47-1) for the appearance of her soft and hard tissues. Given the narrative, were the findings what you expected?

RADIOGRAPHIC EXAMINATION
Review Ms. Cronin's radiographs (Fig. 47-2) for evidence of pathological conditions, existing restorations, and periodontal findings. Do the radiographs reflect the disease patterns you expected to see?

PERIODONTAL CHARTING
Review Ms. Cronin's periodontal charting (Figs. 47-3 and 47-4). Associate findings on the periodontal charting, clinical photographs, and radiographic images that present evidence of periodontal disease or other oral conditions.

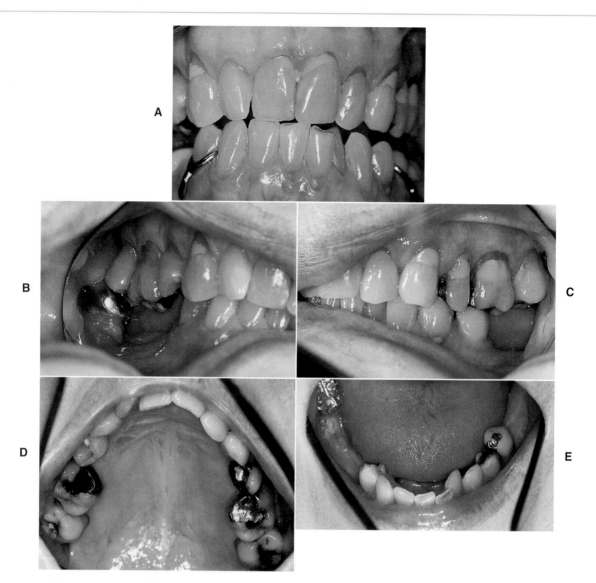

FIG. 47-1 Intraoral images. **A,** Direct facial. **B,** Right facial. **C,** Left facial. **D,** Maxillary occlusal. **E,** Mandibular occlusal.

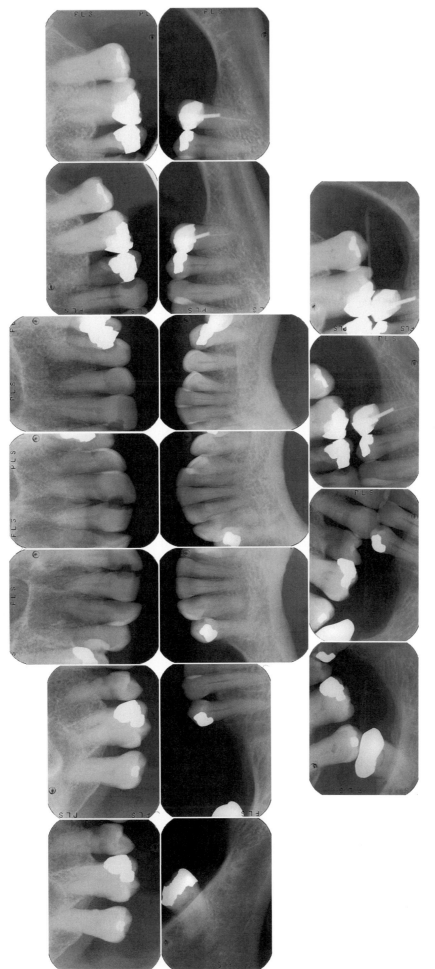

FIG. 47-2 Full-mouth radiographic images.

Ann Cronin

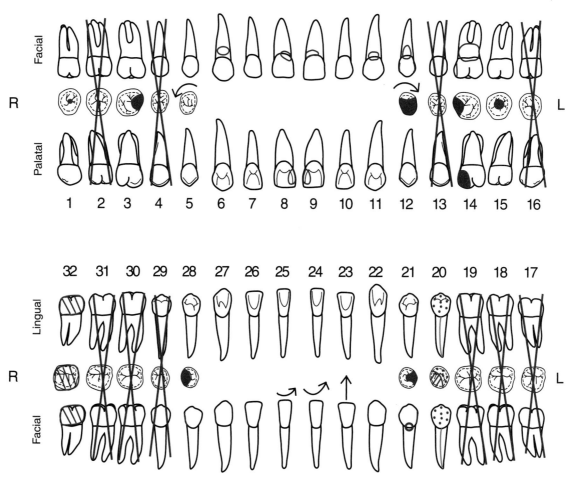

FIG. 47-3 Dental chart.

Patient Name: _Cronin, Ann_

Last   First   MI

Key:

Horizontal lines on chart are placed in 2-mm increments.

Probe Depth	6	4	2
*FGM to CEJ	-3	0	1
Attachment Loss	3	4	3

*Free gingival margin to the cementoenamel junction (CEJ): measurements coronal to the CEJ are noted as negative numbers.

• To note bleeding on probing, circle probing depth in red (or place a red dot above the number).

To calculate plaque score:

$$\frac{\text{Total \# surfaces w/plaque}}{6 \times \text{\# of teeth present}} \times 100 = \text{Score \%}$$

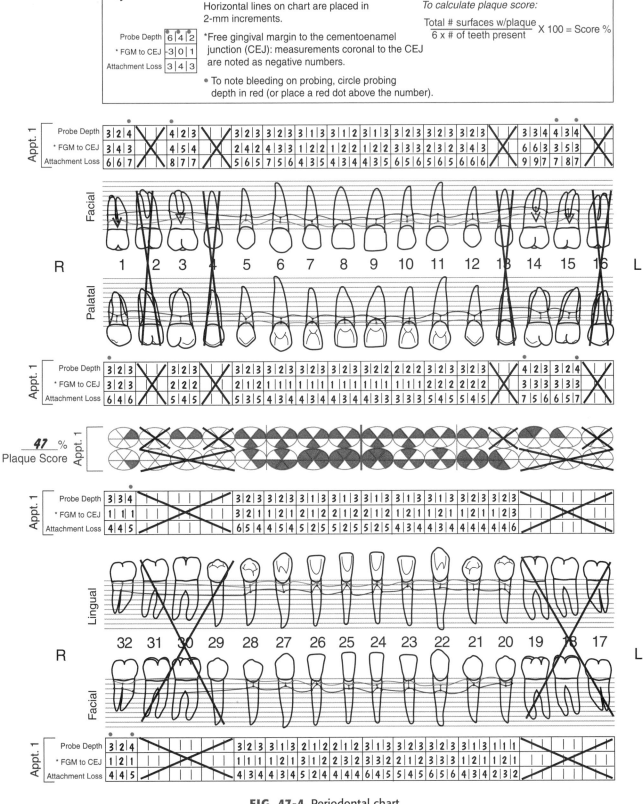

FIG. 47-4 Periodontal chart.

RITICAL THINKING ACTIVITIES

1. From your family of patients, identify those that present with oral and systemic diseases whose condition would warrant documentation. Select an audience for the presentation of your documentation.

2. Role-play with a peer the discussion you would have with a patient to request permission to document his or her case.

 REVIEW QUESTIONS

1. All *except* which of the following are ethical examples of how a case documentation and presentation can be used?
   a. Education of peers and patients
   b. Patient education and motivation
   c. Third-party payer reimbursement
   d. Advertising for increased profit
   e. Evaluation of the outcome of care

2. Which of the following must be considered before a case is developed?
   a. Purpose of developing case
   b. Intended audience
   c. Goal of development efforts
   d. All the above

3. Which of the following is *not* part of the patient profile section of case development?
   a. Current and historical health information
   b. Current and historical dental information
   c. Treatment strategies
   d. Age, gender, ethnicity
   e. Professional or familial roles

4. Which of the following presentation formats is the most widely used?
   a. Written
   b. Oral
   c. Electronic
   d. All the above

 SUGGESTED AGENCIES AND WEB SITES

Because of the ever-changing nature of the Internet, some of the web sites listed here may have changed since publication. Please refer to Mosby's Evolve web site for the most current information.

College of Dental Sciences [India] ("Case study archive"):
   http://omr-cods.tripod.com
DH Net: ("Clinical practice; Case study clearinghouse"):
   http://jeffline.tju.edu
National Center for Case Study Teaching in Science:
   http://ublib.buffalo.edu
Procter & Gamble, Dental Resource Net:
   http://www.dentalcare.com
The University of Iowa College of Dentistry ("Web cases"):
   http://uiowa.edu

UCLA Interactive Case Studies ("On-line courses"):
   http://dent.ucla.edu
University at Buffalo School of Dental Medicine ("Case studies in dentistry"): http://research.sdm.buffalo.edu
University of California, San Francisco ("Dental case-related tutorials"): http://itsa.ucsf.edu

Dental Hygiene Case Studies
East Tennessee State University: http://www.etsu.edu
Marquette University: http://www.marquette.edu

 ADDITIONAL READINGS AND RESOURCES

Case-based methods for dental hygiene faculty, *J Dent Educ* 62(3), 1998 (special section).

REFERENCES

1. Belcher JV: Improving managers' critical thinking skills: student-generated case studies, *J Nursing Admin* 30(7-8):351-3, 2000.
2. Bowen DM: Integrating case-based instruction into dental hygiene curricula, *J Dent Educ* 62(3):253-6, 1998.
3. Clark GT, Koyano K, Nivichanov A: Case-based learning for orofacial pain and temporomandibular disorders, *J Dent Educ* 57:815-20, 1996.
4. Coleman PW: An overview of case-based test construction, *J Dent Educ* 62(3):242-7, 1998.
5. Daniel SJ: Case-based methods for dental hygiene faculty, *J Dent Educ* 62(3):230, 1998.
6. Dowd SB, Daviodhizer R: Using case studies to teach clinical problem-solving, *Nurse Educator* 24(5):42-6, 1999.
7. Engel FE, Hendricson WD: A case-based learning model in orthodontics, *J Dent Educ* 58:762-7, 1994.
8. Hendricson WD, Berlocher WC, Herbert RJ: A four year longitudinal study of dental students learning styles, *J Dent Educ* 41:175-81, 1987.
9. Jones DC, Sheridan ME: A case study approach: developing critical thinking skills in novice pediatric nurses, *J Cont Ed Nursing* 30(2):75-8, 1999.
10. Kassebaum KD, Averbach RE, Fryer GE: Student preference for a case-based vs. lecture instructional format, *J Dent Educ* 44:781-4, 1991.
11. Lindesman HM, Bilan JP: Dental education and practice in the 21st century: opportunities for excellence, *J Prosthet Dent* 75:660-5, 1996.
12. Miller L: Presenting your case: solid verbal skills lay out the facts for periodontal treatment, *RDH* 17(5):26-8, 30,58, 1997.
13. Norman GR, Schmidt HG: The psychological basis of problem-based learning: a review of the evidence, *Acad Med* 67:557-65, 1992.
14. Vaughan DA, DeBiase CB, Gibson-Howell JC: Use of case-based learning in dental hygiene curricula, *J Dent Educ* 62(3): 257-9, 1998.
15. Woodall IR, Dafoe B: Case documentation. In Woodall IR: *Comprehensive Dental Hygiene Care*, ed 4, St Louis, 1993, Mosby.

PART XI

Chapter 48
Professional Development

Chapter 49
Insight and Commitment

Competency Statements

The learner is expected to possess knowledge, skills, judgments, values, and attitudes to develop the listed competencies.

Core Competencies
- Apply a professional code of ethics in all endeavors.
- Adhere to state and federal laws, recommendations, and regulations in the provision of dental hygiene care.
- Provide dental hygiene care to promote patient health and wellness using critical thinking and problem solving in the provision of evidence-based practice.
- Use evidence-based decision making to evaluate and incorporate emerging treatment modalities.
- Assume responsibility for dental hygiene actions and care based on accepted scientific theories and research as well as the accepted standard of care.

Courtesy American Dental Education Association, Washington, DC.

Professional Development and Vision

- Continuously perform self-assessment for lifelong learning and professional growth.
- Promote the profession through service activities and affiliations with professional organizations.
- Provide quality assurance mechanisms for health services.
- Communicate effectively with individuals and groups from diverse populations both verbally and in writing.
- Provide care to all patients using an individualized approach that is humane, empathetic, and caring.

Health Promotion and Disease Prevention

- Promote the values of oral and general health and wellness to the public and organizations within and outside the profession.
- Respect the goals, values, beliefs, and preferences of the patient while promoting optimal oral and general health.
- Identify individual and population risk factors and develop strategies that promote health related quality of life.

- Evaluate and utilize methods to ensure the health and safety of the patient and the dental hygienist in the delivery of dental hygiene.

Community Involvement

- Provide screening, referral, and educational services that allow clients to access the resources of the healthcare system.
- Provide community oral health services in a variety of settings.

Professional Growth and Development

- Identify alternative career options within healthcare, industry, education, and research and evaluate the feasibility of pursuing dental hygiene opportunities.
- Develop management and marketing strategies to be used in nontraditional health care settings.
- Access professional and social networks and resources to assist entrepreneurial initiatives.

CHAPTER 48

Professional Development

Susan J. Daniel

Chapter Outline

Case Study: Embracing the Dental Hygiene
  Profession
Professional Self
  Values
  Philosophy of practice
  Interpersonal needs
  Career goal setting
  Measurement of goals
  Development of a professional credo

Working with Other Professionals
  Position on the dental health team
  Position within health care
  Information exchange
Maintaining Competence
  Professional portfolio
  Evaluation

Key Terms

Communication	Empower	Maintaining competence	Portfolio
Continuing education	Goal setting	Philosophy	Professional development

Learning Outcomes

1. Develop professional goals based on assessed values, philosophy, and needs, and determine attainment measures.
2. Establish a respectful working relationship within the healthcare environment and on a dental team by empowering self and others.
3. Continue pursuit of competence.
4. Evaluate career paths.
5. Review the student portfolio for attainment of competence.

Professional development is an integral part of being a healthcare professional and cannot exist without attention to the whole person. This chapter explores elements of professional development and the components that aid in personal development. Healthcare providers are held to a somewhat higher standard than individuals in other occupations. This public expectation requires one to examine one's values and *philosophy* as a healthcare provider and to assess and evaluate personal and professional goals, *communication* skills, and treatment of others.

PROFESSIONAL SELF

VALUES

48-A Values are established early in life by a person's environment. Valuing quality of life is part of being human and certainly essential to the competent dental hygienist, who plays an important role in health promotion and disease prevention as a member of the healthcare team. Value for life and health is a prerequisite for embarking on a healthcare career.

Providing health care also requires a desire to serve humankind, driven by the value for life and health. Not all people share the same values for health. Values determine a person's response in a given situation. Healthcare providers may experience internal conflict when providing health care to someone who does not value health in the same manner. Providing the service in a caring, professional manner is still essential. Learning to recognize this conflict and the cause of the conflict may assist the healthcare provider in self-improvement and professional growth.

PHILOSOPHY OF PRACTICE

In addition to valuing quality of life and providing compassionate care, dental hygienists must examine their 48-B

Embracing the Dental Hygiene Profession

Case Study

Allyson Freeman, a 28-year-old dental hygienist, has been in practice for 4 years. She is the only dental hygienist in the mature (25-year) practice. Her primary responsibilities consist of performing clinical and radiographic assessments and preventive and therapeutic interventions. She is not a member of the American Dental Hygienists' Association and seldom attends professional meetings. She obtains the necessary **continuing education** hours required to maintain an active license. Allyson has become complacent with her position (provides the same treatment to all patients), is no longer satisfied with her job, and is questioning her career choice.

Reflect on Allyson's situation. What elements is Allyson missing in her professional life? What can she do to develop satisfaction in her career?

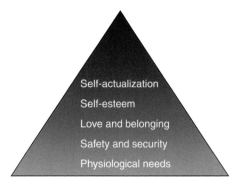

FIG. 48-1 Maslow's hierarchy of needs.

BOX 48-1

Description of Maslow's Hierarchy of Needs

Self-actualization: the need for fulfillment
Self-esteem: the need for recognition
Love and belonging: the needs for communication, affection, identity, modesty, companionship, and dependence
Safety and security: the needs for safety and accident prevention, religion and philosophy, and feelings of well-being
Physiological needs: needs for personal hygiene, activity, sexuality, viral functions, eating and drinking, sleeping, and resting

---

philosophy about the healthcare system. Various work environments and payment methods have led many healthcare providers to assess their philosophy about the delivery of health care. Many questions abound. Where should care be provided; who should provide the services; who should receive care; and at what costs are questions being raised around healthcare issues? Each healthcare professional has to identify a personal philosophy about some of these issues. Typically, the philosophy will be based on personal values. When the chosen philosophy is not based on professional values, any performance or delivery of care will be compromised. Either an individual must pursue this direction, or that person will begin to adjust what is valued. Adjusting one's values will begin to erode self-image and self-worth. As a care provider, the dental hygienist must examine the philosophy of practice and weigh interpersonal needs into this examination.

INTERPERSONAL NEEDS

48-C Each person has certain needs that feed the soul, body, and mind. Maslow's hierarchy of needs is indeed true (Fig. 48-1 and Box 48-1).[1]

Professional growth mandates an examination of interpersonal needs. A dental hygienist may consider the following questions:
1. What are my needs?
2. Are they being met?
3. What adjustments are needed to have my needs met?
4. Are my social outlets enough or the type I want?
5. Can I adjust my professional setting or work responsibilities to meet my needs?

Exploring questions such as these may assist in the achievement of personal fulfillment. One of the primary steps in the development of the professional self requires the meeting of interpersonal needs.

CAREER GOAL SETTING

48-D In the pursuit of professional development, the establish-
48-E ment of goals is essential for success and personal satis-

faction. Generating professional goals is impractical without also addressing components of personal life, such as family. **Goal setting** is the first step in the measurement of professional growth or accomplishments. Establishing both short- and long-term goals is appropriate and necessary. A professional who has identified deficits in interpersonal needs and has a vision for future attainment may begin setting goals. Sometimes immediate changes must be made in pursuit of goals. Small changes or steps toward a larger goal may need to occur first. Outlining these steps is often necessary to achievement of the anticipated change.

A professional may want to focus on more than one area of growth or change. Once these areas have been identified, writing a goal statement complete with action terms and measurable criteria is necessary. Development of a goal may involve an action plan and/or identification of strategies to reach the goal. Implementation of the strategies can be driven by a timeline.

MEASUREMENT OF GOALS

Often articulation of professional goals to others may be helpful in the quest for professional growth. Some individuals perform best when they are accountable to others. Additionally, other persons may offer assistance, encouragement, and feedback during the process. An employer, coworker, peer, spouse, parent, or anyone with whom the professional has a respectful, nurturing relationship can be a coach or mentor.

A Creed for Relationships with Others

You and I are in a relationship, which I value and want to keep, yet each of us is a separate person with unique needs and the right to meet those needs.

When you are having problems meeting your needs I will try to listen with genuine acceptance in order to facilitate your finding your own solutions instead of depending on mine. I also will try to respect your right to choose your own beliefs and develop your own values, different though they may be from mine.

However, when your behavior interferes with what I must do to get my own needs met, I will openly and honestly tell you how your behavior affects me, trusting that you respect my needs and feeling enough to try to change the behavior that is unacceptable to me. Also, whenever some behavior of mine is unacceptable to you, I hope you will openly and honestly tell me your feelings. I will then listen and try to change my behavior.

At those times when we find that neither of us can change a behavior to meet the other's needs, let us acknowledge that we have a conflict of needs that requires resolving. Let us then commit ourselves to resolve each such conflict without either of us resorting to the use of power or authority to try to win at the expense of the other's losing. I respect your need, but I also must respect my own. So let us always strive to search for a solution that will be acceptable to both of us. Your needs will be met, but so will mine—neither will lose, both will win.

In this way, you can continue to develop as a person through satisfying your needs, but so can I. Thus, ours can be a healthy relationship in which each of us can strive to become what each is capable of being. And we can continue to relate to each other with mutual respect, love and peace.

Modified from materials copyright 2000 by Thomas Gordon, PhD, Founder, Gordon Training International, Solana Beach, Calif. [http://www.gordontraining.com].

DEVELOPMENT OF A PROFESSIONAL CREDO

Developing nurturing relationships with professionals and others is an important part of developing the professional self. Establishing for oneself respectful, caring relationships with others is part of fully living one's values and philosophy and meeting interpersonal needs. Some have devised professional credos or codes for interacting with others. Box 48-2 provides an example of one of these. Each professional should establish a unique style of personal interaction based on personal values, philosophy, and needs.

WORKING WITH OTHER PROFESSIONALS

Being a healthcare professional and providing caring service requires effective communication within dentistry and other disciplines. Poor relationships with healthcare professionals may weaken the healthcare delivery system and may cause unnecessary use of services and financial expenditures.

POSITION ON THE DENTAL HEALTH TEAM

Identifying an individual's role and position on the dental healthcare team may benefit patients, employees, coworkers, and employers. The clinical dental hygienist is a prevention specialist, providing direct patient care, and is well educated in disease prevention and health promotion. These roles are enhanced by knowledge of what each person brings to the dental health team and by respectful communication among the team members.

POSITION WITHIN HEALTH CARE

With the growing association between oral disease and systemic disease, the dental hygienist's role is of greater significance than ever before. The dental hygienist's identification of gingival and periodontal diseases and knowledge of the association to systemic diseases may assist patients in the prevention of systemic diseases, many of which have yet to surface.

INFORMATION EXCHANGE

Providing information to patients, peers, coworkers, and the community about the relationship that exists between oral disease and systemic diseases *empowers* the dental hygienist and those receiving the information to become better health promoters and to prevent disease. The most important aspect of this exchange is the potential impact on the reduction of disease.

MAINTAINING COMPETENCE

PROFESSIONAL PORTFOLIO

Throughout this text and the CD-ROM, development of **48-F** the educational *portfolio* has been encouraged. In Chapter 1, the concept of the portfolio was identified as a mechanism for documentation of the process of *maintaining competence*. The process and responsibility of maintaining competence to perform quality health care is continuous. The portfolio documents these pursuits.

EVALUATION

Documenting all aspects of continuing competence can be used for evaluation, promotion, and renewal of the professional license. Goal setting is the first part of the process; following a plan to attain the goals and documenting each step in the process are necessary to evaluate continuing competence. Periodically, the hygienist should review the portfolio contents and assess whether the contents reflect the attainment of goals and continued competence. Once goals are met, new goals should be established.

Materials from the portfolio may be used to verify mandatory continuing education requirements for licensure; however, the portfolio should contain more of the rich evidence of professional growth. Participation in community service projects, publications, educational presentations, the formation of study groups, oral care product inquiry, professional correspondence, mentoring, problem solving with staff, and developing patient communication materials and/or more efficient office patterns should all have a place within the portfolio. Interesting patient cases that have provided new insights into health and disease may be documented and added to the portfolio. The hygienist may choose to record ethical or legal dilemmas encountered, strategies implemented, and the respective outcomes as a means of self-assessment.

Professional development is the responsibility of each healthcare professional. The desire to maintain competence and to maximize potential within the confines of their discipline is incumbent upon all providers of patient care. Dental hygienists have the responsibility of being the most competent and professionally respected oral health direct-care providers in disease prevention and health promotion.

 48-G

RITICAL THINKING ACTIVITIES

1. Establish three professional goals for yourself for the next year.
2. Develop a plan for how you will meet these goals that includes measurable outcomes as follows, for example:

   I will improve my knowledge of the relationship between periodontal diseases and systemic diseases by attending a continuing education course on the topic or reading at least one article each month on this topic.

3. Evaluate the effect of this knowledge to your clinical practice and interpersonal relationships with patients and colleagues.

REVIEW QUESTIONS

1. Which of the following aspects provides the foundation for the way we treat others?
   a. Interpersonal needs
   b. Philosophy
   c. Values
   d. Goals
2. Which of the following best describes the dental hygienist's role within health care?
   a. Efficient healthcare provider
   b. Direct-care provider
   c. Disease prevention, health promotion
   d. *a* and *b*
   e. *b* and *c*
3. Which of the following best describes the intent of the portfolio?
   a. Retain documentation of continuing education for licensure

   b. Documentation for the evaluation of continued competence
   c. Maintain interesting cases for review and learning
   d. Keep personal notes for review and evaluation
4. Which of the following is the most effective way to empower oneself and others?
   a. Compliment others on their performance
   b. Communicate effectively with others
   c. Providing education about the relationship of oral and systemic disease
   d. Keeping track of assistance of others in the office

 SUGGESTED AGENCIES AND WEB SITES

Because of the ever-changing nature of the Internet, some of the web sites listed here may have changed since publication. Please refer to Mosby's Evolve web site for the most current information.

ADA Hygiene Survey: http://www.members.aol.com
American Dental Education Association: http://www.adea.org
[The] American Dental Hygienists' Association:
   http://www.adha.org
[The] American Dental Hygienists' Association ("Dental hygiene association participates in ethics summit I"):
   http://www.adha.org
British Columbia Ministry of Health:
   http://www.moh.hnet.bc.ca/library

Dental Directory: http://www.dentaldirectory.virtualave.net
Dental Globe ("Continuing education"):
   http://www.dentalglobe.com
Health Professions Council Recommendation on the Designation of Dental Hygiene: http://www.moh.hnet.bc.ca
Medical Library Association ("Dental hygiene education"):
   http://www.mlanet.org
Procter & Gamble ("Global dental resources"):
   http://www.dentalcare.com

ADDITIONAL READINGS AND RESOURCES

Maslow AH: Toward a humanistic biology, *Am J Psychol* 24:724, 1969.

Shortell SM, Kaluzny AD: *Health care management: organization design and behavior,* Albany, NY, 1994, Delmar.

Reece SM, Pearce CW, Melillo KD, Beaudry M: The faculty portfolio: documenting the scholarship of teaching, *J Prof Nurs* 17:180, 2001.

REFERENCES

1. Maslow AH: *Toward a psychology of being,* ed 2, New York, 1968, Van Nostrand Reinhold.

CHAPTER 49

Insight *and* Commitment

Susan J. Daniel

Chapter Outline

Case Study: Vision of Oral Care in 2010
Disease Prevention and Health Promotion
Future Direction
    Education and licensure
    Research

Clinical practice
Public health
The Future

Key Terms

Accreditation
Commitment

Distance learning
GENOME

Licensing exams
Vision

Learning Outcomes

1. Generate discussion of trends and future directions for the profession of dental hygiene in the following:
   Clinical practice
   Education and licensure
   Research
   Public health

2. Identify the relationship of technology to the profession of dental hygiene.
3. Suggest changes in content within the learning package based on changes in the practice of dental hygiene.

Planning professional growth is an important step in ensuring a person's future as a dental professional. This type of planning helps hygienists reach higher levels of competence both as individuals and as a profession. Some happenings may appear to be serendipitous, but *vision* and *commitment* to a vision are essential to producing successful outcomes. Dental hygienists may take the first step in achieving their vision by visualizing themselves in a particular situation or at a particular place and time. Major developments in health care have occurred because some individuals had a strong vision, idea, or theory that they unwaveringly pursued. Some risk-takers failed but learned from their mistakes and continued to pursue their goals. Successful individuals attribute their ability to persevere to others who encouraged or mentored them.

Gifted visionaries are not the only contributors to the field of dental hygiene. On the contrary, individuals who share the same vision and who commit to seeing the vision materialize are necessary for the implementation of strategies to reach the vision. This chapter presents future trends in clinical practice, education and licensure, research, and public health.

DISEASE PREVENTION AND HEALTH PROMOTION

Healthcare delivery has been founded on the knowledge and understanding of basic sciences such as biology, anatomy and physiology, chemistry, physics, microbiology, and the psychosocial sciences. These sciences have provided information through scientific inquiry by those committed to improving human life. Without this information founded by scientists and practitioners, the field of dental hygiene would not be where it is today. The profession is still growing in all areas of identification and prevention of disease and health promotion. The role of the healthcare professional encompasses many facets of administration and practice to further advancements in the identification of diseases, to develop new methodologies for preventing and curing disease, and to promote health.

Technological advances coupled with basic and clinical scientific inquiry are critical to future practice. A greater understanding now exists of the human body and the function of the immune system. The technology to locate specific enzymes and markers associated with specific diseases will move health care and dental hygiene to another level. Identification of suspected disease before the manifestation of clinical signs and symptoms will be the next frontier.

Dental hygienists must always pay attention to the patient. Listening to the patient and conducting a thorough assessment inquiry can provide invaluable information for the professional to be a more accurate diagnostician, provide appropriate healing arts, and monitor progress toward health.

The *GENOME*[4] project has provided science with the DNA pattern for life, unlocking the doors of human discovery. Surrounding this incredible finding is controversy over the ethical application of the knowledge—another frontier to explore. Many unanswered questions exist about the affective human component such as the development of a person's soul, compassion, and heart or caring. The affective component of development is clearly not as certain as the physiological development.

FUTURE DIRECTION

The literature is replete with publications on healthcare practices, association between systemic and oral disease, patient practices and trends in seeking healthcare, and present and future healthcare needs. Trends and current practices can provide insight into the future role of the

dental hygienist. Insight can assist the profession in establishing vision and seizing opportunities to improve human life.

To establish a framework of categories to address future direction, a traditional academic model will be used. The "three-legged stool" model subscribed to in academic institutions is that of teaching, service, and research. This model has been stabilized in some institutions with a fourth leg of patient care. The four-component academic model—teaching, service, research, and patient care—will morph into the framework for future directions in dental hygiene education, clinical practice, research, and public health (Table 49-1). Technological advances have made and will continue to make major contributions to each component of the model.

EDUCATION AND LICENSURE

Educational oversight agencies will continue to demand accountability from educational institutions and programs for the product produced (student/graduate). The American Dental Association's (ADA) Commission on Dental and Allied Dental *Accreditation* requires accountability from accredited educational programs. Additionally, to become licensed in 49 of the 50 states students must successfully complete the National Board Dental Hygiene Examination administered by the ADA and pass the clinical and jurisprudence licensure examination for the state/region. Only students who have graduated from an ADA-accredited program can sit for the National Board Dental Hygiene Examination.[1]

Educational accountability occurs in primary, secondary, and higher education in the liberal arts and in the sciences. Holding educational institutions accountable for a competent end product (graduation) is one method of ensuring student outcomes and quality in health care and bettering the quality of life and society.

The Commission on Dental and Allied Dental Accreditation requires each dental hygiene educational program meet certain standards. Dental hygiene, like other healthcare professional educational programs, must be accountable for the type of product or student graduating from each program. The accreditation standards have undergone numerous revisions over the years. Currently, dental hygiene programs are required to establish competence for specific areas of education.[1] Students must be provided competency statements when entering the program, and these statements must be used as a measure for evaluating

Case Study Vision of Oral Care in 2010

Use your imagination as you journey into the future. Make written notes after each question has been presented.

You have walked into a healthcare facility in the year 2010. Dental and medical care is being provided in the same facility. Imagine what the surroundings would look like.

- What type of healthcare equipment would be in this facility?
- What is the reception area like?
- What does the business area look like?
- What type of personnel would you see in this environment?
- What forms of health promotion and disease prevention would be performed in this healthcare environment?
- What would your role(s) be and what types of personnel would you interact with to provide patients with the best possible healthcare?

TABLE 49-1

Use of the academic model for categories of future direction

Academic model	Framework model for direction
Teaching	Education
Service	Public Health
Research	Research
Patient care	Clinical practice

student performance. Documentation of each competency by course and evaluation methodology is required. The portfolio is one such mechanism for documentation and evaluation of student competence. For this reason the portfolio was incorporated within this text and its accompanying CD-ROM to document each student's professional development.

Another trend in higher education in general and specifically in dental hygiene education is *distance learning.* Continuing education may lead to career change and upward mobility. Individuals who want to pursue careers requiring additional education and skill development need flexibility in the procurement of this education. Technology has paved an avenue for those who cannot put aside job and family responsibilities to pursue education from institutions at a distance or on a school-established schedule.

Distance learning is available in dental hygiene. Video-conferencing and the use of the Internet have increased opportunities for those who wish to pursue a dental hygiene career. The use of these technologies now and in the future will change the way traditional dental hygiene education is delivered. Accredited dental hygiene educational programs are currently offering distance learning programs, and a listing of these can be obtained through the ADHA web site (see the suggested agencies and web sites near the end of this chapter).

Flexibility is characteristic of the portability of dental and dental hygiene licenses. The need for mobility in today's society has prompted change in state dental practice acts, affording professionals the option for licensure by credentials or reciprocity rather than requiring an additional examination of clinical skills.

The need for flexibility in today's mobile society has also created a number of regional licensing examination boards representing numerous states in each region. Some regional boards recognize and grant licensure to individuals licensed by other regional boards. At this time, only 12 states administer independent clinical licensure examinations. See Box 1-4 for a listing of state and regional boards.[2] The number of independent state *licensing exams* will probably continue to decline with a movement toward national licensure.

As dental professionals look toward the future, the concept of current clinical examinations for licensure will become passé. With the accountability of competencies established for educational institutions, the need for a clinical examination for licensure will no longer be necessary. Couple this action with a simulated national board examination, and only the need for a jurisprudence and ethical examination will be necessary for licensure. Ethics and law will continue to be the determining factors for licensure. Holding to a high ethical standard would make a dental hygienist less likely to perform functions that the professional is not competent to perform. Additionally, practicing outside the laws governing the dental hygiene profession would not be acceptable conduct of an ethical professional.

Clinical skills are taught, performed, and evaluated by each program, and students are deemed competent at graduation. The standards of competence and accountability are only as good as those who teach and evaluate students and those professionals who evaluate the accountability of educational programs and institutions. With the advent of this new pathway to licensure, dental hygiene faculty members would be given a greater responsibility for ensuring that those persons entering the profession are indeed competent healthcare professionals.

RESEARCH

Research has provided evidence to support practice of certain clinical preventive and therapeutic procedures and methods. Evidence-based research is not limited to clinical techniques but also may be used to support the best time and location for oral care delivery and the most economical methods for that delivery. Continued research across the breadth of oral care provides a basis for improved oral care delivery resulting in optimal oral and systemic health for all.

Further biological and immunological research provide the foundation for future clinical practice. Determining the presence of diseases, both oral and systemic, without invasive procedures may exist by simply obtaining saliva or crevicular fluid samples and may be part of the dental hygienists' future clinical practice. Markers for diseases have been noted in both fluids.

As technologies for identifying components of the immune system advance, markers for diseases will continue to be discovered. These discoveries will lead to further investigations of the presence of markers within saliva and crevicular fluids because they provide a noninvasive mechanism for diagnosis. The dental hygienist, the preventive professional providing direct patient care, is positioned with both scientific knowledge of the oral environment and systemic diseases to be the professional who screens for oral and systemic diseases by obtaining a sample of one or more oral fluids. This link in the healthcare system could indeed place the dental hygienist at the forefront of health care and the dental office as the first line to the healthcare system with referrals to the medical side of the system.

CLINICAL PRACTICE

Technology has changed every area of health care. In dental hygiene practice the use of computers for the demonstration of patient oral self-care has provided greater reliability than traditional techniques and paper records.[3] Patient recall of historical data often may be flawed, and clinician notes may be sketchy or incomplete. A permanent record of health history findings and clinical data maintained in a data base for future access assist the clinician in providing more efficient and effective patient care. Periodontal and dental chartings may be recorded at each visit and easily compared with previous findings for evaluation of oral conditions and assessment of oral risks, preventive and intervention strategies, implementation, and evaluation.

Maintaining clinical and radiographic images electronically reduces the need for physical storage space and provides a ready comparison for the assessment of disease and patient oral care needs. These same images also provide an excellent means of educating and motivating the patient to perform better oral self-care and accept the professional interventions needed to prevent further oral and systemic disease.

Could the oral healthcare provider possibly become the gatekeeper to entry into the healthcare environment? In other words, the person now known as the *dental hygienist, the preventive professional,* would become the individual who screens for diseases at supportive care intervals. Referrals to appropriate healthcare providers would be based on the results of such screening tests.

If the mouth is the portal through which the body receives nourishment, might it also hold the keys to help detect disease and monitor health? With this information in mind, who is more suited to screen, refer, and monitor patients than the oral care prevention specialist, now known as the *dental hygienist?* Perhaps the name of this professional would change to *health promotion disease prevention specialist (HPDP)* or a similar title that encompasses the expanded healthcare concept.

Patients would come in at regular intervals and, by way of either a saliva, plaque, or crevicular fluid sample, would leave the visit knowing whether they required further healthcare evaluations. The technology and science of dentistry are rapidly approaching the day when whole-health screening through an oral assessment will be a reality.

Dental hygienists currently screen for disease with vital signs; health histories; and clinical, periodontal, and radiographic examinations. This information is beginning to be used to link oral health status with total health but not to the extent that will be possible in the future.

Screening by dental hygienists does not mean that the provision of professional oral care would be delegated to another dental healthcare professional. It means that the role of the dental hygienist will expand to more fully use the special knowledge, skills, abilities, and commitment that these professionals already possess.

The ability to screen for total body health can be performed in many settings in which dental hygienists are currently employed. This function would have an impact on public health dentistry, with an increase in the need for more HPDP specialists. Moreover, the opportunity to reach a larger portion of the population with healthcare screening would revolutionize the nation's health and healthcare system. The result would be a healthier society—one in which illness and disease are diagnosed early, resulting in decreased morbidity and mortality.

PUBLIC HEALTH

Public health dentistry offers an exciting and challenging future. Providing access to care, determining oral needs, and providing preventive and restorative services to the half of the population who do not receive consistent oral care are indeed part of the challenges. Although fluoride has significantly reduced dental caries, this disease is still the most prevalent disease in society. Periodontal diseases are also prevalent and exist in some form and extent in nearly all adults. Both diseases are considered infectious and have multifactorial etiologies. Emerging knowledge about the etiology of each results in new innovations, prevention methodologies, techniques, and treatments. The dental hygienists' education includes content on the etiology, prevention, and treatment for these widespread diseases.

Historically, the public and the dental profession have looked upon these oral diseases as less serious than heart disease and stroke. Current focus, however, is on the relationship between oral and systemic disease. Imagine what the future holds for the prevention of systemic diseases and conditions such as heart disease, stroke, diabetes, and low–birth-weight babies. Could it be possible that prevention of caries and periodontal diseases could reduce and perhaps prevent life-threatening conditions?

This question gives those in public health dentistry and dental hygiene something exciting to explore. The public health dental hygienists could be the primary preventive healthcare professional. Programs once geared to prevention of oral disease could now focus on disease prevention and true whole-body health promotion.

School and community oral screening programs could expand to include other types of screening for those presenting with caries and evidence of gingival and periodontal concerns. Individuals could be referred for cholesterol and triglyceride screenings if the oral conditions related to systemic diseases were noted. Additionally, vital signs could be assessed to determine need for referral to a physician for follow-up. Integrating systemic and oral health into public health dentistry and dental hygiene creates an exciting future and integrates the dental hygienist into an interdisciplinary approach to health care.

THE FUTURE

What tools and methods are needed for a future that holds great promise for the delivery of preventive care, monitoring of disease, and provision of appropriate interventions and referrals? Well-educated dental hygienists are needed with knowledge of healthcare delivery, economics, and human needs. They must have well-developed communication skills, insight, and a commitment to capturing the opportunities that lie ahead. Dental hygienists are needed who believe that the oral environment is the portal to the body through which discoveries and advances in diagnosis and treatment of oral and systemic disease lie. Dental hygienists must present themselves as educated professionals to obtain respect within and outside the profession. Self-respect, values for health care, and continued competence are required to obtain respect from others. To embrace this future in health care, the successful dental hygienist will be one with the following:

- Vision to generate ideas, concepts, and strategies
- The ability to organize and implement strategies to see visions come to fruition
- Interpersonal skills to encourage, support, evaluate, provide mentoring, and question the visionaries

Leaders in the future of dental hygiene must possess sound self-assessment skills and a keen awareness that vision cannot materialize unless others value the vision and are willing to work. Leaders are required in research and administration, education, public health, legislation, and clinical practice. Leadership, personal insight, and commitment are necessary for dental hygiene and, more specifically, for the advancement of oral and systemic health care, resulting in a better quality of life for all.

Motivation and risk taking are part of the development and implementation of a vision. With today's tremendous scientific advances, this is an opportune time to continue developing the path set by earlier dental hygiene professionals. This is the time to embrace the vision of the future in health care by recognizing that the future lies in perhaps the yet-undiscovered components of the human body—the immune system in health and disease. As dental hygiene professionals support the continued advancement of technology and research to unlock the mysteries of human health, the future will be limited only by those professionals' vision and wisdom. Insight and commitment to make changes and seize opportunities that present themselves will prove to be vital to the dental hygiene profession. Dental hygiene is now established as an integral component of health care, and the dental hygienist is clearly a valued professional integral to the identification and prevention of oral and systemic diseases.

CRITICAL THINKING ACTIVITIES

1. Working in a small group, research trends or markers for future opportunities in dental hygiene education, clinical practice, public health, administration and management.
2. Projecting yourself to a future world of dental hygiene, imagine yourself at a conference with the authors from your textbook. For each of the following sections, what types of revisions/additions would you need to make as a result of *a change in technology, change in educational requirements, or a change in the role of the dental hygienist?*

Environmental Ergonomics
- Which chapters would change the most? The least?
- Would the chapter on exposure control be more or less relevant to the future dental healthcare worker?
- Judging from the pace of the change in workstation design from past years, will the future delivery be the way in which dental hygienists practice? What way(s)?

Anxiety and Pain Control and Operative Therapies
- Which of these sections would require the most revision? From what standpoint?
- Which of these chapters is more likely to be affected by changes in product development?

Patient Assessment
- Which chapters will require the most revision as the result of developments in technology? As a result of the potential role of the dental hygienist?
- Will the chapter on tobacco cessation be more or less relevant to the next generation of patients?
- Will the chapter discussing the clinical manifestations of common medications need to be increased or downsized?
- What role will new technology play in revisions to the chapter on supplementary aids?
- Will additional chapters need to be added to this section? If yes, what titles?
- Will any chapters need to be deleted from this section?

Care Modifications for Special Needs Patients
- Based on the human GENOME project, which of these chapters will need the most revision?
- Would you advise expanding this section? If yes, in what ways?

- Are there any chapters in this section that will no longer fit under this section title in that these types of patient needs will no longer exist? In that these types of patient needs are no longer "special" but exist on most all patients treated?
- What type of active role do you see in the future in caring for the head and neck cancer patient?

3. Using Chapters 29 and 48 as guidelines, develop a set of professional goals. Include a mission statement (what you feel passionate about in your professional career), a vision statement (what your role will look like now and then in 5 years), and specific goals. Remember that a goal is an accomplishment that can be measured in some dimension.
   Unclear goal statement: I want to be the best dental hygienist in the world. (This might serve as a mission statement, as long as the goal statements that follow can be measured).
   Clear goal statement: I want to maintain my dental hygiene licensure by attending appropriate continuing education courses. I want to share my knowledge with my office staff within two weeks after taking a new course. (This sets a specific measurable goal.)
4. You have been asked to define the ideal dental hygiene educator of the future. What qualities do you see will be necessary in assuming that role?
5. You have accepted the position as the President of the American Dental Hygienists' Association. As part of the role, you have been asked to address all the incoming dental hygiene students for the year (5 years from today's date). Your message will be beamed by satellite into every school of dental hygiene across the world, and downloaded to each student's personal laptop or palmtop computer. All students will hear your message at one time. What message would you like to deliver to them at this initial stage of their career paths? If you could tell them just one motivational element, one influence that has been an inspiration to you during your dental hygiene education, what would it be? What would you tell them to expect for their futures?

REVIEW QUESTIONS

1. Which of the following has had the greatest impact on the future of dental hygiene practice?
   a. Political association funding
   b. Patient needs
   c. Educational requirements
   d. Advancements in technology
2. The association between systemic and oral diseases is important to healthcare delivery, but the application of this knowledge should be in a private medical facility.
   a. Both parts of the statement are true.
   b. The first part is true, and the second part is false.
   c. The first part is false, and the second part is true.
   d. Both parts of the statement are false.
3. Leaders for future development need all of the following characteristics *except* which one?
   a. Insight and commitment
   b. Vision and self-assessment skills
   c. Willingness to work alone
   d. Respect for others
4. Identification of systemic diseases may be as simple as obtaining a saliva and/or crevicular fluid sample. This concept and process can increase the value of the dental hygienist within the healthcare environment.
   a. Both statements are correct.
   b. The first statement is true, and the second statement is false.
   c. The first statement is false, and the second statement is true.
   d. Both statements are false.
5. Which of the following are the most likely characteristics required of an individual to effect change?
   a. Compassion and integrity
   b. Insight and commitment
   c. Energy and a sense of humor
   d. Organization and support

 SUGGESTED AGENCIES AND WEB SITES

Because of the ever-changing nature of the Internet, some of the web sites listed here may have changed since publication. Please refer to Mosby's Evolve web site for the most current information.

American Association for Public Health Dentistry (AAPHD): http://www.aaphd.org
American Association of Dental Examiners (AADE): http://www.ada.org/prof/prac/licensure/lic-aade.html
American Dental Association (ADA): http://www.ada.org
American Dental Education Association (ADEA): http://www.adea.org

American Dental Hygienists' Association (ADHA): http://www.adha.org
American Society of Allied Health Professions (ASAHP): http://www.asahp.org
International American Association for Dental Research (IADR): http://www.iadr.org

 ADDITIONAL READINGS AND RESOURCES

Access
ADA Commission on Dental and Allied Dental Accreditation: *Accreditation standards for dental hygiene programs,* Chicago, 2000, American Dental Association.
Association of Schools of Allied Health Professions
Dental Education at the Crossroads
Journal of Community Dentistry and Epidemiology

Journal of Dental Education
Journal of Dental Hygiene
Journal of Dental Research
Journal of Public Health Dentistry
PEW Allied Health Professions
Surgeon General's Report 2000

 REFERENCES

1. ADA Commission on Dental and Allied Dental Accreditation: *Accreditation standards for dental hygiene programs,* Chicago, 2000, American Dental Association.
2. American Association of Dental Examiners: Listing of regional board examinations for licensure, reciprocity and licensure by credentials, Chicago, 2001, The Association [http://www.ada.org/prof/prac/licensure/lic-change.html].
3. Berthelsen CL, Stilley KR: Automated personal health inventory for dentistry: a pilot study. *J Am Dent Assoc* 131(1):59-66, 2000.
4. Scott B: Impact of the Human GENOME Project on oral health care, *Access* 15: 36-46, 2001.

ANSWER KEY

CHAPTER 1

1. **D** All of these components have changed in the last 100 years, but the need for better communication with patients is always present.

2. **B** Alfred Fones is attributed with having founded formal dental hygiene education. The three other individuals are important historical figures in the development of dental hygiene education and the profession, but they are not credited with the founding of the profession.

3. **B** More dental hygienists are employed in private general dental practices than in any dental specialty or other employment or job scenario.

4. **C** *Modified direct* is not a form of supervision identified in the chapter. Dental hygienists are licensed to practice under various forms of supervision, including *direct* and *general,* which this chapter discusses. *Independent* practice is another form of business in which a dental hygienist may work; however, this is rare.

5. **A** Although all of the items listed have some association with oral and systemic health, it is the immune components that are found in both systemic and oral health. These immune components are part of the body's immune response that maintains health.

6. **D** Dental hygiene programs are located in all of these institutions and must be accredited by the American Dental Association Commission on Dental and Allied Dental Accreditation.

CHAPTER 2

1. **E** All of the prevention methods listed have significantly reduced the incidence, prevalence, and severity of dental caries (see Box 2-1).

2. **C** Health is defined not only by physical aspects of disease or quality of life but by *all* aspects—physical, mental, and social well-being.

3. **D** In healthy, noncompromised oral tissues, pathogens within the oral cavity are overpowered by the body's natural immune system. If these common oral pathogens come into contact with compromised tissues, they have the opportunity to cause infection.

4. **A** Harald Löe defined periodontitis as the sixth complication of diabetes, as reported in *Diabetes Care* in 1993.

5. **F** Recent studies have linked periodontal disease as a causal factor to oral cancer; preterm, low–birth-weight infants; stroke; and diabetes.

6. **A** Dental caries is prevalent in 58.6% of children ages 5 to 17, compared with asthma, which is prevalent in only 11.1%.

7. **F** General health is reflected in oral health. Oral infections are linked to systemic conditions. The association between oral disease and systemic health is becoming more clearly defined. As reflected in Boxes 2-3, 2-7, 2-8, and 2-9, the poor and certain racial and ethnic groups have higher rates of dental problems.

CHAPTER 3

1. **D** Although informed consent may save a dentist or dental hygienist from an unfavorable judgment in a lawsuit, the true purpose of informed consent is to provide the patient with all material information necessary to make treatment decisions.

2. **B** Option A refers to contract law rather than tort law. For a patient/plaintiff to prevail in a lawsuit involving tort law, he or she must prove the following: (1) the dentist or dental hygienist had a duty to help (a professional relationship was established), (2) the duty was breached (lack of due care), and (3) as a result of the breach of duty the patient/plaintiff suffered actual harm or injury.

3. **B** Informed consent is required for risky or invasive procedures, not routine procedures such as dental examinations or routine prophylaxis. When informed consent is required, it applies to all patients being treated by the procedure, regardless of the person's age or competency.

4. **F** It is the duty of a healthcare provider to inform the patient of the treatment; alternatives to the recommended treatment, including the risks and benefits of alternatives; cost of treatment; prognosis of treatment; and the risks and benefits of no treatment, in terms that the patient understands.

5. **C** It is a well-established legal precedent that patients have the right to control decisions relative to their healthcare treatment choices. This is expressed as a *right to self-determination.*

6. **E** It is important to document *what, why,* and *how* treatment was provided to clearly communicate to any third party who reads the record. It is also critical for the person making the entry to have this information to ensure continuity of care.

7. **E** Although dental hygiene licensure is a matter of state statutory law, dental hygienists are also bound by federal, local, and common (case) law.

8. **C** Although exceptions are increasing, most states continue to regulate the practice of dental hygiene through a state board of dentistry.

9. **D** To avoid malpractice, all healthcare providers must minimally *meet* a basic standard of care when treating patients.

CHAPTER 4

1. **D** Clearly, Options A, B, and C discount the patient's affect. Option A will put Mr. Truman on the defense and assumes that he is fully knowledgeable of the need for the surgery. Option B, although it considers Mr. Truman's emotional state, labels his response perhaps inappropriately. Option C assumes that Mr. Truman is concerned about the potential pain involved in the surgery, which is also assumptive. Dr. Jones' empathy is indicated by the statement "Mr. Truman, you seem to be concerned about the surgery." Although Dr. Jones is assuming concern, the response also allows Mr. Truman to comment further. This form of active listening opens avenues

for even deeper discussion of Mr. Truman's concerns, whether they relate to pain, cost, time, or other issues.

2. **C** Options A, B, and D are harsh and punitive. They will make Ms. Buffington respond defensively. Option C recognizes the time demand for flossing regularly. It suggests that Ms. Buffington is doing well and can do even better at flossing regularly with more attention. This response is far more motivating than the other three.

3. **D** Effective communication is far from a passive process. It involves both the sender and receiver in a dynamic interchange. All senses are operating when communication is effective. Hearing seems to dominate the interaction, but subtle clues to meaning are picked up visually.

4. **E** Note the use of "I" statements in this message. In this example, the dental hygienist is taking accountability for her professional knowledge and beliefs. Understandably, this is a difficult situation for the hygienist, so "owning" the problem, so to speak, and using "I" statements is a powerful method to tackle uncomfortable issues. Although the other person may disagree, the message is clear. The dental hygienist is also being genuine, and the "I" message reinforces that value.

CHAPTER 5

1. **A** *Autogenous* refers to self-infection as a result of introducing a microorganism from one area of the body to another. This includes the bacteremia induced during subgingival scaling and is a concern because it may cause infective endocarditis in susceptible individuals. *Aerosol* or *droplet* refers to the transmission of microorganisms incorporated into materials that become airborne from a host source to a person or another host. This can be either cross-infection or autogenous infection (back to the source), however, *autogenous* is the specific term used by definition. *Direct* refers to the transmission of microorganisms from a specific person or source directly to another person or host. *Indirect* refers to the transmission of microorganisms from a specific person or source to an inanimate object (e.g., contaminated surface or item) and then to another person or host. Because the microorganisms leave the host, indirect transmission does not describe self-infection.

2. **D** The dose or quantity of microorganisms transmitted is a significant factor. Some are highly pathogenic in a small dose, whereas others require a large dose exposure before infection is likely. However, if the host has a resistance to the specific microorganisms, then the risk of infection is reduced. Host susceptibility is affected by the individual's general state of health and ability to resist infection. This can alter the impact of dose and virulence of the specific microorganisms. The virulence of a microorganism determines its pathogenicity, how infectious the organism is, and the conditions necessary for infection to occur. Virulence will have a great impact on the outcome of infection, however, it can be altered by dose and susceptibility. After exposure and transmission of pathogenic microorganisms, each of these factors has an impact on whether infection occurs. Altering any one or all of these factors can alter the course of infection.

3. **B** Candidiasis is caused by a fungal agent; hepatitis and influenza are caused by viral agents. Legionella and tuberculosis are caused by bacterial agents; pneumonia may be caused by either a bacterial or viral agent.

4. **D** Neither alcohol nor products approved for use as disinfectants are capable of sterilization. Some products approved as chemical sterilants can be used for disinfection if used according to manufacturer's directions for that purpose. Products approved only for use as disinfectants are not capable of sterilization.

5. **C** Correct terminology for hazard abatement strategies defined by the OSHA bloodborne pathogens (BBP) standard are *universal precautions (UP)*, *work practice controls (WPC)*, and *record keeping*. *Universal controls (UC)* is not a term used in the BBP standard.

CHAPTER 6

1. **C** The dental hygienist worked in an environment that required her to reach for the instruments, suction device, and air/water syringe. The stool was not designed for use at the dental chair. The entire work area was not ergonomically designed for dental hygiene procedures.

2. **A** Of the three syndromes identified by McKenzie, derangement syndrome is the most difficult to treat. At this stage, tearing of tissues has occurred and medical intervention is required.

3. **B** There are three normal curves in the spine when in proper static alignment.

4. **A** The spine has two lordosis curves in the lumbar and cervical regions and only one kyphosis curve in the thoracic region. The two lordosis curves are convex toward the anterior of the body, and the kyphosis curve in the thoracic region is convex toward the posterior of the body.

5. **C** The operator's head should be between 14-16 inches from the patient's oral cavity. Any further or closer positioning would indicate the operator either has not correctly positioned the operator chair or is leaning over the patient.

6. **D** The dental light should be at arm's length for maximum illumination of the oral cavity. This is approximately 36 inches from the oral cavity.

CHAPTER 7

1. **B** The design feature unique to sickle scalers is its two straight cutting edges and pointed toe. Curets have a rounded toe, although hoes have a beveled toe. Files have multiple cutting edges, and explorers have no cutting edges.

2. **A** Curets in general have rounded toes. However, a distinct difference between the cutting edges of universal curets and Gracey curets is that the universal curet has two *straight* cutting edges, whereas the Gracey curet has two *curved* cutting edges but only one usable edge.

3. **D** Explorers have no cutting edges, and hoes have only one cutting edge. Sickles and curets have two cutting edges, and files have multiple edges.

4. **D** Research has indicated that hollow handles permit improved transmission of vibrations to the clinician's fingers. The use of wider handles results in less finger fatigue because the grasp is lighter, which allows for improved instrument control.

5. C   Thicker shanks have increased strength, which prevents the instrument from flexing when heavy calculus deposits are removed.

6. E   In the modified pen grasp, the thumb and first three fingers have a specific placement on the instrument and a specific function to aid in proper handling and use.

7. D   A fulcrum or finger rest is considered a point of stability. Therefore it is designed to control clinician and instrument movements.

8. A   The modified pen grasp requires the index finger and thumb to be placed opposite each other on the handle of the instrument. Because these fingers do not touch one another, they are responsible for rolling the instrument to keep the toe against the tooth when activating an exploring, scaling, or root-planing stroke.

9. E   To engage a piece of calculus, the face of the working end should be just less than a 90-degree angle to the tooth surface. This angle provides maximum cutting ability for the working edge to remove the deposit.

10. E   Scaling strokes are designed to be short and firm to effectively remove calculus deposits. By engaging the edge of the deposit, the clinician can effectively remove the deposit piece by piece rather than attempting to remove the entire deposit with a shaving method. Overlapping strokes ensure the removal of the entire deposit.

11. E   An ultrasonic scaler is appropriate and often the instrument of choice for debridement.

CHAPTER 8

1. E   Sharpened instruments create an edge rather than a rounded surface. This edge enhances tactile sensation and calculus removal, and it bites into the deposit rather than gliding over it.

2. B   Instruments can become dull during treatment rendering them useless for calculus removal. By keeping sterile sharpening devices readily available, the clinician can sharpen as needed.

3. D   Before activation, the stone needs to be positioned to create an edge when moved across the lateral side. An angle of 100 to 110 degrees helps attain that edge.

4. C   The stone must be drawn in small portions across the cutting edge to maintain the curvature of the cutting edge. If the stone is laid against the entire cutting edge, the curvature will be lost and the cutting edge will be ineffective.

5. C   An edge has no surface and cannot reflect light. However, a dull edge has roundness and a surface that can reflect light.

6. B   By starting at a 90-degree angle, it is visually easier for the clinician to establish the 100- to 110-degree angle.

7. E   All of these principles are required to effectively sharpen a hoe. The hoe has one straight cutting edge that can lie flat against the stone. By angling the handle away from the stone, proper edge-to-stone contact is made to ensure the beveled toe is flat against the stone. Holding the instrument in a modified pen grasp with a finger rest assures stability of the instrument against the stone.

8. A   Because the universal curet has two straight cutting edges, the stone can lie against the entire length of the cutting edge. There is no curve to be maintained.

9. A   Only one cutting edge is used and sharpened on an area-specific curet. Therefore it is necessary to round the toe from the cutting-edge side.

10. B   An area-specific curet has a curved cutting edge. To maintain its curvature, the clinician should start the sharpening stroke at the heel and rotate around to the toe.

CHAPTER 9

1. C   Teenagers generally comply with healthcare recommendations if given a specific reason. Because appearance is important to many teenagers, if the dentist focuses on an improved beauty-related outcome, the likelihood that a teenage patient will adhere to a healthcare regimen increases.

2. B   The healthcare model presented in this chapter was based on the biological components of health and the impact that sociological and psychological issues have on the overall health status.

3. D   Oral health status can alter the perception of self either positively or negatively, depending on the patient's degree of health. If health is good, the person is likely to have a positive self-image. However, if patients have significant disease, they may have feelings of worthlessness, hopelessness, and general negative feelings about themselves. They also may feel out of control of their health (locus of control), which can have a negative impact on their well-being. Clearly visible dental disease has a negative impact during social interactions. A patient may experience embarrassment, withdrawal, and a diminished sense of self.

4. D   The core of anticipatory guidance theory is based on the need to anticipate patient needs. To do so the clinician should understand the patient's particular life circumstances and know what events in the various life stages affect health.

5. A   All of the other options can lead to early childhood caries (ECC).

6. D   Nonnutritive sucking provides children with a means to calm themselves and to control self-regulation and emotions.

7. E   Dental disease can cause persistent dental pain and therefore make it difficult to eat comfortably. This can lead to poor nutrition if the patient eats only soft foods, which are usually high in carbohydrates and sucrose. Additionally, dental disease often results in unsightly teeth, which may cause embarrassment in social situations.

8. E   It is well proven that alcohol consumption, illegal drug use, and poor nutrition during pregnancy increase the risk of abnormal fetal development, including improper development of the teeth.

9. B   Demanding a behavior change is ineffective for a patient of any age.
    A   Adolescents generally are self-focused and desire attention. By listening to the concerns of their adolescent patients, clinicians can show that they are interested in them.
    C   By expressing an interest in an adolescent's life outside the dental office, clinicians can demonstrate to the adolescent patient that he or she is important and that others can relate to him or her.
    D   Identifying something positive about the behavior of adolescent patients is a greater motivator than focusing on what they do poorly.

CHAPTER 10

1. **A** The essential elements of a health history are (1) patient identification (biographical data), (2) history of past and present illnesses (medical history), (3) history of present oral condition (chief complaint), (4) family history, (5) social history, (6) review of organ systems, and (7) vital signs. A full-mouth radiographic survey is an important component of a comprehensive *dental* examination.

2. **C** Dull, constant pain in the upper right molar is a description of the patient's present oral condition or the chief complaint. The use of glipizide (Glucotrol) by mouth for diabetes mellitus belongs in the past and present illness portion of the medical history; blood pressure of 180/98 is a vital sign; and a 40-year history of cigarette smoking is part of the social history.

3. **D** Age is a component of the patient identification (biographical data). Alcohol use, emotional status, occupation, and level of education are components of the social history.

4. **C** A prosthetic heart valve has a high risk for the development of infectious endocarditis, and thus it is imperative that patients with this condition be premedicated for invasive dental procedures. A history of rheumatic fever (with no rheumatic heart disease) and functional HM are classified as negligible-risk conditions; therefore premedication is not necessary for any dental procedures. A history of a myocardial infarction is not included in any of the stratified cardiac conditions for infectious endocarditis.

5. **D** The presence of the mycobacterium tuberculi in the sputum indicates that this patient has active TB. A positive PPD means the individual has been exposed to the TB organism; a positive PPD by itself does not imply that this individual has the disease. A history of taking isoniazid (INH) for 6 to 9 months is consistent with the prophylactic approach for a person younger than 35 who has been exposed to the TB organism but does not have the disease. A negative chest radiograph denotes that there is no damage to the lung tissue. (TB would result in visible areas of lung damage on the radiograph.)

6. **E** Fluorosis is related to the ingestion of fluoride at levels above the recommended level for caries control. This can be caused by fluoride supplements or naturally occurring sources of fluoride. Xerostomia, candidiasis, periodontal disease, and caries can all occur in patients with diabetes mellitus. These oral findings can be directly related to the metabolic and microangiopathy components of diabetes.

CHAPTER 11

1. **A** *Palpation* is the examination technique used to examine the structures of the neck, lymph nodes, thyroid gland, salivary glands, tongue, muscles of mastication, and the movements of the condyles. *Auscultation* is used to listen to the temporomandibular joint for crepitus or popping, to measure the blood pressure, and to assess for the presence of bruits in the carotid artery. *Percussion* is used to examine muscles, bones, and teeth. *Probing* in the dental setting refers to examination of the dental sulcus with a periodontal probe.

2. **C** The examination technique of palpation is used in examine the structures of the neck, lymph nodes, thyroid gland, salivary glands, tongue, the muscles of mastication, and evaluating the movements of the condyles. Auscultation is used to listen to the TMJ for crepitus or popping, measuring the blood pressure, and assessing for the presence of bruits in the carotid artery.

3. **B** The submandibular lymph nodes are reactive when there are inflammatory or neoplastic processes in the salivary glands, lips, buccal mucosa, gingiva, teeth, anterior palate, soft palate, and the anterior two thirds of the tongue. The structures associated with the submental nodes are the tip of the tongue, anterior floor of the mouth, anterior lower gingiva, and mid-lower lip. The jugulodigastric nodes are associated with the posterior tongue, posterior floor of the mouth, and maxillary lips. The mandibular nodes are associated with the mucous membranes of nose and cheek.

4. **B** The submandibular lymph nodes will be reactive when there are inflammatory or neoplastic processes in the salivary glands, lips, buccal mucosa, gingiva, teeth, anterior palate, soft palate, and the anterior two-thirds of the tongue. The structures associated with the submental nodes are the tip of tongue, anterior floor of mouth, anterior lower gingiva, and mid-lower lip. The mandibular nodes are associated with the mucous membranes of nose and cheek; and the jugulodigastric nodes are associated with the posterior tongue, posterior floor of mouth, and maxillary lips.

5. **B** In the midline of the neck lies the thyroid gland. The thyroid gland produces hormones that regulate the body's metabolic activities. Enlarged thyroid gland tissue may be clinically significant in the identification of patients with hyperthyroidism or hypothyroidism.

6. **D** The submandibular glands are located in the posterior part of the mandible and below the floor of the mouth (mylohyoid muscle). These glands are easily palpated even when normal. The ducts of the submandibular glands (Wharton's ducts) exit lingual to the anterior mandibular incisors.

7. **B** An infectious process results in an elevated temperature. The temperature elevation in temperature then causes an increase in the heart rate (5-10 beats/minute for each Fahrenheit degree increase in temperature) and an increase in the respirations (2-4/minute for each Fahrenheit degree).

8. **C** The correct sequence for the five A's of tobacco treatment are ask, advise, assess, assist, and arrange.

9. **B** Hypertension
   Stage 1: Systolic 140 to 159 or diastolic 90 to 99
   Stage 2: Systolic 160 to 179 or diastolic 100 to 109
   Stage 3: Systolic ≥180 or diastolic ≥ 110
   Do not provide elective procedures for patients at blood pressure Stage 3.

10. **A** Orthostatic hypotension is syncope brought on by a sudden change from the horizontal position to the upright position or by prolonged standing (peripheral pooling). Patients at risk for orthostatic hypotension are those who take narcotics, tranquilizers, or antihypertensive agents or those with diabetic neuropathy or Addison's disease.

CHAPTER 12

1. **E** Nicotine mimics acetylcholine, which is a neurotransmitter that works throughout the body. Pharmacological texts, nicotine replacement pharmaceutical product materials, and other references describe this general action in more detail.

2. **C** Option C is a conservative statement, in terms of the number of individuals exposed to nicotine who later develop dependence. More people who try nicotine become dependent—approximately half—compared with lesser percentages among those who try other substances.

3. **D** Nicotine is a peripheral vasoconstrictor. Indeed, the absence of or modest gingival bleeding often masks the development of serious periodontal problems.

4. **E** Almost daily, new evidence is reported about how smoking adversely impacts the quality of life. In dentistry, all aspects of patient care are affected to a higher degree among smokers.

5. **B** Evidence presented in both the 1996 Agency for Health Care Policy and Research clinical practice guideline, "Smoking Cessation," and in the 2000 Public Health Service clinical practice guideline, "Treating Tobacco Use and Dependence," makes it clear that the methods used—not the discipline of the user—are the key factor in effective treatment of those who attempt to stop tobacco use.

6. **C** The "attack" step is the exception. This chapter emphasized the use of a supportive approach, which requires the clinician to ask, advise, assist, and arrange.

7. **D** Option D is the only answer that lists the FDA-approved methods presented in this chapter but is not meant to be all-inclusive. For example, the nasal spray form of nicotine replacement therapy is not mentioned.

8. **E** Most people require multiple attempts to quit. The experience of relapse actually increases the chance of achieving long-term abstinence.

9. **B** The most critical contact should occur shortly after the quit date when individuals reach their peak withdrawal symptoms. Recovery from acute conditions, such as from toxic gases, is measured in days. Some effects, such as cognitive and motor functions, may require weeks to recover. A few effects, such as craving precipitated by environmental cues, may remain throughout life.

10. **C** The ADA does not associate with the tobacco industry.

CHAPTER 13

1. **C** *Leukoedema* is an abnormality found on the buccal mucosa that appears as a white filmy corrugated surface. *Leukoplakia* appears as a smooth white film. *Candidiasis* is a fungal infection that appears white and patchy and is associated with denture use. *Erythema multiforme* is initially a red-colored lesion that may ulcer.

2. **A** The *retromolar pad* is the area of tissue just distal to the most posterior mandibular molar. *Raphe* are located on the palate. *Tuberosity* is a bone prominence. *Buccal mucosa* is the internal lining of the cheek surface.

3. **D** After drying the surface of the buccal mucosa with gauze, normal salivary flow may be observed from the parotid and other minor salivary glands.

4. **E** Fordyce granules are associated with sebaceous glands, which are not located on the palate.

5. **C** Sublingual caruncles are located under the tongue along the sides of the lingual frenum and contain the *Wharton's duct,* which drains from the sublingual salivary gland. *Carabelli's duct* is a lingual cusp of the maxillary first molar. *Stenson's duct* drains from the parotid gland and is located on the buccal mucosa adjacent to the maxillary first molars.

6. **B** *Foramen cecum* is located on the dorsal surface of the tongue at the apex of the sulcus terminalis. *Mental foramen* is located on the mandible. *Sella turcica* is a depression located on the sphenoid bone. *Median lingual sulcus* divides the dorsal surface of the tongue in half.

7. **F** The gauze and air remove excess saliva, which allows a clearer intraoral observation. A mouth mirror allows retraction, and an overhead light provides intraoral illumination and visibility.

8. **D** *Linea alba* is a white line, which only appears parallel to the occlusal plane, often associated with trauma. *Leukoedema* appears as a white filmy corrugated surface on the buccal mucosa that disappears when the mucosa is stretched. *Candidiasis* appears white and patchy, typically on surfaces of denture-bearing tissues. Candidiasis is also evident in AIDS/HIV-infected individuals. *Lichen planus* is a plaquelike lesion that appears more generalized throughout the mucosal surfaces and skin.

9. **A** *Filiform*, the most numerous papilla, cover the dorsal surface of the tongue. *Fungiform* are smaller, mushroom-shaped papilla scattered throughout the filiform papilla. *Circumvallate* papilla, which are large and distinct, form a V-shaped line at the posterior of the dorsal surface. *Foliate* papilla are sparsely scattered on the lateral borders of the tongue.

10. **A** Rugae are located on the anterior portion of the palate, just posterior to the incisive papilla. The palatine fovea are small depressions located anterior to the vibrating line. The vibrating line separates the hard and soft palate.

CHAPTER 14

1. **B** *Erythema multiforme (EM)* is a disorder related to numerous factors, including exposure to antimicrobial agents. EM can occur at any age; however, it is more common in men who are in the second and third decades of life. *Lichenoid drug reactions* generally occur in older adults, and the oral presentation is not as severe or debilitating as EM. *Candidiasis* has a pseudomembranous form, atrophic form, and/or hypertrophic form. Ulcerative lesions are not consistent with candidiasis. The ulcerations caused by xerostomia generally are of traumatic origin.

2. **D** Prozac, to date, has not been implicated with gingival enlargement. Phenytoin (Dilantin), calcium channel blockers, and cyclosporine have a history of causing gingival enlargement.

3. **B** Pilocarpine is prescribed to increase salivary activity. Ibuprofen, fluoxetine (Prozac), and lisinopril (Zestril) all report xerostomia as an adverse effect.

4. **B** The gingival enlargement associated with the use of calcium channel blockers is reversible when the medication is no longer taken. The tissues return to normal within 8 weeks after the medication has been stopped.

5. **B** *Candida albicans* can be part of the normal flora. The organism is in a commensal relationship with the other normal inhabitants of the oral cavity. *Candida albicans* becomes a pathogen when the patient's immune status changes if there is an alteration of the normal flora caused by antibiotics, nutritional deficiencies, or anemias.

6. **C** Angioedema is a painless, nonpitting swelling of the face, cheeks, eyelids, lips, tongue, floor of the mouth, soft palate, uvula, and pharynx.

7. **C** Stevens-Johnson syndrome is the severe form of erythema multiforme (EM) characterized by skin lesions resembling EM, an associated stomatitis, and a severe conjunctivitis with visual impairment.

8. **A** Xerostomia is a dryness in the mouth that may be related to a decrease in the normal salivary secretions; however, xerostomia often is a subjective complaint that is not correlated to an actual decrease in salivary gland activity.

9. **A** According to Table 14-1, the most prescribed drugs are in the cardiovascular disease category. Of the responses, xerostomia is the adverse effect most often encountered.

CHAPTER 15

1. **B** The patient's clinical examination revealed generalized accumulations of plaque and calculus with accompanying pocket formation and bone loss, which are standard characteristics of adult periodontitis. She also stated increased spacing between her maxillary right central and lateral incisors, which indicates the presence of the disease for some time (chronic periodontitis).

2. **C** Occlusal trauma is a result of malpositioned teeth, including teeth not in occlusion, clenched teeth, and bruxism. This patient's health history should rule out pregnancy gingivitis and postmenopausal periodontitis. Aspirin-associated bleeding when probed is a result of chronic high doses of aspirin. Propanolol (Inderal) does not induce gingival overgrowth.

3. **C** When probing with 25 g of force, a probe tip with a diameter of 0.5 mm will penetrate into the junctional epithelium in healthy tissue and through the junctional epithelium and into the underlying connective tissue in inflamed gingival tissue.

4. **D** The *2N Nabors probe* has a curved shank with millimeter markings, which allows access to and measurement of furcations. A *Maryland/Moffitt probe* is straight and unable to access furcation areas. The *explorers* may be appropriate for calculus detection in furcation areas, but they have no millimeter markings and thus cannot provide measurements.

5. **B** A Class II furcation involvement, as noted on the periodontal chart by the solid triangle, is a loss of bone that extends underneath the roof of the furca approximately 3 mm horizontally.

6. **B** Tooth mobility Degrees 1 and 2 (as noted by the numeral printed on the crown of the tooth) are measured as movement in a horizontal direction. The numeral 3 indicates Degree 3, which includes movement when the tooth is vertically depressed.

7. **B** Based on the patient's health history, her mitral valve prolapse with no regurgitation or audible murmur may be classified as a functional murmur. Functional murmurs do not require premedication according to the American Heart Association's guidelines published in 1999. The patient's physician should be consulted to verify that the information provided by the patient is correct.

8. **D** To determine bone loss on a radiograph, the normal pattern of the alveolar crest must be identified on the radiographs. The normal crest of bone runs parallel to a line drawn between the cementoenamel junction (CEJ) of adjacent teeth. This line runs 1 to 1½ mm apically to the CEJs. Any deviation in this line indicates some bone loss. Now note the presence of radiolucencies in the furcations of the molars, which indicate bone loss. Using the crest of the interproximal/alveolar bone, determine the approximate depth of the bone loss in the furca areas. (The radiographic images of bone loss show less bone loss than there actually may be clinically.)

CHAPTER 16

1. **A** Healthy teeth are not sensitive, and the absence of a carious lesion does not mean that the tooth is healthy.

2. **A** Use of the explorer for caries detection is less than 60% accurate; accuracy is closer to 42%. Relying on the explorer for caries detection can be misleading in the pit and fissure areas, can potentially harm the smooth surfaces of the tooth, can damage newly erupted teeth and cause cavitations, and can spread pathogens to previously unaffected teeth.

3. **C** *Attrition* is tooth wear caused by tooth-to-tooth contact, and it occurs on the incisal and occlusal surfaces. An exogenous substance does not have to be present for the wear associated with attrition to occur. Loss of tooth structure caused by chemical action is called *erosion. Abfraction* is flexure at the cervical region of the tooth that causes mineral loss.

4. **A** *Abrasion* is the process of tooth wear caused by movement of a substance across the tooth surface during cleaning functions. Chemical wear is called *erosion,* and wear not caused by exogenous material is *attrition. Abfraction* is flexure at the cervical region of the tooth that causes mineral loss.

5. **C** The initial fluorosis-type lesion is seen clinically as a white spot on the enamel, but these spots are formed from increased levels of fluoride during the formation process with no demineralization of the enamel surface. The initial white spot demineralization of the tooth surface is evident as a result of the loss of tooth mineral that produces porosities in the tooth surface changing the way light is reflected through the enamel. Infusion of exogenous proteins into the demineralized enamel surface turns the white demineralization brown.

CHAPTER 17

1. **D** Exposure errors can affect the contrast and density of the film and decrease diagnostic quality. Technique errors can result in distortion and/or loss of structures, which makes diagnosis difficult. Selection of the wrong film series can result in incomplete diagnostic information.

2. **D** According to the criteria, this patient should have a posterior bitewing film series every 2 to 3 years because there is no sign of clinical caries and no high risk factors are present.

3. **C** A posterior vertical bitewing survey is appropriate for this patient. The vertical bitewing shows the most accurate view of the crestal bone and shows any remaining deposits.

4. **D** Film contrast is the difference between the dark and light areas on the film. Increasing the kVp increases the penetrating quality of the beam and results in a radiographic image with more shades of gray.

5. **C** When horizontal alignment is incorrect and the beam is not directed through the spaces in the teeth, the interproximal enamel of adjacent teeth are superimposed (overlapped) on one another.

6. **B** Foreshortening of the image is caused by vertical angulation that is too steep.

7. **A** An overhanging amalgam can trap food debris, plaque, and bacteria, which results in inflammation and ultimately bone resorption in the area directly below the overhang.

8. **B** Studies have shown that smoking increases bone loss in adult patients.

9. **D** The walls and floor of the maxillary sinus consist of bone and appear as a thin radiopaque line above the roots of the maxillary molar and premolar teeth.

10. **A** The charged-coupled device is an image receptor found in the intraoral sensor in some types of digital imaging systems.

CHAPTER 18

1. **B** A 3-to-7 day diet survey is more reflective of the patient's actual food consumption. A 24-hour recall does not contain the variety of foods that truly represent the patient's dietary intake. Evaluation of food texture provides only one tool by which caries risk can be evaluated. Evaluation of the type and frequency of carbohydrate consumption are also important to the dietary data collection process.

2. **B** Nuts, fats, and foods that contain xylitol are noncariogenic and may actually assist to prevent caries (see Box 18-3). Saccharin, although noncariogenic, does not provide caries protection. Raisins and peanut butter are retentive foods and may lower the plaque pH for more than 40 minutes.

3. **E** Depression and diabetes are treated with medications commonly known to contribute to xerostomia. A liquid diet reduces the amount of the patient's daily chewing action; therefore if the patient does not chew as much, salivary flow will be reduced.

4. **E** Infants require proper nutrition to supply calcium and phosphorus for bone and tooth mineralization. Osteoporosis in older patients is an indication that they have experienced bone loss as a result of the lack of calcium in their daily diets. Alcoholics consume many empty calories, and they do not ingest a balanced diet. Alcohol also affects the absorption and digestion of many nutrients. Pregnant and lactating women have increased nutritional needs. Their diet must be adequate to provide the essential building materials for the developing fetus or nursing infant and to protect and promote the oral health of the mother.

5. **A** The frequency of consumption and the physical form of fermentable carbohydrates pose the greatest demineralization potential of a posteruptive tooth. Vitamins, minerals, and proteins provide needed building tools to teeth in the preeruptive state.

6. **D** Although inadequate nutrition does not cause periodontal disease, optimal nutrition is associated with the host defense mechanisms. Therefore nutrition is a factor that influences periodontal disease severity and posttherapy healing time.

7. **A** The consumption of a fermentable carbohydrate causes a drop in the pH of plaque within 2 to 4 minutes.

8. **B** The consumption of a fermentable carbohydrate causes a drop in the pH of plaque within 2 to 4 minutes and can last for 20 to 30 minutes until the buffering capabilities of saliva return the pH to a neutral level.

9. **F** A dental hygienist should not try to eliminate all carbohydrates in a patient's dietary intake. Information should be tailored to each patient's individual needs. Nonnutritive sweeteners and sugar alcohols may not promote caries but can cause caries in patients with xerostomia. Both nonnutritive sweeteners and sugar alcohols contain a small amount of carbohydrate and, without the protective action of saliva, can create an acidic environment.

10. **B** Neutral pH of plaque is approximately 7.0. A fermentable carbohydrate lowers the oral pH to a critical 5.5, which allows enamel to demineralize.

CHAPTER 19

1. **A** A 105-mm macro lens allows a longer focal length for a better working distance and creates a more comfortable distance between the clinician and patient.

2. **E** A film speed of 100 or 200 is desirable for intraoral photography. A speed of 400 or 1000 is more sensitive to light.

3. **C** A pointlight is best used when shape, contour, and depth are important, such as in profile photographs or orthodontic anterior views.

4. **D** *Analog image storing* means that the image on the video monitor needs to be printed to be saved. Second-generation intraoral video imaging systems feed the analog output into a computer system for permanent image storage.

5. **A** Although the focal depth values are factory set for maximum clarity, a focal-length control ring is located on the wand handpiece to allow for one-handed focusing.

6. **E** All IPI systems have desirable qualities, and all of their functions should be evaluated for the clinician's specific use. Diagnostic quality of the resulting image should be the first consideration.

CHAPTER 20

1. **E** Each of the diagnostic aids listed in this question can be used to identify carious lesions.

2. **C** This statement describes diascopy. The other selections are diagnostic techniques that require a different type of examination.

3. **B** *Auscultation* is the process of listening for sounds that are emitted from the area being examined. The tooth does not emit sounds.

4. **B** The bitewing radiograph does not provide an image with much of the surrounding tissue. The intent of a bitewing is to view proximal surfaces of the teeth and interdental bone.

5. **C** *Transillumination* is a technique in which light is reflected with a mouth mirror through a thin surface to detect caries. This technique would not be appropriate to diagnose periapical or pupal infections.

6. **E** A profile of an anemic patient can include a decrease in red blood cells (RBCs), mean corpuscular volume (MCV), oral vasculature, and hemocrit.

7. **D** All laboratory values stated are within normal limits.

8. **B** Iron deficiency is not associated with the patient's ability to stop bleeding. The other selections are important in maintaining hemostasis.

9. E   Folate and B_{12} deficiencies are not associated with diabetes. All other conditions listed are associated with diabetes.

10. C   The use of selective pressure with a rubber wheel is the most definitive of the aids listed. A radiograph and electric pulp tester might be used to determine the problem with tooth #13. The signs and symptoms of this patient are those associated with cracked tooth syndrome.

CHAPTER 21

1. *A*   Mrs. Cronin needs a large-handled toothbrush because of painful arthritis and the dexterity issues with her hands. She also needs a small head to accommodate some of the more difficult-to-clean areas in her mouth, particularly in the posterior regions. A small handle would not be appropriate for her.

2. A   An important aspect of interdental cleaning is that the patient actually does it. Waxed or unwaxed, thick or thin, is of little importance as long as the technique is correct and the plaque is removed.

3. A   All the options are correct. Toothbrushes begin to show signs of wear within 3 months of use. If wear begins to show before that, the brush should be replaced. The brush should also be discarded after any illness.

4. B   Based on the patient's tight contacts and rotated teeth, waxed floss would slide between the contacts with less breakage and shredding than unwaxed floss. Woodsticks and proximal brushes would probably not fit interproximally.

5. *C*   A soft, nylon bristle is preferred for every patient.

6. D   Because of the anatomical considerations in Mrs. Cronin's oral architecture, helping her to properly angle the toothbrush to be certain the bristles reach the sulcular area would be the best idea. Ideally, using a sulcular brushing technique would be the best recommendation. Given her lack of dexterity, however, the next best solution is to observe and correct the tooth-brushing method.

7. B   The Fones' method is preferable for a young child. Children do hot have the dexterity or cognitive abilities to understand angulations or to perform the techniques required with more sophisticated brushing methods.

8. *A*   Since Peter likes to use a wooden toothpick, it is important to assist him in its proper use to avoid tissue damage and to ensure thorough plaque removal. Changing his interproximal cleaning method to one of the other choices may be counterproductive.

CHAPTER 22

1. D   Tooth mineral is a highly soluble carbonated apatite. The carbonate ion *does not* strengthen the enamel, but it makes it soluble to acids in the environment.

2. A   The hydroxide ion is substituted by the fluoride ion to form fluorapatite, the most resistant of each of the minerals to dissolution by acid.

3. A   Both statements are true. The actions of fluoride are both antibacterial and anticariogenic. Fluoride in quantities greater than prescribed can produce acute illness and even death if the quantity is great enough. The amount of fluoride in water supplies is regulated, as is the percentage and quantity in other oral care products.

4. A   Placing a restoration in a carious lesion is a surgical intervention to stop the caries process in that tooth only and with that lesion. The restoration makes the tooth functional again. The restoration does not provide a reduction in the bacteria responsible for caries development; therefore another intervention must be adopted to reduce the bacterial load for caries control.

5. B   The antibacterial effect of fluoride inhibits the bacterial plaque, and the anticariogenic effect is responsible for the decrease in the demineralization process while it aids in the remineralization process. Fluoride has no effect on stain reduction of the enamel surface.

6. B   Demineralization is caused by a low pH of 5.2 or below. A high pH is not acidic but basic and is not responsible for demineralization. The teeth are constantly going through the process of demineralization and remineralization given the changes of salivary pH throughout the day.

7. B   Salivary proteins are present in the pellicle. These proteins and minerals consist of calcium, phosphate, fluoride, and bicarbonate that buffer acids. Antifungal and antibacterial components and immuno-globulins are also present in salivary proteins.

8. D   Small molecules and ions are driven along a concentration gradient by passive diffusion into the porous enamel. These ions and minerals consist of calcium, phosphate, fluoride, and organic acids. Demineralization occurs when the enamel is dissolved by the influx of the organic acids onto and within the enamel surface.

9. C   Saliva is correct because it is filled with not only fluoride ions but also phosphate, calcium, immunoglobulins, and other anticariogenic and antibacterial components.

10. C   Dental caries is an infectious, multifactorial, site-specific disease that is transmissible from mother to child and is measured by use of the DMF index in the population. Dental caries cannot spread from the inside of one tooth (iatrogenically) to another site.

11. B   Caries is caused by several factors. Bacteria (MS and LB) must be present for the carious process to develop. If these bacteria were present in one strain of animals when placed with the other group without caries, the bacteria were spread to the unaffected group through salivary contact.

CHAPTER 23

1. B   Controlled studies have been conducted on anti-gingivitis, anticaries, and antisensitivity agents but not on the development of periodontitis. Although gingivitis is a precursor to periodontitis, not all gingivitis turns into periodontitis; therefore controlling for effects is more difficult.

2. **C** A dentifrice is either in paste, gel, or powder form because of the abrasive contents. A rinse does not have an abrasive effect.

3. **C** Flavoring agents, detergents, and preservatives are the components within dentifrices that have been found to cause allergic reactions.

4. **C** The Council on Scientific Affairs administers the ADA's Seal of Acceptance.

5. **C** The FDA requires manufacturers to provide evidence of no carcinogenicity, no allergenicity, and proof of effectiveness for approval to market.

6. **B** The type of group in which one product ingredient is compared with another is a *superiority study*. A large clinical trial of this sort is not a pilot study because of the study's size.

7. **C** Stannous fluoride has been found effective in the prevention of caries, dentinal sensitivity, and gingivitis. It has not been found to decrease salivary flow.

8. **C** The most effective anticalculus ingredient to date is 3.3% pyrophosphate, which is found in three forms: tetrasodium, disodium dihydrogen, and tetrapotassium.

9. **D** All of the salts listed are included in some antisensitivity formulations except sodium bicarbonate.

10. **A** Nonperoxide tooth whiteners found in dentifrices are formulations of mild abrasives with a tartar-control ingredient.

CHAPTER 24

1. **C** Although none of the other options is actually wrong, C is the preferred answer. If the patient will do the therapy, pulsed irrigation is the simplest method of the choices provided. *Option A:* Ms. Tevus can probably do more for herself at home to improve her plaque control. She is too busy to have to return to the office every 2 months, which also increases the expense of her care. *Option B:* Taking a culture is an option but also raises the expense of care. Although Ms. Tevus would need to purchase a pulsed irrigator, pulsed water irrigation may stop the bleeding without any further intervention. *Option D:* Nonsurgical care and daily, good home care are effective on probe depths ≥5mm. However, if her periodontal condition continues to worsen, a periodontal referral and a medical check-up may be necessary. Tooth #7 needs additional care and may require referral again, but this question is only concerned about her bleeding problem in general.

2. **B** A sufficient amount of plaque arouses suspicion that the bleeding is plaque-associated, but do not discount the possible effect of stress on Ms. Tevus. *Option A:* The reported symptoms do not include pain, ulceration, or a particularly descriptive aspect of the tissue, such as cratering. *Option C:* This case provided no description of linear gingival erythema, nor did the health history reveal any problem, such as HIV infection, that could contribute to this choice. *Option D:* Her health history and age, the quantity of plaque, and the disposition of her gingivitis do not indicate a sex hormone influence.

3. **A** Her plaque index is higher than acceptable. *Option B:* Nothing indicates that Ms. Tevus is not trying at home; indications are only that her efforts are not sufficiently effective to control bleeding. *Option C:* Her health history does not reflect an immunocompromised system. *Option D:* This may be a subtle reason—but not the obvious reason—for the reduced host resistance and the increased bleeding.

4. **B** Ms. Tevus first needs to try daily marginal irrigation. She can do this at home. *Option A:* Supragingival irrigation may not reach far enough into the pockets but does provide some help if marginal irrigation is too difficult for the patient. There is every reason to think Ms. Tevus can perform marginal irrigation. *Option C:* Subgingival irrigation usually refers to professional administration of an antimicrobial.

5. **D** When water irrigation is able to control bleeding, it is the easiest, most economical method and has no side effects. Always recommend the most innocuous agent first.

6. **A** Chlorhexidine is the current gold standard for antimicrobial irrigation. In this question an essential oil was not provided as an option, but this would certainly be another reasonable step if oral irrigation with water is still not adequate. Essential oils do not require a prescription, yet chlorhexidine does, so essential oils are more accessible for patients because they are less expensive and easier to obtain. *Option B:* Because the patient has no evidence of root decay, an irrigant with a fluoride is probably not needed. *Options C and D:* Site-specific therapy is not recommended because the bleeding is still rather generalized.

7. **A** This is the preferred answer in the order listed. None of the others are incorrect procedures; it is the sequence of care that is important. In reality, when the patient continued to exhibit bleeding and gingivitis problems, intervention with irrigation and then chemotherapeutics should have been considered at least 1 year earlier. *Option C:* Because irrigation has not been used, it is prudent to see its effect on tooth #10. Also, debridement is necessary at this appointment because the patient may have a local irritant, such as calculus or a popcorn husk, in the pocket. Because Ms. Tevus received professional debridement regularly, calculus with its accompanying plaque should not be the cause of the flare-up. Additionally, the location and shape of the cingulum and lingual groove on this tooth, and on the tooth itself, should be reevaluated. *Option D:* If oral irrigation and chemotherapeutics do not reverse the trend Ms. Tevus has experienced since surgery, she should be referred back to the periodontist.

8. **C** More research is indicated to determine the effect of fluoride irrigation on inflamed or debrided pockets. *Option A:* Tetracycline is effective as an irrigant but requires a period of 5 minutes of continuous flooding of the area to produce an antimicrobial effect. *Option B:* Chlorhexidine is the gold standard for irrigants, but better results are achieved when used daily rather than professionally. *Option D:* Water is innocuous when used professionally. It is in a pulsed system that is used daily and that yields positive results.

CHAPTER 25

1.   **D**   The facial surfaces at the cervical region of the tooth are most sensitive from various forms of stimuli. This is caused by dentin exposure from gingival recession, abrasion, erosion, and abfraction, most of which are more prevalent on the facial surfaces and affect the cervical region of the tooth.

2.   **D**   Periodontal instrumentation, surgery, and cosmetic polishing all have the potential to cause dentinal sensitivity. Periodontal probing does not cause dentinal sensitivity, although in cases of dentinal sensitivity, probing may produce a painful stimulus.

3.   **C**   Several factors are responsible for *dentinal sensitivity,* such as abrasion, erosion, abfraction, gingival recession, certain periodontal procedures, defective restorations, and dental caries. Stimuli responsible for eliciting a *painful response* are thermal, tactile, chemical, or osmotic.

4.   **A**   Although interfering with the nerve fibers at the dentinal-pulpal junction is believed by some to be the mechanism of action of potassium nitrate, it is not the most accepted theory for the effectiveness of desensitizing agents. Occlusion of the dentinal tubules is the most accepted theory.

5.   **C**   When plaque-control measures are improved, acid within the plaque that precipitates dentinal sensitivity is reduced or removed, which results in less sensitivity. Individuals who have been controls in experimental studies have had reductions in dentinal sensitivity. This has been attributed to the placebo effect.

CHAPTER 26

1.   **A**   Mechanical bonding results when the resin sealant material becomes physically entrapped within the widened enamel pores. The application of a phosphoric acid solution removes inorganic materials and creates micropores that increase the surface area of the enamel to form a strong bond between the resin and the enamel.

2.   **D**   Clinical research has shown sealants to be effective when adequately evaluated, maintained, and replaced. Research has shown that early carious lesions can be safely arrested. Research regarding the use and effectiveness of sealants as a cost-effective preventive measure is overwhelming when compared with the cost and time required for operative treatment.

3.   **C**   Air polishing used during a regular prophylaxis has been shown to increase the amount of wear on resin sealants. Air polishing can create resin surface roughness, leading to future material breakdown. The amount of wear is increased with the time and exposure to air abrasion.

4.   **A**   A routine clinical evaluation is necessary to determine whether resealing of teeth is necessary in cases of sealant loss caused by poor retention. This issue is reflective of the sensitivity with the technique used to apply sealants to the surfaces of teeth. Any form or amount of moisture contamination can influence the overall effectiveness and resultant use of a sealant. Short-term sealant loss is often a result of technical application error rather than inadequate mechanical bonding. The inability to maintain a dry field is the most frequent reason sealants fail; poor isolation and improper acid-etching contribute to short-term loss.

5.   **E**   Inadequate enamel preparation increases the chances for marginal leakage and stains. Contamination of the field allows for marginal microleakage that leads to material breakdown and extrinsic stain trapping. Excessive material placement provides an area for the accumulation of plaque and stain. The stress from occlusion forced at the marginal sites allows the material to flex, which leads to marginal breakdown.

6.   **B**   If replacement of sealant materials becomes necessary as a result of inadequate bond strength or wear, any residual sealant material should be removed if possible, then the tooth should be cleansed, etched again, and treated by placing and curing new resin. Cleansing oils and fluoride ions have been shown to inhibit the mechanical bond between the resin and the enamel pores if applied too early in the sequence of treatment.

CHAPTER 27

1.   **E**   Prevention is not limited to the prevention of dental caries and periodontal disease. Primary care prevention should also include the prevention of traumatic dental injuries through the use of proper protective equipment and recognizing and reporting of suspected child abuse and neglect.

2.   **A**   Time is the most critical factor in successful reimplantation of avulsed teeth. This is directly related to the maintenance of the viability of the periodontal ligament cells.

3.   **C**   Percussion only increases the traumatic insult to the already traumatized tooth and does not yield any useful diagnostic information.

4.   **D**   Oral self-care is essential for the successful reattachment of tissue. Bacterial plaque must be removed even though the tissues may be tender. This is accomplished through the use of a soft toothbrush and is enhanced with an oral rinse.

5.   **C**   Prevention is the key. An athlete is more likely to use a properly fitted mouthguard than one that is ill-fitting, causes gagging, inhibits speech, or obstructs breathing.

CHAPTER 28

1.   **D**   Commercial denture cleansers contain powerful bleaching agents (sodium hypochlorite and sodium perborate) that leave a dull gray deposit on the chrome-cobalt framework of partial dentures if the prostheses are left in the solution for more than 15 minutes a day.

2.   **B**   Many patients find objectionable the somewhat metallic aftertaste of stannous fluoride products, which is caused by tin ion.

3.   **B**   Although the introduction of a fluoride product raises the fluoride concentration throughout the mouth, this patient should use the carrier on the mandibular arch, because this is the location of the teeth most susceptible to root caries, and these teeth need the most intense exposure to fluoride.

4.   **B**   Splint bars often are in direct contact with the adjacent oral mucosa, either because they were designed this way or because poor oral hygiene leads to edema. Unless the patient has been educated on the use of a floss threader or an interproximal cleansing brush, the surface of the bar adjacent to the soft tissue will probably harbor undisturbed plaque that irritates the mucosa.

5. **D** Saliva possesses antifungal and buffering properties; it is an effective lubricant. In a patient with a denture who has a dry mouth, candidal infection is likely to occur because the commensal pathogens are not inhibited from proliferating. The lower oral pH caused by the absence of acid buffers is favorable for candidal growth. The soft tissue, traumatized as the denture shifts against it, is more prone to irritation by the metabolic by-products of the fungal colonies.

6. **D** The patient displays healthy gingival tissue despite his dry mouth; he clearly is effectively controlling plaque with his current regimen. His fixed bridgework likely necessitates use of an interproximal cleaning aid or a floss threader anyway—and the more complex regimens are, the less likely they are to be followed than straightforward ones. The patient displays functional limitations (as a result of hand and shoulder arthritis) that impair his abilities to floss.

CHAPTER 29

1. **B** Understanding each patient's unique clinical, biological, psychological, and sociological needs is critical to plan and implement appropriate therapeutic strategies. Prevention needs are individualized; however, clinicians do build from the knowledge base and increase patients to a level of understanding appropriate to their needs and abilities. Meeting expressed patient needs can increase compliance; however, it is not the basis of appropriate care planning.

2. **D** Oral risk assessment holds to the principles of health promotion (see also Chapter 2) and obviously, to the principles of risk and risk assessment. Based on the findings, intervention and prevention strategies are designed.

3. **D** Although insurance coding is based on the therapy provided, a system-based gathering tool will not aid in predetermining which insurance codes to use.

4. **D** Patient assessment includes the review of *all* forms of patient data to complete the assessment phase of the ORA System.

5. **B** The concern surfaced in the listing of medications that can cause gingival hyperplasia—not because the patient reported a symptom or because the symptoms were clinically evident. This concern is further addressed in Chapter 30.

6. **E** Bleeding on probing is not a clinical evaluation tool for any of these listed conditions.

7. **A** The type of diet indicated in the patient example is most consistent in leading to an oral risk concern of caries. This information coupled with the clinical and radiographic findings indicates an oral risk concern (actual) for root caries and a potential for coronal caries.

8. **A** Although intervention and prevention can indeed be defined exclusive of one another, they can and do overlap in both the design of intervention strategies and the personalization of prevention strategies.

9. **E** Discussing the oral manifestations of current prescription medication is an example of personalization of a prevention plan, not of a therapeutic intervention. Remember, the patient in the case study did not have any oral manifestations from current prescription medications.

10. **B** Both the statement and rationale are false; planning patient care *is* a complex process and is *not* built on the application of a standard set routine for patients.

CHAPTER 30

1. **E** Personalizing patient instruction is the cornerstone of prevention strategy today and is vitally important to both the patient and the clinician.

2. **C** The steps of the ORA process are *review, analyze, plan, recommend,* and *evaluate/reevaluate.* Step 4 is *recommend.*

3. **D** It is critical to review all aspects of the oral care process: therapeutic intervention; prevention strategies; patient understanding, appreciation, and compliance; and outcomes.

4. **E** The only oral risk concerns for the patient example are an increase in plaque and gingival hyperplasia.

5. **D** Raising someone's awareness of an oral concern (a strategy) can occur through demonstration, discussion, example, or a variety of methods. For the case presented in the chapter, the patient needs to be made aware that the medication she takes has several potential oral side effects.

6. **E** The history and data provided for this patient do not validate any of the factors listed.

7. **B** Any therapy initiated should be completed to facilitate better wound healing, and reevaluation should occur as soon as possible after initial therapy.

8. **E** Any demonstration, either within the mouth or a visual aid, that supports an understanding of the signs and symptoms of gingival disease meets this goal. However, pointing out areas of stain does not directly speak to this goal.

9. **E** Although clinician satisfaction can be enhanced through the use of an organizational tool such as ORA, it is not a measure or step in the system.

10. **D** All of these factors are important and must be considered in the personalization of the oral care plan to ensure optimal oral health. All factors, when evaluated together, provide the basis for the personalization of prevention strategies.

CHAPTER 31

1. **B** Only magnetostrictive instruments have an insert with a metal stack. The sonic and piezoelectric tips screw on, and a manual instrument is not a powered instrument.

2. **A** *Lavage* is the process of providing water or chemotherapeutic to the area during debridement with an ultrasonic instrument. All other selections can cause either gouging of the tooth surface or damage to the pulp, resulting from excessive heat generation.

3. **B** Before placement of the tip, the water line should be bled of air bubbles so the stack properly cools and heat buildup is reduced during activation. Final adjustment of water flow and power settings occur after the insert has been placed.

4. **C** The 4910 code is used for patients who return for periodic (every 3 months) supportive periodontal care. This code also includes the examination, oral hygiene instructions, and polishing. The other codes listed are used in supportive care treatments but for different situations.

5. **C** Magnetostrictive and sonic instruments are less powerful or have fewer cycles per second than piezoelectric-powered instruments. The piezoelectric instrument functions up to 50,000 cps, whereas the maximum for the sonic instrument is 8000, and the magnetostrictive instrument is 45,000.

6. **D** The powered instrument tips function best when angled close to 0 degrees but not exceeding 15 degrees. There is no cutting edge as is found on manual instruments, which require a specific angulation for debridement.

7. **B** *Microstreaming* is an action that occurs within the water as it surrounds the activated tip. The cavitational action that occurs as water hits the tip produces the microstreaming that surrounds the tip. It is this action that destroys bacterial cell walls.

CHAPTER 32

1. **D** All of the suggested polishing agents are indicated for Mr. Smith. Air-powder polisher is appropriate for stain removal on lingual and palatal surfaces with heavy stain. Coarse prophylaxis paste may also be used for these surfaces. Diamond polishing paste is indicated for polishing aesthetic restorations on maxillary anterior facial surfaces.

2. **C** Anterior aesthetic porcelain surfaces should be polished first with diamond polishing paste. This can then be followed by coarser paste for the remaining surfaces or the air-powder polisher. Aesthetic restorations should always be polished first to reduce the possibility of coarse abrasives that remain in the rubber cup, which is likely to scratch the aesthetic surface.

3. **A** Mr. Smith's stain classification is considered environmental exogenous because it is most likely attributed to his smoking. Developmental endogenous tetracycline stains are also present but have been cosmetically treated with facial porcelain veneers placed on teeth #6 to #11.

4. **C** Asthma and other respiratory illnesses are a contraindication for the use of air-powder polishing because of the amount of aerosols produced by the procedure. Diabetes, mitral valve prolapse, and chronic migraines are not included in the list of health concerns associated with air polishing.

5. **A** Green stain is a stain acquired from chromogenic bacteria and gingival hemorrhage that forms on the external surface of the tooth near the gingival hemorrhage.

6. **D** Factors that determine the abrasiveness and polishing potential of an agent include particle size, shape, hardness, and concentration.

7. **B** Reduce the speed of the engine polisher and make sure there is plenty of paste in the rubber cup. All others options listed actually increase the frictional heat on the tooth surface.

8. **C** Disadvantages of the porte polisher are that the technique requires considerable hand strength and control and is a slow, tedious process.

9. **B** Polishing of unexposed root surfaces produces a therapeutic effect because it is done to remove toxins from the unexposed root surfaces, which should result in a decrease in disease parameters.

CHAPTER 33

1. **D** Gut sutures are categorized as natural absorbable sutures and are digested by body enzymes and macro-

phages. In contrast, synthetic absorbable sutures are broken down by hydrolysis, a process whereby water penetrates into the suture and contributes to its breakdown.

2. **C** Black silk sutures were used to closely adapt the free soft tissue graft to its underlying nutrient supply and to help stabilize the graft.

3. **B** Nonabsorbable silk sutures are commonly used in dentistry because of their exceptional handling characteristics, including flexibility, pliability, easy manipulation, and superior knot-holding capability.

4. **E** Although no one suture material is considered perfect for every dental need, the ideal suture material inhibits bacterial growth and adverse tissue reactions, maintains strength with decreasing size, is comfortable and easy to manipulate, can be sterilized and conveniently packaged, knots easily, is not adversely affected by products within the oral cavity, and is noncarcinogenic and nonallergenic.

5. **A** Literature has documented that eugenol-containing periodontal dressings contribute to delayed healing, inflammatory/allergic reactions, and tissue necrosis. Therefore modern periodontal dressings are usually formulated as noneugenol-containing products.

6. **D** The use and selection of a periodontal dressing is a personal choice of the dental healthcare worker. Ideal periodontal dressings set with dimensional stability, allow easy manipulation, taste acceptable, are nonirritating and nonallergenic, and discourage accumulation of debris and bacteria.

7. **A** The continuous interlocking suture used in case study #2 incorporates both the facial and lingual flap into the suturing technique and the primary closure of the mesial and distal edentulous ridge adjacent to the remaining molar.

CHAPTER 34

1. **E** All of these behaviors and conditions are characteristic of individuals who have dental fear. Fearful individuals are more likely than individuals without fear to cancel appointments on short notice, to appear indifferent, to avoid preventive care, and to display poor oral health status.

2. **C** Assessment of the patient's anxiety through the use of a valid and reliable dental anxiety inventory or questionnaire is the first step in treatment. Many questionnaires are formulated to ascertain a patient's level of anxiety and to determine a patient's anxiety-provoking stimuli. Questionnaires also identify which anxiety reduction strategy to use.

3. **A** Children between the ages of 3 to 5 do not have the cognitive ability to understand detailed explanations nor to engage in paced breathing. Coaxing is not recommended for children. Because children learn by watching others, modeling is the most effective strategy for a mild-to-moderately anxious 3- to 5-year-old child. The most effective model is a peer of the same age.

4. **B** In systematic desensitization, a hierarchy of fear-producing situations related to the specific fear is generated. Starting with the least feared stimulus, patients gradually progress through all items in the hierarchy while maintaining a relaxed state, which eventually enables them to effectively cope with the previously feared situation.

5. **C** The interpersonal relationship between the patient and provider has the greatest effect on the patient's perceptions of the oral care experience. Once rap-

port and trust have been established, detailed information about the proposed treatment can assist with anxiety reduction and continued development of the patient-provider relationship.

CHAPTER 35

1. **C** Persons with a deficiency of pseudocholinesterase cannot hydrolyze ester-type local anesthetics and would have an increased probability of toxicity. A history of hypertension or a previous hysterectomy do not preclude the use of an ester-type local anesthetic. This patient currently takes captopril, which has no effect on ester-type local anesthetics.

2. **A** Epinephrine is a vasoconstrictor and increases blood pressure. An anesthetic agent with a low concentration of vasoconstrictor was selected because of the patient's history of hypertension. A previous hysterectomy, deficiency of pseudocholinesterase, and current medications (captopril) do not prevent the use of epinephrine.

3. **D** Patient anxiety is the only factor that could cause the patient to feel faint.

4. **A** The vasoconstrictor, epinephrine, is added to the local anesthetic solution to prolong the depth of anesthesia. Epinephrine would not increase the toxicity of the local anesthetic and would have no effect on the pH of the injection area. Epinephrine does not reduce patient anxiety.

5. **A** Local anesthetic must be in the free base form (nonionized form) to have nerve-blocking effects. Infection produces acidic products that lower the pH, and the amount of the effective form of the drug is reduced. The low pH of the infected area keeps the drug in the salt form (ineffective form).

CHAPTER 36

1. **B** Quadrant II is the maxillary left quadrant, and all five of the injections listed in Option B are necessary to fully anesthetize this quadrant.

2. **B** Because the average insertion depth is approximately 16 mm, a short needle is used to avoid overinsertion, which increases the risk of hematoma. A 25- or 27-gauge needle are the gauges of choice that provide the best results when aspirating to avoid intravascular injection. 25-gauge short is not listed as a choice in this question; therefore 27-gauge short is the best choice.

3. **D** In a small number of patients, ingredients in the topical anesthetic solution, such as benzocaine or flavorings, may cause sloughing of tissues in the area of placement.

4. **D** A complete chart entry should include date, type of anesthetic and amount, vasoconstrictor and amount, injections given, any or no reactions, and a signature.

5. **B** Option B acknowledges the patient's anxiety and provides empathetic reassurance that all will be done to make the procedure comfortable without promising that it will be pain-free.

6. **D** Increased heart rate is a symptom of an intravascular injection of a solution that contains a vasoconstrictor.

CHAPTER 37

1. **B** The scavenging nasal hood cannot prevent waste gas from being eliminated when the patient is talking.

2. **A** This is one source of waste gas that cannot be controlled with the equipment. The operator must inform the patient to breathe through the nose and refrain from talking.

3. **D** Because nitrous oxide is nonirritating to mucosa, it does not initiate asthmatic attacks.

4. **C** The reservoir bag expands and contracts concurrently with the patient's inhalations and exhalations.

5. **C** Nitrous oxide is almost completely eliminated via the lungs. No significant amount of the drug is metabolized in the body.

6. **D** When assessing recovery, the patient must feel normal. Continue to administer 100% oxygen until the patient reports "feeling fine." Postoperative vital signs also must be within close range of preoperative values.

7. **C** It is always recommended to follow manufacturers' instructions regarding their specific equipment; however, a general guideline of 2 years has been suggested for equipment evaluation.

8. **B** Recirculating ventilation systems only move the air to another area within the office and do not effectively remove the trace gas.

CHAPTER 38

1. **C** By definition, a Class II lesion/restoration is located on the proximal surface of a posterior tooth.

2. **C** The development of new dental materials has afforded dental clinicians the opportunity to be much more conservative of natural tooth structure in the restorative process. Options A, B, and D are all results of this more conservative approach. Only Option C is the result of a less conservative, "traditional" dental cavity preparation technique.

3. **A** By definition, amalgam is an alloy of mercury with any other metal. Silver (50%-70%) and tin (15%-30%) generally represent the largest percentage by weight of the remaining components in dental amalgam. Copper content varies widely depending on whether the amalgam is a "low copper" dental amalgam (2%-5%) or a "high copper" dental amalgam (12%-30%).

4. **A** Resin composite was specifically designed to be a tooth-colored restorative material. Because it is adhesively bonded to tooth structure, it generally results in lower microleakage than an amalgam restoration.

5. **B** The use of a wedge has no influence on the setting time of dental amalgam. The primary purpose of the wedge is to prevent amalgam from being overpacked beyond the gingival cavosurface margin that, if not confined to the preparation itself, would create an "overhang" of the metallic material. This would, in effect, create a plaque and bacteria trap that could initiate or perpetuate dental caries and/or periodontal disease.

CHAPTER 39

1. **B** Only the 10% carbamide peroxide solution has gained the ADA Seal of Acceptance. Several concentrations and materials have been clinically researched but have not sought ADA approval.

2. **B** The scalloped tray is trimmed following the contour of the tooth at the gingival-tooth interface. Therefore the solution is less likely to have direct contact with the gingival tissues.

3. **B** In-office bleaching uses a higher concentration of solution, and heat is used to produce a quick "power" bleaching effect.

4. **D** Hydrogen peroxide is the correct answer. The other items are popular ingredients in bleaching gels.

5. **A** Whitening strips are convenient, easy use, more economical, and better tolerated. An inherent disadvantage of whitening strips is that they only cover the facial surface of the anterior teeth.

6. **C** Because of the fluidlike consistency of Proxigel, it provided poor substantivity or retention in bleaching trays because of its rapid oxygen release. A more viscous gellike material with better retention replaced Proxigel.

7. **D** Research has shown that bleaching does not cause any nonresolvable problems. Gingival irritation has been the only consistent side effect of cosmetic whitening.

8. **D** Patient expectations should be realized *before* dental whitening is begun. During treatment, the dental hygienist and dentist should be readily available for additional questions and concerns that might arise. After dental bleaching, the patient should be reminded that several factors determine how long the results will last including consumption of chromogenic foods and tobacco use.

9. **D** Any of the options listed can help the sensitivity associated with tooth-bleaching procedures.

10. **A** No safety concerns are associated with glycerine, carbopol, or fluoride.

11. **B** The stain has been present since eruption, and the case information reveals that Jimmy has lived in region typical of high levels of water fluoridation.

12. **D** A nonscalloped, nonreservoir tray can hold the bleaching agent against the neck of the tooth.

13. **C** Third-degree tetracycline stains are dark, gray-blue banding stains

14. **A** A nonscalloped, nonreservoir tray design holds the bleaching agent against the gingival third of the tooth.

15. **C** Cosmetic dental procedures should be completed after the whitening procedures are complete.

16. **B** Refer to the posttreatment intraoral photographs for Case #2, Kathleen O'Bryan.

17. **B** The use of Professional Crest Whitestrips is a good recommendation for Ms. Randall, given her lack of personal free time and the area most noticeably yellow (six anterior teeth). The strip technology available through Crest Whitestrips covers approximately six anterior teeth and can be worn during normal daily activities. Although tray bleaching is an option that might work for Ms. Randall, her busy schedule makes her a good candidate for the strip technology. A whitening dentifrice should be recommended for Ms. Randall, especially after the completion of a whitening procedure to help maintain her whiter smile. A whitening dentifrice, however, is not considered a tooth-whitening system. Although laser bleaching may be appropriate for Ms. Randall, the new professional-strength strip technology may be a better option for her due to convenience.

CHAPTER 40

1. **D** The many properties of saliva are listed in the introduction of this chapter. These properties include normal digesting, tasting, swallowing, speaking, and chewing.

2. **B** Saliva has numerous protective properties that include lubrication, antimicrobial activity, maintenance of pH and tooth integrity, debridement, maintenance of healthy mucous membranes, and maintenance of the oral flora.

3. **C** The parotid gland, the largest of the three glands, contributes approximately 25% of the total salivary secretions, is innervated by cranial nerve IX (glossopharyngeal nerve), and is serous in salivary secretions. The submandibular gland secretions have a mucous component, and the sublingual gland is predominantly mucous secretion. The majority of the minor salivary glands secrete only mucus.

4. **C** Patients with decreased salivary gland function usually avoid eating spicy foods because the spicy foods exacerbate or increase the pain and burning of the tissues in the oral cavity.

5. **D** The patient with decreased salivary function has diminished protective activities from the saliva. Collectively, the end result can be an increased risk and rate of caries. To prevent this, the dental hygienist must (1) insist on meticulous oral hygiene from this patient, including the daily use of fluoride; (2) provide nutritional counseling to decrease the patient's carbohydrate intake; and (3) establish a frequent patient recall program, such as every 3 months or more frequently.

6. **A** Of the 200 most-prescribed medications in 1998, 55 list xerostomia as an expected adverse effect; 8 medications list the subjective complaint of glossodynia/glossitis; and another 15 list dysgeusia, or altered taste.

CHAPTER 41

1. **D** Use of a mouth prop is simple, quick, noninvasive, and usually works. If not, then pursue further options.

2. **D** Taking the steps in Options A, B, and C should minimize the development of new problems or the exacerbation of pressure points and reduce the possibility of decubitus ulcer formation.

3. **C** Air polishing generates significant amounts of dry, powdered aerosols (generally sodium bicarbonate), which irritate the bronchi and may trigger a respiratory crisis.

4. **D** Either a kink in the line or a collection bag placed higher than the patient's bladder may impede urinary drainage. (This condition may also be exacerbated by the diuretic.) Option B is certainly permissible but generally not as appropriate as Option D.

5. **A** If the patient frequently forgets basic personal care, another source should be incorporated. Options B, C, and D are likely to be of little or no help.

6. **A** Radiographs are known to contribute to the formation of cataracts when the lens of the eye is directly exposed, so the operator should use caution (for both medical and legal reasons) when the patient is exposed to the x-rays. A well-collimated positioning indicating device (PID) and careful direction of the beam away from the lens is indicated. Air polishing should only be used with adequate eye protection as with any other patient.

7. **E** Options A and C are easy to try, and they maintain the patient's dignity. Pencils, notepads, and picture boards should only be offered after the initial attempts to communicate fail.

8. **E** Attention to these and other factors ensure compliance with the Americans with Disabilities Act regulations and facilitate the delivery of routine dental care to the broadest possible patient population.

CHAPTER 42

1. **B** Progesterone levels increase after ovulation, which results in changes in the endometrium in preparation for implantation of the fertilized egg and development of the placenta and mammary glands.
2. **D** Progesterone alters both the rate and pattern of collagen production in the gingiva, which results in a reduced ability to repair and maintain the structure of the gingiva.
3. **A** Puberty gingivitis is characterized by enlarged, bluish red, and distinctively bulbous gingival tissues.
4. **A** Estrogen replacement therapy is prescribed only for women who have had their uteruses removed, because estrogen alone causes hyperplasia of the uterine lining, which leads to endometrial cancer.
5. **D** Surgical procedures should be scheduled during the nonestrogen days of the oral contraceptive cycle (days 23-28) to avoid possible osteitis.

CHAPTER 43

1. **C** Sertraline (Zoloft) is the only SSRI. Bupropion (Wellbutrin) and nefazodone (Serzone) are atypical; phenelzine sulfate (Nardil) is an MAO inhibitor; and imipramine (Tofranil) is a tricyclic.
2. **C** *Mysophobia* is the fear of germs; *acrophobia* is the fear of heights; *claustrophobia* is the fear of confinement; *demophobia,* also known as *ochlophobia,* is the fear of crowds; *haptephobia* is the fear of being touched.
3. **D** Posttraumatic stress disorder (PTSD) occurs when a person experiences a negative life event beyond that individual's ability to cope.
4. **D** In bulimia nervosa the patient consumes large quantities of food, followed by purging of that food in an effort to prevent weight gain.
5. **B** A hallucination is a perceptual experience in the absence of external stimulation, such as hearing voices that do not actually exist.
6. **A** *Diagnostic and Statistical Manual of Mental Disorders*, ed 4, Text Revision, American Psychiatric Association.
7. **C** Antipsychotic medications have been shown to cause tardive dyskinesia in approximately 25% of patients within 3 months of treatment initiation.
8. **C** A sense of entitlement is one of the diagnostic criteria for narcissistic personality disorder, not for a major depressive episode.

CHAPTER 44

1. **B** This definition is accepted for cancer. Cancer ignores all the normal controls that healthy cells follow during growing and replicating.
2. **A** Each year the American Cancer Society determines the top new cancer diagnoses; for the year 2000, for example, the top diagnoses in descending order were breast, lung, colon, and rectal cancers.
3. **D** All the roles listed are important in the care of a cancer patient.
4. **C** This guideline is established for an absolute neutrophil count (ANC) before dental treatment commences.

5. **C** This guideline is established for platelet count before dental treatment commences.
6. **B** This guideline is necessary to prevent an infection from developing around the catheter site.
7. **C** HIV has been found predominately in semen, blood, and breast milk.
8. **C** The current most effective treatment for HIV infection requires the use of multiple drugs in combination.
9. **D** All these oral manifestations are present in a patient with HIV/AIDS.
10. **A** Periodontal disease progresses more rapidly in patients with HIV/AIDS because of their immune system dysfunction.

CHAPTER 45

1. **C** Oral mucosal cells have a life span of 10 to 14 days. Radiation terminates the growth and replication of cancer cells by destroying the cell nucleus. Normal cells may also be affected, thereby dying at a faster rate than they are produced.
2. **C** The mandible is more susceptible to osteoradionecrosis because it is denser and less vascular than the maxilla and consequently absorbs more radiation. Patients undergoing radiation doses in excess of 7000 cGy are at greater risk also. As in the case presented, the greatest risk is the patient whose mandible has received extensive radiation and requires tooth extractions after the completion of radiation therapy.
3. **B** Because of the patient's prior exposure to radiation, hyperbaric oxygen treatments were scheduled to flood the tissues with oxygen and increase the blood supply, particularly to the extraction sites to decrease the risk of osteoradionecrosis.
4. **A** 1.23% acidulated phosphate fluoride is a relatively high concentration of fluoride that is recommended for application only once every 6 months.
5. **B** A $T_2N_0M_0$ tumor is classified as stage II because the neoplasm has increased in size, but it has no lymph node involvement and no metastasis.
6. **D** The brain, muscles, and spinal cord are the least affected by radiation. Cells of the bone marrow and alimentary tract divide rapidly and are easily destroyed by radiation.

CHAPTER 46

1. **B** Calcium channel blockers, prescribed for persons with high blood pressure, can cause gingival hyperplasia, and this would hamper Mrs. Lightfoot's plaque control access. A controlled person with non–insulin-dependent diabetes mellitus should exhibit no oral changes that would interfere with plaque control. Naproxen, prescribed for Mrs. Lightfoot's osteoarthritis, should not interfere with her plaque control.
2. **D** Gingival hyperplasia makes plaque removal a challenge, and therefore can cause an increase in gingival bleeding. Options B and C are also likely to result in increased bleeding. In addition, clinical evidence exists that a change in diuretic medication would cause gingival bleeding.
3. **B** If Mrs. Lightfoot has no increased attachment loss, then the pocket reading is deeper because of swelling in the gingiva. Although probe readings may be deeper in the presence of inflammation, an experienced dental hygienist should use appropriate

probing pressure and angulation, so Option A is not the most likely answer. Because her attachment level is currently stable, Option C is incorrect. Option D, poor plaque control, is an incomplete response because just the presence of plaque is not sufficient. The plaque must produce a change in the gingiva, which changes probe measurements.

4. **A**   Bleeding 16% or more should result in a 1-month shorter interval of maintenance care, so Mrs. Lightfoot should be seen before she leaves on her trip. If she is taking an extended trip, Option B is a necessary recommendation. Option C would lengthen her next preventive maintenance appointment, when the interval needs to be shortened. Option D is the least advisable because it is not based on the patient's risks or level of periodontal health.

5. **D**   Although all three other choices are good reasons for concern, Mrs. Lightfoot does not appear to be personally involved in her care other than maintaining her office visits every 3 months. It can be inferred that her indifference to the maintenance procedures includes the instructions for her daily, personal, oral self-care. The reasons for Option D may be many. For example, for some reason she may not have understood everything she has been told. She could have a language barrier or a slight hearing or sight impairment that nobody has detected. If her teeth are sensitive, she may not be able to accomplish her home care as well as she should, or she may have inadequate time, support, or money for oral self-care aids, although she has faithfully kept her 3-month appointments.

6. **C**   Osteoarthritis could be why Mrs. Lightfoot's plaque control is not as thorough as should be expected. Watch her technique, get her to talk about how much time she spends on her teeth, and observe and ask whether oral care is difficult to do with her fingers, hands, or arms. She may have misunderstood previous oral care instructions or she may have difficulty with manual deplaquing aids. If her diabetes and blood pressure are under control, these illnesses would not hamper her plaque control efforts.

CHAPTER 47

1. **D**   All the choices are appropriate methods for use in a case documentation, however, using a case documentation to increase the practice's profit is not ethical. A case documentation could be used ethically to educate peers, motivate patients, evaluate the outcomes of care, and provide third-party payers with information, and some of these options may increase the practice's profits indirectly. The original intent was not designed for this purpose.

2. **D**   The purpose of developing the case, the intended audience, and the goal of the development and doc-

umentation efforts need to be evaluated before actual case development. When these three issues are addressed, the information or answers can act as an outline for organization, thoroughness, precision, and objectivity in the design, documentation, and presentation of the case.

3. **C**   Treatment strategies are generally introduced in the section dedicated to details of case management and proceedings. The patient profile section provides basic information about the individual, which will introduce the patient to the audience.

4. **B**   Oral presentations are the most widely used case-presentation format. Oral delivery can be presented (1) on an individual basis, such as clinician to patient; (2) to small groups, such as a gathering of colleagues or patients; or (3) to large audiences, such as professional or public meetings.

CHAPTER 48

1. **C**   Values are the foundation for which all other components of behavior are built.

2. **E**   The dental hygienist is not only a direct care provider but also a disease prevention and health promotion specialist. He or she may also be an efficient healthcare provider, but this is not the best choice.

3. **B**   The professional portfolio may contain all the other components listed, but the intent is that of documentation to evaluate continued competence.

4. **C**   The greatest feeling a dental hygienist can have and the best thing a dental hygienist can do for patients is to educate them as to the association between oral and systemic diseases. This information empowers others to prevent disease and to promote wellness among even more people.

CHAPTER 49

1. **D**   Although all the other choices have made impacts on either dentistry or dental hygiene, technological advances will have the greatest impact on future dental hygiene practice.

2. **B**   The association between systemic and oral diseases is important to healthcare but will be applied in dental, medical, and public health settings.

3. **C**   Leaders are needed with all of the listed characteristics, but they should not work alone. Vision and implementation of ideas require more than just a leader to accomplish.

4. **A**   Both statements are true as the future of the dental hygienist is projected.

5. **B**   Although all the characteristics in each option are appropriate for a leader to possess, affecting change is almost impossible without insight and commitment.

GLOSSARY

Abandonment: Once a healthcare professional establishes a relationship with a patient, services must continue to be provided for the patient. If the healthcare provider does not provide services and the patient's health is jeopardized, a legal action of *abandonment* may be commenced against the healthcare provider.

Abfraction: The pathological loss of hard tooth substance caused by biomechanical loading forces. Such loss is thought to be a result of flexure and chemical fatigue degradation of enamel and/or dentin at some location distant from the actual point of loading.

Abfraction lesions: Lesions thought to be caused by excessive facial or lingual occlusal load through either compression or tension in the cervical region of the tooth just above the bony support.

Abrasion: The wearing away of surface material as a result of friction.

Abrasive: A material that consists of particles of sufficient hardness and sharpness that cut or scratch a softer material when drawn across its surface. Abrasives are available in various particle sizes.

Abutment: A tooth, a root, or an implant used for the retention of a fixed or removable prosthesis.

Accreditation: The processes of approval, certification, or endorsement. For example, a dental education program can be accredited by the American Dental Association.

Acellular cementum: The first layers of cementum deposited without many embedded cementocytes.

Acid etchant: A 35% to 50% phosphoric acid concentration applied to the occlusal pits and fissures to open the enamel tubules for receipt of a liquid sealant resin.

Acquired immunodeficiency syndrome (AIDS): A syndrome involving a defect in cell-mediated immunity that has a long incubation period, follows a protracted and debilitating course, is manifested by various opportunistic infections, and has a poor prognosis.

Acromegaly: A condition caused by hyperfunction of the pituitary gland in adults. It is characterized by enlargement of the skeletal extremities, including the feet, hands, mandible, and nose.

Acrophobia: The fear of heights.

Acrylic test rod: A plastic rod-shaped device used to check for instrument sharpness.

Active caries: A condition in which a lesion leads to cavitation of the tooth structure. It can be seen radiographically and feels "mushy" or "leathery" to the touch.

Active periodontal therapy: Therapy to bring periodontal disease into remission. It includes professional debridement and personal care instruction that may or may not be used in conjunction with periodontal surgery.

Acute necrotizing ulcerative gingivitis (ANUG): A recurrent periodontal disease that primarily involves the interdental papillae, which undergo necrosis and ulceration.

Addiction: Compulsive behavior. See *"Dependence."*

Addison's disease: A chronic adrenocortical insufficiency caused by bilateral tuberculosis, aplasia, atrophy, or degeneration of the adrenal glands. Symptoms include severe weakness, weight loss, low blood pressure, digestive disturbances, hypoglycemia, lowered resistance to infection, and abnormal pigmentation (bronze color of the skin, with associated melanotic pigmentation of the oral mucous membranes, particularly of the gingival tissues).

Adenoid cystic carcinoma: A pseudoadenomatous basal cell carcinoma originating from salivary glands, the cells of which resemble basal cells and form ductlike or cystlike structures. It grows slowly but is malignant.

Adenoma: A benign epithelial neoplasm or tumor with a basic glandular structure that suggests derivation from glandular tissue.

Adherence: The willingness and ability of a patient to perform those tasks specifically necessary to attain and maintain health.

Adrenocorticotropic hormone (ACTH): The hormone produced by basophilic cells of the anterior lobe of the pituitary gland, which exerts a reciprocal regulating influence on the production of corticosteroids by the adrenal cortex.

Advanced directive: Indicating in advance of the need; a person's wishes regarding his or her health care.

Agoraphobia: An anxiety about, or avoidance of, places or situations from which escape might be difficult or embarrassing or in which help may not be available in the event of experiencing paniclike symptoms.

Air powder polisher: An air-powered device using air and water pressure to deliver a controlled stream of specially processed sodium bicarbonate slurry through the handpiece nozzle; also called *air abrasive, air polishing,* or *air-powered abrasive.*

Air turbine: A handpiece with a turbine powered by compressed air.

Ala: A wing or a winglike anatomical part or process.

Alginate: A flexible impression material in which the alginate in water (sol) reacts chemically with calcium ions to form insoluble calcium alginate (gel).

Algophobia: A fear of pain.

Alopecia: The normal or abnormal deficiency of hair; baldness.

Alveolar bone proper: The bone lining the alveolus.

Alveolar crestal fibers: These fibers run from the crest of the alveolar bone to the cementum in the region of the cementoenamel junction. Their primary function is to retain the tooth in the socket and to oppose lateral forces.

Alveolar mucosa: The portion of the oral mucosa immediately apical to the mucogingival junction.

Alveolar process: The extension of the maxilla and mandible that surrounds and supports the teeth to form the dental arches. It is also known as the *alveolar ridge*.

Amalgam: An alloy in which mercury is one of the metals.

Anatomic crown: The portion of crown covered by enamel.

Anatomical charting forms: The charts used to indicate conditions of the mouth. In all charts, the teeth are presented as if looking into the patient's mouth.

Anemia: A reduction to less than normal of the number of red blood cells, quantity of hemoglobin, or the volume of packed red blood cells in the blood.

Angina pectoris: Frequently a symptom of cardiovascular diseases; characterized by a severe, viselike pain behind the sternum that sometimes radiates to the arms, neck, or mandible. It may also consist of a sense of constriction or pressure of the chest. It is caused by exertion or excitement and is relieved by rest.

Angioma: A benign tumor of vascular nature.

Angle's classification: The system used to initially and simply classify malocclusion.

Angles: *90-degree (right) angle:* The joining of a horizontal line to a vertical line from the same point; *110-degree angle:* a line that is 20 degrees to the right or left of the right angle; *45-degree angle:* an angle less than 90 degrees. These angles are used in periodontal instrumentation, instrument sharpening, radiology, and other dental applications.

Angular cheilosis: An inflammation of the lip or lips with redness and the production of fissures that radiate from the angles of the mouth.

Anionic: Pertaining to a negatively charged ion.

Ankylosed: A joint or tooth that is immobile or abnormally fused as a result of injury, disease, or a surgical procedure.

Anorexia: The partial or complete loss of appetite for food.

Anterior palate: The front or forward part of the palate that is hard and bony.

Antibodies: The protein molecules that are produced by plasma cells and react with a specific antigen.

Anticipatory guidance: The psychological preparation of a person to help relieve fear and anxiety of an event expected to be stressful. An example is the preparation of a child for surgery by explaining what will happen and what it will feel like and by showing equipment or the area of the hospital where the child will be. It is also used to prepare parents for the normal growth and development of their child.

Anticoagulant: A drug that delays or prevents coagulation of blood.

Antifungal agents: Agents that inhibit, control, or kill fungi. The most common yeastlike fungus that occurs in or near the oral cavity is *Candida albicans*.

Antigens: Substances that are able to induce a specific immune response.

Antimicrobial: An agent or substance that kills or inhibits the growth or replication of microorganisms.

Anxiety: A diffuse emotional reaction disproportional to the issue at hand and typically directed at future problems and not toward present circumstances.

Apex: The anatomical end of a tooth root.

Apexification: The process in which an environment is created within the root canal and periapical tissues after death of the pulp, which allows a calcified barrier to form across the open apex.

Apexogenesis: The normal development of the apex of a root of a tooth.

Aphthous ulcers: A recurring condition characterized by the eruption of painful sores (commonly called *canker sores*) on the mucous membranes of the mouth. The cause is unknown, but there is evidence to suggest that aphthous ulcers are an immune reaction. Heredity, some foods, overenthusiastic toothbrushing, and emotional stress are also possible causes.

Apical fibers: Fibers pertaining to the periodontal ligament. These fibers radiate around the apex of the tooth at approximately right angles to their cementum attachment, extending into the bone at the bottom of the alveolus. These fibers resist forces that may lift the tooth from the socket and also help stabilize the tooth against tilting movements.

Area-specific: A specific area on the tooth or a specific group of teeth (i.e., an area-specific dental instrument indicates the instrument can only be used on a specific tooth surface).

Arkansas stone: A type of sharpening stone made of natural stone used to sharpen periodontal instruments.

Arrested caries: Dental decay in which the area of decay has stopped progressing and infection is not present but in which the demineralized area in the tooth remains.

Arthrograms: A radiograph of a joint usually with the introduction of a contrast compound into the joint capsule. In dentistry, an arthrogram usually involves the temporomandibular joint.

Asbestosis: Inflammation and/or fibrosis of the lungs caused by inhalation of asbestos fibers, sometimes complicated by pleural mesothelioma or bronchogenic carcinoma.

Aspiration: The ingestion of a foreign body into the airway tree; also, negative pressure in a hypodermic syringe.

Assessment: Evaluation of a potential or actual problem.

Astraphobia: A fear of thunder, lightning, winds, and heavy rain.

Atherosclerotic plaque: The yellowish deposits containing cholesterol, lipids, and lipophages that form within the intima and inner media of large and medium-sized arteries.

Atrial dysrhythmia: An abnormal cardiac rhythm or a disturbance of rhythm that occurs in an atrium or heart chamber.

Atrophic: Characterized by a wasting of tissues, usually associated with general malnutrition or a specific disease state.

Attached gingiva: The gingiva that tightly adheres to the alveolar bone around the roots of the teeth.

Attachment apparatus: A general term used to designate the cementum, periodontal ligament, and alveolar bone.

Attending: Paying attention to a patient. It involves observation, warmth, empathy, and interest.

Attrition: The wearing away of a tooth surface as a result of tooth-to-tooth contact.

Auscultation: The process of determining the condition of various parts of the body by listening to the sounds they emit.

Autoimmune: Pertaining to the development of an immune response to a person's own tissues.

Autoimmune deficiency syndromes: One of a large group of diseases characterized by the subversion or alteration of the function of the immune system of the body.

Avoidant personality disorder: A long-standing pattern that is characterized by significant social discomfort, fear of negative social evaluation, and timidness. People with this disorder tend to be socially isolated although they want to be liked by others and are often hurt by even the slightest sign of disapproval.

Avulsed: Torn away; extracted by force.

BANA: The acronym for *benzol-arginine napthylamide,* which is an enzyme-based assay.

Basal lamina: Superficial portion of the basement membrane.

Bass method: Refers to a toothbrushing method named for Dr. C.C. Bass, an early pioneer in preventive dentistry. The Bass technique is the most generally recommended method for routine patients with and without periodontal involvement.

Battered child syndrome: Specific injury patterns involving the skin and skeletal system and internal organ damage.

Battery: Committing bodily harm to another individual. Battery can be a civil or criminal offense.

Beliefs: Anything believed or accepted as true.

Beneficence: The promotion of well-being of both individuals and the public by engaging in health promotion and disease prevention activities.

Benign: Not malignant or recurrent; remains localized; favorable for recovery.

Beveled edge: A design feature of specific periodontal instruments in which the toe is flat and angled.

Bidi (*pronounced* "beede"): A crude, unprocessed form of cigarette commonly manufactured in India. Cut tobacco is rolled in a temburni leaf and secured with a thread.

Bidigital palpation: Palpation of the tissue with two fingers.

Bifurcation: The site where a single structure divides into two parts, as in two roots of a tooth.

Bilateral: Having or pertaining to two sides.

Bimanual palpation: The examination of soft tissue between the hands.

Bioburden: Any visible organic debris. In dentistry this is most often blood or saliva.

Biocentric technique: A technique used by a dental professional to position the body while seated in the dental chair.

Biocompatibility: The degree to which the body's defense system tolerates the presence of foreign material. If something is biocompatible there are no toxic or injurious effects on biological function.

Biofeedback: The instrumental process or technique of learning voluntary control over automatically regulated body functions.

Biologic width: The combined width of connective tissue and epithelial attachment superior to the crestal bone.

Biopsy: The removal and examination, usually microscopic, of tissue from the living body. It is usually done to determine if a tumor is malignant or benign.

Biopsychosocial: Pertaining to the complex of biological, psychological, and sociological aspects of life.

Bipolar mood disorder: A mood disorder characterized by episodes of mania and depression.

BIS-GMA: The acronym for bisphenol A-glycidyl methacrylate.

Blepharitis: An inflammatory condition of the lash follicles and meibomian glands of the eyelids, characterized by swelling, redness, and crusts of dried mucus on the lids.

Bond: The linkage or adhesive force between atoms, as in a compound.

Bone: Rigid calcified connective tissue.

Borderline personality disorder: An enduring pattern of instability of mood, self-image, and interpersonal relationships. This disorder is often characterized by frantic efforts to avoid real or perceived abandonment. People with this disorder often hold views of significant others that vacillate between unrealistically positive and negative extremes.

Branchial cleft cyst: This typically occurs as the persistence of the second branchial groove, which forms a space lined by squamous epithelium. It is most commonly seen in children less than 10 years of age.

Breach of duty: The failure to observe the legal and ethical duties as described by law.

Brown spot lesion: Decalcification of enamel discolored by environmental pigmentation.

Bruit: An abnormal blowing sound or murmur heard during auscultation of a carotid artery, organ, or gland, such as the liver or thyroid.

Bruxism: The involuntary grinding or clenching of the teeth that damages both tooth surface and periodontal tissues.

Buccal: Pertaining to or adjacent to the cheek.

Buccal frenula: The area that passes from the oral mucosa of the outer surface of the maxillary arch to the inner surface of the cheek.

Buccal mucosa: The mucosa that lines the inner cheek.

Buccinator: The main muscle of the cheek. It is one of the 12 muscles of the mouth. The buccinator, innervated by buccal branches of the facial nerve, compresses the cheek, acting as an important accessory muscle of mastication by holding food on the chewing surfaces of the teeth.

Bulimia nervosa: A type of eating disorder characterized by episodes of binge eating followed by purging.

Bulimic: Pertaining to bulimia.

Bupropion: A nonnicotine aid to smoking cessation originally developed and marketed as an antidepressant. It is chemically unrelated to other known antidepressant agents.

Burning mouth syndrome: A burning sensation in one or several parts of the mouth that occurs often with no obvious cause.

Burnished calculus: An extrinsic tooth deposit that has been smoothed by improper instrument adaptation, dullness, or inadequate pressure on the working stroke.

Burnishing: Smoothing the surface of a dental amalgam after initial carving, or adapting margins of gold restorations by rubbing with a broad-surfaced metal instrument. This term also refers to the rubbing of a medication into the dentinal tubules.

Calculus: Mineralized, hard deposits developed from plaque and salivary salts found on tooth surfaces above and below the gingiva and on dental appliances.

Calibration: The process of measuring or calibrating against an established standard, such as a deciliter or kilogram. This term also is applied to the process by which consistency is established among examiners.

Cancer: A neoplasm characterized by the uncontrolled growth of anaplastic cells that tend to invade surrounding tissue and to metastasize to distant body sites, or any of a large group of neoplastic diseases characterized by the presence of malignant cells.

Candidiasis: A fungal infection caused by *Candida albicans* that appears as thrush or denture stomatitis in the mouth.

Cannula: A narrow bore (metal) cylinder similar in appearance and size to a needle that permits entry of a fluid into a body opening.

Capillary action: The surface force that draws aqueous liquids into and along the lumen of a capillary tube.

Carcinoma: A malignant tumor of epithelial origin.

Cariogenic: Tending to produce caries.

Carious lesion: A tooth tissue that has sustained a loss of function or a discontinuity caused by dental caries, or decay.

Carotid artery: Either of the two main right and left arteries of the neck.

Catatonia: Motor symptoms including either immobility and extreme muscular rigidity or overactivity.

Catatonic type: A type of schizophrenia that is characterized by symptoms of motor immobility or excessive and purposeless motor activity.

Cationic: Pertaining to a positively charge ion.

Causal factors: Factors or variables that directly cause an event to occur.

Cavitation: The formation of cavities within the body or any cavity within the body, such as the pleural cavities.

Cavity sealers, liners, bases: Materials placed over the pulpal area of the preparation to soothe irritated or sensitive pulp.

Cavosurface: The surface of a cavity, as of a tooth.

Cellular cementum: Outer layers of cementum that contain embedded cementocytes.

Cementum: The thin calcified tissue of ectomesenchyme origin that covers the root of a tooth.

cGy (centigray): A unit of absorbed radiation dose; 1 cGy = 1 rad.

Chancre: The primary lesion of syphilis, located at the site of entrance of the spirochete into the body, that occurs approximately 3 weeks after contact. It begins as a papule and develops into a clean-based shallow ulcer.

Charters' method: The method of toothbrushing in which the toothbrush is held horizontally, with the bristles lying against the teeth and gingivae and pointed in a coronal direction at 45 degrees so that the bristles lie half on the teeth and half on the gingivae. A vibratory cycle of a constricted diameter is negotiated so that the brush head moves circularly but the brush bristles remain fairly stationary while being agitated. The circular vibration loosens debris and pumps the bristles into interproximal areas to massage the tissues.

Charting: The use of a system that allows uniform interpretation of a patient's dental chart information. Symbols are used that indicate certain oral conditions.

Chemotherapeutic: Refers to agents that affect microbial activity. *Chemotherapeutic* is used interchangeably with *pharmacotherapeutics,* which also includes agents that affect host response.

Chemotherapy: The treatment of an illness by chemical means (i.e., by drugs or medications).

Child abuse: The physical, sexual, or emotional maltreatment of a person less than 18 years of age. Child abuse occurs predominantly with children under the age of 3. Symptoms include bruises, contusions, medical records of repeated trauma, radiographic evidence of fractures, emotional distress, and failure to thrive.

Chlorhexidine: A disinfectant with broad antibacterial action.

Chronic obstructive pulmonary disease (COPD): A progressive and irreversible condition characterized by diminished inspiratory and expiratory capacity of the lungs. The person complains of dyspnea with physical exertion, difficulty in inhaling or exhaling deeply, and sometimes a chronic cough.

Circular fibers: Any one of the many fibers in the free gingiva that encircle the teeth.

Circumferential: To carry around the perimeter of the tooth; also with respect to scaling, the use of a horizontal stroke to moves around the tooth.

Circumvallate: Surrounded by a trench or ridge.

Claustrophobia: A fear of confinement or closed areas.

Cleft lip: Developmental disturbance of the upper lip caused by failure of fusion of the maxillary processes with the medial nasal process.

Cleft palate: Developmental disturbance caused by failure of fusion of the palatal shelves with the primary palate or with each other.

Clinical crown: The portion of the anatomic crown that is visible in the oral cavity and not covered by the gingiva.

Clinical trial: An organized study to provide large bodies of clinical data for statistically valid evaluation of treatment.

Clinician: A professional directly providing healthcare assistance.

Collagenase: An enzyme that degrades body protein collagen in connective tissue.

Commissure: A point of union or junction, especially between two anatomical parts.

Commitment: Civil commitment; the legal proceeding by which a person is involuntarily confined to a mental hospital or made to undergo outpatient treatment.

Communication: The act of giving or exchanging information through speech, gestures, or written text.

Competence: A measure of the degree of a person's ability to cope with all aspects of the environment.

Complaint: In law, it denotes the legal document that is filed with a court of law that initiates a lawsuit against an individual. It also can denote the instance in which an individual contacts a dental board with a concern about treatment of a licensee.

Complete dentures: A removable dental prosthesis that replaces the entire dentition and associated structures of the maxilla or mandible.

Compliance: See *Adherence.*

Composite: The resinous filling material formed by a reaction of an ether bisphenol A with acrylic resin monomers. It is initiated by a benzoyl peroxide amine system to which inorganic fillers (e.g., glass beads and rods of either aluminum, silicate, quartz, or tricalcium phosphate) are added.

Comprehensive dental history: Provides information about previous treatment and dental experiences and is often a component of the health questionnaire.

Comprehensive health history: Collection of data provided by the patient about his or her general health. It is an important means of preventing medical emergencies.

Computer-assisted charting: Digital charting of hard tissue and periodontal findings printed out as computer images.

Condyle: An articular prominence of a bone (i.e., in the mandible, an ellipsoidal projection of bone) usually for articulation with another bone.

Confidentiality: A principle that demands that a health-care professional hold in strict confidence all information gained regarding a patient in the course of treatment.

Congestive heart failure: An abnormal condition characterized by circulatory congestion (retention of fluids) caused by cardiac or kidney disorders. This condition usually develops chronically in association with the retention of sodium and water by the kidneys. Acute congestive heart failure may result from myocardial infarction of the left ventricle.

Congruity: The agreement of verbal and nonverbal cues.

Conjunctiva: The mucous membrane lining the inner surfaces of the eyelids and anterior part of the sclera.

Connective tissue: A tissue of mesodermal origin rich in interlacing processes that supports or binds together other tissues.

Consistency: Coherence among parts; reliability of successive events or results.

Context: The whole situation or background relevant to a particular event.

Contraangle: Angles that deviate from a vertical line.

Controlled delivery device: Refers to delivery systems and agents that are pharmaceutically active for more than 1 day.

Convenience form: The methods and space needed to gain access to the cavity preparation to insert and finish the restorative material.

Coping skills: Mechanisms that assist individuals in adjusting to changes in their lives and environments. Includes helping patients to identify sociological, psychological, and environmental conditions that stimulate a desire to use tobacco and helping to develop a way to manage each. Examples include helping the patient resolve living with someone who smokes, stress, weight management, avoidance of places and events where tobacco use is common.

Coronal polishing: The polishing of the tooth surface coronal to the gingival margin to remove bacterial plaque and extrinsic stains. This does not involve calculus removal.

Corrosion: The action, process, or effect of corroding; a product of corroding; the loss of elemental constituents to the adjacent environment.

Cracked tooth syndrome: Transient acute pain that is difficult to locate and to reproduce and is experienced occasionally while chewing. Usually a vertical crack or split in the tooth extends across a marginal ridge through the crown and into the root involving the pulp. Cracked teeth are visible by transilluminated light or with the use of disclosing dyes.

Cracking: An incomplete splitting or breaking.

Crepitus: A cracking or popping sound, such as that produced by the rubbing together of fragments of a fractured bone or by air moving in a tissue space.

Crevicular fluid: The fluid that seeps through the crevicular epithelium. This is usually increased in the presence of inflammation.

Cricoid cartilage: The lowest cartilage of the larynx.

Crohn's disease: A chronic inflammatory bowel disease of unknown origin that usually affects the ileum, the colon, or another part of the gastrointestinal tract.

Cross-section: A view of an object cut through at a right angle to visualize the object internally.

Crossover studies: Multipart research projects, tests, or experiments in which each subject is tested with each (or most) of the treatments being compared in turn, in random order.

Crown elongation: The surgical process by which gingival tissue is removed to increase the crown length. It is usually performed before a crown preparation to obtain enough tooth structure to allow the crown to seat properly.

Crown fracture: Microscopic or macroscopic cleavage in the coronal portion of a tooth.

CT (computed tomography) scans: A radiographic body scanning technique in which thin or narrow layer sections of the body can be imaged for diagnostic purposes. The technique uses a computer-linked x-ray machine to focus the radiographs on a particular section of the body to be viewed.

Cultural sensitivity: The recognition, understanding, and consideration of customs, norms, and behaviors different from a person's own.

Culture: The ideas, customs, and skills of a given people.

Curet: A periodontal scaling instrument designed to remove calculus from above and below the gingival margin and to remove endotoxins from the root surface.

Curing: To process a material from a plastic or raw state to a hard state or finish, usually by means of heat or chemical treatment, such as polymerization.

Cushing's disease (primary aldosteronism): A complex syndrome associated with an excess of adrenal steroids of all types that results from hyperplasia of the adrenal cortex, malignant neoplasms, pituitary basophilia, or prolonged administration of adrenal cortical thyroid hormone. Manifestations include hypertension, buffalo obesity, diabetes mellitus, osteoporosis, purple striae of the skin in areas of tension, and disorders of glucose tolerance.

Cusp fracture: A crack or break in a notably pointed or rounded eminence on or near the masticating surface of a tooth.

Custodial: When an individual is given legal authority and responsibility to care for another.

Custom-fabricated: A term used to describe a prosthesis made specifically for an individual based on that person's specific anatomy.

Cutting edge: Found on the working end of periodontal scaling instruments. The joining of the face of the blade with the lateral side of the working end forms the cutting edge.

Cyanosis: The characteristic bluish tinge or color of the skin and mucous membranes associated with reduction in hemoglobin brought about by inadequate respiratory change.

Cycles per second (CPS): A unit of measurement of wave frequency equal to 1 cycle per second; also called *hertz*.

Cynophobia: A fear of dogs.

Cysts: Abnormal pathological sacs or cavities that are lined with epithelium and are enclosed within a connective tissue capsule.

Cytokines: One of a large group of low-molecular-weight proteins secreted by various cell types. They are involved in cell-to-cell communication, coordination of antibody and T-cell immune interactions, and amplification of immune reactivity. Cytokines include colony stimulating factor, interferons, interleukins, and lymphokines, which are secreted by lymphocytes.

Darkfield microscopy: Examination with a darkfield microscope, in which the specimen is illuminated by a peripheral light source. Organisms in specimens that have been prepared for use with a darkfield microscope appear to glow against a dark background.

Debonding: Removal of the attachment and all the adhesive resin from the tooth and restoration of the surface as closely as possible to its pretreatment condition without inducing iatrogenic damage.

Defendant: The individual or party against whom a lawsuit for recovery is brought in a civil case, or the accused in a criminal case.

Delivery system: The means by which an agent is made available to the body, which includes the drug carrier, the route, and the target.

Demineralization: The removal of minerals from tooth structures.

Demophobia: A fear of crowds.

Dental caries: An infectious disease resulting in the demineralization of the teeth by microbial acids.

Dental history: A record of all aspects of a person's oral health, previous evaluations, and treatments, as well as the state of general physical and mental health.

Dental neglect: Lack of attendance to oral-care needs.

Dental sealant: A plastic film coating that is applied to pits and fissures of teeth to prevent plaque, food, and bacteria from entering.

Dental trauma: The result of injury by force to the oral cavity.

Dentifrice: A pharmaceutical abrasive preparation provided as a paste, gel, or powder and used in conjunction with a toothbrush to clean and polish the teeth.

Dentin: The portion of the tooth that lies subjacent to the enamel and cementum. Dentin consists of an organic matrix on which mineral (calcific) salts are deposited. It can be pierced by tubules that contain filamentous protoplasmic processes of the odontoblasts that line the pulpal chamber and canal. It is of mesodermal origin.

Dentinal sensitivity: A common intermittent pain sensation that affects many people when they eat or drink or touch the teeth. The pain can be caused by mechanical, chemical, thermal, or bacterial stimuli.

Dentinal tubule: Microscopic channels that extend from the pulp through the dentin.

Dentoalveolar fibers (dentoperiosteal): Fibers that extend facially and lingually from the cementum. These fibers pass over the crest of the alveolar bone and then insert into the periosteum of the alveolar process. Their primary function is to support the tooth and gingiva.

Denture adhesive: A material used to adhere a denture to the oral mucosa.

Denture stomatitis: Irritation and inflammation of the palate covered by the denture.

Dependence: The compulsive reliance on a drug after a period of use, with consequences of use being, in part, adverse.

Dependent personality disorder: A pattern of submissive and dependent behavior. Those who exhibit this disorder depend on others for advice and reassurance and often have difficulty making everyday decisions on their own.

Depression: A mood disorder characterized by feelings of profound sadness, despair, loss of energy, sleeping difficulties, and change in eating habits that are persistent and significantly interfere with social, work, and personal activities.

Dermoid cyst: A tumor, derived from embryonic tissues, consisting of a fibrous wall lined with epithelium and a cavity containing fatty material, hair, teeth, bits of bone, and cartilage.

Desensitizing: The depriving of sensation; paralyzing of a sensory nerve by section or blocking.

Diabetes mellitus (DM): A chronic syndrome of impaired carbohydrate, protein, and fat metabolism owing to insufficient secretion of insulin or to target tissue insulin resistance. It occurs in two major forms: type 1 or type 2, which differ in etiology, pathology, genetics, age of onset, and treatment.

Diastema: A space between teeth that is *not* the result of a missing tooth.

Differential diagnosis: The distinguishing between two or more diseases with similar symptoms by systemically comparing their signs and symptoms.

Digastrics: Having two bellies. In dentistry, digastrics refers to the anterior belly and posterior belly of the facial nerve (cranial nerve VII). The anterior belly originates from the lower border of the mandible, and the posterior belly originates from the mastoid process of the temporal bone.

Diopter magnification: Magnification device that helps the eyes focus at a close range. Diopter magnification is available in three basic types: handheld, headband, and clip-on. It is also called *first generation*.

Discipline: In regard to dentistry, it is the corrective action taken by a state dental board against a licensee.

Disclosing tablet: A coloring agent that, when chewed, adheres to the teeth to reveal dental plaque.

Disclosure: The act of revealing facts that were unknown or not understood.

Disease: An abnormal body condition that impairs functioning. Disease exhibits a group of clinical signs, symptoms, and laboratory findings peculiar to a sickness.

Disease prevention: Activities designed to protect patients or other members of the public from actual or potential health threats and their harmful consequences.

Disorder: An abnormal state of mind or body.

Distance: A comfortable distance or space between communicants.

Distance learning: Learning derived from a source that is not originating in the learner's physical presence.

Distraction: In dentistry, an unusual width of the dental arch; the placement of the teeth or other maxillary or mandibular structures farther than normal from the median plane.

Documentation: Documentation is the act or an instance of furnishing or authenticating with documents. It refers to the process by which events and words and/or images are recorded reflect aspects of preventive and/or therapeutic care.

Dorsal surface: Pertaining to the back or to the posterior part of a surface.

Double-blind design: An experimental design for drug testing in which neither the patients receiving the drugs nor the persons conducting the test know which subjects are receiving a new drug and which are getting a placebo, or sugar pill.

Drifted teeth: Teeth that have migrated from their normal positions in the dental arches as a result of factors such as loss of proximal support, loss of functional antagonists, occlusal traumatic tooth relationships, inflammatory and retrograde changes in the attachment apparatus, and oral habits.

Duty: An obligation of care that one party owes to another.

Dysgeusia: The distortion of the taste of sense.

Dysphagia: Difficulty in swallowing.

Dysplasia: An abnormality of development; in pathology, alteration in size, shape, and organization of the adult cells.

Dyspnea: Difficulty breathing.

Dysuria: Painful urination that is usually caused by a bacterial infection or obstructive condition in the urinary tract.

Ecchymosis: A small, flat, hemorrhagic patch, larger than a petechia, on the skin or mucous membrane.

Edema: Swelling that is usually caused by accumulation of fluid in the tissues.

Edentulism: The condition of being without teeth. It usually means having lost all natural teeth.

Efficacy studies: Clinical studies designed to determine the outcome of a specific procedure, drug, intervention, or other similar event to determine whether the entity being observed does what it was intended to do.

Electric pulp tester: A diagnostic device used to determine tooth vitality.

Embrasure: An opening, as in a wall. The space between the curved proximal surfaces of the teeth.

Empathy: The ability to share in another's feelings or emotions.

Empowerment: The giving to others the authority to perform, or the provision to an individual what that person needs to perform a certain act or job.

Enamel: The hard outer layer of the crown of a tooth.

Enamel flaking: The process by which layers of enamel separate and fall off.

Endocrine: Pertaining to a process in which a group of cells secrete into the blood or lymph circulation a substance (e.g., insulin) that has a specific effect on tissues in another part of the body.

Endodontics lesion: A pathological or traumatic injury or loss of function to the dental pulp, tooth root, or periapical tissue.

Endogenous: Produced within or caused by factors within.

Endosteum: The lining of the medullary cavity of bone.

Enzyme-linked immunosorbent assay (ELISA): A laboratory technique for detecting specific antigens or antibodies that uses enzyme-labeled immunoreactants and a solid-phase binding support, such as a test tube. ELISA is nearly as sensitive as radioimmunoassay and more sensitive than complement fixation, agglutination, and other techniques. It is commonly used in the diagnosis of human immunodeficiency virus infections.

Epidermal cyst: An abnormal closed cavity in the epidermis, which is lined by epithelium that contains a liquid or semisolid material.

Epistaxis: Bleeding from the nose.

Epithelium: The basic tissue type that covers and lines the external and internal body surfaces.

Ergonomics: A scientific discipline devoted to the study and analysis of human work, especially as it is affected by individual anatomical, psychological, and other human characteristics.

Erosion: The chemical or mechanical destruction of tooth tissue. The action can create concavities of various shapes at the cementoenamel junction of teeth.

Erythema: A redness of the skin or mucosa.

Erythroplakia: Clinical red mucosal lesions that are not inflammatory and that cannot be otherwise diagnosed clinically by location, specific morphology, or history.

Essential oil: A volatile oil that emits a distinctive odor or flavor.

Esthetics: A branch of philosophy that deals with beauty, especially with the components of color and form.

Estrogen: A natural or artificial substance that induces the development of female sex characteristics.

Estrogenicity: Affects the production, metabolism, and activity of estrogens.

Ethics: A code of morals or standards of conduct. Each health profession defines professional ethics in written standards of professional behavior (see Box 3-2).

Ethyl chloride: A colorless liquid local anesthetic of short duration. Its action is accomplished by rapid vaporization from the skin, producing superficial freezing. It is used occasionally in inhalation therapy as a rapid, fleeting general anesthetic, comparable with nitrous oxide but somewhat more dangerous.

Evidence-based practice: The provision of clinical care based on documented efficacious treatment, procedures, and techniques.

Evidence-based teaching: Teaching using documented effective methodologies to deliver content based on efficacious clinical outcomes.

Exfoliating: The peeling and shedding of tissue cells. In dentistry, it refers to the loss of the primary dentition.

Exocrine glands: A gland having a duct associated with it.

Exofoliatve cytology: A nonsurgical technique that is helpful in the diagnosis of oral lesions. The surface of the lesion is scraped or wiped to gather a sample of the cells. The cells are then spread onto a glass slide for microscopic examination.

Exogenous: Originating outside or caused by factors outside.

Exophthalmos: An abnormal protrusion of the eyeball.

Explorer: A diagnostic instrument used to examine and evaluate tooth structure irregularities and defective margins of restorations.

Exposure: The concept that one may be vulnerable to legal action.

Extension for prevention: The principle of cavity preparation stated by G.V. Black in 1891. To prevent the recurrence of decay, he advocated extension of the preparation subgingivally and axially and occlusally into an area that is readily polished and cleaned.

External auditory meatus: The canal of the external ear that consists of bone and cartilage and extends from the auricle to the tympanic membrane.

Extrinsic: Derived from or situated on the outside; external.

Eye loupes: A convex lens used for low magnification of minute objects at close range; it may be monocular, binocular, or mounted on spectacles.

Face: A portion of the working end of a periodontal scaling instrument that joins with the lateral side to create the cutting edge.

Facet joint: The synovial joint between articular processes (zygapophytes) of the vertebrae.

Facial prosthesis: A removable prosthesis that artificially replaces a portion of the face lost as a result of surgery, trauma, or congenital absence.

Fainting (syncope):   Loss of consciousness because of transient cerebral hypoxia. It is usually preceded by a sensation of light-headedness and often may be prevented by lying down or by sitting with the head between the knees. It may be caused by many different factors, including emotional stress, vascular pooling in the legs, or sudden change in environmental temperature or body position.

Fallible: Liable to be mistaken; capable of error.

Family history: An essential part of a patient's medical history in which he or she is asked about the health of members of the immediate family in a series of specific questions to discover any disorders to which the patient may be susceptible. Hereditary and familial diseases are especially noted. The age and health of each person, age at death, and causes of death are charted. The family health history is obtained from the patient or family in the initial interview and becomes a part of the permanent record.

Fauces: An opening posteriorly from the oral cavity proper into the pharynx.

Fear: An emotion, generally considered negative and unpleasant, that is a reaction to a real or threatened danger; fright. Fear is distinguished from anxiety, which is a reaction to an unreal or imagined danger.

Feedback: A loop of command-action. An idea is demonstrated, questions are posed, or input is solicited; then action is accomplished.

Fiberoptics: The technical process by which an internal organ or cavity can be viewed through the use of glass or plastic fibers to transmit light through a specially designed tube and reflect a magnified image.

Fibrinolysis: The continual process of fibrin decomposition by fibrinolysin, which is the normal mechanism for the removal of small fibrin clots. It is stimulated by anoxia, inflammatory reactions, and other kinds of stress.

Fibromyalgia: A form of nonarticular rheumatism characterized by musculoskeletal pain, spasm and stiffness, fatigue, and severe sleep disturbance. Common sites of pain or stiffness can be palpated in the lower back, neck, shoulder region, arms, hands, knees, hips, thighs, legs, and feet. These are known as trigger points.

File: A periodontal scaling instrument designed to crush and remove heavy calculus deposits.

Filiform: Thread-shaped; in dentistry, it refers to thread-like elevations that cover most of the tongue's surface.

Filled resin: Contains fillers such as glass, quartz, and silica. It is used in composite restorations to make sealants more resistant to wear.

Fixed bridge: A partial denture that is luted or otherwise securely retained to natural teeth, tooth roots, and/or dental implant abutments that furnish the primary support for the prosthesis.

Flap (periodontal/surgical):   Oral tissue that has, by incision, been partially detached from its surrounding vasculature and nutrient supply.

Floss: Waxed or unwaxed dental tape used to clean the interproximal tooth surfaces, subgingivally and supragingivally.

Fluconazole: An oral antifungal tablet used in the treatment of oral candidiasis.

Fluctuant: Pertaining to a wavelike motion that is detected when a structure that contains a liquid is palpated.

Folate: A salt of folic acid; any of a group of substances found in some foods and in mammalian cells that act as coenzymes and promote the chemical transfer of single carbon units from one molecule to another. Folates are often used as a dietary supplement during pregnancy to prevent birth defects such as spina bifida.

Follow-up: Scheduled contacts made by the clinician with patients who have agreed to quit using tobacco.

Fones' method: A toothbrushing technique named after Dr. Alfred Fones.

Foramen cecum: A small pitlike depression located where the sulcus terminalis points backward toward the pharynx.

Fordyce granules: Normal variations sometimes appearing on the buccal mucosa and lips caused by the entrapment of fat cells clinically seen as small yellowish elevations.

Fractionation: The division of the total dose of radiation into small doses given at intervals.

Free gingival groove: A shallow line or depression on the gum surface at the junction of the free and attached gingiva.

Free gingival margin: The unattached gingiva surrounding the teeth in a collarlike fashion and demarcated from the attached gingiva by a shallow curvalinear depression that mirrors the gingival margin.

Free soft-tissue graft: Living tissue detached from its vascular and nutrient supply, removed from its origin, and transplanted to a recipient site within the oral cavity.

Frena: A restraining portion or structure. See also *Frenum.*

Frenectomy: The excision or removal of a frenum.

Frenum: A fold of mucous membrane attaching the cheeks and lips to the upper and lower arches, in some instances limiting the motions of the lips and cheeks.

Fulcrum: The stabilization of an instrument; the pad of the ring finger serves as a finger rest.

Full denture: A removable dental prosthesis that replaces the entire dentition and associated structures of the maxillae or mandible.

Full gold crown (FGC):   A gold crown that completely covers the anatomic crown of an individual tooth to restore the tooth to its original contour and function.

Full-mouth disinfection: The process within a 24-hour period whereby the oral cavity is debrided and the oral tissues, including the pharyngeal area, are scrubbed, rinsed, and/or irrigated with an antimicrobial. It results in a total bacterial count drop throughout the oral cavity.

Full-thickness periodontal flap (mucoperiosteal flap):   A surgical flap that includes epithelium, connective tissue, periosteum, and their components. A full-thickness flap reflection exposes the underlying osseous structure.

Fungiform: Papilla on the dorsum of the tongue that is shaped like a mushroom.

Furcation: The area between two or more root branches before they divide from the root trunk.

Galvanic reaction: A shock that occurs when there is an electrical current present in the oral cavity as a result of the coming together of several conditions: (1) saliva that contains salt, which makes it a good conductor of electricity; (2) two metallic components of different composition that act as the battery (two restorations or a metal object such as a fork placed in the mouth); (3) electrical current, which occurs through the saliva.

Generalized anxiety disorder: A persistent and excessive anxiety or worry that lasts for at least 6 months.

GENOME: The complete set of genes in the chromosomes of each cell of a specific organism.

Genuine: Sincere, frank, and honest.

Geometric angle: The figure formed by two lines that extend from the same point.

Geometric charting forms: Charting forms that use a geometric design to represent a tooth, with each surface represented.

Gingiva: The mucous membrane tissue that immediately surrounds a tooth.

Gingiva/implant interface: Space where the implant and gingival tissue intersect.

Gingival recession: The apical migration of the gingiva from the cementoenamel junction, resulting in root surface exposure.

Gingival sulcus: The shallow furrow formed from the gingival margin to the junctional epithelium between the tooth and the sulcular epithelium.

Gingivitis: Inflammation of the gingiva.

Glass ionomer: A cement, luting, or restorative agent consisting of an acid-soluble glass, polyacrylic acid, and water that sets via an acid-base reaction.

Glossitis: The inflammation of the tongue.

Glossodynia: Painful sensations in the tongue; a sensation of burning in the tongue; a sore tongue.

Glycosaminoglycans: Any of several high molecular weight linear heteropolysaccharides that have disaccharide-repeating units that contain an N-acetylhexosamine and a hexose or hexuronic acid. Either or both residues may be sulfated.

Glycosylated hemoglobin: A hemoglobin A molecule with a glucose group on the *N*-terminal valine amino acid unit of the beta chain. The glycosylated hemoglobin concentration represents the average blood glucose level during the previous several weeks. In controlled diabetes mellitus, the concentration of glycosylated hemoglobin is within the normal range, but in uncontrolled cases, the level may be three to four times the normal concentration.

Goal setting: Determining what a clinician wishes to accomplish, both personally and professionally, based on talents, values, and personal philosophy.

Goiter: An enlarged thyroid gland.

Gold foil (GF):   Pure gold that has been thinned to a small thickness and is used in direct-gold cavity restorations.

Gold inlay (GI):   An intracoronal cast restoration of gold alloy that restores one or more tooth surfaces.

Gold onlay (GO):   An extracoronal cast restoration of gold alloy that restores the occlusal surface extending over the cusp and marginal ridges.

Grade: An attempt to describe the extent to which tumor cells resemble their normal counterparts in histological appearance and biological behavior.

Gram-negative infections: Infections caused by gram-negative bacteria. Some of the most common gram-negative pathogenic bacteria include *Bacteroides fragilis, Brucella abortus, Escherichia coli, Haemophilus influenzae, Klebsiella pneumoniae, Neisseria gonorrhoeae, Proteus vulgaris, Pseudomonas aeruginosa, Salmonella typhi, Shigella dysenteriae,* and *Yersinia pestis.*

Grit: With reference to abrasive agents, grit is the particle size.

Ground substance: A basic substance from which a specific organ or kind of tissue develops.

Guardian ad litem: An individual appointed by a court of law to act on behalf of another who is not capable legally of making decisions (e.g., a minor).

Gutta-percha: A plastic type of filling material used in endodontic treatment.

G.V. Black Caries Classification: A caries and cavity classification system developed by G.V. Black that is still used. Carious lesions are categorized as Class I, II, III, IV, V, or VI.

Gynecomastia: An abnormal enlargement of one or both breasts in men.

Halitosis: An offensive odor of the breath resulting from local and metabolic conditions (e.g., poor oral hygiene, periodontal disease, sinusitis, tonsillitis, suppurative bronchopulmonary disease, acidosis, uremia).

Handle: The portion of a dental hygiene instrument that is held by the clinician.

Hard palate: The anterior portion of the palate.

Health: A complete state of physical, mental, emotional, spiritual, and social well-being and not just the absence of infirmity. It includes actions taken to protect or enhance health and legal, fiscal, educational, and social measures.

Health education: Any combination of learning experiences designed to facilitate voluntary actions conducive to health.

Health promotion: Any planned combination of educational, political, regulatory, and organizational support for actions and conditions of living conducive to the health of individuals, groups, or communities. One component of health promotion also includes actions to protect or enhance health and legal, fiscal, educational, and social measures.

Hematuria: Blood in the urine.

Hemidesmosomal attachment: The mechanism that attaches epithelial cells to the tooth surface.

Hemodialysis: A procedure in which impurities or wastes are removed from the blood. It is used to treat renal failure and various toxic conditions.

Hemolysis: The breakdown of red blood cells and the release of hemoglobin that normally occur at the end of the life span of a red cell.

Hemostasis: The stoppage or cessation of bleeding.

Hepatitis: An inflammation of the liver.

Herniated or slipped disk: A rupture of the fibrocartilage surrounding an intervertebral disk, releasing the nucleus pulposus that cushions the vertebrae above and below. The resultant pressure on spinal nerve roots may cause considerable pain and damage to the nerves. The condition most frequently occurs in the lumbar region.

Hertz (Hz): A unit of frequency equal to 1 cycle per second.

Hirsutism: Increased body or facial hair, which is especially noted in women.

Histoplasmosis: A disease caused by the fungus *Histoplasma capsulatum* that affects the reticuloendothelial system. Ulceration of the oral mucosa may occur.

History of past and present illness: An account obtained during the interview with the patient of the onset, duration, and character of the present illness, as well as of any acts or factors that aggravate or ameliorate the symptoms. The patient is asked what he or she considers to be the cause of the symptoms and whether a similar condition has occurred in the past.

History of present oral condition: The history of the chief concern or complaint.

HIV infection: An infection of the host with the human immunodeficiency virus-1.

Honing machine: A bench-type device in which sharpening stones are mechanically rotated across an instrument blade.

Horizontal fibers: Fibers that run at right angles to the long axis of the tooth, from the cementum to the bone. Their primary function is to restrain lateral tooth movement.

Hormonal gingivitis: An inflammation of the gingiva (gums) relating to hormones.

Host response: The immune response of a host when cells receive an invader or insult.

Human immunodeficiency virus (HIV): A retrovirus that causes acquired immunodeficiency syndrome (AIDS).

Hydrodynamic theory: The theory most accepted for the transmission of a pain stimulus with dentinal tubules.

Hydrolysis: The reaction between the ions of salt and those of water to form an acid and a base, one or both of which is only slightly dissociated. A process whereby a large molecule is split by the addition of water.

Hyoid: Pertaining to the hyoid bone.

Hyperbaric oxygen: Placing a patient in a sealed chamber and administering pure oxygen through a face mask. At the same time, compressed air is introduced into the chamber to raise the atmospheric pressure to several times normal. This equalizes the pressure inside and outside the body and thereby floods the tissues with oxygen. An increase in oxygen to the irradiated tissues can temporarily compensate for the reduction in circulation.

Hyperkeratinization: An abnormal thickening of the epithelium from excessive friction, trauma, or use.

Hypertelorism: An abnormally increased distance between two organs or parts. *Orbital* or *ocular hypertelorism* is an abnormally increased distance between the orbits.

Hypertension: An abnormal elevation of systolic and/or diastolic arterial pressure.

Hyperthyroidism: Metabolic abnormality resulting from an elevation of thyroid hormone.

Hyperventilation: Abnormally prolonged, rapid, and deep breathing; also the condition produced by overbreathing of oxygen at high pressures.

Hypnosis: A condition of artificially induced sleep or of a trance resembling sleep induced by drugs, psychological means, or both. It generally creates a condition of heightened suggestibility in the subject.

Hypochromic microcytic anemia: A group of anemias characterized by a decreased concentration of hemoglobin in the red blood cells.

Hypofunction: A diminished or inadequate level of activity of an organ system or its parts.

Hypomineralized: Pertaining to a deficiency of mineral elements in the body.

Hypoplasia: Incomplete development or underdevelopment of an organ or tissue.

Hypothyroidism: The diminished activity of the thyroid gland with decreased secretion of thyroxin that results in lowered basal metabolic rate, lethargy, sleepiness, dysmenorrhea in women, and a tendency toward obesity.

Hypoxia: Low oxygen content or tension.

Hyptephobia: A fear of being touched.

Icteric: Jaundiced.

Imaging: The production of diagnostic images, including radiography, ultrasonography, photography, or scintigraphy.

Immune system: A biochemical complex that protects the body against pathogenic organisms and other foreign bodies. The system incorporates the humoral immune response, which produces antibodies to react with specific antigens, and the cell-mediated response, which uses T cells to mobilize tissue macrophages in the presence of a foreign body.

Immunoassays: Competitive-binding assays in which the binding protein is an antibody.

Immunocompromised: Weakened immune response caused by a disease or an immunosuppressive agent.

Immunological and inflammatory response: A tissue reaction to injury or an antigen. The response may include pain, swelling, itching, redness, heat, loss of function, or a combination of symptoms.

Immunosuppression: The act or action of lowering or reducing the immune response.

Implant abutments: The portions of dental implants that serve to support and retain any prosthesis.

Implant-borne prostheses: A prosthesis that fits onto a dental implant, such as an overdenture.

Implementation: A deliberate action performed to achieve a goal, such as carrying out a plan in the care of a patient.

Implied consent: On agreement to a treatment, the patient is presumed to have consented to all procedures required for such treatment.

In situ: In its normal place; confined to the site of origin.

In vitro: Occurring in a laboratory apparatus.

Inactive caries: A condition in which lesions do not progress; it may remineralize and appear small on radiographs.

Incidence: The number of times an event occurs.

Incision: A cut or wound created by the separation of adjacent tissue with a sharp instrument.

Incisive canal: Opening in the anterior palate through which the nasopalatine nerve and blood vessels exit.

Incompetent: Descriptor referring to an individual who does not possess the knowledge or skills necessary to perform a professional function to the expected standard.

India stone: A type of sharpening stone made of man-made materials and used to sharpen periodontal instruments.

Indices: A method by which clinical disease parameters are quantitatively recorded.

Inferior: Situated below or lower than a point of reference.

Informed consent: A patient's consent to medical/dental treatment given after the patient understands the nature of his or her condition, treatment options, the risks involved in treatment, and the risks if no treatment is sought.

Informed refusal: A person's election not to accept treatment after being fully educated about the risks and benefits associated with the treatment.

Insulin: A peptide hormone produced in the pancreas by the beta cells in the islets of Langerhans. Insulin regulates glucose metabolism and is the major fuel-regulating hormone.

Insulin-dependent diabetes mellitus (IDDM): An inability to metabolize carbohydrate caused by an absolute insulin deficiency. It occurs in children and adults. It is characterized by excessive thirst, increased urination, increased desire to eat, loss of weight, diminished strength, and marked irritability.

Interdental: Between the proximal surfaces of the teeth within the same arch.

Interdental papilla: A projection of the gingiva filling the space between the proximal surfaces of two adjacent teeth.

Interexaminer reliability: The consistency of measurement between two or more examiners who are evaluating the same event.

Interleukins: The large groups of cytokines produced mainly by T cells or in some cases by mononuclear phagocytes or other cells. Most interleukins direct other cells to divide and differentiate. Each acts on a particular group of cells that express receptors specific for that interleukin.

Internal jugular: One of a pair of veins in the neck. Each internal jugular vein is continuous with the transverse sinus in the posterior part of the jugular foramen at the base of the skull.

International normalized ratio (INR): A comparative rating of a patient's prothrombin time (PT) ratio that is used as a standard for monitoring the effects of warfarin. The INR indicates what the patient's PT ratio would have been if measured by using the primary World Health Organization International Reference reagent.

International system: A system used in more than one country; in dentistry, it is a specific charting system.

Interproximal: Between the proximal surfaces of adjoining teeth.

Interradicular fibers: Fibers that are found only in multirooted teeth. They run from the cementum of the root and insert into the interradicular septum. Their primary function is to aid in the resistance of tipping and twisting.

Interval: A specified period or length of time between healthcare visits when patients manage their chronic conditions. In periodontal maintenance, the most common interval is 3 months between visits, although any interval should be tailored to the patient's current health status.

Intervention: A step or measure designed to halt or significantly alter the current course of an event.

Intimate: Close physical proximity (0 to 18 inches).

Intraexaminer reliability: The internal consistency of one individual during the rating or evaluation of a specific event more than once.

Intrinsic: Situated entirely within.

Irreversible hydrocolloid impression material: Material that cannot return to the sol state after it becomes a gel. The change in the physical state results from a chemical change in the material.

Irrigation: The flushing of an area. Irrigation can be a steady stream of liquid or pulsed. A daily pulsed or a fractionated, intermittent stream of water has been shown to be of therapeutic benefit in the treatment of gingivitis.

ISO: The International Standards Organization designation system.

Jargon: Vocabulary specific to a profession.

Jugulodigastric: Name for a lymph node, based on its location within the neck.

Junctional epithelium: A single or multiple layer of nonkeratinizing cells that adhere to the tooth surface at the base of the gingival crevice by hemidesmosomes.

Juvenile periodontitis: A distinct form of periodontal disease that may exhibit either localized or generalized inflammatory changes in the periodontium at prepubescence and adolescence.

Keratinized: Formation of a protein layer (keratin) on the surface of some epithelia.

Keratoconjunctivitis sicca: Dryness of the cornea caused by a deficiency of tear secretion in which the corneal surface appears dull and rough and the eye feels gritty and irritated.

Ketoacidosis: An accumulation of acid in the body resulting from the accumulation of ketone bodies.

Ketoconazole: A broad-spectrum synthetic antifungal agent applied to the skin to inhibit the growth of dermatophytes and yeasts. It is effective in *Candida* infections and in the treatment of seborrheic dermatitis.

Keyes' technique: The use of salt, baking soda, and hydrogen peroxide to prevent or control periodontal disease.

Knurl: One in a series of small ridges or beads on a metal surface that aids in gripping.

Koch's postulates: The prerequisites for experimentally establishing that a specific microorganism causes a particular disease.

Kretek: Clove and tobacco mixed product.

Kyphosis: An abnormal curvature of the spine with the convexity backward.

Labial mucosa: The mucosal lining of the inner portions of the lips.

Lactobacillus: Any one of a group of nonpathogenic, gram-positive, rod-shaped bacteria that produce lactic acid from carbohydrates.

Lamina densia: A layer of epithelial basal lamina that appears dark in electron micrographs.

Lamina lucida: A layer of epithelial basal lamina that appears light or clear in electron micrographs.

Lamina propria: A layer of connective tissue that lies just under the epithelium of the mucous membrane.

Lateral: Toward the side.

Lateral jaw: A radiographic image of one side of the jaw obtained via external film placement.

Lateral pressure: A force activated by wrist motion that is applied to secure the instrument's working end against the tooth surface.

Lateral sides: The portion of the working end of a periodontal scaling instrument located on either side of the face. The lateral sides join the face at either side to form the cutting edges.

Legal accountability: Legal responsibility for one's actions.

Leukodema: An innocuous oral condition characterized by a filmy, opalescent, white covering of the buccal mucosa that consists of a thickened layer of parakeratotic cells. It is most commonly associated with mechanical and chemical irritation.

Liability: Responsibility for a breach of duty.

Licensing examinations: Practical examinations administered to graduates of professional schools to determine whether each individual is qualified to practice the profession.

Licensure: The process whereby a competent authority issues permission to perform a certain act or engage in a specific business that would otherwise be unlawful.

Ligaments: Tough, fibrous connective tissue bands that connect bones or support viscera.

Line angle: The point where two lines join. In dentistry, the point where the facial surface joins to form the mesial surface of a tooth.

Linea alba: The white ridge of raised keratinized epithelial tissue on the facial mucosa that extends horizontally at the level where the teeth occlude.

Lingual tonsils: The irregular mass of tonsillar tissue located posteriorly on the lateral surfaces of the tongue.

Lipoma: A benign tumor characterized by fat cells.

Lipopolysaccharides: Part of the outer layer of the cell wall in gram-negative bacteria.

Listening: An element of communication that involves hearing, speaking, and paying attention to the spoken word.

Litigation: Court proceedings to determine legal issues regarding the rights and responsibilities between the parties.

Long axis: An imaginary straight line with respect to which a body is symmetrical; the axis of a tooth divides the tooth in half from crown to apex.

Lordosis: An anteroposterior curvature of the spine with the convexity facing forward.

Loss of attachment: A term describing the placement of the junctional epithelium apical to the cementoenamel junction.

Lumen: An opening. Oral irrigators have a lumen at the end of the tip or on the side of the tip.

Lupus: An autoimmune disease of the skin and mucous membrane.

Lupus erythematosus: A chronic inflammatory disease of unknown etiology affecting the skin, joints, kidneys, nervous system, serous membranes, and often other organs of the body.

Luxation: The dislocation or displacement of the condyle in the temporomandibular fossa or a tooth from the alveolus.

Lymph nodes: Bean-shaped bodies grouped in clusters along the connecting lymphatic vessels that are positioned to filter toxic products from the lymph.

Lymphadenectomy: Excision of one or more lymph nodes.

Lymphatic system: A vast, complex network of capillaries, vessels, valves, ducts, nodes, and organs that helps to protect and maintain the internal fluid environment of the entire body by producing, filtering, and conveying lymph and by producing various blood cells. The lymphatic network also transports fats, proteins, and other substances to the blood system and restores 60% of the fluid that filters from the blood capillaries into interstitial spaces during normal metabolism.

Lymphocytes: Leukocytes (white blood cells) found in large numbers in lymphoid tissues that contribute to immunity.

Lymphoma: Any neoplasm consisting of lymphoid tissue.

Macrophages: Phagocytic leukocytes found in tissues.

Magnetostrictive: The mechanism used to convert electrical energy into ultrasonic movement.

Maintaining competence: The act of keeping one's skills and knowledge current to continue quality performance.

Major depression: A severe form of depression that interferes with concentration, decision making, and social functioning.

Malignant: Term used to describe a cancerous tumor.

Malpractice: Negligent conduct of professional individuals or a breach of a standard of care.

Mandibular: Pertaining to the lower jaw.

Mandibular tori: The bony, hard, painless lesions that attach to the jaws and are frequently lobulated. They are usually bilateral and attached to the mandible, lingual to the bicuspid roots.

Mandrel-mounted stones: Small cylindrical or conical stones mounted to a slow-speed handpiece that is used to sharpen periodontal instruments.

Mania: A mood disturbance characterized by symptoms such as elation, inflated self-esteem, hyperactivity, and accelerated speaking and thinking. Mania is often associated with bipolar disorder.

Marginal breakdown: The breakdown of the integrity of the margin of a restoration, creating a trap for bacterial and potential caries activity.

Marginal irrigation: Flushing the pocket area by insertion of a soft, flexible rubber tip approximately 3 mm below the gingival margin; it is used daily at home.

Masseter: One of the four muscles of mastication. The thick rectangular muscle in the cheek that functions to close the jaw.

Masticatory mucosa: The mucosa associated with keratinized stratified squamous epithelium.

Materia alba: A soft white deposit around the necks of the teeth, usually associated with poor oral hygiene. It is composed of food debris, dead tissue elements, and purulent matter and serves as a medium for bacterial growth.

Maxillary tuberosity: A bony extension posterior to the maxillary teeth.

Mechanical: Pertaining to or accomplished by mechanical or physical forces; performed by means of some artificial mechanism.

Medial: In a direction toward or forward of the midline or middle of an object or the body.

Median lingual sulcus: A midline depression on the dorsal surface of the tongue.

Median palatine raphe: Ridge of tissue covering the palatine suture.

Medical history: A record of the state of health and medical history of a patient.

Megaloblastic anemia: An anemia characterized by hyperplastic bone marrow changes and maturation arrest that results from a dietary deficiency, impaired absorption, impaired storage and modification, or impaired use of one or more hematopoietic factors.

Melanocytes: Dendritic cells of the gingival epithelium that, when functional, cause pigmentation regardless of race.

Menopause: The period that marks the permanent cessation of menstrual activity, usually occurring between the ages of 35 and 58.

Mesothelioma: A rare, malignant neoplasm derived from the lining cells of the pleura and peritoneum, which grows as a thick sheet covering the viscera.

Metastasis: The transfer of disease from one organ or part to another not directly connected with it (e.g., regional or distant spread of cancer cells from the site primarily involved).

Microcrystals: Extremely minute crystals.

Microleakage: The seepage of fluids, debris, and microorganisms along the interface between a restoration and the walls of a cavity preparation.

Micron: The one-thousandth part of a millimeter, or the one-millionth part of a 0 symbol: μm.

Microradiography: A process by which a radiograph of a small object is produced on fine-grained photographic film under conditions that permit subsequent microscopic examination.

Microstreaming: A phenomena associated with ultrasonic scaling instruments whereby the water hitting the lip causes a hydrodynamic shear stress close to the oscillating tip.

Microvasculature: That portion of the circulatory system composed of the capillary network.

Minor: An individual who has not reached the age of legal competence (usually 21 years of age).

Mobility: The distance beyond normal physiological movement that the tooth moves in its socket.

Modified Stillman's method: A toothbrushing technique developed to simply massage the gingiva; the modified Stillman's method now includes cleaning the entire tooth.

Monofilament: Made of a single strand of material.

Monomer: The simplest molecular form of a substance.

Mononucleosis: An acute infectious viral disease that most commonly affects young adults and older children.

Monophobia: The fear of being alone.

Monostotic: Affecting a single bone.

Mood disorder: Disturbances in emotions severe enough to interfere with normal living.

Motivation: The provision of encouragement, support, and direction.

Mount and Hume classification system: A proposed classification for cavity designs that allows the introduction of smaller, more conservative caries than are possible with G.V. Black classification while allowing for the more extensive cavities that are the inevitable end-result of continuing replacement restorative dentistry.

Mouthguard: A resilient intraoral device worn during participation in contact sports to reduce the potential for injury to the teeth and associated tissue.

MRI: Acronym for *magnetic resonance imaging*.

Mucocutaneous: Of or pertaining to the mucous membrane and the skin.

Mucoepidermoid carcinoma: A malignant neoplasm of glandular tissues, especially the ducts of the salivary glands. The tumor contains mucinous and epidermoid squamous cells.

Mucogingival junction: The line that separates the attached gingiva from the alveolar mucosa. It is relatively loose, thin, and moveable.

Mucoperiosteal full-thickness flap: All soft tissue in an area is incised and elevated.

Mucoperiosteal split-thickness flap: Epithelium and part of the underlying connective tissue are incised and separated from the remaining connective tissue and periosteum.

Mucositis: An oral inflammation.

Mucous membrane: A membrane composed of epithelium and lamina propria that lines the oral cavity and other canals; also cavities of the body that communicate with external air.

Multiaxial: The classification system developed by the American Psychiatric Association in which the person is evaluated with regard to multiple variables rather than from a single aspect of assessment.

Multifilament: Consisting of several filaments or strands that are braided or twisted together.

Multilevel brush design: Toothbrush in which the head contains bristles of varying lengths.

Muscles of mastication: The powerful muscles that elevate and rotate the mandible so that the opposing teeth may occlude for mastication.

Musculoskeletal disorders (MSD):   Disorders affecting muscle and skeletal tissues resulting from inappropriate positioning, usually during repetitive use.

Mutans streptococci: A group of *Streptococcus* specifically with properties similar to *S. mutans (S. mutans, S. sobrinus, S. cricetus, S. rattus, S. ferus, S. macacae).*

Myasthenia gravis: An abnormal condition characterized by chronic fatigability and muscle weakness, especially in the face and throat, as a result of a defect in the conduction of nerve impulses at the myoneural junction.

Mylohyoid muscle: One of a pair of flat triangular muscles that form the floor of the cavity of the mouth. It is innervated by the mylohyoid nerve and acts to raise the hyoid bone and the tongue.

Myocardial infarction: An occlusion or blockage of arteries supplying the muscles of the heart that results in injury or necrosis of the heart muscle.

Mysophobia: A fear of germs.

Nadir: The lowest point, such as the blood count after it has been depressed by chemotherapy, of the item being measured.

Narcissistic personality disorder: A pattern of thinking and behavior characterized by a person's sense of grandiosity and preoccupation with his or her own achievements and abilities.

Nasal septum: The thin, vertical, bony septum separating the right and left nasal cavities.

Nasogastric tube: A tube placed through the nose into the stomach to introduce nutrients in a liquid form or to relieve gastric distension by removing gas, gastric secretions, or food or to obtain a specimen for laboratory analysis.

Nasolabial sulcus: The groove formed by the labial surface of the upper lip at the midline and the inferior border of the nose. It is a measure of the relative protrusion of the upper lip.

Necrotizing ulcerative periodontitis: Massive tissue destruction of the bone and connective tissue attachment in which the gingiva appears red and ulcerative, with punched-out papilla.

Neglect: The failure to do something that one is bound to do; lack of due care.

Negligence: The failure to use such care as a reasonable and careful person would use under similar circumstances.

Neonatal: The period of time covering the first 28 days after birth.

Neoplasia: The process of the formation of tumors by the uncontrolled proliferation of cells.

Neoplasm: Any new and abnormal growth, specifically one in which cell multiplication is controlled and progressive; may be benign or malignant.

Neuroleptic: A type of antipsychotic medication with associated side effects that resemble Parkinson's disease.

Neurotoxicity: The ability of a drug or other agent to destroy or damage nervous tissue.

Neurotransmitters: Chemicals that are activated to transmit signals from one neuron to another (neural pathways) and to other tissues. The neurotransmitters primarily activated by nicotine are acetylcholine, norepinepherine, dopamine, serotonin, vasopressin, beta-endorphin, growth hormones, and adrenal cortical thyroid hormone.

Neutral position: Position of a dental clinician in which an appendage is not moved from or directed toward the body's midline, including during monitoring or twisting.

Nicotine: A tertiary amine composed of a pyradine and a pyrrolidine ring. It is the chief alkaloid in tobacco products. It is absorbed rapidly through the skin and respiratory tract.

Nicotine replacement agents/products/drugs: Nicotine in a form that is free of tobacco and can be taken as a gum, transdermal patch through the skin, nasal spray, or oral inhaler to supply nicotine to the central nervous system so the intensity and duration of some withdrawal symptoms can be reduced.

Nicotinic stomatitis: A whitish lesion on the hard palate caused by the heat from smoking or consuming hot liquid.

Nightguard: Any removable artificial occlusal surface used for diagnosis or therapy that affects the relationship of the mandible to the maxillae. It may be used for occlusal stabilization, treatment of temporomandibular disorders, or prevention of dentition wear.

Non–insulin-dependent diabetis mellitus (NIDDM):   A type of diabetes mellitus in which patients are not insulin-dependent or ketosis-prone, although they may use insulin for correction of symptomatic or persistent hyperglycemia and can develop ketosis under special circumstances, such as infection or stress. Onset is usually after 40 years of age but can occur at any age. Two subclasses are the presence or absence of obesity.

Nonkeratinized: Moveable and compressible; soft and smooth to the touch.

Nonmaleficence: An obligation to provide services in a manner that protects the patient and results in the prevention of harm.

Nonspecific plaque hypothesis: A hypothesis associated with the cause of periodontal disease based on the quality of plaque present, *not* on specific organisms.

Nonverbal cues: Gestures, facial expressions, or body posture used to convey a message.

Normochromic normocytic anemia: An anemia associated with disturbances of red cell formation and related to endocrine deficiencies, chronic inflammation, and carcinomatosis.

Nuchal: Referring to the neck.

Nucleic acid probes: A microbiological assay that uses DNA and RNA to identify oral microorganisms.

Nucleus pulposus: The central part of each intervertebral disk consisting of a pulpy elastic substance that loses some of its resiliency with age. The nucleus pulposus may be suddenly compressed and squeezed out through the annular fibrocartilage, which causes a herniated disk and extreme pain.

Nyctophobia: A fear of darkness or night.

Nystagmus: The state of oscillatory movements of an organ or part, especially the eyeballs; irregular jerking movement of the eyes. Each movement of the cycle consists of a slow component in one direction and a rapid component in the opposite direction.

Oblique: Neither perpendicular or parallel; inclined.

Oblique fibers: Any of the collagenous filaments that are bundled together obliquely in the periodontal ligament, inserted into the cementum, and extended more occlusally in the alveolus. These fibers compose approximately two thirds of the periodontal fibers.

Observing: To notice or pay attention to; watching in a nonverbal manner.

Obsessions: Ideas or thoughts that involuntarily and constantly intrude into awareness and are generally pointless thoughts.

Obsessive-compulsive disorder: Characterized by obsessions that provoke clinically significant anxiety and by compulsions that act to neutralize the anxiety.

Obturator: A device used to restore the continuity of the hard or soft palate or both.

Occipital: Referring to the back part of the head

Occlude: To close or bring the teeth together.

Occlusal plane: The average plane established by the incisal and occlusal surfaces of the teeth. Generally, it is not a plane but represents the planar mean of the curvature of these surfaces.

Occlusal radiograph: An intraoral radiograph made with occlusal film placed on the occlusal surfaces of one of the arches. It shows the relationship of teeth to the underlying structures in the alveolar process, such as cysts and abscesses.

Odontoblast: A cell that forms the surface layer of the dental papilla that forms dentin of the tooth. Odontoblasts continue production for years after eruption.

Omohyoid: Pertaining to the shoulder and the hyoid bone.

Oncology: The sum of knowledge regarding tumors; the study of tumors.

Operator positioning: The operator's chair position changes in relation to the area of the mouth that is being treated. A change in the position of the operator within the zone of activity can improve visibility and reduce back and neck strain caused by bending and leaning.

Oral candidiasis: An infection caused by a species of *Candida*, usually *Candida albicans*. It is characterized by pruritus (a white exudate), peeling, and easy bleeding. Oral candidiasis without a history of recent antibiotic therapy, chemotherapy, corticosteroid therapy, or radiation therapy to the head and neck or other immunosuppressive disorder may indicate the possibility of human immunodeficiency virus infection.

Oral human papillomavirus infection: Warts caused by the human papillomavirus (HPV) that may be scattered throughout the mouth or localized in one area. They frequently recur. Oral warts are associated with acquired immunodeficiency syndrome infection.

Oral irrigator: A powered device for personal use that delivers an intermittent stream of water or an antimicrobial agent at the tooth or below the gingival margin.

Oral nystatin: An antifungal antibiotic taken by mouth.

Oral physiotherapy aids: Any oral cleaning device, such as a toothbrush, floss, etc.

Organ system: A part of the body having a special or specific function.

Orofacial: Pertaining to the mouth and face.

Oropharyngeal isthmus: The narrow opening between the mouth and the pharynx.

Oropharynx: The oral division of the pharynx that is located between the soft palate and the opening of the larynx.

Orthopnea: An inability to breathe except in an upright position.

OSHA: Acronym for Occupational Safety and Health Administration.

Osmolarity: The osmotic pressure of a solution expressed in osmols or milliosmols per liter of the solution.

Osmotic: Pertaining to osmosis.

Osseous: Bony.

Osseous defect: An imperfection, failure, or absence of bone.

Osseous surgery: A portion of periodontal surgery that modifies bone in an attempt to correct osseous defects and deformities.

Osteoblast: Cuboidal cells associated with the growth and development of bone. In active growth, osteoblasts form a continuous layer on old bone similar to a sheet of epithelial cells; when the bone growth is arrested, the cells assume an elongated appearance like fibroblasts.

Osteoporosis: A disease process that results in reduction in the mass of bone.

Outline form: The shape of the area of the tooth surface included within the cavosurface margins of a prepared cavity.

Overbite: A vertical overlapping of maxillary over mandibular teeth that is usually measured perpendicular to the occlusal plane.

Overdenture: A complete or partial removable denture supported by retained roots to provide improved support, stability, and tactile sensation and to reduce ridge resorption.

Overjet: The horizontal projection of maxillary teeth beyond the mandibular teeth, usually measured parallel to the occlusal plane.

Pain: A subjective unpleasant sensory and emotional experience associated with actual or potential tissue damage or described in terms of such damage.

Pain stimulus: An event that precipitates the conduction of the pain response.

Palatal lift: The vault-shaped muscular structure forming the soft palate between the mouth and the nasopharynx.

Palatine fovea: Small pits in the mucosa on each side of the midline where the soft and hard palates meet.

Palatine rugae: Irregular ridges or folds of masticatory mucosa extending laterally from the incisive papilla and the anterior part of the palatine raphe.

Palatine tonsil: One of a pair of almond-shaped masses of lymphoid tissue between the palatoglossal and the palatopharyngeal arches on each side of the fauces. They are covered with mucous membrane and contain numerous lymph follicles and various crypts.

Palatopharyngeal fold: A sphincteric action sealing the oral cavity from the nasal cavity by the synchronous movement of the soft palate superiorly, the lateral pharyngeal wall medially, and the posterior wall of the pharynx anteriorly.

Palliative: Affording relief but not curing.

Palmer's tooth notation: A tooth numbering system that codes the teeth with numbers and letters using brackets to indicate the arch.

Palpation: The act of feeling with the hand.

Panic attack: A sudden, overwhelming sense of terror. Unlike anxiety, which involves a more generalized stimulus for onset, a panic attack has a more focused precipitant.

Panoramic: A radiographic method in which a continuous image of both maxillary and mandibular dental arches and associated structures are obtained.

Papilla: Gingiva filling the interproximal spaces between adjacent teeth; projections located on the dorsum of the tongue that contain receptors for the sense of taste.

Parallel: Two straight lines of equal distance apart that will never meet.

Paranoid personality disorder: A pattern of thinking and behavior characterized by inappropriate suspiciousness of the motives and behaviors of others.

Paranoid type: A type of schizophrenia characterized by persecutory delusions.

Paraphrase: Rewording of the meaning expressed in something spoken.

Parathormone (PTH): The trade name for parathyroid hormone.

Paresis: A progressive psychosis associated with neurosyphilis.

Paresthesia: An extended time period of numbness.

Parotid: Pertaining to the parotid gland, which is one type of salivary gland.

Partial denture: A prosthetic device containing artificial teeth supported on a framework and attached to natural teeth by means of clasps.

Partial gold crown (¾ GC): A gold crown that does not cover the entire anatomic crown. The tooth is prepared so the facial surface of the tooth is unchanged. When the crown is placed, the natural enamel on the facial surface is visible and the prepared portion is covered by the crown.

Partial/split-thickness periodontal flap: See *Mucoperiosteal full-thickness flap* and *Mucoperiosteal split-thickness flap*.

Partially erupted tooth: A tooth that has only a portion of the anatomic crown exposed in the oral cavity.

Pastille: A gelatin-based sweetened and molded medication impregnated with a therapeutic substance intended to be sucked. Also, a chemically-treated paper disk that undergoes color changes when exposed to radiation.

Pathogenesis: The source or cause of an illness or abnormal condition.

Pathophobia: A fear of disease.

Patient positioning: Arrangement of the patient in the dental chair and the relationship of the chair to the workspace and clinician.

Pellagra: A nutritional deficiency resulting from faulty intake or metabolism of nicotinic acid, a vitamin B complex factor. It is characterized by glossitis, dermatitis of sun-exposed surfaces, stomatitis, diarrhea, and dementia.

Pellicle: The thin, saliva-based, protein layer that coats the teeth and forms the base over which dental plaque develops.

Percussion: Examination by striking an area and evaluating the sounds and sensations.

Performance Logic positioning: Clinician positioning during patient care, based on the elimination of musculoskeletal strain.

Periapical radiolucency (PAR): A translucent area observed at the apex of a tooth, depicting reduced calcification, usually due to infection.

Pericoronitis: An inflammation of the tissue flap over a partially erupted tooth, commonly a third molar.

Perimenopause: The phase before the onset of menopause.

Periodontal debridement: The removal of plaque, calculus, and endotoxins from the root surface of the tooth.

Periodontal disease: An infectious disease that results in destruction of the soft tissue and/or bone that support the teeth (e.g., gingivitis, periodontitis).

Periodontal dressing (pack): A protective material applied postoperatively to the surface of a wound created by a periodontal surgical procedure.

Periodontal ligament: The connective tissue fibers that surround the root of the tooth and attach it to the alveolar process.

Periodontal maintenance (PM): A term accepted by the American Academy of Periodontology in 2000 to replace the term *supportive periodontal therapy*.

Periodontal surgery: A surgical procedure used to modify the periodontium in an attempt to treat or prevent periodontal disease.

Periodontitis: An inflammation of the supporting tissues of the teeth, resulting in attachment loss.

Periodontium: The tissues that invest (or help to invest) and support the teeth (i.e., the gingiva, cementum of the tooth, periodontal ligament, and alveolar and supporting bone).

Pernicious anemia: A macrocytic-normochromic, megaloblastic anemia associated with achlorhydria and a lack of a gastric intrinsic factor necessary for the binding and absorption of vitamin B_{12} (an erythrocyte-maturing factor).

Perpendicular: Two straight lines that meet at a right angle.

Personal space: The distance between two people that is neither threatening nor too distant so as not to be heard.

Personality disorder: Maladaptive patterns of personality that result in either social or occupational problems and in significant distress to the person.

Petechiae: Minute red spots on the skin or mucous membranes resulting from escape of a small amount of blood.

Pharyngeal: Pertaining to the pharynx.

Phase-contrast microscopy: A microscope with a special condenser and objective, which contains a phase-shifting ring by which small differences in the index of refraction become visible. The use of phase-contrast capabilities allows for direct viewing of transparent live cells and tissues.

Philtrum: The vertical groove on the midline of the upper lip that extends downward from the nasal septum to the tubercle of the upper lip.

Phobia: A persistent and irrational fear associated with a specific object or situation.

Photodynamic therapy (PDT): A cancer treatment modality that uses a photosensitizing drug and a laser.

Piezoelectric: Term pertaining to a type of ultrasonic powered scaler used in dentistry. The conversion of electrical power to tip motion is by way of ceramic crystal vibrations.

Pilocarpine (Salagen): An alkaloid that causes parasympathetic effects (e.g., secretion of the salivary, bronchial, and gastrointestinal glands). It stimulates the sweat glands and also causes vasodilation and cardiac inhibition.

Pits and fissures: A result of noncoalescence of enamel during tooth formation.

Plaintiff: The party who sues in a civil action and is named on the record of the lawsuit. In a criminal action the plaintiff would be the people of the state in a state action or the people of the United States in a federal action.

Plaque: A microcosm of bacteria, various food particles, salivary proteins, and polysaccharides that accumulates on the teeth.

Plaque-associated gingivitis: An inflammation of the gingivae directly related to the presence of bacterial plaque on the tooth surface and the amount of time during which the plaque is allowed to remain undisturbed.

Plaque index: A standardized mechanism used to categorize or quantify the amount and/or location of plaque within the oral cavity.

Plica fimbriata: Fringelike projections on the ventral surface of the tongue in the location of the lingual veins.

Plica lingualis: Fingerlike tissue projections along the top of the sublingual fold.

Point angle: An angle formed by the junction of three walls at a common point; designated by combining the names of the walls forming the angle.

Polarized light microscopy: Microscopy where polarized light is used for special diagnostic purposes, such as examining crystals of chemicals found in patients with gout and related disorders. Polarized light is light where the radiation waves occur in only one direction in the vibration plane and not at random.

Polishing: The production, especially by friction, of a smooth, floss, mirrorlike surface that reflects light; a fine agent is used for polishing after a coarser agent is used for cleaning.

Polishing agent: Any material used to impart luster to a surface.

Polycythemia: An increase in the total red blood cell mass in the blood.

Polydipsia: Abnormally increased thirst.

Polymer: The product formed by joining together many small molecules (monomers).

Polymerization: A reaction in which a complex molecule of relatively high molecular weight is formed by the union of a number of simpler molecules, which may or may not be alike.

Polymerization shrinkage: Pulling away or contraction of polymerized composite resins.

Polymyositis: An inflammation of many muscles, usually accompanied by deformity, edema, insomnia, pain, sweating, and tension. Some forms of polymyositis are associated with malignancy.

Polyostotic: Affecting more than one bone.

Polyphagia: Excessive uncontrolled eating.

Polyuria: The passage of an abnormally increased volume of urine. It may result from increased intake of fluids, inadequate renal function, uncontrolled diabetes mellitus or diabetes insipidus, diuresis of edema fluid, or ascites.

Pontic: An artificial tooth on a fixed partial denture that replaces a missing natural tooth, restores its function, and usually fills the space previously occupied by the clinical crown.

Porcelain fused to metal (PFM): A fixed restoration that uses a metal substructure on which a ceramic veneer is fused.

Porcelain jacket crown (PJC): A ceramic crown made on a platinum matrix.

Porte polisher: A hand instrument constructed to hold a wooden point. It is used in a dental engine to burnish and to apply polishing paste to teeth.

Postauricular: Term referring to a portion posterior to the ear.

Postmenopause: The phase following the completion of menopause.

Postprandial: After a meal.

Posttraumatic stress disorder: The reexperiencing of an extremely traumatic event accompanied by increased arousal and by avoidance of stimuli associated with the trauma.

Postural syndrome: A condition that occurs from the maintenance of muscles in a position other than the neutral position for long periods of time repetitively, ultimately resulting in pain.

Potassium nitrate: A compound occurring as a white granular or crystalline powder or as colorless transparent prisms; used as a food preservative and formerly used as an oral diuretic. Called also *niter* and *saltpeter*.

Power-driven: Energy of movement from an external source, such as electricity.

Powered toothbrush: A toothbrush using one or several motions such as back and forth, up and down, or circular that is powered by batteries or electricity.

Practice act: The combined state statutory regulations and agency laws.

Practice philosophy: A way of thinking that underpins an individual's clinical practice or patient care.

Preauricular: Located anterior to the auricle of the ear.

Preceptorship: Learning a new career on the job. The role of teacher is assumed by the employer. Commonly called *"on-the-job training."* In dentistry, this relates to the training of a dental hygienist by a dentist.

Precipitate: An insoluble solid substance that forms from chemical reactions between solutions.

Premature ventricular contractions (PVCs): A cardiac sinus conducted dysrhythmia characterized by ventricular depolarization that occurs earlier than expected. It is shown on the electrocardiogram as an early, wide QRS complex without a preceding related P wave.

Prepubertal periodontitis: A disease of the periodontium that occurs early in life, affecting both deciduous and permanent teeth and usually resulting in early edentulism. Patients with this condition often have white blood cell defects.

Presentation: (1) Something presented as a symbol or image that represents something; (2) something offered or given (e.g., gift); (3) something set forth for the attention of the mind; (4) a descriptive or persuasive account. Case presentation is a symbol that represents a case and a persuasive account of the strategies within the case for the intent of learning more about the actual care of a patient.

Prevalence: The number of people infected with a particular disease at any one time.

Prevention: A method that prevents an expected or anticipated event from occurring.

Prevention strategy: An action plan directed to prevent illness and promote health so as to eliminate the need for secondary or tertiary health care.

Primary care provider: A practitioner in one of the health professions (e.g., medicine; nursing; psychology; dentistry/oral health; physical, occupational, and respiratory therapy) who provides healthcare services.

Principal fibers: Collagen fibers organized into groups based on their orientation to the tooth and related function.

Professional portfolio: A method by which an individual's achievements, work, or performance is documented.

Progesterone: A steroid hormone responsible for changes in the endometrium in the second half of the menstrual cycle.

Prognosis: A forecast of the probable course and outcome of an attack of disease and the prospects of recovery as indicated by the nature of the disease and the symptoms of the case.

Prophylaxis: Term pertaining to the cleaning and polishing of the teeth.

Proprioceptive: Term used describe the feeling of muscle movement associated with operator positioning and movement during patient care.

Prostaglandins: A group of potent hormonelike substances that produce a wide range of body responses such as changing capillary permeability, smoothing muscle tone, clumping of platelets, and endocrine and exocrine functions. They may be used in some instances to terminate a pregnancy.

Proteinase: A proteolytic enzyme that splits protein molecules at central linkages.

Proteoglycans: Any of a group of polysaccharide-protein conjugates occurring primarily in the matrix of connective tissue and cartilage. Proteoglycans are composed mainly of polysaccharide chains—particularly glycosaminoglycans—and minor protein components.

psi: Abbreviation for pounds per square inch.

Psychoactive chemicals/drugs: Substances that produce signals in the brain's limbic and cortical systems and produce strong sensations of "liking," "well-being," or "pleasure." Such signals, needed for thriving and survival, are reinforcing so, when artificially stimulated, tend to upset and distort natural balances of consciousness, reason, and behavior.

Pterygoid: Term pertaining to a winglike structure. Pterygoid plates are part of the sphenoid bone of the skull.

Pterygomandibular raphe: A tendinous line between the buccinator and the constrictor pharynges superior muscles, from which the middle portions of both muscles originate.

Ptosis: An abnormal condition of one or both upper eyelids in which the eyelid droops because of a congenital or acquired weakness of the levator muscle or paralysis of cranial nerve III.

Puberty: The stage in life when members of both sexes become functionally capable of reproduction.

Public: Term used to express a formal status.

Pulpitis: An inflammation of the pulp of a tooth.

Pulsating: An intermittent or fractionated stream of water or irrigant.

Pulse rhythm: The rhythmic expansion of an artery as the heart beats; it can be felt with slight finger pressure on the surface of the skin in several areas of the body.

Pumice: A type of volcanic glass used as an abrasive. It is prepared in various grits and used for finishing and polishing.

Purpura: A group of disorders characterized by purplish or brownish-red discolorations caused by bleeding into the skin or tissues.

Purulent: Containing or forming pus.

Purview: The body and scope of an act or bill.

Pyogenic granuloma: A small nonmalignant mass of excessive granulation tissue usually found at the site of an injury. Most often a dull red color, it contains numerous capillaries, bleeds readily, and is tender. It may be attached by a narrow stalk.

Pyrophobia: A fear of fire.

Quiescence: A state of inactivity, quiet, or rest; latency or dormancy.

Quit day: The day of a given cessation attempt during which a patient tries to abstain totally from tobacco use.

Radiation caries: Decay, mostly at the cervical margins, caused by the loss of minerals that results from radiation therapy.

Radiation modifiers: Agents such as beta-carotene and 13 cis-retinoic acid believed to have value as chemopreventives in the reduction of tumors.

Radiation osteomyelitis/osteonecrosis: The damage or destruction of the blood supply to the bone, resulting from radiation therapy.

Radiolucency: A characteristic of materials of relatively low atomic number that have low attenuation characteristics, which allows most x-rays to pass through them and thus produces relatively dark images.

Radiolucent: A substance that allows radiant energy to pass through it, producing black areas on radiographs.

Radiopacity: The quality of being radiopaque, or having the ability to stop or reduce the passage of radiation.

Radiopaque: A substance that does not allow radiant energy to pass through it, producing light areas on radiographs.

Radiotherapy: The treatment of disease by ionizing radiation; may be external megavoltage or internal by use of interstitial implantation of an isotope (radium).

Radium: A highly radioactive chemical element found in uranium minerals. It is used in the treatment of malignant tumors in the form of needles or pellets for interstitial implantation.

Radon: A colorless gas produced by the disintegration of radium.

Rapidly progressive periodontitis: A condition that occurs in young adults ages 20 to 30 years that is characterized by gingival inflammation and rapid loss of bone and supporting tissues.

Rapport: The creation and enhancement of a positive relationship.

Recession: Loss of part or all of the gingiva over the root of a tooth.

Reciprocity: Professional licensure valid in one state based on the fact that the individual requesting the license is validly licensed in another state.

Recurrent or secondary caries: Caries occurring at the restoration-tooth interface or under an existing restoration.

Refractory periodontitis: A progressive inflammatory destruction of the periodontal attachment that resists conventional mechanical treatment.

Regulation: A criterion described in laws that outlines what a practitioner can do under that act or statute.

Relapse: A return to tobacco use after a period of hours, days, weeks, months, or years by an individual who had at one time been a tobacco user (100 or more cigarettes in one's life, or a regular user of any tobacco product or combination of tobacco products).

Relaxation: A reduction of tension, as when a muscle relaxes between contractions.

Remineralization: The process of restoring minerals to a mineralized tissue that has been demineralized.

Removable partial denture: A prosthesis that replaces one or more teeth in a partially dentate arch and is removable from the mouth.

Reparative dentin: Dentin of an irregular nature formed below a carious lesion as a means of preserving pulpal integrity.

Repetitive strain injuries (RSI): Tissue damage to the neck and arms associated with tasks that require repeated manipulations of the hands, such as meat cutting, computer keyboarding, playing musical instruments, or practicing dentistry or dental hygiene.

Resistance form: A shape that is given to a cavity to provide a filling that has the ability to withstand the stress brought on it in mastication.

Respect: To look at with or to show consideration, regard, or esteem.

Retainer: A device used to hold something in place; the attachment or abutments of a fixed or removable prosthesis; an appliance for maintaining the positions of the teeth and jaws immediately after the completion of orthodontic treatment.

Retention: The act of retaining or holding back; the fixation or stabilization.

Retention form: Shaping the remaining enamel and dentin to strengthen the tooth and restoration.

Retinopathy: A noninflammatory eye disorder resulting from changes in the retinal blood vessels.

Retroauricular: Pertaining to a location behind the ear.

Retromolar pad: A dense pad of tissue just distal to the last tooth of the mandibular arch.

Revocation: The act of terminating an individual's license to practice a profession such as dental hygiene. This action is delegated to the regulatory agency that governs a profession.

Reynaud's phenomenon: Intermittent attacks of ischemia of the extremities of the body, especially the fingers, toes, ears, and nose, caused by exposure to cold or by emotional stimuli. The attacks are characterized by severe blanching of the extremities, followed by cyanosis, then redness; they are usually accompanied by numbness, tingling, burning, and often pain. Normal color and sensation are restored by heat.

Rheumatic heart disease (RHD): Damage to heart muscle and heart valves caused by episodes of rheumatic fever. When a susceptible person acquires a group A beta-hemolytic streptococcal infection, an autoimmune reaction may occur in heart tissue, which results in permanent deformities of heart valves or chordae tendineae.

Rhomboidal: Resembling the shape of an oblique equilateral parallelogram, as in a rhomboid muscle.

Rinsing: The act of vigorously forcing liquid from side to side in the oral cavity by closing the lips and flexing the cheeks and tongue.

Risk: The probability of an event occurring, such as a loss or injury.

Risk assessment: A survey designed to determine the degree to which an individual is placed at risk for developing a condition or a disease.

Risk factors: Those conditions or behaviors associated with risk occurrence.

Risk in a health event: The probability of experiencing a change in health status over time.

Rolling stroke: A toothbrushing method characterized by the rolling of the brush head to clean the facial and lingual tooth surfaces.

Root canal (RC): The space occupied by the nerves, blood vessels, and lymph in the radicular part of the tooth, or the procedures associated with the removal of the components within the canal and filling with a material.

Rotated teeth: The movement of teeth to the left or right from normal alignment.

Rounded edge: An instrument edge that may or may not be sharp and contains no angles.

rpm: Abbreviation for revolutions per minute.

Rubber dam: A material used in the patient's mouth for protection, to ensure access and visibility in the operating field, and for efficient use of operating time.

Rubber dam clamp: A device made of spring metal that is used to retain a rubber dam in place or to improve the operating field by isolating it from the oral environment.

Salivary gland acini: Any small saclike structure found in the salivary glands.

Salivary glands: Glands that produce saliva.

Sanguinarine: A benzophenanthridine alkaloid thought to be useful in reducing plaque and gingivitis.

Schizoid personality disorder: Pattern of thinking and behavior characterized by indifference to other people, coupled with a diminished range of emotional experience and expression.

Scleroderma: A collagen disease of unknown etiology; skin lesions are characterized by thickening, rigidity, and pigmentation in patches or diffuse areas.

Sclerosis: Hardening. As applied to the jaws, sclerosis usually indicates an increased calcification centrally, with radiopacity. Tracts of increased density in the dentin are called *areas of dentinal sclerosis.* Sclerosis occurs beneath caries and with abrasion, attrition, or erosion.

Sclerotic dentin: Hardening or induration of the chief material of teeth, which surrounds the pulp and is situated inside the enamel and cementum.

Sealant: Resin that bonds to enamel surface by mechanical retention via tiny openings created by acid etching the enamel surface.

Sebaceous cyst: A misnomer for *epidermoid cyst* or *pilar cyst.*

Self-help: Treatment methods that are not aided by a clinician.

Self-regulation: A profession's assumption of the responsibility for controlling its members through licensure and enforcement of the rules and regulations governing it.

Semisupine position: Pertaining to a posture that is between a midposition and the supine position.

Sensitivity: A state of responsiveness to external influences or sensations such as heat or trauma; susceptibility to a substance, such as drug or antigen.

Sequelae: Any abnormal condition that follows and is the result of a disease, treatment, or injury, such as paralysis after poliomyelitis, deafness after treatment with an ototoxic drug, or scar formation after a laceration.

Shank: The portion of a dental hygiene instrument that joins the handle with the working end. The shank can be straight or contraangled.

Sharpey's fibers: The collagen fibers from the periodontal ligament that are partially inserted into the cementum and bone.

Sialadenitis: Any inflammation of one or more of the salivary glands.

Sialadenopathy: A disease of a salivary gland.

Sialograms: Radiographic films taken after injection of a radiopaque medium that determine the presence or absence of calcareous deposits in a salivary gland or its ducts.

Sialolith: A calcification within the salivary gland.

Sicca syndrome: An abnormal dryness of the mouth, eyes, or other mucous membranes. The condition is seen in patients with Sjögren's syndrome, sarcoidosis, amyloidosis, and deficiencies of vitamins A and C.

Sickle: A periodontal scaling instrument designed to remove calculus deposits from the coronal tooth surface.

Side-port: The location of the lumens on the irrigator tip are on the side of the tip.

Single-blind study: An experiment in which the person collecting data knows whether the subject is in the control group or the experimental group yet the subjects do not.

Sinus bradycardia: The slow beating of the sinus node at rates of fewer than 60 beats/min.

Sinus rhythm: A cardiac rhythm stimulated by the sinus (sinoatrial) node. A rate of 60 to 100 beats/min is normal.

Sinus tachycardia: A rapid heartbeat generated by discharge of the sinoatrial pacemaker. The rate is generally 100 to 180 beats/min in the adult, 140 to 200 beats/min in a child, and greater than 200 beats/min in an infant.

Site-specific: Localized to a particular area.

Sjögren's syndrome: A condition related to deficient secretion of salivary, sweat, lacrimal, and mucous glands (xerostomia, keratoconjunctivitis, rhinitis, dysphagia), increased size of salivary glands, and polyarthritis.

Slow-speed handpiece: A dental handpiece used to hold rotary instruments that operates at 6,000 to 10,000 rpms.

Sludge: Collection of metal fragments and oil from grinding a stone against an instrument.

Smear layer: A thin (5 to 10 microns) organic film of organic debris that adheres to dentin as a result of cavity preparation, or burnishing action on exposed dentin.

Snyder colorimetric test: A method of determining the concentration of acid-producing bacteria in the saliva by use of bromcresol green in a culture medium.

Social history: A patient's activities that could have an effect on disease risk.

Social phobia: A clinically significant anxiety provoked by exposure to certain types of social or performance situations that often leads to avoidance behavior.

Sodium benzoate: The sodium salt of benzoic acid used as an antifungal preservative in pharmaceutical preparations and foods. It may also be used as a test for liver function, administered orally or intravenously.

Sodium bicarbonate: An antacid, electrolyte, and urinary alkalinizing agent. It is prescribed in the treatment of acidosis, gastric acidity, peptic ulcer, and indigestion.

Sodium citrate: The trisodium salt of citric acid that is used as an anticoagulant for blood or plasma that is to be fractionated or for blood that is to be stored.

Sodium fluoride: A dental caries preventive agent, occurring as a white powder. It is used in the fluoridation of water and applied topically to the teeth.

Sodium laurel sulfate: An anionic surfactant that is used as a wetting agent, emulsifying aid, and detergent in various cosmetic and dermatological preparations and as an ingredient in toothpastes.

Soft palate: Posterior portion of the palate.

Solubility: The extent to which a substance (solute) dissolves in a liquid (solvent) to produce a homogeneous system (solution).

Sonic scaler: A type of instrument for scaling that is air-driven, which produces vibrations in the sonic range of 2,300 to 6,300.

Specific phobia: Avoidance behavior and clinically significant anxiety provoked by exposure to a specific feared object or situation.

Specific plaque hypothesis: A hypothesis associated with the cause of specific forms of periodontal disease based on a specified form or forms of bacteria.

Specificity: The quality of being distinctive. Kinds of specificity may include group, species, and type.

Specificity rate: Statistical rates in which the events in both the numerator and the denominator are restricted to a specific subgroup of a population.

Sphygmomanometer: A blood pressure cuff used to indirectly measure the systolic and diastolic blood pressure.

Spinal accessory: Either of a pair of cranial nerves essential for speech, swallowing, and certain movements of the head and shoulders. Each nerve has a cranial and a spinal portion, communicates with certain cervical nerves, and connects to the nucleus ambiguous of the brain.

Spit tobacco: Also called "smokeless tobacco" by the tobacco industry and in most scientific forums. It is tobacco that is not burned but used primarily in the oral cavity, where nicotine and other chemicals are absorbed through the oral mucosa.

Staging: The classification of neoplasms according to the extent of the tumor.

Stannous fluoride: A fluoride salt of tin, used in toothpaste and mouthrinses to reduce dental caries incidence and as an antiplaque agent.

Staphylococcus: A species of spherical, gram-positive bacteria that grows in grapelike clusters. It is of low pathogenicity, although occasional strains may be coagulase-positive and produce hemolysis. Staphylococcus is normally present as part of the oral flora and mucosa-lined cavities, such as the mouth and the nasal cavity. It can be isolated, along with *S. aureus*, streptococci, pneumococci, fusiform bacilli, *Borrelia vincentii*, molds, and yeasts, from the gingival crevice by cultural examination.

Statutes: Laws enacted and written by federal and state legislatures.

Stensen's duct: The excretory duct of the parotid gland; it passes lateral to the masseter muscle and enters the oral cavity through the buccal tissues adjacent to the maxillary first and second molars.

Sternocleidomastoid: A muscle of the neck that is attached to the mastoid process of the temporal bone and superior nuchal line and by separate heads to the sternum and clavicle. They function together to flex the head.

Stimuli: Chemical, thermal, electrical, or mechanical influences that change the normal environment of irritable tissue and create an impulse.

Stimulus generalization: A tendency to give conditioned, or learned, responses to stimuli (situations or objects) that are similar to the original stimulus.

Stippling: Pin-point depressions present on the surface of the attached gingiva.

Stock: A security certificate that represents an equity ownership in a corporation.

Stratified: Arranged in layers.

Stratified squamous: Epithelial cells that include the superficial layers of the skin and oral mucosa.

Stratum basale: The deepest of the five layers of the epidermis, which is composed of tall cylindrical cells. This layer provides new cells by mitotic cell division.

Stratum corneum: The horny, outermost layer of the skin, composed of dead flat cells converted to keratin that continually flake away. The thickness of the layer is correlated with the normal wear of the area it covers. The stratum corneum is thick on the palms of the hands and the soles of the feet but relatively thin over most areas.

Stratum granulosum: One of the layers of the epidermis situated just below the stratum corneum.

Stratum spinosum: One of the layers of the epidermis situated just beneath the stratum granulosum.

Streptococcus mutans: A cariogenic bacteria found in dental plaque and one of two of the index organisms (lactobacillus) used to assess caries susceptibility.

Strontium chloride: The chloride salt of strontium 89, a calcium analog that concentrates in areas of increased osteogenesis; used as a local radiation source for palliative treatment of bone pain in patients with metastatic bone lesions; administered intravenously.

Subgingival: Below the gingival margin.

Subgingival irrigation: Delivery of water or an antimicrobial agent to a deep periodontal pocket, usually by insertion of a cannula.

Sublingual: Pertaining to the region or structures located beneath the tongue.

Sublingual caruncle: Small papilla at the anterior end of each sublingual fold that contains openings of the submandibular glands.

Subluxation: Partial dislocation of both temporomandibular joints.

Submandibular: Below the mandible.

Submargination: When a deficiency of contour at the margin of a restoration or pattern is present.

Submental: Situated below the chin.

Substantivity: The ability of an agent to adhere to oral soft tissues, thereby permitting continued antimicrobial action; resists dilution by salivary action or gingival crevicular fluid.

Sulci: The grooves or depressions on the surface of a tooth. Grooves in a portion of the oral cavity.

Sulcular epithelium: Epithelium that stands away from the tooth, creating a gingival sulcus.

Supererupted teeth: Teeth where the projection lies beyond the normal occlusal plane.

Superior: In a direction above or higher than a specified point.

Supervision: In dental hygiene practice, this term is used to denote that the dentist must accept responsibility for the services provided by the dental hygienist. The term implies that the dentist will review or evaluate the procedures performed depending on the level of supervision required.

Supine position: Lying on the back.

Supporting alveolar bone: That part of the bone considered best suited to bear the forces of mastication with functioning dentures.

Supportive care: The practice of frequent professional supervision and monitoring of a person with a chronic disease.

Supportive periodontal care (SPC):   Describes three levels of periodontal care: (1) preventive, (2) posttreatment, and (3) palliative. *Preventive care* preserves the healthy periodontium; *posttreatment care* is specific and regular professional care after periodontal treatment; and *palliative care* is the optimal possible treatment for patients who are not adherent. Supportive periodontal care was defined at the first European Workshop on Periodontology in 1989.

Supportive periodontal therapy (SPT):   Described at the 1989 World Workshop in Clinical Periodontics; replaced by the term *periodontal maintenance* in 2000. The terms mean the same as SPC, which is used in Europe.

Suppurating: Producing or discharging pus.

Suppuration: The formation and discharge of pus.

Supraclavicular: Pertaining to the area above the clavicle, or collar bone.

Supragingival: Pertaining to the area above the gingival margin.

Supragingival irrigation: Flushing of the gingival sulcus by directing a stream of water or irrigant at right angles to the long axis of the tooth. This is accomplished with the use of an irrigating tip with a lumen at the end.

Surgeon's knot: A mechanical technique that unites opposite ends of suture material.

Surgical stent: A device used to hold a skin graft placed to maintain a body orifice, cavity, or space. A surgical stent is also an acrylic resin appliance used as a positioning guide or support.

Survival rate: The time period describing years alive after diagnosis; normally defined as 5 years.

Sustained release device: Refers to delivery systems and agents that are pharmaceutically active for less than 24 hours.

Suture: Material (e.g., silk, gut) used to approximate or unite surfaces.

Synaptic junction: The space between two nerve cells where the release of neurotransmitters from a transmitting (presynaptic) neuron briefly allows an ion flow that activates a signal in the receiving (postsynaptic) neuron.

Synovial joints: Freely movable joints in which contiguous bony surfaces are covered by articular cartilage and connected by a fibrous connective tissue capsule lined with synovial membrane.

Systemic: Pertains to the entire body.

Systemic desensitization: A technique used in behavior therapy for eliminating maladaptive anxiety associated with phobias. The procedure involves the construction by the person of a hierarchy of anxiety-producing stimuli and the general presentation of these stimuli until they no longer elicit the initial response of fear.

Tachypnea: Excessively rapid respiration; a respiratory neurosis marked by quick, shallow breathing.

Tactile sensitivity: Sensitivity relating to the sense of touch.

Taste buds: Barrel-shaped organs of taste associated with certain lingual papilla of the tongue.

Telangietasia: Dilation of the capillaries and small arteries of a region. A hereditary form (hereditary hemorrhagic telangiectasia) may appear intraorally. Also, it is a disorder characterized by cutaneous and mucosal vascular macules, nodules, and arterial spiders that tend to bleed sporadically.

Telescopic loupes: Surgical telescopes that can improve visual activity.

Temporalis: It is a broad radiating muscle that acts to close the jaws and retract the mandible.

Temporomandibular disorders: Abnormal, incomplete, or impaired function of the temporomandibular joint(s). The symptoms can include headache around the vertex and occiput, tinnitus, pain around the ear, impaired hearing, and pain around the tongue.

Temporomandibular joint: The joint formed by the two condyles of the mandible. The structures that make up the temporomandibular joint include the mandibular fossae of the temporal bones, articular disks, mandibular condyles, and articular tubercles of the zygomatic process of the temporal bone.

Teratogens: Drugs or substances that cause congenital deformities.

Terminal shank: The portion of a periodontal scaling instrument just above the working end.

Therapeutic alliance: Cooperation and contribution between the patient and the oral care professional in achieving health stability for the patient.

Therapeutic intervention strategy: A specific procedure or set of procedures designed to intervene in the disease process to produce a therapeutic benefit.

Therapeutic polishing: Polishing of the tooth surface to remove or disrupt bacterial agents responsible for disease.

Therapeutic privilege: An exception to informed consent; based on disclosure harming the emotional well-being of the patient and contraindicated from a medical point of view.

Thermal stimulus: Causing a pain sensation with either heat or cold.

Thoracic outlet syndrome (TOS):   An abnormal condition and a type of mononeuropathy characterized by paresthesia. It may be caused by a nerve root compression by a cervical disk.

Thrombocytopenia: A reduction in the number of platelets. There may be decreased production of platelets, decreased survival of platelets, and increased consumption of platelets or splenomegaly. Thrombocytopenia is the most common cause of bleeding disorders.

Thromboxane: A compound synthesized by platelets and other cells that cause platelet aggregation and vasoconstriction.

Thyroglossal duct cyst: A tube that connects the thyroid gland with the base of the tongue during prenatal development and later becomes obliterated.

Thyroid cartilage: Includes the midline prominence of the larynx.

Thyroid gland: An endocrine gland in the neck.

Tinnitus: A noise in the ears, often described as ringing or roaring.

Tip: The portion of the working end of a periodontal instrument that should be placed against the tooth at all times to ensure proper instrument adaptation.

Tobacco abstinence: State of being tobacco-free either as a never-user or an ex-user.

Tobacco user: An individual who regularly uses tobacco, usually measured as daily use among adults (age 18 and older) and as any use within the past month among children and youths (less than age 18).

Toe: The end portion of the working end of a curet. The toe is usually round.

Tofflemire universal matrix system: A mechanism composed of two components: (1) a retainer and (2) a band; it is used to hold and form the restorative material (amalgam) during the packing and carving of the amalgam restoration.

Tomograms: A radiograph made with a tomograph.

Tongue: The muscular organ that is the main articulatory element in the production of speech and accounts for the clarity and fluidity of speech.

Tonsillectomy: Surgical removal of the tonsils, which are a rounded mass of tissue, usually of a lymphoid nature (especially the palatine tonsil).

Tooth-colored restoration (TC): A restorative material that matches the color of a tooth, usually a resin or ceramic.

Topical: On the surface.

Tort: A civil wrong or injury, other than a breach of contract, for which the plaintiff is compensated monetarily for the unreasonable harm he or she has sustained.

Trabecular: An irregular meshwork of joined matrix pieces forming a lattice in cancellous bone or when bands of connective tissue in a lymph node separate the node into lymphatic nodules.

Tragus of the ears: A prominence in front of the opening of the external ear.

Transdermal nicotine: Nicotine diffusion through the skin, usually by the use of a "nicotine patch."

Transient ischemic attacks (TIAs): Episodes of cerebrovascular insufficiencies, usually associated with partial occlusion of an artery by an atherosclerotic plaque or an embolism. The symptoms vary with the site and the degree of occlusion. Disturbance of normal vision in one or both eyes, dizziness, weakness, dysphasia, numbness, or unconsciousness may occur. The attacks are usually brief, lasting a few minutes; symptoms rarely continue for several hours.

Transmucosal nicotine: Nicotine diffusion through the oral mucosa, usually by the use of a nicotine gum (nicotine polacrilex) or oral inhaler.

Transseptal fibers: A part of the gingival fiber system that extends from the supraalveolar cementum of one tooth horizontally through the interdental attached gingiva above the septum of the alveolar bone to the cementum of the adjacent tooth.

Trapezius: A large, flat triangular muscle of the shoulder and upper back. It arises from the occipital bone, the ligamentum nuchae, and the spinous processes of the seventh cervical and all the thoracic vertebrae. It acts to rotate the scapula, raise the shoulder, and abduct and flex the arm.

Triage: A process in which a group of patients is sorted according to their need for care. The kind of illness or injury, the severity of the problem, and the facilities available govern the process, as in a hospital emergency room.

Triclosan: An antibacterial effective against gram-positive and most gram-negative organisms and exhibiting slight activity against yeasts and fungi; used as a detergent in surgical scrubs, soaps, and deodorants.

Trifurcation: The areas in a three-rooted tooth where the roots divide.

Trigeminal neuralgia (cranial nerve V): The fifth cranial nerve, which provides motor innervation to the muscles of mastication and sensory innervation to the face, jaws, and teeth.

Trismus: Limitations of opening because of spasm and/or fibrosis of the muscles of mastication and/or temporomandibular joint.

Tuberculosis: An infectious disease caused by *Mycobacterium tuberculosis* and characterized by the formation of tubercles in the tissues.

Tubule: A nodule or a small eminence, such as that on a bone. Also, a tubule is a nodule that is especially elevated from the skin and is larger than a papule.

Tumor necrosis factor alpha: A natural body protein, also produced synthetically, with anticancer effects. The body produces it in response to the presence of toxic substances such as bacterial toxins. Adverse effects are toxic shock and cachexia.

Type 1 diabetes: See *Insulin-dependent diabetes mellitus.*

Type 2 diabetes: See *Non–insulin-dependent diabetes mellitus.*

Type II herpes: An infection caused by a herpes simplex virus (HSV), which has an affinity for the skin and nervous system and usually produces small, transient, irritating, and sometimes painful fluid-filled blisters on the skin and mucous membranes. Type II herpes *(herpes genitalis)* infections are usually limited to the genital region.

Ulcerative stomatitis: Periodic episodes of aphthous lesions (canker sores) ranging from 1 week to several months. Trauma, menses, immunological factors, upper respiratory tract infections, herpes simplex, and other causes have been suggested. The single or multiple discrete or confluent ulcers have a well-defined marginal erythema and central area of necrosis with sloughing. The herpetic appearance suggests a common mechanism with herpes simplex, but no known infectious agents have been demonstrated.

Ultrasonic instruments: The use of high frequency sound waves, instrument vibrations, and a water lavage to remove plaque, calculus, and endotoxins from the root surface.

Unerupted teeth: Teeth not having perforated the oral mucosa. In dentistry, used with reference to a normal developing tooth, an embedded tooth, or an impacted tooth.

Unilateral: One-sided.

Universal: The ability to be used on all tooth surfaces.

Upper respiratory infections (URIs): Any infectious disease of the upper respiratory tract. URIs include the common cold, laryngitis, pharyngitis, rhinitis, sinusitis, and tonsillitis.

Urticaria: A pruritic skin eruption characterized by transient wheels of varying shapes and sizes with well-defined erythematous margins and pale centers. It is caused by capillary dilation in the dermis that results from the release of vasoactive mediators, including histamine, kinin, and the slow reactive substance of anaphylaxis associated with antigen-antibody reaction. It may be caused by drugs, food, insect bites, inhalants, emotional stress, exposure to heat or cold, and exercise. Urticaria is also called *hives.*

Uvula: A midline muscular structure that hangs down from the posterior margin of the soft palate.

Values: The social principles, goals, or standards accepted by a society.

Varnish: A resin surface coating formed by evaporation of a solvent.

Vasovagal syncope: A sudden loss of consciousness, resulting from cerebral ischemia; secondary to decreased cardiac output, peripheral vasodilation, and bradycardia; and associated with vagal activity. The condition may be triggered by pain, fright, or trauma and is accompanied by symptoms of nausea, pallor, and perspiration.

Ventral surface: Denoting a position more toward the belly surface than some other object of reference; the anterior surface.

Ventricular fibrillation: A cardiac arrhythmia marked by rapid disorganized depolarizations of the ventricular myocardium. The condition is characterized by a complete lack of organized electric activity, as well as ventricular contraction. Blood pressure falls to zero, resulting in unconsciousness. Death may occur within 4 minutes. Cardiopulmonary resuscitation must be initiated immediately with defibrillation and resuscitative medications given per advance cardiac life support protocol.

Vermilion border (or zone):   Transition zone where the lips are outlined from the surrounding skin.

Vertical: Upright; perpendicular to the horizon.

Vesiculo-bullous disease (desquamative gingivitis): A gingival inflammation characterized by peeling of the surface epithelium. In its chronic state it is most frequently associated with menopause caused by hormonal changes. It may also be associated with any biological stress, such as trauma to the epithelium.

Vestibule: A space or a cavity that serves as the entrance to a passageway, such as the vestibule of the vagina or the vestibule of the ear.

Vibrating line: An imaginary line across the posterior part of the palate marking the division between the movable and immovable tissues of the soft palate. This can be identified when the movable tissues are functioning.

Videofluoroscopy: Dynamic radiographs recorded on videotape.

Viscosity: The resistance that a liquid exhibits to the flow of one layer over another.

Vision: Sight; the faculty of seeing.

Vital signs: The measurement of pulse rate, respiration rate, body temperature, and tobacco use.

Vital staining: A dyeing process used to impart color to tissues or cells of living organisms.

Wall: The outside layer of material surrounding an object or space; a paries.

Wharton's duct: The excretory duct of the submandibular glands; opens into the oral cavity at the sublingual caruncle of the mucous membrane of the floor of the mouth behind the lower incisor teeth.

White spot lesion: Lesions found on the mucosa that have a white coating. They require differential diagnosis because they may indicate trauma, infection, or a cancerous process.

Wire edge: Unsupported metal fragments extending beyond the cutting edge.

Within normal limits (WNL):   Term referring to clinical measurements and radiographs that are within the health parameters; findings are noncontributory to disease.

Working end: That portion of the instrument that comes in contact with the tooth and performs the intended task.

Work-related musculoskeletal disorders (WMSD): Musculoskeletal disorders of the neck, back, and shoulder, as well as carpal tunnel syndrome and thoracic outlet syndrome, resulting from repetitive appropriate body mechanics during the performance of work activities.

Xerostomia: Dry mouth caused by a decreased production of saliva.

Zoophobia: A fear of animals.

Zygomatic: Term pertaining to the cheekbone, or malar bone of the face.

APPENDIX A

Health Insurance Portability *and* Accountability Act (HIPAA) *of* 1996

The Health Insurance Portability and Accountability Act (HIPAA) of 1996 was signed into law by former President Bill Clinton on August 21, 1996. Conclusive regulations were issued on August 17, 2000, to be instated by October 16, 2002. HIPAA requires that the transactions of all patient health care information be formatted in a standardized electronic style. In addition to protecting the privacy and security of patient information, HIPAA includes legislation on the formation of medical savings accounts, the authorization of a fraud and abuse control program, the easy transport of health insurance coverage, and the simplification of administrative terms and conditions.

HIPAA COVERAGE

HIPAA encompasses three primary areas, and its privacy requirements can be broken down into three types—privacy standards, patients' rights, and administrative requirements.

1. Privacy Standards. A central concern of HIPAA is the careful use and disclosure of protected health information (PHI), which generally is electronically controlled health information that is able to be distinguished individually. PHI also refers to verbal communication although the HIPAA Privacy Rule is not intended to hinder necessary verbal communication. The U.S. Department of Health and Human Services (USDHHS) does not require restructuring, such as soundproofing, architectural changes, and so forth, but some caution is necessary when exchanging health information by conversation.

An Acknowledgment of Receipt Notice of Privacy Practices, which allows patient information to be used or divulged for treatment, payment, or health care operations (TPO), should be procured from each patient. A detailed and time-sensitive authorization can also be issued, which allows the dentist to release information in special circumstances other than TPOs. A *written consent* is also an option. Dentists can disclose PHI *without* acknowledgement, consent, or authorization in very special situations, for example, perceived child abuse, public health supervision, fraud investigation, or law enforcement with valid permission (i.e., a warrant). When divulging PHI, a dentist must try to disclose only the *minimum necessary* information, to help safeguard the patient's information as much as possible.

It is important that dental professionals adhere to HIPAA standards because health care providers (as well as health care clearinghouses and health care plans) who convey *electronically* formatted health information via an outside billing service or merchant are considered *covered entities*. Covered entities may be dealt serious civil and criminal penalties for violation of HIPAA legislation. Failure to comply with HIPAA privacy requirements may result in civil penalties of up to $100 per offense with an annual maximum of $25,000 for repeated failure to comply with the same requirement. Criminal penalties resulting from the illegal mishandling of private health information can range from $50,000 and/or 1 year in prison to $250,000 and/or 10 years in prison.

2. Patients' Rights. HIPAA allows patients, authorized representatives, and parents of minors, as well as minors, to become more aware of the health information privacy to which they are entitled. These rights include, but are not limited to, the right to view and copy their health information, the right to dispute alleged breaches of policies and regulations, and the right to request alternative forms of communicating with their dentist. If any health information is released for any reason other than TPO, the patient is entitled to an account of the transaction. Therefore, it is important for dentists to keep accurate records of such information and to provide them when necessary.

The HIPAA Privacy Rule determines that the parents of a minor have access to their child's health information. This privilege may be overruled, for example, in cases where there is suspected child abuse or the parent consents to a term of confidentiality between the dentist and the minor. The parents' rights to access their child's PHI also may be restricted in situations when a legal entity, such as a court, intervenes and when a law does not require a parent's consent. For a full list of patient rights provided by HIPAA, be sure to acquire a copy of the law and to understand it well.

3. Administrative Requirements. Complying with HIPAA legislation may seem like a chore, but it does not need to be so. It is recommended that you become appropriately familiar with the law, organize the requirements into simpler tasks, begin compliance early, and document your progress in compliance. An important first step is to evaluate the current information and practices of your office.

Dentists will need to write a *privacy policy* for their office, a document for their patients detailing the office's practices concerning PHI. The ADA's *HIPAA Privacy Kit* includes forms that you (the dentist) can use to customize your privacy policy. It is useful to try to understand the role of health care information for your patients and the ways in which they deal with the information while they are visiting your office. Train your staff; make sure they are familiar with the terms of HIPAA and your office's privacy policy and related forms. HIPAA requires that you designate a *privacy officer,* a person in your office who will be responsible for applying the new policies in your office, fielding complaints, and making choices involving the minimum necessary requirements. Another person with the role of *contact person* will process complaints.

A *Notice of Privacy Practices*—a document detailing the patient's rights and the dental office's obligations concerning PHI—also must be drawn up. Further, any role of a third party with access to PHI must be clearly documented. This third party is known as a *business associate* (BA) and is defined as any entity who, on behalf of the dentist, takes part in any activity that involves exposure of PHI. The *HIPAA Privacy Kit* provides a copy of the USDHHS "Business Associate Contract Terms," which provides a concrete format for detailing BA interactions.

The main HIPAA privacy compliance date, including all staff training, was April 14, 2003, although many covered entities who submitted a request and a compliance plan by October 15, 2002, were granted one-year extensions. It is recommended that dentists prepare their offices ahead of time for all deadlines, which include preparing privacy polices and forms, business associate contracts, and employee training sessions.

FOR MORE INFORMATION ON HIPAA

For a comprehensive discussion of all of these terms and requirements, a complete list of HIPAA policies and procedures, and a full collection of HIPAA privacy forms, contact the American Dental Association for a *HIPAA Privacy Kit.* The relevant ADA Web site is www.ada.org/goto/hipaa. Other Web sites that may contain useful information about HIPAA are:

- USDHHS Office of Civil Rights www.hhs.gov/ocr/hipaa
- Work Group on Electronic Data Interchange www.wedi.org/SNIP
- Phoenix Health www.hipaadvisory.com
- USDHHS Office of the Assistant Secretary for Planning and Evaluation http://aspe.os.dhhs.gov/admnsimp/

Sources used:
1. *HIPAA Privacy Kit*
2. http://www.ada.org/prof/prac/issues/topics/hipaa/index.html

APPENDIX B

Update *to the* Summary *of* Significant Infectious Diseases (Table 5-3)

SARS (severe acute respiratory syndrome) was first identified in late 2002 in Asia. The virus responsible for SARS is a unique coronavirus named the SARS-associated coronavirus (SARS-CoV). There are no diagnostic tests to date that can definitively diagnose the SARS-CoV; therefore diagnosis is made from clinical data. The illness manifests as respiratory distress ranging from mild to extreme (cough, difficulty breathing, hypoxia) with fever and radiographic evidence of pneumonia. The virus is spread by close contact with someone who is infected with SARS through droplets from coughing, sneezing, kissing, embracing, sharing eating and drinking utensils, and from close conversation.

West Nile Virus (WNV) is transmitted by the bite of an infected mosquito. The virus may be asymptomatic (mild infection) in some to severe (1 in 150 infections) resulting in encephalitis, meningitis, or meningoencephalitis. The incubation period in humans is from 3 to 14 days after exposure. Symptoms are fever, headache, body aches, sometimes a skin rash, swollen lymph nodes, and in more severe cases high fever, neck stiffness, stupor, disorientation, coma, tremors, headache, muscle weakness, and paralysis. There is no specific treatment for WNV unless the illness is severe, at which time hospitalization is often necessary due to the symptoms. Treatment can include IV fluids, pain control, respiratory support, and the prevention of secondary infections.

CARIES RISK ASSESSMENT FORM FOR CHILDREN 6 YEARS AND OLDER/ADULTS

Instructions on reverse

Patient Name: _____ I.D. # _____ Age _____ Date _____

Initial/baseline exam date _____ Recall/POE date _____

Respond to each question in sections 1, 2, and 3 with a check mark in the yes or no column	Yes	No	Notes
1. High Risk Factors**			
(a) Visible cavitation (carious) or caries into dentin by radiograph			
(b) Caries restored in past three years			
(c) Readily visible heavy plaque on teeth			
(d) Frequent (greater than three times daily) between-meal snacks of sugars/cooked starch			
(e) **Saliva-reducing factors:**			
1. Hyposalivatory medications			
2. Radiation to head and neck			
3. Systemic reasons, e.g., Sjogren's			
(f*) Visually inadequate saliva flow. (If yes, measure) less than 0.7 ml/min by test = low salivary flow or dry mouth			Amount: _____ ml/min
(g) Appliances present, fixed or removable, e.g., orthodontic brackets/bands/retainer or removable partial denture(s)			
2. Moderate Risk Factors			
(a) Exposed roots			
(b) Deep pits & fissures/developmental defects			
(c) Interproximal enamel lesions/radiolucencies			
(d) Other white spot lesions or occlusal discoloration			
(e) Uses recreational drugs			
3. Protective Factors			
(a) Lives/works/school in fluoridated community			
(b) Uses fluoride toothpaste daily			Type _____
(c) Uses fluoride mouthwash/rinse/gel daily			Type _____
(d*) Salivary flow visually adequate >1 ml/min by test			
(e) Uses xylitol gum or mints 4x day			Type _____ and % xylitol _____
(f) Mother/caregiver has no caries activity			Brand _____ Frequency _____

If yes to 1 (a) or any two of 1 (b)-(g), perform bacterial culture	High Count Date: _____	Moderate Count Date: _____	Low Count Date: _____	
(a) Mutans streptococci				(Place a check in the box below the count)
(b) Lactobacillus				(Place a check in the box below the count)
Caries risk overall* (see over)	High	Moderate	Low	Circle High, Moderate or Low
Recommendations given: yes _____ no _____ Date given: _____			or Date follow up: _____	

*Indicates that test descriptions for these procedures are on the following pages

Competencies *for* Entry *into the* Profession *of* Dental Hygeine

(As approved by the 2003 House of Delegates)

FOREWORD

The American Dental Education Association (ADEA), Section on Dental Hygiene Education Competency Development Committee, drafted the competency statements presented in this document. This committee had representation from both baccalaureate and associate degree dental hygiene programs. It also included representation from dental hygiene, clinical, social, and basic sciences, and the American Dental Hygienists' Association. A separate committee, the Dental Hygiene Education Competency Draft Review Committee, further reviewed and provided feedback on the document once developed. Following these reviews, the competency statements were presented for public comment at the 1998 ADEA Annual Session, the 1998 Dental Hygiene Directors' Conference, and the ADEA Section on Dental Hygiene Education homepage on the World Wide Web.

The competency statements have been presented in five domains. These domains were defined during a consensus exercise that was conducted at the 1997 Annual Session of the ADEA, Section on Dental Hygiene Education program session. Individuals representing various facets of dental hygiene and dental hygiene education participated in this exercise.

INTRODUCTION

This document describes the abilities expected of a dental hygiene entering the profession. These competency statements are meant to serve as guidelines. It is important for individual programs to further define the competencies they want their graduates to possess, describing (1) the desired combination of knowledge, psychomotor skills, communication skills, and attitudes, and (2) the standards used to measure the hygienist's independent performance. The following should help to assess the competence of dental hygiene students and to improve the dental hygiene curriculum. Given the dynamic nature of science and the health professions, these suggestions should be reviewed and updated periodically.

As a participating member of the health care team, the dental hygienist plays an integral role in assisting patients to achieve and maintain optimal oral health. Dental hygienists provide educational, clinical, and consultative services to individuals and populations of all ages, including the medically compromised, mentally or physically challenged, and socially or culturally disadvantaged.

As defined in this document, dental hygienists must exhibit competence in the following five do-mains:

(1) The dental hygienist must first possess the *Core Competencies* (C), the ethics, values, skills, and knowledge integral to all aspects of the profession. These core competencies are foundational to all of the roles of the dental hygienist.

(2) Second, inasmuch as *Health Promotion (HP)/Disease Prevention* is a key component of health care; changes within the health care environment require the dental hygienist to have a general knowledge of wellness, health determinants, and characteristics of various patient/client communities. The hygienist needs to emphasize both prevention of disease and effective health care delivery.

(3) Third is the dental hygienist's complex role in the *Community* (CM). Dental hygienists must appreciate their role as health professionals at the local, state, and national levels. This role requires the graduate dental hygienist to assess, plan, and implement programs and activities to benefit the general population. In this role, the dental hygienist must be prepared to influence others to facilitate access to care and services.

(4) Fourth is *Patient/Client Care* (PC), requiring competencies described here in ADPIE format. Because the dental hygienist's role in patient/client care is ever-changing, yet central to the maintenance of health, dental hygiene graduates must use their skills to assess, diagnose, plan, implement, and evaluate treatment.

(5) Fifth, like other health professionals, dental hygienists must be aware of a variety of opportunities for *Professional Growth and Development* (PGD). Some opportunities may increase clients' access to dental hygiene; others may offer ways to influence the profession and the changing health care environment. A dental hygienist must possess transferable skills (e.g., in communication, problem-solving, and critical thinking) to take advantage of these opportunities.

CORE COMPETENCIES (C)

C.1 Apply a professional code of ethics in all endeavors.

C.2 Adhere to state and federal laws, recommendations, and regulations in the provision of dental hygiene care.

C.3 Provide dental hygiene care to promote patient/client health and wellness using critical thinking and problem solving in the provision of evidence-based practice.

C.4 Use evidence-based decision making to evaluate and incorporate emerging treatment modalities.

C.5 Assume responsibility for dental hygiene actions and care based on accepted scientific theories and research as well as the accepted standard of care.

C.6 Continuously perform self-assessment for life-long learning and professional growth.

C.7 Promote the profession through service activities and affiliations with professional organizations.

C.8 Provide quality assurance mechanisms for health services.

C.9 Communicate effectively with individuals and groups from diverse populations both verbally and in writing.

C.10 Provide accurate, consistent, and complete documentation for assessment, diagnosis, planning, implementation, and evaluation of dental hygiene services.

C.11 Provide care to all clients using an individualized approach that is humane, empathetic, and caring.

HEALTH PROMOTION AND DISEASE PREVENTION (HP)

HP.1 Promote the values of oral and general health and wellness to the public and organizations within and outside the profession.

HP.2 Respect the goals, values, beliefs, and preferences of the patient/client while promoting optimal oral and general health.

HP.3 Refer patients/clients who may have a physiological, psychological, and/or social problem for comprehensive patient/client evaluation.

HP.4 Identify individual and population risk factors and develop strategies that promote health-related quality of life.

HP.5 Evaluate factors that can be used to promote patient/client adherence to disease prevention and/or health maintenance strategies.

HP.6 Evaluate and utilize methods to ensure the health and safety of the patient/client and the dental hygienist in the delivery of dental hygiene.

COMMUNITY INVOLVEMENT (CM)

CM.1 Assess the oral health needs of the community and the quality and availability of resources and services.

CM.2 Provide screening, referral, and educational services that allow clients to access the resources of the health care system.

CM.3 Provide community oral health services in a variety of settings.

CM.4 Facilitate client access to oral health services by influencing individuals and/or organizations for the provision of oral health care.

CM.5 Evaluate reimbursement mechanisms and their impact on the patient's/client's access to oral health care.

CM.6 Evaluate the outcomes of community-based programs and plan for future activities.

PATIENT/CLIENT CARE (PC)

Assessment PC.1 Systematically collect, analyze, and record data on the general, oral, and psychosocial health status of a variety of patients/clients using methods consistent with medico-legal principles.

This competency includes:

a. Select, obtain, and interpret diagnostic information recognizing its advantages and limitations.

b. Recognize predisposing and etiologic risk factors that require intervention to prevent disease.

c. Obtain, review, and update a complete medical, family, social, and dental history.

d. Recognize health conditions and medications that impact overall patient/client care.

e. Identify patients/clients at risk for a medical emergency and manage the patient/client care in a manner that prevents an emergency.

f. Perform a comprehensive examination using clinical, radiographic, periodontal, dental charting, and other data collection procedures to assess the patient's/client's needs.

DIAGNOSIS

PC.2 Use critical decision making skills to reach conclusions about the patient's/client's dental hygiene needs based on all available assessment data.

This competency includes:

a. Determine a dental hygiene diagnosis.

b. Identify patient/client needs and significant findings that impact the delivery of dental hygiene services.

c. Obtain consultations as indicated.

Planning PC.3 Collaborate with the patient/client, and/or other health professionals, to formulate a comprehensive dental hygiene care plan that is patient/client-centered and based on current scientific evidence.

This competency includes:

a. Prioritize the care plan based on the health status and the actual and potential problems of the individual to facilitate optimal oral health.

b. Establish a planned sequence of care (educational, clinical, and evaluation) based on the dental hygiene diagnosis; identified oral conditions; potential problems; etiologic and risk factors; and available treatment modalities.

c. Establish a collaborative relationship with the patient/client in the planned care to include etiology, prognosis, and treatment alternatives.

d. Make referrals to other health care professionals.

e. Obtain the patient's/client's informed consent based on a thorough case presentation.

Implementation PC.4 Provide specialized treatment that includes preventive and therapeutic services de-

signed to achieve and maintain oral health. Assist in achieving oral health goals formulated in collaboration with the patient/client.

This competency includes:

a. Perform dental hygiene interventions to eliminate and/or control local etiologic factors to prevent and control caries, periodontal disease, and other oral conditions.

b. Control pain and anxiety during treatment through the use of accepted clinical and behavioral techniques.

c. Provide life support measures to manage medical emergencies in the patient/client care environment.

EVALUATION

PC.5 Evaluate the effectiveness of the implemented clinical, preventive, and educational services and modify as needed.

This competency includes:

a. Determine the outcomes of dental hygiene interventions using indices, instruments, examination techniques, and patient/client self-report.

b. Evaluate the patient's/client's satisfaction with the oral health care received and the oral health status achieved.

c. Provide subsequent treatment or referrals based on evaluation findings.

d. Develop and maintain a health maintenance program.

PROFESSIONAL GROWTH AND DEVELOPMENT

PGD.1 Identify career options within health care, industry, education, and research and evaluate the feasibility of pursuing dental hygiene opportunities.

PGD.2 Develop practice management and marketing strategies to be used in the delivery of oral health care.

PGD.3 Access professional and social networks to pursue professional goals.

APPENDIX E

Summary *of the* Guidelines *for* Infection Control *in* Dental Healthcare Settings—2003

The 2003 report consolidates recommendations for preventing and controlling infectious diseases and managing personnel health and safety concerns related to infection control in dental settings. The report (1) updates and revises previous CDC recommendations regarding infection control in dental settings, (2) incorporates relevant infection-control measures from other CDC guidelines, and (3) discusses concerns not addressed in previous recommendations for dentistry. These updates and additional topics include the following:

- Application of standard precautions rather than universal precautions
- Work restrictions for health-care personnel (HCP) infected with or occupationally exposed to infectious diseases
- Management of occupational exposures to bloodborne pathogens, including postexposure prophylaxis (PEP) for work exposures to hepatitis B virus (HBV), hepatitis C virus (HCV), and human immunodeficiency virus (HIV)
- Selection and use of devices with features designed to prevent sharps injury
- Hand-hygiene products and surgical hand antisepsis
- Contact dermatitis and latex hypersensitivity
- Sterilization of unwrapped instruments
- Dental water-quality concerns (e.g., dental unit waterline biofilms, delivery of water of acceptable biological quality for patient care, usefulness of flushing waterlines, use of sterile irrigating solutions for oral surgical procedures, handling of community boil-water advisories)
- Dental radiology
- Aseptic technique for parenteral medications
- Preprocedural mouth rinsing for patients
- Oral surgical procedures
- Laser/electrosurgery plumes
- Tuberculosis (TB)
- Creutzfeldt-Jakob disease (CJD) and other prion-related diseases
- Infection-control program evaluation
- Research considerations

Some infection-control practices routinely used by health-care practitioners cannot be rigorously examined for ethical or logistical reasons. In the absence of scientific evidence for such practices, certain recommendations are based on strong theoretical rationale, suggestive evidence, or opinions of respected authorities based on clinical experience, descriptive studies, or committee reports. In addition, some recommendations are derived from federal regulations. No recommendations are offered for practices for which insufficient scientific evidence or lack of consensus supporting their effectiveness exists.

To view the 2003 guidelines, refer to www.cdc.gov/OralHealth/infectioncontrol/guidelines/index.htm

Adapted from Kohn WG, Collins AS, Cleveland JL, et al: Guidelines for infection control in dental healthcare settings, *MMWR*, Dec. 19, 2003, 52(RR-17).

APPENDIX F

Glove Types *and* Indications

Gloves	Indication	Comment	Commercially available glove material*	Attributes†
Patient examination gloves‡	Patient care, examinations, other nonsurgical procedures involving contact with mucous membranes, and laboratory procedures	Medical device regulated by the Food and Drug Administration (FDA). Nonsterile and sterile single-use disposable. Use for one patient and discard appropriately.	Natural-rubber latex (NRL)	1, 2
			Nitrile	2, 3
			Nitrile and chloroprene (neoprene) blends	1, 2, 3
			Nitrile and NRL blends	2, 3
			Butadiene methyl methacrylate	4
			Polyurethane	4
			Styrene-based copolymer	4, 5
Surgeon's gloves‡	Surgical procedures	Medical device regulated by the FDA. Sterile and single-use disposable. Use for one patient and discard appropriately.	NRL	1, 2
			Nitrile	2, 3
			Chloroprene (neoprene)	2, 3
			NRL and nitrile or chloroprene blends	2
			Synthetic polyisoprene	4, 5
			Styrene-based copolymer Plyurethane	4
Nonmedical gloves	Housekeeping procedure (e.g., cleaning and disinfection) Handling contaminated sharps or chemicals Not for use during patient care	Not a medical device regulated by the FDA. Commonly referred to as utility, industrial, or general purpose gloves. Should be puncture- or chemical-resistant, depending on the task. Latex gloves do not provide adequate chemical protection. Sanitize after use.	NRL and nitrile or chloroprene blends	2, 3
			Chloroprene (neoprene)	2, 3
			Nitrile	2, 3
			Butyl rubber	3, 4, 6
			Fluroelastomer	3, 4, 6
			Polyethylene and ethylene vinyl alcohol copolymer	

*Physical properties can vary by material, manufacturer, and protein and chemical composition.
†*1*, Contains allergenic NRL proteins
 2, Vulcanized rubber, contain allergenic rubber processing chemicals
 3, Likely to have enhanced chemical or puncture resistance
 4, Nonvulcanized and does not contain rubber processing chemicals
 5, Inappropriate for use with methacrylates
 6, Resistant to most methacrylates
‡Medical and dental gloves include patient-examination gloves and surgeon's (i.e., surgical) gloves and are medical devices regulated by the FDA. Cleared medical or dental patient-examination gloves and surgical gloves can be used for patient care.

INDEX

A

AADR. *See* American Association for Dental Research (AADR).
Abandonment, 52
Abdominal pain in health history, 205
Abfraction of tooth (teeth), 318
Abrasion of tooth (teeth), 317-318
Abrasive system in anticaries dentifrice, 410
Abuse, allegations of, prevention of, 465
Abutments for fixed partial dentures, 470
Accreditation, 7
Acellular cementum, 288
Acetylcholine as neurotransmitter, 229
Acid etching in sealant application, 441-442
Acidogenic bacteria in caries process, 391
Acquired immunodeficiency syndrome (AIDS), 83, 725-727
   CDC definitions of, 84b
   herpes lesions in, 81
Acrylic test rod in testing instrument sharpness, 160, 161f
Action potential in nerve conduction, 587
Actisite, 423
Activation in instrumentation, 154-155
Active immunity, 91
Acute brain attack, neurological/sensory impairment from, 672-673
Acute necrotizing ulcerative gingivitis (ANUG), 289
Addiction
   in chemical dependency, 229
   in social history, 198
   nicotine, diagnosis of, 233
Addison's disease
   immune system dysfunction in, 719
   in health history, 207
   vitiligo in, 199
ADHA. *See* American Dental Hygienists' Association (ADHA).
Adherence, 748
Adolescence, 181-183
Adrenal hyperfunction in health history, 207
Adrenal hypofunction in health history, 207
Adrenocorticotropic hormone (ACTH) overproduction, hyperpigmentation from, 199
Adulthood
   early, 183-184
   late, 186-189
   mature, 184-186
   young, 181-183
Aerosol transfer of microorganisms, 76-77
Aesthetic dentistry, 632

Age
   in health history, 195
   in risk assessment, 747
Aging
   immune system dysfunction in, 716
   in oral cavity, 187-188
Agoraphobia, 700
AIDS. *See* Acquired immunodeficiency syndrome (AIDS).
Air-powder polishing, 553-558
Air turbine units, sonic scalers as, 528
Alcohols, sugar, cariogenicity of, 349
Allergic reactions to dentifrices, 407
Allergy(ies)
   in health history, 199
   latex, gloves and, 96
Alliance, therapeutic, 748
Alveolar bone structure, 287-288
Alveolar crestal fibers, 288
Alveolar mucosa
   epithelium covering, 285
   structure of, 287
Alzheimer's disease
   in health history, 209
   neurological/sensory impairment from, 676
Amalgam
   as restorative material, 638-639
   placement techniques for
      for Class I, V, and VI preparations, 639-642
      for Class II preparations, 642-645
Amalgam-sealant combinations in minimally invasive dentistry, 630-631
Ameloblast, nutrition and, 347
American Association for Dental Research (AADR), 12
American Dental Hygienists' Association (ADHA), 12
Amides
   clinical actions of, 591-592
   local anesthetics as, 588
Amnesia from nitrous oxide/oxygen sedation, 611
Amyotrohic lateral sclerosis, neurological/sensory impairment from, 675
Analgesic agent(s)
   nitrous oxide as, discovery of, 610-611
   topical, for erythema multiforme, 270-271
Analog technology for intraoral video imaging systems, 358
Anatomical charting of hard tissues, 311, 312f
Anemia
   diagnostic aids for, 371-372
   in health history, 208
   pernicious
      immune system dysfunction in, 717-718
      vitiligo in, 199
Anesthetic(s), 585-621
   absorption of, 589
   chemistry of, 588

Page numbers followed by *f* indicate illustrations; *t* indicates tables; *b* indicates boxes.

Anesthetic(s)—cont'd
  distribution of, 589
  excretion of, 589
  history of, 586
  ionization factors in, 588-589
  local, 595-608
    administration of
      chart entry for, 606
      equipment for, 596-598
      myths about, 606-607
      techniques for, 599-600b, 601t, 602-603f, 604t,
        605-606f, 606
    clinical actions of, 591-592
    systemic actions of, 589-590
  mechanism of action of, 588
  metabolism of, 589
  nitrous oxide as, discovery of, 610-611
  pharmacokinetics of, 589
  selection of, 586b
  solutions of, vasoconstrictors in, 590-591
  topical, 598-599
Angina pectoris, 194
  in health history, 202
Angioedema, 276-277
Angle's classification in occlusal analysis, 328-329
Angles of working end of instrument, sharpening and,
  159
Angular cheilosis, 194
Angulation in instrumentation, 153-154
Anions, 586
Ankle swelling in health history, 202
Annulus fibrosus, 118
Anorexia nervosa, 707-708
Anthropometric evaluation in nutritional assessment,
  351
Anticariogenic properties, nutrients with, 347
Anticipatory guidance in life stages, 178
Antidepressants, 704
Antifungal agents for oral candidiasis, 278
Antimicrobials, 420
  systemic delivery of, 424-425
Antipsychotics, atypical, for schizophrenia, 711
Antisepsis, hand, in infection control program, 94
Antisocial personality disorder, 705
ANUG. *See* Acute necrotizing ulcerative gingivitis
  (ANUG).
Anxiety
  control of, 576-583
    nitrous oxide/oxygen sedation in, 610-621. *See also*
      Nitrous oxide/oxygen sedation.
    psychological management in, 580-581
  definition of, 577, 698
  etiology of, 577-578
  in dental patient, 695b
  rebound, 702
  related to dental hygiene care, 578-580
    assessment of, 578
    care planning in, 579-580
    creating positive relationship in, 580
Anxiety disorder, 698-702
  definition of, 699
  dental considerations on, 702
  etiology of, 699

Anxiety disorder—cont'd
  generalized, 701
  obsessive-compulsive disorder as, 701
  panic attack as, 699
  panic disorder as, 69-700
  phobic disorders as, 700-701
  posttraumatic stress disorder as, 701-702
  treatment of, 702
Anxiolytic properties of nitrous oxide, 612
Apatite, carbonated, as tooth mineral, 392
Aperture setting of 35-mm camera, 357
Apexification, 456
Apexogenesis, 456
Aphthous ulcers, recurrent, data on, 28
Apical fibers of periodontal ligament, 288
Appliances
  dental. *See also* Dentures.
    care and cleaning of, 478-481
    care of, 469-482
    oral tissues associated with, evaluating, 476-478
    overview of, 470-476
    wear of, conditions associated with, 476-478
  orthodontic, 474
Arestin, 424
Armrests in reducing fatigue, 128
Arrested caries, 320
Arteriosclerosis in health history, 205
Arteriovenous malformation (AVM), stroke from, 672
Arthritis
  in health history, 199
  rheumatoid, immune system dysfunction in, 716-717
Articaine, methemoglobinemia from, 589
Artificial immunity, 91
Asbestosis, 570
Aspirating syringe in local anesthetic administration,
  596
Aspiration in physical examination, 216, 367
Assessment, patient, 174-375
  hard tissue examination in, 309-331. *See also* Hard
    tissue examination.
  health history in, 192-198
  history in, 192-212. *See also* History.
  intraoral photographic imaging in, 355-364
  life stage changes in, 176-189. *See also* Life stage
    changes.
  nutritional, 344-354. *See also* Nutritional assessment.
  physical and extraoral examinations in, 214-226. *See
    also* Physical examination.
  radiographic, 338-340
  supplementary aids in, 366-375. *See also* Supplemen-
    tary diagnostic aids.
Asthma in health history, 201
Ataxic cerebral palsy, 674
Atherosclerosis in health history, 205
Athetoid cerebral palsy, 674
Atrial dysrhythmia, 194
Atrigel, 423-424
Attachment apparatus of periodontium, 287-288
Attachment loss in risk assessment, 747
Attending in communication, 61-62
Attrition of tooth (teeth), 318
Auditory meatus, external, examination of, 217
Auscultation in physical examination, 214, 216, 222f, 367

Autism, neurological/sensory impairment from, 677
Autoclaves in sterilization, 104-105
Autogenous transfer of microorganisms, 77
Autoimmune diseases, 716-719
Autoimmune thyroid diseases, 719
Automatic iris in intraoral video imaging system, 359
Avoidance behavior in anxiety disorders, 699
Avoidant personality disorder, 706
Avulsed teeth, 457-458

B

Bacteria
    acidogenic, in caries process, 391
    cariogenic, fluoride and, 347
    diseases caused by, 79t, 85-86
Bactericidal activity, inhibition of, fluoride in, 395
Baking soda
    in antigingivitis dentifrices, 411
    in dentifrices, 423
Balanced reference posture, 122b
Barrier protection, in infection control program, 98
Basal lamina, 287
Bass tooth-brushing method, 381, 382t
Battered child syndrome, 458
Battery, 47
Bedsores in neurological/sensory impairment, 681
Behavior
    avoidance, in anxiety disorders, 699
    grossly disorganized, in schizophrenia, 710
    health, in ORA worksheet, 499
    observations of, in evaluation of child abuse, 459-460
Behavioral management in anxiety control, 580-581
Bell's palsy, neurological/sensory impairment from, 676
Beneficence, 46
Benign lesions, 734
Benzocaine topical anesthetics, 598
Benzodiazepines for anxiety disorders, 702t
Benzonatate, clinical actions of, 592
Beveled edges of instruments, 159
Bifurcations, 294
Bill of rights, patient's, 43-44b
Binge eating, 707
Binge eating/purging type of anorexia nervosa, 708
Bioburden
    on instruments, cleaning to reduce, 106
    reduction of, periodontal debridement in, 523
    removal of, in environmental surface preparation, 101
Biocentric technique of positioning, 122, 123b
Biofeedback in anxiety control, 581
Biofilm in waterline management, 99
Biohazardous materials, handling of, 75
Biologic width, 287
Biological indicators in sterilization, 105-106
Biopsy
    in cancer diagnosis, 734
    in oral mucosal lesion diagnosis, 371
Biopsychosocial model, 178
Biotin deficiency, oral symptoms of, 346t
Bipolar disorder, 704-705
    in health history, 209
Birth defects, periodontal disease and, 20
BIS-GMA in sealants, 443
Bladder dysfunction in neurological/sensory impairment, 680-681

Bleaching. *See also* Whitening.
    agents for, 653-654
    dentist-prescribed, home-applied, 656-657
    evolution of, 653
    in-office, 656
    laser, 656
    nightguard vital, 653
        technique for, 656-657
    power, 656
    side effects of, 657-658
    techniques for, 656-657
Bleaching trays, care of, 474-475
Bleeding
    complicating chemotherapy, 724
    excessive, in health history, 208
    indices of, in periodontal examination, 298, 299t
    on probing, detection of, 293-294
Bleeding problems, diagnostic aids for, 372, 373b
Blood
    exposure to, CDC recommendations for management following, 108t
    in sputum in health history, 201
    in urine in health history, 206
    OSHA definition of, 88
Blood pressure
    abnormal, in health history, 202
    determination of, 115
    evaluation of, 224-225
Bloodborne pathogens, OSHA definition of, 88
Body language in establishing rapport, 64
Bonding in sealant application, 441-442
Bone(s)
    deformity/fracture of, in health history, 200
    loss of, 339
        vertical, 339
    periodontal, 285
Bowel
    dysfunction of, in neurological/sensory impairment, 680-681
    inflammatory disease of, immune system dysfunction in, 718
Bradycardia, sinus, 223
Brain injury in neurological/sensory impairment, 673
Breach of duty in tort, 47
Breast cancer in health history, 207
Breath, shortness of, in health history, 202
Bronchitis in health history, 201
Brown spot lesion, 325
Bruising, easy, in health history, 208
Bruxism, 318
Buccal frenula, 253
Buccal mucosa
    epithelium covering, 285
    examination of, 252-254
Buffering role of saliva, 392
Bulimia nervosa, 708-709
Bupivacaine, clinical actions of, 592
Bupropion (Zyban) in tobacco cessation, 237b
Burning mouth syndrome, 692
Burnishing
    for desensitizing agent application, 435
    of amalgam restoration, 642
Burns, inflicted, in child abuse, 460

C

Calcium carbonate, as dental abrasive, 550
Calcium channel blockers, gingival hyperplasia form, 273-274
Calcium deficiency, oral symptoms of, 346t
Calcium hydroxide to decrease dentinal sensitivity, 435
Calculi, urinary, in health history, 206
Calculus, 283
    assessment of, 296-298
    dentifrices to control, 410-411
    indices of, in periodontal examination, 298, 300t
    periodontal disease and, 8
    removal of, instruments for, 138
    supragingival, 298
Caliculus angularis, 252
Camera
    35-mm, for intraoral photography, 356-357
    digital, for intraoral photography, 359-360
    in intraoral video imaging system, 359
Cancer, 719-725
    breast, in health history, 207
    chemotherapy for, 721-722
    definition of, 719-720
    dental hygienist and, 722-723
    emotional aspects of, 722
    head and neck, 731-742. *See also* Head and neck cancer.
    incidence of, 720
    oral
        data on, 24, 27b
        self-exam procedures for, 735-736b
    patient with
        oral care considerations for, 718b
        oral self-care for, 719-720b
    pharyngeal, data on, 24, 27b
    prevalence of, 720
    prostate, in health history, 207
    risk factors for, 720-721
    squamous cell, in AIDS, 726
    treatment of, 721-722
Candida infection associated with appliance wear, 477-478f
Candidiasis, 86
    associated with appliance wear, 477-487f
    complicating xerostomia, 665
    in AIDS, 726
    oral, 277-278
        data on, 28
        etiology of, 277
        signs and symptoms of, 277-278
        systemic drugs associated with, 278
        treatment of, 278
    salivary gland dysfunction and, 667
    summary of, 79t
Candidosis associated with appliance wear, 477
Canker sores in health history, 201
Cannula shape for irrigation tips, 418
Carbamazepine for bipolar disorder, 705
Carbamide peroxide as bleaching agent, 653-654
Carbocaine. *See* Mepivacaine.
Carbohydrates, fermentable
    dental caries and, 348-351
    dental decay and, 347

Carbohydrates, fermentable—cont'd
    frequency of intake of, 350-351
    nutritive sweeteners as, 349-350
    physical forms of, 350
Carbonated apatite as tooth mineral, 392
Carcinoma, 732. *See also* Cancer.
Carcinoma in situ, 733
Cardiac dysrhythmias in health history, 204
Cardiovascular system
    in review of organ systems, 202-205
    local anesthetics and, 590
Career goal setting, professional self and, 771
Caries
    active, 320
    approximal, 326
    arrested, 320
    charting of, 318-319
    classification systems for, 311, 316
        new, 320-321
    dentifrices to control, 410
    detection of
        changes in, 8
        conductance measurements in, 327
        current methods of, 323-324
        dyes in, 326
        fluorescence in, 328
        future technologies in, 327-328
        impedance measurements in, 327-328
        new advances in, 327
        optical coherence tomography in, 328
        ultrasound in, 328
        with dental radiographs, 326-327
    diet and, 348-351
    food protecting against, 347b
    in adults, 21, 23b, 23f, 24b
    in children, 21-22f, 22b
    in salivary gland dysfunction, 666-667
    interproximal, detection of, errors in, 337
    management of, 395-399
        by risk assessment, 396
        carious lesion management in, 397-399
        patient involvement in, 397
        reevaluation period in, 399
        salivary analysis in, 397
        team approach to, 395-396
    nutrition and, 347
    oral hygiene and, 391
    prevention of
        changes in, 8
        fluoride supplements in, 403
    process of, 391-393
    recurrent, 324-325
    secondary, 324-325
    supportive care for, 752-753
    tooth sensitivity from, 368-369
Cariogenic bacteria, fluoride and, 347
Carious lesion management, 397-399
Carpal tunnel syndrome (CTS), 117b
Cartridges for local anesthetic administration, 597
Case development, documentation, and presentation, 756-766
    applications of, 756-757
    guidelines for, 759-761, 762-765f

Case development, documentation, and
  presentation—cont'd
  theory of, 757-759
  uses of, 756-757
Casts, study, 368
Cataracts in health history, 200
Catastrophizing, 578
Cationic bisbiguanide, chlorhexidine as, 421
Cations, 586
Causal factors of oral disease, 18
Causation in tort, 47
Cavitation, 320
Cavitational action created by powered instruments, 523
Cavity bases, 639
Cavity/cavitation in caries process, 392
Cavity liners, 639
Cavity preparation
  Class I, 627-628, 628-629f
    amalgam restorations for, 639-642
    composite restorations for, 646
  Class II, 629-630f
    amalgam restorations for, 642-645
    composite restorations for, 646
  Class III, 629-630
    composite restorations for, 646
  Class IV, 630, 631f
  Class V, 630, 631f
    amalgam restorations for, 639-642
  Class VI
    amalgam restorations for, 639-642
    composite restorations for, 646
  components of, 627
Cavity sealers, 639
Cavosurface of cavity preparation, 627
CDC. *See* Centers for Disease Control and Prevention
  (CDC).
Cellular cementum, 288
Cementum, 285
  color changes in, 326
  structure of, 288-289
Centers for Disease Control and Prevention (CDC),
  86-87
Centigray, 737
Central nervous system, local anesthetics and, 590
Centric relation-centric occlusion shift, 329
Cerebral palsy, neurological/sensory impairment from,
  674
Cerebrovascular accident, neurological/sensory impair-
  ment from, 672-673
Cervical-enamel projections, periodontal disease risk
  and, 301, 302f
Cevimeline (Evoxac) for Sjögren's syndrome, 667
Chair, operator, 120-121
  armrests of, 128
Chancre in health history, 206
Channel scaling, 155
Charged-coupled device (CCD), 340-341
Charters' tooth-brushing method, 381, 382t
Charting
  of caries, 318-319
  of existing conditions, 316
  of hard tissue examination, 310-311
  periodontal, 292f

Chayes-Siemon apparatus to decrease dentinal
  sensitivity, 436-437
Cheilosis, angular, 194
Chemical disinfection, 104
Chemical factors in skin disorders, 199
Chemical sterilization, 105
Chemical stimuli in dentinal sensitivity, 431
Chemical vapor sterilizers, 105
Chemotherapeutic agents in dentifrices, 406-407
Chemotherapeutics, 416-427
  antimicrobial, 420
  delivery systems for, 417-420
    controlled, 423-424
  irrigation with, 418-420
  quality assurance for, 425
  rinsing with, 417-418
  selection of, based on need, 417b
  site-specific, 417
  success of, evaluation of, 425
  sustained release, 417
  systemic delivery of, 424-425
  topical, 417
Chemotherapy
  for cancer, 721-722
  for head and neck cancer, 736
  oral complications related to, 723-725
Chest pain/pressure in health history, 202
CHF. *See* Congestive heart failure (CHF).
Chickenpox, summary of, 79t
Child(ren)
  caries in, 21-22f, 22b
  fearful, management of, 582
Child abuse
  and neglect, dental trauma from, 458-463
    definitions on, 459
    demographic factors on, 459
    documentation of, 462
    evaluation of, 459-462
    historical perspective on, 458-459
    legal considerations on, 463
    legislative efforts on, 458-459
    reporting of, 462-463
  definition of, 459
Childhood
  early, 178-180
  late, 180-181
Chisels, 142, 143f
  design features of, 148
  sharpening of, 169, 170f
Chlorhexidine
  as oral antimicrobial, 421
  in antigingivitis dentifrices, 411
  treatment of carious lesion with, 399
Chronic obstructive pulmonary disease (COPD), 194
  in health history, 201
Circular fibers, 287
Circumferential strokes, 155
Circumvallate papillae, 257
Citanest. *See* Prilocaine.
Citanest Forte. *See* Prilocaine.
Clinical practice, future direction of, 777-778
Closing pathway, 329
CMV. *See* Cytomegalovirus (CMV).

Cobalamin deficiency, oral symptoms of, 346t
Cocaine, 586
  clinical actions of, 592
Cocaine hydrochloride as topical anesthetic, 598
Code of ethics for dental hygienists, 44-46b
Coe-Pak Periodontal Dressings, 570-571
Cognitive deficits in neurological/sensory impairment, 681-682
Cold, common, 83-85
  summary of, 79t
Cold sores in health history, 201
Cold sterilization, 103
Colitis, ulcerative, immune system dysfunction in, 718
Commitment to vision in professional development, 775
Common law, 41
Communication, 57-70
  assets for, 60-61
  attending in, 61-62
  being concrete in, 66
  being direct in, 66
  being genuine in, 66
  better, recognizing need for, 61
  deepening rapport in, 65
  deficits in, in neurological/sensory impairment, 682-683
  definition of, 60
  demonstrating respect in, 65-66
  effective, 53, 62b
  establishing ongoing relationships in, 65
  establishing rapport in, 62-65
  expressing emotional warmth in, 66
  feedback in, using "I" message, 67-69
  habits of, poor, unlearning, 61
  key elements of, 61-69
  learned, models for, 60
  listening in, 61
  observing in, 61-62
  responding with empathy in, 65
  self-disclosure in, 67
  self-evaluation on, 58, 60
  team approach to, 59-60b
  verbal, regulating, in establishing rapport, 64
Communicators, influential, 60
Competence
  in professional development, 772-773
  maintaining, 12-13
Complaint in health history, 195
Compliance, patient, 748-749
Composite materials for minimally invasive dentistry, 631
Composite restorations, direct resin, 645-647
Computer-assisted charting of hard tissues, 311, 313f
Computer-based caries classification system, 321, 322-323f
Computers, changes related to, 9
Concreteness in communication, 66
Condensing osteitis, radiographic appearance of, 339
Conductance in caries detection, 327
Confidentiality, 42b
Congenital abnormalities, sports dentistry related to, 465
Congestive heart failure (CHF), 194
  in health history, 204

Connective tissue
  gingival, fibers of, 287
  periodontal, 285, 287
Consent
  implied, 47-48
  informed, 9, 41, 46-49
    for nitrous oxide/oxygen sedation, 615
    form for, 48f
    therapeutic privilege as exception to, 47
Consultations from physical examination, 225-226
Contaminated, OSHA definition of, 88
Context in establishing rapport, 63
Continuous sutures, 568
Contraceptives, oral, 689
  oral effects of, 689-690
Controlled drug delivery systems, 423-424
Convenience form, 627
COPD. *See* Chronic obstructive pulmonary disease (COPD).
Corticosteroids to decrease dentinal sensitivity, 437
Cosmetic whitening, 650-660
Cost of care resources in social history, 198
Costs, of tobacco habit, 230-231
Cough in health history, 201
Cracked tooth syndrome, diagnosis of, 369
Cracking of enamel, 318
Credentials, licensure by, 9-10
Crest Whitestrips, 653, 654
  technique for use of, 657
Crohn's disease, 198
  immune system dysfunction in, 718
Crown fracture, 319
  emergency management of, 456
CTS. *See* Carpal tunnel syndrome (CTS).
Cultural sensitivity in establishing rapport, 63
Culture techniques in periodontal disease diagnosis, 370
Cumulative trauma disorders (CTDs), 116. *See also* Repetitive strain injuries (RSIs).
Curets, 138, 141, 142f
  area-specific
    design features of, 145, 146t, 147-148
    sharpening of, 166-167
  universal, 148
    sharpening of, 167-168
Cushing's syndrome in health history, 207
Cusp fracture, 319
Cyanoacrylate to decrease dentinal sensitivity, 437
Cycles per second in operation of sonic scalers, 528
Cyclosporine, gingival hyperplasia from, 274
Cystitis in health history, 206
Cytomegalovirus (CMV), 83
  summary of, 79t

D

Debridement
  in periodontal disease treatment, 8
  in periodontal supportive care, 752
  periodontal, 522-536. *See also* Periodontal debridement.
Decontamination
  in infection control program, 102-103
  OSHA definition of, 88
  thermal, 103

Defibrillator in health history, 204
Delusions in schizophrenia, 710
Demineralization, 319
   fluoride in inhibition of, 394
   fluoride inhibiting, 347
   in caries process, 391-392
Demyelinating disease in health history, 209
Dental caries. *See* Caries.
Dental endoscope, 536-537
Dental floss, 384
Dental history, 209-210
   in nutritional assessment, 351
Dental hygiene
   clinical practice patterns for, 7-9
   development of, 3-5, 4f
   practice environment for, changes in, 7-8f
Dental hygiene professional, 1-71. *See also* Dental
        hygienist(s).
Dental hygienist(s)
   accreditation of, 7
   as educator, 11
   career mobility and choices for, 11-12
   code of ethics for, 44-46b
   competence of, maintaining, 12-13
   education of, 5-7
   entry level for, 7
   functions of, 10
   in care of appliances and dental prostheses, 470
   in cosmetic whitening, 658-659
   in dental caries management, 395-396
   in dental product sales and marketing, 11
   in dental research, 11-12
   in insurance industry, 11
   in prevention of traumatic dental injuries, 464-466
   in private practice, 11
   in public health, 11
   origin of term, 5
   positioning for, 116
   practice of, within limits of law, 53
   professional portfolio of, 12-13
   responsibilities of, in providing dental hygiene care,
      52-55
   risk management for, 53
   supervision of, types of, 10, 11b
   workstation for, 116
Dentifrices, 406-414
   adverse effects of, 407
   antigingivitis, 411-412
   clinical studies on, evaluating, 409
   composition of, 407, 408f
   desensitizing, 433, 435
   efficacy claims for, 409
   efficacy of, 407-407
   formulations of, 409-412
      anticaries, 410
      calculus control, 410-411
      sensitivity control, 410
   safety of, 407-408
   selection of, 407b
   whitening, 411
Dentin, 285
   affected versus infected, 325-326
   carious, removal of, 627
   color changes in, 325-326

Dentin—cont'd
   fracture of, 456
   infected, radiography and, 326-327
   sensitivity of, 429-437
      agents for
         criteria for, 432
         studies of, factors influencing, 432
      dentifrices to control, 410
      etiology of, 429-430
      natural defense mechanisms and, 431-432
      stimuli eliciting, 430-431
      to cold stimuli, treatment of, 430b
      treatment of, 432-437
         personal oral hygiene in, 432-433
         professional products in, 434f, 435-437
Dentistry
   aesthetic, 632
   history of, 3-5, 4f
   human health and, 17
   minimally invasive, 630-631
Dentoalveolar fibers, 287
Dentogingival fibers, 287
Dentoperiosteal fibers, 287
Denture stomatitis, data on, 28
Dentures
   complete, 472-473
   full, 472
   partial
      fixed, 470-472
      removable, 473
Dependency, tobacco, 228-243
Dependent personality disorder, 706, 707b
Deplaquing in periodontal supportive care, 752
Depression in health history, 209
Depressive disorder, major, 703-704
Depth of field in intraoral video imaging system, 359
Derangement syndrome, 120
Dermatitis in health history, 198
Desensitization, systematic, in anxiety control, 581
Desensitizing agents
   commercially available, 433, 435
   criteria for, 432
   professional, 434f, 435-437
   studies of, factors influencing, 432
Desensitizing toothpastes, 433, 435
Desquamation associated with appliance wear,
      478, 479f
Developmental anomalies
   data on, 28
   from radiotherapy, 740-741
Diabetes mellitus (DM)
   age of onset of, 195
   diagnostic aids for, 373, 374b, 374f
   immune system dysfunction in, 716
   in health history, 207
   periodontal disease and, 19-20
DIAGNOdent, 327, 369
Diagnostic quality of radiographs, 334
Dialysis, renal, in health history, 206
Diascopy in physical examination, 216, 367
Dibasic calcium phosphate to decrease dentinal
      sensitivity, 435

Diet
  dental caries and, 348-351
  oral health problems associated with, 348b
Diet survey in ORA worksheet, 499
Dietary intake evaluation in nutritional assessment, 351-352
Diffusion channels in caries process, 392
Diffusion hypoxia in nitrous oxide/oxygen sedation, 617
Diflucan (fluconazole) for oral candidiasis from salivary dysfunction, 667
DiFOTI, 327
Digital fiberoptic transillumination (DiFOTI) in caries detection, 327
Dilantin (phenytoin), gingival hyperplasia from, 273
Dioptre magnification, 127
Diplopia in health history, 200
Direct resin composite restorations, 645-647
Directness in communication, 66
Disaccharides as fermentable carbohydrates, 349-350
Disclosing agents
  in caries diagnosis, 369
  in oral self-care, 386
Discoid lupus erythematosus, 717
Disease transmission
  dental healthcare providers and, 78-86
  factors in, 75-77
  microbial resistance and, 78
  prevention of. *See also* Infection control program.
  risk of exposure in, 77-78
  routes of, 76-77
  theory of, 75-98
Disinfectants, chemical classifications of, 103-104
Disinfection
  chemical, 104
  full-mouth, 749
  in infection control program, 103-104
Disorganized thinking in schizophrenia, 710
Distance in establishing rapport, 62
Distance learning, 777
Distraction in anxiety control, 581
Dizziness in health history, 209
DM. *See* Diabetes mellitus (DM).
DNA probe assays in periodontal disease diagnosis, 370
Documentation
  as dental hygienist's responsibility, 53-54
  case, 756-766. *See also* Case development, documentation, and presentation.
  legal, 757
  of child abuse and neglect, 462
  of patient care, 9
Domestic violence prevention, hygienist in, 464-465
Dopamine as neurotransmitter, 229
Dorsal surface of tongue, 256
Dressings, periodontal, 570-572
Dri-Clave sterilizers, 105
Droplet transfer of microorganisms, 76-77
Drug-induced lupus, 717
Drug interactions, 268
Drugs. *See* Medications.
Durable Power of Attorney for Health Care, 51f
Duty in tort, 47
Dyclone. *See* Dyclonine.

Dyclonine
  as topical anesthetic, 598
  clinical actions of, 592
Dyes, caries-indicating, 326
Dysarthria, 677-678
Dysfunction syndrome, 120
Dysgeusia, 274-275
  from radiotherapy, 739
Dysphagia, 677-678
  in health history, 205
Dysphasia from radiotherapy, 739
Dysplasia, 733
Dyspnea, 224
  in health history, 201
Dysrhythmias, cardiac, in health history, 204
Dysuria in health history, 206

E

Ears
  examination of, 217
  in review of organ systems, 200
Eating disorders, 707-709
EBV. *See* Epstein-Barr virus (EBV).
ECP. *See* Exposure control plan (ECP).
ECs. *See* Engineering controls (ECs).
Eczema in health history, 198
Edema
  associated with appliance wear, 478
  gingival, 283
  in polymyositis, 199
Edentulism, data on, 24, 26f
Education
  as dental hygienists' responsibility, 52-53
  case development, documentation, and presentation in, 757
  continuing, 12, 53
  dental hygienist in, 11
  future direction of, 776-777
  of dental hygienists, 5-7
    formal, development of, 6
    institutional settings for, 6-7
    programs for, 6-7
  patient
    in anxiety control, 580
    on fluoride applications, 400
Educational status as risk factor for cancer, 721
Electric pulp tester, 369-370
Embrasure, 287
Emotion, expressing, in establishing rapport, 65
Emotional disturbances, 694-713. *See also* Mental/emotional disturbances.
Emotional factors in social history, 197
Empathy
  in communication, 62
  responding with, 65
Emphysema in health history, 201
Enamel, 285
  color changes in, 325
  cracking of, 318
  flaking of, 318, 319f
  fracture of, 456
  hypoplasia of, nutrition and, 346-347

Enamel—cont'd
  mottled, 545
  walls of, finishing, 627
Enameloplasty, 324
Encephalitis, herpes, 82
Endocarditis
  history of, in health history, 205
  prevention of, guidelines for, 203b
Endocrine factors in skin disorders, 199
Endocrine system in review of organ systems, 207-208
Endogenous progesterone, hyperpigmentation from, 199
Endogenous tooth staining, 542
  developmental, 543f, 543t
  drug induced, 543-545, 544t
  enamel hypoplasia with, 544-545, 544t
  environmental, 544t, 545-546
Endosteum, 288
Engine-driven polishing, 550-553
Engineering controls (ECs)
  implementing, in infection control program, 98-99
  OSHA definition of, 89
Environmental ergonomics, 72-172
  disease transmission prevention in, 74-112
  exposure control in, 74-112
  instrument design in, 137-149. *See also* Instrument(s), design of.
  instrument sharpening in, 158-172. *See also* Sharpening, instrument.
  instrumentation in, 150-156. *See also* Instrumentation.
  workstation design and positioning in, 115-135
Environmental factors in social history, 198
Environmental procedures, in infection control program, 100-102
Environmental Protection Agency (EPA), 87
Enzyme-based assays in periodontal disease diagnosis, 370
Enzyme inhibitor, 586b
EPA. *See* Environmental Protection Agency (EPA).
Epidemiological surveys, 21
Epilepsy in health history, 209
Epinephrine, mepivacaine with, 586b
Epistaxis in health history, 200-201
Epithelium
  junctional, 287
  periodontal, 285
  sulcular, 287
Epstein-Barr virus (EBV), 83
Equipment
  dental, position of, 125-126
  musculoskeletal problems resulting from, 116b
Equipment procedures in infection control program, 100-102
Ergonomics, environmental, 72-172. *See also* Environmental ergonomics.
Erosion of tooth, 316-317
Erythema
  associated with appliance wear, 478
  gingival, 283
  skin, from radiotherapy, 741
Erythema multiforme, 268-271
  drug-associated, 270
  epidemiology of, 269
  etiological factors of, 269

Erythema multiforme—cont'd
  factors precipitating, 270
  herpes-associated, 270
  history of, 268-269
  mycoplasma-associated, 270
  signs and symptoms of, 269
  systemic drugs associated with, 269t
  treatment of, 270-271
Essential oils in mouthrinses, 421
Esters
  clinical actions of, 592
  local anesthetics as, 588
Esthetics, dental stains and, 542-543
Estrogen, 689
Ethical considerations on risk management, 40-55
Ethics
  code of, for dental hygienists, 44-46b
  law and, 42b
Ethnicity as risk factor for cancer, 721
Ethyl chloride in pulp testing, 370
Ethylene oxide sterilizers, 105
Evaluation of care, 744-766
  case development, documentation, and presentation in, 756-766
  for initial therapy, 749-750
  patient compliance in, 748-749
  risk assessment in, 747
  supportive care and, 746-755
Evidence-based practice, 9
Evidence-based teaching, 9
Evoxac (cevimeline), for Sjögren's syndrome, 667
Examination(s)
  for licensure, 9, 10b
  hard tissue, 309-331. *See also* Hard tissue examination.
  head, eyes
    ear, nose and throat (HEENT). *See also* Physical examination, HEENT.
    ears, nose and throat (HEENT), 214-222
  intraoral, 245-265. *See also* Intraoral examination.
  periodontal, 282-307. *See also* Periodontal examination.
  physical and extraoral, in patient assessment, 214-226. *See also* Physical examination.
Excursions, initial contacts in, 330
Exercises in prevention/treatment of musculoskeletal disorders, 128-134
  isometric, 131, 132f
  postural, 129-130
  strengthening, 131-134
  stretching, 130-131
Exocrine glands, salivary glands as, 664
Exogenous progesterone, hyperpigmentation from, 199
Exogenous tooth staining, 542
Explorers, 138, 142, 143f
  design features of, 145
  sharpening of, 169-170
Exposure control plan (ECP), OSHA definition of, 89
Exposure incident, OSHA definition of, 88
Extraoral findings in disease, 19, 20b
Extremities, in review of organ systems, 199-200
Extrinsic staining, 546
Eye contact in establishing rapport, 64
Eyelids, drooping, in health history, 200

Eyes
examination of, 217
in review of systems, 200
Eyewear, protective, in infection control program, 96-97

F

F-stop of 35-mm camera, 357
Face, examination of, 216-217
Face masks in infection control program, 97
Face shields in infection control program, 96
Faces of instruments, 138
Facet joint, spinal, 119
Facial expressions in establishing rapport, 64
Fainting in health history, 202, 209
Family history, 197
Fatigue, reducing, 127-128
Fauces of oral cavity, 261
Fear
definition of, 577, 698
dental, 576
in children, management of, 582
in dental patient, 695b
signs associated with, 580b
Federal agencies, 86-87
Feedback using "I" message in communication, 67-69
Female sex hormones, 687-689
Fermentable carbohydrates
dental caries and, 348-351
dental decay and, 347
frequency of intake of, 350-351
nutritive sweeteners and, 349-350
physical forms of, 350
Fever blisters in health history, 201
Fiber optics, 125
Fibromyalgia, 195
in health history, 200
Files, 138, 141, 142f
design features of, 148-149
sharpening of, 169, 170f
Filiform papillae, 256
Film for 35-mm camera, 357
Flaking, enamel, 318, 319f
Flap(s)
periodontal, 563
full-thickness, 564b
surgical, 563
Flash of 35-mm camera, 357-358f
Floss, dental, 384
Floss threaders for interdental cleaning, 384
Fluconazole (Diflucan) for oral candidiasis from salivary dysfunction, 667
Fluorapatite as tooth mineral, 393, 394-395
Fluorescence in caries detection, 328
Fluoridation, water, community, 17
Fluoride(s), 390-404
carriers for, care of, 474-475
deficiency of, oral symptoms of, 346t
delivery systems for, 399-400
in saliva, 393-394
mechanisms of action of, 394-395
professional applications of, 400-401
self-applied topical products with, 401
supplements of, in caries prevention, 402

Fluoride(s)—cont'd
to decrease dentinal sensitivity, 436
topical
treatment of carious lesion with, 398
versus systemic uptake of, 393
toxicity of, 401
traditional paint-on technique for, 400
Fluoride level detection kits in caries diagnosis, 369
Fluoride trays, 400-401
Fluoride varnish, 400
Fluorosis, 393
cosmetic whitening for, 651b, 655
dental, 544, 545f
Focal length, with 35-mm camera, 357
Focusing mechanism in intraoral video imaging system, 359
Folic acid deficiency, oral symptoms of, 346t
Fones' tooth-brushing method, 381, 382t
Food, dental stains from, 547t, 548
Food and Drug Administration (FDA), 87
Food intake, oral health problems associated with, 348b
Foramen cecum, 257-258
Fordyce granules, 253
Formalin to decrease dentinal sensitivity, 435
Fractionation of radiation, 737
Fracture(s)
crown, 319
emergency management of, 456
cusp, 319
in health history, 200
mandibular, 458
root, emergency management of, 456-457
tooth, types of, 318-319
Free gingival groove, 285
Free gingival margin, 285, 286
location of, recession and, 291
Free soft tissue graft for lost tooth, 564b
Frenectomy, 564b
Frenula, buccal, 253
Frenum(a), 287
labial, 250
removal of, suturing after, 564b
Fulcrum, 151-152
Fungal diseases, 79t, 86
Fungiform papillae, 256
Furcation(s)
exploration of, 294-295
grades of, 295t
Furcation involvement, 339
Furcation probe, 283
Future, 778-779
Future direction, 776-778

G

GAD. *See* Generalized anxiety disorder (GAD).
Gag reflex reduction, nitrous oxide/oxygen sedation in, 612
Galvanic reaction from amalgam restorations, 639
Gantrez in calculus control dentifrices, 410
Garments, protective, in infection control program, 97-98
Gastroesophageal reflux in health history, 206
Gastrointestinal system in review of organ systems, 205-206

Gauge of needle for local anesthesia, 596-597
Gauze stripe for interdental cleaning, 384
Generalized anxiety disorder (GAD), 701
Genital herpes in health history, 206
Genitourinary system in review of organ systems, 206-207
GENOME project, 776
Genuineness in communication, 66
Geographical tongue, 257
Geometrical charting of hard tissues, 311, 313f
Gingiva
    attached, 286
        amount of, 293
    components of, 286-287
    connective tissue fibers of, 287
    erythema of, linear, in AIDS, 727
    indices of, in periodontal examination, 298, 300t
    inflammation of. *See* Gingivitis.
    interface of
        with implant, 474
        with tooth, 286
    keratin in, 285
    keratinized, amount of, 293
    visual characteristics of, 289-290
Gingival hyperplasia, 273-274
Gingival retractor clamp, application of, 636-637
Gingival sulcus, 287
Gingivitis
    acute necrotizing ulcerative, 289
    dentifrices to control, 411-412
    erythema in, 289
    from oral contraceptives, 690
    identifying, 303
    necrotizing ulcerative, in AIDS, 727
    pregnancy, 689
    puberty, 689
Gingivopalatal groove, periodontal risk and, 301, 302f
Gingivostomatitis, herpes, 82
Gland(s)
    parotid, examination of, 218
    salivary, 664-670. *See also* Salivary glands.
    thyroid, examination of, 218
Glass ionomers as restorative material, 638
Glasses, safety, 96
Glaucoma in health history, 200
Global assessment of functioning (GAF) scale, 696, 697-698t
Glossitis
    in xerostomia, 665
    wandering, 257
Glossodynia in xerostomia, 665
Gloves, in infection control program, 95-96
Glucometer, 373, 374f
GLUMA to decrease dentinal sensitivity, 437
Goals
    patient, in ORA system, 508, 510
    professional self and, 771
Goggles, safety, 96
Gonorrhea, 85
    summary of, 79t
Government agencies, 86-88
Gracey curet(s), 145, 146t, 147-148
    sharpening of, 166-167

Grafts, soft tissue, free, for lost tooth, 564b
Granuloma, pyogenic, in pregnancy, 689
Grits of polishing materials, 558
Ground substance of gingiva, 287
Guidelines, definition of, 86

H

Habits
    dietary, dental caries and, 348-351
    in social history, 198
Hair care in infection control program, 91-92
Hairy tongue, 276
Hallucinations in schizophrenia, 710
Hand care in infection control program, 92-94
Hand-held stones for instrument sharpening, 161-163
Hand-washing facilities, OSHA definition of, 88
Handles, instrument, 138-139
Hard palate, 259-260
Hard tissues
    assessment of, in child abuse, 461-462
    examination of, 309-331
        caries classification systems and cavity design in, 311, 316
        caries in, 319-328. *See also* Caries.
        charting existing conditions in, 316
        charting of, 310-311
        conditions modifying teeth in, 316-318
        in periodontal supportive care, 751
        infection control in, 311
        occlusal analysis in, 328-330
        tooth fracture types in, 318-319
        tooth numbering systems for, 311, 314-315f
    formation of, nutrition and, 346-347
Harm in tort, 47
Hazard abatement
    in infection control program, 90-109
    OSHA definition of, 88-89
Head, examination of, 216-217, 219, 222f
Head and neck cancer, 731-742
    clinical diagnosis of, 733
    contributing factors for, 732-733
    early detection of, 733-734, 735-736b
    etiology of, 732-733
    radiation therapy for, 737-741
        developmental anomalies complicating, 740-741
        dysgeusia complicating, 739
        dysphasia complicating, 739
        fractionation of, 737
        infections complicating, 739
        mucositis complicating, 738
        nutritional deficiency complicating, 740
        oral care protocol in, 741
        oral complications of, 738-741
        osteoradionecrosis complicating, 740
        skin erythema complicating, 741
        trismus complicating, 740
        xerostomia complicating, 738-739
    staging of, 733, 734b
        postoperative irradiation and, 737
    treatment of, 734
Headaches, frequent, in health history, 208-209
Healing, wound, periodontal, 526-527

Health
  definition of, 18
  dentistry and, 17
  promotion of, 16-38
    barriers to, 18b
    broadening paradigm of, 18-19
    community strategies for, 17b
    definition of, 18-19
    guidelines for, 29-36
      Healthy People 2010 as, 29-31
    guidelines for, surgeon general's report as, 31,
      32-36b
    historical perspective on, 17-18
    obstacles to, 18
Health behavior in ORA worksheet, 499
Health beliefs in ORA worksheet, 500
Health history
  age in, 195
  family history in, 197
  gender in, 193, 195
  history of illness in, 196-197
  in evaluation of child abuse, 459
  in infection control program, 91
  in nutritional assessment, 351
  in ORA worksheet, 498
  in patient assessment, 192-198
  in sports-related injury evaluation, 455
  patient identification in, 193, 195
  present oral condition in, 195-196
  race in, 195
  review of organ systems in, 198-209. *See also* Review of
    organ systems.
  social history in, 197-198
  thorough, significance of, 194
Health promotion
  individualizing preventive and therapeutic strategies
    in, 507-519
  oral risk assessment in, 486-506. *See also* Risk assess-
    ment, oral.
Healthy People 2010 as health promotion guidelines,
  29-31
Hearing aid in health history, 200
Hearing loss in health history, 200
Heart
  disease of, rheumatic, in health history, 202-203
  disorders of, congenital, in health history, 203
  dysrhythmias of, in health history, 204
  failure of, congestive, 194
  murmur in, in health history, 203-204
  valves of, prosthetic, in health history, 205
Heart attack in health history, 205
Heartbeats, abnormal, in health history, 204
HEENT examination, 214-222. *See also* Physical
  examination, HEENT.
Hematopoietic system in review of organ systems, 208
Hematuria in health history, 206
Hemidesmosomal attachment, 287
Hemophilia in health history, 208
Hemorrhagic stroke, 672
Hemostasis, laboratory tests for, 373b
Hepatitis A virus, 80-81
Hepatitis B virus, 81
Hepatitis C virus, 81

Hepatitis D virus, 81
Hepatitis E virus, 81
Hepatitis G virus, 81-82
Hepatitis infections, 78, 79t, 80-82, 80t
  comparison of, 80t
  in health history, 206
  summary of, 79t
Herniated disc, 118, 119f
Herpes, genital, in health history, 206
Herpes conjunctivitis, 82
Herpes encephalitis, 82
Herpes gingivostomatitis, 82
Herpes labialis, 82
Herpes simplex virus infections
  in AIDS, 726
  oral, data on, 28
  summary of, 79t
  type 1, 82
  type 2, 82-83
Herpetic whitlow, 82
Hertz, 528
High-intensity lights, eye protection for, 97
High-velocity evacuation (HVE), 98
History
  accident, in sports-related injury evaluation, 455
  dental, 209-210
    in nutritional assessment, 351
    in ORA worksheet, 498-499
  fluoride, in ORA worksheet, 499
  health, 192-209. *See also* Health history.
  of illness, 196-197
  of present oral condition, 195
  social, in nutritional assessment, 351
Histrionic personality disorder, 705
HIV. *See* Human immunodeficiency virus (HIV).
Hoarseness in health history, 201
Hoes, 141-142, 143f
  design features of, 148
  sharpening of, 168-169
Honing machine, 161
Horizontal fibers of periodontal ligament, 288
Horizontal strokes, 155
Hormone replacement therapy (HRT), 689, 691
Hormones
  female sex, 687-689
  imbalances in, 687-693
    dental hygiene supportive care in, 691-692
    osteoporosis from, 691
  imbalances of, effects of, on oral flora, 689
Host immunity
  disease transmission and, 77
  in infection control program, 90-91
Host response, periodontal debridement and, 523, 526
Host susceptibility in disease transmission, 77
Housekeeping, OSHA definition of, 89
Human immunodeficiency virus (HIV), 725-727
  disease caused by, 83
    summary of, 79t
  virulence of, 77
Human papillomavirus infections, oral, data on, 28
Hydrocephalus, neurological/sensory impairment form,
  676
Hydrodynamic theory of dentinal sensitivity, 430

Hydrogen peroxide
   in antigingivitis dentifrices, 411
   in Crest Whitestrips, 653
Hydrophilic amino group in local anesthetics, 588
Hydrophobic component of local anesthetics, 588
Hydroxyapatite, 392
Hygiene
   dental
      anxiety related to, 578-580
      polishing in, 559
   oral
      caries and, 391
      personal, in dentinal sensitivity management,
         432-433
   personal, in infection control program, 91-94
Hygienist. *See* Dental hygienist(s).
Hyperbaric oxygen in cancer management, 732b
Hypermelanosis, 199
Hyperpigmentation, 199
Hypertension, 194
   causes of, 224
   guidelines for
   in health history, 202
Hyperthermia, causes of, 223
Hyperthyroidism
   in health history, 207
   vitiligo in, 199
Hyperventilation, 224
Hypnosis in anxiety control, 581
Hypomania in bipolar disorder, 704
Hypoplasia, enamel
   endogenous staining with, 543-544, 544t
   from tetracycline, 543
Hypotension
   causes of, 224
   in health history, 202
   orthostatic, 224-225
Hypothermia, causes of, 223
Hypothyroidism in health history, 207
Hypoxia, diffusion, in nitrous oxide/oxygen sedation,
   617

I

ICP. *See* Infection control policy (ICP).
Illness, restricting healthcare employee duties during, 91
Immersion burns in child abuse, 460
Immune system
   dysfunction of, 715-729, 716-719
      in acquired immunodeficiency syndrome, 725-727
      in Addison's disease, 719
      in aging, 716
      in autoimmune diseases, 716-719
      in autoimmune thyroid diseases, 719
      in diabetes, 716
      in inflammatory bowel diseases, 718
      in lupus erythematosus, 717
      in multiple sclerosis, 718
      in myasthenia gravis, 718
      in pernicious anemia, 717-718
      in psoriasis, 718
      in rheumatoid arthritis, 716-717
      in scleroderma, 718-719
   function of, 716

Immunity, host
   disease transmission and, 77
   in infection control program, 90-91
Immunizations in infection control program, recom-
      mendations for, 91, 92t
Immunological assays in periodontal disease diagnosis,
   370
Impedance measurements in caries detection, 327-328
Implants, 473-474
   dental, examination and evaluation of, 303
   polishing of, 559
Incident, exposure, OSHA definition of, 88
Incontinence in neurological/sensory impairment, 680
Infarction, stroke from, 672
Infection(s)
   Candida, associated with appliance wear, 477-478f
   complicating chemotherapy, 724
   control of, in hard tissue examination, 311
   from radiotherapy, 739
   hepatitis, 78, 79t, 80-82, 80t
   human papillomavirus, oral, data on, 28
   kidney, in health history, 206
   oral, heart disease and stroke and, 20
   periodontal, laboratory assays of, 304
Infection control policy (ICP), OSHA definition of, 89
Infection control program, 89-109
   decontamination procedures in, 102-103
   dental unit waterline management in, 99
   disinfection in, 103-104
   environmental and equipment procedures in, 100-102
   goal of, 89-90
   hazard abatement in, 90-109
   implementing work practice and engineering controls
      in, 98-99
   personal protective equipment in, 90f, 94-98
   sanitization in, 102-103
   standard operating procedures in, 90-109
   universal precautions in, 90-94
Infectious agents
   nature of, 76
   risk of exposure to, 77-78
   sources of, 76
Infectious disease, dental healthcare providers and,
      78-86
Infectious mononucleosis, summary of, 79t
Inferior fold of lower lip, 250
Infiltration versus nerve block for local anesthesia, 596
Inflammation, gingival. *See* Gingivitis.
Inflammatory bowel disease, immune system
      dysfunction in, 718
Influenza, 85
   summary of, 79t
Information and training, OSHA definition of, 89
Informed consent, 9, 41, 46-49
   for nitrous oxide/oxygen sedation, 615
   form for, 48f
   therapeutic privilege as exception to, 47
Injections
   guidelines for, 599-600b
   mandibular, technique guide for, 604t, 605-606f
   maxillary, technique guide for, 601t, 602-603f
   techniques for, myths about, 606-607
Injury. *See* Trauma.

Insomnia in depression, 703
Inspection in physical examination, 214, 216, 220f, 367
Instrument(s)
    classification of, 141-142
    cleaning of, to reduce bioburden, 106
    dental mirrors as, 142, 144-145
    design name of, 142, 144f
    design number of, 142, 144f
    design of, 137-149
    evolution of, 138
    grasp of, 150
    handles of, 138-139
    identification of, 141-149
    management of, 106-107
    parts of, 138-141
    shanks of, 139, 140f, 141
    sharp
        care and maintenance of, 171
        maintenance of, goals for, 159-160
    sharpening of, 158-172. *See also* Sharpening,
            instrument.
    sharpness of, testing for, 160, 161f
    sterilization of, 106
    sterilized, storage of, 106-107
    ultrasonic, 138, 142
    working end of, 140f, 141
Instrumentation
    activation in, 154-155
    adaptation in, 153
    angulation for insertion and activation in, 153-154
    fulcrum in, 151-152
    fundamentals of, 150-155
    instrument grasp in, 150
    operator positioning during, 124
    powered, 522-536. *See also* Powered instrumentation.
Insulin resistance, 716
Insurance, submission of, case documentation for, 757
Insurance industry, dental hygienist in, 11
Integumentary deficits in neurological/sensory impair-
        ment, 681
Interdental cleaning, 383-386
Interest in discussion, reflecting, in establishing rapport,
        64-65
International normalized ratio (INR), 194
International Organization for Standardization (ISO),
        380
International Standard Organization (ISO) number for
        film, 357
International system of tooth numbering, 311, 314t,
        315f
Interproximal cleaning devices, 378
Interproximal contacts, periodontal disease risk and, 302
Interradicular fibers of periodontal ligament, 288
Interrupted sutures, 567-568
Intervention
    definition of, 488b
    strategies for, 487
    therapeutic
        individualizing, 507-519
        planning of, in ORA system, 501-502
Intervertebral disc(s), 118, 119f
    herniated/slipped, 118, 119f

Intimate distance in establishing rapport, 62
Intraoral examination, 245-265
    buccal mucosa in, 252-254
    floor of mouth in, 254-256
    hard and soft palates in, 259-261
    labial mucosa in, 246-252
    lips in, 246-252
    oropharynx in, 261-263
    palatine tonsils in, 261-263
    tongue in, 256-259
    vestibular folds in, 252-254
Intraoral findings in disease, 19, 20b
Intrinsic factor deficiency in pernicious anemia,
        717-718
Intrinsic stains, 542
Ionization factors in anesthetics, 588-589
Ionized proteins in extracellular fluid, 586
Iontophoresis to decrease dentinal sensitivity, 436-437
Iris, automatic, in intraoral video imaging system, 359
Iron deficiency, oral symptoms of, 346t
Irrigation with chemotherapeutics, 418-420
Irritable mood in depression, 703-704
Ischemic stroke, 672
Isocaine. *See* Mepivacaine.
Isolation of teeth, 632-638
    rubber dam in, 632-638. *See also* Rubber dam.
Itching in health history, 198

J

Jargon, 63
Jaundice in health history, 206
Jewelry, personal, in infection control program, 92
Joint(s)
    facet, spinal, 119
    prosthetic, in health history, 200
    stiff and swollen, in health history, 199
    synovial, in spine, 118
Junctional epithelium, 287
Justice and fairness, 46-47

K

Kaposi's sarcoma in AIDS, 726
Keratinized epithelium, 285
Keratinized gingiva, amount of, 293
Keratitis, 82
Keratoconjunctivitis sicca in Sjögren's syndrome, 666
Ketoacidosis, 195
Ketoconazole (Nizoral) for oral candidiasis from salivary
        dysfunction, 667
Ketone topical local anesthetic, 592
Kidney infections in health history, 206
Knitting yarn for interdental cleaning, 384
Knurled handles, 139
Koch's postulates, 296
Kwashiorkor, hair in, 199
Kyphosis, 118

L

Labial mucosa
    alveolar mucosa continuous with, 287
    anatomical landmarks on, 247, 250
    examination technique for, 250-252

Labial mucosa—cont'd
  lesions of
    elevated, 248f
    flat, 248f
    red, isolated, 250f
    white, 249f
  topography, 247, 250
Laboratory evaluations in nutritional assessment, 351
Laboratory procedures, infection control and, 109
Lacerations associated with appliance wear, 478
Lactobacilli in caries process, 391
Lamina propria, 287
Language in establishing rapport, 64
Laser bleaching, 656
Laser detection device in caries diagnosis, 369
Laser lights, eye protection for, 97
Lasers to decrease dentinal sensitivity, 437
Lateral labial fold, 250
Lateral pressure on instrument, 152
Latex allergy
  gloves and, 96
  in health history, 199
Law
  common, 41
  ethics and, 42b
Leaders in future of dental hygiene, 778
Learned communication models, 60
Learning, distance, 777
Legal considerations on risk management, 40-55
Legionnaire's disease, 85
  summary of, 79t
Lemonstron apparatus to decrease dentinal sensitivity, 437
Lens of 35-mm camera, 356-357
Leukemia in health history, 208
Liability of dental hygienist, 41
Licensing exams, state, future of, 777
Licensure, 9-10
  as dental hygienists' responsibility, 52-53
  future direction of, 776-777
Lichenoid drug reaction, 272-273
Lidocaine (Xylocaine, Octocaine), 586
  as topical anesthetic, 598
  clinical actions of, 591
Life stages
  anticipatory guidance in, 178
  physical-physiological characteristics of, 178
  psychosocial-behavioral characteristics of, 178
Ligament, periodontal
  principal fibers of, 287
  structure of, 288
Light polymerization of direct resin composite restorations, 645
Lighting
  dental, position of, 125-126
  for intraoral video imaging, 359
Lights
  high-intensity, eye protection for, 97
  laser, eye protection for, 97
Line angles, of cavity preparation
  Class I, 628-629f
  Class II, 629, 630f
Line angles of cavity preparation, 627

Linea alba, 252
Linear gingival erythema, in AIDS, 727
Liners, cavity, 639
Lingual tonsils, 258
Lipopolysaccharides, periodontal disease and, 523
Lips
  anatomical landmarks on, 247, 250
  examination technique for, 250-252
  lesions of
    elevated, 248f
    flat, 248f
    red, isolated, 250f
    white, 249f
  topography of, 247, 250
Listening, in communication, 61
Lithium for bipolar disorder, 705
Living Will Declaration, 51f
Local tissue toxicity of local anesthetics, 590
Long axis of handle, 139, 140f
Lordosis, 118
Lotions, hand, in infection control program, 93
Lou Gehrig's disease, neurological/sensory impairment from, 675
Loupes, telescopic, 127-128
Low-birth-weight babies, periodontal disease and, 20
Lumen of irrigation tip, 418
Lupus erythematosus
  immune system dysfunction in, 717
  systemic, 195
Lupus in health history, 199
Luxation, intrusive, in primary dentition, 453
Luxation injuries, 457
Lyme disease in health history, 209
Lymph node examination, 217-218
Lymphoma, non-Hodgkin's, in AIDS, 726

M

Magnesium deficiency, oral symptoms of, 346t
Magnetostrictive ultrasonic scalers, 528-529
Magnification systems, 127-128
Malignant tumors, 731-732
Malpractice allegations, prevention of, 465
Mandibular fracture, 458
Mandibular tori, 255-256
Mandrel-mounted stones for instrument sharpening, 161, 162f
Mania in bipolar disorder, 704
Manic-depressive illness, 704-705
Marcaine. *See* Bupivacaine.
Marginal breakdown of amalgam restorations, 639
Marginal irrigation, 418-419
Marketing, dental product, dental hygienist in, 11
Masks, face, in infection control program, 97
Masticatory mucosa, 259
Materia alba, 296
Mattress sutures, 569, 570f
Maxillofacial prostheses, 475-476
Maximum incisal opening, 329, 330f
McCall's festoon, 289
Meador's biocentric technique of positioning, 122, 123b
Measles, 83
  summary of, 79t
Mechanical pain stimuli in dentinal sensitivity, 430-431

Medial, 253
Medications
 adverse reactions to, in health history, 199
 clinical manifestations of, 267-280
  angioedema as, 276-277
  candidiasis as, 277-278
  dysgeusia as, 274-275
  erythema multiforme as, 268-271
  gingival hyperplasia as, 273-274
  hairy tongue as, 76
  lichenoid drug reaction as, 272-273
  oral pigmentation as, 275-276
  xerostomia as, 271-272
 endogenous tooth staining induced by, 543-545, 544t
 extrinsic dental stains from, 547t, 548
 interactions of local anesthetics with, 590
 neuroleptic, for schizophrenia, 710-711
 xerostomia from, 665, 666b
Melanocytes in gingival epithelium, 286-287
Membrane potential, resting, in nerve conduction, 586-587
Menopause, 689
 oral changes in, 691
 supportive care in, 688b
Menstrual cycle, 687, 688f
 oral changes in, 689
Mental/emotional disturbances, 694-713
 anxiety disorder as, 698-702
 classification of, 696-698
 definitions of, 696-698
 eating disorders as, 707-709
 mood disorders as, 703-705
 personality disorders as, 705-707
 schizophrenia as, 709-711
Mepivacaine (Carbocaine, Isocaine)
 clinical actions of, 591
 with epinephrine, 586b
Mesothelioma, 570
Metabolic factors in skin disorders, 199
Metals, adverse reactions to, in health history, 199
Methemoglobinemia, articaine and prilocaine causing, 589
Methyl red-plaque-sugar test in caries diagnosis, 369
Microorganisms
 environmental survival of, 78t
 methods of escape of, 76
 nature of, 76
 reducing load of, 98
 resistance of, 78
 risk of exposure to, 77-78
 sources of, 76
 virulence of, in disease transmission, 77
Microscopic techniques in periodontal disease diagnosis, 370
Microstreaming phenomena, acoustic, from power instruments, 523
Minerals, tooth, composition of, caries process and, 392-393
Minimally invasive dentistry, 630-631
Minocycline, dental stains from, whitening for, 655
Minute ventilation in nitrous oxide/oxygen sedation administration, 616

Mirrors
 dental, design features of, 142, 144-145
 for intraoral photography, 360-361
Mobility
 deficits in, in neurological/sensory impairment, 683
 detection of, 295-296
 disorders of, from stroke, 673
 in periodontal examination, 289
 tooth, in risk assessment, 747
Modeling in anxiety control, 580-581
Models, study, 368
Monitor in intraoral video imaging system, 359
Monomers in sealants, 443
Mononucleosis, infectious, summary of, 79t
Monosaccharides as fermentable carbohydrates, 349
Mood disorders, 703-705
Motor control deficits in neurological/sensory impairment, 677-678
Mount and Hume caries classification system, 320-321
Mounted stones for instrument sharpening, 161, 162f
Mouth
 floor of, examination of, 254-256
 ulcers of, in health history, 201
Mouthguards, 463-464
 care of, 474
MSDs. *See* Musculoskeletal disorders (MSDs).
Mucogingival junction, 285
Mucoperiosteal flap, 564b
Mucosa
 alveolar
  epithelium covering, 285
  structure of, 287
 buccal
  epithelium covering, 285
  examination of, 252-254
 labial, 247-252. *See also* Labial mucosa.
  alveolar mucosa continuous with, 287
Mucositis, oral
 complicating chemotherapy, 723
 from radiotherapy, 738
Mulling, 639
Multilevel brush designs, 380
Multiple sclerosis
 immune system dysfunction in, 718
 in health history, 209
 neurological/sensory impairment from, 675
Mumps, 85
 summary of, 79t
Murmur, heart, in health history, 203-204
Muscle tone deficits in neurological/sensory impairment, 678-679
Muscle weakness in health history, 200
Muscular dystrophy
 in health history, 209
 neurological/sensory impairment from, 676
Musculoskeletal deficits in neurological/sensory impairment, 679
Musculoskeletal disorders (MSDs), 116-118
 definition of, 117-118
 in health history, 199-200
 prevalence of, 116-117
 prevention and treatment of, exercises in, 128-134. *See also* Exercises in prevention/treatment of musculoskeletal disorders.

Mutans streptococci in caries process, 391
Myasthenia gravis
  immune system dysfunction in, 718
  in health history, 200

N

Nails in infection control program, 93
Narcissistic personality disorder, 705-706
National Board Examination, 9
National Health and Nutrition Examination Survey
    (NHANES), 21
National Health Interview Survey (NHIS), 21
National Institute of Dental and Craniofacial Research
    (NIDCR), 21
Natural defense mechanisms, dentinal sensitivity and,
    431-432
Natural immunity, 90-91
Neck
  cancer of, 731-742. *See also* Head and neck cancer.
  examination of, 218, 219, 220-222f
Neck extension, 129, 130f
Neck retraction, 129, 129f, 130f
Necrotizing ulcerative gingivitis, in AIDS, 727
Needle guards, 597
Needle holders, 597-598
Needles
  for local anesthetic administration, 596-597
  suture, 566
Needs, interpersonal, professional self and, 771
Neglect, definition of, 459
Negligence, 42b
Neonatal lupus, 717
Neoplasms. *See also* Tumor(s).
  in AIDS, 726
Nerve block versus infiltration for local anesthesia, 596
Nerve conduction
  peripheral, local anesthetics and, 590
  physiology of, 586-587
Nervous system
  central, local anesthetics and, 590
  impairment of, 671-685. *See also* Neurological/sensory
    impairment.
  in review of organ systems, 208-209
  sympathetic, vasoconstrictors released by, in anes-
    thetic solutions, 590-591
Nervousness in health history, 209
Neuralgia in health history, 209
Neuritis in health history, 209
Neurofibromatosis in health history, 199
Neuroleptic drugs for schizophrenia, 710-711
Neurological/sensory impairment, 671-685
  bowel and bladder dysfunction in, 680-681
  cognitive deficits in, 681-682
  communication deficits in, 682-683
  from Alzheimer's disease, 676
  from amyotrophic lateral sclerosis, 675
  from autism, 677
  from Bell's palsy, 676
  from brain injury, 673
  from cerebral palsy, 674
  from hydrocephalus, 676
  from multiple sclerosis, 675
  from muscular dystrophy, 676

Neurological/sensory impairment—cont'd
  from Parkinson's disease, 674
  from spina bifida, 675
  from spinal injury, 674-675
  from stroke, 672-673
  integumentary deficits in, 681
  mobility deficits in, 683
  motor control deficits in, 677-678
  muscle tone deficits in, 678-679
  musculoskeletal deficits in, 679
  neuromuscular deficits in, 677-679
  perceptual deficits in, 681-682
  respiratory deficits in, 679-680
  visual deficits in, 682
Neuromuscular blockade from local anesthetics, 590
Neuromuscular deficits in neurological/sensory impair-
    ment, 677-679
Neurotoxicity complicating chemotherapy, 725
Neurotransmitters, 229
NHANES. *See* National Health and Nutrition Examina-
    tion Survey (NHANES).
NHIS. *See* National Health Interview Survey (NHIS).
Niacin deficiency, oral symptoms of, 346t
Nicotine dependence, 228-243. *See also* Tobacco, depen-
    dency on.
Nicotine replacement in tobacco cessation, 237-238b
Nicotinic stomatitis, 194
NIDCR. *See* National Institute of Dental and Craniofacial
    Research (NIDCR).
Nightguard vital bleaching, 653
  technique for, 656-657
Nightguards, care of, 474
Nitrous oxide/oxygen sedation, 610-621
  administration of, 611, 614-617
    equipment for, 612-614
    oversedation in, 615
    stages of anesthesia in, 614-615
    technique of, 615-617
  biological effects of, 618-620
  effects of, 611
  exposure levels in, 619
  indications for, 612
  issues related to, 618-620
  pharmacology of, 611-612
  recovery from, 617-618
  relative contraindications to, 612
  trace contamination from, 619-620
Nizoral (ketoconazole) for oral candidiasis from salivary
    dysfunction, 667
Nodule, 252
Non-Hodgkin's lymphoma in AIDS, 726
Nonionized form of anesthetic, 588
Nonkeratinized epithelium, 285
Nonmalficence, 46
Nonnutritive sucking in early childhood, 180
Nonspecific plaque hypothesis, 296
Nonsteroidal antiinflammatory agents in periodontal
    disease management, 422
Nonverbal cues in establishing rapport, 64
Norepinephrine
  as neurotransmitter, 229
  in anesthetic solutions, 590-591
Nose

examination of, 217
in review of organ systems, 200-201
Nosebleeds, frequent, in health history, 200-201
Novocain. *See* Procaine.
Nucleus pulposus, 118
Nutrition
as risk factor for cancer, 721
effects of, on oral cavity, 345-348
oral complications and, 348
Nutritional assessment, 344-354
anthropometric evaluation in, 351
dental history in, 351
dietary intake evaluation in, 351-352
evaluation and, 352
health history in, 351
laboratory evaluations in, 351
social history in, 351
treatment plan based on, 352
Nutritional deficiency from radiotherapy, 740
Nutritional factors in skin disorders, 199

O

Oblique fibers of periodontal ligament, 288
Oblique strokes, 154-155
Observation in communication, 61-62
Obsessive-compulsive disorder (OCD), 701
Obsessive-compulsive personality disorder, 706-707
Obturator in maxillofacial prosthesis, 475
Occlusal analysis, 328-330
Occlusion, traumatic, 330
Occupation in social history, 198
Occupational exposure, OSHA definition of, 89
Occupational Safety and Health Administration (OSHA), 87
ergonomic standards of, 116-117
terms of, 88-89
OCD. *See* Obsessive-compulsive disorder (OCD).
Octocaine. *See* Lidocaine.
Odontoblasts
in hydrodynamic theory of dentinal sensitivity, 430
nutrition and, 347
Opening, pathway of, 329
Operative therapies, 622-661
aesthetic, 632
application of, 625b
classification and nomenclature for, 625-630
cosmetic whitening as, 650-660
evaluation criteria for, 638
in minimally invasive dentistry, 630-631
isolation of teeth in, 632-638
restorative, 639-647
restorative materials for, 638-639
Operator chair, 120-121
armrests of, 128
Operator positioning, 118, 120-123
during instrumentation procedures, 124
for ultrasonic scaling, 124-125
OPIM. *See* Other potentially infectious materials (OPIM).
Optical coherence tomography in caries detection, 328
ORA system, 488-502
application of, to case study, 498-502
case summary in, 502, 503-504f
ORA system—cont'd
prevention survey of, 489-490f, 494-495f
recommend in, 508-514
reevaluation in, 514, 515-517t
worksheet for, 491, 492-493f, 496-498f
Oral cancer, data on, 24, 27b
Oral cavity
as pathogenic port of entry, 19
in health and disease, 19-20
infection of, heart disease and stroke and, 20
nutritional effects on, 345-348
Oral contraceptives, 689
oral effects of, 689-690
Oral disease
burden of, 21-29
systemic manifestations of, 18
Oral health
in adolescence, 182
in early adulthood, 184
in early childhood, 179-180
in late adulthood, 187
in late childhood, 181
in mature adulthood, 185
in young adulthood, 182
Oral hygiene, personal, in dentinal sensitivity management, 432-433
Oral motor deficits, 677-678
Oral mucosal lesions, supplementary diagnostic aids for, 370-371
Oral mucositis complicating chemotherapy, 723
Organ systems, review of, 198-209. *See also* Review of organ systems.
Orofacial pain, data on, 28-29
Orofacial trauma, 453. *See also* Trauma.
Oropharyngeal isthmus, 261
Oropharynx, examination of, 261-263
Orthostatic hypotension, 224-225
in health history, 202
OSHA. *See* Occupational Safety and Health Administration (OSHA).
Osmotic stimuli in dentinal sensitivity, 431
Osseous defects, recontouring of, 564b
Osseous surgery, 564b
Osteitis
condensing, radiographic appearance of, 339
localized, from oral contraceptives, 690
Osteoblasts in periosteum, 288
Osteoporosis, 691
in health history, 199
Osteoradionecrosis from radiotherapy, 740
Other potentially infectious materials (OPIM), OSHA definition of, 89
Overbite, 329
Overdenture, 472
Overgloves in infection control program, 95
Overjet, 329
Oversedation with nitrous oxide/oxygen sedation, 615
Oxalate solutions to decrease dentinal sensitivity, 436
Oxygen, hyperbaric, in cancer management, 732b
Oxygenating agents, 422

P

PABA. *See* Paraaminobenzoic acid (PABA).
Pacemaker in health history, 204

Pain
  abdominal, in health history, 205
  control of, 585-621. *See also* Anesthetics.
    nitrous oxide/oxygen sedation. *See also* Nitrous
      oxide/oxygen sedation.
    nitrous oxide/oxygen sedation in, 610-621
  orofacial, data on, 28-29
Palatal hyperplasia associated with appliance wear, 477,
  478f
Palatal lift in maxillofacial prosthesis, 475
Palate, examination of, 259-261
Palatine fovea, 260, 261f
Palatine tonsils, examination of, 261-263
Palatoglossal fold, 261
Palliative treatment of mucositis, 738
Palm grasp, 150
Palmer's notation for tooth numbering, 311, 314t, 315f
Palpation
  bilateral, of mucosal surfaces, 250
  in physical examination, 214, 216, 220-222f, 367
  in sports-related injury evaluation, 455
Panic attack, 69
Panic disorder, 699-700
Papillae
  interdental, 287
  of tongue, 256-257
Papillomavirus infections, human, oral, data on, 28
Paraaminobenzoic acid (PABA), 589
Parafunction, 318
Parallel orientation of wire edge, 161
Paralysis in health history, 209
Paranoid personality disorder, 705
Parathyroid hormone (PTH), bone integrity and, 200
Parenteral, OSHA definition of, 89
Paresis of third cranial nerve, drooping eyelids from, 200
Parkinson's disease
  in health history, 209
  neurological/sensory impairment from, 674
Parotid duct, 253
Parotid glands, 665
  examination of, 218
Passive immunity, 91
Pathogens, bloodborne, OSHA definition of, 88
Patient
  and practitioner, relationship between, respect for, 54
  as clinical partner, 507-508
  assessment of, 174-375. *See also* Assessment, patient.
  bill of rights of, 43-44b
  control of, in anxiety control, 580
  duties and responsibilities of, 52
  in caries management, 397
  positioning of, 118, 123-124
    semisupine, 124
    supine, 123
  record on, review of, 750-751
  rights of
    and responsibilities of, in dental care, 41, 42-46b,
      46-52
    First Amendment, 50
  self-determination for, 50
  special needs, 662-742. *See also* Special needs patient.
Pattern burns in child abuse, 460

Pellagra, skin in, 199
Pellicle, 287
Pen grasp, 150
Perceptual deficits in neurological/sensory impairment,
  681-682
Percussion
  in physical examination, 214, 216, 367
  in sports-related injury evaluation, 455
Performance based, OSHA definition of, 89
Performance logic (PL) positioning, 122-123
Periapical lesions, radiographic diagnosis of, 338-339
Periimplantitis, 474
Perimenopause, 689
PerioChip, 423
Periodontal care, supportive, 747
Periodontal chart, 292f
Periodontal debridement, 522-536
  case study on, 524-525f
  charting of, 525f
  coding for, 537
  evaluation of, 536
  goals of, 523, 526
  instrument design and, 138
  mechanical root planing in, 523
  posttherapy evaluation of, at 4 to 6 weeks, 536
Periodontal disease(s)
  adverse birth defects and, 20
  classification of, 304, 305-306b
  data on, 21, 24, 25-26f
  diabetes and, 19-20
  diagnostic aids for, 370
  etiology of, changes in, 8
  in AIDS, 727
  nutrition and, 347-348
  pathogenesis of, 526-527
  risk assessment for, 747
  risk of, dental factors in, 301-303
  treatment of, changes in, 8
  wound healing in, 526-527
Periodontal dressings, 564b, 570-572
Periodontal examination, 282-307
  attachment loss calculation in, 293
  calculus assessment in, 296-298
  components of, 289-290
  imaging technology in, 303-304
  in periodontal supportive care, 751
  indices in, 298, 299-301t, 301
  laboratory assays of periodontal infections in, 304
  mobility detection in, 295-296
  plaque assessment in, 296-298
  technology in, 303-304
Periodontal flap, 563
  full-thickness, 564b
Periodontal ligament
  principal fibers of, 287
  structure of, 288
Periodontal maintenance, 747
Periodontal pocket, probing of, 290-291, 292f
  bleeding on, detection of, 293-294
Periodontal probes, design features of, 143f, 145
Periodontal procedures, dentinal sensitivity and, 431
Periodontal surgery, dressing after, 572

Periodontal therapy
  active, 747
  supportive, 747
    appointment scheduling in, 752
    elements of, 751-752
    intervals for, 750
Periodontitis, erythema in, 289
Periodontium
  anatomical landmarks of, 285-287
  anatomy of, 285
  attachment mechanisms of, 287-289
  connective tissue of, 287
  diseases of. *See also* Periodontal disease(s).
  evaluation of, 283
Perioscopy, 536-537
Periosteal sutures, 569
Periosteum, 288
PerioTemp, 303
Periotron 8000, 303
Peripheral nerve conduction, local anesthetics and,
    590
Pernicious anemia
  immune system dysfunction in, 717-18
  vitiligo in, 199
Perpendicular light in transillumination, 144-145
Perpendicular orientation of wire edge, 161
Personal characteristics, describing, in establishing
    rapport, 65
Personal distance in establishing rapport, 62
Personal factors in social history, 198
Personal hygiene in infection control program, 91-94
Personal protective equipment (PPE)
  face masks as, 97
  gloves as, 95-96
  in infection control program, 90f, 94-98
  OSHA definition of, 88
  protective eyewear as, 96-97
  protective garments as, 97-98
Personal space in establishing rapport, 62-63
Personality disorders, 705-707
Peutz-Jegher's disease in health history, 199
Pharmacologic sedation, 615
Pharyngeal cancer, data on, 24, 27b
Pharyngeal wall, 262
Pharyngitis in health history, 201
Phenytoin (Dilantin), gingival hyperplasia from, 273
Philosophy of practice, professional self and, 770-771
Phobia, definition of, 577
Phobic disorders, 700-701
Phosphorus deficiency, oral symptoms of, 346t
Photodynamic therapy (PDT) for head and neck cancer,
    736-737
Photographic imaging, intraoral, 355-364
  accessories for, 360-361
  exposures for, 361-363f
  future trends in, 361, 364
  systems for
    35-mm camera, 356-357
    digital camera, 359-360
    selection process for, 360
    video imaging, 357-359
  theory of, 356
Photopolymerized system for sealant delivery, 443

Physical examination, 214-226
  blood pressure in, 224-225
  consultations from, 225-226
  HEENT
    blood vessels in, 219
    bones in, 219
    cartilage in, 219
    components of, 216-219
    documentation form for, 247f
    ears in, 217
    eyes in, 217
    face in, 216-217
    head in, 216-217, 219, 222f
    lymph nodes in, 217-218
    muscles in, 219
    neck in, 218, 219, 220-222f
    nose in, 217
    principles of, 216
    salivary glands in, 218
    supplemental diagnostic aids in, 219, 222
    temporomandibular joint in, 219
  observations in, general, 215
  principles and techniques of, 215-222
  pulse in, 223-224
  referrals from, 225-226
  respiration in, 224
  temperature in, 223
  tobacco assessment in, 225
  vital signs in, 222-225
Physical-physiological characteristics
  in adolescence, 182
  in early adulthood, 183-184
  in late adulthood, 186-188
  in late childhood, 181
  in mature adulthood, 185
  in young adulthood, 182
  of early childhood, 179-180
  of life stages, 178
Piezoelectric ultrasonic scalers, 529-530
Pigmentation
  in health history, 199
  oral, abnormal, from tetracycline, 275-276
Pilocarpine (Salagen) for salivary dysfunction, 667
Pipe cleaners for interdental cleaning, 384
Pits and fissures, sealants for, 440-449. *See also*
    Sealants.
Plaque
  assessment of, 296-298
  indeces of
    in oral self-care, 386
  indices of
    in periodontal examination, 298, 299-300t
  removal of, in educational program, 6
Plaque hypotheses, 296
Plica fimbriata, 258, 259f
Plica sublingualis, 254, 256f
Pneumonia
  bacterial, 85
    summary of, 79t
  in health history, 202
  viral, 85
    summary of, 79t

Point angles of cavity preparation, 627
  Class I, 628, 629f
  Class II, 629, 630f
Polishing, 541-561
  agents in, 549-550
  air-powder, 553-558
    clinical technique of, 556-557
    indications for, 553-555
    operator preparation for, 555-556
    patient selection and preparation for, 555
    precautions for, 557-558
    safety issues for, 557-558
    unit preparation for, 555-556
  engine-driven, 550-553
    clinical technique of, 551-552, 553t
    indications for, 551
    operator preparation for, 551
    patient selection and preparation for, 551
    precautions for, 553
    safety issues for, 553
    unit preparation for, 551
  in dental hygiene care, 559
  in maintaining aesthetic restorations, 558-559
  in periodontal supportive care, 752
  mechanical devices for, 550-558
  need for, assessment of, 542
  of implants, 559
  of restorative materials, 558-559
  porte polisher for, 550
  therapeutic, 559
Polycythemia, epistaxis and, 201
Polydipsia in health history, 207
Polymerization of sealants, 443
Polymerization shrinkage of direct resin composite restorations, 645
Polymers in sealants, 443
Polymyositis in health history, 199
Polysaccharides as fermentable carbohydrates, 350
Polyuria in health history, 206
Pontic, 470
Pontocaine. *See* Tetracaine.
Porte polisher, 550
Position(s)
  neutral, 121-122, 123b
  of dental equipment, 125-126
  supine, for patient, 123
  working
    alternative, 121-123
    traditional, 121, 123f, 125t
Positioning, 120-127
  biocentric technique of, 122, 123b
  equipment, 126
  errors in, recognition of, 126-127
  operator, 118, 120-123
    for powered debridement, 533-534
  patient, 118
    for powered debridement, 533-534
  performance logic, 122-213
Posterior boundary of buccal mucosa, 253
Postmenopause, 689
Postsurgical stents, 476
Posttraumatic stress disorder (PTSD), 701-702

Postural exercises in prevention/treatment of musculoskeletal disorders, 129-130
Postural syndrome, 120
Posture, balanced reference, 122b
Potable water, 99
Potassium ferrocyanide to decrease dentinal sensitivity, 435-436
Potassium nitrate
  in bleaching process, 657
  in desensitizing toothpastes, 433, 435
Povidone-iodine in mouthrinse, 422
Power bleaching, 656
Powered instrumentation in periodontal debridement, 522-536
  adaptation of, 534-535
  cavitational action of, 523
  fulcrum of, 534
  fundamentals of, 533-536
  grasp of, 534
  indications for use of, 533
  insertion and activation of, 535-536
  instrument selection in, 533
  patient and operator positioning for, 533-534
  preparation of, 532-533
  scaling, 527-536. *See also* Scalers.
  therapeutic use of, 532
  tip selection and application for, 530-532
PPE. *See* Personal protective equipment (PPE).
Practice
  clinical, future direction of, 777-778
  health promotion as basis of, 16-37
  private, dental hygienist in, 11
Practice act, 41
Prebrushing rinse, 423
Pregnancy
  hormonal imbalances in, 687, 689
  in health history, 206-207
  oral changes in, 689
  supportive care in, 688b
Pressure, selective, in cracked tooth syndrome diagnosis, 369
Pressure sores in neurological/sensory impairment, 681
Prevention
  chemotherapeutics in, 416-427. *See also* Chemotherapeutics.
  definition of, 488b
  dentifrices in, 406-414. *See also* Dentifrices.
  extension for, 627
  fluoride in, 390-404. *See also* Fluoride(s).
  of dental trauma, 463-467. *See also* Trauma, dental.
  of sports-related dental trauma, 463-464
  oral self-care in, 378-387. *See also* Self-care, oral.
  sealants in, 440-449. *See also* Sealants.
  strategies for, 487
    implementation of, 511-514
    individualizing, 507-519
Prilocaine (Citanest, Citanest Forte)
  clinical actions of, 591-592
  methemoglobinemia from, 589
Printer in intraoral video imaging system, 359
Private practice, dental hygienist in, 11

Probes, 142, 143f
    periodontal, design features of, 143f, 145
Probing, periodontal, 290-291, 292f, 367
    automated systems for, 303
    bleeding on, detection of, 293-294
Procaine, 586
    clinical actions of, 592
Product recommendation in ORA system, 510-511
Professional associations, 87-88
Professional development, 768-780
    competence in, 772-773
    insight and commitment in, 775-780
    professional self in, 770-772
    working with other professionals in, 772
Professional organizations in maintaining competence,
    12
Professional self, 770-772
Progesterone, 689
    skin and, 199
Prognosis in cancer, 733
Prophylaxis angle in engine-driven polishing, 550-553
Propoxycaine, clinical actions of, 592
Proprioceptive self-derivation method of operator chair
    height determination, 121, 121b, 122b
Prostate cancer in health history, 207
Prostheses
    dental, care of, 469-482
    implant-borne, 473-474
    maxillofacial, 475-476
Prosthetic joints in health history, 200
Protein deficiency, oral symptoms of, 346t
Proxigel as bleaching agent, 654
Pseudocholinesterase deficiency, 586b
Psoriasis
    immune system dysfunction in, 718
    in health history, 198
Psychiatry in review of organ systems, 209
Psychological-behavioral characteristics
    in adolescence, 182-183
    in early adulthood, 184
    in late adulthood, 188-189
    in late childhood, 181
    in mature adulthood, 185-186
    in young adulthood, 182-183
    of early childhood, 180
Psychomotor assessment after nitrous oxide/oxygen se-
    dation administration, 617
Psychosocial-behavioral characteristics, of life stages, 178
Psychosocial factors in social history, 197-198
Psychosocial treatments for schizophrenia, 711
Ptosis in myasthenia gravis, 200
PTSD. *See* Posttraumatic stress disorder (PTSD).
Puberty, 687
    oral manifestations of, 689
Public distance in establishing rapport, 62
Public health
    dental hygienist in, 11
    future of, 778
Pulp in crown fracture, 456
Pulpal disease, diagnostic aids for, 369-370
Pulpitis, diagnosis of, 370
Pulsating irrigation stream, 418
Pulse, evaluation of, 223-224

Pulse oximeter in nitrous oxide/oxygen sedation
    monitoring, 617
Pumice as dental abrasive, 550
Pyelitis in health history, 206
Pyelonephritis in health history, 206
Pyogenic granuloma in pregnancy, 689
Pyridoxine deficiency, oral symptoms of, 346t
Pyrophosphate in calculus control dentifrices, 410

Q

Quadriplegic patients. *See also* Neurological/sensory
    impairment.
    supportive care challenges in treatment of, 672b
Quaternary ammonium compounds, 423
Quiescence in periodontal disease, 296

R

Race in health history, 195
Radiation modifiers for head and neck cancer, 736
Radiation therapy
    as risk factor for cancer, 721
    for head and neck cancer, 737-741. *See also* Head and
        neck cancer, radiation therapy for.
    xerostomia from, 666
Radiographs, 333-342
    caries detection with, 326-327
    diagnostic quality of, 334
    digital, 340-341
    elongation on, 337
    evaluation of, 334
    exposure errors in, 337
    film contrast in, 337, 338f
    film density in, 337
    foreshortening on, 337
    full-mouth series of, 336f
    guidelines for prescribing, 335t
    in oral mucosal lesion diagnosis, 371, 372f
    in patient assessment, 338-340
    in patient education, 340
    in sports-related injury evaluation, 455
    in treatment planning, 340
    indications for, clinical, 336b
    new techniques with, 340-341
    overlapped teeth in, 337
    pathological findings on, 338-339
    patient protection and, 337-338
    periodontal findings on, 339-340
    processing errors in, 337
    selection of, 334
    structural findings on, 338
    technical errors in, 337
    vertical bitewing, 334
Radiotherapy, 732b. *See also* Radiation therapy.
Rapport
    deepening, 65
    establishing, 62-65
        context in, 63
        cultural sensitivity in, 63
        describing personal characteristics in, 65
        expressing emotion in, 65
        language in, 64
        nonverbal cues in, 64
        personal space in, 62-63

Rapport—cont'd
  establishing—cont'd
    reflecting interest in discussion in, 64-65
    reflecting status in, 65
    regulating verbal communication in, 64
    time in, 63-64
RCRA. *See* Resource Conservation and Recovery Act (RCRA).
Rebound anxiety, 702
Recession, location of free gingival margin and, 291
Reciprocity, licensure by, 9-10
Recommendations, definition of, 86
Record(s)
  dental treatment, ownership and access to, 54
  patient, review of, 750-751
Record keeping, OSHA definition of, 89
Referrals, from physical examination, 225-226
Refractory, 304
Regional licensure examinations, 9, 10b
Regulated waste, OSHA definition of, 89
Regulations, definition of, 86
Regulatory terminology, 86
  explanations of, 88-89
Relaxation in anxiety control, 581
Remineralization, 320
  fluoride enhancing, 347
  fluoride in enhancement of, 394-395
  in caries process, 391b, 392
Renal dialysis in health history, 206
Repetitive strain injuries (RSIs), 116
  definition of, 117
Reporting of child abuse and neglect, 462-463
Research, 9
  dental, dental hygienist in, 11-12
  future direction of, 777
Resistance, microbial, 78
Resistance form, 627
Resource Conservation and Recovery Act (RCRA), 87
Respect, demonstrating, 65-66
Respiration, evaluation of, 224
Respiratory system
  deficits in, in neurological/sensory impairment, 670-680
  diseases of, 83-85
  in review of organ systems, 201-202
Resting membrane potential in nerve conduction, 586-587
Restorations
  amalgam, placement techniques for
    for Class I, V, and VI preparations, 639-642
    for Class II preparations, 642-645
  direct resin composite, 645-647
Restorative approaches, surgical differing views on, 327
Restorative lesions, Black's classification of, 625, 626f
Restorative materials, 638-639
  amalgam as, 638-639
  periodontal risk and, 302
  polishing of, 558-559
Restorative procedures, dentinal sensitivity and, 431
Retainers for fixed partial dentures, 470
Retention form, 627
Retention of sealants, 442
Retractors for intraoral photography, 360
Retromolar pad, 253, 254f

Review of organ systems, 198-209
  cardiovascular system in, 202-205
  ears in, 200
  endocrine system in, 207-208
  extremities in, 199-200
  eyes in, 200
  gastrointestinal system in, 205-206
  genitourinary system in, 206-207
  hematopoietic system in, 208
  neurological system in, 208-209
  nose in, 200-201
  psychiatry in, 209
  respiratory system in, 201-202
  skin in, 198-199
  throat in, 200-201
Rheumatic fever in health history, 202-203
Rheumatic heart disease in health history, 202-203
Rheumatoid arthritis
  immune system dysfunction in, 716-717
  in health history, 199
Rhinitis in health history, 201
Rhythm, sinus, 223
Riboflavin, deficiency of, oral symptoms of, 346t
Risk, definition of, 487
Risk assessment
  caries, 396-397
    management by, 396
  caries prevention and, 8
  for periodontal disease, 747
  oral, 486-506. *See also* ORA system.
    application of, to medicine and dentistry, 487-488
    concept of, 487
  total, 8-9
Risk factors
  definition of, 487
  for oral disease, 18
Risk management, 40-55
  for dental hygienist, 53
Risk taking in future of dental hygiene, 779
Rolling stroke tooth-brushing method, 381, 382t
Root fracture, emergency management of, 456-457
Root planing. *See* Debridement.
Rounded edges of instruments, 159
RSIs. *See* Repetitive strain injuries (RSIs).
Rubber dam, 98, 632-638
  armamentarium for, 632-633f
  clamps for, 632, 633f
    placement of, 633-634
    selection of, 633
  examination of mouth for, 633
  patient preparation for, 632-633
  placement of, 635-636
  preparation of, 634-635
  removal of, 637-638
Rubella, 83
  summary of, 79t
Rubeola, 83
  summary of, 79t

S

Safety of local anesthetic, 597-598
Salagen (pilocarpine) for xerostomia, 667
Sales, dental product, dental hygienist in, 11

Saliva
  analysis of, in caries management, 397
  buffering role of, 392
  fluoride in, 393-394
  nutrition and, 348
Salivary flow in caries diagnosis, *369*
Salivary glands, 664-670
  accessory, 250
  classification of, 664-665
  development of, 664
  dysfunction of, 665-666. *See also* Xerostomia.
    caries in, 666-667
    dental management of, 666-667
  examination of, 218
  stimulators of, for xerostomia, 271
Salivary reductase test in caries diagnosis, 369
Sanguinarine
  in dentifrices, 412
  in gingivitis management, 422
Sanitization in infection control program, 102-103
Scalers
  sickle
    design features of, 145
    sharpening of, 166
  sonic, 528
    tip selection and application for, 530-531
  ultrasonic, 149, 528-536. *See also* Ultrasonic scalers.
Scaling. *See also* Debridement.
  channel, 155
  ultrasonic, operator positioning during, 124
  zone, 155
Scavenging devices in nitrous oxide/oxygen sedation administration, 615
Schizoid personality disorder, 705
Schizophrenia, 709-711
Schizotypal personality disorder, 705
Scleroderma
  immune system dysfunction in, 718-719
  in health history, 199
Scoop technique for recapping needles, 597
Sealants, 440-449
  action and effectiveness of, 441-443
  application of, 443-446
    future, 447
    pediatric considerations on, 441b
    technique for, 444-446
  armamentarium for, 443-446
  composition of, 443
  estrogenicity of, potential, 447
  filled resin, 446
  placement of
    contraindications to, 443
    indications for, 442-443
  replacement of, 447
  retention of, 446-447
  types of, 443
  wear of, 447
Sealers, cavity, 639
Seborrhea in health history, 198
Sedation
  nitrous oxide/oxygen, 610-621. *See also* Nitrous oxide/oxygen sedation.
  pharmacologic, 615

Seduction in chemical dependency, 229
Seizure disorder in health history, 209
Selective pressure in cracked tooth syndrome diagnosis, 369
Selenium deficiency, oral symptoms of, 346t
Self, professional, 770-772
Self-care, oral, 378-387
  devices for, evaluating effectiveness of, 386
  guidelines for, 378-380
  interdental cleaning in, 383-386
  interproximal cleaning devices in, 378
  toothbrushes in, 380-383
Self-disclosure in communication, 67
Self-evaluation on communication skills, 58, 60
Sensitivity
  cultural, in establishing rapport, 63
  dentinal. *See also* Dentin, sensitivity of.
    dentifrices to control, 410
  tactile, instrument handle and, 139
  tooth, supplementary diagnostic aids for, 368-370
Sensory impairment, 671-685. *See also* Neurological/sensory impairment.
Serotonin as neurotransmitter, 229
Sex hormones, female, 687-689
Sexually transmitted diseases (STDs) in health history, 206
Shank, instrument, 139, 140f, 141
Sharpening, instrument, 158-172
  devices for, 161-163
  equipment for, 163
  for sickles, 166
  goals of, 159-160
  manual methods of, 163-166
    stationary instrument/moving stone method as, 163-166
  needs for, 160
  technique errors in, 170-171f
  workstation for, 163
Sharpey's fibers of periodontal ligament, 287
Sharps
  contaminated, OSHA definition of, 88
  injury from, 107, 108t
  managing, 107
Shoulder retraction, 129, 130f
Shutter release of 35-mm camera, 357
Sickle cell anemia in health history, 208
Sickle scalers
  design features of, 145
  sharpening of, 166
Sickles, 138, 141, 142f
Sideported tip for irrigation, 418
Signs and labels, OSHA definition of, 89
Silver nitrate, basic or ammoniated, to decrease dentinal sensitivity, 435
Sinus bradycardia, 223
Sinus rhythm, 223
Sinus tachycardia, 224
Sinusitis in health history, 201
Sjögren's syndrome
  data on, 29
  in health history, 199
  management of, 667
  xerostomia in, 666

Skin
  breakdown of, in neurological/sensory impairment, 681
  broken, on hands, in infection control program, 93
  erythema of, from radiotherapy, 741
  in review of organ systems, 198-199
Sleep apnea devices, 476
Sling sutures, 568-569
Slipped disc, 118, 119f
Slouching, 118, 119f, 120f. *See also* Postural syndrome.
Smear layer, occlusion of, dentinal sensitivity and, 431
Snyder colorimetric test in caries diagnosis, 369
Soaps for hand washing in infection control program, 93
Social distance in establishing rapport, 62
Social history, 197-198
  in nutritional assessment, 351
Social phobia, 700-701
Socioeconomic status as risk factor for cancer, 721
Sodium bicarbonate
  in antigingivitis dentifrices, 411
  in dentifrices, 423
Sodium citrate in desensitizing toothpastes, 435
Sodium fluoride
  in anticaries dentifrice, 410
  to decrease dentinal sensitivity, 436
Sodium silicofluoride to decrease dentinal sensitivity, 436
Soft palate, 259, 260-261
Soft tissues
  assessment of, in child abuse, 460-461
  formation of, nutrition and, 346-347
  graft of, free, for lost tooth, 564b
Sonic scalers, 528. *See also* Powered instrumentation in periodontal debridement.
  preparation of, 532-533
  therapeutic use of, 532
  tip selection and application for, 530-531
SOP. *See* Standard operating procedures (SOP).
Sore throat in health history, 201
Source individual, OSHA definition of, 89
Space, personal, in establishing rapport, 62-63
Spastic cerebral palsy, 674
Special needs patient, 662-742
  with head and neck cancer and radiation, 731-742. *See also* Head and neck cancer; Radiation therapy.
  with hormonal imbalances, 687-693. *See also* Hormones, imbalances in.
  with immune system dysfunction, 715-729. *See also* Immune system, dysfunction of.
  with mental/emotional disturbances, 694-713. *See also* Mental/emotional disturbances.
  with neurological and sensory impairment, 671-685. *See also* Neurological/sensory impairment.
  with salivary dysfunction, 664-670. *See also* Salivary glands.
Specific phobias, 701
Specific plaque hypothesis, 296
Spina bifida, neurological/sensory impairment from, 675
Spinal cord injury, neurological/sensory impairment from, 674-675
Spine, normal anatomy and anatomical changes in, 118-120
Splash burns in child abuse, 460

Splints, 474
Sports-related dental injury
  case report on, 453b
  community activities related to, 465-466
  dental evaluation of, 455-456
  dentistry related to, 465
  patient assessment in, 454-455
  predictive index for, 454
  prevention of, 463-464
  risk assessment for, 454
Sputum, blood in, in health history, 201
Squamous cell carcinoma in AIDS, 726
Staining, vital, in oral mucosal lesion diagnosis, 370
Stains, dental, 542-550
  endogenous, 542
    developmental, 543f, 543t
  evaluation of, 449
  extrinsic
    abrasive agents for, 549
    in examination for cosmetic whitening, 655-656
    polishing for. *See also* Polishing.
      agents in, 549-550
      mechanical devices for, 550-558
    professional treatment of, 549-558
Standard operating procedures (SOP)
  in infection control program, 90-109
  OSHA definition of, 89
Standards, definition of, 86
Stannous fluoride
  in anticaries dentifrice, 410
  in antigingivitis dentifrices, 411
  in antigingivitis irrigation, 422
  to decrease dentinal sensitivity, 436
Staphylococcal infections, 85
  summary of, 79t
State agencies, 87
State licensure examinations, 9
Status, reflecting, in establishing rapport, 65
Statutes, 41
Stensen's duct, 253
Stents, postsurgical, 476
Sterilization, 104-106
  autoclaves in, 104-105
  chemical, 105
  chemical vapor in, 105
  cold, 103
  Dri-Clave in, 105
  ethylene oxide in, 105
  monitors of, 105-106
  of instruments, 106
Steroids, topical, for erythema multiforme, 271
Stillman's cleft, 289
Stillman's tooth-brushing method, modified, 381, 382t
Stimulus generalization in phobic disorders, 700
Stippling effect on gingiva, 286
Stomatitis
  denture, data on, 28
  nicotinic, 194
Stones for instrument sharpening
  care of, 162-163
  hand-held, 161-163
  mounted, 161, 162f
Stratified squamous epithelium, 285

Stratum basale, 285
Stratum corneum, 285
Stratum granulosum, 285
Stratum spinosum, 285
Strengthening exercises in prevention/treatment of
          musculoskeletal disorders, 131-134
Streptococcal infections, 85
      summary of, 79t
Streptococcus mutans count in caries diagnosis, 369
Stretching exercises in prevention/treatment of muscu-
          loskeletal disorders, 130-131
Stroke
      in health history, 205
      neurological/sensory impairment from, 672-673
      oral infection and, 20
Strokes in instrumentation, 154-155
Strontium chloride in desensitizing toothpastes, 435
Study casts, 368
Subgingival irrigation, 418-419
Sublingual gland(s), 665
      examination of, 218
Sublingual ridge/fold, 254, 256f
Submandibular duct, 254
Submandibular gland(s), 665
      examination of, 218
Substance abuse, 228-243
Substantivity of antimicrobials, 420
Sucking, nonnutritive, in early childhood, 180
Sugar alcohols, cariogenicity of, 349
Sulcular epithelium, 287
Sulcus terminalis, 257
Superior constructor muscle of pharynx, 253
Supervision, dental, types of, 10, 11b
Supine position for patient, 123
Supplementary diagnostic aids, 366-375
      for anemia, 371-372
      for caries, 368-369
      for cracked tooth syndrome, 369
      for oral mucosal lesions, 370-371
      for periodontal disease, 370
      for pulpal disease, 369-370
      for tooth sensitivity, 368-370
      study casts as, 368
      systemic, 371-374
Supportive care
      for chronic oral conditions, 753
      for dental caries, 752-753
      intervals of, for periodontal patients, 750
      periodontal, 747
            appointment scheduling in, 752
            elements of, 751-752
            rationale for, 748
Supportive periodontal therapy, 747
Suppuration
      detection of, 294
      in periodontal examination, 289
Supragingival calculus, 298
Supragingival irrigation, 418-419
Surgeon general's report as health promotion guidelines,
          31, 32-36b
Surgical flap, 563
Survival rate, 737
Suture(s)
      continuous, 568

Suture(s)—cont'd
      interrupted, 567-568
      materials for, 563, 565-566
      mattress, 569, 570f
      monofilament, 565-566
      multifilament, 565
      natural absorbable, 566
      nonabsorbable, 565-566
      packaging of, 566, 567f
      periosteal, 569
      removal of, 570
      size of, 566
      sling, 568-569
Suture needles, 566
Suturing, 563-570
      after frenum removal, 564b
      techniques of, 567-569, 570f
Swallowing, difficulty in, in health history, 205
Sweeteners
      nonnutritive, 350
      nutritive, 349-350
Sympathetic nervous system, vasoconstrictors released
          by, in anesthetic solutions, 590-591
Syncope in health history, 202
Synovial joints, in spine, 118
Syphilis, 86
      summary of, 79t
Syringe(s)
      aspirating, in local anesthetic administration, 596
      in local anesthetic administration, 597
Systemic disease, oral manifestations of, 18
Systemic lupus erythematosus, 717

T

Tachycardia, sinus, 224
Tachypnea, 224
Tactile sensitivity, instrument handle and, 139
Tardive dyskinesia from neuroleptic drugs, 710-711
Teaching, evidence-based, 9
Team approach
      to communication, 59-60b
      to dental caries management, 395-396
      to tobacco cessation, 240
Telescopic loupes, 127-128
Temperature, evaluation of, 223
Temporomandibular joint, disorders of, data on, 29
Teratogens, 198
Terminal shank, 139, 140f
Tertiary amine, 599
Tessalon. *See* Benzonatate.
Tetanus, 86
Tetracaine, 599
      clinical actions of, 592
Tetracycline
      oral pigmentation abnormalities from, 275-276
      tooth discoloration from, 543, 545f
            cosmetic whitening for, 651b, 652f
      topical application of, 421-422
Therapeutic alliance, 748
Therapeutic implementation, 520-573
      polishing in, 541-561. *See also* Polishing.
      powered instrumentation in, 522-536. *See also* Powered
            instrumentation in periodontal debridement.
      suturing in, 563-570. *See also* Suture(s); Suturing.

Therapeutic interventions, periodontal dressings in, 570-572
Therapeutic polishing, 559
Therapeutic privilege, 47
Thermal decontamination, 103
Thermal stimuli in dentinal sensitivity, 431
Thiamin deficiency, oral symptoms of, 346t
Thinking, disorganized, in schizophrenia, 710
Thirst, excessive, in health history, 207
Thoracic outlet syndrome (TOS), 117b
Throat in review of organ systems, 200-201
Thrombocytopenia, epistaxis and, 200-201
Thrush associated with appliance wear, 477
Thyroid gland
    diseases of, autoimmune, 719
    examination of, 218
    problems of, in health history, 207
Tidal volume in nitrous oxide/oxygen sedation
        administration, 615-616
Time in establishing rapport, 63-64
Tinnitus in health history, 200
Tip, ultrasonic, handle of, 139
Titration of nitrous oxide/oxygen sedation, 615
Tobacco
    dental stains from, 547t
    dependency on, 228-243
        addiction in, 229
        as intended consequence, 229-230
        costs of, 230-231
        diagnosis of, 233
        environmental stimuli in, 233
        initiation of, 232
        patient history of, 232-234
        progression of, 232
        quitting, 234-240
            advice on, 235
            arrangements for, 239
            assessment for, 235-236
            assistance for, 236-239
            follow-up visits for, 239-240
            methods of, helpful, 235
            pharmaceutical agents in, 237-238b
            referral for, 240
            relapse in, 239-240
            team approach to, 240
        relapse in, 232-233
        results of, 230
        risks of, 232
        rituals associated with, 233
        seduction in, 229
    oral conditions induced by/associated with, 231b
    oral lesions related to, data on, 24, 27f
    smokeless/spit, 231
    use of
        in health history, 201
        in risk assessment, 747
Tobacco assessment, 225
Tobacco-cessation services, 234
Tofflemire universal matrix system, 642, 643f
Toluidine, 591
Tomography, optical coherence, in caries detection, 328
Tongue
    examination of, 256-259
    geographical, 257

Tongue—cont'd
    hairy, 276
    inflammation of. *See* Glossitis.
Tonsillitis in health history, 201
Tonsils
    lingual, 258
    palatine, examination of, 261-263
Tooth-brushing methods, 381-383
Tooth (teeth)
    abfraction of, 318
    abrasion of, 317-318
    attrition of, 318
    avulsed, 457-458
    conditions modifying, 316-318
        caries as. *See* Caries.
    discoloration of, 542-549
    diseased, surgical repair of, Black's principles for, 625, 627
    erosion of, 316-317
    fracture of, types of, 318-319
    interface of, with gingiva, 286
    isolation of, 632-638. *See also* Rubber dam.
    loss of, data on, 24, 26f
    lost, aesthetic treatment for, 564b
    minerals of, composition of, caries process and, 392-393
    mobility of
        detection of, 295-296
        in periodontal examination, 289
    numbering system for, 311, 314t
    overlapped, in radiographs, 337
    sensitivity of, supplementary diagnostic aids for, 368-370
Toothbrushes, 380-383
    design of, 380, 381t
    powered, 383t
Toothpastes. *See* Dentifrices.
Toothpicks for interdental cleaning, 386
Topical anesthetics, 598-599
Tort, 47
Torus palatinus, 259
TOS. *See* Thoracic outlet syndrome (TOS).
Toxic shock syndrome, 85
Transient ischemic attacks (TIAs), 194
    in health history, 205
Transillumination
    digital fiberoptic, in caries detection, 327
    in caries diagnosis, 369
    in sport-related injury evaluation, 455
Transseptal fibers, 287
Trauma
    brain, neurological/sensory impairment from, 673
    dental, 452-467
        developmental etiology of, 453-454
        emergency management of, 465-458
        epidemiology of, 453
        from child abuse and neglect, 458-463
            definitions on, 459
            demographic factors on, 459
            documentation of, 462
            evaluation of, 459-462
            historical perspective on, 458-459
            legal considerations on, 463

Trauma—cont'd
  dental—cont'd
    from child abuse and neglect—cont'd
      legislative efforts on, 458-459
      reporting of, 462-463
    incidence of, 453
    prevalence of, 453
    sports-related, 454-456
      case report on, 453b
      community activities related to, 465-466
      dental evaluation of, 455-456
      dentistry related to, 465
      patient assessment in, 454-455
      predictive index for, 454
      prevention of, 463-464
      risk assessment for, 454
    orofacial, 453
      data on, 28
    spinal, neurological/sensory impairment from, 674-675
Traumatic occlusion, 330
Treatment room
  cleanup of, 102
  preparation of, 101-102
Triclosan, in antigingivitis dentifrices, 411-412, 422
Trifurcations, 294
Trismus from radiotherapy, 738, 740
Tuberculosis, 86
  exposure to, in health history, 201-202
  summary of, 79t
Tubules in dentinal sensitivity, 429
Tumor(s)
  in AIDS, 726
  malignant, 731-732
  pregnancy, 689

U

Ulcer(s)
  aphthous, recurrent, data on, 28
  gastrointestinal, in health history, 205
  mouth, in health history, 201
Ulcerations, associated with appliance wear, 478
Ulcerative colitis, immune system dysfunction in, 718
Ultrasonic instrumentation in periodontal disease treatment, 8
Ultrasonic instruments, 138, 142
Ultrasonic scalers, 149, 528-536. *See also* Powered instrumentation in periodontal debridement.
  magnetostrictive, 528-529
  piezoelectric, 529-530
  preparation of, 532-533
  therapeutic use of, 532
  tip selection and application for, 530-532
Ultrasonic scaling, operator positioning during, 124
Ultrasonic tip, handle of, 139
Ultrasound in caries detection, 328
Universal precautions (UP)
  in infection control program, 90-94
    extraoral and intraoral examination in, 91
    host immunity in, 90-91
    immunizations in, 91, 92t
    patient health history in, 91
    personal hygiene and appearance in, 91-94
  OSHA definition of, 88

Universal system of tooth numbering, 311, 314f, 314t
UP. *See* Universal precautions (UP).
Urethritis in health history, 206
Urinary calculi in health history, 206
Urination
  difficulty and pain on, in health history, 206
  excessive, in health history, 206
Urine, blood in, in health history, 206
Uvula, 260, 261f

V

Valproate for bipolar disorder, 705
Values, professional self and, 770
Valves, heart, prosthetic, in health history, 205
Varicella-zoster virus (VZV), 83
Vasoconstrictors, 586b
  in anesthetic solutions, 590-591
Venereal disease in health history, 206
Ventilation, minute, in nitrous oxide/oxygen sedation administration, 616
Ventral surface of tongue, 254
Ventricular fibrillation in health history, 204
Verbal communication, regulating, in establishing rapport, 64
Vertical strokes, 154
Vertigo in health history, 200
Vestibular folds, examination of, 252-254
Video imaging systems, intraoral, 357-359
Videoconferencing, 777
Violence, domestic, prevention of, hygienist in, 464-465
Virulence of microorganisms in disease transmission, 77
Virus(es)
  as risk factor for cancer, 721
  diseases caused by, 79t
    dental healthcare providers and, 78-85
  Epstein-Barr, 83
  herpes simplex, in AIDS, 726
  human immunodeficiency. *See* Human immunodeficiency virus (HIV).
  varicella-zoster, 83
Viscosity of resin sealant, 442
Vision in professional development, 775
Visual deficits in neurological/sensory impairment, 682
Vital signs
  in nitrous oxide/oxygen sedation, 617
  in physical examination, 222-225
Vital staining in oral mucosal lesion diagnosis, 370
Vitality tests in sports-related injury evaluation, 455
Vitamin deficiencies, oral symptoms of, 346t
Vitiligo in health history, 199
VZV. *See* Varicella-zoster virus (VZV).

W

Wall(s)
  enamel, finishing of, 627
  of cavity preparation, 627
    Class I, 627, 628f
    Class II, 629
    Class III, 630
    Class V, 630, 631f
Wandering glossitis, 257
Washing, hand, in infection control program, 94
Waste management in infection control program, 109

Water
   fluoridation of, community, 17
   for irrigation, 420-421
   potable, 99
Waterborne transfer of microorganisms, 77
Waterline, dental, management of, 99
Weight changes in health history, 207
Wharton's duct, 254, 256f
Wheezing in health history, 201
White spot lesion, 320, 325
   in caries process, 392
Whitening. *See also* Bleaching.
   cosmetic, 650-660
      data collection on, 655-656
      delivery methods for, 656-657
      hygienist in, 658-659
      patient instructions for, 656
      patient selection for, 654-655
      side effects of, 657-658
   dentifrices for, 411
Whitestrips, Crest, 653, 654
   technique for use of, 657
Whitlow, herpetic, 82
Wire edges of instruments, 159
   from hand methods of instrument sharpening, 161
Woodsticks for interdental cleaning, 386
Work practice controls (WPCs)
   daily preparation as, 100-101
   implementing, in infection control program, 98-99
   OSHA definition of, 88
Work-related musculoskeletal disorders (WMSDs), 116. *See also* Repetitive strain injuries (RSIs).
Work zones, 100, 101f

Working end of instrument, 140f, 141
   angles of, sharpening and, 159
Worry, definition of, 698
Wound healing, periodontal, 526-527
WPCs. *See* Work practice controls (WPCs).

X

X-ray equipment, 98-99
Xerostomia, 271-272. *See also* Salivary glands, dysfunction of.
   clues to presence of, 667, 668b
   complicating chemotherapy, 724-725
   definition of, 665
   from benzodiazepines, 702
   from radiotherapy, 738-739
   in Sjögren's syndrome, 666
   indications for, 348b
   management of, 667
   medications causing, 665, 666b
   radiation therapy causing, 666
Xylidine, 591
Xylocaine. *See* Lidocaine.

Y

Yarn, knitting, for interdental cleaning, 384
Yellowing, cosmetic whitening for, 651-652b

Z

Zinc chloride to decrease dentinal sensitivity, 435-436
Zinc deficiency, oral symptoms of, 346t
ZOE dressings, 570
Zone Periodontal Pak, 570-571
Zone scaling, 155
Zyban (bupropion) in tobacco cessation, 237b